Contents

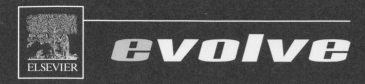

PHYSICAL EXAMINATION & Health Assessment

First Canadian Edition

Carolyn Jarvis, PhD, APN, CNP

Adjunct Associate Professor of Nursing   and   Family Nurse Practitioner
School of Nursing   Chestnut Health Systems
Illinois Wesleyan University   Bloomington, Illinois
Bloomington, Illinois

Canadian Editors

Annette J. Browne, PhD, RN

Associate Professor
New Investigator, Canadian Institutes
of Health Research
Scholar, Michael Smith Foundation
for Health Research
School of Nursing
University of British Columbia
Vancouver, British Columbia

June MacDonald-Jenkins, RN, BScN, MSc

Professor, School of Health and
Community Studies
Durham College
Assistant Adjunct Professor
Faculty of Health Science
University of Ontario Institute
of Technology
Oshawa, Ontario

Marian Luctkar-Flude, RN, BScN, MScN

Nursing Laboratory Coordinator
Faculty of Health Sciences Patient
Simulation Laboratory
Queen's University, School of Nursing
Nursing Research Program Coordinator
Nursing Research Unit
Kingston General Hospital
Kingston, Ontario

Original Illustrations by Pat Thomas, CMI, FAMI
Oak Park, Illinois

Assessment Photographs by Kevin Strandberg
Professor of Art
Illinois Wesleyan University
Bloomington, Illinois

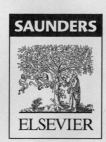

SAUNDERS

ELSEVIER

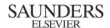

Notice

Knowledge and best practice in this field are constantly changing. As new research and experience broaden our knowledge, changes in practice, treatment, and drug therapy may become necessary or appropriate. Readers are advised to check the most current information provided (1) on procedures featured or (2) by the manufacturer of each product to be administered, to verify the recommended dose or formula, the method and duration of administration, and contraindications. It is the responsibility of the practitioner, relying on his or her own experience and knowledge of a patient, to make diagnoses, to determine dosages and the best treatment for each individual patient, and to take all appropriate safety precautions. To the fullest extent of the law, neither the Publisher nor the Authors assume any liability for any injury and/or damage to persons or property arising out of or related to any use of the material contained in this book.

The Publisher

Library and Archives Canada Cataloguing in Publication

Jarvis, Carolyn
　　Physical examination & health assessment / Carolyn Jarvis; Canadian editors: Annette J. Browne, June MacDonald-Jenkins, Marian Luctkar-Flude; original illustrations by Pat Thomas; assessment photographs by Kevin Strandberg. — 1st Canadian ed.

Includes bibliographical references and index.
ISBN 978-1-897422-18-2

　　1. Physical diagnosis. 2. Nursing assessment. I. Browne, Annette J. II. MacDonald-Jenkins, June, 1965- III. Luctkar-Flude, Marian, 1961- IV. Title. V. Title: Physical examination and health assessment.
RC76.J37 2008a　　　　616.07'5　　　C2008-902121-5

Vice President, Publishing: Ann Millar
Managing Developmental Editor: Martina van de Velde
Managing Production Editor: Lise Dupont
Copy Editor: Susan Harrison
Cover, Interior Design: Paula Catalano; Adapted by Olena Sullivan
Typesetting and Assembly: Jansom
Printing and Binding: Transcontinental

Elsevier Canada
905 King Street West, 4th Floor
Toronto, ON, Canada M6K 3G9
Phone: 1-866-896-3331
Fax: 1-866-359-9534

Printed in Canada

3 4 5　　　　13 12 11 10

To Paul,
Still and always.

About the Author

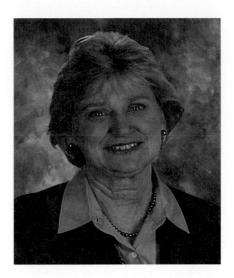

Carolyn Jarvis received her BSN cum laude from the University of Iowa, her MSN from Loyola University (Chicago), and her PhD from the University of Illinois at Chicago, with a research interest in the physiological effect of alcohol on the cardiovascular system. She has taught physical assessment and critical care nursing at Rush University (Chicago), the University of Missouri (Columbia), and the University of Illinois (Urbana), and she has taught physical assessment, pharmacology, and pathophysiology at Illinois Wesleyan University (Bloomington).

Dr. Jarvis is a recipient of the University of Missouri's Superior Teaching Award; has taught physical assessment to thousands of baccalaureate students, graduate students, and nursing professionals; has held 150 continuing education seminars; and is the author of numerous articles and textbook contributions. Dr. Jarvis has maintained a clinical practice in advanced practice roles— first as a cardiovascular clinical specialist in various critical care settings and as a certified family nurse practitioner in primary care. She is currently an associate professor at Illinois Wesleyan University; is a nurse practitioner at Chestnut Health Systems, Bloomington, Illinois; and is licensed as an advanced practice nurse in the state of Illinois.

About the Canadian Editors

Annette J. Browne's career began as an outpost nurse, living and working in northern First Nations and Inuit communities in Canada. She holds a master's degree as a family nurse practitioner from the University of Rhode Island and a PhD in nursing from the University of British Columbia (UBC). She is a faculty member at the UBC School of Nursing and has taught advanced health assessment to nurse practitioners and post-RNs for many years. Dr. Browne is an active researcher whose work focuses on the complex sociopolitical factors that shape health and health care. She has published extensively on First Nations women's health, healthcare inequities, and access to health care. Dr. Browne holds a New Investigator award from the Canadian Institutes of Health Research and a Scholar award from the Michael Smith Foundation for Health Research. In 2008 she received the Award of Excellence in Nursing Research from the College of Registered Nurses of British Columbia.

June MacDonald-Jenkins is a recognized expert in hybrid course delivery e-learning, having worked in this field for many years. As a nursing professor in the Durham College/University of Ontario Institute of Technology (UOIT) BScN program and an instructor in the critical care certificate program at Durham College, Ms. MacDonald-Jenkins brings strong education experience to the team. She has taught health assessment to hundreds of students, from those enrolled in diploma to advanced practice programs. She is also an accomplished practitioner and researcher on the subject of technology and hybrid course delivery use in nursing education. Ms. MacDonald-Jenkins's research interests are primarily in the areas of simulation and in assessing core competencies across curriculum and e-learning course delivery. She is the recipient of the 2007 Elsevier Canada Resource Award, which recognizes exemplary use of technology resources in the academic environment. Ms. MacDonald-Jenkins has presented at international conferences and is looking forward to building future research partnerships to evaluate the effectiveness of e-learning as a means of customizing the student experience.

Marian Luctkar-Flude received her BScN summa cum laude from the University of Ottawa, her critical care nursing diploma with distinction from St. Lawrence College (Kingston), and more recently her MScN from the University of Ottawa. She has over 20 years' medical–surgical nursing experience in various clinical settings and, in particular, in general surgery and urology nursing. She has taught clinically in the St. Lawrence College and Queen's University (Kingston) nursing programs and is currently a course coordinator for the Health Assessment Course at Queen's University School of Nursing, where she has been involved in the introduction of the use of human patient simulation and standardized patients in health assessment. She is also involved in interprofessional education, including teaching interprofessional cardiac resuscitation rounds.

Ms. Luctkar-Flude is currently the nursing laboratory coordinator for the Faculty of Health Sciences Patient Simulation Laboratory at Queen's University and a program coordinator in the Nursing Research Unit at Kingston General Hospital. Her research interests include older persons with cancer, with a specific focus on fatigue and physical activity, and the use of human patient simulation in undergraduate nursing, with a focus on interprofessional education. She has presented at local, national, and international nursing conferences and has acted as a peer reviewer for several nursing and medical journals. She is an editor of *The Nursing Journal* and an active member of the Nursing Research Conference Planning Committee of the Nursing Research Council of Southeastern Ontario Health Sciences Centre.

Contributors

Ian M. Camera, MSN, ND, RN

Ian Camera is an associate professor in the Division of Nursing Education at Holyoke Community College in Massachusetts, where he teaches the fundamentals and advanced medical–surgical courses. His work experience includes long-term care, summer camp nursing, and inpatient medical–surgical nursing. His doctoral research has focused on the impact of for-profit penetration into the home healthcare market in Ohio, using a human ecology framework.

Chapter 28: Reassessment of the Hospitalized Adult

Kim Campbell, RM, RN, BScN, MN

Kim Campbell holds dual certification as a registered midwife and RN. She is a lecturer in the Division of Midwifery within the Faculty of Medicine at the University of British Columbia. In addition to maintaining an active midwifery practice for the past 10 years, Ms. Campbell had extensive experience in labour and delivery prior to obtaining her midwifery certificate. She has also served on the boards of the Midwives Association of British Columbia, the College of Midwives of British Columbia, and the Canadian Association of Midwives.

Chapter 29: Pregnancy

Martha Driessack, PhD, ARNP

Martha Driessack is a pediatric nurse practitioner with over 25 years of experience in teaching, practice, and research. She received her BSN from the Ohio State University, her MSN from Yale University, and her PhD from Oregon Health and Science University. She also completed a postdoctoral research fellowship in clinical genetics from the University of Iowa. She is currently an assistant professor in the College of Nursing at the University of Iowa.

Promoting Health feature boxes

Dana S. Edge, PhD, RN

Dana Edge received her BSN from the University of Iowa, her MSN from University of North Carolina at Chapel Hill, and her doctorate in epidemiology from University of Toronto. She has taught health assessment to undergraduate students at Memorial University of Newfoundland and at the University of Northern British Columbia, and to both undergraduate and graduate students at the University of Calgary. Dr. Edge practised nursing in Minnesota, Colorado, Alaska, and North Carolina before moving to Newfoundland and Labrador in 1986. In Canada she has practised in nursing stations in Labrador and in a rural hospital in northern British Columbia. She is currently an associate professor at Queen's University in Kingston, Ontario.

Chapter 2: Developmental Tasks and Health Promotion Across the Lifespan

Carla Graf, MS, RN, APRN-BC

Carla Graf is a board-certified geriatric clinical nurse specialist at the University of California, San Francisco (UCSF) and is an assistant clinical professor at the UCSF School of Nursing. She has experience in nursing administration, critical care, and medical–surgical nursing. She is currently a doctoral student at UCSF, with a research focus on functional decline in hospitalized older adults.

Chapter 30: Functional Assessment of the Older Adult

Dianne Groll, PhD, RN, BA, BScH, MScH

Dianne Groll is an assistant professor with the Faculty of Medicine at Queen's University in Kingston and an adjunct professor with the University of Ottawa School of Nursing. Her research interests include factors affecting physical function and patient quality of life and the impact of comorbid illness on patient outcomes. Her doctoral research focused on the influence of comorbidity on physical function and how best to quantify the impact of chronic illness. She is involved with studies of older patients in orthopedics, oncology, cardiology, and psychiatry. She is also involved in several studies funded by the Registered Nurses' Association of Ontario, measuring and evaluating nursing best practices. She received her undergraduate and master's degrees from Queen's University and her PhD from the University of Toronto.

Chapter 30: Functional Assessment of the Older Adult

Joyce K. Keithley, DNSc, RN, FAAN

Joyce Keithley is a professor in the Department of Adult Health Nursing, Rush University College of Nursing and Rush University Medical Center in Chicago. Because she has worked in both clinical and instructional settings, she is an experienced and well-known practitioner, teacher, researcher, and author in the area of clinical nutrition.

Chapter 11: Nutritional Assessment

Melissa A. Lee, MS, RN, APRN-BC

Melissa Lee is a medical–surgical clinical nurse specialist at the University of California San Francisco (USCF) Medical Center. She has experience in medical–surgical and telemetry nursing, education, and staff development. She graduated from UCSF in the geriatric clinical nurse specialist program and is certified in geriatrics by the American Nurses Credentialing Center.

Chapter 30: Functional Assessment of the Older Adult

Shawna S. Mudd, MSN, CRNP

Shawna Mudd is a pediatric nurse practitioner in the Pediatric Emergency Department at the Johns Hopkins Hospital. She is also a member of the hospital's child protection team, which provides inpatient and outpatient consultation for cases of suspected child abuse and neglect. Additionally, she is adjunct faculty at Johns Hopkins University School of Nursing.

Chapter 7: Interpersonal Violence Assessment (US Fifth Edition)

Mona Sawhney, RN, MN, ACNP, PhD(Cand.)

Mona Sawhney is an advanced practice nurse with the acute pain service at Sunnybrook Health Sciences Centre in Toronto. She holds a BScN from Ryerson University and an MN and ACNP certificate from the University of Toronto. She is currently a PhD student at the University of Toronto. Mona has published and presented at conferences in the area of pain management both nationally and internationally.

Chapter 10: Pain Assessment: The Fifth Vital Sign

Daniel Sheridan, PhD, RN, CNS, FNE-A, FAAN

Daniel Sheridan is an associate professor in the Johns Hopkins University School of Nursing, where he coordinates a forensic clinical nurse specialist graduate degree program. Dr. Sheridan has almost 25 years of experience working with survivors of family abuse and sexual assault, and he lectures and consults nationally and internationally on these topics.

Chapter 7: Interpersonal Violence Assessment (US Fifth Edition)

Rachel E. Spector, PhD, RN, CTN, FAAN

Rachel Spector has been a student and teacher of culturally diverse health and illness beliefs and practices for more than 35 years and has retired from the Connell Boston College School of Nursing, Chestnut Hill, Massachusetts. In 2006 she was a Lady Davis Fellow in the Henrietta Zold-Hadnassah Hebrew University School of Nursing in Jerusalem, Israel. The sixth edition of her text *Cultural Diversity in Health and Illness* was translated into Spanish and published in Madrid as *Las Culturas de la SALUD* in 2003. She is a fellow in the American Academy of Nursing and a scholar in transcultural nursing.

Chapter 3: Cultural Competence: Cultural Care (US Fifth Edition)

Wendy Stanyon, RN, Ed(D)

Wendy Stanyon is an assistant professor in the Faculty of Health Science at the University of Ontario Institute Technology. An educator for more than 25 years, she has extensive classroom and practicum expertise in a wide variety of core nursing subjects, including mental health. Her research interests involve mental health and vulnerable populations as well as educational strategies, in particular the use of simulations and practicum models in nursing. Ms. Stanyon has developed strong links with practicum partners and a variety of local health and social service organizations through her commitment to community-based research.

Chapter 6: Mental Status Assessment

Deborah E. Swenson, MSN, ARNP

Deborah Swenson is a women's healthcare nurse practitioner with OBSTETRIX Medical Group of Washington, Inc., P.S., in Seattle, Washington. She holds certification from the NCC as a women's healthcare nurse practitioner. She is the author of *Telephone Triage for the Obstetric Patient: A Nursing Guide* and a contributing author for *All-In-One Care Planning Resource*. She is an editorial advisory board member for the magazine *ADVANCE for Nurse Practitioners* and is a certified medical–legal nurse consultant.

Chapter 29: Pregnancy

Denise Tarlier, PhD, MSN, NP(F)

Denise Tarlier is a family nurse practitioner in British Columbia and has also held national U.S. NP certification since 1998. Her clinical practice over many years has been primarily in remote and northern Aboriginal communties across Canada. Her recent doctoral research explored nurses' practice in primary care roles, maternal–infant health outcomes, and continuity of care in a remote First Nations community. She is currently an assistant professor in the School of Nursing at Thompson Rivers University in Kamloops, British Columbia. The focus of her scholarship and teaching continues to be guided by a strong clinical practice orientation to primary health care, rural and remote healthcare services, Aboriginal health issues, and primary care and nurse practitioner nursing roles. She also maintains a part-time clinical practice as a family nurse practitioner in an urban setting and teaches health assessment to nurse practitioner students.

Chapter 17: Breasts and Regional Lymphatics

Christina Vaillancourt, RD, CDE

Christina Vaillancourt completed her bachelor's degree in applied science at Ryerson University. She is a registered dietitian and a certified diabetes educator, currently working in the area of nephrology. She has taught nutrition courses for Durham College and is currently a teaching assistant at the University of Ontario Institute of Technology.

Chapter 11: Nutritional Assessment

Colleen Varcoe, PhD, RN

Colleen Varcoe teaches at undergraduate and graduate levels with a focus on culture, ethics, inequity, and policy at the University of British Columbia. Her research focuses on women's health, with an emphasis on violence and inequity; and on the culture of health care, with an emphasis on ethical practice. Her program of research is aimed at promoting ethical practice and policy in the context of violence and inequity. She recently completed a study of the interacting risks of violence and human immunodeficiency virus infection for rural and Aboriginal women and another study relating to ethical practice in nursing. In 2008 she completed a participatory study of rural Aboriginal maternity care with women in four communities. She is currently co-leader of a team studying the health and economic effects of violence against women after women have left abusive partners. She has over 50 peer-reviewed publications and recently co-edited a book titled *Women's Health in Canada: Critical Perspectives on Theory and Policy.*

Chapter 3: Cultural and Social Considerations in Health Assessment; and Chapter 7: Interpersonal Violence Assessment

Ellen Vogel, PhD, RD, FDC

Ellen Vogel is an assistant professor in the Faculty of Health Sciences at the University of Ontario Institute of Technology, located in Oshawa, Ontario. Dr. Vogel completed a PhD in nutrition and metabolism at the University of Alberta (2001). In 2003 she was awarded a postdoctoral fellowship from the Office of the Chief Scientist at Health Canada. Dr. Vogel is a fellow with Dietitians of Canada; a past chair of the Dietitians of Canada's Board of Directors; and the recipient of numerous awards for leadership and innovation in dietetics practice. Currently Dr. Vogel is a principal investigator on a groundbreaking interdisciplinary study on nutritional genomics and dietetics practice. In 2008 a new text titled *Nutrition and Genomics: Issues of Ethics, Law, Regulation and Communication* (Elsevier) will feature a chapter by Dr. Vogel on the role of the dietetics professional in diet–gene interactions.

Chapter 11: Nutritional Assessment

Barbara Wilson-Keates, RN, MS

Barbara Wilson-Keates has experience in adult medicine and cardiac and critical care nursing in acute care hospitals across Canada and the United States. Over the past 20 years, she has worked in a variety of nursing positions, including clinical nurse and nursing instructor for clinical and classroom courses for undergraduate and graduate nursing students. Ms. Wilson-Keates has assisted in the development and implementation of nursing and interprofessional simulation teaching modules for numerous Ontario colleges and universities. Currently she is a course coordinator for the Nursing Health Assessment Course and is an instructor for Health Sciences Interprofessional Simulation Resuscitation Rounds at the Faculty of Health Sciences Patient Simulation Laboratory at School of Nursing, Queen's University, in Kingston, Ontario. Ms. Wilson-Keates is also a full-time PhD student and research assistant at the Faculty of Nursing, University of Toronto, with an interest in the impact of work environment on nurse retention.

Chapter 16: Nose, Mouth, and Throat

Reviewers of the US Fifth Edition

Pier A. Broadnax, PhD, RN
Assistant Professor
Howard University
Children's National Medical Center
Washington, D.C.

Janice S. DuBrueler, DNSc, RN
Assistant Professor of Nursing
Division of Nursing
Shenandoah University
Winchester, Virginia

Elizabeth E. Hand, MS, RN, BSN
Education Specialist, Author and Consultant
Hands-on Nursing
Broken Arrow, Oklahoma

Anne M. Hautamaki, MSN, RN
Adjunct Nursing Faculty
Oakland Community College
Bloomfield Hills, Michigan

Helen Jackson-Ruiz, RN, MSN
Assistant Professor
Nebraska Methodist College
Omaha, Nebraska

Pameula S. Johnson, RN, BSN, FNE
Nash Healthcare Systems, Inc.
Elm City, North Carolina

Karen C. Johnson-Brennan, BSN, MSN, EdD
Professor and Associate Director
San Francisco State University
School of Nursing
San Francisco, California

Patricia Ketchum, RN, MSN
Adjunct Assistant Professor
Oakland University
School of Nursing
Rochester, Michigan

Jenifer Markowitz, ND, RNc, WHNP
Consultant, Program Development and Clinical Education
The DOVE Program
Summa Health System
Cleveland Heights, Ohio

Lora McGuire, RN, MS
Professor of Nursing and Pain Consultant
Joliet Junior College
Joliet, Illinois

Barbara Pascoe, RN, BA, MA
Director of Maternity/Pediatrics/Women's Health
Concord Hospital
Concord, New Hampshire

Reviewers of the First Canadian Edition

Annette J. Browne, PhD, RN
Associate Professor, School of Nursing
University of British Columbia
Vancouver, British Columbia

Kim Campbell, RM, BSN, BScN, MN
Instructor, Midwifery Program
University of British Columbia
Vancouver, British Columbia

Dana S. Edge, PhD, RN
Associate Professor, School of Nursing
Queen's University
Kingston, Ontario

Dianne Groll, PhD, RN, BA, BScH, MScH
Assistant Professor, Department of Psychiatry
Queen's University
Kingston, Ontario

Marian Luctkar Flude, RN, BScN, MScN
Nursing Laboratory Coordinator, Faculty of Health
    Sciences Patient Simulation Laboratory
Queen's University, School of Nursing
Kingston, Ontario

June MacDonald-Jenkins, RN, BScN, MSc
Learning Technologies Facilitator
Innovation Centre DC/University of Ontario
    Institute of Technology
Oshawa, Ontario

Mona Sawhney, RN, MN, ACNP, PhD(Cand.)
Acute Pain Service
Sunnybrook Health Sciences Centre
Toronto, Ontario

Wendy Stanyon, RN, Ed(D)
Assistant Professor, Faculty of Health Sciences
University of Ontario Institute of Technology
Oshawa, Ontario

Denise Tarlier, PhD, MSN, NP(F)
Assistant Professor, School of Nursing
Thompson Rivers University
Kamloops, British Columbia

Christina Vaillancourt, RD, CDE
Clinical Dietitian
University of Ontario Institute of Technology
Oshawa, Ontario

Colleen Varcoe, PhD, RN
Associate Professor and Associate Director, Research
School of Nursing, University of British Columbia
Vancouver, British Columbia

Ellen Vogel, PhD, RD, FDC
Assistant Professor, Faculty of Health Sciences
University of Ontario Institute of Technology
Oshawa, Ontario

Barbara Wilson-Keates, RN, MS
Sessional Lecturer, School of Nursing
Queen's University
Kingston, Ontario

Preface

It is important that students develop, practise, and then learn to trust their health history and physical examination skills. In this book we give you the tools to do that. Learn to listen to the patient—most often he or she will tell you what is wrong (and right) and what you can do to meet his or her healthcare needs. Then learn to inspect, examine, and listen to the person's body. The data are all there and are accessible to you by using just a few extra tools. High-technological machinery is a smart and sophisticated adjunct, but it cannot replace your own bedside assessment of your patient.

Whether you are a beginning examiner or an advanced-practice student, this book holds the content you need to develop and refine your clinical skills. The **First Canadian Edition** of *Physical Examination & Health Assessment* is a comprehensive textbook of health history-taking methods, physical examination skills, health promotion techniques, and clinical assessment tools.

Thank you for your enthusiastic anticipation of this first-ever Canadian edition. We are excited to be able to bring you an established, successful text with a new focus on Canadian issues and content to further meet the needs of both novice and advanced practitioners in Canada.

DUAL FOCUS AS TEXT AND REFERENCE

Physical Examination & Health Assessment is a **text for beginning students** of physical examination as well as a **text and reference for advanced practitioners such as nurse practitioners and clinical nurse specialists.** The chapter progression and format permit this scope without sacrificing one use for the other.

Chapters 1 through 7 focus on **health assessment of individuals and families**, including developmental tasks and health promotion for all age groups, the importance of relational practice in health assessment, cultural and social considerations in assessment, interviewing and complete health history gathering, and the social context of mental status assessment and interpersonal violence assessment.

Chapters 8 through 11 begin the approach to the **clinical care setting,** describing physical data-gathering techniques, how to set up the examination site, body measurement and vital signs, pain assessment, and nutritional assessment.

Chapters 12 through 26 focus on the **physical examination and related health history** in a body systems approach. This is the most efficient method of performing the examination and is the most logical method for student learning and retrieval of data. **Each chapter has five major sections:** Structure and Function, Subjective Data (history), Objective Data (examination skills and findings), Documentation and Critical Thinking, and Abnormal Findings. The novice practitioner can review anatomy and physiology and learn the skills, expected findings, and common variations for generally healthy people and selected abnormal findings in the Objective Data sections.

Chapters 27 through 30 **integrate the complete health assessment.** Chapters 27 and 28 present the choreography of the head-to-toe examination for a complete screening examination in various age groups and for the focused examination of a hospitalized adult. Special populations are addressed in Chapters 29 and 30—the health assessment of the pregnant woman and the functional assessment of the older adult.

Students continue to use this text in subsequent courses throughout their education and well into advanced practice. Since each course demands more advanced skills and techniques, students can review the detailed presentation and the additional techniques in the Objective Data sections as well as variations for different age levels. Students can also study the extensive pathology illustrations and detailed text in the Abnormal Findings sections.

This text is valuable to both advanced practice students and experienced clinicians because of its comprehensive approach. *Physical Examination & Health Assessment* can help clinicians learn the skills for advanced practice, refresh their memory, review a specific examination technique when confronted with an unfamiliar clinical situation, and compare and label a diagnostic finding.

NEW TO THE FIRST CANADIAN EDITION

All chapters are **revised and updated** to include Canadian terminology, statistics, standards and guidelines, and assessment tools commonly used in Canadian healthcare settings. Two newly written chapters and several new features that span various chapters are presented in this First Canadian Edition. Fifteen new **Promoting Health** boxes are presented—one in each of the physical examination chapters. These boxes describe an important health promotion topic related to the system discussed in each chapter—a topic you can use to enhance patient education initiatives.

The **Cultural and Social Considerations** sections have been newly written in each chapter to reflect issues relevant to Canada. The cultural and social factors that influence health, illness, and access to health care are discussed, and implications requiring consideration in the context of health assessment are identified. Highlights of Canadian content in each chapter are outlined below.

Chapter 1, **Critical Thinking in Health Assessment,** includes a discussion of relational approaches to nursing practice and the relevance of these approaches to health assessment. The leading role that Canada has played in the area of health promotion is emphasized.

Chapter 2, **Developmental Tasks and Health Promotion Across the Lifespan,** provides the latest Canadian guidelines for health promotion, disease prevention, screening, patient counselling, and immunizations across the lifespan.

Chapter 3, **Cultural and Social Considerations in Health Assessment,** is newly written to reflect the ethnocultural and social diversity within the Canadian population. Examples of current trends in health, social, and gender inequities are reviewed and discussed in terms of the implications for health assessment. Guidelines are provided for assessing culturally based understandings and the social and economic contexts shaping people's lives.

Chapter 6, **Mental Status Assessment,** offers new content reflecting Canadian perspectives on the social factors that shape mental health and illness and provides Canadian guidelines for screening and assessment across the lifespan.

Chapter 7, **Interpersonal Violence Assessment,** has also been newly written to include guidelines for assessing intimate partner violence, sexual assault, child abuse, and elder abuse as important problems for healthcare professionals to recognize and respond to. The long-term effects of violence on health and the implications in the context of health assessment are discussed.

Chapter 8, **Assessment Techniques and the Clinical Setting,** focuses on assessment techniques and includes the Canadian Hypertensive Education Program guidelines for diagnosis. The chapter will help both novice and advanced practitioners make clinical decisions based on accurate assessment techniques.

Chapter 10, **Pain Assessment: The Fifth Vital Sign,** has been updated to include assessment tools for both conscious and unconscious patients. These additions reflect a growing trend toward caring for palliative patients in the community setting and the increased complexity of caring for the patient found outside the intensive care environment.

Chapter 11, **Nutritional Assessment,** has been updated to reflect the content that appears in the new publication, *Eating Well with Canada's Food Guide.*

Chapter 29, **Pregnancy,** incorporates Canadian screening and diagnostic tests for the pregnant woman and guidelines for health promotion.

Chapter 30, **Functional Assessment of the Older Adult,** includes Canadian statistics on aging, guidelines for screening for elder abuse and prevention of falls, and content related to caregiver, environmental, and spiritual assessments. Tools for assessment of activities of daily living, instrumental activities of daily living, and advanced activities of daily living are discussed.

APPROACHES USED IN THIS EDITION

The First Canadian Edition of *Physical Examination & Health Assessment* is built on the strengths of the US Fifth Edition and is designed to engage students and enhance learning:

1. **Method of examination** (Objective Data section) is clear, orderly, and easy to follow. Hundreds of original examination illustrations are placed directly with the text to demonstrate the physical examination in a step-by-step format.

2. **Two-column format** begins in the Subjective Data section, where the running column highlights the rationales for asking various history questions. In the Objective Data section, the running column highlights selected abnormal findings to show a clear relationship between normal and abnormal findings.

3. **Abnormal Findings tables** organize and expand on material in the examination section. The atlas format of these extensive collections of pathology and original illustrations helps students recognize, sort, and describe abnormal findings. When applicable, the text under a table entry is presented in a Subjective Data–Objective Data format.

4. **Developmental approach** in each chapter presents prototypical content on the adult, then age-specific content for the infant, child, adolescent, pregnant woman, and older adult so that students can learn common variations for all age groups.

5. **Cultural and social considerations** are discussed throughout as factors that shape health, illness, and access to health care. In addition to Chapter 3, where these issues are discussed in depth, cultural and social considerations are included throughout the chapters to orient readers to relevant issues in the Canadian context.

   Readers will note that literature citations based on US or British research continue to use the terms "Black" (to refer to people of African American descent) and "White" (for people of European descent). In Canada, there has been a shift away from identifying people on the basis of "race," and these issues are discussed in more depth in Chapter 3. When US or British literature is cited, however, the terms "Black" and "White" are retained in keeping with the original reference sources.

6. **Stunning full-colour art** shows detailed human anatomy, physiology, examination techniques, and abnormal findings.

7. **Health history** (Subjective Data) appears in two places: Chapter 4, The Interview, has the most complete discussion available on the process of communication and on interviewing skills, techniques, and traps. This chapter includes guidelines for communicating with people whose primary language differs from yours and for working with interpreters to conduct respectful and accurate health assessments. In Chapter 5, The Complete Health History, and in pertinent history questions that are repeated and expanded in each chapter, history questions are included that highlight health promotion and self-care. This presentation helps students understand the relationship between subjective and objective data. Because the history and examination data are considered together, as you would do in the clinical setting, each chapter can stand on its own if a person has a specific problem related to that body system.

8. **Summary checklists** toward the end of each chapter provide a quick review of examination steps to help you develop a mental checklist.

9. **Sample recordings** of normal findings show the written language you should use to ensure that charting is complete yet succinct.

10. **Focused assessment and clinical case studies** of frequently encountered situations demonstrate the application of assessment techniques to patients of different ages in differing clinical situations. These case histories, in subjective-objective-analysis-plan (SOAP) format, ending in diagnosis, are presented in the language actually used during recording.

11. **Integration of the complete health assessment** for the adult, infant, and child is presented as an illustrated essay in Chapter 27. This approach integrates all the steps into a choreographed whole. Included is a complete write-up of a health history and physical examination.

12. **User-friendly design** makes the book easy to use. Frequent subheadings and instructional headings help readers to easily retrieve content.

13. Reassessment of the Hospitalized Adult, in Chapter 28, provides a unique photo sequence that **illustrates a head-to-toe assessment** suitable for each daily shift of care. It would be neither possible nor pertinent to perform a complete head-to-toe examination on every patient during every 24-hour stay in the hospital. Therefore, this sequence shows a consistent specialized examination for each 8-hour shift that focuses on certain parameters pertinent to areas of medical, surgical, and cardiac step-down care.

The Canadian content that appears in the book, particularly the content dealing with hospitalized patients, older adults, and pain assessment, and the content relating to interpersonal violence and to cultural and social considerations, are part of the standard repertoire of knowledge that Canadian examiners can draw on.

CONCEPTUAL APPROACH

The First Canadian Edition of *Physical Examination & Health Assessment* reflects a commitment to the following approaches:

- **Relational practice** in clinical practice recognizes that health, illness, and the meanings they hold for people are shaped by one's gender, age, ability, and social, cultural, familial, historical, and geographical contexts. These contexts influence how nurses and other healthcare professionals view, relate, and work with patients and families. By practising relationally, healthcare professionals will be optimally prepared to conduct accurate health assessments and to respond meaningfully to the patient's health, illness, and health promotion needs.

- **Health promotion** is presented in the health history questions—which explore peoples' various health practices—and in the age-specific charts for periodic health examinations (Chapter 2), the Promoting Health boxes, and patient education guidelines for skin, breast, testicles, and nutrition.

- Engaging with the patient as an **active participant in health care** involves encouraging discussion of what the person currently is doing to promote his or her health and supporting people to participate in health promoting practices given the social contexts of their lives.

- **Cultural and social considerations** take into account our global society and the wide range of ethnocultural and social diversity within Canada.

- Assessing individuals **across the lifespan** reflects the understanding that a person's state of health must be considered in light of his or her developmental stage. Chapter 2 presents a baseline of developmental tasks and topics expected for each age group, and subsequent chapters integrate relevant developmental content. Developmental anatomy, modifications of examination techniques, and expected findings for infants and children, adolescents, pregnant women, and older adults are provided.

ANCILLARIES

- The *Companion CD-ROM* presents realistic patient **case studies**—including a variety of developmental variables—to help you apply your health assessment skills and knowledge. It includes 20 in-depth case studies with critical thinking questions and answer guidelines, as well as printable **health promotion handouts.**

  Also included is a complete **head-to-toe video examination** of the adult that can be viewed in its entirety or by systems and a new printable section on Quick Assessments for 20 Common Conditions.

- **Instructor resources** on the Evolve site include an Instructor's Manual, PowerPoint slides, Image Collection, and Computerized Test Bank. The *Instructor's Manual* provides annotated learning objectives; key terms; teaching strategies for the classroom, skills laboratory, and clinical setting; and critical thinking exercises. The PowerPoint slides include over 600 integrated images and new animations, as well as 50 new questions for use in the classroom with audience-response systems. A separate 1000-illustration **Image Collection** is featured; and, finally, the **ExamView Computerized Test Bank** has over 850 multiple choice questions with coded answers and rationales. Instructors also have access to the accompanying online course, Health Assessment Online.

- The *Pocket Companion for Physical Examination & Health Assessment* continues to be a handy and current clinical reference that provides pertinent material in full colour including more than 150 illustrations from the textbook.

- The *Student Laboratory Manual* with physical examination forms is a workbook that includes for each chapter a student study guide, glossary of key terms, clinical objectives, regional write-up forms, and review questions. The pages are perforated so that students can use the regional write-up forms in the skills laboratory or in the clinical setting and turn them in to the instructor.

- The new revised *Health Assessment Online* resource is an innovative and dynamic teaching and learning tool with over **8000 electronic assets,** including video clips, animations, audio clips, interactive exercises, laboratory and diagnostic tests, review questions, and Weblinks to accompany each chapter. New to this version are comprehensive

Self-Paced Learning Modules, which offer increased flexibility to faculty who wish to provide students with tutorial learning modules and in-depth capstone cases for each body system chapter in the text. Animations, sounds, images, interactive activities, and video clips are embedded in the learning modules and cases to provide a dynamic, multimodal learning environment for today's learners.

- *Physical Examination & Health Assessment DVD Series* is a 17-disc package developed in conjunction with the text. There are 12 body system videos and five head-to-toe videos, with the latter containing complete examinations of the neonate, child, adult, older adult, and pregnant woman. This series is available in DVD or streaming online formats. Over 5 hours of all-new video footage is included with highlighted Cross-Cultural Care Considerations, Developmental Considerations, and Health Promotion Tips, as well as Instructor Booklets with video overviews, outlines, learning objectives, discussion topics, and questions with answers.

- The *EVOLVE Student Web site* (located at http://evolve.elsevier.com/Canada/Jarvis/examination/) contains learning objectives, over 150 multiple choice review questions, new system-by-system examination summaries and bedside examination summaries that are downloadable into audio CD or MP3 player files, a comprehensive physical examination form for the adult, 2000 Weblinks for further research, and numerous **reference appendices** from previous editions that have been updated and moved online, including immunization schedules, standard precautions, growth charts, blood pressure levels, and more—in effect, a comprehensive online student resource that takes advantage of the dynamic nature of electronic content and online delivery.

IN CONCLUSION

Throughout all stages of manuscript preparation and production, every effort has been made to develop a book that is readable, informative, instructive, and vital. Your comments and suggestions have been important to this task and continue to be welcome for this new Canadian edition.

Carolyn Jarvis
Annette J. Browne
June MacDonald-Jenkins
Marian Luctkar-Flude
c/o Elsevier Canada
905 King Street West, 4th Floor
Toronto, ON M6K 3G9

Acknowledgements for the US Fifth Edition

It is my pleasure to recognize the many wonderful friends and colleagues who helped make the revision of this textbook possible. For their help and support I send my gratitude:

To my colleagues, who were a willing resource of information and constructive comments. I am particularly grateful to Joyce Keithley, DNSc, RN, FAAN, who contributed the chapter on nutritional assessment and who was always willing and responsive to my queries about content and photographs. Rachel Spector, PhD, RN, CTN, FAAN, contributed the chapter on cultural care in assessment, sharing a wealth of pertinent content on diversity and a global perspective. Daniel Sheridan, PhD, RN, CNS, FNE-A, FAAN, and Shawna Mudd, MSN, CRNP, provided a thoughtful and important chapter on domestic violence assessment. Finally, my thanks to Deborah Swenson, MSN, ARNP, who brought her knowledge and years of experience to the revised chapter on The Pregnant Female.

To my colleagues who provided advice on specific topics in this edition: Vickie Folse, RN, PhD; Donna Hartweg, RN, PhD; Paul Jarvis, PhD; Sharie Metcalfe, RN, PhD; Mariann Piano, RN, PhD; Marilyn Prasun, RN, PhD; and Kathy Scherck, RN, DNSc.

To my artistic colleagues, who made this book the vibrant visual display it is. Pat Thomas, medical illustrator, is a gifted artist with an eye for detail and clarity. Kevin Strandberg is a clever and careful photographer who has endless patience for capturing the images of children and adults in just the right moment of the examination. Our team has worked together for five editions, providing an artistic unity and clarity to this latest textbook.

To my research assistants, whose tireless help enabled me to survive and proceed through manuscript preparation and revision. Caitlin Zindars read and reread endless copies of galley and page proofs, making astute suggestions and correcting errors. Susan Kuretski retrieved countless articles.

To the faculty and students who took the time to write letters of encouragement and suggestions—your comments are gratefully received and are very helpful. To the reviewers who spent considerable time reading the chapter manuscript and filling out response questionnaires—your suggestions and ideas are very important for this fifth edition.

Thank you to the remarkable professional team at Elsevier. I am grateful to Sally Schrefer, executive vice president for Nursing and Health Professions, for her guidance and support for the book and its ancillaries. Sally knows the text well and has been personally involved in its advancement and promotion. Robin Carter, executive editor, has been a beacon of support for me and for the book. Robin always has sound suggestions for new ideas for the book and is everlastingly prompt and positive. Mary Parker, senior editorial assistant, has spent countless research hours in our quest for fresh new photographs for examples of abnormalities in the book.

Many people worked very hard to guide this book through production. I am grateful to Debbie Vogel, publishing services manager, for supervising the schedule for book production and making all the contacts to keep everyone on schedule. My thanks go to Steve Ramay and especially to Jodi Willard, senior project managers, who have been great point persons in our day-to-day production schedule. I am grateful to Paula Catalano, senior designer, for the beautiful interior design. The design draws the reader into the book and guides one through all the subsections. The dramatic cover is the work of Paula and Max Fischer as well. The individual page layout is the wonderful work of Leslie Foster, illustrator/designer. Leslie crafts every page, always planning how the page can be made even better. Finally, I am so fortunate to have the support of Deanna Davis, developmental editor. Deanna has worked tirelessly and efficiently to keep the manuscript moving. Deanna anticipates and provides answers to questions before the questions themselves arise. Deanna has seen to so many details that I could not work without her. Thank you for everything, Deanna.

Most important are the members of my wonderful family for their help, love, and complete support. Their constant belief in me and their encouragement have kept me going throughout this process.

Carolyn Jarvis

Acknowledgements for the First Canadian Edition

Carolyn Jarvis's text has been a constant companion throughout my clinical and teaching career; providing Canadian perspectives, content, and guidelines in the form of a First Canadian Edition has therefore been an honour. I have thoroughly enjoyed thinking critically about the range of content to include, especially given the diverse range of students, clinicians, and faculty who may use this text. I want to thank Sally Thorne, professor and director at the University of British Columbia School of Nursing, for encouraging me to take on this project, and Ann Millar at Elsevier, for her guidance throughout this process. I am also grateful to June MacDonald-Jenkins and Marian Luctkar-Flude, who worked so diligently to ensure this book's timely completion. I was fortunate to have been able to draw on the expertise of Colleen Varcoe, Denise Tarlier, Dana Edge, and Wendy Stanyon as chapter authors and contributors, and I thank them for investing their knowledge and time. A special thank you goes to Denise Tarlier, whose extensive knowledge of clinical assessment in the Canadian context was invaluable, and who spent countless hours reviewing clinical guidelines and various other aspects of the chapters. Finally, thank you to my partner, John, for providing support in so many ways.

Annette J. Browne

What a pleasure to have been given the opportunity to potentially influence the learning of students across the country. My thanks to every student who risked taking a stance of inquiry, looked for more, and sought the answers; you are the reason that editing this text was such a pleasure. I, too, would like to thank the editorial team at Elsevier Canada; they have been gracious and supportive while ensuring that we met timelines for publication of the First Canadian Edition. I would like to thank my colleagues Ellen Vogel and Christina Vaillancourt for contributing to Chapter 11, Nutritional Assessment, and to Mona Sawhney for her work on Chapter 10, Pain: The Fifth Vital Sign. Their expertise in these areas allowed a seamless transition to Canadian content. I extend my thanks to these three people for hours of collaboration and consultation to ensure the inclusion of a truly national perspective. Thanks of course to my co-editors Annette and Marian; your knowledge and insight have truly shaped the new perspective of this text. Finally, I, too, would like to thank my family for their endless support and indulgence of my "adventures:" my husband, Dean, and my three daughters, Sarah, Emily, and Mackenzie.

June MacDonald-Jenkins

I am truly grateful for having had the opportunity to participate in the development of the First Canadian Edition of Jarvis's *Physical Examination & Health Assessment*. The support of the Elsevier Canada staff throughout this challenging process has been invaluable. In particular, I would like to thank the publisher, Ann Millar, the managing developmental editor, Martina van de Velde, and the managing production editor, Lise Dupont, for their guidance and for keeping us on track with the tight timelines. I would also like to thank my colleagues Barbara Wilson-Keates and Dianne Groll for their contributions to the Nose, Mouth, and Throat, and Functional Assessment of the Older Adult chapters; and Kim Campbell for contributing to the Pregnancy chapter, since these are not my areas of expertise. I would like to thank my Canadian co-editors, Annette J. Browne and June MacDonald-Jenkins, for their long-distance collaboration, for sharing their knowledge, contacts, and resources, and for providing helpful feedback on my revisions. It has been a pleasure and a great learning experience to work with each of you. And, finally, I would like to acknowledge the patience, understanding, and support of my wonderful family: my husband, Richard, my sons, Curtis, Cameron, and Corey, and my daughter, Brianna, who all took on additional responsibilities so that I could complete my MScN degree and contribute to this exciting project.

Marian Luctkar-Flude

Companion CD-ROM Reference Guide

CASE STUDIES

Case Study	Related Clinical Chapters*	Cultural and Developmental Variables
Case Study #1	Chapter 11: Nutritional Assessment Chapter 21: Abdomen	Nikki Age: 16
Case Study #2	Chapter 18: Thorax and Lungs	Tommy Age: 4
Case Study #3	Chapter 9: General Survey, Measurement, Vital Signs Chapter 15: Ears	Molly and Maggie Ages: 2 months and 11 years
Case Study #4	Chapter 5: The Complete Health History Chapter 15: Ears Chapter 14: Eyes Chapter 22: Musculoskeletal System	Mr. Emerson Age: 68
Case Study #5	Chapter 19: Heart and Neck Vessels Chapter 18: Thorax and Lungs	Mrs. Lee Age: 80
Case Study #6	Chapter 6: Mental Status Assessment	Mr. Fletcher Age: 77
Case Study #7	Chapter 4: The Interview Chapter 17: Breasts and Regional Lymphatics	Mrs. Reynaldo Age: 40
Case Study #8	Chapter 19: Heart and Neck Vessels Chapter 20: Peripheral Vascular System and Lymphatic System	Mr. Madison Age: 49
Case Study #9	Chapter 12: Skin, Hair, and Nails Chapter 18: Thorax and Lungs	Joe Age: 30
Case Study #10	Chapter 26: Female Genitourinary System Chapter 29: The Pregnant Female	Rosie Age: 25
Case Study #11	Chapter 7: Domestic Violence Assessment Chapter 29: The Pregnant Female	Sue Li Age: 20
Case Study #12	Chapter 12: Skin, Hair, and Nails Chapter 24: Male Genitourinary System	Jason Age: 26
Case Study #13	Chapter 3: Cultural Competence: Cultural Care Chapter 10: Pain Assessment: The Fifth Vital Sign Chapter 19: Heart and Neck Vessels	Esperanza Vasquez Age: 39
Case Study #14	Chapter 16: Nose, Mouth, and Throat Chapter 18: Thorax and Lungs	Daniel Little Bear Age: 14
Case Study #15	Chapter 9: General Survey, Measurement, Vital Signs Chapter 14: Eyes Chapter 19: Heart and Neck Vessels	Ruby Jones Age: 78
Case Study #16	Chapter 6: Mental Status Assessment Chapter 20: Peripheral Vascular System and Lymphatic System Chapter 23: Neurologic System	Kurt Age: 48
Case Study #17	Chapter 12: Skin, Hair, and Nails Chapter 13: Head, Face, and Neck, Including Regional Lymphatics Chapter 23: Neurologic System	Mr. de Gail Age: 68

*Content in Chapters 1 to 8 is integrated throughout the case studies.

Continued

Case Study	Related Clinical Chapters*	Cultural and Developmental Variables
Case Study #18	Chapter 11: Nutritional Assessment	Melku Age: 2
Case Study #19	Chapter 4: The Interview Chapter 18: Thorax and Lungs Chapter 19: Heart and Neck Vessels	LaToya Age: 51
Case Study #20	Chapter 12: Skin, Hair, and Nails Chapter 21: Abdomen Chapter 25: Anus, Rectum, and Prostate	Leroy Age: 61

*Content in Chapters 1 to 8 is integrated throughout the case studies.

HEALTH PROMOTION GUIDES

Breast Cancer *(relates to Chapter 17)*
Cancer of the Cervix *(relates to Chapter 26)*
Chewing Tobacco *(relates to Chapter 16)*
Child Safety and Health *(relates to Chapter 2)*
Colon and Rectal Cancer *(relates to Chapter 25)*
Depression *(relates to Chapter 6)*
Diabetes (Type 2) *(relates to Chapter 11)*
Heart Disease *(relates to Chapter 19)*
High Blood Pressure *(relates to Chapter 20)*
Prostate Cancer *(relates to Chapter 25)*
Sexually Transmitted Infections *(relates to Chapters 24 and 26)*
Skin Cancer *(relates to Chapter 12)*
Smoking Cessation *(relates to Chapter 18)*
Testicular Cancer *(relates to Chapter 24)*

ADULT HEAD-TO-TOE EXAMINATION VIDEO

- Complete full-length video
- Video clips organized by body system

QUICK ASSESSMENTS FOR 20 COMMON CONDITIONS

Alzheimer's Disease *(relates to Chapters 6, 9, and 30)*
Asthma *(relates to Chapter 18)*
Benign Prostatic Hypertrophy *(relates to Chapters 24 and 25)*
Brain Attack (stroke or cerebral vascular accident) *(relates to Chapter 23)*
Cellulitis *(relates to Chapter 12)*
Congestive Heart Failure (CHF) *(relates to Chapter 19)*
Deep Vein Thrombosis *(relates to Chapter 20)*
Degenerative Joint Disease (Osteoarthritis) *(relates to Chapter 22)*
Depression *(relates to Chapter 6)*
Fracture *(relates to Chapter 22)*
Hyperlipidemia *(relates to Chapter 19)*
Iron Deficiency Anemia *(relates to Chapters 9 and 29)*
Osteoporosis *(relates to Chapter 22)*
Otitis Media *(relates to Chapter 15)*
Peptic Ulcer Disease *(relates to Chapter 21)*
Premenstrual Syndrome (PMS) *(relates to Chapter 26)*
Renal Calculus (Urolithiasis) *(relates to Chapters 24 and 26)*
Rhinovirus (Common Cold) *(relates to Chapter 16)*
Sickle Cell Anemia *(relates to Chapters 3 and 10)*
Urinary Tract Infection *(relates to Chapter 24 and 26)*

PHYSICAL EXAMINATION
&
Health Assessment

First Canadian Edition

Critical Thinking in Health Assessment

Written by **Carolyn Jarvis**, PhD, APN, CNP
Adapted by **Annette J. Browne**, PhD, RN

Ellen K. is a 23-year-old unemployed woman who entered a substance abuse treatment program because of numerous drug-related driving offenses (Fig. 1-1).

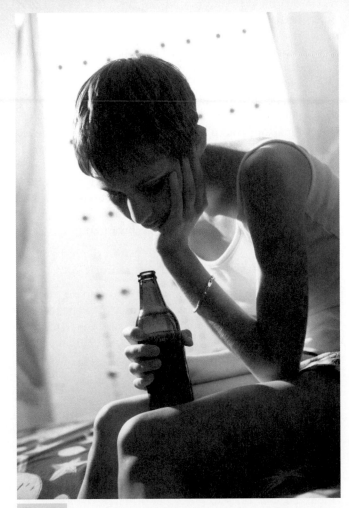

Fig. 1-1

After her admission, the examiner collected a health history and performed a complete physical examination. The actual preliminary list of significant findings looked like this:

- High-school academic record strong (A−/B+) in first 3 years, grades fell in Grade 12 but did graduate
- Alcohol use, started age 16, heavy daily usage × 3 years prior to admission (PTA), last drink 4 days PTA
- Smoked two packs per day (PPD) × 2 years, prior use one PPD × 4 years
- Elevated blood pressure (BP; 142/100 at end of examination today)
- Diminished breath sounds, with moderate expiratory wheeze and scattered rhonchi at both bases
- Grade ii/vi systolic heart murmur, left lower sternal border
- Resolving hematoma, 2 to 3 cm, right (R) infraorbital ridge
- Missing R lower first molar, gums receding on lower incisors, multiple dark spots on all teeth
- Well-healed scar, 28 cm long × 2 cm wide, R lower leg, with R leg 3 cm shorter than left (L), sequelae of auto accident at age 12
- Altered nutrition—omits breakfast, daily intake has no fruits, no vegetables, meals at fast food restaurants most days
- Oral contraceptives for birth control × 3 years, last pelvic exam 1 year PTA
- Unemployed × 6 months, previous work as cashier, bartender
- History of physically abusive relationship with boyfriend, today has orbital hematoma as a result of being hit, states, "It's OK, I probably deserved it"
- History of sexual abuse by father when Ellen was 12 to 16 years of age
- Relationships—estranged from parents, no close women friends, only significant relationship is with boyfriend of 2 years whom Ellen describes as physically abusive and alcoholic

The examiner analyzed and interpreted all the data; clustered the information, sorting out which data to refer and which to treat; and identified the diagnoses. Although the diagnostic process is discussed later, it is interesting now to note how many significant findings are derived from data the examiner collected. Not just physical data but cognitive, psychosocial, and behavioural data are significant for an analysis of Ellen's health state. Also, the findings are interesting when considered from a life cycle perspective; that is, Ellen is a young adult who normally should be concerned with the developmental tasks of emancipation from parents, building an independent lifestyle, establishing a vocation, and choosing a mate (see Chapter 2, p. 24). Many factors are important for a complete health assessment.

ASSESSMENT—POINT OF ENTRY IN AN ONGOING PROCESS

Assessment is the collection of data about the individual's health state. Throughout this text, you will be studying the techniques of collecting and analyzing **subjective data** (i.e., what the person *says* about himself or herself during history taking) and **objective data** (i.e., what you as the healthcare professional *observe* by inspecting, percussing, palpating, and auscultating during the physical examination). Together with the patient's record and laboratory studies, these elements form the **database.**

From the database, you make a clinical judgement or diagnosis about the individual's health state or response to actual or risk health problems and life processes, as well as diagnoses about higher levels of wellness. Thus, the purpose of assessment is to make a judgement or diagnosis.

An organized assessment is the starting point of every approach to clinical reasoning. Because all healthcare treatments and decisions are made based on the data you gather during assessment, it is paramount that your assessment be factual and complete. Discussed below are these considerations to healthcare delivery: diagnostic reasoning, the nursing process, and critical thinking.

Diagnostic Reasoning in Clinical Judgement

The step from data collection to diagnosis can be a difficult one. Most beginning examiners perform well in gathering the data, given adequate practice, but then treat all the data as being equally important. This makes decision making slow and laboured.

Diagnostic reasoning, the process of analyzing health data and drawing conclusions to identify diagnoses, is based on the scientific method. It has four major components: (1) attending to initially available cues; (2) formulating diagnostic hypotheses; (3) gathering data relative to the tentative hypotheses; and (4) evaluating each hypothesis with the new data collected, thus arriving at a final diagnosis. A *cue* is a piece of information, a sign or symptom, or a piece of laboratory data. A *hypothesis* is a tentative explanation for a cue or a set of cues that can be used as a basis for further investigation.

For example, consider Ellen K., the case study presented at the beginning of this chapter. Ellen presents with a number of initial cues, one of which is the resolving hematoma under her eye. (1) You can recognize this cue even before history-taking begins. Is it significant? (2) Ellen says she ran into a door, although she mumbles as she speaks and avoids eye contact. At this point, you formulate a hypothesis of trauma. (3) During the history and physical examination, you gather data to support or reject the tentative hypothesis. (4) You synthesize the new data collected, which support the hypothesis of trauma but eliminate the accidental cause. The final diagnoses are resolving right orbital contusion and risk for trauma.

Diagnostic hypotheses are activated very early in the reasoning process. Consider this a "hunch" that Ellen has suffered physical trauma. A hunch helps diagnosticians adapt to large amounts of information because it clusters cues into meaningful groups and directs subsequent data collection. Later, you can accept your hunch or rule it out.

Once you complete data collection, develop a preliminary list of significant signs and symptoms and all patient health needs. This is less formal in structure than your final list of diagnoses will be and is in no particular order. (Such a list for Ellen is found on p. 1.) In some institutions, it is easier to generate such a list if you use a conceptual model. Examples of conceptual models are described later in this chapter.

Cluster or group together the assessment data that appear to be causal or associated. For example, with a person in acute pain, associated data may include rapid heart rate and anxiety. Organizing the data into meaningful clusters is slow at first; experienced examiners cluster data more rapidly because they recall proven results of earlier patient situations (Benner et al., 1996). Use of a conceptual model helps to organize data.

Validate the data you collect to make sure they are accurate. As you validate your information, look for gaps in data collection. Be sure to find the missing pieces, as identifying missing information is an essential critical thinking skill. How you validate your data depends on experience. If you are unsure of the BP, validate it by repeating it yourself. Eliminate any extraneous variables that could influence BP results, such as recent activity or anxiety over admission. If you have less experience analyzing breath sounds or heart murmurs, ask an expert to listen. Even with years of clinical experience, some signs always require validation (e.g., a breast lump).

Nursing Process in Clinical Judgement

Also based on the scientific method, the **nursing process** includes six phases: assessment, diagnosis, outcome identification, planning, implementation, and evaluation (American Nurses Association, 2004). In the 1970s and 1980s, the nursing process was considered a clear, stepwise, linear approach that started with assessment and ended with evaluation. Now we consider it to be a more dynamic, interactive process; in today's complex clinical setting, practitioners move back and forth within the steps (Fig. 1-2).

Although the nursing process is a problem-solving approach to clinical judgements, the way in which we apply the process depends on our level and time of experience. The *novice* nurse has no experience with a specified patient population and uses rules to guide performance (Benner et al., 1996). It takes time, perhaps 2 to 3 years in similar clinical

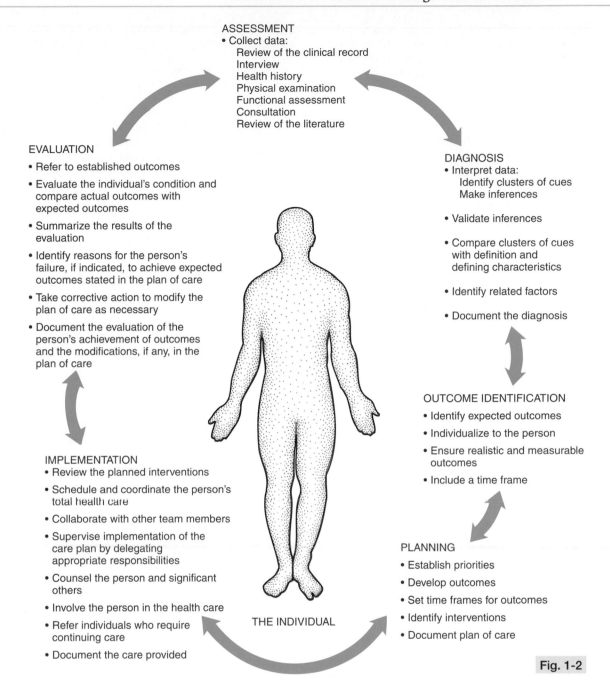

ASSESSMENT
• Collect data:
    Review of the clinical record
    Interview
    Health history
    Physical examination
    Functional assessment
    Consultation
    Review of the literature

EVALUATION

• Refer to established outcomes

• Evaluate the individual's condition and compare actual outcomes with expected outcomes

• Summarize the results of the evaluation

• Identify reasons for the person's failure, if indicated, to achieve expected outcomes stated in the plan of care

• Take corrective action to modify the plan of care as necessary

• Document the evaluation of the person's achievement of outcomes and the modifications, if any, in the plan of care

IMPLEMENTATION
• Review the planned interventions

• Schedule and coordinate the person's total health care

• Collaborate with other team members

• Supervise implementation of the care plan by delegating appropriate responsibilities

• Counsel the person and significant others

• Involve the person in the health care

• Refer individuals who require continuing care

• Document the care provided

THE INDIVIDUAL

DIAGNOSIS
• Interpret data:
    Identify clusters of cues
    Make inferences

• Validate inferences

• Compare clusters of cues with definition and defining characteristics

• Identify related factors

• Document the diagnosis

OUTCOME IDENTIFICATION
• Identify expected outcomes

• Individualize to the person

• Ensure realistic and measurable outcomes

• Include a time frame

PLANNING
• Establish priorities

• Develop outcomes

• Set time frames for outcomes

• Identify interventions

• Document plan of care

Fig. 1-2

situations to achieve *competency*, where the nurse sees actions in the context of arching goals or daily plans for patients. With more time and experience, the *proficient* nurse understands a patient situation as a whole rather than as a list of tasks. This nurse sees long-term goals for the patient and how today's nursing actions apply to achieving those goals in, for example, 6 weeks. Finally, it seems that *expert* nurses vault over the steps and arrive at a clinical judgement in one leap. The expert nurse has an intuitive grasp of a clinical situation and zeroes in on the accurate solution (Benner et al., 1996).

This is true particularly with expert nurses in critical care situations in which patient status changes rapidly and accurate decisions are paramount. The stakes are high, and nursing autonomy is strong. In these cases, the expert focuses on patient responses and prevents complications with vigilant

monitoring (Hanneman, 1996). The expert has well-developed physical assessment skills and trusts these physical assessment skills, even if this conflicts with technologically driven data. For example, consider the expert's actions in assessing a woman with a drug overdose who had an endotracheal tube and was receiving mechanical ventilation.

The expert nurse examined the woman's posterior chest during medical rounds. She said to the medical team, "Mrs. Potter has bronchial breath sounds and dullness to percussion here and here (pointing to an area the size of a nickel and to another area the size of a quarter over the right lower lobe). Do you think she aspirated?" The physicians said, "No, her chest x-ray is normal." Three physicians took turns auscultating and percussing Mrs. Potter's chest. None of them could hear the changes, even when the expert drew circles around the areas. The medical conclusion was that Mrs. Potter had not aspirated. Undaunted, the expert nurse initiated a regimen of pulmonary interventions. On rounds the next day, the medical team ordered antibiotics and frequent pulmonary treatments based on the early morning chest x-ray findings of right lower lobe consolidation. (Hanneman, 1996, p. 332)

Functioning at the level of expert in clinical judgement includes using intuition—that is, knowledge received as a whole. Intuition is characterized by immediate recognition of patterns—expert practitioners learn to attend to a pattern of assessment data and act without consciously labelling it. Whereas the beginner operates more from a set of defined, structured rules, the expert practitioner uses intuitive links, has the ability to see salient issues in a patient situation, and knows instant therapeutic responses (Benner et al., 1997). The expert has a storehouse of experience about which interventions have been successful in the past.

For example, compare the actions of the nonexpert and the expert nurse in the following situation of a young man with *Pneumocystis jiroveci (P. carinii)* pneumonia.

He was banging the side rails, making gurgling sounds, and pointing to his endotracheal tube. He was diaphoretic, gasping, and frantic. The nurse put her hand on his arm and tried to ascertain whether he had a sore throat from the tube. While she was away from the bedside retrieving an analgesic, the expert nurse strolled by, hesitated, listened, went to the man's bedside, reinflated the endotracheal cuff, and accepted the patient's look of gratitude because he was able to breathe again. The nonexpert nurse was distressed that she had misread the situation. The expert reviewed the signs of a leaky cuff with the nonexpert and pointed out that banging the side rails and panic help differentiate acute respiratory distress from pain. (Hanneman, 1996, p. 333)

Critical Thinking

The way of moving from novice to becoming an expert practitioner is through the use of critical thinking. We all start as novices, when we need the familiarity of clear-cut rules to guide actions. Critical thinking is the means by which we learn to assess and modify, if indicated, before acting.

Critical thinking is required for sound diagnostic reasoning and clinical judgement. During your career, you will need to sort through vast amounts of data and information in order to make the sound judgements to manage patient care. This data will be dynamic, unpredictable, and ever changing. There will not be any one protocol you can memorize that will apply to every situation.

Critical thinking enables you to (Oermann, 1999):
- Analyze complex data about patients
- Make decisions about the patients' problems and alternate possibilities
- Evaluate each problem to decide which applies
- Decide on the most appropriate interventions for the situation

What is critical thinking? Paul (1993) calls it "thinking about your thinking while you're thinking in order to make your thinking better." This sounds like circular feedback, but

it means that a critical thinker is simultaneously problem-solving and self-improving his or her thinking ability.

The ideal critical thinker is habitually inquisitive, well-informed, trustful of reason, open-minded, flexible, fair-minded in evaluation, honest in facing personal biases, prudent in making judgments, willing to reconsider, clear about issues, orderly in complex matters, diligent in seeking relevant information, reasonable in the selection of criteria, focused in inquiry, and persistent in seeking results that are as precise as the subject and the circumstances of the inquiry permit. (American Philosophical Association, 1990, p. 3)

Picture critical thinking ability as having three overlapping dimensions (Fig. 1-3). Your critical thinking ability grows as you develop (1) a critical thinking character (a commitment to learning critical thinking characteristics, attitudes, and dispositions); (2) the theoretical and experiential knowledge (what to do, when to do it, why to do it); and (3) the intellectual and manual skills (assessing systematically and psychomotor skills) (Alfaro-LeFevre, 1999). Watson and Glaser (1991) have a similar definition of the three dimensions of critical thinking: an attitude of inquiry, knowledge of the subject, and skills in using this knowledge in problem situations.

Alfaro-LeFevre (2004) presents the following 17 critical thinking skills, organized in the logical progression of the ways the skills might be used in the nursing process. Although each skill here is described separately, they are not used that way in the clinical area. Rather than a step-by-step linear process, critical thinking is a multidimensional thinking process. With experience, you will be able to apply these skills in a rapid, dynamic, and interactive way. For now, follow Ellen's case study through the steps.

1. **Identifying assumptions.** That is, recognize that you could take information for granted or see it as fact when actually there is no evidence for it. Ask yourself, what am I taking for granted here? For example, in

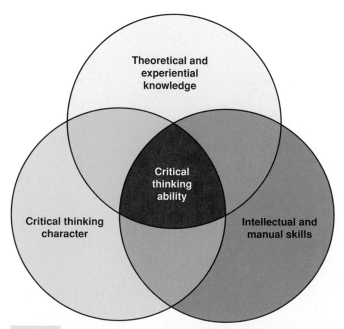

Fig. 1-3   *Adapted from Alfaro-LeFevre, 1999.*

Theoretical and experiential knowledge

Critical thinking ability

Critical thinking character

Intellectual and manual skills

Ellen's situation, you might have assumptions of a "typical profile" of a person with alcohol abuse, based on your past experience or exposure to media coverage. However, the facts of Ellen's situation are unique.

2. Identifying an **organized and comprehensive approach** to assessment. This depends on the patient's priority needs and your personal or institutional preference. Ellen has many problems, but at her time of admission, she is not acutely physically ill. Thus, you may use any organized format for assessment that is feasible for you: a head-to-toe approach, a body systems approach (e.g., cardiovascular, gastrointestinal), a regional area approach (e.g., pelvic examination), or the use of a preprinted assessment form developed by the treatment facility.

3. **Validating** or checking the accuracy and reliability of data. For example, in addictions treatment, a clinician will corroborate data with a family member or friend in order to verify the accuracy of Ellen's history. In Ellen's particular case, her significant others are absent or nonsupportive, and the corroborative interview may need to be with a social worker.

4. Distinguishing **normal from abnormal** when identifying signs and symptoms. This is the first step to problem identification, and your ease will grow with study, practice, and experience. Increased BP, wheezing, and heart murmur are among the many abnormal findings in Ellen's case.

5. **Making inferences,** or drawing valid conclusions. This involves interpreting the data and deriving a correct conclusion about the health status. This presents a challenge for the beginning examiner, because it needs a baseline amount of knowledge and experience. Is Ellen's increased BP due to the stress of admission or a chronic condition? Is the heart murmur innocent or due to heart valve pathology?

6. **Clustering** related cues, which will help you see relationships among the data. For example, heavy alcohol use, social consequences of alcohol use, academic consequences, and occupational consequences are a clustering of cues that suggest a maladaptive pattern of alcohol use.

7. Distinguishing **relevant from irrelevant.** A complete history and physical examination furnish a vast amount of data. Look at the clusters of data, and consider which data are important for a health problem or a health promotion need. This skill is also a challenge for beginning examiners, and one area where a clinical mentor can be invaluable.

8. **Recognizing inconsistencies.** When Ellen gives the explanation that she ran into a door (subjective data), it is at odds with the location of the infraorbital hematoma (objective data). With this kind of conflicting information, you can investigate and further clarify the situation.

9. **Identifying patterns.** This helps to fill in the whole picture and discover missing pieces of information. You need to know usual function of the heart, characteristics of innocent murmurs, and risk factors for abnormal or pathological murmurs in order to decide if the systolic murmur is a problem for Ellen.

10. Identifying **missing information,** gaps in data, or a need for more data to make a diagnosis. Ellen will need more interviewing regarding any increasing tolerance to alcohol, any withdrawal signs or symptoms, and laboratory data regarding liver enzymes and blood count, in order to name a diagnosis.

11. **Promoting health** by identifying risk factors and considering a patient's social contexts. This applies to generally healthy people and concerns disease prevention and health promotion. To accomplish this skill, you need to identify and work with each patient to manage known risk factors for the individual's age-group and social context. This will drive your wellness diagnosis. For example, counselling for injury prevention is an important intervention for Ellen because motor vehicle and other unintentional injuries are a leading cause of death for this age group.

12. Diagnosing **actual and potential (risk) problems** from the assessment data. A full list of diagnoses (both medical and nursing) derived from Ellen K.'s health history and physical examination is found in Chapter 27.

13. **Setting priorities** when there is more than one diagnosis. In the hospitalized, acute care setting, the initial problems are usually related to the reason for admission. However, the acuity of illness often determines the order of priorities of the person's problems (Table 1-1).

For example, **first-level priority problems** are those that are emergent, life threatening, and immediate, such as establishing an airway or supporting breathing.

Second-level priority problems are those that are next in urgency—those requiring your prompt intervention to forestall further deterioration, for example, mental status change, acute pain, acute urinary elimination problems, untreated medical problems, abnormal laboratory values, risks of infection, or risk to safety or security. Ellen has abnormal physical signs that fit in the category of untreated medical problems. For example, Ellen's adventitious breath sounds are a cue to further assess respiratory status to determine the final diagnosis. Ellen's mildly elevated blood pressure needs monitoring also.

Third-level priority problems are those that are important to the patient's health but can be addressed after more urgent health problems are addressed. In Ellen's case, the data indicating diagnoses of knowledge deficit, social isolation, risk for other-directed violence, and risk for situational low self-esteem fit in this category. Interventions to treat these problems are more long term, and the response to treatment is expected to take more time.

Collaborative problems are those in which the approach to treatment involves multiple disciplines. Collaborative problems are certain physiological complications in which nurses have the primary responsibility to diagnose the onset and monitor the changes in status (Carpenito-Moyet, 2004). For example, the

TABLE 1-1	A Common Approach to Identifying Immediate Priorities

Treatment for first- and second-level priorities is usually initiated in rapid succession or simultaneously. At times, the order of priority might change, depending on the seriousness of the problem and relationship between the problems. For example, if abnormal laboratory values are life threatening, they become a higher priority; if the patient is having trouble breathing because of acute pain, treating the pain might become the highest priority. It is important to consider the relationship between the problems; for example, if *Problem Y* causes *Problem Z*, *Problem Y* takes priority over *Problem Z*.

1. First-level priority problems (immediate priorities; remember the ABCs):
   - Airway problems
   - Breathing problems
   - Cardiac/circulation problems
   - Signs (vital signs concerns)
2. Second-level priority problems (immediate, after treatment for first-level problems is initiated).
   Note: To help you remember, the mnemonic MAA-U-AR provides the first letter of each of the second-level priority problems):
   - Mental status change
   - Acute pain
   - Acute urinary elimination problems
   - Untreated medical problems requiring immediate attention (e.g., a diabetic who has not had insulin)
   - Abnormal laboratory values
   - Risks of infection, safety, or security (for the patient or for others)
3. Third-level priority problems (later priorities):
   - Health problems that do not fit into the above categories (e.g., problems with lack of knowledge, activity, rest, family coping)

From Alfaro-LeFevre, R. (2008). *Critical thinking in nursing: a practical approach* (4th ed.). Philadelphia, PA: Saunders.

data regarding alcohol abuse represent a collaborative problem. With this problem, the sudden withdrawal of alcohol has profound implications on the central nervous and cardiovascular systems. During detoxification, Ellen's response to the rebound effects of these systems is managed.

14. Determining **patient-centred expected outcomes.** What specific, measurable results will you expect that will show an improvement in the person's problem after treatment? The outcome statement should include a specific time frame.

15. Determining **specific interventions** that will achieve your outcomes. These interventions aim to prevent, manage, or resolve health problems. This is the healthcare plan. For specific interventions, state who should perform the intervention, when and how often, and the method used.

16. **Evaluating and correcting thinking.** Look at the expected outcomes, and apply them for evaluation. Do the stated outcomes match the individual's actual progress? Then, analyze whether your interventions were successful or not. Continually think, "What could I be doing differently or better?"

17. Determining a **comprehensive plan** or evaluating and updating the plan. Record the revised plan of care and keep it up to date. Communicate the plan to the multidisciplinary team. Be aware that this is a legal document, and accurate recording is important for evaluation, insurance reimbursement, and research.

USING A CONCEPTUAL FRAMEWORK TO GUIDE NURSING PRACTICE

Nursing conceptual models and frameworks provide nurses with a perspective to view patient situations, a way to organize assessment data, and a method to analyze and interpret information (Thorne, 2006). There are many different conceptual frameworks and models in nursing; however, each is concerned with addressing four common metaparadigm concepts: person, environment, health, and nursing.

Examples of conceptual models or frameworks that Canadian nurses have drawn on include: Dorothea Orem's self-care theory (2001); Rosemary Parse's theory of human becoming (1999); Jean Watson's caring theory (1999); Betty Neuman's systems model (1982); and the McGill Model's focus on engaging the person or family to actively participate in learning about health (Gottlieb et al., 1987). Although each framework organizes nursing knowledge and systematic reasoning in differing ways, each aims to promote the ideal of excellent decision making in nursing practice. Although nursing frameworks and models are no longer considered useful as prescriptive tools for clinical practice, drawing on a model, or a blend of models, can be helpful for organizing your thinking, gaining insights into the contexts of patients' lives, determining priorities for health, and engaging meaningfully with patients (Thorne, 2006).

Nursing diagnoses are clinical judgements about a person's response to an actual or potential health state. The most recently approved North American Nursing Diagnosis Association (NANDA) 2007–2008 list is provided on the Evolve Web site. The NANDA listing has become popular as a device to organize nursing care because it allows for efficient categorization of patient problems or diagnoses into computer databases that can then articulate with standardized nursing care plans (Thorne, 2006). Despite its popularity with healthcare administrators in some jurisdictions, the NANDA list is not used uniformly and can create challenges for nurses who prefer to develop more individualized ways of identifying and responding to unique patient problems. Note that the list includes (1) *actual diagnoses,* existing problems that are amenable to independent nursing interventions; (2) *risk diagnoses,* potential problems that an individual does not currently have but is particularly vulnerable to developing; and (3) *wellness diagnoses,* which focus on strengths and reflect an individual's transition to a higher level of wellness. Throughout this book, appropriate diagnoses from this list are presented and developed as they pertain to related content in each chapter. In Chapter 27, the list of findings for Ellen K. is analyzed and rewritten as diagnoses.

Regarding Ellen's case study, the medical diagnosis is used to evaluate the etiology (cause) of disease. The nursing diagnosis is used to evaluate the response of the whole person to actual or potential health problems. For example, both the admitting nurse and later the physician auscultate Ellen's lung sounds and determine that they are diminished and that wheezing is present. This is both a medical and a nursing clinical problem. The physician or nurse practitioner listens to diagnose the cause of the abnormal sounds (in this case, asthma) and to order specific drug treatment. The nurse listens to detect abnormal sounds early, to monitor Ellen's response to treatment, and to initiate supportive measures and health education; for example, you might ask Ellen if she is interested in learning about ways to reduce her alcohol intake, or in developing a safety plan to ensure she has a safe place to go to if her boyfriend becomes abusive. Or you might refer Ellen to a dentist who can provide low-cost or no-cost dental care at a community health clinic.

The medical and nursing diagnoses should not be seen as isolated from each other. **Nurse practitioners (NPs)**, for example, have expanded scopes of practice. NPs are registered nurses who typically have master's degrees and have advanced education in health assessment and diagnosis and management of illnesses and injuries, including the ability to prescribe medications. NPs provide a direct point of entry to the healthcare system for case management, diagnosis, treatment, prevention and promotion, and, in some cases, palliative care (Canadian Nurses Association [CNA], 2002; Canadian Nurse Practitioner Initiative, 2005). It makes sense that the medical diagnosis of asthma be reflected in the nursing diagnoses, as interpreted by the nurse's knowledge of the person's response to asthma. In this book, common nursing diagnoses are presented along with medical diagnoses to illustrate common abnormalities. Please observe how these two types of diagnoses are interrelated.

EXPANDING THE CONCEPT OF HEALTH

Assessment is the collection of data about an individual's health state. A clear idea of health is important because this determines which assessment data should be collected. In general, the list of data that must be collected has lengthened as our concept of health has broadened.

The **biomedical model** of Western tradition views health as the absence of disease (Fig. 1-4). Health and disease are opposites, extremes on a linear continuum. Disease is caused by specific agents or pathogens. Thus, the biomedical focus is the diagnosis and treatment of those pathogens and the curing of disease. Assessment factors are a list of biophysical symptoms and signs. The person is certified as healthy when these symptoms and signs have been eliminated. When disease does exist, medical diagnosis is worded to identify and explain the cause of disease.

The accurate diagnosis and treatment of illness is an important part of health care. But the medical model has limiting boundaries. The **behavioural model** moves health beyond treating disease to include secondary and primary preventions, with emphasis given to changing behaviours and lifestyles (e.g., quitting smoking or eating nutritiously) (Doane et al., 2005). The **socioenvironmental model** incorporates sociological and environmental aspects as well as the biomedical and behavioural ones. The socioenvironmental perspective articulates with the definition provided by the World Health Organization (WHO, 1986), which defines *health* as a resource for living and as the ability to realize goals or aspirations, meet personal needs, and change or cope with everyday life. Building on these ideas, the *Ottawa Charter for Health Promotion* in 1986 identified the prerequisites to health as peace, shelter, education, food, income, a stable ecosystem, sustainable resources, social justice, and equity. More than 20 years have passed since the writing of the *Ottawa Charter*, but many people in Canada still lack these basic prerequisites, and their health is profoundly compromised as a result.

By taking the lead in developing the *Ottawa Charter for Health Promotion*, Canada has played a leading international role in emphasizing the importance of the **social determinants of health.** Social determinants are the social, economic, and political conditions that shape the health of individuals, families, and communities (CNA, 2005; Raphael, 2007). For example, some of the best predictors of adult-onset diabetes, mental illness, heart attack, and stroke are low income, inability to afford nutritious foods, and crowded housing or lack of affordable housing. These are issues that also impact patients' and families' abilities to engage in health promoting practices.

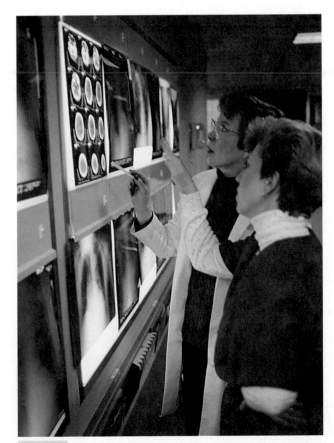

Fig. 1-4

Canada has also been a major international leader in the area of **health promotion**. *Health promotion* can be defined as a comprehensive social and political process of enabling people to increase control over the determinants of health and therefore improve their health (Raphael et al., 2006). Health promoting actions focus on strengthening the skills and capabilities of individuals and families and are directed toward changing social, economic, and environmental conditions to improve health.

The concept of "relational" is increasingly used to describe the complex, interrelated nature of health, people, society, and nursing practice (Doane et al., 2005). *Relational* is not the same as *relationships*: although relationships between people are important, relational practice refers to more than interpersonal relationships. A **relational approach in nursing practice** recognizes that health, illness, and the meanings they hold for a person are shaped by one's social, cultural, family, historical, and geographical contexts as well as one's gender, age, ability, and so on. Relational approaches focus nurses' attention on what is significant to people in the context of their everyday lives and how capacities and socioenvironmental limitations shape people's choices. One of the central skills of relational practice is *reflectivity*, a process of continually examining how you view and respond to patients based on your own assumptions, cultural and social orientation, past experiences, and so on. Practising from a relational stance is therefore critical to "connecting across differences"—meaning differences in your own and your patients' values, beliefs, privileges, practices, concerns, and experiences. Approaching difference relationally promotes understanding rather than defensiveness, and responsiveness rather than a sense of frustration or powerlessness. These concepts are discussed further in Chapters 3, 4, and 7.

Nurses need to draw on a variety of perspectives. For example, if you were working with Ellen, the young woman in the case study, you would use a medical perspective to assess and treat her underlying respiratory infection. From a behavioural perspective, you might focus on providing information and teaching Ellen about how to eat a more nutritious diet. The socioenvironmental model would attune you to assessing Ellen's risks for violence and helping her to develop a safety plan should she need to quickly remove herself from a violent situation at home. Considering the social determinants of health, you would focus attention on whether Ellen could afford fresh fruits or vegetables or pay for the prescription required to treat her respiratory infection. A relational stance would prompt you to consider what biases or assumptions you might be drawing on in relation to Ellen, and would involve you exploring with her those issues she felt were most important at this point in her life. For example, the health assessment process might indicate that the most important health promoting intervention would be a referral to a women's social support agency in the community.

COLLECTING FOUR TYPES OF DATA

Every examiner needs to collect four different kinds of data depending on the clinical situation: complete, episodic or problem-centred, follow-up, and emergency.

1. Complete (Total Health) Database

The complete database includes a complete health history and a full physical examination. It describes the current and past health state and forms a baseline against which all future changes can be measured. It yields the first diagnoses.

In primary care, the complete database is collected in a primary care setting, such as a pediatric or family practice clinic, independent or group private practice, college health service, women's healthcare agency, visiting nurse agency, or community healthcare agency. When you work in these settings, you are the first healthcare professional to see the patient and have primary responsibility for monitoring the person's health care. For the well person, this database must describe the person's health state, perception of health, strengths or assets such as the ability to engage in health maintenance or health promoting practices, support systems, current developmental tasks, and any risk factors or social issues. For the ill person, the database also includes a description of the person's health problems, perception of illness, and response to the problems.

For well and ill people, the complete database must screen for pathology as well as determine the ways people respond to that pathology or to any health problem. You must screen for pathology because you are the first, and often the only, healthcare professional to see the patient. You will screen for pathology in order to refer the patient to another professional, to help the patient make decisions, and to perform appropriate treatments. But this database also notes the human responses to health problems. This factor is important because it provides additional information about the person that leads to nursing diagnoses.

In acute hospital care, the complete database also is gathered following admission to the hospital. In the hospital, data related specifically to pathology may be collected by the admitting physician. You will collect additional information on the patient's perception of illness, functional ability or patterns of living, activities of daily living, health maintenance behaviours, response to health problems, coping patterns, interaction patterns, and health goals. This approach completes the database from which the nursing diagnoses can be made.

2. Episodic or Problem-Centred Database

The episodic database is for a limited or short-term problem. Here, you collect a "mini" database, smaller in scope and more focused than the complete database. It concerns mainly one problem, one cue complex, or one body system. It is used in all settings—hospital, primary care, or long-term care. For example, 2 days following surgery, a hospitalized person suddenly has a congested cough, shortness of breath, and fatigue. The history and examination focus primarily on the respiratory and cardiovascular systems. Or, in an outpatient clinic, a person presents with a rash. The history and examination follow the direction of this presenting concern, such as whether the rash had an acute or chronic onset, was associated with a fever, and was localized or generalized. History and examination must include a clear description of the rash.

3. Follow-Up Database

The status of any identified problems should be evaluated at regular and appropriate intervals. What change has occurred? Is the problem getting better or worse? What coping strategies are used? The follow-up database is used in all settings to follow up short-term or chronic health problems.

4. Emergency Database

The emergency database calls for a rapid collection of the data, often compiled concurrently with life-saving measures. Diagnosis must be swift and sure. For example, in a hospital emergency department, a person is brought in with suspected substance overdose. The first history questions are, "What did you take?" "How much did you take?" and "When?" The person is questioned simultaneously while his or her airway, breathing, circulation, level of consciousness, and disability are being assessed. Clearly, the emergency database requires more rapid collection of data than the episodic database.

FREQUENCY OF ASSESSMENT

The frequency of assessment varies with the person's age, gender, social context, and illness and wellness needs. Most ill people seek care because of pain or some abnormal signs and symptoms they have noticed. This prompts an assessment—gathering a complete, an episodic, or an emergency database.

But for the well person, opinions are changing about assessment intervals. The term *annual checkup* is vague. What does it constitute? Is it necessary or cost effective? Does it sometimes give an implicit promise of health and thus provide false security? What about the classic situation of a person suffering a heart attack 2 weeks after a routine checkup and normal findings on electrocardiogram? The timing of some formerly accepted procedures is now variable—for example, the annual Papanicolaou (Pap) test for cervical cancer in women. The same annual routine physical examination cannot be recommended for all persons because health priorities vary among individuals, different age groups, and risk categories.

In Canada, there are various guidelines for disease prevention and health promotion. New national guidelines are developed regularly for particular populations, for example, the 2007 human papillomavirus (HPV) vaccine guidelines for adolescents (HPV Consensus Guidelines Committee, 2007). Many of these are outlined in Chapter 2.

National standards for **immunizations** are contained in the *Canadian Immunization Guide* (Public Health Agency of Canada, 2006). Each province and territory adapts these standards slightly according to its population's needs. In addition, there are ongoing updates posted by the National Advisory Committee on Immunizations (2008). It is important to check the provincial or territorial guidelines where you practise.

Periodic health examinations are designed to prevent morbidity and mortality by identifying modifiable risk factors and early signs of treatable conditions (Milone et al., 2006). In 1980 the Canadian Task Force on the Periodic Health Examination produced its first evidence-based clinical practice guide-

lines. The task force was renamed the Canadian Task Force on Preventive Health Care (CTFPHC) in 1984, and many of the guidelines were updated in 2006 (CTFPHC, 2008).

Since 2006 the Public Health Agency of Canada (2008) has taken the lead in developing and distributing health promotion, disease prevention, and other guidelines for children, adults, pregnant women, and seniors. The Canadian Medical Association (CMA) *Clinical Practice Guidelines* (CMA, 2008) are also updated regularly and include prevention, promotion, and treatment guidelines for use by nurses, NPs, and physicians.

For infants and children, there are clinical practice guidelines developed at the provincial and territorial level that you can access, including:

- Developmental screening tools
- Schedules for periodic well-child assessments
- Health promotion and injury and disease prevention strategies for various age groups
- Depression screening tools for adolescents
- Strategies to promote healthy parenting
- Strategies to support psychosocial and emotional development in children

For example, the *Rourke Baby Record* (Rourke et al., 2006) is an evidence-based health maintenance and prevention guide that can be used by community health nurses, NPs, and physicians caring for children in the first 5 years of life. The Canadian Paediatric Society (2008) and WHO (2008) also have evidence-based developmental and preventative screening guidelines.

The United States has taken a lead in developing evidence-based guidelines for age-specific periodic health visits and preventive services in the *Guide to Clinical Preventive Services, Second Edition* (U.S. Preventive Services Task Force, 2006). Aspects of these guidelines can be adapted for use with Canadian populations, for example:

- Screening for major risk factors
- Age-specific and gender-specific items for physical examination and laboratory procedures
- Health promotion guidelines
- Health education and counselling topics

However, you will need to follow the Canadian rather than the American immunization schedule.

ASSESSMENT THROUGHOUT THE LIFE CYCLE

It makes good sense to consider health assessment from a life cycle approach. First, you must be familiar with the usual and expected developmental tasks for each age group (see Chapter 2). This alerts you to which physical, psychosocial, cognitive, and behavioural tasks are currently important for each person. For example, an adult in Ellen K.'s age group has developmental tasks that include growing independent from the parents' home and care, establishing a career, forming an intimate bond with another, making friends, and establishing a social group (see complete list on p. 24).

Next, once assessment skills are learned, they are more meaningful when considered from a developmental perspective. Your knowledge of communication skills and health history content is enhanced as you consider how they apply to individuals throughout the life cycle. The physical examination also is more relevant when you consider age-specific data about anatomy, the method of examination, normal findings, and abnormal findings. For example, an average normal blood pressure for a woman Ellen K.'s age is 116/70 mm Hg (see Fig. 9-18 on p. 171).

For each age group, the approach to health assessment arises from an orientation toward wellness and health maintenance. One learns to capitalize on the person's strengths. What is the person already doing that promotes health? What other areas are ripe for health teaching so that the person can further build his or her potential for health?

CULTURAL AND SOCIAL CONSIDERATIONS

Cultural and social considerations are critical to health and physical assessments. An introduction to key concepts is provided in Chapter 3. These concepts are threaded throughout the text as they relate to specific chapters. Importantly, a relational stance in your clinical practice will help you to attend to the varying contexts that shape people's health and well-being.

Canada's population, estimated at 33 million in 2007, is very diverse. The Canadian population grew more rapidly between 2001 and 2006 (+5.4%) than it did in the previous 5-year interval, and this acceleration was due primarily to an increase in international migration (Statistics Canada, 2007a, 2007b). During this 5-year time frame, it was estimated that just over one million people immigrated to Canada. Canada's Aboriginal population is also relatively large, accounting for almost 4% of the total population (Statistics Canada, 2008).

Aboriginal people in Canada include the First Nations, Métis, and Inuit groups, which are recognized as three separate groups with unique histories, cultural backgrounds, and languages spoken.

Disturbingly, Canada is also experiencing increasing divisions between people who are wealthy and those who are poor (Beiser et al., 2005). At least 15% of Canadians live in impoverished circumstances, and these rates are dramatically higher for lone-mother families (51%) (Raphael, 2007). Of concern is the fact that, as poverty rates increase, health status declines (Raphael et al., 2006). Nurses and other healthcare professionals therefore require the skills and knowledge to effectively—and respectfully—explore these interrelated biological, social, cultural, and economic factors.

HIGH-LEVEL ASSESSMENT SKILLS

This attention to life cycle, social and cultural contexts, and relational approaches to practice, does not detract from the importance of the assessment skills themselves. Assessment skills must be practised with hands-on experience and refined to a high level. In many community settings, the nurse is the first and often the only healthcare professional to see an individual. In the hospital, the nurse is the only healthcare professional continually present at the bedside.

Current efforts of cost containment result in a hospital population composed of people who have increased acuity, a shorter stay, and an earlier discharge than in the past. This situation requires faster, more efficient assessments from the nurse. Procedures that used to require a standard hospital stay of several days (e.g., surgery for inguinal hernia, insertion of a central intravenous line for total parenteral alimentation) now are done on an outpatient basis. As a result, nurses go to people's homes for follow-up assessment and diagnosis. These situations require first-rate assessment skills that are grounded in a relational approach and a knowledge of age-specific problems.

BIBLIOGRAPHY

Alfaro-LeFevre, R. (2004). *Critical thinking and clinical judgment: A practical approach* (3rd ed.). Philadelphia, PA: W.B. Saunders.

Alfaro-LeFevre, R. (2006). *Applying nursing process—a tool for critical thinking* (6th ed.). Philadelphia, PA: Lippincott Williams & Wilkins.

Alfaro-LeFevre, R. (2007). *Critical thinking indicators—2006 evidence-based version, 2006.* Retrieved March 4, 2007, from http://www.AlfaroTeachSmart.com

American Nurses Association. (2004a). *Nursing scope and standards of performance and standards of clinical practice.* Washington, DC: American Nurses Publishing.

American Nurses Association. (2004b). *Standards of clinical nursing practice.* Washington, DC: Author.

American Philosophical Association. (1990). *Critical thinking: A statement of expert consensus for purposes of educational assessment and instruction.* Millbrae, CA: The Delphi Report. (ERIC Document Reproduction Service. No. ED315-423)

Beiser, M., & Stewart, M. (2005). Reducing health disparities: A priority for Canada. *Canadian Journal of Public Health, 96*(2), 4–5.

Benner P. (1984). *From novice to expert—excellence and power in clinical nursing practice.* Menlo Park, CA: Addison-Wesley Publishing Company.

Benner, P., Hooper-Kyriakidis, P., & Stannard, D. (1999). *Clinical wisdom and interventions in critical care.* Philadelphia, PA: W.B. Saunders.

Benner, P., Tanner, C. A., & Chesla, C. A. (1996). *Expertise in nursing practice.* New York, NY: Springer.

Benner, P., Tanner, C. A., & Chesla, C. A. (1997). Becoming an expert nurse. *American Journal of Nursing, 97*(6), 16BBB–16DDD.

Budd, G. M., & Hayman, L. L. (2006). Childhood obesity, determinants, prevention, and treatment. *Journal of Cardiovascular Nursing, 21,* 437–441.

Canadian Medical Association. (2008). *Clinical practice guidelines.* Retrieved February 11, 2008, from http://mdm.ca/cpgsncw/cpgs/search/english/help/recent_add.htm

Canadian Nurse Practitioner Initiative. (2005). *Frequently asked questions about nurse practitioners.* Retrieved February 7, 2008, from http://www.cnpi.ca/faq.asp

Canadian Nurses Association. (2002). *Fact sheet: Role of the nurse practitioner around the world.* Ottawa, ON: Author.

Canadian Nurses Association. (2005). *Social determinants of health and nursing: A summary of the issues.* Ottawa, ON: Author.

Canadian Pediatric Society. (2008). *News and publications.* Retrieved February 11, 2008, from http://www.cps.ca/english/index.htm

Canadian Task Force on Preventive Health Care. (2008). *Evidence-based clinical prevention.* Retrieved February 11, 2008, from http://www.ctfphc.org

Carpenito-Moyet, L. (2004). *Nursing diagnosis: Application to clinical practice* (10th ed.). Philadelphia: Lippincott Williams & Wilkins.

DiCenso, A., Guyatt, G., & Ciliska, D. (2005). *Evidence-based nursing—a guide to clinical practice.* St. Louis, MO: Elsevier/Mosby.

Doane, G. H., & Varcoe, C. (2005). *Family nursing as relational inquiry: Developing health-promoting practice.* Philadelphia, PA: Lippincott, Williams & Wilkins.

Frisch, N. (2002). Nursing diagnosis and nursing theory—exploration of factors inhibiting and supporting simultaneous use. *Nursing Diagnosis, Apr–June,* 1–8.

Gordon, M. (1994). *Nursing diagnosis: process and application* (3rd ed.). St Louis, MO: Mosby.

Gottlieb, L. N., & Rowat, K. (1987). The McGill model of nursing: A practice-derived model. *Advances in Nursing Science, 9,* 51–61.

Hanneman, S. K. (1996). Advancing nursing practice with a unit-based clinical expert. *Image, 28,* 331–337.

HPV Consensus Guidelines Committee. (2007). Canadian consensus guidelines on human papillomavirus. *Journal of Obstetrics and Gynaecology Canada, 29*(8 Suppl. 3).

Hunter, A., Denman-Vitale, S., & Garzon, L. (2007). Global infections: Recognition, management and prevention. *Nurse Practitioner, 32*(2), 34–41.

Jackson, M., Ignatavicius, D. D., & Case, B. (2004). *Conversations in critical thinking and clinical judgment.* Pensacola, FL: Pohl Publishing.

Joint Commission on Accreditation of Healthcare Organizations. (2004). *National patient safety goals, 2004.* Retrieved March 5, 2007, from http://www.jcaho.org/accredited organizations/patient safety/npsg

Katz, J. R. & Hirsch, A. M. (2003). When global health is local health—Infectious diseases travel easily. *American Journal of Nursing, 103*(12), 75–79.

Leininger, M. (2002). *Transcultural nursing: Concepts, theories, and practice* (3rd ed.). New York, NY: McGraw-Hill.

Melnyk, B. M., & Fineout-Overholt, E. (2005). *Evidence-based practice in nursing and healthcare.* Philadelphia, PA: Lippincott Williams & Wilkins.

Milone, D., & Lopes Milone, S. (2006). Evidence-based periodic health examination of adults: Memory aid for primary care physicians. *Canadian Family Physician, 52*(1), 40–47.

National Advisory Committee on Immunizations. (2008). *About NACI.* Retrieved February 12, 2008, from http://www.phac-aspc.gc.ca/naci-ccni/index-eng.php

Neuman, B. (1982). *The Neuman systems model: Application in nursing education and practice.* Norwalk, CT: Appleton-Century Crofts.

Niederhauser, V. P., & Arnold, M. (2004). Assess health risks and risk status for intervention reduction. *Nurse Practitioner, 29*(2), 35–42.

Oermann, M. H. (1999). Critical thinking, critical practice. *Nursing Management, 30*(4), 40C–40I.

Orem, D. E. (2001). *Nursing: Concepts of practice* (6th ed.). New York, NY: McGraw Hill.

Orem, D. E., Taylor, S. G., & Renpenning, K. M. (2001). *Nursing: Concepts of practice* (6th ed.). St Louis, MO: Mosby.

Parse, R. R. (1999). Nursing science: the transforming of practice. *Journal of Advanced Nursing, 30,* 1383–1387.

Paul, R. (1993). *Critical thinking: How to prepare students for a rapidly changing world.* Santa Rosa, CA: Foundation for Critical Thinking.

Paul, R. W., & Heaslip, P. (1995). Critical thinking and intuitive nursing practice. *Journal of Advanced Nursing, 20,* 40–47.

Peden-McAlpine, C., & Clark, N. (2002). Early recognition of client status changes—The importance of time. *Dimensions in Critical Care Nursing, 21*(4), 144–151.

Pender, N., Murdaugh, C. L., & Parsons, M. A. (2006). *Health promotion in nursing practice* (5th ed.). Paramus, NJ: Prentice Hall.

Pesut, D. J., & Herman, J. (1999). *Clinical reasoning: The art and science of critical and creative thinking.* Albany, NY: Delmar.

Public Health Agency of Canada. (2006). *Canadian immunization guide* (7th ed.). Retrieved February 12, 2008, from http://www.phac-aspc.gc.ca/publicat/cig-gci/index-eng.php

Public Health Agency of Canada. (2008). *Health promotion topics.* Retrieved February 11, 2008, from http://www.phac-aspc.gc.ca/hp-ps/index-eng.php

Raphael, D. (2007). *Poverty and policy in Canada: Implications for health and quality of life.* Toronto, ON: Canadian Scholars' Press.

Raphael, D., Bryant, T., & Rioux, M. (2006). *Staying alive: Critical perspectives on health, illness and health care.* Toronto, ON: Canadian Scholars' Press.

Rourke, L., Leduc, D., & Rourke, J. (2006). *Rourke baby record: Evidence-based infant/child health maintenance record.* Retrieved

February 14, 2008 from, http://www.cfpc.ca/local/files/Programs/Rourke%20Baby/RBR_National_EN.pdf

Roy, C., & Andrews, H. A. (1999). *The Roy adaptation model: The definitive statement* (2nd ed.). Stamford, CT: Appleton & Lange.

Royal Commission on Aboriginal Peoples. (1996). *Report of the Royal Commission on Aboriginal Peoples: Vol. 3. Gathering strength.* Ottawa, ON: Author.

Scheffer, B. K., & Rubenfeld, M. G. (2000). A consensus statement on critical thinking in nursing. *Journal of Nursing Education, 39,* 352–359.

Spector, R. E. (2004). *Cultural diversity in health and illness.* Upper Saddle River, NJ: Prentice Hall.

Statistics Canada. (2007a). *Immigration in Canada: A portrait of the foreign-born population, 2006 census.* Retrieved February 28, 2008, from http://www.statcan.ca/bsolc/english/bsolc?catno=97-557-XIE2006001#formatdisp

Statistics Canada. (2007b). *Portrait of the Canadian population in 2006. Population and dwelling counts.* Retrieved March 10, 2008, from http://www12.statcan.ca/english/census06/analysis/popdwell/index.cfm

Statistics Canada. (2008). *Aboriginal peoples in Canada in 2006: Inuit, Métis and First Nations, 2006 census.* Retrieved March 10, 2008, from http://www12.statcan.ca/english/census06/analysis/aboriginal/pdf/97-558-XIE2006001.pdf

Thorne, S. (2006). Theoretical foundations of nursing. In P. Potter, A. G. Perry, J. Ross-Kerr, M. Wood (Eds.), *Canadian fundamentals of nursing* (3rd ed., pp. 67–79). Toronto, ON: Elsevier.

U.S. Bureau of the Census. (2000). *General population characteristics.* Washington, DC: U.S. Government Printing Office.

U.S. Preventive Services Task Force. (2006). *Guide to clinical preventive services.* Baltimore, MD: Williams & Wilkins.

Watson, G., & Glaser, E. M. (1991). *Critical thinking appraisal manual.* Kent, UK: Psychological Corporation.

Watson, J. (1999). *Postmodern nursing and beyond.* Edinburgh, Scotland: Churchill Livingstone.

World Health Organization. (1986). *Ottawa charter for health promotion.* Retrieved February 2008, from http://www.who.int/healthpromotion/conferences/previous/ottawa/en/

World Health Organization. (2008). *The WHO child growth standards.* Retrieved February 2008, from http://www.who.int/childgrowth/en/

Chapter Two

Developmental Tasks and Health Promotion Across the Lifespan

Written by **Carolyn Jarvis**, PhD, APN, CNP

Adapted by **Dana S. Edge**, PhD, RN

Much of this book details the method of collecting subjective and objective data about a person to construct a database. The **database** is used to assess the health state; to applaud health strengths and assets; and to uncover, diagnose, and treat health problems. To fit this database into a meaningful frame, we must consider the developmental stage of that individual at that particular time. Appraising the life tasks that currently absorb the individual lets us appreciate the holistic frame of reference.

Consider Randy, a 45 year old single male who seeks health care for recurrent early morning insomnia. He falls asleep easily at night but awakens around 3:00 A.M. and spends hours unable to fall back asleep, sitting in front of the television in his armchair. As the interview proceeds, Randy indicates that he was a chief engineer at a major automobile assembly plant but was "let go" 4 weeks ago; he isn't sure how he will be able to pay his bills or his mortgage. His aging parents who live in another province are not aware of his situation. Randy reveals that he has lost 5 kg in the past month and isn't interested much in eating. The diagnosis and treatment of Randy's presenting symptom of insomnia is affected by the knowledge that the suicide rate among Canadians is highest between ages 45 and 54 (17.5 per 100,000; Public Health Agency of Canada [PHAC], 2008a). Randy is experiencing the loss of a valued occupational role as well as social isolation, which increase the risk. What interventions would you use if this same symptom were presented by a 60-year-old woman considering early retirement who reported continuing hot flashes?

Growth is continuous and change is perpetual throughout the life cycle. Development is lifelong, not only in biological growth but also in maturation of the physiological systems, in cognitive development, and in personality development. Developmental stages are "qualitative changes in thinking, feeling, and behaving that characterize particular time periods of development" (Berk, 2006). During each of the stages, certain issues are dominant and consume more of the individual's attention and energy. The stages are not precisely distinct; transitions occur and overlap exists between stages.

The following sections combine data to give a general portrayal of the individual in each age period of the life cycle. Each portrayal considers the physical, psychosocial, cognitive, and behavioural developments of the person. The stages are:

1. Infancy (birth to 1 year)
2. Early childhood: toddler (1 to 3 years)
3. Early childhood: preschooler (3 to 5 or 6 years)
4. School child (6 to 10 or 12 years)
5. Preadolescent (10 to 12 or 13 years)
6. Adolescent (12 or 13 to 19 years)
7. Early adult (20 to 40 years)
8. Middle adult (40 to 64 years)
9. Late adult (65+ years)

Infancy (Birth to 1 Year)

The first year is the most dramatic and rapid period of growth and development. The baby changes from a totally dependent being into a person who interacts with the environment and forms close relationships with other people (Fig. 2-1).

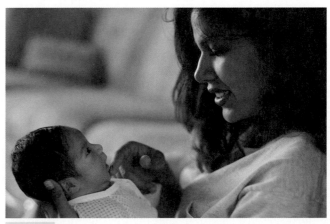

Fig. 2-1

Physical Development

Weight, height, and head circumference reflect physical growth and are sensitive indicators of the infant's general health. The average healthy term infant weighs 3.4 kg, with 95% of full-term infants ranging from 2.5 to 4.6 kg. During the first few days, the baby loses a little weight but regains the birth weight by 10 days. Growth spurts double the birth weight by 4 to 6 months and triple the birth weight by 1 year. Length increases 50% by 1 year.

Head circumference reflects brain size; head growth shows brain growth. At birth, the average head circumference is 35 cm, with about 95% of infants within the range of 32.6 to 37.2 cm. Brain growth occurs rapidly during the first 2 years. Nutrition is essential, with the proper type and amount of calories from fat and essential fatty acids required for brain development (see Chapter 11).

The central nervous system is the organ system that makes the most dramatic gains. Tremendous brain growth occurs during infancy. Also, the baby has numerous primitive reflexes that are present at birth or soon after and persist for specific time periods. These are under subcortical control; as the cerebral cortex grows and matures, it inhibits their expression. In a healthy infant, these reflexes should disappear at specific times during the first year (see Chapter 23). Certain protective reflexes (cough, gag, sneeze, eye-blink) are always present. Visual acuity is very poor at birth (about 20/800) and for the first few months because of immature and widely spaced foveas (i.e., the area on the retina of keenest vision). But acuity develops rapidly and is close to adult levels by the end of the first year.

Psychosocial Development

Erik Erikson (1902 to 1994) focused on cultural and societal influences as determinants of behaviour. Erikson was concerned with the growth of the **ego,** the conscious, organized, rational part of the personality. He described eight stages of **ego development** that encompass the lifespan (Erikson, 1963).

Each stage is characterized by a distinct conflict relating to the person's physiological maturation and to what society expects of a person at that age. Each conflict is a bipolar issue, a point at which personality development may go one way or another through the choices made by the infant's caregivers, or later, by the individual. The bipolar aspect means that the conflict can be resolved along a continuum, and have a more positive or a more negative outcome.

Erikson's first stage, **trust versus mistrust,** has a broad psychosocial dimension. The crucial element in this stage is the *quality* of the parent–child relationship. The infant is completely helpless and depends on the parent for food, warmth, comfort, and companionship. When the parent is responsive and consistent in nurturing, the psychological conflict is resolved on the positive side and the infant learns **trust.** The security from this trust extends to trust in others and in the self. The infant learns that the world is a safe and reliable place and that he or she is welcome in it. If the parent is unresponsive, unnurturing, haphazard, or abusing, the infant learns **mistrust.** Since the infant never feels secure, he or she experiences anxiety and alienation and may protect him- or herself by withdrawing. Without a trusting foundation, this individual will flounder in attempts to resolve future crises.

Absolute trust is not actually the healthy goal of this conflict. When resolution of this crisis is successful, the infant holds *relatively* more trust than mistrust. Total trust would impede survival in later years because not everyone or everything in the world *should* be trusted.

Cognitive Development

Jean Piaget (1896 to 1980) described stages of cognitive development in the growing child. Cognition is defined as how the individual perceives and processes information about the world; it is the ability to know. Piaget believed that a child's thinking develops progressively from simple reflex behaviour into complex logical and abstract thought. This development is biologically inherent in each maturing child and occurs independently of any special training.

The child's cognitive development proceeds through four definite and sequential stages. Each stage demonstrates a *qualitative* change, representing a new way of thinking and behaving. Although the ages of reaching the stages are approximate, the sequence of stages never varies. All children move through the same stages in the same order; no stage is skipped. Each stage is the foundation for the next, and the next stage builds on the stage before it. At each stage, the child's *scheme* (how the child views the world) becomes more intricate and complex.

According to Piaget, the first stage of **sensorimotor skills** (birth to 2 years) is a time of intelligent activity, although full language skill has not yet developed. Infants perceive information through the five senses and learn to modify their behaviour in response to these environmental stimuli. At birth, the only response is an array of reflexes (crying, rooting, sucking, grasping) that occur automatically. Gradually, the infant learns the important concept of **object permanence,** that objects and people continue to exist even when they are no longer in sight.

Piaget believed that object permanence begins around 7 months, when the infant searches for an object that is *partly* hidden but does not search for one *completely* out of sight. By 9 to 10 months, the infant looks behind a screen for an object, but only if it was seen to be hidden there. By 18 to 24 months, the concept is fully developed and the child conducts a true search in many places for objects hidden from sight. As this concept develops, the infant also learns that he or she is *separate* from objects in the environment. Last, by age 2 the infant has acquired **mental representation** (or thought) and can think of an external event without actually experiencing it.

Piaget's work stimulated tremendous research and formed the base of our practice of providing developmentally stimulating environments for children. However, recent research indicates Piaget underestimated the cognitive capacity of infants and toddlers, perhaps because he lacked today's sophisticated experimental techniques (Berk, 2006). Infants as young as 3 months old appear to have an abstract understanding of the world as a real and predictable place. Spelke et al. (1992) showed that babies acted surprised and looked longer at "magical" events, such as an object disappearing through a hidden trapdoor, or an object stopping in midair without support. Spelke et al. concluded that infants know that objects continue to exist even when you do not look at them, and they know that objects cannot pass through barriers. Infants have an awareness of real physical events even though they lack the motor coordination to demonstrate this.

Behavioural Development

Gross Motor Skills. Gross motor skills include posture, head balance, sitting, crawling, and walking. Their development is predictable because it follows the direction of myelinization (laying down of myelin) in the nervous system; cephalocaudal (head-to-foot direction) and proximodistal (central-to-peripheral direction, or midline before extremities).*

Some head balance already is present at birth for protection; when prone, the baby can turn the head to the side to avoid suffocation. Otherwise there is marked head lag, as when pulled to a sitting position from a lying position. By 3 months of age, the baby can raise the head *and* chest from a prone position with the arms extended for support. By 4 months of age, the head and chest are raised 90 degrees with only slight head lag when pulled to a sitting position. Sitting alone without support occurs at 6 to 7 months of age.

After 7 months, the baby ventures from the sitting position to explore the environment, and crawling begins. At 8 months, the baby pulls to a stand and stands while holding onto an object for support. Between 9 and 11 months, the baby starts to "cruise" the room, walking upright while holding onto the furniture. Usually, the child can stand independently around 11 months, and by 12 months the child walks alone.

Fine Motor Skills. The development of fine motor skills involves using the hands and fingers for **prehension,** or the act of grasping. The infant is born with a grasp reflex; it fades at 2 months of age and is absent at 3 months of age. At 3 months the infant expresses interest in an object more with the eyes than with the hands. At 4 months, the infant inspects his or her hands, looks from object to hands and back, and may try to grasp an object with the hands but overshoots the mark. The voluntary two-handed grasp is present at 4 to 5 months.

Further distal refinement follows at 8 to 10 months with a crude pincer grasp using the index, fourth, and fifth fingers. By 10 months, the index finger is an apposition with the thumb for a neat pincer grasp, and the baby is absorbed in picking up raisins, finger foods, and toys (Fig. 2-2). By 11 months the baby puts objects into a container and removes them, and at 13 months the baby builds a tower of two blocks.

Language Skills. Crying is the infant's first means of communication. Cries are undifferentiated at first, but by 1 month of age the infant alters the pitch and intensity of the cry to communicate different needs, such as hunger, discomfort, or loneliness. Vocal sounds build rapidly; the baby laughs out loud at 3 months, coos when he or she awakens or when someone talks to him or her at 2 to 4 months, and babbles at 6 months. At 9 to 10 months, the baby can imitate the sounds of others, although he or she may not necessarily understand them. At 12 months, a baby usually can say the first recognizable word with meaning.

Personal–Social Skills. Throughout the first year, the infant learns more and more social ties that bind her or him to other people. Early on, the baby shows a visual preference for the human face, and even in the first 30 to 60 minutes following birth watches the mother intently (see Fig. 2-1). The social smile erupts at 6 to 8 weeks, to the family's delight and continual reinforcement. At 4 months, the baby laughs and enjoys other people, and at 6 months extends arms to the parent to be picked up.

Imitation, or the copying of another person's behaviour, is present in a limited way in newborns. Even the young baby will copy adult facial expressions such as opening the mouth, protruding the tongue, and pursing the lips. As the neurological system develops, at 7 months the baby imitates others' actions, at 9 months their sounds, and at 10 months waves bye-bye and enjoys interactive games such as pat-a-cake and peek-a-boo. At 11 months the baby can help with feeding and dressing and follows simple directions. Emotions develop during the first year, and by 12 months the baby will give a hug or kiss and show jealousy, fear, or anger.

Infant's Periodic Health Examination

Table 2-1 lists the immunization, counselling, and screening services that should be addressed during the infant's well-baby checkups. Note the parent counselling items regarding diet and injury prevention, as well as aspects of screening at birth. In Canada, the National Advisory Committee on Immunization (NACI) provides national recommendations on all immunizations, including those in infancy and childhood. Despite this, vaccine schedules vary slightly across the country, and the publicly funded immunization programs differ among provinces (PHAC, 2008b). The Canadian Task Force on Preventive Health Care (CTFPHC) first set guidelines for 78 target conditions in 1979 and established standards for evidence ("Obituary," 2003). The task force devolved in 2005, and currently PHAC maintains the Canadian Best Practices Portal for

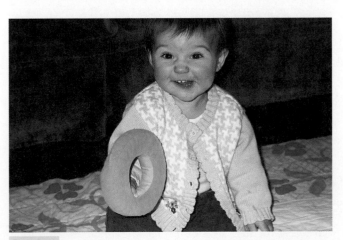

Fig. 2-2

*Tables summarizing growth and development milestones for infancy and for other age-groups can be found in *Student Laboratory Manual for Physical Examination and Health Assessment,* 1st Canadian ed.

TABLE 2-1 | Clinical Preventive Healthcare Recommendations: Birth to 9 Years

Leading Causes of Death (2004)[1]

Conditions originating in perinatal period
Congenital anomalies
Sudden infant death syndrome (SIDS)
Unintentional injuries
Cancer

INTERVENTIONS FOR THE PEDIATRIC POPULATION[2]

Screening

Hip examination, serial (first year)
Eye examination (infants)
Hearing examination, serial (first year)
Vision screen (age 3–4 yr)
Serial height, weight, head circumference measurements (infants)
Phenylalanine level (birth)
TSH (birth)

Counselling

Injury prevention:
  Child safety car seats (<5 yr)
  Seatbelts (≥5 yr)
  Smoke detector, flame retardant sleepwear
  Hot water heater temperature <48.8–54.4°C
  Window and stair guards, pool fence
  Poison control phone number (see http://www.capcc.ca/index.html)
Diet and exercise:
  Breastfeeding, iron-enriched formula and foods (infants and toddlers)
  Regular exercise—60 min of moderate physical activity (bike riding, skating) and 30 min of vigorous activity (running, basketball, soccer) per day[3]
Anticipatory guidance:
  Enquiries about developmental milestones
  Night-time crying

Skin cancer:
  Sun exposure and protective clothing
Substance abuse:
  Effects of passive smoking
  Anti-tobacco message
Dental health:
  Community fluoridation
  Regular visits to dental care professional
  Floss, brush with fluoride toothpaste daily

Immunizations

Diphtheria-tetanus–acellular pertussis–inactivated polio virus (DTaP-IPV)[4]
Haemophilus influenzae type b (Hib) conjugate[5]
Measles-mumps-rubella (MMR)[6]
Varicella (Var)[7]
Hepatitis B (HB)[8]
Pneumococcal conjugate (Pneu-C-7)[9]
Meningococcal C conjugate (Men-C)[10]
Influenza (Inf)[11]

Chemoprophylaxis

Ocular prophylaxis (birth)

INTERVENTIONS FOR HIGH-RISK POPULATIONS[2]

Population	Potential Interventions
First-time mothers of low SES, lone parents or teenage mothers at risk for child maltreatment	Home visitation by nurses during perinatal period through infancy
Dental caries in high-risk children	Fissure sealants
Infants at high risk for iron deficiency anemia	Routine hemoglobin
High-risk children for exposure to lead	Blood lead screening
Recent immigrants from endemic areas; Canadian-born Aboriginal children; parental history of IV drug use, HIV-positive status, or alcohol abuse	Tuberculin (TB) skin test

[1]From Public Health Agency of Canada. (2008a). [2]From Canadian Task Force on Preventive Health Care. [3]From Public Health Agency of Canada. *Canada's Physical Activity Guides for Children and Youth.* Retrieved from http://www.phac-aspc.gc.ca/pau-uap/paguide/child_youth/index.html. Source of immunization schedule: Public Health Agency of Canada. (2006, pp. 93–95). [4]2, 4, 6 mo, 18 mo, and 4–6 yr. [5]2, 4, 6 mo, 18 mo. [6]12 mo and 18 mo or 4–6 yr. [7]12 mo. [8]Three doses in infancy or 2 or 3 doses as preteen or teen. [9]2, 4, 6 mo, and 12–15 mo. [10]Infancy—2 mo, 6 mo or 12 mo. At least one dose in primary infant series should be given after 5 months of age. If the provincial policy is to give the vaccine at 12 months or older, then only one dose is required. [11]6–23 months, 1 dose.
TSH, thyroid-stimulating hormone; *SES,* socioeconomic status; *IV,* intravenous, *HIV,* human immunodeficiency virus.

Health Promotion and Chronic Disease Prevention (http://cbpp-pcpe.phac-aspc.gc.ca/system/index_e.cfim). Content in Tables 2-1 to 2-4 reflects recommendations from this portal and specifically from the CTFPHC-linked Web site (http://www.ctfphc.org). Note that these tables are not intended to be a complete list of all the steps that *should* be included in the health examination. Rather, the tables list preventive services that received either an A or a B recommendation, indicating good to fair clinical evidence from the CTFPHC.

Early Childhood, Toddler (1 to 3 Years)

With successful completion of first-year tasks, the child enters the second year secure in a basic sense of trust. That security plus maturing muscles and developing language enable the child to launch into the process of exploring the environment (Fig. 2-3). The toddler explores everything, inhaling the world with the zeal of all first-time adventurers. Developmental tasks of this next stage include:

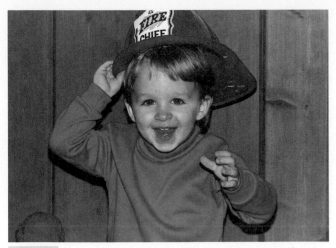

Fig. 2-3

1. Differentiating self from others, particularly the mother
2. Tolerating separation from mother or parent
3. Withstanding delayed gratification
4. Controlling bodily functions
5. Acquiring socially acceptable behaviour
6. Acquiring verbal communication
7. Interacting with others in a more empathic way (i.e., understanding another person's emotional state)

Physical Development

The rate of growth decelerates during the second year, with the child gaining an average of 2.5 kg in body weight and 12 cm in length.

Toddler lordosis describes the normal upright posture of the toddler, with the potbelly, sway back, and short, slightly bowed legs. The increase in head circumference slows, and the head circumference equals the chest circumference between 1 and 2 years. After the second year, the chest circumference exceeds individual head and abdominal measurements, and the extremities grow faster than the trunk.

Maturation of the physiological systems is detailed in the corresponding physical examination chapters in this text. Neurological advances are cited now because they permit developmental changes during the toddler years. For example, most brain growth occurs during the first 2 years, and changes in certain cortical areas permit language and motor development. In the spinal cord, myelination is almost complete by age 2, matching the gross motor achievements in locomotion. Visual acuity is close to 20/40 at 2 years and close to 20/30 by age 3 (Barnard & Edgar, 1996). The maturing convergence–accommodation mechanism matches the toddler's fascination with minute objects.

Psychosocial Development

Autonomy is the goal of all daily activities. The pursuit of independence occupies the toddler. For example, muscle maturation allows walking, exploring, and some self-care in feeding and dressing; refined visual acuity enhances close scrutiny and attention span; and language advances so the child can make known independent demands, such as "me out." Between 12 and 18 months, the toddler ventures away from the parent to explore the immediate environment, still using her or him as a home base to come back to for support. Practice builds confidence, which encourages more exploration. Between 18 months and 3 years, it occurs to the child that he or she really has become quite separate from the parent. This creates some anxiety, which is manifested in the negativism, or the "terrible twos" behaviour, normally seen at this age.

Autonomy Versus Shame and Doubt (1 to 3 Years). The quest for autonomy characterizes the psychological conflict of Erikson's second stage. The toddler wants to be autonomous and to govern his or her own body and experiences. The child wants to apply newly attained skills to explore the world. However, the child has not yet attained any sense of discrimination or judgement. The parent must find a balance between letting the child explore and protecting the child from experiences that are dangerous or frustrating at the child's current ability level. This conflict is resolved favourably when the parent uses patience and appropriate guidance and has reasonable expectations of the toddler's capabilities and attention span. A parent who is overcontrolling or undercontrolling may foster a negative outcome. Then the child may feel shame and experience doubts about his or her own ability.

Erikson believed that toilet training symbolizes this stage. The toddler's muscle maturation has progressed to the "holding on" and "letting go" of things; this naturally extends to the sphincter muscles.

Cognitive Development

During the second year, the toddler is still considered to be in Piaget's **sensorimotor period.** The readiness for independence is demonstrated between 12 and 18 months as the child now tries out new activities and new experiments to reach a goal. To reach a desired toy in her toybox, a girl at this age may try the various routes of taking out each object one by one, overturning the box and dumping the contents out, or climbing into the box herself. Learning comes by trial and error.

Between 18 and 24 months, the child develops **mental representation** for external events. This is a major achievement because the toddler can *think* through plans to reach a goal rather than merely perform them and observe the results by trial and error.

The concept of **object permanence** now is fully developed. The toddler comprehends both visible and invisible *displacements.* That means the child can search for an object in several places, even though it was not seen as it was hidden.

Around age 2, Piaget's **preoperational** stage begins. This use of symbols to represent objects and experiences is discussed in the next section on preschoolers.

Behavioural Development

Motor Skills. Locomotion advances as the toddler usually walks alone at 12 months, runs stiffly at 18 months, and runs well without falling at 2 years. At 2 years, the child also can walk up and down stairs. The child jumps with both feet by 2 years.

Fine motor development shows increasing manual dexterity. At 15 months, the child can drop a pellet into a narrow-neck container and can hurl and retrieve objects. Fourteen-month-old hands can hold a pencil and make scribbles, whereas by 2 years, the child can reproduce a vertical line from a demonstration.

Language Skills. Language progresses from a vocabulary of about two words at 1 year to a spurt of about 200 words by 2 years. Then the 2-year-old combines words into simple two-word phrases—"all gone," "me up," "baby crying." This is called **telegraphic speech,** which is usually a combination of a noun and a verb and includes only words that have concrete meaning. Interest in language is high during the second year, and a 2-year-old seems to understand all that is said to him or her. A 3-year-old uses more complex sentences with more parts of speech.

Personal–Social Skills. Toddlers are usually compliant and co-operative with parents who are warm and sensitive and have reasonable expectations (Berk, 2006). However, parents often are surprised at the swift transformation of their loving affectionate child into a determined toddler who resists requests. Toddlers want their parents' approval but also want to assert themselves and do as many things for themselves as they can. As they test their powers, they sometimes clash with parents' restrictions, and a battle of wills results. "No" seems to be a favourite word.

This **negativism** is a normal part of the quest for autonomy. Although they protest vigorously, toddlers seem to fare better with firm, consistent limits. The thought of a limitless world and of personal untested powers is disabling to the child. Knowing where they stand, even if they disagree, is reassuring to toddlers.

Ritualism emerges along with the negativity. A 2-year-old wants things done in the same way; any change in schedule or habit is upsetting. A consistent routine assures the child that the world is predictable and orderly. Ritualism is heightened at age 2½, especially at bedtime, when the child insists on the same order of nighttime tasks or the same order of coloured blankets on the bed.

Although attachment to the parent is still strong, the toddler begins to play alone. Children 1 and 2 years of age venture away to explore but still need the reassurance of the parent's being there. Play with peers can be comical to the observer. Toddlers engage in **parallel** play—that is, playing the same thing side by side without interaction and without trying to influence each other's behaviour. The two children seemingly ignore each other yet unobtrusively check the other out to note what is happening. Imitation in play is apparent, both of peer activities and especially of parent activities such as sweeping, lawn mowing, or cooking. As the toddler is increasingly able to form mental images, play reveals increased imagination.

Toddler Periodic Health Examination

Study Table 2-1 for the immunization schedule, examination, screening, and counselling measures to address with parents of young children. Of note during this age is the need to review with parents the proper installation and use of car and booster seats with growing toddlers. Injuries are the leading cause of death among Canadian children 1 to 4 years of age.

Early Childhood, Preschooler (3 to 5 or 6 Years)

Successful mastery of the toddler tasks plus a highly energized state make the preschooler ready for this time of developing initiative and purpose. Although parental relationships are still the most important, the preschooler begins to turn to other children and adults to broaden learning and play. Tasks during this period include:

1. Realizing separateness as an individual
2. Identifying gender role and its functions
3. Developing a conscience
4. Developing a sense of initiative
5. Interacting with others in socially acceptable ways
6. Growing use of language for social interaction
7. Developing readiness for school

Physical Development

The rate of growth continues at a slower pace, and the average child gains about 2 kg in weight and 7 cm in height per year. The appearance changes as the "baby face" matures, the potbelly slims, and the legs elongate more than the trunk does. The preschooler looks taller, slimmer, and more graceful.

Most physiological systems are now mature, but the musculoskeletal system is still developing. Muscles are growing, and cartilage is changing to bone at a faster rate than before. Nutrition is crucial for bone growth. A serious nutrient loss at this age alters the shape, thickness, and growth of bones. Conversely, the rise of childhood obesity is linked to poor diet choices and physical inactivity, with Canada receiving an overall failing "D" grade in the *Report Card on Physical Activity for Children and Youth—2007* (Active Healthy Kids Canada, 2008).

Psychosocial Development

Although still primarily egocentric, the preschooler now broadens the scope to include some awareness of other people's interests, needs, and values. As this happens, the **conscience** or **superego** develops. The child learns right from wrong and their corresponding rewards and punishments.

Identifying the Gender Role. As children become aware of their separateness, they also learn that they belong to a further differentiated category—male or female. They are learning **gender,** or how males and females *do* differ. As early as age 2, children label themselves as "girl" or "boy" and assign their family members and pets to these basic gender categories. Then children begin to develop gender roles by a process called **gender typing,** or how society says males and females *should* differ. Children learn the behaviours and attitudes that their culture says are right for a man or a woman. The parents have a strong influence in gender typing, as is seen, for example, when a preschool girl imitates words and actions she has observed in her mother. But her social circle is enlarging, and the girl also picks up important messages from peers, teachers, books, and television about how girls and boys should differ. These messages can forge strong gender stereotyping, and the preschooler often develops rigid rules about what boys and girls should wear and about what roles they can "be" when they play make-believe (Berk, 2006).

Learning at this stage has a broader scope, though, than just learning the appropriate gender role. As the girl mentioned earlier identifies with her mother, she assimilates and internalizes the mother's ideals and values. She learns the standards of society presented to her by the words and deeds of the mother. This is the development of the conscience, which now will direct the girl's behaviour. Interaction with peers helps to develop the conscience too, as in play in which children construct notions of justice and fair play.

Initiative Versus Guilt (4 to 5 Years). For this stage of ego development, Erikson believed that the child's chief task is to develop a sense of initiative. With increasing locomotor and mental powers, the child now has an energy surplus, resulting in determination and enterprise. The child plans and attacks a new task with gusto and wants to stay with it. Any failures are easily forgotten in the quest to test the world. When the parent encourages, reassures, and cheers the child on (while protecting him or her from harm), the child learns self-assertion, spontaneity, self-sufficiency, direction, and purpose. But if the parent ridicules, punishes, or prevents the child from following through on tasks that could be done, the child feels guilty. The guilt exists not only when the child acts inappropriately but also when he or she is thinking of goals that the child would like to accomplish.

By nurturing successes and promoting a healthy self-image, the parents help the preschooler develop *self-esteem.* Self-esteem is the judgement the child makes about his or her own worth as well as any feelings about the judgement (Berk, 2006). Self-esteem is most important because it becomes the way we value our own competence. Our self-esteem affects our emotional experiences, future behaviour, and long-term psychological adjustment (Berk, 2006).

Cognitive Development

Piaget's **preoperational stage** covers age 2 to 7 years, a longer span than the preschool years. It is characterized by **symbolic function,** because the child now uses symbols to represent people, objects, and events. This process is liberating. Now the child can conjure up thoughts of the father, for example, without actually seeing him or hearing his voice. The symbolic function is revealed in child's play, as in **delayed imitation.** That means a child can witness an event, form a mental representation of it, and imitate it later in the absence of the model. For example, a little boy watches his father dress and leave for work, then later in the day the boy wraps a tie around his neck, packs his "briefcase," and heads for the door.

Although representational thought is a great milestone, the preschooler's thinking continues to be limited. Thinking is concrete and literal. The preschooler focuses on only one aspect of a situation at a time and ignores others, a characteristic known as **centration.** For example, given a pile of blocks, a preschooler will sort by colour (red, blue, yellow), or by shape (square, triangle, circle), but not by both. According to

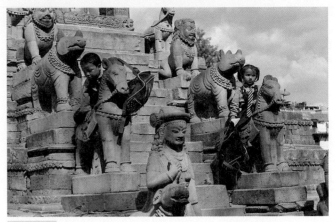

Fig. 2-4

Piaget, a child in the preoperational stage is **egocentric.** This child cannot see another's point of view and feels no need to elaborate his or her own point of view, because the child assumes everyone else sees things as he or she does (Piaget, 1968). However, recent research suggests that 4-year-olds *can* have an awareness of another's view (Berk, 2006).

Behavioural Development

Motor Skills. The physical bumbling of the toddler fades, and the preschool child demonstrates admirable gross motor and fine motor control (Fig. 2-4). A 4-year-old child can hop on one foot. A 5-year-old child can skip on alternate feet and jump rope and may begin to swim and skate. Girls often achieve fine motor milestones ahead of boys of the same age. A 3-year-old child can draw a circle; a 4-year-old child can cut on a line with scissors, draw a person, and make crude letters. A 5-year-old can string beads, control a crayon well, and copy a square and letters and numbers, and has a demonstrated preference for the right or left hand.

Language Skills. Between 3 and 4 years of age, the child uses three- to four-word **telegraphic** sentences containing only essential words. By 5 to 6 years, the sentences are six to eight words long, and grammar is well developed.

Piaget labelled the earlier speech pattern as egocentric (Piaget, 1975). Children at this age talk incessantly. They are wrapped up in their own thoughts and talk to themselves merely for the pleasure of hearing their own voices say the words. Piaget believed this speech is in the form of a *monologue* to the self, or a *collective monologue* between two children, in which they talk at each other but are still absorbed in themselves, and no communication has occurred.

However, more recent research challenges Piaget's views and demonstrates that this **private speech** is a problem-solving tool that is beneficial to all children as they try new tasks or work through unfamiliar situations (Berk, 1994). Children chatter to themselves between the ages of 4 and 6; this chatter becomes inaudible muttering during early elementary school, and then it mostly drops away. Researchers noted that when a child undertakes a new task, an adult usually explains the steps needed to perform the task, often in detail, as directions or strategies. When the child next works through the task alone, he or she uses private speech as a way of repeating the adult's expert advice as his or her own independent guidelines. This evolves into muttering because one often uses verbal shorthand with oneself; that is, the child omits saying the words that refer to familiar steps and verbalizes only the words that refer to the still-confusing steps. Finally, as the child has mastered the skill, he or she is silent because the mind has internalized the private speech into thinking inner speech. Private speech re-emerges throughout life as we confront new tasks or unfamiliar or stressful situations (Berk, 1994).

Personal–Social Skills. The preschooler is self-assertive, but the negativism of the toddler years has diminished. This child wants to please others. By taking on the values of the family and developing a conscience, the child monitors his or her own behaviour to maximize acceptance. The preschooler is proud of his or her self-sufficiency and accomplishes everyday self-care (dressing, feeding, toileting) almost completely. The world enlarges because the child's anxiety toward strangers and fear of separation decreases; the at-home preschooler is able to tolerate brief separations from the parents to enjoy visiting peers or preschool. Some preschoolers have already been in daycare from an early age, and parental separations are less of an issue.

With their growing social regard, preschoolers enjoy **co-operative play** with each other. This means that they play the same game and interact while doing it. The child's imagination runs rampant, and this factor shows in the play. Preschoolers love to dress up and imitate the sex role behaviours of their parents, as well as adult role models such as teachers, firefighters, nurses, police officers, physicians, and sports and media heroes. Often this make-believe or fantasy play is a coping strategy: a sheltered workshop in which the preschooler can work out conflicts and fears or master life experiences.

It is easy for fantasy and reality to blur. Children experience the greatest number of new fears between 2 and 6 years of age. Visions of ghosts and monsters, fear of the dark, fear of being lost—all arise from the child's increased imagination as well as from actual frightening experiences that the child has had. Also, beginning around age 2½ or 3 years, children often invent imaginary playmates. The imaginary friend often serves as an alter ego and tries out behaviours that the child yearns to try or takes the blame when the child misbehaves. Although it is important for a time, the imaginary friend is easily given up when the child enters school.

Middle Childhood, School-Age Child (6 to 10 or 12 Years)

The best preparation for middle childhood is a firm foundation in trust, autonomy, and initiative (Fig. 2-5). Secure in these attributes, the child is able to move into a larger world and tackle these tasks:
1. Mastering skills that will be needed later as an adult
2. Winning approval from other adults and peers
3. Building self-esteem and a positive self-concept
4. Taking a place in a peer group
5. Adopting moral standards

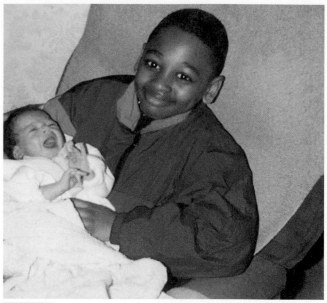

Fig. 2-5

Physical Development

Physical growth is slow but steady during the school years. The average child gains about 3 kg and grows about 5.5 cm per year. The growth rates in boys and girls are basically the same, with boys only slightly heavier and taller than girls. The preadolescent growth spurt occurs earlier in girls, at about age 10, as compared with age 12 for boys.

Physically the school-age child is relatively slimmer than that of the younger child because of the older child's proportionately longer legs, diminishing body fat, and a lower centre of gravity. Although the cranium achieved most of its growth in the early years, now the bones of the face and jaw grow faster. During these years, primary teeth are lost, which the child hails as a big event and developmental milestone. The eruption of large permanent teeth into a mouth and face that looks too small for them gives this child the ungainly, so-called ugly duckling appearance.

Body carriage is more agile and graceful. Bones continue to ossify during these years, and bone replaces cartilage. Muscles are stronger and more developed, though not yet fully mature. Neuromuscular control is more coordinated. All these refinements ready the school child for the pursuit of activities requiring fine motor skills, such as writing, drawing, needlework, small model building, and playing instruments, and large-muscle activities, such as running, throwing, jumping, cycling, and swimming.

Psychosocial Development

Erikson highlighted the directing of energy into learning skills when he characterized middle childhood as a period focused on **industry versus inferiority.** In this stage, age 6 to 11 years, the child focuses much of the time on school. Now, the approval and esteem of people outside the immediate family become important. The child wins this recognition by working and producing. Play and fantasy give way to mastering the skills that the child will need later to compete in the adult world. This child values independence in tackling a new task and takes pleasure in carrying it through to completion. The young worker is eager, diligent, and absorbed. Also, the value of social relationships emerges as the child sees the benefits of working in an organized group. Children learn to divide labour and to co-operate to achieve a common goal.

Real achievement at this stage builds a feeling of confidence, competence, and industry. The child is rewarded by his or her own inner sense of satisfaction in achieving a skill and, more importantly at this age, by external rewards such as approval from teachers, parents, and peers in the form of grades, allowance, or special gifts. Problems arise when the child feels inferior. If the child believes that he or she cannot measure up to society's expectations, the child loses confidence and does not take pleasure in the work. A gnawing feeling of inferiority and incompetence grows and will continue to haunt this child.

The reality is that no one can master everything. There is bound to be something at which each child will feel inferior. Caring parents and teachers will try to balance these weaker skills with areas in which the child can excel. The problem is that, in some cultures, success in certain areas has a higher social value, particularly among peers. For example, in some Western cultures, team sports are admired more than playing chess, or success in reading may be rewarded more than in drawing. The challenge to adults is to provide the successful experiences and positive reinforcement so that each child can achieve.

At this age, peer approval is beginning to be significant. During middle childhood, it is important to belong to a peer group. The peer group is a key socializing agent. Group solidarity is enhanced by secret codes or strict rules. The child conforms to group rules because acceptance is paramount. The child begins to prefer peer group activities to activities with the parents.

Cognitive Development

Piaget labels the stage of middle childhood, age 7 to 11 years, as the period in which the child focuses on **concrete operations.** At this age, the child can use symbols (mental representations) of objects and events in more logical ways. This means a child can experience mentally what she or he would have had to do physically before. For example, to describe the classic hopscotch manoeuvres to you, a girl now can articulate them ("first you hop on one foot . . .") rather than merely performing them.

Armed with the ability to use thinking to experience things or events, the school-age child can:
- *Use numbers.* While counting with numbers begins in preschool years, the school-age child has the combinational skill to add and subtract, multiply and divide.
- *Read.* By using printed symbols (words) for objects and events, the child can process a significant amount of information. Also, reading fosters independence in learning.
- *Serialize.* While this begins in preschool years, the school-age child can order objects by an increasing or decreasing scale, such as according to number size (smallest to largest) or weight (lightest to heaviest).
- *Classify.* This is the ability to sort objects by something they have in common. While young children can do this, the school-age child is able to organize a hierarchy of classes and subclasses. It shows in the school-age child's penchant for collections: rocks, shells, novelty cards, cars, and dolls. A child spends many hours sorting the collections, and the logic of the classification system gets more complex as the child grows.
- *Understand conservation principles.* Understanding conservation of matter is the ability to tell the difference between how things seem and how they really are. It is the ability to see that mass or quantity stays constant even though shape or position is transformed. For example, the child who can conserve sees that two equal amounts of water remain the same even if one is poured into a beaker with a different shape.

At this age, thinking is more stable and logical. The school-age child can *decentre* and consider all sides of a situation to form a conclusion. The school-age child is able to reason, but this reasoning capacity still is limited because he or she cannot yet deal with abstract ideas.

Preadolescence (10 to 12 or 13 Years)

Preadolescence covers the fifth to eighth grades, ending with puberty (Fig. 2-6). Although this stage is still part of childhood, children in this group have common skills and interests that set them apart. It becomes more difficult now to typify characteristics of a single year. Because of rapid growth, the age levels start to blend and overlap. A child may be at one level physically and intellectually but at another level socially. Children of the same age show a range of development levels.

Physical Development

Physical growth is markedly different at this stage; boys show slow and steady growth, whereas girls have rapid growth. On the average, the growth spurt begins in girls at age 10 years and reaches its greatest velocity at 12, whereas in boys the growth spurt begins at 12 and attains its maximum velocity at 14 years.

Even among girls, growth is varied. In a group of 11-year-old girls, each girl looks different from the others. Some look

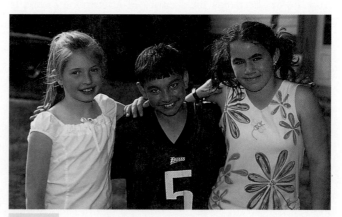

Fig. 2-6

like children, and some are starting to look like adolescents. At 10 years, some girls have begun their growth spurt and have begun to grow pubic hair and to have breast development. At 12 years, girls demonstrate the most rapid growth in height and weight. The breasts enlarge, the areolae darken, growth of axillary hair begins, and menarche occurs.

Physical size among 11-year-old boys is fairly uniform. At 12 years, boys show a wider range of growth. Most demonstrate the onset of secondary sex characteristics with initial genital growth, appearance of pubic hair, and the occurrence of erections and nocturnal emissions.

Boys and girls both exhibit a great amount of physical restlessness. Their activity is well directed into individual and team sports. Their percolating energy makes it hard for them to sit still, and it shows by tapping the foot or drumming the finger.

Psychosocial Development

Parent–child ties exhibit some strain as the child gradually starts to drift away from the family. The parents continue to set standards and values, but the child begins to challenge authority and to reject their standards. Parents decrease in stature in the child's eyes as the child learns that parents are not perfect and do not know everything. Yet the child loves the parents. He or she needs and wants some restrictions. Making up one's own rules is too frightening.

At 9 to 10 years, the child demonstrates a new ability to love by establishing a relationship with a best friend. This is important because the best friend is the first one outside the family that the child loves as being *as* important as himself or herself. By sharing interests, goals, and secret ideas with the best friend, the child learns a lot about himself or herself. This is comforting because the child realizes that he or she is not so different from other children after all. This yields a valuable lesson in self-acceptance.

Preadolescents demonstrate social interest outside the family. There is strong identity with the peer group by a small *clique* or a larger, more loosely organized *crowd* formation. Girls and boys stay within their own gender group. The clique has an exclusive membership, and one is privileged to belong. The code of the clique is important, with rules for dressing, speaking, and behaving in common. The child merges his or her identity with that of the peer group. The child is substituting conformity with the family to that with the peers because he or she needs the security of a temporary identity before formulating a clear sense of self (Berk, 2006).

Despite the fact that peer groupings are composed of the same gender, some preadolescents show an emerging interest in mixed groups, an interest that will flourish in adolescence.

Adolescence (12 or 13 to 19 Years)

Adolescence is a transition stage between childhood and adulthood (Fig. 2-7). Beginning at puberty and extending through the teenage years, the most important task of adolescence is the **search for identity**—"who I really am." With successful mastery of skills from the previous stage, childhood ends. Now the adolescent must process the information from earlier stages and assume a personal identity that is

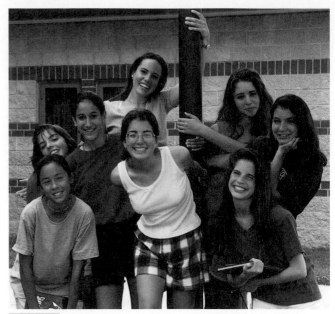

Fig. 2-7

more than just the sum of childhood experiences. The search for identity is the motive behind all the other tasks of the period. The eight main tasks of adolescence are:
1. Searching for one's identity
2. Appreciating one's achievements
3. Growing independent from parents
4. Forming close relationships with peers
5. Developing analytical thinking
6. Evolving one's own value system
7. Developing a sexual identity
8. Beginning to choose a career

Physical Development

Adolescence begins with puberty. Puberty is a time of dramatic physiological change. It includes the growth spurt—rapid growth in height, weight, and muscular development; development of primary and secondary sex characteristics; and maturation of the reproductive organs.

A changing body affects a person's self-concept. With bodies that are changing so rapidly, it is difficult for boys and girls to adjust. Their self-awareness peaks; they continually compare their bodies with those of their peers and to some ideal standard of attractiveness. They are keenly attuned to the appearance of secondary sex characteristics but are embarrassed if these appear too early or too late. It is best when their own development parallels that of close friends and peers. Being an early maturer or, especially, a late maturer adds to normal self-doubts that they experience.

Physical health is generally good. Childhood illnesses are behind them, and the risks of adult illnesses are not yet present. What does place their health at risk are episodes of poor or immature judgement resulting in accidents, drug or alcohol abuse, driving a car while impaired with drugs or alcohol, sexually transmitted infections (STIs), and unwanted pregnancy. Psychological dysfunction may occur, such as anorexia nervosa or depression. Suicide acts and attempts affect an increasing number of adolescents. Suicide is a leading cause of death in this age-group. Its incidence would probably be higher if more accidental deaths were investigated.

Adolescent's Periodic Health Examination

Study Table 2-2 for screening procedures and counselling measures. The physical examination now should include self-care on skin self-examination, breast self-examination or testicular self-examination, and frequency of pelvic examinations (see Chapters 12, 17, 24, and 26 for details). It is particularly important to include counselling on substance use, unwanted pregnancy prevention, and STI risk reduction.

Psychosocial Development

Erikson believed the main psychological conflict of adolescence (the fifth stage in his theory) to be **ego identity versus identity confusion.** The adolescent is preoccupied with how he or she looks to others, and how that image fits with his or her own view of the self. If this process is successful, a sense of ego identity emerges, culminating in what Erikson terms a *career choice.* If unsuccessful—if the teen is unsure of his or her skills, self-worth, or sexual identity—identity confusion results. The adolescent feels cut adrift and experiences anxiety about being a social outcast.

Finding one's own identity is stressful. In the search for identity, teens often form cliques; wear fad clothing; and follow rock singers, movie stars, or charismatic heroes in an attempt to siphon identity from them. Falling in love also feeds the quest for personal identity; the teen projects his or her own ego qualities onto another person and tries to understand them as they are reflected by the loved one.

Cognitive Development

Adolescence corresponds to Piaget's fourth stage, in which the person focuses on **formal operations** and the ability to develop abstract thinking, deal with hypothetical situations, and make logical conclusions from reviewing evidence. Now, thinking is no longer confined to the concrete or the real but encompasses all that is possible. Abstract thinking is liberating. The adolescent is no longer limited to the present but can

---

TABLE 2-2	Clinical Preventive Healthcare Recommendations: 10 to 19 Years

Leading Causes of Death (2004)[1]

Unintentional injuries
Suicide
Cancer
Homicide
Nervous system diseases

INTERVENTIONS FOR THE PREADOLESCENT AND ADOLESCENT POPULATION[2]

Screening
Height, weight measurements
Blood pressure
Papanicolaou (Pap) test[3] (females)
Assess for problem drinking

Counselling
Injury prevention:
 Seatbelts
 Avoidance of the combination of alcohol and drug use and
  driving, swimming, boating, etc.
 Smoke detector
Diet and exercise:
 Limit fat and cholesterol; maintain caloric balance; emphasize
  grains, fruits, vegetables
 Adequate calcium intake
 Regular exercise—60 min of moderate physical activity (bike
  riding, skating) and 30 min of vigorous activity (running,
  basketball, soccer) per day[4]

Skin cancer:
 Sun exposure and protective clothing
Substance abuse:
 Anti-tobacco message
 Avoid underage drinking and illicit drugs
Sexual behaviour:
 STI prevention: avoid high-risk behaviour; abstinence;
  use condoms and female barrier with spermicide
 Unintended pregnancy: contraception
Dental health:
 Regular visits to dental care professional
 Floss, brush with fluoride toothpaste daily
Immunizations
Diphtheria-tetanus–acellular pertussis (Tdap)[5]

INTERVENTIONS FOR HIGH-RISK POPULATIONS[2]

Population	Potential Interventions
Recent immigrants from endemic areas; Canadian-born Aboriginal children; parental history of IV drug use, HIV-positive status, or alcohol abuse	Tuberculin (TB) skin test

[1,1]Public Health Agency of Canada. (2008a). [2]Canadian Task Force on Preventive Health Care (CTFPHC). According to CTFPHC, insufficient evidence exists to recommend routine individual counselling on bicycle helmet use; sufficient evidence does exist for helmet legislation. [3]Cervical cytology screening should be initiated within 3 years of first vaginal sexual activity. Screening should be done annually until there are three consecutive negative Pap tests. [4]Public Health Agency of Canada. *Canada's Physical Activity Guides for Children and Youth.* Retrieved from http://www.phac-aspc. gc.ca/pau-uap/paguide/child_youth/index.html. Source of immunization schedule: Public Health Agency of Canada (2006, pp. 93–95). [5]14–16 yr; "adult-like" preparation.
STI, sexually transmitted infection; *IV,* intravenous; *HIV,* human immunodeficiency virus.

ponder the lessons of the past and the possibilities of the future. The adolescent now can analyze and use scientific reasoning. One can imagine hypotheses and then set up experiments to test them. One learns to use logic and solve problems by methodically eliminating each possibility, one by one. This opens the doors to new academic achievements such as mastering advanced mathematical concepts, chemistry, physics, or logic (Fig. 2-8).

This analytical thinking extends to values. Developing personal values is a part of the search for identity. The adolescent does not accept packaged values of parents or institutions but can reason through his or her inconsistencies and recognize injustices. The adolescent is sensitive to hypocrisy and notes when an adult professes a value (such as honesty) and then acts counter to it (such as cheating on income tax).

Behavioural Development

Socially, the adolescent is in limbo, because he or she rejects identity with the parents but is not yet sure of his or her own individual identity. The perfect solution to this dilemma is immersion in a peer group. Pressure to belong to a peer group intensifies at this age. The adolescent is influenced strongly by the group's norms for dress and behaviour. By identifying with peers, the adolescent joins a sheltered workshop in which he or she feels safe and can experiment with various roles. Group members are allies in the universal goal of seeking freedom from parental domination.

Group identity means the adolescent spends more time away from home and the parents. Adolescents often feel ambivalent toward the parents. They desperately want to be independent from the parents but realize that economically, and even emotionally, this is impossible. Their stated desire to escape from parental dominance conceals their anxiety about leaving the safety of the family. The conflict is exacerbated when the parents try to maintain rigid control and use the protective stance that worked during earlier childhood. Often, things go smoother when the parents are not as strict; allow privacy; respect the adolescent's budding identity; and, above all, take the adolescent seriously.

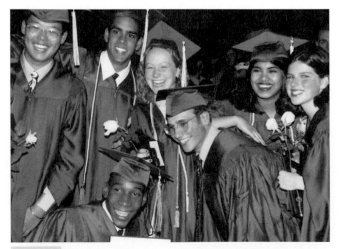

Fig. 2-8

Developing close friendships is important to personal identity. In preadolescence the experience of the relationship with the best friend is valuable in teaching intimacy, trust, and regard for another person. These lessons become a link in the new quest of developing close relationships with the opposite sex. Finding a girlfriend or boyfriend enables the adolescent to learn his or her own sex role identity. In many settings, group dating (youth groups, teen dances) is the norm at first. This decreases stress from paired dating. When adolescents do pair off, the healthy goal is a monogamous relationship involving affection and fidelity.

Most adolescents worry that an occasional homosexual thought or act means that they are homosexual. These adolescent experiences are common and do not turn a person into a gay or lesbian. Of course, some teenagers do discover that they have a homosexual orientation and that this lifestyle feels natural for them.

The end of adolescence is more difficult to define. Some societies have recognized rites of passage, usually at puberty, when the young person earns a place in the adult world with its attendant responsibilities. But in complex Western societies, the adolescent remains dependent on the parents through the teen years and into the 20s for economic and educational reasons. This extends the period of adolescence. Consequently, the role is not well defined in our society, and this is a source of conflict.

Early Adulthood (20 to 40 Years)

The young adult is concerned with emancipation from his or her parents and building an independent lifestyle. The young adult has finished most formal schooling and is ready to embark on a chosen path (Fig. 2-9). The tasks of this era include:
1. Growing independent from the parents' home and care
2. Establishing a career or vocation
3. Forming an intimate bond with another and choosing a mate
4. Learning to co-operate in a marriage relationship
5. Setting up and managing one's own household
6. Making friends and establishing a social group
7. Assuming civic responsibility and becoming a citizen in the community
8. Beginning a parenting role
9. Forming a meaningful philosophy of life

Physical and cognitive developments now are steady and do not affect the young adult as much as they have before. Rather, sociocultural factors and values buffet the novice adult.

Physical Development

By early adulthood, the body reaches its maximum potential for growth and development. All body systems now operate at peak efficiency. The young adult enjoys maximum muscle tone and coordination, a high energy level, and optimum mental power. This person exudes freshness and vitality.

Since growth is finished, nutritional needs depend on maintenance and repair requirements and on activity levels. If activity decreases from its level during adolescence, calories must be reduced. Eating sensibly is a major challenge for

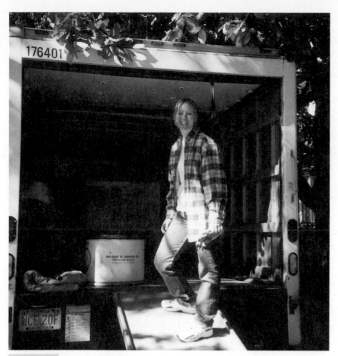

Fig. 2-9

many adults; overweight and obesity are currently at epidemic levels. The diet should be high in fruits, vegetables, and grain but all too often is high in sugar, salt, and fat. A sedentary lifestyle adds further problems. However, more adults are learning that frequent steady exercise maintains weight, muscle strength, and joint flexibility; builds heart and lung capacity; and reduces stress. Table 2-2 lists these and other preventive counselling measures to address during healthcare visits.

Cognitive Development

During adolescence, cognitive functioning reached the new level of formal operations, or the capacity for abstract thinking. This level continues, but the young adult's thinking is different from the adolescent's. The young adult is less egocentric and operates in a more realistic and objective manner. Now the young adult is close to maximum ability to acquire and use knowledge. The potential for sophisticated problem solving and creative thinking is at a new height.

Education continues for many young adults, from formal courses in college or university to on-the-job training, military service, and continuing education classes. Usually, this education prepares the young adult to do some type of work. Work is an important factor in the young adult's life because it is tied closely with ego identity. A person with job satisfaction feels challenged, rewarded, and fulfilled. One who is frustrated with work feels bored and apathetic. Similarly, when young adults cannot find work and are unemployed, loss of self-esteem, loss of social status, and poorer health may ensue (Frankish et al., 2005).

Psychosocial Development

Erikson's sixth stage covers the first years of early adulthood, from 20 to 24 years. He believed the major psychological conflict to be resolved is that of **intimacy versus isolation.**

Once self-identity is established after adolescence, it can be merged with another's in an intimate relationship. During the early 20s, the adult seeks the love, commitment, and intimacy of an intense lasting relationship. This mature relationship includes mutual trust, co-operation, sharing of feelings and goals, and complete acceptance of the other person. Although Erikson had a heterosexual union in mind, this intimacy could be satisfied through a homosexual relationship or through a bond with a cause or an institution.

Erikson believed that without a secure personal identity, a person cannot form a love relationship. The result is the negative outcome of a person who is isolated, withdrawn, and lonely. This person may fill the void with numerous transient liaisons or promiscuity, but Erikson believed that these experiences will be found to be shallow and the person will feel remote and alone.

Daniel Levinson's (1986, 1996) time frame of early adulthood is much broader than Erikson's. It encompasses 22 to 40 years. Levinson believes that an adult's life alternates between periods of **structure building,** in which a lifestyle is fashioned, and periods of **transition,** in which this lifestyle is evaluated, appraised, and modified.

Levinson's era of Early Adulthood has two structure-building periods. In the 20s (about 22 to 28 years), the novice adult establishes the "entry structure," a first provisional lifestyle linking him or her to adult society. He or she is building a home base. During this time, the first set of important choices are made concerning a mate, friends, an occupation, values, and lifestyle. In making these choices, the person must juggle the conflicting drives of (1) *exploring* many possibilities and keeping options open on the one hand, and (2) securing some *stability* on the other hand (Levinson et al., 1986).

The Age Thirty Transition, age 28 to 33 years, is a time of self-reflection. Questions asked include, "Where am I going?" and "Why am I doing these things?" This is the first major reassessment in life. A person ponders aspects that he or she wants to add, exclude, or modify in life. The person feels, "If there is anything I want to change I better start now, or it will be too late" (Levinson et al., 1986).

According to Levinson, the rest of the 30s (33 to 40 years) is characterized by settling down. A person takes the reforms or the reaffirmations established during the transitional period of the 30s and fashions a culminating life structure, one that realizes his or her youthful aspirations. During these years, the adult strives to establish a niche in society and to build a better life in all the choice points. This person is building a nest, using deliberation, and seeking order and stability.

Sometimes, the reforms include having children. The addition of children brings a major readjustment to an adult's or couple's life. Roles are reshaped in the new family unit. For some couples, the father is more involved in child care than most fathers were in past generations. The mother's role may include a choice between full-time parenting or a return to employment outside the home, a decision that is often stressful. The focus shifts from having few choices years ago to today, having to make the decision that is right for the family.

However, for many women, the luxury of having options does not exist. Single parents struggle to support themselves and their children. Often they have neither the time nor the financial resources to provide the basic needs for their children or for themselves.

Middle Adulthood (40 to 64 Years)

At some point in the 40s, the realization dawns and grows that life is half over. No longer does the dream of young adulthood seem fully attainable. To some, it seems that there is more time to look back on than to look forward to. How the person deals with these feelings and builds a meaningful life structure is the task of middle adulthood (Fig. 2-10). Its composite tasks include:
1. Accepting and adjusting to the physical changes of middle age
2. Reviewing and redirecting career goals
3. Achieving desired performance in career
4. Developing hobby and leisure activities
5. Adjusting to aging parents
6. Helping adolescent children in their search for identity
7. Accepting and relating to the spouse as a person
8. Coping with an empty nest at home

Physical Development

A look in the mirror brings rueful recognition of the beginning of aging effects on the body. The skin loses its taut surface and forms wrinkles around the eyes, mouth, and forehead. Some notice sagging jowls and pouches under the eyes. The hair thins a little, starts to lose pigment, and turns grey, and in men the hairline often recedes. An abdominal paunch grows from increased fat deposits and decreased physical activity. Internally, most organ systems hold constant, with some small decrease in respiratory capacity and cardiac function. Sensory function remains intact except for some visual changes (e.g., decreased accommodation for near vision, or presbyopia). Bone mineralization peaks in one's 20s; with increasing age, bone mass decreases and the potential for osteoporosis rises (see Chapter 22).

In the late 40s and early 50s, females experience **menopause,** the decreasing frequency and finally the cessation of menstruation. This involves a decrease in the female hormones, estrogen and progesterone, which brings attendant symptoms such as atrophy of reproductive organs, vasomotor disturbances, and mood swings (see Chapter 26). Although men do not have such an abrupt halt to reproductive ability, they experience a decrease in the production of testosterone, which causes decreased sperm and semen production and less intense orgasms.

Middle-aged adults are suddenly aware of the occasional death of their peers. This is a rude reminder of their own mortality. The leading causes of death among Canadians during middle adulthood are cancer, circulatory system diseases, unintentional injuries, and suicide (Table 2-3). Morbidity also is increased, probably caused most often by obesity. Obesity is associated primarily with hypertension and also with cardiovascular disease, diabetes, and mobility dysfunction such as arthritis. Chronic smoking leads to health problems in middle adulthood.

Cognitive Development

Intelligence levels remain generally constant during middle adulthood. Intelligence is further enhanced by the knowledge that comes with life experience, self-confidence, a sense of humour, and flexibility. The middle-aged adult is interested in how new knowledge is applied, not just in learning for learning's sake. Continuing education courses meet the need to keep knowledge current in occupational and personal interest areas. Many middle-aged adults are seeking college degrees for the first time or are pursuing advanced degrees.

Psychosocial Development

Physical, personal, and social forces all interact during the era of middle adulthood. How a person reacts to the physical cues of aging affects his or her personality and self-perception. A success or disappointment in the career affects a person's self-image, stress level, and interpersonal relationships.

Erikson believed that the most important task for personality development at this stage is resolution of the conflict of **generativity versus stagnation.** Erikson believed that during the middle years adults have an urge to contribute to the next generation. This need can be fulfilled either by producing the next generation or by producing something to pass on to the next generation. Thus, middle-aged adults want to rear their own children or to engage in other creative, socially useful work. The motivation is to create and/or nurture those who will follow.

The middle-aged adult needs to be needed, to leave something behind, to leave his or her mark on the world. Generativity is sharing, giving, and contributing to the growth of others. If this need is not fulfilled, the negative outcome is stagnation. Stagnation means experiencing boredom and a sense of emptiness in life, which leads to being inactive, self-absorbed, self-indulgent, and a chronic complainer.

Levinson (1986) describes the era of middle adulthood as beginning with a midlife transition. Roughly between 40 and 45 years, the person starts a major reassessment: "What have I done with my life?"

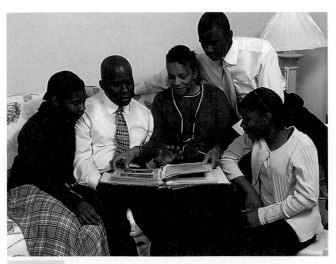

Fig. 2-10

TABLE 2-3 | Clinical Preventive Healthcare Recommendations: 20 to 64 Years

Leading Causes of Death (2004)[1]

Ages 20–44
Unintentional injuries
Cancer
Suicide

Ages 45–64
Cancer
Circulatory system diseases
Endocrine, nutritional, and metabolic diseases

INTERVENTIONS FOR THE ADULT POPULATION[2]

Screening
Height, weight measurements
Blood pressure
Papanicolaou (Pap) test (women)[3]
Fecal occult blood test[4] (≥50 yr)
Mammography ± clinical breast examination[5] (women ≥50 yr)
Screening for depression[6]
Clinical and risk factor screening for osteoporosis (≥50 yr)[7]
Assess for problem drinking

Counselling
Injury prevention:
  Seatbelts
  Avoidance of the combination of alcohol and drug use and driving,
    swimming, boating, etc.
  Smoke detector
Diet and exercise:
  Limit fat and cholesterol; maintain caloric balance; emphasize
    grains, fruits, vegetables
  Adequate calcium intake
  Regular physical activity

Sexual behaviour:
  STI prevention: avoid high-risk behaviour; use condoms
    and female barrier with spermicide
  Unintended pregnancy: contraception
Skin cancer:
  Sun exposure and protective clothing
Substance abuse:
  Smoking cessation
Dental health:
  Regular visits to dental care professional
  Floss, brush with fluoride toothpaste daily

Immunizations
Diphtheria-tetanus (Td)[8]

Chemoprophylaxis
Multivitamin with folic acid (women planning or capable
  of pregnancy)
Calcium and vitamin D supplements (≥50 yr)

INTERVENTIONS FOR HIGH-RISK POPULATIONS[2]

Population	Potential Interventions
Recent immigrants from endemic areas; Canadian-born Aboriginal children; parental history of IV drug use, HIV-positive status, or alcohol abuse	Tuberculin (TB) skin test
High-risk individuals susceptible to type 2 diabetes (e.g., hypertension, hyperlipidemia)	Fasting plasma glucose test

[1]Public Health Agency of Canada. (2008a). [2]Canadian Task Force on Preventive Health Care (CTFPHC). According to CTFPHC, insufficient evidence exists to recommend routine individual counselling on bicycle helmet use; sufficient evidence does exist for helmet legislation. [3]Cervical cytology screening should be initiated within 3 years of first vaginal sexual activity. Screening should be done annually until there are three consecutive negative Pap tests; screening then continues every 2–3 years until after the age of 70. Women who have not been screened in more than 5 years should be screened annually until there are three consecutive negative Pap tests. [4]At least once every 2 years. [5]Mammography every 12–18 months; current evidence regarding effectiveness does not suggest the inclusion of the procedure during, or its exclusion from, the periodic examination of women ages 40–49. Canadian women should be informed at age 40 of the potential benefits and risks of screening mammography and assisted in determining what age they wish to initiate the procedure. Note: Some provincial screening plans recommend and cover the cost of screening mammography at age 40 (e.g., British Columbia). [6]Fair evidence for screening adults in general population for depression in settings with integrated feedback and treatment systems. [7]The four key predictors of fracture related to osteoporosis are low bone mineral density (BMD), prior fragility fracture, age, and family history. BMD testing is appropriate for targeted case-finding among people under age 65 and for all women 65 and older. [8]Td booster every 10 years.
STI, sexually transmitted infection; *IV*, intravenous; *HIV*, human immunodeficiency virus.

The rest of the 40s, according to Levinson, involves making choices and building a new life structure. The person confronts reality; some goals simply cannot be met. This must be accepted and goals adjusted. The person takes stock and emerges with a new perception of the self and the environment. For those who have come through the midlife transition and have found inner meaning, life will be "less tyrannized by the ambitions, passions, and illusions of youth" (Levinson, 1986).

For women, the midlife transition includes the issue that the biological boundary of child-bearing is now in sight. Women feel a time pinch that forces a survey of their life.

Aging and biology force women to review options that were set aside and that will be closed off in the now-foreseeable future. Even those satisfied with the number of children that they have or those without children will face this review.

Whatever the central issue, all those in midlife transition explore the meaning of their career, their family, and their personal identity. In terms of career, people who spent their 30s searching for power and responsibility now may pursue more personally meaningful goals (Levinson, 1986). Also, the middle-aged adult is aware of the time left until retirement. This may result in a reordering of career goals or in a new career path.

Career reassessment is intertwined with personal and family reassessment. New roles emerge as the middle-aged adult deals with growing children and aging parents. This popularly is termed the "sandwich generation." The adult often is caught in a "squeeze" between the simultaneously changing needs of adolescent children and aging parents.

Role realignment occurs in the individual's relationship with aging parents. Even if the parents are healthy and active, a role reversal occurs. The middle-aged adult gradually starts to take the parent's place as the one in charge. When one of the parents dies, the middle-aged adult is confronted with loss of the protective myth that "Death cannot happen to me or my loved ones" (Gould, 1979). The parent was a shield between the self and death. Once the parent dies, the middle-aged adult is more vulnerable and realizes the limited quantity of time left.

Another family task facing the middle-aged adult is to help the adolescent child in his or her search for identity. The parent must adjust to the adolescent's desire to be independent and less involved in the family activities and the need for increased responsibility. Some parents nurture the independence and delight in the budding individual. Others tend to be overprotective and controlling. They may feel that their adolescent is too immature, or they do not want the adolescent to make the same mistakes that they did. The adolescent resents the parent's attempt to relive life through his or her own. Also, some parents dread the empty nest.

Once the youngest child does leave home, the parent faces an empty nest. If the parent (often the mother) has focused only on the children, she may feel left with little to live for. Will she find something as important as the children to replace them? This dilemma is more poignant now than it was in the past when adult children stayed fairly close to home. With society's current mobility, the grown child often starts a new family far away.

The empty nest leaves parents alone as a couple again. They may face a relationship that is devoid of meaning apart from their children. They may find themselves dissatisfied, that they do not know each other, that they have drifted apart. Divorce may result and loom as a major crisis. Other couples find this a positive and liberating phase. Their marriage is happier, with shared activities, increased freedom, and more time to travel. They look back on the shared memories of parenting with a satisfied smile.

Late Adulthood (65+ Years)

Although negative stereotypes exist for each age-group, none is more prevalent than the one for aging adults. **Ageism** means discrimination based on age. It is a derogatory attitude that characterizes older adults as sick, senile, and useless, and as a burden on the economy. It reveals our society's anxiety about aging. The attitude stems in part from our cultural emphasis on youth, beauty, and vigour. Other cultures respect and revere their aging members.

This ageist attitude is changing, partly because late adulthood now is the fastest-growing segment of our population and its members command attention. Older adults should be seen not as a homogeneous group with predictable reactions but as individuals with specific needs and widely divergent responses (Fig. 2-11). Developmental tasks of this group include:

1. Adjusting to changes in physical strength and health
2. Forming a new family role as an in-law or grandparent
3. Affiliating with one's age-group
4. Adjusting to retirement and reduced income
5. Developing postretirement activities that enhance self-worth and usefulness
6. Arranging satisfactory physical living quarters
7. Adjusting to the death of spouse, family members, and friends
8. Conducting a life review
9. Preparing for the inevitability of one's own death

Physical Development

Everyone does not age at the same rate. One person at 60 years can look older and feel weaker than another at 75 years. The widely divergent response depends on subjective attitude, physical activity, nutrition, personal habits, and the occurrence of physical illness. Although aging is known to be a lifelong process, its mechanism is not fully understood. An inevitable decline occurs in body functions that seems to be independent of stress, trauma, and disease. The degenerative effects of normal aging are described for each organ system in the corresponding chapters on physical examination.

Illness affects aging people more than those in other age-groups. Incidence of chronic disease increases, resistance to illness decreases, and recuperative power decreases. That is, after an acute illness an aging person does not recover as quickly or as completely as a younger person. Everyday body aches and pains increase. Some older people become preoccupied with their physical discomfort, whereas others adjust to a few aches with equanimity. All these events mean that the aging person is increasingly dependent on the healthcare system for advice, health teaching, and physical care (Table 2-4).

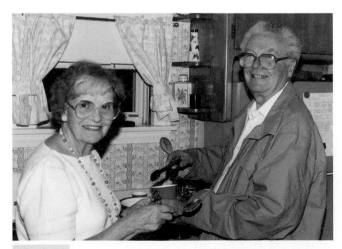

Fig. 2-11

TABLE 2-4 | Clinical Preventive Healthcare Recommendations: 65+ Years

Leading Causes of Death (2004)[1]

Circulatory system diseases
Cancer
Respiratory system diseases
Nervous system diseases
Endocrine, nutritional, and metabolic diseases

INTERVENTIONS FOR THE LATE ADULT POPULATION[2]

Screening

Height, weight measurements
Blood pressure
Papanicolaou (Pap) test (women)[3]
Fecal occult blood test[4]
Mammography ± clinical breast examination[5]
Screening for depression[6]
Visual screening (Snellen sight card)
Hearing screening
Fall prevention (postfall multidisciplinary team assessment)
Bone mineral density (BMD)[7]
Assess for problem drinking

Counselling

Injury prevention:
  Seatbelts
  Avoidance of the combination of alcohol and drug use and driving, swimming, boating, etc.
  Smoke detector
Diet and exercise:
  Limit fat and cholesterol; maintain caloric balance; emphasize grains, fruits, vegetables
  Adequate calcium intake
  Regular physical activity

Sexual behaviour:
  STI prevention: avoid high-risk behaviour; use condoms
Skin cancer:
  Sun exposure and protective clothing
Substance abuse:
  Smoking cessation
Dental health:
  Regular visits to dental care professional
  Floss, brush with fluoride toothpaste daily

Immunizations

Diphtheria-tetanus (Td)[8]
Influenza[9]
Pneumococcal vaccine[10]

Chemoprophylaxis

Calcium and vitamin D supplements[11]

INTERVENTIONS FOR HIGH-RISK POPULATIONS[2]

Population	Potential Interventions
Informants or caregivers describe cognitive decline of individual or corroborate self-reported memory complaint	Cognitive assessment and careful follow-up required
Vascular risk factors for dementia (elevated systolic blood pressure, hyperlipidemia)[12]	Management of hypertension; physical exercise
High-risk individuals susceptible to type 2 diabetes (e.g., hypertension, hyperlipidemia)	Fasting plasma glucose test
Recent immigrants from endemic areas; Canadian-born Aboriginal children; parental history of IV drug use, HIV-positive status, or alcohol abuse	Tuberculin (TB) skin test

[1] Public Health Agency of Canada. (2008a). [2]Canadian Task Force on Preventive Health Care. [3]Cervical cytology screening every 2–3 years for all women who are or have been sexually active and who have a cervix. Consider discontinuation after age 70 if previous regular screening produced consistently normal results. [4]At least once every 2 years. [5]Mammography every 12–18 months to age 69. [6]Fair evidence for screening adults in general population for depression in settings with integrated feedback and treatment systems. [7]The four key predictors of fracture related to osteoporosis are low bone mineral density (BMD), prior fragility fracture, age, and family history. BMD testing is appropriate for targeted case-finding among people under age 65 and for all women 65 and older. [8]Td booster every 10 years. [9]Annually. [10]Given once over age 65. [11]Premenopausal women, 1000 mg calcium; menopausal women and men >50, 1500 mg calcium. Vitamin D: < age 50, 400 IU; > age 50, 800 IU. From Brown et al. (2006). [12]From Patterson et al. (2008).
STI, sexually transmitted infection; IV, intravenous; HIV, human immunodeficiency virus.

Cognitive Development

Aging does not have a predictable effect on intelligence. Intellectual function depends on various factors, such as motivation, interest, sensory impairment, educational level, general health, social concerns, involvement in community activities or stimulating leisure activities, as well as a compensatory tendency to conserve time and emotional energy. Older adults do have a slower reaction time. They often have decreased ability for complex decision making and decreased speed of performance, but no decrease in general knowledge occurs. Older adults experience little or no loss in verbal comprehension or in the application of experience. Age-related memory decline is usually related to tasks that need deliberate processing (i.e., problems remembering names, where they placed their keys or other objects, appointments, or medication schedules) (Berk, 2006).

Psychosocial Development

Levinson (1986) suggests a relationship between physical changes of the body and personality. By 60 years, most people are aware of some body decline. Although variations exist, most aging persons have at least one serious illness or limiting condition and have experienced the death of peers. These issues, coupled with society's negative connotation of aging, lead to a fear that the person has lost all vestiges of youth, even those to which he or she had a tenuous hold during middle adulthood. The person fears that the youth within is dying. The task, then, is to look for a new form of youthfulness, a new force of inner growth to sustain the last era.

The era of late adulthood directs this inner youthfulness toward new creative endeavours. The older adult has stepped off centre stage both in formal employment and in the family clan. This can be traumatic because it means a loss of recognition and authority. But now the person can direct energy inward. When financially and socially secure, the older adult can pursue whatever activity is important. One has paid one's dues to society and now can pursue whatever is pleasing. The person creates a new balance with society; he or she is less interested in society's extrinsic rewards and more interested in using inner resources (Fig. 2-12).

Confronting Tasks. How an older adult responds to retirement depends largely on job satisfaction. If the job was rote and meaningless, the person may welcome the release provided by retirement. But if the job signified power and status, or had high complexity, retirement may have a devastating effect. The retired person feels the loss of title and authority. A loss of professional associates who had common interests and were intellectually stimulating also occurs, and a social outlet is lost when co-workers constituted a friendship group.

It is important to develop postretirement activities that enhance self-worth and give a feeling of usefulness. These activities may include developing a new "semiretired" career, or a hobby, sport interest, or community service activity. The transition to retirement is eased if these activities are well in place before the last formal day on the job.

Having the retired person spend more time at home affects the marriage relationship. Traditionally, it was the husband who was suddenly at home and "underfoot." Now more employed women face the same retirement adjustment. Some couples do find that having one or both at home more means an invasion of previously held "turf," such as the kitchen, garden, or workshop. Other couples develop a more egalitarian relationship. They are now free of earlier sex role definitions and are able to share household tasks and leisure activities equally.

Family roles also are adjusted with the marriage of grown-up children and the addition of in-laws. How the sons- or daughters-in-law are absorbed into the family affects the older adult. This often involves a new role as grandparent. Being able to indulge and provide moral support to a grandchild is usually positive for all, unless the caregiving becomes a burden to the grandparent.

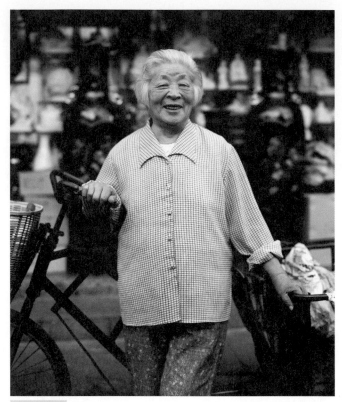

Fig. 2-12

Retirement often involves financial adjustment. This may involve a reduced income, perhaps only Canada Pension Plan (CPP) and a small pension. This may be hard if the person is used to a higher standard of living. Even if the retired person owns his or her own home, the cost of maintaining it may exceed the income.

Establishing suitable living arrangements has both financial and family significance. For many in North America, the extended family has largely disappeared. Rarely do three generations live under one roof. In the past, the older adult contributed light household tasks that gave a sense of personal worth. Now, the contributions to the extended family that were made by the older family member have been replaced by advances in household mechanization, food processing, and daycare centres.

Thus most older adults choose to live independently, either as couples or alone. When it becomes difficult to manage self-care, they face the choice of moving in with grown children or moving into a retirement home or assisted living home. All of these choices involve some disbursement of personal belongings and the relinquishing of some privacy.

Through the late adult years, each person is reminded of one's own limited time left by the increasing frequency of death and serious illness of friends, colleagues, siblings, or other family members, perhaps including the spouse.

The Life Review. One important task of late adulthood is performing a life review. Older adults have finished all or most of their life's work. Their contributions to society and to their own immortality are mostly completed (Levinson et al.,

1986). The life review is a cataloguing of life events, a considering of one's successes and failures with the perspective of age. The objective of the task is to gain a sense of integrity while reviewing one's life as a whole (Fig. 2-13).

This period relates to Erikson's last ego stage, with its key psychological conflict of **ego integrity versus despair.** A successful resolution to this final conflict occurs when the adult accepts "one's one and only life cycle as something that had to be and that, by necessity, permitted of no substitutions" (Erikson, 1963). The adult feels content with his or her one life on earth, satisfied that if it were possible to do it over again, he or she would live it the same way. The older adult reviews events, experiences, and relationships and realizes that these have been mostly rewarding. There are cherished memories. The person feels as though he or she had a meaningful role in human history and can meet death with equanimity.

Failure to resolve this last conflict leaves the person with a sense of despair, resentment, futility, hopelessness, and a fear of death. However, a successful outcome completes the cycle. The contented older adult who does not fear death serves as proof to younger adults that life holds promise.

Levinson believes everyone has a sense of utter despair at some point during this time. To gain a sense of integrity, one has to confront the *lack* of integrity (Levinson, 1986). Some goals have not been achieved, and what is worse is that the damage is done and it is too late to set it right. The person realizes that whatever values were held, he or she cannot fully live up to them. This must be reconciled; it is an imperfect world. The task is to make peace with the self.

This final sense of what life is about is a close parallel to Erikson's last stage. Levinson likens the person's perspective at this time to a "view from the bridge" at the end of the life cycle (Levinson, 1986). One "must come finally to terms with the self—knowing it and loving it reasonably well, and being ready to give it up."

DEVELOPMENTAL SCREENING TESTS

Prior to its revision in 1989, the Denver Developmental Screening Test (DDST), a professionally administered test, was used extensively by public health nurses in Canada. By the early 1990s, however, CTFPHC reported insufficient evidence for the routine developmental screening of children. With the lack of effectiveness evidence, as well as funding cuts in public health, the routine use of the DDST ceased. In its place, several provincial programs now use the Nipissing District Developmental Screen™ (NDDS), a parent-report screening tool (see Appendix F).

The NDDS originated in 1993 from the work of a multidisciplinary committee of healthcare professionals within the Nipissing District of Ontario; by 1997 the screen was being used across Canada, and since that time the tool has been revised and analyzed for cultural sensitivity, grade 5 literacy level, and reliability. Currently Ontario, New Brunswick, and the Northwest Territories have endorsed the NDDS as the screening tool of choice in provincial programs (http://www.ndds.ca/history.html), and the forms are free of charge to Ontario residents. Translated versions in French, Spanish, and Vietnamese are available, and the tool can be accessed electronically, with interactive screens. The NDDS elicits a "yes" or "no" response from parents for a set of developmental milestones appropriate to the age of the child; a "no" response highlights a potential developmental delay. Other parent-report developmental screening tools available that were developed in North America include the Ages and Stages Questionnaires® (ASQ), the Child Development Inventory (CDI), and the Parents' Evaluation of Developmental Status (PEDS).

Adult Life Stress Measures

Some tools are available that attempt to quantify the impact of life change on a person's health. They are based on the assumption that a relationship exists between daily life stress and a person's susceptibility to physical and psychological problems. Many of the life change events are the developmental tasks discussed earlier in the chapter.

The Hassles and Uplifts Scale

This is a 53-item self-administered questionnaire whose purpose is to assess day-to-day stress (Table 2-5). Take this test yourself just before you go to bed one day. Consider each item on the list, and circle a number on the left-hand side regarding how much of a hassle the item was for you that day. On the right-hand side, circle a number regarding how much of an uplift the same item was for you that day. Total scores are obtained by summing across ratings given to all items.

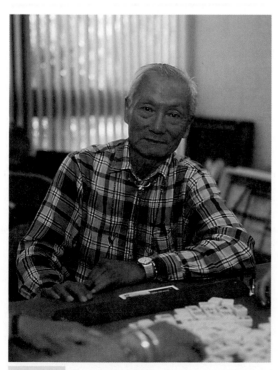

Fig. 2-13

TABLE 2-5	The Hassles and Uplifts Scale

HASSLES are irritants—things that annoy or bother you; they can make you upset or angry. UPLIFTS are events that make you feel good; they can make you joyful, glad, or satisfied. Some hassles and uplifts occur on a fairly regular basis and others are relatively rare. Some have only a slight effect; others have a strong effect.

This questionnaire lists things that can be hassles and uplifts in day-to-day life. You will find that during the course of a day some of these things will have been only a hassle for you and some will have been only an uplift. *Others will have been both a hassle AND an uplift.*

DIRECTIONS: Please think about how much of a hassle and how much of an uplift each item was for you today. Please indicate on the left-hand side of the page (under "HASSLES") how much of a hassle the item was by circling the appropriate number. Then indicate on the right-hand side of the page (under "UPLIFTS") how much of an uplift it was for you by circling the appropriate number.

Remember, circle one number on the left-hand side of the page *and* one number on the right-hand side of the page for *each* item.

PLEASE FILL OUT THIS QUESTIONNAIRE JUST BEFORE YOU GO TO BED.

HASSLES AND UPLIFTS SCALE

HOW MUCH OF A HASSLE WAS THIS ITEM FOR YOU TODAY?	HOW MUCH OF AN UPLIFT WAS THIS ITEM FOR YOU TODAY?
HASSLES	UPLIFTS
0 = *None or not applicable*	0 = *None or not applicable*
1 = *Somewhat*	1 = *Somewhat*
2 = *Quite a bit*	2 = *Quite a bit*
3 = *A great deal*	3 = *A great deal*

DIRECTIONS: Please circle one number on the left-hand side and one number on the right-hand side for each item.

Hassles	Item	Uplifts
0 1 2 3	1. Your child(ren)	0 1 2 3
0 1 2 3	2. Your parents or parents-in-law	0 1 2 3
0 1 2 3	3. Other relative(s)	0 1 2 3
0 1 2 3	4. Your spouse	0 1 2 3
0 1 2 3	5. Time spent with family	0 1 2 3
0 1 2 3	6. Health or well-being of a family member	0 1 2 3
0 1 2 3	7. Sex	0 1 2 3
0 1 2 3	8. Intimacy	0 1 2 3
0 1 2 3	9. Family-related obligations	0 1 2 3
0 1 2 3	10. Your friend(s)	0 1 2 3
0 1 2 3	11. Fellow workers	0 1 2 3
0 1 2 3	12. Clients, customers, patients, etc.	0 1 2 3
0 1 2 3	13. Your supervisor or employer	0 1 2 3
0 1 2 3	14. The nature of your work	0 1 2 3
0 1 2 3	15. Your workload	0 1 2 3
0 1 2 3	16. Your job security	0 1 2 3
0 1 2 3	17. Meeting deadlines or goals on the job	0 1 2 3
0 1 2 3	18. Enough money for necessities (e.g., food, clothing, housing, health care, taxes, insurance)	0 1 2 3
0 1 2 3	19. Enough money for education	0 1 2 3
0 1 2 3	20. Enough money for emergencies	0 1 2 3
0 1 2 3	21. Enough money for extras (e.g., entertainment, recreation, vacations)	0 1 2 3
0 1 2 3	22. Financial care for someone who doesn't live with you	0 1 2 3
0 1 2 3	23. Investments	0 1 2 3
0 1 2 3	24. Your smoking	0 1 2 3
0 1 2 3	25. Your drinking	0 1 2 3
0 1 2 3	26. Mood-altering drugs	0 1 2 3
0 1 2 3	27. Your physical appearance	0 1 2 3
0 1 2 3	28. Contraception	0 1 2 3
0 1 2 3	29. Exercise(s)	0 1 2 3
0 1 2 3	30. Your medical care	0 1 2 3
0 1 2 3	31. Your health	0 1 2 3
0 1 2 3	32. Your physical abilities	0 1 2 3
0 1 2 3	33. The weather	0 1 2 3
0 1 2 3	34. News events	0 1 2 3
0 1 2 3	35. Your environment (e.g., quality of air, noise level, greenery)	0 1 2 3
0 1 2 3	36. Political or social issues	0 1 2 3
0 1 2 3	37. Your neighbourhood (e.g., neighbours, setting)	0 1 2 3
0 1 2 3	38. Conserving (gas, electricity, water, gasoline, etc.)	0 1 2 3
0 1 2 3	39. Pets	0 1 2 3
0 1 2 3	40. Cooking	0 1 2 3
0 1 2 3	41. Housework	0 1 2 3
0 1 2 3	42. Home repairs	0 1 2 3
0 1 2 3	43. Yardwork	0 1 2 3
0 1 2 3	44. Car maintenance	0 1 2 3
0 1 2 3	45. Taking care of paperwork (e.g., paying bills, filling out forms)	0 1 2 3
0 1 2 3	46. Home entertainment (e.g., TV, music, reading)	0 1 2 3
0 1 2 3	47. Amount of free time	0 1 2 3
0 1 2 3	48. Recreation and entertainment outside the home (e.g., movies, sports, eating out, walking)	0 1 2 3
0 1 2 3	49. Eating (at home)	0 1 2 3
0 1 2 3	50. Church or community organizations	0 1 2 3
0 1 2 3	51. Legal matters	0 1 2 3
0 1 2 3	52. Being organized	0 1 2 3
0 1 2 3	53. Social commitments	0 1 2 3

Received March 21, 1986
Revision received July 20, 1987
Accepted August 4, 1987

From DeLongis, A., Folkman, S., & Lazarus, R.S. (1998). The impact of daily stress on health and mood: psychological and social resources as mediators. *Journal of Personality and Social Psychology, 54*, 486–495. © 1988 by the American Psychological Association. Used with permission.

Relatively minor but frequently experienced stresses, termed *hassles* in this tool, have been found to correlate strongly with negative health status (Weinberger et al., 1987). DeLongis, Folkman, & Lazarus (1988) found a significant relationship between daily stress and concurrent or later occurrence of physical health problems, such as flu, sore throat, headaches, and backaches. There was great individual variation, however, with one third of the respondents reporting a somewhat improved health and mood with increased stress levels! Regarding daily stress and psychological disturbance, they found that individuals with unsupportive social relationships and low self-esteem had a greater risk of psychological and somatic health problems, both on their stressful days and following their stressful days, than did individuals with positive social networks and high self-esteem (DeLongis et al., 1988).

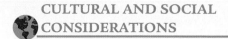

CULTURAL AND SOCIAL CONSIDERATIONS

Much of the developmental content of this chapter is based on research findings and experience with people from dominant European cultures. Given the rate of demographic change, it is imperative to consult with cultural brokers and/or advocates from the patient's cultural heritage who have a deeper understanding of the expected norms associated with various developmental tasks.

The immunization protocols in Canada differ from those of other nations and careful examinations of health records must be undertaken. When assessments are conducted, competent interpreters must be used.

BIBLIOGRAPHY

Abdullah, A. S. M., & Simon, J. L. (2006). Health promotion in older adults: Evidence-based smoking cessation programs for use in primary care settings. *Geriatrics, 61*(3), 30–34.

Active Healthy Kids Canada. (2007). *Older but not wiser, Canada's future at risk. Canada's report card on physical activity for children and youth—2007.* Retrieved February 27, 2008, from http://www.activehealthykids.ca/Ophea/ActiveHealthyKids_v2/upload/Full-English-Report-Card-2007.pdf

Arnett, J. J. (2000). Emerging adulthood: a theory of development from the late teens through the twenties. *American Psychologist, 55,* 469–480.

Barnard, S., & Edgar, D. (1996). *Pediatric eye care.* Oxford, UK: Blackwell Science.

Berk, L. E. (1994). Why children talk to themselves. *Scientific American, 271*(5), 60–65.

Berk, L. E. (2006). *Development through the lifespan* (4th ed.). Boston, MA: Allyn and Bacon.

Bos, R. (2006). Health impact assessment and health promotion. *Bulletin of the World Health Organization, 84,* 914–915.

Bryant, L. L., Altpeter, M., & Whitelaw, N. A. Evaluation of health promotion programs for older adults: An introduction. *Journal of Applied Gerontology, 25,* 197–213.

Brown, J. P., Fortier, M., & Osteoporosis Guidelines Committee. (2006). Canadian consensus conference on osteoporosis, 2006 update. *Journal of Obstetrics and Gynecology of Canada, 172,* S95–S112.

Brown, J. P., & Josse, R. G., for Scientific Advisory Council of the Osteoporosis Society of Canada. (2002). 2000 clinical practice guidelines for the diagnosis and management of osteoporosis in Canada. *Canadian Medical Association Journal, 167*(10 Suppl.), S1–S34.

Budd, G. M., & Hayman, L. L. (2006). Childhood obesity: determinants, prevention, and treatment. *Journal of Cardiovascular Nursing, 21,* 437–441.

Canadian Task Force on Preventive Health Care. Retrieved from http://www.ctfphc.org

Canadian Task Force on Preventive Health Care. (2003). New grades for recommendations from the Canadian Task Force on Preventive Health Care. *Canadian Medical Association Journal, 169,* 207–208.

Centers for Disease Control and Prevention, National Center for Injury Prevention and Control. (2002). *Suicide prevention fact sheet.* Retrieved March 27, 2002, from http://www.cdc.gov/ncipc/factsheets/suifacts.htm

Christie, D., & Viner, R. (2005). ABC of adolescence: Adolescent development. *British Medical Journal, 330,* 301–304.

de Onis, M., Onyango, A. W., Borghi, E., Siyan, A., Nishida, C., & Siekmann, J. (2007). Development of a WHO growth reference for school-aged children and adolescents. *Bulletin of the World Health Organization, 85,* 660–667.

DeLongis, A., Folkman, S., & Lazarus, R. S. (1988). The impact of daily stress on health and mood: Psychological and social resources as mediators. *Journal of Personality and Social Psychology, 54,* 486–495.

Durocher, H. J. (2006). As they grow. 4–5 years: "I'll get it right!" *Parents, 81*(8), 123–124.

East, L., Jackson, D., O'Brien, L. (2006). Father absence and adolescent development: A review of the literature. *Journal of Child Health Care, 10,* 283–295.

Erikson, E. H. (1963). *Childhood and society.* New York: WW Norton.

Erikson, E. H. (1968). *Identity: Youth and crisis.* New York: WW Norton.

Ertem, I. O., Atay, G., Bingoler, B. E., Dogan, D. G., Bayhan, A., & Sarica, D. (2006). Promoting child development at sick-child visits: a controlled trial. *Pediatrics, 118*(1), e124–e131.

Feig, D. S., Palda, V. A. Lipscombe, L., with the Canadian Task Force on Preventive Care. (2005). Screening for type 2 diabetes mellitus to prevent vascular complications: Updated recommendations from the Canadian Task Force on Preventive Health Care. *Canadian Medical Association Journal, 172,* 177–180.

Fitzgerald, B. (2005). An existential view of adolescent development. *Adolescence, 40*(160), 793–799.

Frankish, C. J., Hwang, S. W., & Quantz, D. (2005). Homelessness and health in Canada: Research lessons and priorities. *Canadian Journal of Public Health, 96,* S23–S29.

Fulkerson, J. A., Story, M., Mellin, A., Leffert, N., Neumark-Sztainer, D., & French, S. A. (2006). Family dinner meal frequency and adolescent development: A relationship with developmental assets and high-risk behavior. *Journal of Adolescent Health, 39,* 337–345.

Girolami, G., et al. (2006). Parent's knowledge and perception about child development: evidence from a practice-based survey. *Pediatric Physical Therapy, 18*(1), 91–92.

Gould, R. L. (1979). *Transformations: Growth and change in adult life.* New York: Simon & Schuster.

Haines, J., & Neumark-Sztainer, D. (2006). Prevention of obesity and eating disorders: A consideration of shared risk factors. *Health Education Research, 21,* 770–782.

Klaff, L. G. (2006). As they grow. 1 year: Walk on! *Parents, 81*(8), 115–116.

Lee, L. L. S., & Harris, S. R. (2005). Psychometric properties and standardization samples of four screening tests for infants and young children: A review. *Pediatric Physical Therapy, 17*(2), 140–147.

Levinson, D. J. (1986). A conception of adult development. *American Psychologist, 41,* 3–13.

Levinson, D. J. (1996). *The seasons of a woman's life.* New York, NY: AA Knopf.

Levinson, D. J., Darrow, C. N., & Klein, E. B. (1986). *The seasons of a man's life* (2nd ed.). New York: Ballantine.

Long, R., & Boffa, J. (2007). Why internationally adopted children should be screened for tuberculosis. *Canadian Medical Association Journal, 177,* 172–173.

Moninger, J. (2006). As they grow. 6–8 years: Funny business. *Parents, 81*(8), 127–128.

Nakasato, Y. R., & Carnes, B.A. (2006). Health promotion in older adults: Promoting successful aging in primary care settings. *Geriatrics, 61*(4), 27–31.

Neumark-Sztainer, D., van den Berg, P., Hannan, P. J., & Story, M. (2006). Self-weighing in adolescents: Helpful or harmful? Longitudinal associations with body weight changes and disordered eating. *Journal of Adolescent Health, 39,* 811–818.

Niemeier, H. M., Raynor, H. A., Lloyd-Richardson, E. E., Rogers, M. L., & Wing, R. R. (2006). Fast food consumption and breakfast skipping: Predictors of weight gain from adolescence to adulthood in a nationally representative sample. *Journal of Adolescent Health, 39,* 842–849.

Nilsson, M., Stenlund, H., Bergström, E., Weinehall, L., & Janlert, U. (2006). It takes two: Reducing adolescent smoking uptake through sustainable adolescent–adult partnership. *Journal of Adolescent Health, 39,* 880–886.

Obituary: The Canadian Task Force on Preventive Health Care [Editorial]. (2003). *Canadian Medical Association Journal, 169*(11), 1137.

Olds, D. L. (2004). Effects of nurse home-visiting on maternal life course and child development: Age 6 follow-up results of a randomized trial. *Pediatrics, 114,* 1550–1559.

Padula, C. A., & Sullivan, M. (2006). Long-term married couples' health promotion behaviors: Identifying factors that impact decision making. *Journal of Gerontological Nursing, 32*(10), 37–47.

Piaget, J. (1968). *Judgment and reasoning in the child.* Totowa, NJ: Littlefield, Adams.

Piaget, J. (1975). *The construction of reality in the child.* New York: Ballantine.

Patterson, C., Feightner, J. W., Garcia, A., Hsiung, G-Y. R., MacKnight, C., & Sadovick, A. D. (2008). Diagnosis and treatment of dementia: 1. Risk assessment and primary prevention of Alzheimer disease. *Canadian Medical Association Journal, 178,* 548–556.

Position Paper Working Group. (2004). The use of growth charts for assessing and monitoring growth in Canadian infants and children. *Canadian Journal of Dietetic Practice and Research, 65,* 22–32.

Public Health Agency of Canada. (2006). *Canadian immunization guide* (7th ed). Retrieved from http://www.phac-aspc.gc.ca/publicat/cig-gci/index-eng.php

Public Health Agency of Canada. (2008a). *Leading causes of death and hospitalization in Canada, 2004* (Table 1). Retrieved February 12, 2008, from http://phac-asc-aspc.gc.ca/publicat/lcd-pcd97/table1-eng.php

Public Health Agency of Canada. (2008b). *Publicly funded immunization programs in Canada—Routine schedule for infants and children.* Retrieved February 11, 2008, from http://www.phac-aspc.gc.ca/im/ptimprog-progimpt/table-1_e.html

Rydz, D., et al. (2006). Screening for developmental delay in the setting of a community pediatric clinic: A prospective assessment of parent-report questionnaires. *Pediatrics, 118,* e1178–e1186.

Smith, J., & McSherry, W. (2004). Spirituality and child development: a concept analysis. *Journal of Advanced Nursing, 45,* 307–315.

Smith, L.M., LaGasse, L. L., Derauf, C., Grant, P., Shah, R., Arria, A., et al. (2006). The infant development, environment, and lifestyle study: Effects of prenatal methamphetamine exposure, polydrug exposure, and poverty or intrauterine growth. *Pediatrics, 118,* 1149–1156.

Spelke, E.S., Breinlinger, K., Macomber, J., & Jacobson, K. (1992). Origins of knowledge. *Psychological Review, 99,* 605–632.

Srof, B. J., & Velsor-Friedrich, B. (2006). Health promotion in adolescents: A review of Pender's health promotion model. *Nursing Science Quarterly, 19,* 366–373.

Struck, B. D., & Ross, K. M. (2006). Health promotion in older adults: Prescribing exercise for the frail and home bound. *Geriatrics, 61*(5), 22–27.

Thomas, H. (2006). Obesity prevention programs for children and youth: Why are their results so modest. *Health Education Research, 21,* 783–795.

Thomas, S., & Stewart, J. (2005). Optimising health promotion activities. *Journal of Community Nursing, 19*(1), 9–10, 12.

Timmons, B. W., Naylor, P-J., & Pfeiffer, K. A. (2007). Physical activity for preschool children—How much and how? *Canadian Journal of Public Health, 98*(Suppl. 2), 5122–5134.

To, T., Guttmann, A., Rosenfield, J. D., Parkin, J. D., Tassoudji, M., Vydykhan, T.N., et al. (2004). Risk markers for poor development attainment in young children: Results from a longitudinal national survey. *Archives of Pediatrics and Adolescent Medicine, 158,* 643–649.

U.S. Department of Health and Human Services. *Healthy People 2010.* Retrieved from http://www.health.gov/healthypeople

U.S. Preventive Services Task Force. (2006). *Guide to clinical preventive services, 2006.* Retrieved from http://www.ahrq.gov/clinic/uspstfix.htm

van Beek, Y., et al. (2006). Maternal expectations about infant development of pre-term and full-term infants: A cross-nation comparison. *Infant and Child Development, 15*(1), 41–58.

Van Breeman, C. (2006). Adolescent development amidst progressive illness: A support group model. *Journal of Palliative Care, 22,* 240–241.

van Mechelen, W., & Verhagen, E. (2005). Injury prevention in young people—Time to accept responsibility [Special issue]. *Lancet, 366,* S46.

Wagner, J., Jenkins, B., & Smith, J. C. (2006). Nurses' utilization of parent questionnaires for developmental screening. *Pediatric Nursing, 32,* 409–412, 452–454.

Weinberger, M., Hiner, S. L., & Tierney, W. M. (1987). In support of Hassles as a measure of stress in predicting health outcomes. *Journal of Behavioral Medicine, 10*(1), 19–31.

Woolf, S. H., Jonas, S., & Lawrence, R. S. (1996). *Health promotion and disease prevention in clinical practice.* Baltimore, MD: Williams & Wilkins.

Worsham, N. L., & Crawford, E. K. (2005). Parental illness and adolescent development. *The Prevention Researcher, 12*(4), 3–6.

Zehle, K., Wen, L. M., Orr, N., & Rissel, C. (2007). "It's not an issue at the moment": A qualitative study of mothers about childhood obesity. *American Journal of Maternal Child Nursing, 32*(1), 36–41.

Web Sites of Interest

Canada's Physical Activity Guides for Children and Youth—http://www.phac-aspc.gc.ca/pau-uap/paguide/child_youth/index.html

Canadian Best Practices Portal for Health Promotion and Chronic Disease Prevention—http://cbpp-pcpe.phac-aspc.gc.ca/index_e.cfm

Canadian Immunization Recommendations—http://www.phac-aspc.gc.ca/im/is-cv/index-eng.php#a

Canadian Task Force on Preventive Health Care—http://www.ctfphc.org/

Health Promotion, Public Health Agency of Canada—http://www.phac-aspc.gc.ca/hp-ps/index-eng.php#pa

Nipissing District Developmental Screen™—http://www.ndds.ca/

Ontario Cervical Screening Guidelines: McLachlin, C. M., Mai, V., Murphy, J., Fung Kee Fung, M., Chambers, A. & members of the Cervical Screening Guidelines Development Committee of the Ontario Cervical Screening Program and the Gynecology Cancer Disease Site Group of Cancer Care Ontario. (2005). *Cervical screening: A clinical practice guideline.* Program in Evidence-Based Care, a Cancer Care Ontario Program—http://www.cancercare.on.ca/pdf/pebc_cervical_screen.pdf

Cultural and Social Considerations in Health Assessment

Written by **Annette J. Browne**, PhD, RN, and **Colleen Varcoe**, PhD, RN
Based on the original chapter by **Rachel E. Spector**, PhD, RN, CTN, FAAN

Who is the person you are meeting for the first time? Where does he or she come from? What is the person's heritage? What is the person's cultural, social, and family background—his or her ethnicity and religion? Does the person understand, speak, and read English or French? What language does the person understand, speak, and read? What are the person's health* and illness beliefs and practices? Operating from a relational† standpoint, you would also want to ask—Who am I? Where do I come from? What is my social, cultural, or family background? What is my heritage, ethnicity, and religion? What is my primary language? Do I understand, speak, and read a language other than English? What are my health and illness beliefs and practices?

A relational approach to health assessment prompts you to ask, "How do my social, cultural, and professional backgrounds shape my ability to relate to, and my assumptions about, the various people I encounter in my practice?" Approaching cultural and social considerations in health assessment from a relational stance will help you understand and attend to the contexts that shape patterns of health and illness. These contexts include people's past experiences, culture, heritage, socioeconomic status, history, and understandings of health, illness, and pathways to healing. By recognizing and attending to these contexts, you will be optimally prepared to conduct accurate health assessments and respond meaningfully to people's health, illness, and health promotion needs.

---

*The World Health Organization (WHO) defines health as "a state of complete physical, mental and social well-being and not merely the absence of disease or infirmity" (WHO, 2008).
†As introduced in Chapter 1, a "relational" approach refers to more than interpersonal relationships among people (Doane et al., 2005). A relational approach recognizes that health, illness, and the meanings they hold for people are shaped by one's gender, age, ability, and social, cultural, family, historical, and geographical contexts. Similarly, these contexts influence how nurses and other healthcare professionals view, relate, and work with patients and families. It is therefore imperative that nurses and other healthcare professionals remain critically attuned to the significance of these contexts during the process of health assessment.

Over the course of your professional education, you will study the developmental tasks and the principles of health promotion across the lifespan and learn to conduct numerous assessments, such as a complete health history, a mental health assessment, risks for violence, a nutritional assessment, a pain assessment, and a physical examination on a patient. As a healthcare professional, you will continually experience similarities and differences between you and the people and families with whom you come in contact. These differences are based on a wide range of factors: life experiences, opportunities and circumstances, and the linguistic, social, and cultural traditions of all persons, including you. A relational approach seeks to make similarities and differences more transparent to us so that we can be as responsive as possible to people's varying needs.

The purpose of this chapter is as follows:
1. To describe concepts that are central to understanding cultural and social considerations in health assessment
2. To distinguish between cultural sensitivity and cultural safety
3. To review demographic trends within the Canadian population
4. To provide examples of ethnocultural diversity within the Canadian population
5. To review trends in health, social, and gender inequities in Canada
6. To identify guidelines for assessing culturally based understandings, and the social and economic contexts shaping people's lives

CULTURAL AND SOCIAL CONSIDERATIONS: CENTRAL CONCEPTS

Culture and Culturalism

No single definition of **culture** exists, and all too often, definitions tend to be so general that they lack any real meaning or erase the complexity and shifting nature of culture.

Culture is not something that is external to us; it is a universal phenomenon that shapes the health and well-being of every person. Yet a person's cultural orientation develops in distinctive and specific ways depending on where he or she lives, family background, socioeconomic circumstances, languages spoken, spiritual orientation, ancestry, and history as an individual and as a member of specific groups. Within any given group, people have varying health practices, differing levels of knowledge about health-related issues, diverse family norms, and so on.

In disciplines such as anthropology, culture is understood as an inherently complex dimension of peoples' lives. In health care, however, culture tends to be viewed in very narrow and prescriptive terms, as the values, beliefs, and customs and practices inherent to particular ethnocultural group members. These assumed "cultural traits" are typically those identified as different from "ours," the unspoken comparison being made with the assumed dominant norm. This narrow view tends to equate culture with ideas about ethnicity or "race," overlooking most sociocultural aspects relevant to health.

Because health care in Canada and the United States has drawn so heavily on narrowly defined ideas about culture, there has been a proliferation of textbooks in nursing and medicine that provide healthcare professionals with systematized descriptions or lists of cultural characteristics for various groups. While these culturally based characteristics are applicable to some people, they most certainly do not apply to all members of a group. For example, Chinese or Iranian communities in Canada are extremely diverse. There is no "recipe" or predefined approach for a Canadian-born person to follow in interacting with people who have recently immigrated from China or Iran. Further, there are often significant differences between generations, including differences post migration. Regardless of country of birth, language, or religion, people have diverse points of view, educational levels, economic levels, and religions (Behjati-Sabet et al., 2005; Yue, 2005). The dangers of applying lists of cultural traits to patients that you encounter lies in drawing on stereotypes and making assumptions about particular people, which, in turn, lead to unsafe health assessment practices. Healthcare professionals must therefore find ways of learning about all their patients, and their contexts, to understand how best to address their health needs (Gustafson, 2008).

This process of conceptualizing culture in fairly narrow terms, or assuming that people act in particular ways because of their culture, is known as **culturalism**. From a culturalist perspective, culture, in the narrow sense, is often given as the primary explanation for certain people or groups experiencing various health, social, or economic problems. For example, research has shown that healthcare professionals frequently attribute people's social problems to their cultural characteristics (Anderson et al., 2003; Browne, 2005, 2007; Varcoe, 2001, 2008). This would lead them to wrongly assume that violence toward women may be acceptable in particular cultural groups, or that some people are more prone to using drugs or alcohol because of "their culture." Similarly, you can-

not make accurate assumptions about people's health beliefs based on their ethnicity—for example, it would be wrong to assume that people from China necessarily embrace the hot–cold theory of health and illness (an explanatory model that views the treatment of illness as requiring cold, heat, dryness, or wetness to restore balance). Such assumptions are culturalist because they (1) are based on popularized (and often stereotypical) ideas about culture as something fixed and inherent to particular groups defined by language, country of origin, or physical characteristics, and (2) assume that culture is the primary explanation for people's health-related practices or decisions. Most importantly, such assumptions do not lead to useful information.

To counter this tendency toward culturalism in health care, it can be useful to define culture from a **critical cultural perspective** (Browne et al., 2006). From a critical cultural perspective, we understand culture as a relational aspect of ourselves that shifts and changes over time depending on our history,

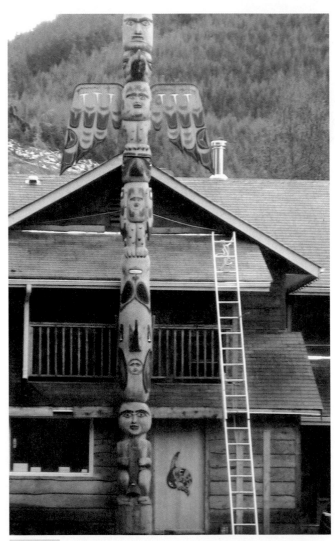

Fig. 3-1   What aspects of culture do you see in this picture? Do you tend to think of the Aboriginal carvings as "cultural" and overlook the ways in which the house's architecture, the logging slash behind the house, and the various items (ladder, chimney) also reflect culture?

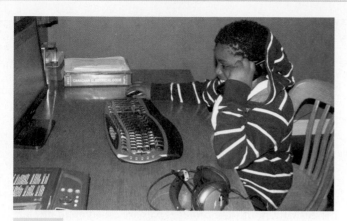

Fig. 3-2   What definition of "culture" comes to your mind when looking at this picture?

social context, past experiences, gender, professional identity, and so on. As Anderson & Reimer Kirkham (1999) explain:

> [Culture] is located in a constantly shifting network of meanings enmeshed within historical, social, economic and political relationships and processes. It is not therefore reduced to an easily identifiable set of characteristics, nor is it a politically neutral concept. (p. 63)

Viewing culture in this way does not imply that one should not pay attention to people's values, beliefs, and practices in healthcare contexts. From a critical perspective of culture, these are viewed as highly significant—not as determining factors in people's lives but as intersecting with broader social determinants of health. For example, rather than seeing people's diet (or other health-related practices) as determined by their "culture," a critical cultural perspective prompts us to see that what people eat is equally influenced by their income, access to food resources, ability to afford fresh fruits and vegetables, geographical location, and educational levels. In many rural or remote communities, it is often less expensive to purchase high-carbohydrate fast foods or drinks than to purchase milk, fresh fruits, and fresh vegetables. This explains why in these communities it can be difficult for people to purchase fresh foods that, for example, would be beneficial for those living with diabetes or heart disease. It also explains, in part, why there are high rates of type 2 diabetes in some Aboriginal communities, where access to traditional foods (e.g., berries, fish, game) has been denied by policies (e.g., the reserve system and land appropriation) and environmental damage (e.g., fisheries collapse). Similarly, people who immigrate to Canada may have difficulty accessing the ingredients with which they are familiar and therefore turn to less healthy, prepackaged foods. Thus, when taking a health history, understanding whether a person or family can afford healthy food choices is as important as understanding their culturally based preferences for particular foods.

Just as each of us has a particular cultural orientation, so does health care have a particular culture. For example, Western-educated healthcare professionals tend to attribute illness to individual behaviours or factors, such as bacteria and viruses, poor lifestyle practices, or failure to exercise (Waxler-Morrison et al., 2005). They also tend to view the individual as responsible for getting well and to value "compliance" with recommended technical diagnostic procedures, medications, and surgeries. However, there is great variation in the extent to which patients and their family members ascribe to the values of the **dominant healthcare culture**. For some patients, the Western-style approach to history-taking (asking questions in quick succession) is not part of their pattern of communication. For some, taking a prescribed medication requires consultations with other members of the family. Healthcare professionals who are alert to and respectful of the wide variety of healthcare practices and understandings about health will more easily find a mutually acceptable way to address people's concerns. This will require you to remain critically reflective about how you may be conveying the dominant culture of health care in ways that can make patients feel uncomfortable or hesitant to share their perspectives.

Culture, Ethnicity, and "Race"

Culture is often wrongly equated with ethnicity, and because ethnicity is often based on ideas about "race," culture is also often confused with "race." **Ethnicity** is a complex concept often inferring geographical and national affiliation. An **ethnic group** is a group or "community maintained by a shared heritage, culture, language or religion" (Henry et al., 2005, p. 350). However, ethnicity is an ambiguous concept because it can encompass multiple different aspects such as "race," origin or ancestry, identity, language, and religion. Statistics Canada (2006a) notes that ethnicity is dynamic and in a constant state of flux, changing as a result of new immigration flows and the development of new identities. In the context of health assessment, it is important to remember that people's ethnic identities depend on how they perceive themselves. In some contexts, people may choose to report that they are Iranian, or Greek, or Sri Lankan, or Jewish. In other situations, they may feel that if they reveal their ethnicity to the healthcare professionals or the admissions clerk, they may be treated differently on the basis of assumptions about them.

In healthcare and other sectors of Canadian society, ethnicity is often used as a substitute for the idea of "race." **"Race"** is defined as:

> A socially constructed category used to classify humankind according to common ancestry and reliant on differentiation by such physical characteristics such as colour of skin, hair texture, stature and facial characteristics. The concept of race has no basis in biological reality and, as such, has no meaning independent of its social definitions. (Henry et al., 2005, p. 351)

Although the United Nations Educational Scientific and Cultural Organization (UNESCO) released its first statement on "race" in 1952, dismissing it as a biological category (UNESCO, 1952) and has continued to do so as recently as 1997, and despite the ongoing scientific evidence that dispels the existence of "races," the tendency in nursing, medicine, and health care is to continue to confuse "race" with genetic characteristics. All people, regardless of the colour of their skin or other physical appearances are a mixture of populations (Henry et al., 2005). As stated in the 1952 UNESCO declaration, "biological differences between human beings within a single [so called] 'race' may be as great as, or greater than, the same biological differences between races" (p. 15). While skin colour, eye shape, and hair texture are genetically determined and reflect heredity and ancestry, those features do not signify any meaningful biological groupings. Rather, "race," like ethnicity, is a way of categorizing people socially.

In the United States, "*race*" and *ethnicity* are often used interchangeably to categorize people, for example, as "Black," "White," "Hispanic," or "Asian." These categories signal social categories rather than genetically linked groups of people. For example, research has demonstrated that the increased incidence of high blood pressure among African Americans is attributable to experiences of discrimination (Krieger et al., 1998). Although "race" is not a biological entity, the social dynamics that occur in our societies because of racialization (in this case, discrimination against people with dark skin or against those who are thought to be descended from people with dark skin) have a profound effect on patterns of health and illness.

Racialization continues to affect people in many ways—in health care and in the wider social world. Racialization is the process whereby racial categories are constructed as different and unequal in ways that lead to social, economic, and political impacts (Galabuzi, 2001). For example, in our research, we have seen situations where healthcare professionals have erroneously assumed that alcoholism is "genetic" among Aboriginal people, leading them to presume that someone is drunk when, in fact, the person is experiencing a cerebral bleed, severe dehydration, a seizure disorder, or ataxia as a side effect of prescription medication.

Racialization is closely linked to culturalism and **discrimination**, the process by which a member or members of a social or ethnocultural group are treated differently (especially unfairly) (Krieger, 2002). Of significance was a recent survey that reported that one in five people aged 15 years and over who were part of a "visible minority"[‡] in Canada said they had experienced discrimination or unfair treatment sometimes or often in the past 5 years because of their ethnicity, culture, "race," skin colour, language, accent, or religion (Perreault, 2004). As a healthcare professional, you will need to think critically about these processes and examine the categories and assumptions that you may be using (sometimes unconsciously) in relation to particular

---

[‡]The concept of **visible minority** applies to persons who are identified according to Canada's Employment Equity Act "as being non-Caucasian . . . or non-white in colour. Under the Act, Aboriginal persons are not considered to be members of visible minority groups" (Statistics Canada, 2006c). Using the term *visible minority* is a classification of people by skin colour or other physical characteristics and is a racializing process.

patients and families. In health assessments, it is usually not necessary to ask people to identify their ethnicity. Rather, focusing on an individual's particular understandings, explanations, values, and practices related to health and illness will help you obtain information relevant to health and avoid making assumptions—in other words, provide culturally safe care.

CULTURAL SENSITIVITY, CULTURAL COMPETENCE, AND CULTURAL SAFETY

Increasingly, healthcare professionals are called on to provide culturally sensitive healthcare services. **Cultural sensitivity** reflects the idea that healthcare professionals should be sensitive to people's values, beliefs, customs, and practices. Being sensitive to people can be useful if it is done in a way that does not demean people or their differences from the dominant norm. However, a critical cultural perspective emphasizes that healthcare professionals must go beyond being passively sensitive to examine how values, beliefs, customs, and practices intersect with broader social determinants and the power relations that shape health and health care. **Cultural competence** is a term that is sometimes used to emphasize a more active role for healthcare professionals, including consideration of these broader contexts (Spector, 2004). In Canada, Srivastava (2007) uses the idea of cultural competence to draw attention to power relations and to consider culture in ways that directly address issues of racism and inequity. Regardless of the school of thought upon which one is drawing, developing knowledge about cultural and social considerations cannot be achieved through quick one-lesson programs or brief "cross-cultural training" alone. Rather, you must develop knowledge in several areas, such as:

1. Your own personal ethnocultural and social background
2. The culture of nursing and related professions
3. The culture of the healthcare system
4. The signifance of social, economic, and cultural contexts
5. Your ability to critically examine your assumptions about each of these areas.

We use the idea of *cultural safety* as a form of cultural competence that assists you to develop in these areas.

Cultural Safety

Cultural safety emerged in the nursing literature in the 1990s in New Zealand as a concept that was developed by Maori nurse leaders and educators who were concerned by the persistent health and healthcare inequities affecting Maori people (the indigenous people of New Zealand) (Papps et al., 1996; Ramsden, 1993, 2002; Wepa, 2005). In Canada, cultural safety is increasingly being used in nursing, medicine, and other healthcare disciplines to provide care that takes into account the social, economic, political, and historical positions of groups within society (Anderson et al., 2003; Reimer Kirkham et al., 2002; Smye et al., 2002; Smye et al., 2006). Cultural safety acknowledges that culturally based meanings and practices must be respected; however, it also directs health-care professionals to change the culture of health care, especially the practices and policies that perpetuate culturalism, racialization, and inequities.

Some of the main principles of cultural safety are as follows:

- The cultural, social, economic, and historical positioning of people intersect to shape their health status and access to health care.
- Individual and institutional discrimination, culturalism, and racialization create risks for patients, particularly when people from a particular group perceive they are "demeaned, diminished or disempowered by the actions and delivery systems" of professionals within the healthcare system. (Ramsden et al., 1994, p. 164)
- How members of a group are treated and perceived within the healthcare system is more important than the cataloguing of culturally specific beliefs or practices. (Polaschek, 1998)
- Nurses and other healthcare professionals must reflect on their own personal and cultural histories, and the values, beliefs, and assumptions that they bring to healthcare encounters, and must avoid uncritically imposing their understandings, assumptions, or beliefs on others. (Anderson et al., 2003).

Because relational approaches are concerned with relationships among professionals and patients within particular historical, economic, social, and cultural contexts, relational approaches are integral to cultural safety. As you approach a new patient who is different from you in terms of skin colour, clothing, socioeconomic status, accent, or primary language spoken, ask yourself:

- What biases, assumptions, or stereotypes am I drawing on?
- What am I paying attention to, and how is that causing me to overlook certain things?
- How does the work environment (e.g., norms, colleagues, workload) contribute to, or challenge, the formation of these stereotypes and assumptions?

DEMOGRAPHIC PROFILE OF CANADA

Canada's population in 2007 was estimated to be approximately 33 million. Canada's population is diverse in terms of where people live, languages spoken, age distributions, and ethnocultural identities. Although the majority of the population is Canadian born, the Canadian population is increasing primarily due to international migration. Of significance is the fact that 70% of people who immigrated to Canada in 2006 reported a mother tongue[§] other than English or French (Statistics Canada, 2007a).

Canada's two official languages, English and French, are entrenched in the country's history, which confers rights and institutional support for anglophones and francophones. In 2006, 58% of the population in Canada reported English and

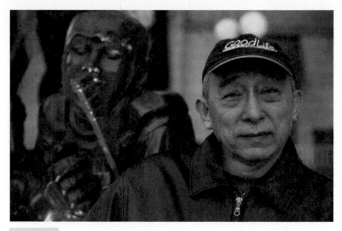

Fig. 3-3   How can you counter your own assumptions?

22% reported French as their mother tongue (Statistics Canada, 2007d). Many distinct Aboriginal language families and dialects also exist. Strategies for communicating effectively with people whose primary language is different from yours are discussed in depth in Chapter 4.

Canadians live primarily in urban areas. In 2006, nearly 25 million people, or more than four fifths of Canadians, lived in urban areas, and six million people lived in rural areas (Canadian Institute for Health Information [CIHI], 2006). Many people reside in large census metropolitan areas, or CMAs.[‖] In 2006, Canada had six Census Metropolitan Areas (CMAs) whose populations were over one million: Toronto, Montréal, Vancouver, Ottawa-Gatineau, and, for the first time, Calgary and Edmonton (Statistics Canada, 2007c). Together, these cities contain 45% of Canada's total population.

Canada's population as a whole is aging (Statistics Canada, 2007b). In 2006, the 65-and-over population hit a record high, comprising 13.7% of the total population. In contrast,

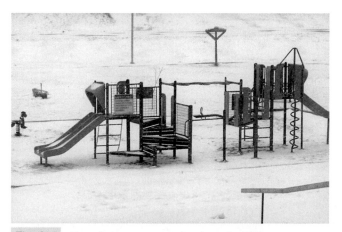

Fig. 3-4   How does our geography shape health?

[‖]A CMA is an area consisting of one or more neighbouring municipalities situated around a major urban core. A CMA must have a total population of at least 100,000, of which 50,000 or more live in the urban core.

[§]*Mother tongue* is defined by Statistics Canada as the first language learned at home in childhood and still understood by the individual.

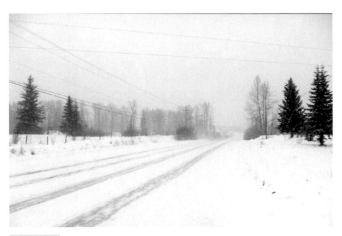

Fig. 3-5   How does our geography shape healthcare access?

the proportion of the under-15 population fell to 17.7%, its lowest level ever. The median age, which divides the population into two groups of equal size, has risen steadily since 1966, reaching 39.5 years in 2006. Since the first national census in 1871, Canada has never had so many persons aged 80 years and over (representing 1.2 million people in 2006). Due to longer life expectancy for women (82.5 years for women

compared with 77.7 years for men), nearly two out of three people aged 80 and over are women.

The increasing ethnocultural, linguistic, and social diversity within society requires healthcare policies and practices that support professionals to work across differences. Box 3-1 outlines guidelines adapted from standards developed in the United States to support services for culturally and linguistically diverse populations (Office of Minority Health, 2001). Many hospitals and healthcare agencies in Canada have similar policies.

ETHNOCULTURAL DIVERSITY WITHIN THE CANADIAN POPULATION

As suggested by the demographic profile in the preceding section, Canada is one of the most diverse countries in the world along many dimensions. Ethnocultural diversity is part of Canada's national identity. As the demographics indicate, the majority of Canadians associate themselves with the dominant linguistic groups (English and French) and with the dominant European ancestry. These patterns create both the potential for "othering" (Canales, 2000; Peternelj-Taylor, 2005) in health care and the potential for modelling culturally safe, actively respectful ways of working across differences in health care. Differences are most evident when members of

---

BOX 3-1 | **Standards for Culturally, Linguistically, and Socially Appropriate Services in Health Care**

1. Promote and support the attitudes, openness, knowledge, behaviours, and skills necessary for staff to work respectfully and effectively with patients and each other in a culturally, linguistically, and socially diverse work environment.

2. Have a comprehensive management strategy to address culturally, linguistically, and socially appropriate services, including strategic goals, plans, policies, procedures, and designated staff responsible for implementation.

3. Use formal mechanisms for community and consumer involvement in the design and execution of service delivery, including planning, policymaking, operations, evaluation, training, and, as appropriate, treatment planning.

4. Develop and implement a strategy to recruit, retain, and promote diverse administrative, clinical, and support staff who are trained and qualified to address the needs of the various communities being served.

5. Require and arrange for continuing education and training for administrative, clinical, and support staff in how to foster respectful and responsive services for culturally, linguistically, and socially diverse people.

6. Provide all patients who have limited English or French proficiency with access to interpretation services.

7. Provide oral and written notices, including translated signage at key points of contact, to patients in their primary languages, and inform them of their right to receive interpreter services free of charge.

8. Translate and make available signage and commonly used written patient educational material and other material for members of the predominant language groups in the local service areas.

9. Ensure that interpreters and bilingual staff can demonstrate bilingual proficiency and receive training that includes the skills and ethics of interpreting, and knowledge of the terms and concepts relevant to clinical or nonclinical encounters. Family and friends are not considered adequate substitutes because they usually lack these abilities.

10. Ensure that the patient's primary language spoken is included in the healthcare organization's information system and in any patient records used by staff or healthcare professionals.

11. Use a variety of methods to collect and make use of accurate demographic, epidemiological, and clinical outcome data for groups and populations in the service area, and become informed about the cultural, linguistic, and social needs, resources, and assets of the surrounding community.

12. Undertake continuing organizational self-assessments, internal audits, and performance improvement programs, and integrate measures of access, quality, and outcomes of services particularly for culturally, linguistically, and socially diverse people.

13. Develop structures and procedures to address ethical and legal conflicts in healthcare delivery and complaints or grievances by patients and staff about unfair, insensitive, or discriminatory treatment, inequities in accessing services, or denial of services.

14. Prepare an annual progress report documenting the organization's progress with implementing services that are culturally, linguistically, and socially responsive, including information on programs, staffing, and resources.

dominant groups provide care to people who are from racialized groups or visible minorities, such as Aboriginal people or some people who have immigrated to Canada, particularly if those persons cannot communicate in the official languages. Therefore, to provide culturally safe care, healthcare professionals require particular knowledge pertaining to Aboriginal people and immigrants.

Aboriginal Peoples in Canada

The term *Aboriginal peoples* is used to refer generally to the indigenous inhabitants of Canada including First Nations, Métis, and Inuit people (Royal Commission on Aboriginal Peoples, 1996, p. xii). These three groups reflect "political and cultural entities that stem historically from the original peoples of North America, rather than collections of individuals united by so-called 'racial' characteristics" (p. xii). Of the 3.8% of the population in Canada who self-identified as Aboriginal, 60% identified as First Nations, 33% identified as Métis, and 4% identified as Inuit (Statistics Canada, 2008). Although the terms *Indian* or *Native* are used in federal legislation (e.g., the *Indian Act*) and by the federal government (e.g., Indian and Northern Affairs Canada [INAC]), the term *First Nations* is often viewed as more respectful than the colonial term *Indian*. *Inuit* replaces the colonial term *Eskimo*, and *Métis* refers to people of mixed European and Aboriginal ancestry. It is important to recognize that there is a great deal of diversity within First Nations, Métis, and Inuit people, reflected, in part, by the more than 50 Aboriginal languages that are currently spoken (Cook et al., 2004).

Increasingly, many Aboriginal people are moving from rural and northern communities into urban areas, often to seek employment that is not available in other regions. In 2006, the proportion of First Nations people living off-reserve (60%) exceeded those living on-reserve (40%) (Statistics Canada, 2008). Winnipeg was home to the largest urban Aboriginal population, and Saskatoon, Regina, Edmonton, Vancouver, Toronto, and Calgary also had high proportions of Aboriginal residents. Among the Inuit population, however, 78% continued to reside in the northern regions of Canada, with 49% living in Nunavut, 19% in Nunavik in northern Quebec, 6%

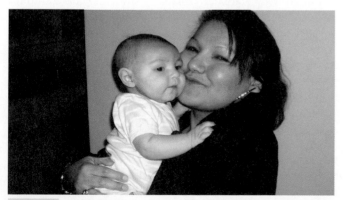

Fig. 3-6   What do you imagine about this woman? She is the grandmother of a great-grandchild of a renowned traditional medicine woman, Mrs. Sophie Thomas.

in the Inuvialuit region of the Northwest Territories, and 4% in Nunatsiavut in northern Labrador (Statistics Canada, 2008).

Policies Affecting Aboriginal Peoples in Canada

In Canada, the complex history of colonialism and current policies and practices have resulted in profound social disruption within many Aboriginal communities. This has contributed to the lack of employment opportunities, limited access to educational programs, inadequate and, often, crowded housing, and high levels of poverty (Waldram et al., 2006). The regulation of First Nations people's lives through the policies of the **Indian Act**, and the ongoing restrictions placed on self-government, land claims, and economic development in Aboriginal communities, continue to shape life opportunities, economic conditions, and the overall health and social status of individuals and families.

The *Indian Act*, originally developed in 1876, was founded on the paternalistic motivation of assimilating and governing "Indians" (now often referred to as First Nations people). The original *Indian Act* has been amended several times, but it remains an actively applied set of legislation and contains all the federal policies and regulations pertaining to "registered status Indians" (a term used in the *Indian Act*). The *Indian Act* classifies First Nations people into registered status Indians or nonstatus Indians to distinguish those people who receive legal recognition in Canada from those who do not (INAC, 2007). The process of obtaining registered status (here on referred to as *status*) is complex and requires a series of paperwork submissions to INAC, the federal department responsible for meeting the government's constitutional, treaty, political, and legal responsibilities to First Nations people.

Some First Nations people do not have status (e.g., approximately 20% of the total First Nations population), but they identify themselves as First Nations and are often members of a First Nation community (Statistics Canada, 2008). They are not, however, recognized by the federal government under the *Indian Act*, either because they are unable to prove their status or because they have lost their status rights. For example, many First Nations women in Canada lost their status when they married nonstatus men. While the Act was changed in 1985 to repeal these discriminatory policies, it is still possible for the grandchildren of status First Nations women to lose their status designation. The issue of who has status and who does not is relevant to healthcare professionals because people who are nonstatus are not entitled to the limited benefits available to people with status.

Currently, First Nations people with status and Inuit people receive limited healthcare benefits (called Non-Insured Health Benefits [NIHBs]) not covered by provincial health insurance plans (Health Canada, 2007). NIHBs are administered by Health Canada and include selected prescription drugs, limited medical supplies and equipment, short-term crisis counselling, limited coverage for glasses and vision care, medical transportation, and dental care (though many dentists do not provide services to people who have status because the dentist must wait to be reimbursed by the federal government versus receiving payment directly from the patient). Unfortunately, many members of the public, including healthcare professionals, are unaware that the services provided through NIHBs are very limited and that these benefits do not apply to nonstatus or Métis people.

Another prevalent misconception is that Aboriginal people in Canada do not pay taxes. This can be a source of resentment for some Canadians. In general, Aboriginal people are required to pay taxes on the same basis as other people in Canada, except where limited exemptions are defined by the *Indian Act* for people with status (INAC, 2007). Status First Nations people are not required to pay provincial or federal taxes for goods, services, income, and property on-reserve. However, this exemption does not apply to 60% of First Nations people in Canada who live off-reserve. Nonstatus and Inuit people are subject to taxation like all other Canadians.

Inequities in Health Status

In the past, discriminatory practices and policies were aimed at assimilating Aboriginal people into the dominant Canadian society. First Nations lands were appropriated and **reserves** were created, often in regions where economic development was limited. Cultural and spiritual practices were outlawed, including the work of traditional healers. Although it is not commonly known among the Canadian public, status First Nations people were not permitted to vote in federal elections until 1960, despite the fact that historically they were among the most intensively governed members of Canadian society (Furniss, 1999). Indoctrination into the dominant culture was attempted through church- or state-run **residential schools.** Residential schools included industrial schools, boarding schools, student residences, and hostels and were located in every province and territory, except New Brunswick and Prince Edward Island. The last residential school, located in Saskatchewan, closed in 1996. In recent years, many individuals and their family members have come forward with painful stories of physical and sexual abuse at residential schools. In response, in 2006, the federal government announced the approval of the Indian Residential Schools Settlement

Agreement and the new Truth and Reconciliation Commission (Indian Residential Schools Resolution Canada, 2008).

The inequities of the past continue to influence people's health status in the present. Despite improvements in recent years, the health of many Aboriginal people continues to lag behind that of the overall Canadian population based on virtually every measure (CIHI, 2004). In the year 2000, life expectancy at birth for the "registered Indian" population was estimated at 68.9 years for men and 76.6 years for women, differences that are 7.4 and 5.2 years less, respectively, than that of the total Canadian population. The poverty rate among First Nations children is at least double the national average (Assembly of First Nations, 2005). Infant mortality rates, one of the most powerful indicators of the social determinants of health, are almost twice as high for status First Nations infants as for other Canadians.

These health and social status indicators cannot be understood outside of their social, historical, and economic contexts, or viewed as "cultural" problems. Rather, they are manifestations of the complex interplay of historical, social, political, and economic determinants influencing health status and access to equitable health care. For example, healthcare professionals often fail to see the ways social conditions, systemic racism, and discrimination have shaped substance use and suicide among Aboriginal people (Kirmayer et al., 2007). Other research shows that prenatal care for Aboriginal women in some settings is hampered by judgemental discriminatory attitudes and, for many, poverty and limited resources in rural settings (Calam et al., 2008). Yet, healthcare professionals may judge these women for not accessing care (Browne, 2005, 2007; Browne et al., 2001). This is where relational approaches in clinical practice can make a difference: it is important for you to remain critically reflective about the assumptions that you may have and to also remain focused on the historical and social contexts and current living conditions that continue to shape people's health, access to health care, and overall well-being.

People Who Immigrate to Canada

Canada's population is becoming increasingly diverse, with immigration contributing to two thirds of our nation's population growth (Statistics Canada, 2007a). Canada continues to be the country of choice for many people, and in 2006, one in five people living in Canada were born outside of Canada. This means you will have the opportunity to work with increasingly diverse groups of patients, particularly if you work in urban areas.

Over the past four decades, patterns of immigration have shifted significantly. In the past, European nations such as the United Kingdom, Italy, Germany, and the Netherlands, as well as the United States, were the primary sources of immigrants to Canada (Badets et al., 2003). In 2006, people immigrating from Asia and the Middle East made up the largest proportion (58.3%) of newcomers to Canada (Statistics Canada, 2007a). People born in Europe comprised the second-largest group (16.1%) of recent immigrants. This was followed by an estimated 11.6% from India, 10.8% from Central and South

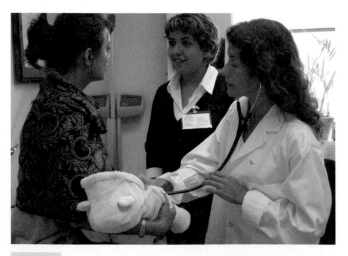

Fig. 3-7   What do you miss when you make assumptions based on appearances about the social influences on health?

America and the Caribbean, 10.6% from Africa, and 7% from the Philippines.

It is important to be aware of the terms used to refer to the diverse groups of people who move to Canada. The term *immigrant* applies to all people who have been granted the right to permanently reside in Canada by Citizenship and Immigration Canada (Statistics Canada, 2006b). Mistakenly, the term *visible minority* is sometimes confused with the term *immigrant*. Many people in Canada who fulfill the definition of visible minority are not immigrants but are from families who have resided in Canada for many generations. Nurses and other clinicians cannot assume that a person's appearance or accent has anything to do with a person's country of birth or citizenship. Rather, they need to remain open to learning about people's unique and multifaceted contexts, including their ethnocultural backgrounds, family origins, and social circumstances. Healthcare professionals should also realize that some people view the term *visible minority* as demeaning because it tends to erase or ignore people's various histories. Recognizing this as an issue, organizations such as the Ontario Human Rights Commission use the term *racialized groups* to acknowledge the dynamic and complex processes by which racial categories are socially produced and used in ways that entrench social inequities (Access Alliance, 2007).

The Longitudinal Survey of Immigrants to Canada asked people why they chose to immigrate to Canada; the largest proportion of people cited improving the future for their family and reuniting with family and close friends (Statistics Canada, 2007a). People's decisions to migrate can be voluntary, involuntary, or a blend of both (Vissandjée et al., 2007). The "push–pull" factors in migration are often due to the need to explore new economic opportunities, family reunification, or forced relocation owing to persecution or ecological disasters. Refugees often come from countries where there is conflict and war, and they seek safer conditions in Canada. The decision and ability to migrate is never easy: immigration involves complex applications, classification, and landing procedures. Immigration applications can take many years to process. With changing eligibility requirements, those who immigrate generally must come with significant economic resources. On the other hand, people who are refugees may come with few or no resources. Following migration, the processes of integration and adaptation into a new society is often lengthy and may take an entire lifetime or many generations. The development of a healthy and vibrant society requires the ongoing commitment of both recent immigrants and Canadians already residing in Canada (Vissandjée et al., 2007).

The vast majority of recent immigrants to Canada (97.2%) live in either a CMA or a census agglomeration, that is, an urban community (Statistics Canada, 2007a). Among these population groups, two thirds reside in Canada's three largest CMAs: Toronto, Montréal, and Vancouver. People who were born in countries other than Canada accounted for 45.7% of Toronto's, 39.6% of Vancouver's, and 20.6% of Montreal's populations (Statistics Canada, 2007a). In these three cities, immigration continues to be the major contributor to population growth. The most common reasons for settling in Toronto, Vancouver, or Montréal were to join social support networks of family and friends or because of the job prospects. Most recently, an increasing number of new immigrants are settling in CMAs other than the three largest, including Calgary, Ottawa-Gatineau, Edmonton, Winnipeg, Hamilton, and London.

The Process of Immigration and Effects on Health

As a clinician, you will need to recognize how the processes of migration and resettlement to another country can impact people's health and social status. Although many people are healthy when they first arrive in Canada, research shows that the health of non-European immigrants, in particular, deteriorates over time compared with that of Canadian-born residents and immigrants from Europe (Pederson et al., 2006). This pattern of declining health status is due to a number of factors. Some health problems are linked to the stress of immigration itself, which involves finding suitable employment and establishing a new social support network (Ng et al., 2005). The likelihood of a deterioration in health is also related to socioeconomic status, specifically, low education and low household income. A recent study showed that immigrant women, in particular, are often vulnerable to the stress that comes from trying to meet the basic needs of their families in a new country, learning a new language, and the social isolation that comes from leaving family and friends behind (Vissandjée et al., 2007).

People who immigrate to Canada often experience difficulties getting the help they need from healthcare professionals, hospitals, and other healthcare agencies (Waxler-Morrison et al., 2005). Immigrants can feel frustrated because few healthcare professionals can communicate in the family's language and few interpreter services are available. Immigrants may also lack a basic understanding of how the Canadian healthcare system works. Some people experience discrimination or prejudice in hospitals and clinics, which can lead to situations of mistrust. Clinicians, in turn, may feel that families are not following their instructions or are not abiding by hospital policies in terms of the numbers of visitors. Despite these

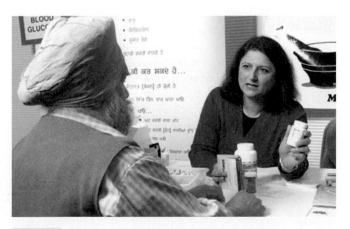

Fig. 3-8   What situations most challenge you when trying to shift from the stance of expert to that of inquirer?

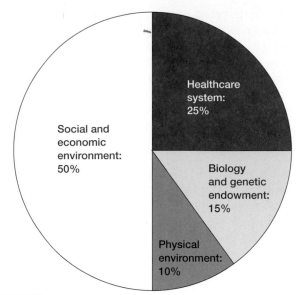

Fig. 3-9 Estimated impact of determinants of health on the health status of the population.

frustrations, most people who immigrate to Canada are very appreciative of the health care they receive, particularly if services were scarce or limited in their countries of origin.

People also face challenges accessing health and social services because they have limited proficiency in English or French, despite their ability to speak other languages (often several). Waiting periods to qualify for provincial healthcare coverage can extend to several years, compromising access to healthcare services for children and families (Caulford et al., 2006). Findings from the literature on immigrants' economic integration in Canada have shown that those with non-European origins are more likely than those with European origins to have low-paid jobs that require little education. It has been shown that despite higher levels of education, immigrants have greater difficulties finding meaningful employment and are often forced to take low paying jobs. These factors, in combination

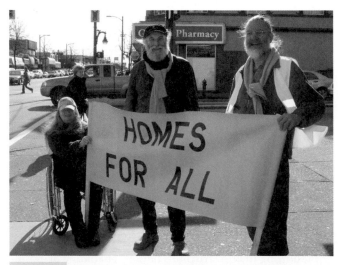

Fig. 3-10 How do gender, disability, and poverty intersect to affect health?

with experiences of racism and discrimination and lower levels of social support, contribute to declining health status. Together, these social and economic trends have a profound effect on health status and can limit access to the resources and services required to maintain health in Canada.

It is important to remember that people who come from the same country are nevertheless very diverse culturally, socially, and linguistically. People have varying levels of education and proficiency in Canada's two official languages, varied socioeconomic backgrounds, and varied understandings of Western healthcare services. Applying relational approaches in clinical practice will help you to assess the unique contexts, histories, and experiences that shape an individual's or a family's overall health and well-being.

HEALTH, SOCIAL, AND GENDER INEQUITIES

To understand how inequities impact health, it is useful to distinguish between concepts such as health inequality and inequity. **Health inequality** is a generic term used to designate differences, variations, and disparities in the health status of individuals and groups (Kawachi et al., 2002). An example of health inequality is the higher incidence of deaths in the prime of life for women in Canada compared with men, largely due to breast and other cancers (Varcoe et al., 2007). **Health inequity** refers to those inequalities in health that are unnecessary and avoidable, and differences that are considered unfair and unjust (Marmot, 2007; Whitehead, 1992). In Canada and elsewhere, many of the healthcare services are inequitable because they reflect an unfair distribution of the underlying social determinants of health, for example, access to educational opportunities and meaningful employment, adequate income for people with physical or intellectual disabilities, access to needed health care, the ability to afford nutritious foods, and respectful treatment free of discrimination.

As indicated in Fig. 3-9, the economic, social, and political conditions in which people live are the major determinants of whether they are healthy or not. Particular groups of people experience especially high rates of ill health because of social, economic, and historical conditions. For example, people living in poverty, lone mothers in low-income brackets, older women, people who experience discrimination or racism, significant proportions of the Aboriginal population, women experiencing abuse, people with severe or persistent mental illnesses or addictions, refugees, and some immigrant groups are more likely than others to become ill and are less likely to receive appropriate healthcare services (CIHI, 2003; Henry et al., 2005; Krieger, 2005; Raphael et al., 2006). Assessing risk factors and promoting health therefore require consideration of the intersecting social and economic factors that go far beyond the immediately identifiable behavioural or biological risk factors (e.g., smoking, a diet high in processed foods, high blood pressure, high cholesterol levels).

Evidence is now conclusive that poverty is a primary cause of poor health among Canadians (Raphael, 2007). Studies have shown that Canadians who live in the poorest 20% of

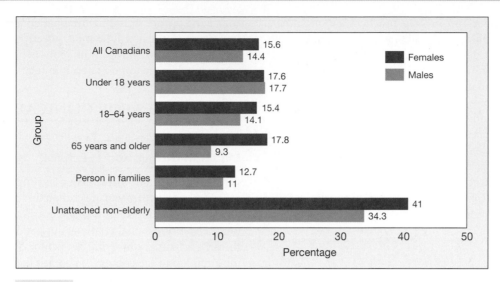

Fig. 3-11   Percentage of Canadians living in poverty, by age, gender, and family situation, 2004

urban neighbourhoods have significantly shorter life expectancies than do other Canadians. Of major concern is the ongoing evidence indicating that inequities in health and social status are continuing to grow, despite Canada's official commitment to equity and access.

In wealthy industrialized nations such as Canada, **poverty** is best understood as "the experience of material and social deprivation that prevents individuals, communities, and entire societies from reaching their full human and societal potential" (Raphael, 2007, p. 7). In 2004, 15.6% of all Canadians were living in poverty (Raphael, 2007). Poverty rates also differ by family type and gender, as shown in Fig. 3-11.

Women's poverty in Canada is of particular concern. For example, for **lone-mother families**, the poverty rate in 2004 was 51%, which is exceptionally high compared with that of other wealthy industrialized nations. Living in poverty is an especially significant threat to the health of children since it has both immediate and long-lasting effects. For women, the main causes of poverty are labour market inequities, family circumstances such as marriage breakdown or lone parenting, clawbacks to welfare payments for women with small children, and wage disparities with men (Reid, 2007). These are important factors to consider in the context of health assessment. Recognizing how health and social inequities intersect to differentially affect people will help you to recognize and be more responsive to the range of factors that influence health and well-being.

HEALTHCARE PRACTICES

Healthcare practices vary among individuals and groups and cannot be determined based on assumptions regarding ethnicity. The extent to which any individual subscribes to the tenets of Western medicine will be shaped by the totality of his or her own life experiences, including experience with and exposure to Western medicine. Today, Canadians of all backgrounds draw upon a range of traditions as part of their health care. Some wholeheartedly ascribe to the full range of allopathic medicine

(referring to the dominant Western practice of medicine), including some aspects (e.g., cosmetic surgery) that many others would not embrace. Most people also draw on other approaches, for example, using chiropractic medicine, massage therapy, vitamins, or herbs such as echinacea.

Perspectives on what are acceptable healthcare practices change over time and are culturally and socially bound. Whereas in the past, few people were familiar with the practice of acupuncture, many today seek the services of qualified acupuncturists or traditional Chinese medicine practitioners. Your responsibility is to inform patients about the potential effects of particular practices (e.g., the potential for some nutritional supplements to potentiate certain anticoagulants) but not to judge the acceptability of those practices.

More and more Canadians are turning to **complementary and alternative health care** (CAHC) and **natural health products** (NHPs) to treat illness and promote health (Health Canada, 2005). As defined by Health Canada (2005), CAHC is an umbrella term that encompasses numerous individual therapies and healthcare approaches, including traditional Chinese medicine, reflexology, homeopathy, therapeutic massage, chiropractic services, relaxation therapy, and Aboriginal

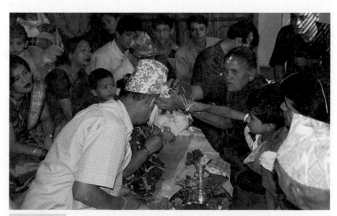

Fig. 3-12   How does a "critical cultural" lens shape your view differently than a "culturalist" lens?

traditional medicines and healing practices, among others. An increasing number of Canadians are also using NHPs, a general term that describes a variety of products, such as herbal medicines, homeopathic remedies, nutritional supplements, vitamins, and minerals.

When conducting a health assessment, remember that people may draw on a combination of approaches. However, the ability to access and engage in complementary and alternative approaches varies greatly depending on people's economic and social resources and their geographic locale. For example, acupuncture, chiropractic medicine, massage, and NHPs can be prohibitively expensive. In general, most of these approaches are not covered by provincial or territorial healthcare plans.

Spirituality and Health

The significance of **spirituality** to people's health and healing has long been recognized. Although spirituality commonly tends to be perceived as an offshoot of religion, it is important to distinguish between religion and spirituality (O'Murchu, 1998). Spirituality has always been more central to the human experience than religion. Religions are often established by formal institutional structures, rituals, and beliefs, whereas spirituality may refer more generally to the search for meaning. Both religion and spirituality can play a significant role in the ways people deal with health and illness (Reimer Kirkham et al., 2004). As a healthcare professional, you do not need to know the specifics of various religious and spiritual traditions. However, it is important to convey openness, interest, and acceptance. First, checking your own assumptions and biases is important. If you call places of worship "churches" in your work with patients, you will be conveying a Christian bias that may discourage those who call their places of worship by other names (e.g., temples, mosques, or synagogues). Second, you need to avoid making assumptions about particular people. A person may be part of an ethnocultural group but not part of an associated religion. During the health assessment,

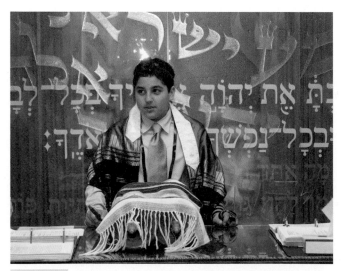

Fig. 3-13 How does your understanding of religion and spirituality shape your health assessments?

conveying openness and inviting patients to identify what is important to them will be most effective. For example, you might ask, "Do you have any religious beliefs or practices that you would like me to know about in relation to your health?"

GUIDELINES FOR CLINICAL PRACTICE

Assess Culturally Based Understandings and Practices

Performing a health assessment can proceed over time. But regardless of whether you are completing a health assessment rapidly in the context of a single encounter or as part of a long-term professional relationship, building trust, engaging through listening, conveying respect for differences, and paying attention to the context of people's lives are key to culturally safe health assessments.

Work to Build Trust

While certain data must be collected in the initial interview to address the patient's presenting health issues, patients should not be expected to share sensitive information until trust has been established (Anderson et al., 2005). Patients may be reluctant to reveal their understandings or beliefs for fear of being dismissed as providing information that is less than legitimate. Clinicians can find out more by asking questions phrased in a nonjudgemental way such as, "Have you found anything else that has helped you?" rather than, "Are you taking medications besides those prescribed by the doctor?" (Anderson et al., 2005, p. 339).

Engage Through Listening

Engaging in conversations with patients or their family members during the process of establishing trust will help you gain a deeper understanding of their explanatory models—that is, how they understand their world and health, illness, and approaches to healing. Kleinman (1980) and colleagues (Kleinman et al., 2006) and Anderson et al. (2005, p. 343) provide some questions that can assist clinicians in assessing patients' culturally based understandings. These are not always asked as direct questions but can be used as cues for listening and, in some cases, as follow-up questions.

- What do you call this health problem? What term or name do you give it?
- What do you think may have brought on this health problem?
- What concerns you most about this illness?
- What do you usually do to stay healthy? Have you been able to continue with those (activities, foods, medications, etc.)?

Convey Respect for Differences

As this chapter discusses, you will engage with a wide range of people from diverse backgrounds. Conveying respect for differences will build trust and welcome patients to share their understandings. Research continues to show that patients are very quick to sense when healthcare professionals are judging them negatively, particularly through verbal and nonverbal communications conveyed to patients. Questions that convey respect while exploring people's varying health practices can focus on what the patients themselves have done to address their health or illness concerns. For example:

- Have you found any treatments or medications that have worked for you in the past?
- How did they help you?
- Are you using them now? If so, are they helping?
- (For people who have recently come to Canada) Did you use any special treatments or medicines in your home country that seemed to work for you?

Questions that convey an interest in hearing about traditional or complementary healing practices include:

- Have you used any traditional medicines or healing methods that you found helpful?
- Are you able to access those medicines or healing methods?

Pay Attention to the Social and Economic Contexts of Patients' and Families' Lives

For all patients and families, it is important to consider how people are managing with jobs, housing, child care, financial resources, care of older parents or relatives, transportation, and access to healthcare services (Anderson et al., 2005). These considerations are relevant whether you are working in a community healthcare setting or in an acute care or long-term care facility. Conveying interest in the circumstances of people's lives with a simple question such as, "How have things been going for you?" is not "small talk" but rather an opportunity for you to assess a person's overall health in a nonjudgemental way.

Assessing a patient's social and economic context requires tact and effective listening and interviewing skills (as discussed in Chapter 4). Depending on the context, it may or may not be appropriate to explore this during your first meeting with a patient or family. Asking direct questions about a person's finances may be seen as intrusive, and many people are embarrassed by such questions. However, inquiring about the person's ability to deal with the health, illness, or health promo-

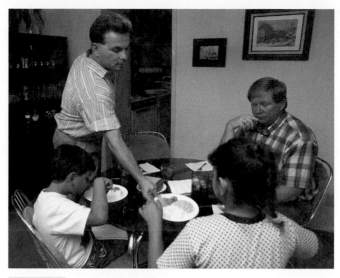

Fig. 3-15   How do dominant ideas about families shape your assessments?

tion issues may be a good way to start the discussion. Questions that have been suggested by Anderson et al. (2005) as helpful for assessing people's social and economic contexts include:

- What is particularly challenging or difficult, or what is needed to manage your health or illness?
- Are you working currently? Can you tell me a bit about the job you have?
- What do you need help with at home in order to manage (with your health or illness issues)?
- Whom do you rely on to help you at home? Do you live alone?
- Do you have family or friends nearby who can help you if needed?
- What kinds of things do you need help with?
- Are you able to afford the things you need to stay healthy, such as medications, glasses, dental work, and assistive devices such as a cane or wheelchair?
- Are you able to travel where necessary to access services or support?

Many families in Canada are required to take on the extra work of caring for family members in their homes because of shortened hospital stays for acutely ill patients; the lack of affordable, quality long-term care facilities; and, in some cases, families' personal commitments to care for older parents in the home (Armstrong et al., 2002). The financial circumstances of the family influence if and how they are able to take on these caregiving responsibilities. Research continues to show that healthcare professionals in hospitals are usually not familiar with patients' home environments and may assume that a family has the resources to care for a sick or older person at home (Anderson et al., 2005). However, you must remember that for many, staying at home to care for a relative most likely means loss of wages, which many families cannot afford. Social circumstances, therefore, have a profound effect on how people can manage illness and the changes that are associated with aging. These are important aspects to consider in the process of health assessment.

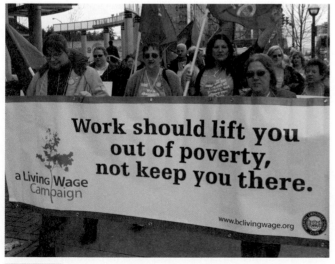

Fig. 3-14   How can healthcare professionals participate in social change?

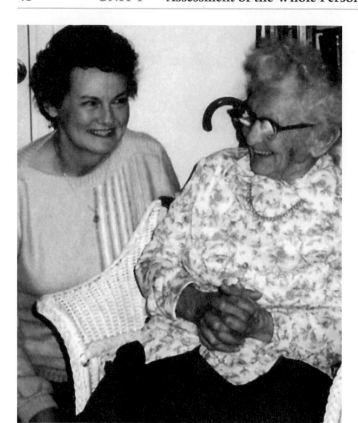

Fig. 3-16 What stereotypes about women, aging, and caregiving does this photo of a 101-year-old woman and her daughter challenge?

SUMMARY: CONNECTING ACROSS DIFFERENCES

The notion of "connecting across differences" comes from Doane and Varcoe (2005), who emphasize that "relational practice requires that you connect across differences by joining people as they are and where they are" (p. 295). This can be easier said than done, and the integration of knowledge and reflection will take time. In preparing to work across differences, the first step is to anticipate your own biases and assumptions by reflecting on your own social, cultural, economic, and family backgrounds relative to health, illness, and health promotion. In the process, you will need to critically examine and, in some cases, challenge your own biases, perceptions, and prejudices about particular groups, practices, and health behaviours.

Secondly, learn to critically reflect on the culture of the healthcare system, how it works, its taken-for-granted practices and policies, and their consequences for patients. Third, become knowledgeable about the social and economic conditions and policies in Canada that influence people's ability to maintain their health or to access the resources required to stay healthy. This includes gaining knowledge about immigration trends, racism, discrimination, socioeconomic trends, gender inequities, welfare reforms, child-care availability, issues affecting older people and so on related to your practice area. Finally, as discussed in Chapter 4, you will need the skills to communicate effectively with people from a variety of backgrounds, including those whose primary language is different from yours.

BIBLIOGRAPHY

Access Alliance. (2007). *Racialization and health inequalities: Focus on children. City of Toronto and neighbourhood highlights.* Toronto, ON: Access Alliance Multicultural Community Health Centre.

Anderson, J., Perry, J., Blue, C., Browne, A., Henderson, A., Khan, K., et al. (2003). "Rewriting" cultural safety within the postcolonial and postnational feminist project. *Advances in Nursing Science 26*(3), 196–214.

Anderson, J. M., & Reimer Kirkham, S. (1999). Discourses on health: A critical perspective. In H. Coward & P. Ratanakul (Eds.), *A cross-cultural dialogue on health care ethics* (pp. 47–67). Waterloo, ON: Wilfrid Laurier University Press.

Anderson, J. M., Reimer Kirkham, S., Waxler-Morrison, N., Herbert, C., Murphy, M., & Richardson, E. (2005). Conclusion. In N. Waxler-Morrison, J. M. Anderson, E. Richardson, & N. Chambers (Eds.), *Cross-cultural caring: A handbook for health professionals* (2nd ed., pp. 323–352). Vancouver, BC: UBC Press.

Armstrong, P., Amaratunga, C., Bernier, J., Grant, K., Pederson, A., & Wilson, K. (Eds.). (2002). *Exposing privatization: Women and health care reform in Canada.* Aurora, ON: Garamond Press.

Assembly of First Nations. (2005). *International reports highlight Canada's lack of progress in addressing First Nations poverty: UNICEF ranks Canada 19th out of 26 countries in child poverty.* Retrieved April 11, 2008, from http://www.afn.ca/article.asp?id=200

Badets, J., Chard, J., & Levett, A. (2003). *Ethnic Diversity Survey: Portrait of a multicultural society* (Catalogue No. 89-593-XIE). Retrieved February 7, 2008, from http://www.statcan.ca/bsolc/english/bsolc?catno=89-593-XIE

Behjati-Sabet, A., & Chambers, N. (2005). People of Iranian descent. In N. Waxler-Morrison, J.M. Anderson, E. Richardson, &

N. Chambers (Eds.), *Cross-cultural caring: A handbook for health professionals* (2nd ed., pp. 127–162). Vancouver, BC: UBC Press.

Browne, A. J. (2005). Discourses influencing nurses' perceptions of First Nations patients. *Canadian Journal of Nursing Research, 37*(4), 62–87.

Browne, A. J. (2007). Clinical encounters between nurses and First Nations women in a Western Canadian hospital. *Social Science and Medicine, 64*(10), 2165–2176.

Browne, A. J., & Fiske, J. (2001). First Nations women's encounters with mainstream health care services. *Western Journal of Nursing Research, 23*(2), 126–147.

Browne, A. J., & Varcoe, C. (2006). Critical cultural perspectives and health care involving Aboriginal peoples. *Contemporary Nurse, 22*(2), 155–167. Also available at http://www.contemporarynurse.com/22.2/

Calam, B., Varcoe, C., Brown, H., Cranmer, B., Edgars, M., Harvey, T., et al. (2008). *Rural Aboriginal maternity care.* Vancouver, BC: University of British Columbia.

Canadian Institute for Health Information. (2003). *The impact of poverty on health. A scan of the literature.* Ottawa, ON: Author.

Canadian Institute for Health Information. (2004). Improving the health of Canadians. Ottawa, ON: Author.

Canadian Institute for Health Information. (2006). *How healthy are rural Canadians? An assessment of their health status and health determinants. Summary report.* Ottawa, ON: Author.

Canales, M. K. (2000). Othering: Toward an understanding of difference. *Advances in Nursing Science, 22*(4), 16–31.

Caulford, P., & Vali, Y. 2006. Providing health care to medically uninsured immigrants and refugees. *Canadian Medical Association Journal, 174*(9), 1253–1254.

Cook, E. D., & Howe, D. (2004). Aboriginal languages of Canada. In W. O'Grady & J. Archibald (Eds.), *Contemporary linguistic analysis* (5th ed, pp. 294–309). Toronto, ON: Addison Wesley Longman.

Doane, G. H., & Varcoe, C. (2005). *Family nursing as relational inquiry: Developing health-promoting practice*. Philadelphia, PA: Lippincott, Williams & Wilkins.

Furniss, E. (1999). *The burden of history: Colonialism and the frontier myth in a rural Canadian community*. Vancouver, BC: UBC Press.

Galabuzi, G. E. (2001). *Canada's creeping economic apartheid: The economic segregation and social marginalization of racialised groups*. Toronto, ON: Social Justice Foundation for Research and Education.

Gustafson, D. L. (2008). Are sensitivity and tolerance enough? Comparing two theoretical approaches to caring for newcomer women with mental health problems. In S. Guruge & E. Collins (Eds.), *Working with immigrant women: Issues and strategies for mental health professionals* (pp. 39–63). Toronto, ON: Canadian Centre for Addiction & Mental Health.

Health Canada. (2005). *Complementary and alternative health care: The other mainstream?* Retrieved March 15, 2008, from http://www.hc-sc.gc.ca/sr-sr/pubs/hpr-rpms/bull/2003-7-complement/intro_e.html#page6

Health Canada. (2007). *Non-insured health benefits*. Retrieved March 15, 2008, from http://www.hc-sc.gc.ca/fnih-spni/nihb-ssna/index_e.html

Henry, F., Tator, C., Mattis, W., & Rees, T. (2005). *The colour of democracy: Racism in Canadian society* (3rd ed.). Toronto, ON: Nelson.

Indian and Northern Affairs Canada. (2007). *Status—Most often asked questions*. Retrieved April 15, 2008, from http://www.ainc-inac.gc.ca/pr/pub/ywtk/index-eng.asp#mript

Indian Residential Schools Resolution Canada. (2008). *Frequently asked questions*. Retrieved March 10, 2008, from http://www.irsr-rqpi.gc.ca/english/truth_reconciliation_commission.html

Kawachi, I., Subramanian, S. V., & Almeida-Filho N. (2002). A glossary for health inequalities. *Journal of Epidemiology and Community Health, 56*(9), 647–652.

Kirmayer, L., Brass, G., Holton, T., Paul, K., Simpson, C., & Tait, C. (2007). *Suicide among Aboriginal people in Canada*. Ottawa, ON: Aboriginal Healing Foundation.

Kleinman, A. (1980). *Patients and healers in the context of culture*. Berkeley, CA: University of California Press.

Kleinman, A., & Benson, P. (2006). Anthropology in the clinic: The problem of cultural competency and how to fix it. *PLoS Medicine—A Peer-Reviewed Open-Access Journal, 3*(1), 1673–1676.

Krieger, N. (2002). A glossary for social epidemiology. *Epidemiological Bulletin, 23*(1), 693–700.

Krieger, N. (2005). Defining and investigating social disparities in cancer: Critical issues. *Cancer Causes and Control, 16*(1), 5–14.

Krieger, N., Sidney, S., & Coakley, E. (1998). Racial discrimination and skin color in the CARDIA study: Implications for public health research. *American Journal of Public Health, 88*(9), 1308–1313.

Marmot, M. (2007). Achieving health equity: From root causes to fair outcomes. *The Lancet, 370*(9593), 1153–1163.

Ng, E., Wilkins, R., Gendron, F., & Berthelot. J. M. (2005). *Dynamics of immigrants' health in Canada: Evidence from the National Population Health Survey*. Ottawa, ON: Statistics Canada.

O'Murchu, D. (1998). *Reclaiming spirituality*. New York, NY: Crossroad.

Office of Minority Health. (2001). *National standards for culturally and linguistically appropriate services in health care. Final report*. Washington, DC: Office of Minority Health, Department of Health and Human Services.

Papps, E., & Ramsden, I. (1996). Cultural safety in nursing: The New Zealand experience. *International Journal for Quality in Health Care, 8*(5), 491–497.

Pederson, A., & Raphael, D. (2006). Gender, race and health inequities. In D. Raphael, T. Bryant, & M. Rioux (Eds.), *Staying alive: Critical perspectives on health, illness and health care* (pp. 159–191). Toronto, ON: Canadian Scholars' Press.

Perreault, S. (2004). *Visible minorities and victimization*. Ottawa, ON: Statistics Canada.

Peternelj-Taylor, C. (2005). An exploration of othering in forensic psychiatric and correctional nursing. *Canadian Journal of Nursing Research, 36*(4), 130–147.

Polaschek, N. R. (1998). Cultural safety: A new concept in nursing people of different ethnicities. *Journal of Advanced Nursing, 27*(3), 452–457.

Ramsden, I. (1993). Kawa Whakaruruhau: Cultural safety in nursing education in Aotearoa (New Zealand). *Nursing Praxis in New Zealand, 8*(3), 4–10.

Ramsden, I. (2002). *Cultural safety and nursing education in Aotearoa and Te Waipounamu*. Wellington, New Zealand: University of Wellington.

Ramsden, I., & Spoonley, P. (1994). The cultural safety debate in nursing education in Aotearoa. *New Zealand Annual Review of Education, 3*, 161–174.

Raphael, D. (2007). *Poverty and policy in Canada: Implications for health and quality of life*. Toronto, ON: Canadian Scholars' Press.

Raphael, D., Bryant, T., & Rioux, M. (2006). *Staying alive: Critical perspectives on health, illness and health care*. Toronto, ON: Canadian Scholars' Press.

Reid, C. (2007). Women's heath and the politics of policy and exclusion. In M. Morrow, O. Hankivsky, & C. Varcoe (Eds.), *Women's health in Canada: Critical theory, policy and practice* (pp. 199–220). Toronto, ON: University of Toronto Press.

Reimer Kirkham, S., Pesut, B., Meyerhoff, H., & Sawatzky, R. (2004). Spiritual care giving at the juncture of religion, culture, and state. *Canadian Journal of Nursing Research, 36*(4), 148–169.

Reimer Kirkham, S., Smye, V., Tang, S., Anderson, J., Browne, A., Coles, R., et al. (2002). Rethinking cultural safety while waiting to do fieldwork: Methodological implications for nursing research. *Research in Nursing and Health, 25*(3), 222–232.

Reutter, L., Neufeld, A., & Harrison, M. J. (2000). A review of the research on the health of low-income Canadian women. *Canadian Journal of Nursing Research, 32*(1), 75–97

Royal Commission on Aboriginal Peoples. (1996). *Report of the Royal Commission on Aboriginal peoples: Vol. 3. Gathering strength*. Ottawa, ON: The Commission.

Smye, V., & Browne, A. J. (2002). Cultural safety and the analysis of health policy affecting Aboriginal people. *Nurse Researcher: The International Journal of Research Methodology in Nursing and Health Care, 9*(3), 42–56.

Smye, V., Rameka, M., & Willis, E. (2006). Indigenous health care. Advances in nursing practice: An introduction. *Contemporary Nurse, 22*(2), 142–154. Retrieved April 15, 2008, from http://www.contemporarynurse.com/22.2/

Spector, R. E. (2004). *Cultural diversity in health and illness* (2nd ed.). Upper Saddle River, NJ: Prentice Hall.

Srivastava, R. H. (2007). *The healthcare professional's guide to clinical cultural competence*. Toronto, ON: Elsevier.

Statistics Canada. (2001). *Canada's ethnocultural portrait: The changing mosaic*. Retrieved February 28, 2008, from http://www12.statcan.ca/english/census01/products/analytic/companion/etoimm/canada.cfm#more_than_200_ethnic_origins

Statistics Canada. (2006a). *Concept: Ethnicity*. Retrieved March 3, 2008, from http://www.statcan.ca/english/concepts/definitions/ethnicity.htm

Statistics Canada. (2006b). *Concept: Immigration*. Retrieved March 3, 2008, from http://www.statcan.ca/english/concepts/definitions/immigration.htm

Statistics Canada. (2006c). *Concept: Visible Minority*. Retrieved March 3, 2008, from http://www.statcan.ca/english/concepts/definitions/vis-minorit.htm

Statistics Canada. (2007a). *Immigration in Canada: A portrait of the foreign-born population, 2006 census*. Retrieved February 28, 2008, from http://www.statcan.ca/bsolc/english/bsolc?catno=97-557-XIE2006001#formatdisp

Statistics Canada. (2007b). *Portrait of the Canadian population in 2006, by age and sex: Findings*. Retrieved February 28, 2008, from http://www12.statcan.ca/english/census06/analysis/agesex/index.cfm

Statistics Canada. (2007c). *Portrait of the Canadian population in 2006: Population and dwelling counts*. Retrieved March 10, 2008, from http://www12.statcan.ca/english/census06/analysis/popdwell/index.cfm

Statistics Canada. (2007d). 2006 census: Immigration, citizenship, language, mobility and migration. *The Daily*, 2007, December 4. Retrieved February 28, 2008, from http://www.statcan.ca/Daily/English/071204/d071204a.htm

Statistics Canada. (2008). *Aboriginal peoples in Canada in 2006: Inuit, Métis and First Nations, 2006 census*. Retrieved March 10, 2008, from http://www12.statcan.ca/english/census06/analysis/aboriginal/pdf/97-558-XIE2006001.pdf

United Nations Educational, Scientific and Cultural Organization. (1952). *The race concept: Results of an inquiry*. Retrieved April 11, 2008, from http://72.14.253.104/search?q=cache:bvtj475yseUJ:unesdoc.unesco.org/images/0007/000733/073351eo.pdf+unesco+race&hl=en&ct=clnk&cd=1&gl=ca

Varcoe, C. (2001). Abuse obscured: An ethnographic account of emergency nursing in relation to violence against women. *The Canadian Journal of Nursing Research, 32*(4), 95–115.

Varcoe, C. (2008). Inequality, violence and women's health. In B. S. Bolaria & H. Dickinson (Eds.), *Health, illness and health care in Canada* (4th ed., pp. 211–230). Toronto, ON: Nelson.

Varcoe, C., Hankivsky, O., & Morrow, M. (2007). Beyond gender matters: An introduction. In M. Morrow, O. Hankivsky & C. Varcoe (Eds.), *Women's health in Canada: Critical theory, policy and practice* (pp. 3–30). Toronto, ON: University of Toronto Press.

Vissandjée, B., Thurston, W., Apale, A., & Nahar, K. (2007). Women's health at the intersection of gender and the experience of international migration. In M. Morrow, O. Hankivsky & C. Varcoe (Eds.), *Women's health in Canada: Critical theory, policy and practice* (pp. 221–243). Toronto, ON: University of Toronto Press.

Waldram, J. B., Herring, A., & Young, T. K. (2006). *Aboriginal health in Canada: Historical, cultural and epidemiological perspectives* (2nd ed.). Toronto, ON: University of Toronto Press.

Waxler-Morisson, N., & Anderson, J. (2005). Introduction: The need for culturally sensitive health care. In N. Waxler-Morrison, J. M. Anderson, E. Richardson, & N. Chambers (Eds.), *Cross-cultural caring: A handbook for health professional* (2nd ed., pp. 1–10). Vancouver, BC: UBC Press.

Wepa, D. (Ed.) (2005). *Cultural safety in Aotearoa New Zealand*. Aukland, New Zealand: Pearson New Zealand Limited.

Whitehead, M. (1992). The concepts and principles of equity and health. *International Journal of Health Services, 22*(3), 429–445.

World Health Organization. (2008). *Frequently asked questions*. Retrieved March 9, 2008, from http://www.who.int/suggestions/faq/en/index.html

Yue, K. K. (2005). People of Chinese descent. In N. Waxler-Morrison, J. M. Anderson, E. Richardson, & N. Chambers (Eds.), *Cross-cultural caring: A handbook for health professionals* (2nd ed., pp. 127–162). Vancouver, BC: UBC Press.

Web Sites of Interest

Aboriginal Nurses Association of Canada—http://www.anac.on.ca/

Access Alliance: Multicultural Health Community Services—http://www.accessalliance.ca/

Canadian Institute for Health Information—http://secure.cihi.ca/cihiweb/dispPage.jsp?cw_page=home_e

Canadian Nurses Association—http://www.cna-nurses.ca/cna/

Centre of Excellence for Women's Health—http://www.cewh-cesf.ca/

Citizenship and Immigration Canada—http://www.cic.gc.ca/english/index.asp

Inuit Tapiriit Kanatami—http://www.itk.ca/

National Aboriginal Health Organization—http://www.naho.ca/english/

Native Women's Association of Canada—http://www.nwac-hq.org/en/index.html

Public Health Agency of Canada: Complementary and Alternative Health—http://www.canadian-health-network.ca/servlet/ContentServer?cid=1047656077028&pagename=CHN-RCS%2FPage%2FGTPageTemplate&c=Page&lang=En

Statistics Canada—http://cansim2.statcan.ca

Status of Women Canada—http://www.swc-cfc.gc.ca/

World Health Organization—http://www.who.int/about/en/

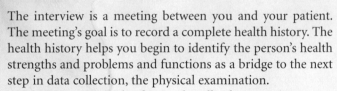

The Interview

Written by **Carolyn Jarvis**, PhD, APN, CNP
Adapted by **Annette J. Browne**, PhD, RN

The interview is a meeting between you and your patient. The meeting's goal is to record a complete health history. The health history helps you begin to identify the person's health strengths and problems and functions as a bridge to the next step in data collection, the physical examination.

The interview is the first and really the most important part of data collection. It collects **subjective data**—what the person says about himself or herself. The interview is the first and the best chance a person has to tell you what *he or she* perceives his or her health state to be. Once people enter the healthcare system, they may relinquish some control. At the interview, however, the patient is still in charge. The individual knows everything about his or her own health state, and you know nothing. Your skill in interviewing will glean all the necessary information as well as build rapport for a successful working relationship. When you have a successful interview, you:

1. Gather complete and accurate data about the person's health state, including the description and chronology of any symptoms of illness
2. Establish rapport and trust so the person feels accepted and thus free to share all relevant data
3. Teach the person about the health state so that the person can participate in identifying problems
4. Build rapport for a continuing therapeutic relationship; this rapport facilitates future diagnoses, planning, and treatment
5. Begin teaching for health promotion and disease prevention

Consider the interview as being similar to forming a contract between you and your patient. A contract consists of spoken or unspoken rules for behaviour. In this case, the contract concerns what the person needs and expects from the healthcare system and what you, the healthcare professional, have to offer. Your mutual goal is optimal health and health care for the patient. The contract's terms include:

- Time and place of the interview and succeeding physical examination

- Introduction of yourself and a brief explanation of your role
- The purpose of the interview
- How long it will take
- Expectation of participation for each person
- Presence of any other people (e.g., patient's family, other healthcare professionals, students)
- Confidentiality and to what extent it may be limited
- Any costs that the patient must pay

Although the patient may know some of this information already through telephone contact with receptionists or the admitting office, the remaining points need to be stated clearly at the outset. Any confusion could produce a mismatch in expectations, rather than the openness and trust you need to facilitate the interview.

THE PROCESS OF COMMUNICATION

The vehicle that carries you and your patient through the interview is communication. Communication is exchanging information so that each person clearly understands the other. If you do not understand each other, if you have not *conveyed meaning,* no communication has occurred.

It is challenging to teach the skill of interviewing because initially most students think little needs to be learned. They assume that if they can talk and hear, they can communicate. But much more than talking and hearing is necessary. Communication is all behaviour, conscious and unconscious, verbal and nonverbal. *All behaviour has meaning.*

The contexts in which we practise can also profoundly shape how we engage in the interview process. To more consciously choose how you will practise requires that you develop the skill of reflectivity. Reflectivity is one of the central skills of relational practice, as discussed in Chapter 1. It involves "a combination of self-observation, critical scrutiny, and conscious participation . . . and paying attention to who, how, and what you are doing in the moment" as you work with patients and families (Doane et al., 2005, p. 150). By paying attention to how you are acting and what you are feeling in any particular situation, you can begin to see how your behaviours and responses affect others. By observing yourself and paying attention to your thoughts, emotions, and bodily responses during the health assessment process, you will more consciously and intentionally choose how to act and respond.

Sending

Likely, you are most aware of *verbal* communication—the words you speak, vocalizations, the tone of voice. *Nonverbal* communication also occurs. This is your body language—posture, gestures, facial expression, eye contact, foot tapping, touch, even where you place your chair. Since nonverbal communication is under less conscious control than verbal communication, nonverbal communication probably is more reflective of your true feelings. A high degree of reflectivity is required to remain attuned to your nonverbal communication during the interview and physical examination.

Receiving

Being aware of the messages you send is only part of the process. Your words and gestures must be interpreted in a *specific context* to have meaning. You have a specific context in mind when you send your words. The receiver has his or her own interpretation of them. The receiver attaches meaning determined by his or her past experiences, social and family contexts, culture, and self-concept, as well as current physical and emotional states. Sometimes these contexts do not coincide. Remember how frustrating it may have been to try to communicate something to a friend, only to have your message totally misunderstood? Your message can be misinterpreted by the listener. It takes mutual understanding by the sender and receiver to have successful communication.

Even greater risk for misunderstanding exists in the healthcare setting than in a social setting. The patient usually has a health problem, and this factor emotionally charges your professional relationship. It *intensifies* the communication because the person feels dependent on you to get better.

Communication and reflectivity are *basic skills* that can be learned and polished when you are a beginning practitioner. It is a tool, as basic to quality health care as the tools of inspection or palpation.

Attending to Power Differentials

Nurses and other healthcare professionals are usually in a position of power relative to patients and families (Doane et al., 2005). They usually have more knowledge about the healthcare system and have influence over the access that patients have to health care. Healthcare professionals also have advantages such as education, language skills, and employment, which can position them as relatively powerful in relation to patients. At the same time, nurses and healthcare professionals are also diverse in terms of their experiences, social contexts, knowledge, and so on. On an ongoing basis, it is important to

be aware of how your power and privilege relative to patients, families, and colleagues are reflected in the way you communicate, both verbally and nonverbally.

Communication Skills

Cultivating the skills of relational practice during the interview involves particular communication skills. These include, among others, the skills of unconditional positive regard, empathy, and active listening.

Unconditional Positive Regard. One essential feature of effective communication is the ability to meet patients, individuals, and families with "unconditional positive regard" (Doane et al., 2005, p. 280). Conveying unconditional positive regard requires a high degree of self-reflectivity, particularly when patients or families seem to be making choices that have negative health effects. Although it may be challenging, you will need to develop the skills and capacity to convey unconditional positive regard to engage therapeutically with people. This means a generally optimistic view of people: an assumption of their strengths and an acceptance of their limitations. An atmosphere of warmth and caring is necessary. The patient must feel that he or she is accepted unconditionally.

The respect for other people extends to respect for their own control over their health. Your goal is *not* to make your patients dependent on you, but to help them to be increasingly responsible for themselves. You wish to promote their growth. Pay attention to the cues you pick up from patients and families and follow their lead. Be prepared to think critically and reflectively about the various contexts that influence people's situations and decisions related to their health.

Empathy. Empathy means viewing the world from the other person's inner frame of reference while remaining yourself. Empathy means recognizing and accepting the other person's feelings or actions without criticism. It is described as "feeling *with* the person rather than feeling *like* the person." It does not mean you become lost in the other person at the expense of your own self. If this occurred you would cease to be helpful. Rather, it is to *understand with* the person how *he or she* understands his or her world.

Active Listening. Listening is not a passive role in the communication process; it is active and demanding. Listening requires your complete attention. You cannot be preoccupied with your own needs or the needs of other patients, or you will miss something important with this one. For the time of this interview, no one is more important than this person. This person's needs are your sole concern.

Active listening is the route to understanding. You cannot be thinking of what you are going to say as soon as the person stops for breath. A vast difference exists between listening and simply waiting to speak (Doane et al., 2005). Listen to *what* the person says. The story may not come out in the order you would expect, or will record it in later. Let the person talk from his or her own outline; nearly everything that is said will be relevant. Listen to *the way* a person tells the story, such as difficulty with language, impaired memory, the tone of the person's voice, and even to what the person is leaving out (Clinical Illustration).

Attending to the Physical Setting

Prepare the physical setting. The setting may be in a hospital room, an examination room in an office or clinic, or in the person's home (where you will have less control). In any location, optimal conditions are important to the completion of a smooth interview.

Ensure Privacy. Aim for geographical privacy—a private room in the hospital, clinic, office, or home. This may involve asking an ambulatory roommate to step out for a while or finding an unoccupied room or an empty lounge. If geographical privacy is not available, "psychological privacy" by curtained partitions may suffice as long as the person feels sure no one can overhear the conversation or interrupt.

Refuse Interruptions. Most people resent interruptions except in cases of an emergency. Inform any support staff of your interview, and ask that they not interrupt you during this time. Discourage other health professionals from interrupting you with *their* need for access to the patient. You need to concentrate and to establish rapport. An interruption can destroy in seconds what you have spent many minutes building up.

Physical Environment
- Set the room temperature at a comfortable level.
- Provide sufficient lighting so that you can see each other clearly. Avoid facing the patient directly toward a strong light where the patient must squint as if on stage.
- Reduce noise. Multiple stimuli are confusing. Turn off the television, radio, and any unnecessary equipment.
- Remove distracting objects or equipment. It is appropriate to leave some professional equipment (oto/ophthalmoscope, blood pressure manometer) in view. However, clutter, stacks of mail, files of other patients, or your lunch should not be seen. The room should convey the professional nature of the interviewer.
- Place the distance between you and the patient at about 1 1/2 m (twice arm's length). If you place the patient any closer, you may invade his or her private space and you may create anxiety. If you place the patient farther away, you seem distant and aloof.
- Arrange equal-status seating. Both you and the patient should be comfortably seated, at eye level. Avoid facing a patient across a desk or table because that feels like a barrier. Placing the chairs at 90 degrees is good because it

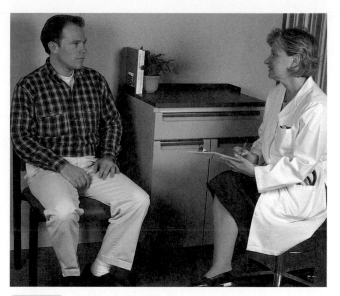

Fig. 4-1   Equal-status seating.

allows the person either to face you or to look straight ahead from time to time (Fig. 4-1). Most important, avoid standing. Standing does two things: (1) it communicates your haste, and (2) it assumes superiority. Standing makes you loom over the patient as an authority figure. When you are sitting, the person feels some control in the setting.
- Arrange a face-to-face position when interviewing the hospitalized bedridden person. The person should not have to stare at the ceiling because this causes him or her to lose the visual message of your communication.

Dress
- The patient should remain in street clothes except in the case of an emergency.
- Your appearance and clothing should be appropriate to the setting and should meet conventional professional standards: a uniform or laboratory coat over conservative clothing, a name tag, and neat hair. Avoid extremes.

Note-Taking. Some use of history forms and note-taking may be unavoidable. When you sit down later to record the interview, you cannot rely completely on memory to furnish details of previous hospitalizations or of the review of body systems, for example. But be aware that note-taking during the interview has disadvantages:
- It breaks eye contact too often.
- It shifts your attention away from the person, diminishing his or her sense of importance.
- It can interrupt the patient's narrative flow. You may say "Please slow down; I'm not getting it all." Or, the patient may see you recording furiously, and in an effort to please you, adjust his or her tempo to your writing. Either way, the patient's natural mode of expression is lost.
- It impedes your observation of the patient's nonverbal behaviour.
- It is threatening to the patient during the discussion of sensitive issues (e.g., amount of alcohol and drug use, number of sexual partners, or incidence of physical abuse).

So keep note-taking to a minimum, and try to focus your attention on the person. Any recording you do should be secondary to the dialogue and should not interfere with the person's spontaneity. With experience, you will not rely on note-taking as much.

Tape and Video Recording. A digital recorder or audio tape documents a complete record of what was said during the interview. You cannot refer to it as easily as you can to your notes, but the recording is an excellent teaching tool to study objectively your abilities as an interviewer. After listening, other students have commented:

"I never realized how much I talked. I really dominated the patient."
"I need to watch my interrupting. I cut her off that time."
"There. That response really worked. She opened up. I want to be that effective more often."

Audio recordings demonstrate how you can improve your communication. And, as you gain experience, the tapes also document your advancing skills. This process is very rewarding.

A video recording takes the teaching-learning tool one step further because you can study both verbal and nonverbal communication at the same time. Initial anxiety is common among students who feel self-conscious and fear "making a fool" of themselves on camera, but the video can detect richer detail in nonverbal behaviour.

"I must have crossed and uncrossed my legs 20 times! I never realized I did that. My fidgeting sure made Mr. J. look distracted."
"It was good that I leaned toward her when she paused that time. I think it helped her continue."
"I talked for 5 minutes nonstop about how to perform a breast self-examination, without ever letting Mrs. S. ask a question!"

If you use any tape recording, some ethical considerations are necessary. Explain to the person the purpose of the recording (whether for teaching, supervision, research), exactly who will hear it (you, your supervisor), and that it will then be destroyed. Obtain consent before you start. Be thoroughly familiar with the equipment; fumbling with the controls is distracting. Arrange the microphone between you and the patient and place the rest of the recording equipment out of sight. It is likely that after a few moments, neither of you will be aware of the recording.

TECHNIQUES OF COMMUNICATION

Introducing the Interview

The patient is here and you are ready for the interview. If you are nervous about how to begin, remember to keep the beginning short. Probably, the patient is nervous, too, and is anxious to start. Address the person, using his or her surname, and shake hands if that seems comfortable. Introduce yourself and state your role in the agency (if you are a student, say so). If you are gathering a complete history, give the reason for this interview:

"Mrs. Singh, I would like to talk about your illness that caused you to come to the hospital."

"Ms. Tang, I want to ask you some questions about your health so that we can identify what is keeping you healthy and explore any problems."
"Mr. Craig, I want to ask you some questions about your health and your usual daily activities so that we can plan your care here in the hospital."

If the person is in the hospital, more than one healthcare team member may be collecting a history. Patients are apt to feel exasperated because they believe they are repeating the same thing unless you give a reason for this interview.

After this brief introduction, ask an open-ended question (see the following section) and then let the person proceed. In most instances, you do not need friendly small talk to build rapport. This is not a social visit; the person has some concern to talk about and wants to get on with it. You will build rapport best by letting him or her discuss the concern early.

The Working Phase

The working phase is the data-gathering phase. Verbal skills for this phase include your questions to the patient and your responses to what the patient has said. Two general types of questions exist: open-ended and closed. Each type has a different place and function in the interview.

Open-Ended Questions

The **open-ended** question asks for narrative information. It states the topic to be discussed but only in **general** terms. Use it to begin the interview, to introduce a new section of questions, and whenever the person introduces a new topic.

"Tell me how I can help you."
"What brings you to the clinic (or) hospital?"
"Tell me why you have come here today."
"How have you been getting along?"
"You mentioned shortness of breath. Tell me more about that."
"How have you been feeling since your last appointment?"
"What has been most challenging?"
"What would you like to be able to do, change, or address?"
"What stands out for you as really important for me to know about your situation?"

The open-ended question leaves the person free to answer in any way. This type of question encourages the person to respond in paragraphs and to give a spontaneous account in any order chosen. It lets the person express herself or himself fully.

As the person answers, stop and *listen*. This will involve "listening to" and "listening for" particular things (Doane et al., 2005). For example, *listening to* involves attending to how people describe their health concerns in the larger context of their lives, observing their nonverbal communication, and listening to their beliefs about health and illness. *Listening for* involves tuning into what is of particular concern to patients and families, and listening for the emotions people convey and for the capacities and strengths that they have (which may be discussed tangentially). Also listen for things that patients may not be saying yet seem relevant given the other issues that have been raised or that you have observed.

What usually happens is that the patient answers with a short phrase or sentence, pauses, and then looks at you expecting to receive some direction of how to go on. What you do next is the key to the interview. If you pose new questions on other topics, you may lose much of the initial story. Instead, respond to the first statement with, "Tell me about it," or "Anything else?" or merely look acutely interested. The person then will tell the story.

Closed or Direct Questions

Closed or **direct** questions ask for specific information. They elicit a short one- or two-word answer, a yes or no, or a forced choice. Whereas the open-ended question allows the patient to have free rein, the direct question limits his or her answer (Table 4-1).

Use the direct questions after the person's opening narrative to fill in any details he or she left out. Also use direct questions when you need many specific facts, such as when asking about past health problems or during the review of systems. You need direct questions to speed up the interview. Asking all open-ended questions would be unwieldy and might take hours. But be careful not to overuse closed questions. Follow these guidelines:

1. Ask only one direct question at a time. Avoid bombarding the person with long lists: "Have you ever had pain, double vision, watering or redness in the eyes?" Avoid double-barrelled questions, such as, "Do you exercise and follow a diet for your weight?" The person will not know which question to answer. And if the person answers "yes," you will not know which question the person has answered.
2. Choose language the person understands. You may need to use regional phrases or colloquial expressions.

Responses: Assisting the Narrative

You have asked the first open-ended question, and the patient answers. As the person talks, your role is to encourage free expression but not let the person wander off course. Your responses help the teller amplify the story.

Some people seek health care for short-term or relatively simple needs. Their history is direct and uncomplicated; for these people, two responses (facilitation and silence) may be all you need to get a complete picture. Other people have a complex story, a long history of a chronic condition, or accompanying emotions. Additional responses help you gather data without cutting them off.

TABLE 4-1	Comparison of Open-Ended and Closed Questions	
Open-Ended	**Direct, Closed**
Use for narrative information	Use for specific information
Calls for long paragraph answers	Calls for short one- to two-word answers
Elicits feelings, opinions, ideas	Elicits facts
Builds and enhances rapport	Limits rapport and leaves interaction neutral

There are nine types of verbal responses in all. The first five responses (facilitation, silence, reflection, empathy, clarification), involve your *reactions* to the facts or feelings the person has communicated. Your response focuses on the patient's frame of reference. Your own frame of reference does not enter into the response. In the last four responses (confrontation, interpretation, explanation, summary), you start to express your *own* thoughts and feelings. The frame of reference shifts from the patient's perspective to yours. In the first five responses, the patient leads; in the last four responses, you lead.

Facilitation. These responses encourage the patient to say more, to continue with the story ("mm-hmm, go on, continue, uh-huh"). Also called general leads, these responses show the person you are interested and will listen further. Simply maintaining eye contact, shifting forward in your seat with increased attention, nodding "yes," or using your hand to gesture, "Yes, go on, I'm with you," encourage the person to continue talking.

Silence. Silence is golden after open-ended questions. Your silent attentiveness communicates that the patient has time to think, to organize what he or she wishes to say without interruption from you. This "thinking silence" is the one healthcare professionals interrupt most often. The interruption destroys the person's train of thought. The patient is often interrupted because silence is uncomfortable to beginning examiners. They feel responsible for keeping the dialogue going and feel at fault if it stops. But silence has advantages. One advantage is letting the person collect his or her thoughts. Also, silence gives you a chance to observe the person unobtrusively and to note nonverbal cues. Finally, silence gives you time to plan your next approach.

Reflection. This response echoes the patient's words. Reflection is repeating part of what the person has just said. In this example, it focuses further attention on a specific phrase and helps the person continue in his own way:

Patient: I'm here because of my water. It was cutting off.
Response: It was cutting off?
Patient: Yes, yesterday it took me 30 minutes to pass my water. Finally I got a tiny stream, but then it just closed off.

Reflection also can help express feeling behind a person's words. The feeling is already in the statement. You focus on it and encourage the person to elaborate:

Patient: It's so hard having to stay flat on my back in the hospital with this pregnancy. I have two more little ones at home. I'm so worried they are not getting the care they need.
Response: You feel worried and anxious about your children?

Think of yourself as a mirror reflecting the person's words or feelings. This helps the person to elaborate on the problem.

Empathy. A physical symptom, condition, or illness often has accompanying emotions. Many people have trouble expressing these feelings, perhaps because of confusion or embarrassment. In the reflecting example above, the person already had stated her feeling and you echoed it. But in the following example, he has not said it yet. An empathic response recognizes a feeling and puts it into words. It names the feeling and allows the expression of it. When the empathic response is used, the patient feels accepted and can deal with the feeling openly.

Patient (sarcastically): This is just great. I have my own business, I direct 20 employees everyday, and now here I am having to call you for every little thing.
Response: It must be hard—one day having so much control, and now feeling dependent on someone else.

Your response does not cut off further communication as would happen by giving false reassurance ("Oh, you'll be back to work in no time"). Also, it does not deny the feeling and indicate that it is not justified ("Now I don't do *every*thing for you. Why, you are feeding yourself"). An empathic response recognizes the feeling, accepts it, and allows the person to express it without embarrassment. It strengthens rapport. The patient feels understood, which by itself is therapeutic, because it eases the feelings of isolation brought on by illness. Other empathic responses are, "This must be very hard for you," "I understand," or just placing your hand on the person's arm (Fig. 4-2).

Clarification. Use this when the person's word choice is ambiguous or confusing (e.g., "Tell me what you mean by 'tired blood'"). Clarification also is used to summarize the person's words, simplify them to make them clearer, then ask if you are on the right track. You are asking for agreement, and the person can confirm or deny your understanding.

Response: Now as I understand you, this heaviness in your chest comes when you shovel snow or climb stairs, and it goes away when you stop doing those things. Is that correct?
Patient: Yes, that's pretty much it.

Confrontation. Recall that in these last four responses, (confrontation, interpretation, explanation, summary), the frame of reference shifts from the patient's perspective to yours. These responses now include your own thoughts and feelings. Use the last four responses only when merited by the situation. If you use them too often, you take over at the patient's expense. In the case of confrontation, you have observed a certain action, feeling, or statement and you now focus the person's attention on it. You give your honest feedback about what you see or feel. This may focus on a discrepancy: "You say it doesn't hurt, but when I touch you here, you grimace." Or, it may focus on the person's affect: "You look sad," or, "You sound angry." Or, you may confront the person when you notice parts of the story are inconsistent: "Earlier you

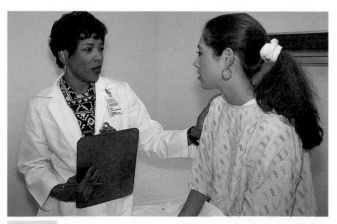

Fig. 4-2

said you were laying off alcohol and just now you said you had a few drinks after work."

Interpretation. This statement is based not on direct observation, as is confrontation, but rather on your inference or conclusion. It links events, makes associations, or implies cause: "It seems that every time you feel the stomach pain, you have had some kind of stress in your life." Interpretation also ascribes feelings and helps the person understand his or her own feelings in relation to the verbal message.

Patient: I have decided I don't want to take any more treatments. But I can't seem to tell my doctor that. Every time she comes in, I tighten up and can't say anything.
Response: Could it be that you're afraid of her reaction?

You do run a risk of making the wrong inference. If this is the case, the person will correct it. But even if the inference is corrected, interpretation helps to prompt further discussion of the topic.

Explanation. With these statements, you inform the person. You share factual and objective information. This may be for orientation to the agency setting: "Your dinner comes at 5:30 P.M." Or, it may be to explain cause: "The reason you cannot eat or drink before your blood test is that the food will affect the test results."

Summary. This is a final review of what you understand the person has said. It condenses the facts and presents a survey of how you perceive the health problem or need. It is a type of validation in that the person can agree with it or correct it. Both you and the patient should participate. When the summary occurs at the end of the interview, it signals that termination of the interview is imminent.

Ten Traps of Interviewing

The verbal skills discussed above are productive and enhance the interview. Now take time to consider nonproductive, defeating verbal messages, or *traps*. It is easy to fall into these traps because you are anxious to help. The danger is that they restrict the patient's response. The following traps are obstacles to obtaining complete data and to establishing rapport.

1. Providing False Assurance or Reassurance. A woman says, "Oh I just know this lump is going to turn out to be cancer." What happens inside you? The automatic response of many clinicians is to say, "Now don't worry; I'm sure you will be all right." This "courage builder" relieves *your* anxiety and gives you the false sense of having provided comfort. But for the woman it actually closes off communication. It trivializes her anxiety and effectively denies any further talk of it. (Also it promises something that may not happen—that is, she may *not* be all right). Consider instead these responses:

"You are really worried about the lump, aren't you?"
"It must be hard to wait for the biopsy results."

These responses acknowledge the feeling and open the door for more communication.

A genuine, valid form of reassurance does exist. You *can* reassure patients that you are listening to them, that you understand them, that you have hope for them, and that you will take care of them.

Patient: I feel so lost here since they transferred me to the medical centre. No one comes to see me. No one here cares what happens to me.

Response: I care what happens to you. I am here today and I want you to know that I'll be here all week.

This type of reassurance makes a commitment to the patient, and it can have a powerful impact.

2. Giving Unwanted Advice. Know when to give advice and when to avoid giving it. Often, people seek health care because they want your professional advice and information on the management of a health problem: "My child has chickenpox; how should I take care of him?" This is a straightforward request for information that you have that the parent needs. You respond by giving a health prescription, a therapeutic plan based on your knowledge and experience.

In other situations, advice is different; it is based on a hunch or feeling. It is your personal opinion. Consider the woman who has just left a meeting with her consultant physician: "Dr. Kline just told me my only chance of getting pregnant is to have an operation. I just don't know. What would you do?" Does the woman really want your advice? If you answer, "If I were you, I'd . . . ," then you would be making a mistake. You are not her. If you give your answer, you have shifted the accountability for decision making from her to you. She has not worked out her own solution. She has learned nothing about herself.

Does the woman really want to know what you would do? Probably not. Instead, a better response is reflection:

Response: Have an operation?
Woman: Yes, and I'm terrified of being put to sleep. What if I don't wake up?

Now you know her *real* concern and can help her deal with it. She will have grown in the process and may be better equipped to meet her next decision.

When asked for advice, other preferred responses are,

"What are the pros and cons of _____ [this choice] for you?"
"What concerns do you have?"
"What is holding you back?"

Although it is quicker just to give advice, take the time to involve the patient in a problem-solving process. When a patient participates, he or she is more likely to learn and to change behaviour.

3. Using Authority. "Your doctor/nurse knows best" is a response that promotes dependency and inferiority. The communication pathway looks something like this:

Interviewer:

Patient:

with your talk coming "down" and little from the patient going back "up." A better approach is to avoid using authority. Although you and the patient cannot have equality of professional skill and experience, you do have equally worthy roles in the health process, each respecting the other.

4. Using Avoidance Language. People use euphemisms such as "passed on" to avoid reality or to hide their feelings. They think if they just say the word "death," it might really happen. So to protect themselves, they evade the issue. Although it seems this will make comfortable potentially fearful topics, it does not. Not talking about the fear does not make it go away; it just suppresses the fear and makes it even more frightening. Using direct language is the best way to deal with frightening topics.

5. Engaging in Distancing. Distancing is the use of impersonal speech to put space between a threat and the self: "My friend has a problem; she is afraid she . . .," or, "There is a lump in the left breast." By using "the" instead of "my," the woman can deny any association with her diseased breast and protect herself from it. Healthcare professionals use distancing, too, to soften reality. This does not work because it communicates to the other person that you also are afraid of the procedure. The use of blunt specific terms actually is preferable to defuse anxiety.

6. Using Professional Jargon. What is called a myocardial infarction in the healthcare profession is called a heart attack by most laypeople. Use of jargon sounds exclusionary and paternalistic. You need to adjust your vocabulary to the person, but avoid sounding condescending.

If a patient uses medical jargon, do not assume he or she always knows the correct meaning. For example, some people think "hypertensive" means that they are very tense. As a result, they take their medication only when feeling stressed and not when they feel relaxed. This misinformation must be corrected. They need to understand that hypertension is a chronic condition that needs consistent medication to avoid side effects. On the other hand, you do not need to feel that it is a moral imperative to correct all misstatements (e.g., when a patient says "prostrate" for prostate gland).

7. Using Leading or Biased Questions. Asking a man, "You don't smoke, do you?" implies that one answer is "better" than another. If the person wants to please you, either he is forced to answer in a way corresponding to your values or he feels guilty when he must admit the other answer. He risks your disapproval. And if he feels dependent on you for care, the last thing he wants to do is alienate you.

8. Talking Too Much. Some examiners positively associate helpfulness with verbal productivity. If the air has been thick with their oratory and advice, these examiners leave thinking they have met the patient's needs. Just the opposite is true. Anxious to please the examiner, the patient lets the professional talk at the expense of his or her need to express himself or herself. A good rule for every interviewer is to *listen more than you talk*.

9. Interrupting. Often, when you think you know what the person will say, you interrupt and cut the person off. This does not show that you are clever. Rather, it signals that you are impatient or bored with the interview.

A related trap is preoccupation with yourself by thinking of your next remark while the person is talking. The communication pathway looks like this:

Patient: ⟶   Interviewer: ⟶

As the patient speaks, you are thinking about what to say next. Thus you cannot fully understand what the person says. You are so preoccupied with your own role as the interviewer that you are not really listening. Aim for a second of silence between the person's statement and your next response. Ideally, your communication pathway should look like this:

with two people talking, and two people listening.

10. Using "Why" Questions. A young child asks, "Why does the moon look like the end of my fingernail?" The motive behind this question is an innocent search for information. This is quite different from that of an adult's "why" question, such as, "*Why* were you so late for your appointment?" The adult's use of why questions usually implies blame and condemnation; it puts the person on the defensive.

Consider your use of "why" questions in the healthcare setting. "Why did you take so much medication?" Or, let's say you ask a man who has just come to the emergency department, "Why did you wait so long before coming to the hospital?" The only possible answer to a "why" question is, "Because . . .," and the man may not know the answer. He may not have worked it out. You sound whining, accusatory, and judgemental. And the man now must produce an excuse to rationalize his own behaviour. To avoid this trap, say: "I see you started to have chest pains early in the day. What was happening between the time the pains started and the time you came to the emergency department?"

Nonverbal Skills

Learn to listen with your eyes as well as with your ears. Nonverbal modes of communication include physical appearance, posture, gestures, facial expression, eye contact, voice, and touch. Nonverbal messages are very important in establishing rapport and in conveying information, especially about feelings. Nonverbal messages provide clues to understanding feelings. When nonverbal and verbal messages are congruent, the verbal is reinforced. When they are incongruent, the nonverbal message tends to be the true one, because it is under less conscious control.

Physical Appearance. In his classic work *The Stress of Life,* Hans Selye (1956) reports his interest in the body's total response to stress began as a student. Unbiased as yet by medical knowledge, he noted that some patients just "looked sick," even though they did not exhibit the specific characteristic signs that would lead to a precise medical diagnosis. Such people simply felt and looked ill or feverish. The same view can work for you. Inattention to dressing or grooming suggests the person is too sick to maintain self-care or has an emotional dysfunction such as depression. Choice of clothing also sends a message, projecting such varied images as role (student, worker, or professional) or attitude (casual, suggestive, or rebellious).

Your own appearance sends a message to the patient. Professional dress varies among agencies and settings. Depending on the setting, the use of a professional uniform may create a positive stereotype (comfort, expertise, or ease of identifica-

tion) or a negative stereotype (distance, authority, or formality). Whatever your personal choice in clothing or grooming, the aim should be to convey a competent, professional image.

Posture. Note the patient's position. An open position with extension of large muscle groups shows relaxation, physical comfort, and a willingness to share information. A closed position with arms and legs crossed looks defensive and anxious. Note any change in posture. If a person in a relaxed position suddenly tenses, it suggests discomfort with the new topic.

Your own calm, relaxed posture creates a feeling of warmth and trust and conveys an interest in the person. Standing and hastily filling out a history form with periodic peeks at your watch communicates that you are busy with many more important things than interviewing this person. Even when your time is limited, appear calm and unhurried. Sit down, even if it is only for a few minutes, and look as if nothing else matters except this person.

Gestures. Gestures send messages. For example, nodding or an open turning out of the hand shows acceptance, attention, or agreement. A wringing of the hands often indicates anxiety. Pointing a finger occurs with anger and vehemence. Also, hand gestures can reinforce a person's description of pain. When a crushing substernal chest pain is described, the person often holds the hand twisted into a fist in front of the sternum. Or, pain that is bright and sharply localized may be shown by pointing one finger to the exact spot: "It hurts right here."

Facial Expression. The face reflects a wide variety of relevant emotions and conditions. The expression may look alert, relaxed, and interested or it may look anxious, angry, and suspicious. Physical conditions such as pain or shortness of breath also show in the expression.

Your own expression should reflect a professional who is attentive, sincere, and interested in the patient. Any expression of boredom, distraction, disgust, criticism, or disbelief is picked up by the other person, and rapport will dissolve.

Eye Contact. Lack of eye contact in some situations or contexts suggests that the person is shy, withdrawn, confused, bored, intimidated, apathetic, or depressed. This applies to examiners, too. You should aim to maintain eye contact, but do not "stare down" the person. Do not have a fixed, penetrating look but rather an easy gaze toward the person's eyes, with occasional glances away. One exception to this is when you are interviewing someone from a culture that avoids direct eye contact (see the section on Cultural and Social Considerations).

Voice. Besides the spoken words, meaning comes through the tone of voice, the intensity and rate of speech, the pitch, and any pauses. These are just as important as words in conveying meaning. For example, the tone of a person's voice may show sarcasm, disbelief, sympathy, or hostility. An anxious person often speaks in a loud, fast voice. A whining voice is similar; it has a high-pitched wavering quality and long, drawn-out syllables. A soft voice may indicate shyness or fear. A hearing-impaired person may use a loud voice.

Even the use of pauses conveys meaning. When your question is easy and straightforward, a patient's long unexpected pause indicates the person is taking time to think of an answer. This raises some doubt as to the honesty of the answer. Unusually frequent and long pauses, when combined with speech that is slow and monotonous and a weak breathy voice, indicate depression.

Touch. The meaning of physical touch is influenced by the person's age, gender, family norms, cultural and social backgrounds, past experience, and current setting. The meaning of touch is easily misinterpreted. In most Western cultures, physical touch is reserved for expressions of love and affection or for clearly defined acts of greeting (for example, shaking hands). Do not use touch during the interview unless you know the person well and are sure how it will be interpreted. When appropriate, touch communicates effectively, such as a touch of the hand or arm to signal empathy.

In sum, an examiner's nonverbal messages that are productive and enhancing to the relationship are those that show attentiveness and unconditional acceptance. Defeating, nonproductive nonverbal behaviours are those of inattentiveness, authority, and superiority (Table 4-2).

Closing the Interview

The session should end gracefully. An abrupt or awkward closing can destroy rapport and leave the person with a negative impression of the whole interview. To ease into the closing, ask the person:

"Is there anything else you would like to mention?"
"Are there any questions you would like to ask?"
"Are there any other areas I should have asked about?"

This gives the person the final opportunity for self-expression. Then, to indicate that closing is imminent, say something like, "Our interview is just about over." No new topic should be introduced now. This is a good time to give your summary or a recapitulation of what you have learned during the interview. The summary is a final statement of what you and the patient agree the health state to be. It should include positive health aspects, any health problems that have been identified, any plans for action, or an explanation of the following physical examination. As you part from patients, thank them for the time spent and for their co-operation.

♥ DEVELOPMENTAL CARE

Interviewing the Parent

When your patient is a child, you must build rapport with two people—the child and the accompanying parent. Greet both by name, but with a younger child (1 to 6 years old), focus more on the parent. By ignoring the child temporarily, you allow the child to size you up from a safe distance. The child can observe your interaction with the parent, see that the parent accepts and likes you, and relax (Fig. 4-3).

Begin by interviewing the parent and child together. If any sensitive topics arise (e.g., the parents' troubled relationship or the child's problems at school or with peers), explore them with the parent later when he or she is alone. Provide toys to occupy the child as you and the parent talk. This frees the parent to concentrate on the history. Also, it indicates the child's level of attention span or independent play. Through the interview, be alert to ways the parent and child interact.

For younger children, the parent will provide all or most of the history. Thus you are collecting the child's health data from the parent's frame of reference. Usually, this viewpoint is reliable because most parents have the child's well-being as a priority and see co-operation with you as a way to enhance this well-being. But the possibilities exist for parental bias. Bias can occur when parents are asked to describe the child's achievements, or whenever their own parenting ability seems called into question. For example, if you say, "His fever was 103 and you did not bring him in?" you are implying a lack of parenting skill. This puts the parent on the defensive and increases anxiety. Instead, use open-ended questions that

TABLE 4-2	Nonverbal Behaviours of the Interviewer	
Positive	**Negative**
Appropriate professional appearance	Appearance objectionable to patient
Equal-status seating	Standing
Close proximity to patient	Sitting behind desk, far away, turned away
Relaxed open posture	Tense posture
Leaning slightly toward person	Slouched back
Occasional facilitating gestures	Critical or distracting gestures: pointing finger, clenched fist, finger-tapping, foot-swinging, looking at watch
Facial animation, interest	Bland expression, yawning, tight mouth
Appropriate smiling	Frowning, lip biting
Appropriate eye contact	Shifty, avoiding eye contact, focusing on notes, personal digital assistant (PDA), or computer screen
Moderate tone of voice	Strident, high-pitched tone
Moderate rate of speech	Rate too slow or too fast
Appropriate touch	Too frequent or inappropriate touch

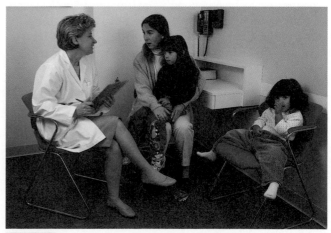

Fig. 4-3

increase description and defuse threat, such as, "What happened when the fever went up?"

A parent with more than one child has more than one set of data to remember. Be patient as the parent sorts through his or her memory to pull out facts of developmental milestones or past history. A comprehensive history may be lacking if the child is accompanied by a family friend or daycare provider instead of the parent.

In collecting developmental data, avoid being judgemental about the age of achievement of certain milestones. Parents are understandably proud of their child's achievements and are sensitive to inferences that these milestones may occur late.

Refer to the child by name—not as "the baby." Refer to the parent by name, and not the demeaning "Mother" or "Dad." Also, be clear when identifying the parents. The mother's present husband may not necessarily be the child's father. Instead of asking about "your husband's" health, ask, "Is Joan's father in good health?"

Although most of your communication is with the parent, do not ignore the child completely. You need to make contact to ease into the physical examination later. Begin by asking about the toys the child is playing with or about a special doll or teddy bear brought from home: "Does your doll have a name?" or, "What can your truck do?" Stoop down to meet the child at his or her eye level. Adult size can be overwhelming to young children and can emphasize their smallness.

Nonverbal communication is even more important to children than it is to adults. Children are quick to pick up feelings, anxiety, or comfort from nonverbal cues. Keep your physical appearance neat and clean, and avoid formal uniforms that distance you. Keep your gestures slow, deliberate, and close to your body. Children are frightened by quick or grandiose gestures. Do not try to maintain constant eye contact; this feels threatening to a small child. Use a quiet, measured voice, and choose simple words in your speech. Considering the child's level of language development is valuable in planning your communication.

The Infant

Nonverbal communication is the primary method. Most infants look calm and relaxed when all their needs are met, and they cry when they are frightened, hungry, tired, or uncomfortable. They respond best to firm, gentle handling and a quiet, calm voice. Your voice is comforting, even though they do not understand the words. Older infants have anxiety toward strangers. They are more co-operative when the parent is kept in view.

The Preschooler

A 2- to 6-year-old is egocentric. He or she sees the world mostly from his or her own point of view. Everything revolves around him or her. It may not work to cite the example of another child's behaviour to get the child to co-operate. It has no meaning. Only the child's own experience is relevant.

Preschoolers' communication is direct, concrete, literal, and set in the present. Avoid expressions such as "climbing the walls," because they are easily misinterpreted by young children. Use short, simple sentences with a concrete explanation. Take time to give a short simple explanation for any unfamiliar equipment that will be used on the child. Preschoolers can have *animistic* thinking about unfamiliar objects. They may imagine that unfamiliar inanimate objects can come alive and have human characteristics (e.g., that a blood pressure cuff can wake up and bite or pinch).

The School-Age Child

A child 7 to 12 years old can tolerate and understand others' viewpoints. This child is more objective and realistic. He or she wants to know functional aspects—how things work and why things are done.

Children of this age-group have the verbal ability to add important data to the history. Interview the parent and child together, but when a presenting symptom or sign exists ask the child about it first, then gather data from the parent. For the well child seeking a checkup, pose questions about school, friends, or activities directly to the child.

The Adolescent

Adolescents want to be adults, but they do not have the cognitive ability yet to achieve their goal. They are between two stages. Sometimes they are capable of mature actions, and other times they fall back on childhood response patterns, especially in times of stress. You cannot treat adolescents as children, yet you cannot overcompensate and assume that their communication style, learning ability, and motivation are consistently at an adult level.

Adolescents value their peers. They crave acceptance and sameness with their peers. Adolescents think no adult can understand them. Because of this, some act with aloof contempt, answering only in monosyllables. Others make eye contact and tell you what they think you want to hear, but inside they are thinking, "You'll never know the full story about me."

This knowledge about adolescents is apt to paralyze you in communicating with them. However, successful communication is possible and rewarding. The guidelines are simple.

The first consideration is your attitude, which must be one of respect. Respect is the most important thing you can communicate to the adolescent. The adolescent needs to feel validated as a human being, accepted, and worthy.

Second, your communication must be totally honest. The adolescent's intuition is highly tuned and can detect phoniness or when information is withheld. Always give them the truth. Play it straight or you will lose them. They will co-operate if they understand your rationale.

Stay in character. Avoid using language or colloquialisms that are not part of your usual way of interacting. It is helpful to understand some of the jargon used by adolescents, but you cannot use those words yourself simply to try to bond with the adolescent. Do not try to be his or her peer. You are not, and the patient will not accept you as such.

Use icebreakers. Focus first on the adolescent, not on the problem. Although an adult often wants to get on with it and talk about the health concern immediately, the adolescent responds best when the focus is on him or her as a person. Show an interest in the adolescent. Ask open, friendly questions about school, activities, hobbies, and friends. Refrain from asking questions about parents and family for now—these issues can be emotionally charged during adolescence.

Do not assume adolescents know *anything* about a health interview or a physical examination. Explain every step and give the rationale. They need direction. They will co-operate when they know the reason for the questions or actions. Encourage their questions. Adolescents are afraid they will sound "dumb" if they ask a question to which they assume everybody else knows the answer.

Keep your questions short and simple. "Why are you here?" sounds brazen to you, but it is effective with the adolescent. Be prepared for the adolescent who does *not* know why he or she is there. Some adolescents are pushed into coming to the examination by a parent.

The communication responses described for the adult need to be reconsidered when talking with the adolescent. Silent periods usually are best avoided. Giving adolescents a little time to collect their thoughts is acceptable, but a silence for other reasons is threatening. Also, avoid reflection. If you use reflection, the adolescent is likely to answer, "What?" They just do not have the cognitive skills to respond to that indirect mode of questioning. Also, adolescents are more sensitive to nonverbal communication than are adults. Be aware of your expressions and gestures. They are also more sensitive to any comment they take to mean criticism from you, and will withdraw.

Later in the interview, after you have developed rapport with the adolescent, you can address the topics that are emotionally charged, including alcohol and drug use, sexual behaviours, suicidal thoughts, and depression. Adolescents will assume that healthcare professionals have similar values and standards of behaviour as most of the other authority figures in their lives, and they may be reluctant to share this information. You can assure them that your questions are not intended to be curious or intrusive, but cover topics that are important for most teens and on which you have relevant health information to share.

If confidential material is uncovered during the interview, consider what can remain confidential and what you feel you must share for the well-being of the adolescent. Provincial and territorial laws vary with respect to confidentiality requirements with minors; several provinces (but not all) observe the "mature minors rule," and healthcare professionals are not required to notify parents about birth control, for example, or treatment for sexually transmitted infections (STIs). However, if the adolescent talks about an abusive home situation, state that you must share this information with other healthcare professionals for his or her own protection. Ask the adolescent, "Do you have a problem with that?" and then discuss it. Tell the adolescent, "You will need to trust that I will handle this information professionally and in your best interest."

Finally, take every opportunity to provide positive reinforcement. Praise every action regarding healthy lifestyle choices: "That's great that you don't smoke. You get lots of gold stars in my book for staying off the cigarettes. It's great for your heart, it will save you lots of money that you can use on other things, and your skin won't be wrinkled when you get older."

The Older Adult

The aging adult has the developmental task of finding the meaning of life and the purpose of his or her own existence, and adjusting to the inevitability of death. Some people have developed comfortable and satisfying answers and greet you with a calm demeanour and self-assurance. Be alert for the occasional person who sounds hopeless and despairing about life at present and in the future. Symptoms of illness are even more frightening when they mean physical limitation or threaten independence.

Always address the person by the last name (e.g., "Hello, Mr. Choi;" "Good morning, Mrs. Smith"). Some older adults resent being called by their first name by younger persons, and almost all cringe at the ignominious "Grandma" or "Pop."

The interview usually takes longer with older adults because they have a longer story to tell. You may need to break up the interview into more than one visit, collecting the most important historical data first. Or certain portions of the data, such as past history or the review of systems, can be provided on a form that is filled out at home, as long as the person's vision and handwriting are adequate. Take time to review these parts with the person during the interview.

It is important to adjust the pace of the interview to the aging person. The older person has a great amount of background material to sort through, and this takes some time. Also, some aging persons need a greater amount of response time to interpret the question and process their answer. Avoid trying to hurry them along. This approach only affirms their stereotype of younger persons in general and healthcare providers in particular—that is, people who are merely interested in numbers of patients and filling out forms. Any urge from you to get on with it will surely make them retreat. You will lose valuable data, and their needs will not be met (Fig. 4-4).

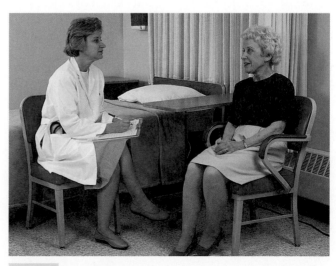

Fig. 4-4

Consider physical limitations when planning the interview. An aging person may fatigue earlier and may require that the interview be broken up into shorter segments. For the person with impaired hearing, face him or her directly so that your mouth and face are fully visible. Do not shout; it does not help and actually distorts speech.

Touch is a nonverbal skill that is very important to older persons. Their other senses may be diminished, and touch grounds you in reality. Also, a hand on the arm or shoulder is an empathic message that communicates you empathize with the person and want to understand his or her problem (see the Cultural and Social Considerations section for exceptions).

INTERVIEWING IN CHALLENGING SITUATIONS

People With Hearing Impairment

Although many people will tell you in advance that they have a hearing deficit, in others it must be recognized from clues, such as staring at your mouth and face, not attending unless looking at you, or speaking in a voice unusually loud or with guttural or garbled sounds. The deaf person may be familiar with some equipment in the hospital or office setting or may have had previous experience with healthcare settings. But without full communication, the person with hearing impairment is sure to feel isolated and anxious. Ask his or her preferred way to communicate—by signing, lip reading, or writing.

A complete health history requires a sign language interpreter. Since most healthcare professionals are not proficient in signing, try to find an interpreter through a social service agency or the person's own social network. You may use family members, but be aware that they sometimes edit for the person. Use the same guidelines as for the bilingual interpreter (see the section on Working With (and Without) an Interpreter).

If the person prefers lip reading, be sure to face him or her squarely and have good lighting on your face. Examiners with a beard, mustache, or foreign accents are less effective. Do not exaggerate your lip movements because this distorts your words. Similarly, shouting distorts the reception of a hearing aid the person may wear. Speak slowly and supplement your voice with appropriate hand gestures or pantomime. Nonverbal cues are important adjuncts because the lip reader understands at best only 50% of your speech when relying solely on vision. Be sure the person understands your questions. Many people with hearing impairment nod "yes" just to be friendly and co-operative but really do not understand.

Written communication is efficient in sections such as past health history or review of systems. For the present history of illness, writing is very time consuming and laborious. The syntax of the person's written words will read normally if the hearing impairment occurred after speech patterns developed. If the deafness occurred before speech patterns developed, the written syntax follows that of signing, which is different from that of English.

Acutely Ill People

An emergency demands your prompt action. You must combine interviewing with physical examination skills to determine life-saving actions. Although life support measures may be paramount, still try to interview the person as much as possible. Subjective data are crucial to determine the cause and course of the emergency. Abbreviate your questioning. Identify the main area of distress and question about that. Family or friends often can provide important data.

A hospitalized person with a critical or severe illness is usually too weak, too short of breath, or in too much pain to talk. First attend to the comfort of the person. Then establish a priority; find out immediately what parts of the history are the most relevant. Explore the first concern the person mentions. Begin to use closed, direct questions earlier. Finally, watch that your statements are very clear. When a person is very sick, even the simplest sentence can be misconstrued. The person will react according to preconceived ideas about what a serious illness means, so anything you say should be direct and precise.

People Under the Influence of Street Drugs or Alcohol

It is common for persons under the influence of alcohol or other mood-altering drugs to be admitted to a hospital; all of these drugs affect the central nervous system, increasing the risk for accidents and injuries. Also, chronic use creates complex medical problems that require increasing care.

Many substance abusers are poly-drug abusers. You may be faced with a wide range of patient behaviours due to current influence. Alcohol and the opioids (heroin, meperidine [Demerol], acetaminophen and hydrocodone [Vicodin], propoxyphene) are central nervous system depressants. Stimulants of the central nervous system (cocaine, amphetamine) can cause an intense high, agitation, and paranoid behaviour. Hallucinogens can cause bizarre, inappropriate, sometimes even violent behaviour.

When interviewing a person currently under the influence of alcohol or illicit drugs, ask simple and direct questions. Take care to make your manner and questions nonthreatening. Avoid confrontation at this point. Further, avoid any display of scolding or disgust, because this person may become belligerent. One priority is to find out the time of the person's last drink and how much he or she drank at this episode as well as the name and amount of other drugs taken. This information will help assess any withdrawal patterns. For your own protection, be aware of hospital security or other personnel who could be called on for assistance.

Once he or she is sober, the hospitalized person should be assessed for the extent of the problem and the meaning of the problem for the person and family. Initially you will likely encounter denial and increased defensiveness; special interview techniques will likely be needed.

Personal Questions

Occasionally, people will ask you questions about *your* personal life or opinions, such as, "Are you married?" "Do you have children?" or, "Do you smoke?" You do not need to answer every question. You may supply brief information when you feel it is appropriate, but be sensitive to the possibility that there may be a motive behind the personal questions such as loneliness or anxiety. Try directing your response back to the person's frame of reference. You might say something like, "No, I don't have children; I wonder if your question is related to how I can help you care for little Jamie?"

Dealing With Sexual Advances

On some occasions, personal questions extend to flirtatious compliments, seductive innuendo, or advances. Your response must make it clear that you are a healthcare professional who can best care for the person by maintaining a professional relationship. At the same time, you should communicate that you accept the person and you understand the person's need to be self-assertive but that you cannot tolerate sexual advances. This may be difficult, considering that the person's words or gestures may have left you shocked, embarrassed, or angry. Your feelings are normal. You need to set appropriate verbal boundaries by saying, "I am uncomfortable when you talk to me that way; please don't." A further response that would open communication is: "I wonder if the way you're feeling now relates to your illness or to being in the hospital?"

Crying

A beginning examiner usually feels horrified when the patient starts crying. But crying actually is a big relief to a person. Health problems come with powerful emotions. Worries about illness, death, or loss take a great amount of energy to keep bottled up inside. When you say something that "makes the person cry," do not think you have hurt the person. You have just hit on a topic that is important. Do not go on to a new topic. Just let the person cry and express his or her feelings fully. You can offer a tissue and wait until the crying subsides to talk. The person will regain control soon.

Sometimes your patient looks as if he or she is on the verge of tears but is trying hard to suppress them. Again instead of moving on to something new, acknowledge the expression by saying, "You look sad." Do not worry that you will open an uncontrollable floodgate. The person may cry but will be relieved, and you will have gained insight to a serious concern (Clinical Illustration).

Anger

Occasionally you will try to interview a person who is already angry. Try not to personalize this anger; usually it does not relate to you. The person is showing aggression as a response to his or her own feelings of anxiety or helplessness. Do ask

---

CLINICAL ILLUSTRATION

Alice P., a 49-year-old divorced woman with chronic alcoholism and skin yellow with jaundice has entered treatment for substance abuse. Today, she needs a pelvic examination and Papanicolaou (Pap) smear.

Alice: I haven't had a pelvic exam in 5 years. I had a hysterectomy 18 years ago. They said I had "preinvasive" cancer cells. (At this, Alice's lips fold in, her eyes squeeze shut; she puts hand to mouth, and breathes in audibly in jerks.)

Response: Alice, you look sad. (Puts hand on upper arm.)

Alice: (Crying freely now.) What if you find more cancer now? They can't operate on me with my liver so big. I'd never survive the anaesthesia. And my father died of cancer. He had cirrhosis too, and they opened him up and he was full of cancer. He never woke up from surgery and he died 2 weeks later.

Response: I understand how worried you are. I think you have done the right thing to come in for treatment. That took courage. As for today, let's take one step at a time. Today we need to do the pelvic exam and Pap smear. There is no reason today to assume you need an operation. I'll do your exam today and I'll be here all week. We'll work together to help you get through this.

Alice: (Breathing deeply, sitting up straight, arms down and open at sides, making eye contact.) All right. I'm better now. Let's go ahead.

---

about the anger and hear the person out. Deal with the angry feelings before you ask anything else. An angry person cannot be an effective participant in a health interview.

Maybe because of an unrelated incident *you* are angry when you come into the interview. When you are angry, say so and tell the patient that you are angry at something or someone else. Otherwise the patient, unusually vulnerable and dependent on you, thinks you are angry at him or her.

Threat of Violence

The healthcare setting is not immune to violent behaviour. An individual may act with such angry gestures that you feel a threat to your personal safety. Other red flag behaviours of a potentially disruptive person include fist clenching, pacing back and forth, a vacant stare, confusion, statements out of touch with reality, statements that do not make sense, a history of recent drug use (alcohol, hallucinogen, cocaine), or perhaps even a recent history of intense bereavement (loss of spouse, loss of job). Trust your instincts. If you sense any suspicious or threatening behaviour, act immediately to defuse the situation. Leave the examining room door open and position yourself between the person and the door. Many departments have a prearranged sign or signal so that a co-worker can call 911 and the security department to send help to the setting. Do not raise your own voice or try to argue with the threatening person. Act quite calm and talk to the person in a soft voice. Act interested in what the person is saying, and behave in an unhurried way. Your most important goal is safety; avoid taking any risks.

Anxiety

Finally, take it for granted that nearly all sick people have some anxiety. This is a normal response to being sick. It makes some people aggressive and others dependent. Remember that the person is not reacting as typically as when he or she is healthy.

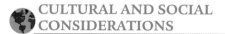

CULTURAL AND SOCIAL CONSIDERATIONS

CROSS-CULTURAL COMMUNICATION

When people come from different cultural and social backgrounds, the probability of miscommunication can increase. Verbal and nonverbal communications are influenced by the cultural, social, and family backgrounds of both the healthcare professional and the patient. *Cross-cultural* or *intercultural communication* refers to the communication process occurring between a healthcare professional and a patient, each with different cultural, social, and historical backgrounds, in which both attempt to understand the other's point of view (Fig. 4-5).

Relational practice requires that you connect across differences by relating with people as they are and where they are, no matter what their context, decisions, or life history (Doane et al., 2005). This does not dismiss the fact that you may sometimes find it challenging to relate to or communicate with patients or family members for a variety of reasons. Some people may be living with severe addictions or substance use issues, or may be harming themselves or others through violence, abuse, or neglect. Some people may be challenging to communicate with because your primary language

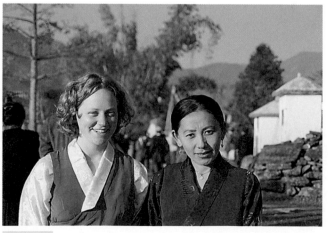

Fig. 4-5

is different from theirs. In all situations, you will need to be highly reflective about your reactions, assumptions, biases, and judgements so that you can be conscious of how you are relating to people, rather than reacting based on habit.

It is particularly important to establish effective communication with people whose primary language is different from yours. Unfortunately, the current patchwork of interpreter services and different levels of understanding about the importance of effective communication in health care have led to inconsistencies in how language barriers are addressed in healthcare settings (Hoen et al., 2006). Repeatedly, studies show that access to health care and the quality of health services are seriously compromised without interpretation services for those who need them. For example, nursing and medical errors such as misdiagnosis and inappropriate treatment, inadequate patient comprehension, and higher readmission rates and emergency room visits can result from poor communication (Anderson et al., 2003; Hoen et al., 2006; Lynam et al., 2003; Tang, 1999).

As was discussed in Chapter 3, people who have limited English and French proficiencies (LEP and LFP) and therefore speak a language(s) other than English or French must be provided with an interpreter who is **not** a family member or friend. Carefully document that the patient and family fully understand what is happening to them; what their diagnosis and the implications of this diagnosis are; what procedures, diagnostic and therapeutic, are going to be done, how the procedures will be done, and what they mean; how medications are to be taken and when; and the prognosis derived from the given problem(s). Later in this chapter, we discuss strategies for working effectively with (and without) an interpreter.

Perspectives on Professional Interactions

The way you interact with patients and families will vary relationally, depending on their and your social, ethnocultural, and historical contexts. Some patients may nod their head in the affirmative or smile a lot to fulfill their assumptions about what is required of "good patients." In this situation, you may need to invite the person to respond frankly to your suggestions or by giving the person "permission" to disagree.

Etiquette

Etiquette refers to the diverse patterns of interaction that are considered to be appropriate in some (though certainly not all) social, familial, or ethnocultural contexts. For example, some people will expect you to engage in conversation of a personal or social nature before they feel comfortable entering into the more personal and intimate aspects of the health history and physical examination. For some people, there is a high value placed on developing interpersonal relationships and getting to know about a person's family, personal concerns, and interests before they allow you to interact therapeutically. Recognizing that time constraints frequently affect the social interchange expected by some individuals, from some cultures, you should strive to incorporate the person's interactional style and needs with the health history data categories. For example, using a conversational tone of voice, you might begin the health history by inquiring about the patient's family members and their health.

You should be prepared for the converse; that is, some people may want to interview *you*. They may ask questions about your family, marital status, salary, home address, telephone number, and so forth. You will need to determine your level of comfort in responding to these questions, but it is respectful to reply to some of the patient's questions. Remember that you aren't obligated to answer questions that you deem too personal and always have a right to protect your personal safety. For example, you are **never** to provide your home address, e-mail, or telephone number. Rather, you should provide the patient with the hospital, clinic, or agency's business number. If you want the patient to be able to contact you while you're at home, you should ask a secretary or other third party at the healthcare facility to call your home number. You may want to consider in advance which categories of questions you are willing to discuss and which ones you will politely avoid. If you refuse to answer certain questions about yourself, remember that the person may perceive your behaviour as aloof and uncaring. Thus, the manner in which you reply to personal inquiries should be carefully worded, sensitive to the needs of the patient, and congruent with your own needs and comfort level.

When meeting a patient for the first time, it is best to be relatively formal, respectful, and polite. Unless a physical disability or handicap prevents you from doing so, you should be standing when you first greet the person and those accompanying him or her. Another aspect of etiquette concerns the use of *names* and *titles*. In order to ensure that a mutually respectful relationship is established, you should introduce yourself and indicate to the person how you prefer to be called—that is, by first name, last name, and/or title. You should elicit the same information from the patient because this enables you to address the person in a manner that is socially and culturally appropriate and could actually spare you considerable embarrassment. Everyone likes to be called by his or her correct name. You must be certain that you know your patients' names and pronounce them correctly. Follow cultural conventions concerning the use of titles. Avoid being unduly casual or familiar. For example, refrain from routinely using the person's first name before you have been invited to do so. The same guidelines should be followed when addressing the family members and other visitors. It is suggested to greet the patient, "Hello, Mr. or Mrs. or Ms., my name is," and to use your last name. The common use of "you guys" and other colloquialisms must be eradicated when talking to patients and family members.

Space and Distance

Both the patient's and your own sense of spatial distance are significant throughout the interview and physical examination, with culturally appropriate distance zones varying widely. For example, you may find yourself backing away from people of Hispanic, East Indian, or Middle Eastern origins who invade your personal space with regularity in an attempt to bring you closer into the space than is comfortable for them. Although you are uncomfortable with their close physical proximity, they are perplexed by your distancing behaviours and may perceive you as aloof and unfriendly.

Considerations Related to Gender

Lack of attention to ethnocultural or family norms related to appropriate male–female relationships may jeopardize your professional relationship with many patients. Among some Arab Canadian families, you may find that an adult male is rarely alone with a woman (except his wife) and is generally accompanied by one or more other men when interacting with women. This is socioculturally very significant; failure to respect norms of behaviour can be viewed as a serious transgression, often one in which the lone man will be accused of sexual impropriety. The best way to ensure that particular norms have been considered is to ask the person about relevant aspects of male–female relationships, preferably at the beginning of the interview. When you have determined that gender differences are important to the patient, you might try strategies such as offering to have a third person present when this is feasible. If a family member or friend has accompanied the patient, you might inquire whether the patient would like that person to be in the examination room during the history or physical examination, or both. It is not unusual for a female to refuse to be examined by a male and vice versa. Modesty is another issue and it is imperative to ensure that all patients are carefully draped at all times, that curtains are closed, and when possible doors are also closed. A room must not be entered without knocking first and announcing yourself.

Among some ethnocultural groups, it is considered an acceptable expression of friendship and affection to openly and publicly hold hands with or embrace members of the same gender without any sexual connotation being associated with the behaviour. For example, you may notice that some women hold hands with female relatives and friends while walking with them.

Considerations Related to Sexual Orientation

In approaching lesbian, gay, bisexual, or transgendered individuals, you should be aware of heterosexist biases and the communication of these biases during the interview and physical examination. *Heterosexism* refers to the institutionalized belief that heterosexuality is the only natural choice and assumes it is the norm. For example, most health histories include a question concerning marital status. Although many same-sex couples are in committed, long-term monogamous relationships, seldom is there a category on the standard form that acknowledges this type of relationship. Although technically and legally the person may be single, this trivializes the relationship with his or her significant other. It also may have health-related implications if the person is diagnosed, for example, with a communicable disease, which may range in severity from a minor sore throat to a life-threatening condition such as HIV or AIDS.

OVERCOMING COMMUNICATION BARRIERS

Healthcare professionals tend to have stereotypical expectations of the patient's behaviour during the interview and physical examination. In general, we expect behaviour to consist of undemanding compliance, an attitude of respect for the healthcare professional, and co-operation with requested behaviour throughout the examination. Although patients may ask a few questions for the purpose of clarification, we generally expect to take the lead in directing the conversation. Some individuals, however, may have significantly different perceptions about the appropriate role of the individual and his or her family when seeking health care. If you find yourself becoming annoyed that a patient is asking too many questions, assuming a defensive posture, or otherwise feeling uncomfortable, you should pause to reflect critically on the source of their concerns. Consider that some patients who have experienced healthcare inequities through discrimination or racialization may be concerned that their health concerns will be dismissed or that they won't be treated respectfully because of past experiences with the healthcare system. In these situations, it is particularly important to convey unconditional positive regard, empathy, and active listening. Remaining reflective will create opportunities for you to make conscious and intentional choices about how best to respond.

Working With (and Without) an Interpreter

In Canada, one in five people in 2006 was born outside of Canada, which reflects the highest proportion in 75 years (Statistics Canada, 2007). Allophones (people whose mother tongue is neither English nor French) comprised one fifth of the population of Canada. This means that you will have the opportunity to work with a wide range of patients and family members whose primary language is different from yours. It is helpful to recognize that language is not only a means of communication; language also connects people to their social, emotional, familial, and spiritual vitality (Statistics Canada, 2008). For these reasons, it is important to develop ways of communicating effectively with people so that you can provide the best care possible.

After English and French, the most common mother tongues spoken in Canada in 2006 were the Chinese languages (e.g., Cantonese, Mandarin) (Statistics Canada, 2007). Italian was the fourth most common mother tongue, with German fifth, and Punjabi sixth, followed by Spanish, Arabic, Tagalog (the national language of the Philippines), and Portuguese.

One of the greatest challenges in cross-cultural communication occurs when you and the patient speak different languages (Fig. 4-6). After assessing the language skills of people who have LEP or LFP, you may find yourself in one of two situations: trying to communicate effectively through an interpreter or trying to communicate effectively when no interpreter is present.

Interviewing the non–English or non–French-speaking person requires a bilingual interpreter for full communication. Even the person from another country who has a basic command of English or French (those for whom English or French is a second language) may need an interpreter when faced with the anxiety-provoking situation of entering a hospital, describing a strange symptom, or discussing sensitive topics such as those related to reproductive or urological concerns.

Although interpreters are employed in many healthcare agencies and hospitals in Canada, current research demonstrates that nurses and doctors tend not to use interpreter services adequately (Anderson et al., 2003; Hoen et al., 2006; Lynam et al., 2003). It is tempting to ask a relative, friend, or even another patient to interpret because this person is readily available and probably would like to help. This is disadvantageous because it violates confidentiality for the patient, who may not want personal information shared with another. Furthermore, the friend or relative, although fluent in ordinary language usage, is likely to be unfamiliar with medical terminology, hospital or clinic procedures, and medical ethics.

Whenever possible, work with a bilingual team member or a trained medical interpreter. This person knows interpreting techniques, has a healthcare background, and understands patients' rights. The trained interpreter also is knowledgeable about culturally specific meanings and practices about health, healing, or illness. This person can help you bridge the communication cultural gap that may exist and can advise you concerning the cultural appropriateness of your recommendations.

Many patients with LEP or LFP do not have access to interpreters. It is your responsibility to ensure that patients have access to a skilled interpreter. You must make sure that your patients (and in some situations, the families) are fully informed of what you are telling them, particularly related to informed consent for procedures, treatments, and discharge or follow-up plans (Abraham et al., 2008). It is well known

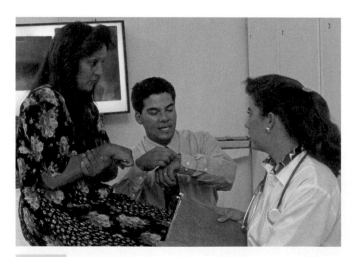

Fig. 4-6

that few clinicians receive the necessary preparation to practice with interpreters. Very few healthcare agencies or hospitals provide this type of training (Tang, 1999). As a first preference, language services should include the availability of a bilingual staff member who can communicate directly with patients in their preferred language and dialect. The services can be handled in person—that is, with an interpreter present—or there are now several resources that you may access to receive the support you and the patient require. **Ad hoc interpreters, such as family members, friends, children, and untrained workers cannot be used**. They do not understand the medical jargon well enough to translate it and issues such as confidentiality are not understood. Errors made in translation can be fatal. In the United States, this issue is serious enough to warrant some states (e.g., California) to develop bills prohibiting children younger than 15 years of age to serve as interpreters, and several states such as Massachusetts and New York are legislating the use of interpreters. Although Canada has a universal healthcare system, no legislative provisions or court precedents effectively require the availability of interpretation services for patients who need them (Hoen et al., 2006). Only the deaf community in Canada has had success in the courts in obtaining the right to access interpreter services in healthcare settings.

Although interpreters are trained to remain neutral, they can influence both the content of information exchanged and the nature of the interaction. Many trained medical interpreters are members of the linguistic community they serve. While this is largely beneficial, it has limitations. For example, interpreters often know patients and details of their circumstances before the interview begins. This is a significant risk in smaller, rural, or northern towns and communities. In these contexts, it is critical to be judicious about who is interpreting for patients. Although acceptance of a code of ethics governing confidentiality and conflicts of interest is part of the training interpreters receive, discord may arise when they relate information that the patient has not volunteered to the examiner.

It should be noted that being bilingual doesn't always mean the interpreter is able to communicate with the patient. Aboriginal languages, for example, are so diverse that an Aboriginal-speaking interpreter from one region of a province or territory may not necessarily understand the language or cultural practices of an Aboriginal person from another region of the same province or territory. Even when an interpreter and patient are from similar ethnocultural backgrounds, trained interpreters may live in urban areas and in an entirely different social context, and may be unaware of particular meanings, practices, or beliefs that are important to the patient for whom they interpret.

Although you will be in charge of the focus and flow of the interview, view yourself and the interpreter as a team. Ask the interpreter to meet the patient beforehand to establish rapport and to garner information about the patient's social, cultural, educational, and family contexts. This enables the interpreter to communicate on the patient's level.

Allow more time for this interview. With the third person repeating everything, it can take considerably longer than interviewing English-speaking people. You need to focus on priority data.

There are two styles of interpreting—line by line and summarizing. Translating line by line takes more time, but it ensures accuracy. Use this style for most of the interview. Both you and the patient should speak only a sentence or two, then allow the interpreter some time. Use simple language yourself, not medical jargon that the interpreter must simplify before it can be translated. Summary translation progresses faster and is useful for teaching relatively simple healthcare techniques with which the interpreter is already familiar. Be alert for nonverbal cues as the patient talks. These cues can give valuable data. A good interpreter also notes nonverbal messages and passes them on to you. Summarized in Table 4-3 are suggestions for the selection and use of an interpreter.

Although use of an interpreter is the ideal, you may find yourself in a situation with a non–English or non–French-speaking patient when no interpreter is available. Table 4-4 summarizes some suggestions for overcoming language barriers when no interpreter is present. Communicating with these patients may require that you combine verbal and nonverbal communication.

Nonverbal Cross-Cultural Communication

Basically, there are five types of nonverbal behaviours that convey information about the person: (1) *vocal cues,* such as pitch, tone, and quality of voice, including moaning, crying, and groaning; (2) *action cues,* such as posture, facial expression, and gestures; (3) *object cues,* such as clothes, jewellery, and hairstyles; (4) *use of personal and territorial space* in interpersonal transactions and care of belongings; and (5) *touch,* which involves the use of personal space and action (Lapierre and Padgett, 1991).

Unless you make an effort to understand the patient's nonverbal behaviour, you may overlook important information such as that conveyed by facial expressions, silence, eye contact, touch, and other body language. Communication patterns vary widely across families and cultural and social groups, even for such conventional social behaviours as smiling and handshaking.

Wide cultural variation exists when interpreting **silence.** Some individuals find silence extremely uncomfortable and make every effort to fill conversational lags with words. Conversely, many Aboriginal people consider silence essential to understanding and respecting the other person. A pause following your question can signify that what has been asked is important enough to be given thoughtful consideration. For some people from various ethnocultural groups, silence may mean that the speaker wishes the listener to consider the content of what has been said before continuing. For others, silence may be used out of respect for another's privacy or to demonstrate respect for elders. It is important to remember that there are no "prescriptions" for how to behave when communicating with people whose background may be different from yours. Rather, what is needed is a high degree of

TABLE 4-3 | Use of an Interpreter

CHOOSING AN INTERPRETER

- Before locating an interpreter, identify the language the person speaks at home. Be aware that it may differ from the language spoken publicly.
- Whenever possible, use a *trained* interpreter, preferably one who knows medical terminology.
- Be aware of gender differences between interpreter and patient. In general, the same gender is preferred.
- Be aware of age differences between interpreter and patient. In general, an older, more mature interpreter is preferred to a younger, less experienced one.
- Be aware of socioeconomic differences between interpreter and patient.

STRATEGIES FOR EFFECTIVE USE OF AN INTERPRETER

- Plan what you want to say ahead of time. Meet privately with the interpreter before the interview. Avoid confusing the interpreter by backing up, hesitating, or inserting a proviso.
- Ask the interpreter to provide a line by line verbatim account of the conversation. Ask for a detailed interpretation when provided with brief summaries of longer exchanges between interpreter and patient.
- Be patient. When using an interpreter, interviews often take two to three times longer.
- Longer-than-expected explanatory exchanges are often required to convey the meaning of words such as *stress, depression, allergy, preventive medicine,* and *physical therapy* because comparable terms may not exist in the language the patient understands.
- When discussing diagnostic tests such as mammography, magnetic resonance imaging, and computed tomography, or those involving body fluids such as blood, urine, stool, spinal fluid, or saliva, be sure to clarify the nature of the test to the interpreter. Indicate the purpose of the test, exactly what will happen to the patient, approximately how long the test will take, whether the procedure is invasive or noninvasive, and what part(s) of the body will be tested.
- Be aware that the interpreter may modify or edit some aspects of the conversation, especially if he or she thinks you might not understand the cultural context of the patient's response (e.g., culturally specific beliefs and practices related to healing).
- Avoid ambiguous statements and questions. Refrain from using conditional or indefinite phrasing such as "if," "would," and "could," especially for target languages, such as Khmer (Cambodia), that lack nuances of conditionality or distinctions of time other than actual past and present. Conditional statements may be mistaken for actual agreement or approval of a course of action.
- Avoid abstract expressions, idioms, similes, metaphors, and medical jargon.
- To ensure confidentiality and privacy, avoid using as interpreters children or strangers who may be visiting other patients.

RECOMMENDATIONS FOR INSTITUTIONS

- Maintain a current, computerized list of interpreters who may be contacted as needed.
- Network with local community healthcare centres, hospitals, colleges, universities, and other organizations that may serve as resources.
- Some private companies, and phone companies, offer over-the-phone interpretation for a fee. Some institutions may consider paying for these services if no interpretation is available.

TABLE 4-4 | Overcoming Language Barriers: What to Do When No Interpreter Is Available

1. Be polite and formal. Be sure to convey unconditional positive regard through nonverbal communication such as facial expressions, body positions, and tone of voice.
2. Pronounce name correctly. Use proper titles of respect, such as "Mr.," "Mrs.," "Ms.," and "Dr." Greet the person using the last or complete name.
   Gesture to yourself and say your name.
   Offer a handshake or nod. Smile.
3. Proceed in an unhurried manner. Pay attention to any effort by the patient or family to communicate.
4. Speak in a low, moderate voice. Avoid talking loudly. Remember that there is a tendency to raise the volume and pitch of your voice when the listener appears not to understand. The listener may perceive that you are shouting and/or angry.
5. Use any words that you might know in the person's language. This indicates that you are aware of and respect his or her culture.
6. Use simple words, such as "pain" instead of "discomfort." Avoid medical jargon, idioms, and slang. Avoid using contractions (e.g., don't, can't, won't). Use nouns repeatedly instead of pronouns.
   Example:
   Do not say: "He has been taking his medicine, hasn't he?"
   Do say: "Does Juan take medicine?"
7. Pantomime words and simple actions while you verbalize them.
8. Give instructions in the proper sequence.
   Example:
   Do not say: "Before you rinse the bottle, sterilize it."
   Do say: "First wash the bottle. Second, rinse the bottle."
9. Discuss one topic at a time. Avoid using conjunctions.
   Example:
   Do not say: "Are you cold and in pain?"
   Do say: "Are you cold (*while pantomiming*)? Are you in pain?"
10. Validate if the person understands by having him or her repeat instructions, demonstrate the procedure, or act out the meaning.
11. Write out several short sentences in English and determine the person's ability to read them.
12. Try a third language. Many Indochinese speak French. Europeans often know two or more languages. Try Latin words or phrases.
13. Ask who among the person's family and friends could serve as an interpreter.
14. Obtain phrase books from a library or bookstore, make or purchase flash cards, contact community healthcare centres or hospitals for a list of interpreters, and use both a formal and an informal network to locate a suitable interpreter.

reflectivity, self-observation, an awareness of peoples' unique contexts and histories, and the intention to ensure that you and the patient (and the family members) are communicating effectively.

Eye contact is perhaps among the most culturally variable nonverbal behaviours. Although you probably have been taught to maintain eye contact when speaking with others, people from some ethnocultural backgrounds may use eye contact in other ways. For example, some people may avert their eyes when talking with you in an effort to convey respect to people in positions of authority. Some Aboriginal people may stare at the floor during conversations to indicate that the listener is paying close attention to the speaker. In some Inuit communities, people raise their eyebrows as a way to signal an affirmative response to a question, or to signal agreement, rather than nodding their head up and down.

Bodily Exposure and Touch

For all people, modesty in relation to bodily exposure (e.g., removing clothing for physical examinations) is particularly important to respect. For some people, because of past negative experiences, family norms, or culturally specific norms, it will be entirely inappropriate for a male examiner to view a woman's body unless she is fully clothed. You will need to remain attuned to the verbal and nonverbal cues conveyed by patients or their families as you proceed. In all cases, provide a clear explanation of why you are asking someone to remove part of his or her clothing for the purpose of examination, and

be prepared to make adaptations or forgo bodily exposure in some cases.

Without doubt, touching the patient is a necessary component of a comprehensive assessment. From a cultural perspective, however, you are urged to give careful consideration to issues concerning **touch.** While recognizing the benefits reported by many in establishing rapport with patients through touch, physical contact with patients can convey various meanings cross-culturally. For some people, depending on their social, cultural, and historical contexts, male healthcare professionals may be prohibited from touching or examining either all or certain parts of the female body. Adolescent girls often prefer female healthcare professionals or refuse to be examined by a male. You should be aware that the patient's significant others also may exert pressure on nurses by enforcing these culturally meaningful norms in the healthcare setting.

Touching children also may have associated meaning in some ethnocultural groups. Some people from areas of Asia believe that one's strength resides in the head and that touching the head is a sign of disrespect. The clinical significance of this is that you need to be aware that patting a child on the head or examining the fontanelle may need to be avoided or done only with parental permission. Whenever possible, you should explore alternative ways to express affection or to obtain information necessary for assessment of the patient's condition (e.g., hold the child on the lap, observe for other manifestations of increased intracranial pressure or signs of premature fontanelle closure, or place one's hand over the mother's while asking for a description of what she feels).

BIBLIOGRAPHY

Abraham, D., & Rahman, S. (2008). The community interpreter: A critical link between clients and service providers. In S. Guruge & E. Collins (Eds.), *Working with immigrant women: Issues and strategies for mental health professionals* (pp. 103–118). Toronto, ON: Canadian Centre for Addiction and Mental Health.

Adubato, S. (2004). Making the communication connection. *Nursing Management, 35*(9), 33–35.

Aita, V., McIlvain, H., Backer, E., McVea, K., & Crabtree, B. (2005). Patient-centered care and communication in primary care practice. *Patient Education and Counseling, 58,* 296–304.

Amerson, R., & Burgins, S. (2005). Hablamos espanol: Crossing communication barriers with the Latino population. *Journal of Nursing Education, 44,* 241–243.

Anderson, J., Perry, J., Blue, C., Browne, A., Henderson, A., Khan, K., et al. (2003). "Rewriting" cultural safety within the postcolonial and postnational feminist project. *Advances in Nursing Science 26,* 196–214.

Arnold, E., & Boggs, K. (2007). *Interpersonal relationships: professional communication skills for nurses* (5th ed.). Philadelphia, PA: W.B. Saunders.

Baker, L. H., O'Connell, D., & Platt, F. W. (2005). "What else?" Setting the agenda for the clinical interview. *Annals of Internal Medicine, 143,* 766–770.

Bernstein, L., & Bernstein, R. S. (1985). *Interviewing: A guide for health professionals* (4th ed.). E. Norwalk, CT: Appleton & Lange.

Branch, W. T., & Gordon, G. H. (2004). Making the most of challenging patient interviews. *Patient Care for the Nurse Practitioner, 7,* July 15. Retrieved December 10, 2006, from http://www.patientcarenp.com/pcnp/article

Doane, G. H., & Varcoe, C. (2005). *Family nursing as relational inquiry: Developing health-promoting practice.* Philadelphia, PA: Lippincott, Williams & Wilkins.

Duxbury, J., & Whittington, R. (2005). Causes and management of patient aggression and violence: staff and patient perspectives. *Journal of Advanced Nursing, 50,* 469–478.

Fallowfield, L., & Jenkins, V. (2004). Communicating sad, bad, and difficult news in medicine. *Lancet, 363*(9405), 312–319.

Flores, G. (2006). Language barriers to health care in the United States. *New England Journal of Medicine, 355,* 229–231.

Gerrish, K., Chau, R., Sobowale, A., & Birks, E. (2004). Bridging the language barrier: the use of interpreters in primary care nursing. *Health and Social Care in the Community, 12,* 407–413.

Goldenring, J. M., & Rosen, D. S. (2004). Getting into adolescent heads: An essential update. *Contemporary Pediatrics, 21*(1), 64–68, 70, 73–74.

Harrahill, M. (2005). Giving bad news gracefully. *Journal of Emergency Nursing, 31,* 312–314.

Hoen, B., Nielsen K., & Sasso, A. (2006). *Health care interpreter services: Strengthening access to primary health care. National report.* Toronto, ON: Access Alliance, Multicultural Community Health Centre.

Instone, S. L. (2002). Developmental strategies for interviewing children. *Journal of Pediatric Health Care, 16,* 304–305.

Lange, N., & Tigges, B. B. (2005). Influence positive change with motivational interviewing. *Nurse Practitioner, 30*(3), 44–45, 48–50, 53.

Lapierre, E. D., & Padgett, J. (1991). How can we become more aware of culturally specific body language and use this awareness therapeutically? *Journal of Psychosocial Nursing and Mental Health Services, 29*(11), 38–41.

Lehna, C. (2005). Interpreter services in pediatric nursing. *Pediatric Nursing, 31,* 292–296.

Lynam, M. J., Henderson, A., Browne, A., Smye, V., Semeniuk, P., Blue, C., et al. (2003). Healthcare restructuring with a view to equity and efficiency: Reflections on unintended consequences. *Canadian Journal of Nursing Leadership, 16*(1), 112–140.

McAleer, M. (2006). Communicating effectively with deaf patients. *Nursing Standard, 20*(19), 51–54.

McAllister, M., Matarasso, B., Dixon, B., & Shepperd, C. (2004). Conversation starters: Re-examining and reconstructing first encounters within the therapeutic relationship. *Journal of Psychiatric and Mental Health Nursing, 11,* 575–582.

Minton, P. R. (2006). Setting the agenda for the clinical interview. *Annals of Internal Medicine, 144,* 306.

Nordby, H. (2006). Nurse-patient communication: Language mastery and concept possession. *Nursing Inquiry, 13*(1), 64–72.

O'Hagen, B., Webb, L., & Moore, K. (2004). Listening and learning from patients. *Emergency Nursing, 12*(7), 12–14.

Price, B. (2004). Conducting sensitive patient interviews. *Nursing Standard, 18*(38), 45–52, 54–55.

Purtilo, R., & Haddad, A. (2002). *Health professional and patient interaction* (6th ed.). Philadelphia, PA: W.B. Saunders.

Selye, H. (1956). *The stress of life.* New York: McGraw-Hill.

Shattel, M., & Hogan, B. (2005). Facilitating communication: How to truly understand what patients mean. *Journal of Psychosocial Nursing and Mental Health Services, 43*(10), 29–32.

Sheldon, L. K., Barret, R., & Ellington, L. (2006). Difficult communication in nursing. *Journal of Nursing Scholarship, 38*(2), 141–147.

Smith, S. (2004). Nurse practitioner consultations: Communicating with style and expertise. *Primary Health Care, 14*(10), 37–41.

Statistics Canada. (2007). *The daily, 2006 census. Immigration, citizenship, language, mobility and migration.* Retrieved February 28, 2008, from http://www.statcan.ca/Daily/English/071204/d071204a.htm

Statistics Canada. (2008). *Aboriginal peoples in Canada in 2006: Inuit, Métis and First Nations, 2006 census.* Retrieved March 10, 2008, from http://www12.statcan.ca/english/census06/analysis/aboriginal/pdf/97-558-XIE2006001.pdf

Tang, S. Y. S. (1999). Interpreter services in healthcare: Policy recommendations for healthcare agencies. *JONA: The Journal of Nursing Administration, 29*(6), 23–29.

Williams, K., Kemper, S., & Hummert, M. L. (2005). Enhancing communication with older adults: Overcoming elderspeak. *Journal of Psychosocial Nursing and Mental Health Services, 43*(5), 12–16.

Web Sites of Interest

Canadian Association for the Deaf—http://www.cad.ca/
Canadian Health Network—http://www.canadian-health-network.ca/
I Love Languages—www.ilovelanguages.com/index/php
Statistics Canada—http://cansim2.statcan.ca

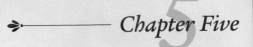

The Complete Health History

Written by **Carolyn Jarvis**, PhD, APN, CNP
Adapted by **Annette J. Browne**, PhD, RN

The purpose of the health history is to collect **subjective data**—what the person says about himself or herself. The history is combined with the **objective data** from the physical examination and with laboratory studies to form the database. The database is used to make a judgement or a diagnosis about the health status of the individual.

The following health history provides a complete picture of the person's past and present health. It describes the individual as a whole and how the person interacts with the environment. It records health strengths and coping skills. The history should recognize and affirm what the person is *doing right:* what he or she is doing to help stay well. For the well person, the history is used to assess his or her health promoting practices, including such factors as exercise, diet, risk reduction, and preventive behaviours, such as health screening.

For the ill person, the health history includes a detailed and chronological record of the health problem. For all, the health history is a screening tool for abnormal symptoms, health problems, and concerns, and it records ways of responding to the health problems.

In many settings the patient fills out a printed history form or checklist. This allows the person ample time to recall and consider such items as dates of health landmarks and relevant family history. The interview is then used to validate the written data and to collect more data on lifestyle management and current health problems.

Although history forms vary, most contain information in this sequence of categories:

1. Biographical data
2. Reason for seeking care
3. Present health or history of present illness
4. Past history
5. Family history
6. Review of systems
7. Functional assessment or activities of daily living (ADLs)

The health history discussed in the following section follows this format and presents a generic database for all practitioners. Those in clinical settings may use all of it, whereas those in a hospital may focus primarily on the history of present illness and the functional, or patterns of living, data.

THE HEALTH HISTORY: THE ADULT

Biographical Data

Include the patient's name, address and phone number, age and birthdate, birthplace, gender, marital status, ethnocultural background, and occupation, usual and present (an illness or disability may have prompted a change in occupation). Note that in some healthcare agencies and institutions, the primary language spoken by the patient is recorded. Therefore, the person's primary language and authorized representative, if any, should be recorded here. This is in response to research showing that differences in language and culture may have an impact on the quality and safety of care (Joint Commission, 2007).

Source of History

1. Record who furnishes the information—usually the person herself or himself, although the source may be a relative or friend.
2. Judge how reliable the informant seems and how willing he or she is to communicate. A reliable person always gives the same answers, even when questions are rephrased or are repeated later in the interview.
3. Note any special circumstances, such as the use of an interpreter. Sample statements include:

Patient herself, who seems reliable.
Patient's son, John Ramirez, who seems reliable.
Mrs. R. Fuentes, interpreter for Theresa Castillo who does not speak English.

Reason for Seeking Care*

The reason for seeking care is a brief, spontaneous statement in the person's own words that describes the reason for the visit. Think of it as the "title" for the story to follow. It states one (possibly two) symptoms or signs and their duration. A **symptom** is a subjective sensation that the person feels from the disorder. A **sign** is an objective abnormality that you as the examiner could detect on physical examination or in laboratory reports. Whatever the person says is the reason for seeking care is recorded, enclosed in quotation marks to indicate the person's exact words.

"Chest pain" for 2 hours.
"Earache and fussy all night."
"Need yearly physical examination for work."
"Want to start jogging and need checkup."

The patient's reason for seeking care should not be used for diagnosis. Avoid translating the patient's statement into the terms of a medical diagnosis. For example, Mr. J. Schmidt enters with shortness of breath, and you ponder writing "emphysema." Even if he is known to have emphysema from previous visits, it is not the chronic emphysema that prompted *this visit,* but rather the "increasing shortness of breath" for 4 hours.

Some people try to self-diagnose based on similar signs and symptoms in their relatives or friends, or based on conditions they know they have. Rather than record a woman's statement that she has "strep throat," ask her what symptoms she has that make her think this is present and record those symptoms.

Occasionally a person may list *many* reasons for seeking care. The most important reason to the person may not necessarily be the one stated first. Try to focus on which is the most pressing concern by asking the person which one prompted him or her to seek help *now.*

Present Health or History of Present Illness

For the well person, present health is a short statement about the general state of health.

For the ill person, this section is a chronological record of the reason for seeking care, from the time the symptom first started until now. Isolate each reason for care identified by the person and say, for example, "Please tell me all about your headache, from the time it started until the time you came to the hospital." If the concern started months or years ago, record what occurred during that time and find out why the person is seeking care *now.*

---

*In the past, this statement was called the "Chief Complaint" (CC). This title is avoided now because it labels the person a "complainer" and, more importantly, does not include wellness needs.

As the person talks, do not jump to conclusions and bias the story by adding your opinion. Collect *all* the data first. Although you want the person to respond in a narrative format without interruption from you, your final summary of any symptom the person has should include these *eight critical characteristics:*

1. **Location.** Be specific; ask the person to point to the location. If the problem is pain, note the precise site. "Head pain" is vague, whereas descriptions such as "pain behind the eyes," "jaw pain," and "occipital pain" are more precise and are diagnostically significant. Is the pain localized to this site or radiating? Is the pain superficial or deep?

2. **Character** or **quality.** This calls for specific descriptive terms such as burning, sharp, dull, aching, gnawing, throbbing, shooting, viselike. Use similes—does blood in the stool look like sticky tar? Does blood in vomitus look like coffee grounds?

3. **Quantity** or **severity.** Attempt to quantify the sign or symptom such as "profuse menstrual flow soaking five pads per hour." The symptom of pain is difficult to quantify because of individual interpretation. What one person may identify as "terrible pain," another may describe as "not too bad." With pain, avoid adjectives and ask how it affects daily activities. Then the person might say, "I was so sick I was doubled up and couldn't move," or "I was able to go to work, but then I came home and went to bed."

4. **Timing** (onset, duration, frequency). When did the symptom first appear? Give the specific date and time, or state specifically how long ago the symptom started prior to arrival (PTA). "The pain started yesterday" will not mean much when you return to read the record in the future. The report must include questions such as: How long did the symptom last (duration)? Was it steady (constant) or did it come and go during that time (intermittent)? Did it resolve completely and reappear days or weeks later (cycle of remission and exacerbation)?

5. **Setting.** Where was the person or what was the person doing when the symptom started? What brings it on? For example, "Did you notice the chest pain after shovelling snow, or did the pain start by itself?"

6. **Aggravating** or **relieving factors.** What makes the pain worse? Is it aggravated by weather, activity, food, medication, standing bent over, fatigue, time of day, season, and so on? What relieves it (e.g., rest, medication, or ice pack)? What is the effect of any treatment? Ask, "What have you tried?" or "What seems to help?"

7. **Associated factors.** Is this primary symptom associated with any others (e.g., urinary frequency and burning associated with fever and chills)? Review the body system related to this symptom now rather than wait for the review of systems.

8. **Patient's perception.** Find out the meaning of the symptom by asking how it affects daily activities. Also ask directly, "What do you think it means?" This is crucial because it alerts you to potential anxiety if the person thinks the symptom may be ominous.

You may find it helpful to organize this same question sequence into the mnemonic **PQRSTU** to help remember all the points. Note that you still need to address the patient's perception of the problem.

P: Provocative or palliative. What brings it on? What were you doing when you first noticed it? What makes it better? Worse?

Q: Quality or quantity. How does it look, feel, sound? How intense or severe is it?

R: Region or radiation. Where is it? Does it spread anywhere?

S: Severity scale. How bad is it (on a scale of 1 to 10)? Is it getting better, worse, staying the same?

T: Timing. Onset—Exactly when did it first occur? Duration—How long did it last? Frequency—How often does it occur?

U: Understand patient's perception of the problem. What do you think it means?

Past Health

Past health events may have residual effects on the current health state. Also, the previous experience with illness may give clues as to how the person responds to illness and to the significance of illness for him or her.

Childhood Illnesses. Measles, mumps, rubella, chicken pox, pertussis, and strep throat. Avoid recording "usual childhood illnesses," because an illness common in the person's childhood (e.g., measles) may be unusual today. Ask about serious illnesses that may have sequelae for the person in later years (e.g., rheumatic fever, scarlet fever, and poliomyelitis).

Accidents or Injuries. Auto accidents, fractures, penetrating wounds, head injuries (especially if associated with unconsciousness), and burns.

Serious or Chronic Illnesses. Diabetes, hypertension, heart disease, sickle-cell anemia, cancer, and seizure disorder.

Hospitalizations. Cause, name of hospital, how the condition was treated, how long the person was hospitalized, and name of the physician.

Operations. Type of surgery, date, name of surgeon, name of hospital, and how the person recovered.

Obstetrical History. Number of pregnancies (gravidity), number of deliveries in which the fetus reached full term (term), number of preterm pregnancies (preterm), number of incomplete pregnancies (abortions), and number of children living (living). This is recorded: Grav _____ Term _____ Preterm _____ Ab _____ Living _____. For each complete pregnancy, note the course of pregnancy; labour and delivery; sex, weight, and condition of each infant; and postpartum course. For any incomplete pregnancies, record the duration and whether the pregnancy resulted in spontaneous (S) or induced (I) abortion.

Immunizations. Measles-mumps-rubella, polio, diphtheria-pertussis-tetanus, hepatitis B, human papillomavirus, *Haemophilus influenzae* type b, pneumococcal vaccine. Note the date of the last tetanus immunization, last tuberculosis skin test, and last flu shot.

Last Examination Date. Physical, dental, vision, hearing, electrocardiogram, chest X-ray examinations.

Allergies. Note both the allergen (medication, food, or contact agent, such as fabric or environmental agent) and the reaction (rash, itching, runny nose, watery eyes, difficulty breathing). With a drug, this symptom should not be a side effect but a true allergic reaction.

Current Medications. Note all prescription and over-the-counter medications. Ask specifically about vitamins, birth control pills, aspirin, and antacids, because many people do not consider these to be medications. For each medication, note the name, dose, and schedule, and ask, "How often do you take it each day?" "What is it for?" and "How long have you been taking it?" Finally, note any herbal remedies.

Family History

Ask about the age and health or the age and cause of death of blood relatives, such as parents, grandparents, and siblings. These data may have genetic significance for the patient. Also ask about close family members, such as spouse and children. You need to know about the person's prolonged contact with any communicable disease or the effect of a family member's illness on this person.

Specifically ask for any family history of heart disease, high blood pressure, stroke, diabetes, blood disorders, cancer, sickle-cell anemia, arthritis, allergies, obesity, alcoholism, mental illness, seizure disorder, kidney disease, and tuberculosis. Construct an accurate family tree, or genogram, to show this information clearly and concisely (Fig. 5-1).

🌎 CULTURAL AND SOCIAL CONSIDERATIONS

Add several questions to the complete health history for people who are new immigrants:
- Biographical data—when did they come to Canada and from what country; if they are refugees, what were the conditions under which they came here, if they underwent particularly challenging experiences, and so forth
  - The older adult may be a person who came to this country after World War II and may be a holocaust survivor—questions regarding family and past history may evoke painful memories and must be asked carefully
- Spiritual resources and religion—assess if certain procedures cannot be done, such as administering blood to a Jehovah's Witness
- Past health—what immunizations were given in their country of origin; for example, was the person given bacille Calmette-Guérin (BCG). This vaccine is used in many countries to prevent tuberculosis. If they have had BCG, they will have a positive tuberculin test and further diagnostic procedures must be done, including a sputum test and chest X-ray

Drawing Your Family Tree

- Make list of all of your family members.
- Use this sample family tree as a guide to draw your own family tree.
- Write your name at the top of your paper and date you drew your family tree.
- In place of the words father, mother, etc., write the names of your family members.
- When possible, draw your brothers and sisters and your parents' brothers and sisters starting from oldest to the youngest, going from left to right across the paper.
- If dates of birth or ages are not known, then estimate or guess ("50s," "late 60s")

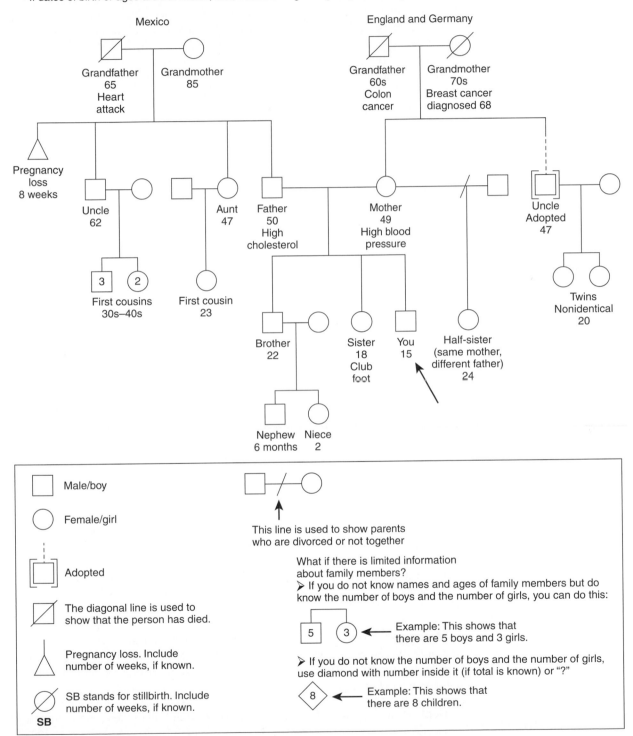

Fig. 5-1   Genogram or family tree.

- Health perception—how do they describe health and illness and what do they see as the problem they are now experiencing?
- Nutritional—what foods and food combinations are taboo?

Review of Systems

The purposes of this section are (1) to evaluate the past and present health state of each body system, (2) to double-check in case any significant data were omitted in the present illness section, and (3) to evaluate health promotion practices. The order of the examination of body systems is roughly head to toe. The items within each system are not inclusive, and only the most common symptoms are listed. If the present illness section covered one body system, you do not need to repeat all the data here. For example, if the reason for seeking care is earache, the present illness section describes most of the symptoms listed for the auditory system. Just ask now what was not asked in the present illness section.

Medical terms are listed here, but they need to be translated for the patient. (Note that symptoms and health promotion activities are merely listed here. These terms are repeated and expanded in each related physical examination chapter, along with suggested ways to pose questions and a rationale for each question.)

When recording information, avoid writing "negative" after the system heading. You need to record the *presence* or *absence* of all symptoms, otherwise the reader does not know about which factors you asked.

A common mistake made by beginning practitioners is to record some physical finding or objective data here, such as "skin warm and dry." Remember that the history should be limited to patient statements, or subjective data—factors that the person *says* were or were not present.

General Overall Health State. Present weight (gain or loss, period of time, by diet or other factors), fatigue, weakness or malaise, fever, chills, sweats or night sweats.

Skin. History of skin disease (eczema, psoriasis, hives), pigment or colour change, change in mole, excessive dryness or moisture, pruritus, excessive bruising, rash, or lesion.

Hair. Recent loss, change in texture. Nails: change in shape, colour, or brittleness.
Health Promotion. Amount of sun exposure; method of self-care for skin and hair.

Head. Any unusually frequent or severe headache, any head injury, dizziness (syncope), or vertigo.

Eyes. Difficulty with vision (decreased acuity, blurring, blind spots), eye pain, diplopia (double vision), redness or swelling, watering or discharge, glaucoma or cataracts.
Health Promotion. Wears glasses or contacts; last vision check or glaucoma test; and how coping with loss of vision if any.

Ears. Earaches, infections, discharge and its characteristics, tinnitus or vertigo.
Health Promotion. Hearing loss, hearing aid use, how loss affects daily life, any exposure to environmental noise, and method of cleaning ears.

Nose and Sinuses. Discharge and its characteristics, any unusually frequent or severe colds, sinus pain, nasal obstruction, nosebleeds, allergies or hay fever, or change in sense of smell.

Mouth and Throat. Mouth pain, frequent sore throat, bleeding gums, toothache, lesion in mouth or tongue, dysphagia, hoarseness or voice change, tonsillectomy, altered taste.
Health Promotion. Pattern of daily dental care, use of prostheses (dentures, bridge), and last dental checkup.

Neck. Pain, limitation of motion, lumps or swelling, enlarged or tender nodes, goitre.

Breast. Pain, lump, nipple discharge, rash, history of breast disease, any surgery on the breasts.
Health Promotion. Performs breast self-examination? Include its frequency and method used, last mammogram.

Axilla. Tenderness, lump or swelling, rash.

Respiratory System. History of lung diseases (asthma, emphysema, bronchitis, pneumonia, tuberculosis), chest pain with breathing, wheezing or noisy breathing, shortness of breath, how much activity produces shortness of breath, cough, sputum (colour, amount), hemoptysis, toxin or pollution exposure.

Health Promotion. Last chest X-ray study.

Cardiovascular System. Precordial or retrosternal pain, palpitation, cyanosis, dyspnea on exertion (specify amount of exertion, e.g., walking one flight of stairs, walking from chair to bath, or just talking), orthopnea, paroxysmal nocturnal dyspnea, nocturia, edema, history of heart murmur, hypertension, coronary artery disease, anemia.

Health Promotion. Date of last electrocardiogram (ECG) or other heart tests.

Peripheral Vascular System. Coldness, numbness and tingling, swelling of legs (time of day, activity), discoloration in hands or feet (bluish red, pallor, mottling, associated with position, especially around feet and ankles), varicose veins or complications, intermittent claudication, thrombophlebitis, ulcers.

Health Promotion. Does the work involve long-term sitting or standing? Avoid crossing legs at the knees. Wear support hose.

Gastrointestinal System. Appetite, food intolerance, dysphagia, heartburn, indigestion, pain (associated with eating), other abdominal pain, pyrosis (esophageal and stomach burning sensation with sour eructation), nausea and vomiting (character), vomiting blood, history of abdominal disease (ulcer, liver or gallbladder, jaundice, appendicitis, colitis), flatulence, frequency of bowel movement, any recent change, stool characteristics, constipation or diarrhea, black stools, rectal bleeding, rectal conditions (hemorrhoids, fistula).

Health Promotion. Use of antacids or laxatives. (Alternatively, diet history and substance habits can be placed here.)

Urinary System. Frequency, urgency, nocturia (the number of times the person awakens at night to urinate, recent change), dysuria, polyuria or oliguria, hesitancy or straining, narrowed stream, urine colour (cloudy or presence of hematuria), incontinence, history of urinary disease (kidney disease, kidney stones, urinary tract infections, prostate), pain in flank, groin, suprapubic region, or low back.

Health Promotion. Measures to avoid or treat urinary tract infections, use of Kegel exercises after childbirth.

Male Genital System. Penis or testicular pain, sores or lesions, penile discharge, lumps, hernia.

Health Promotion. Performs testicular self-examination? How frequently?

Female Genital System. Menstrual history (age at menarche, last menstrual period, cycle and duration, any amenorrhea or menorrhagia, premenstrual pain or dysmenorrhea, intermenstrual spotting), vaginal itching, discharge and its characteristics, age at menopause, menopausal signs or symptoms, postmenopausal bleeding.

Health Promotion. Last gynecological checkup and last Papanicolaou (Pap) test.

Sexual Health. Presently in a relationship involving intercourse? Are the aspects of sex satisfactory to the patient and partner? Any dyspareunia (for female), any changes in erection or ejaculation (for male), and use of contraceptive? Is the contraceptive method satisfactory? Aware of contact with a partner who has any sexually transmitted infection (STI) (e.g., gonorrhea, herpes, chlamydia, venereal warts, HIV or AIDS, or syphilis)?

Musculoskeletal System. History of arthritis or gout. In the joints: pain, stiffness, swelling (location, migratory nature), deformity, limitation of motion, noise with joint motion? In the muscles: any pain, cramps, weakness, gait problems or problems with coordinated activities? In the back: any pain (location and radiation to extremities), stiffness, limitation of motion, or history of back pain or disc disease?

Health Promotion. How much walking per day? What is the effect of limited range of motion on daily activities, such as on grooming, eating, toileting, dressing? Are any mobility aids used?

Neurological System. History of seizure disorder, stroke, fainting, blackouts. In motor function: weakness, tic or tremor, paralysis, or coordination problems. In sensory function: numbness and tingling (paraesthesia). In cognitive function: memory disorder (recent or distant, disorientation). In mental status: any nervousness, mood change, depression, or any history of mental health dysfunction or hallucinations.

Health Promotion. Alternatively, data about interpersonal relationships, coping patterns placed here.

Hematological System. Bleeding tendency of skin or mucous membranes, excessive bruising, lymph node swelling, exposure to toxic agents or radiation, blood transfusion and reactions.

Endocrine System. History of diabetes or diabetic symptoms (polyuria, polydipsia, polyphagia), history of thyroid disease, intolerance to heat and cold, change in skin pigmentation or texture, excessive sweating, relationship between appetite and weight, abnormal hair distribution, nervousness, tremors, and need for hormone therapy.

Functional Assessment (Including Activities of Daily Living)

Functional assessment measures a person's self-care ability in the areas of general physical health or absence of illness; activities of daily living (ADLs), such as bathing, dressing, toileting, eating, walking; instrumental activities of daily living (IADLs), or those needed for independent living, such as housekeeping, shopping, cooking, doing laundry, using the telephone, managing finances; nutrition; social relationships and resources; self-concept and coping; and home environment.

Functional assessment may mean organizing the entire assessment around functional "pattern areas" (Gordon, 2002). Instruments that emphasize functional categories may help in leading to a nursing diagnosis.

Functional assessment may also mean that the health history may be supplemented by a standardized instrument on functional assessment. Instruments such as The Katz Index of Activities of Daily Living (see Fig. 30-1) and the Lawton Instrumental Activities of Daily Living Scale (see Fig. 30-2) objectively measure a person's present functional status and monitor any changes over time (Granger et al., 1995; Mahoney & Barthel, 1965; Pearlman, 1987).

Whether or not you use any of these formalized instruments, functional assessment questions such as those listed in the following section should be included in the standard health history. These questions provide data on the lifestyle and type of living environment to which the person is accustomed. Since some of the data may be judged private by the individual, the questions are best asked at this later point in the interview after you have had time to establish rapport.

Self-Esteem, Self-Concept. Education (last grade completed, other significant training), financial status (income adequate and health or social concerns), value–belief system (religious practices and perception of personal strengths).

Activity and Mobility. A daily profile reflecting usual daily activities: ask, "Tell me how you spend a typical day." Note ability to perform ADLs: independent or needs assistance with feeding, bathing, hygiene, dressing, toileting, bed-to-chair transfer, walking, standing, or climbing stairs. Any use of wheelchair, prostheses, or mobility aids?

Record leisure activities enjoyed and the exercise pattern (type, amount per day or week, method of warm-up session, method of monitoring the body's response to exercise).

Sleep and Rest. Sleep patterns, daytime naps, any sleep aids used.

Nutrition and Elimination. Record the diet by a recall of all food and beverages taken over the last 24 hours (see Chapter 11 for suggested method of inquiry). "Is that menu typical of most days?" Describe eating habits and current appetite. Ask, "Who buys food and prepares food?" "Are your finances adequate for food?" "Who is present at mealtimes?" Indicate any food allergy or intolerance. Record daily intake of caffeine (coffee, tea, cola drinks).

Ask about usual pattern of bowel elimination and urinating including problems with mobility or transfer in toileting, continence, use of laxatives.

Interpersonal Relationships and Resources. Social roles: "How would you describe your role in the family?" "How would you say you get along with family, friends, and co-workers?" Ask about support systems composed of family and significant others: "To whom could you go for support with a problem at work, with a health problem, or a personal problem?" Include contact with spouse, siblings, parents, children, friends, organizations, workplace: "Is time spent alone pleasurable and relaxing, or isolating?"

Spiritual Resources. Many people believe in a relationship between spirituality and health, and they may wish to have spiritual matters addressed in the traditional healthcare setting. Use the faith, influence, community, and address (FICA) questions to incorporate the person's spiritual values into the health history (Post et al., 2000). *Faith:* "Does religious faith or spirituality play an important part in your life? Do you consider yourself to be a religious or spiritual person?" *Influence:* "How does your religious faith or spirituality influence the way you think about your health or the way you care for yourself?" *Community:* "Are you a part of any religious or spiritual community or congregation?" *Address:* "Would you like me to address any religious or spiritual issues or concerns with you?"

Coping and Stress Management. Kinds of stresses in life, especially in the last year, any change in lifestyle or any current stress, methods tried to relieve stress, and if these have been helpful.

Smoking History. "Do you smoke cigarettes (pipe, use chewing tobacco)?" "At what age did you start?" "How many packs do you smoke per day?" "How many years have you smoked?" Record the number of packs smoked per day (PPD) and duration, for example, 1 PPD $\times$ 5 years. Then ask, "Have you ever tried to quit?" and "How did it go?" to introduce plans about smoking cessation.

Alcohol. Healthcare professionals often fail to question about alcohol unless problems are obvious. However, alcohol interacts adversely with all medications; is a factor in many social problems such as assaults, rapes, high-risk sexual behaviour, and child abuse; contributes to half of all fatal traffic accidents and is among the top three risk factors contributing to the burden of disease, disability, and death (compared with tobacco at 12% and high blood pressure at 11%) (National Alcohol Strategy, 2007). Over 30% of alcohol-related motor vehicle collisions involved people under the age of 25 (Canadian Institute for Health Information [CIHI], 2005).

Be alert, then, to early signs of hazardous alcohol use. Ask whether the person drinks alcohol. If yes, ask specific questions about the amount and frequency of alcohol use: "When was your last drink of alcohol?" "How much did you drink that time?" "Out of the last 30 days, about how many days would you say that you drank alcohol?" "Have you ever had a drinking problem?"

You may wish to use a screening questionnaire to identify excessive or uncontrolled drinking, such as the Alcohol Use Disorder Identification Test (AUDIT) (Volk et al., 1997), the Cut down, Annoyed, Guilty, and Eye-opener (**CAGE**) test (Ewing, 1984), or the TWEAK alcohol screening questions (**T**olerance, **W**orried, **E**ye-opener, **A**mnesia, and **K**/Cut down), which includes five questions and is often used to screen for alcohol use in pregnant women (Dell et al., 2006; About.com, Inc., 2007). The CAGE test asks:

- Have you ever thought you should **C**ut down your drinking?
- Have you ever been **A**nnoyed by criticism of your drinking?
- Have you ever felt **G**uilty about your drinking?
- Do you drink in the morning? (i.e., an **E**ye-opener?)

If the person answers "yes" to two or more CAGE questions, you should suspect alcohol abuse and continue with a more complete substance abuse assessment. If the person answers "no" to drinking alcohol, ask the reason for this decision (psychosocial, legal, health). Any history of alcohol treatment? Involvement in recovery activities? History of family member with problem drinking?

Drug Use. Ask specifically about marijuana, cocaine, crack cocaine, amphetamines, heroin, methadone, benzodiazepines, barbiturates, crystal methamphetamine, Ecstasy (3,4-methylenedioxymethamphetamine), phencyclidine (PCP), and other drugs. Indicate frequency of use and how usage has affected work or family.

Environmental Hazards. Housing and neighbourhood (living alone, knowledge of neighbours), safety of area, adequate heat and utilities, access to transportation, and involvement in community services. Note environmental health, including hazards in workplace, hazards at home, use of seatbelts, geographical or occupational exposures, and travel or residence in other countries, including time spent abroad during military service.

Intimate Partner Violence. Begin with open-ended questions. Convey openness and listen in a nonjudgemental manner. "How are things going at home (or at school or work)?" "How are things at home affecting your health?" "Is your home (or work or school) environment safe?" These are valuable questions for all patients. Specifically, in relation to intimate partner violence, people may not recognize their situation as abusive, or may be reluctant to discuss their situation due to guilt, fear, or shame. Follow each person's lead to inquire more specifically. If you sense that violence is an issue, use the strategies discussed in Chapter 7.

Occupational Health. Ask the person to describe his or her job. Ever worked with any health hazard, such as asbestos, inhalants, chemicals, repetitive motion? Wear any protective equipment? Any work programs in place that monitor exposure? Aware of any health problems now that may be related to work exposure?

Note the timing of the reason for seeking care, and whether it may be related to work or home activities, job titles, or exposure history. Take a careful smoking history, which may contribute to occupational hazards. Finally, ask the person what he or she likes or dislikes about the job.

Perception of Health

Ask the person questions such as: "How do you define health?" "How do you view your situation now?" "What are your concerns?" "What do you think will happen in the future?" "What are your health goals?" "What do you expect from us as nurses, nurse practitioners, physicians, or other healthcare professionals?"

 DEVELOPMENTAL CARE

Children

The health history is adapted to include information specific for the age and developmental stage of the child (e.g., the mother's health during pregnancy, labour and delivery, and the perinatal period). Note that the developmental history and nutritional data are listed as separate sections because of their importance for current health.

Biographical Data

Include the child's name, nickname, address and phone number, parents' names and work numbers, child's age and birthdate, birthplace, gender, race, ethnic origin, and information on other children and family members at home.

Source of History

1. Person providing information and relation to child
2. Your impression of reliability of information
3. Any special circumstances, for example, the use of an interpreter

Reason for Seeking Care

Record the parent's spontaneous statement. Because of the frequency of well child visits for routine health care, there will be more reasons such as "time for the child's checkup" or "she needs the next baby shot." Reasons for health problems may be initiated by the child, parent, or by a third party such as the classroom teacher.

Sometimes the reason stated may not be the real reason for the visit. A parent may have a "hidden agenda," such as the mother who brought her 4-year-old child in because "she looked pale." Further questioning revealed that the mother had heard recently from a former college friend whose own 4-year-old child had just been diagnosed with leukemia.

Present Health or History of Present Illness

If the parent or child seeks routine health care, include a statement about the usual health of the child and any common health problems or major health concerns.

Describe any presenting symptom or sign, using the same format as for the adult. Some additional considerations include:

- Severity of pain: "How do you know the child is in pain?" (e.g., pulling at ears alerts parent to ear pain). Note effect of pain on usual behaviour (e.g., does it stop child from playing?).
- Associated factors, such as relation to activity, eating, and body position.
- The parent's intuitive sense of a problem. As the constant caregiver, this intuitive sense is often very accurate. Even if proved otherwise, this factor gives you an idea of parent's area of concern.
- Parent's coping ability and reaction of other family members to child's symptoms or illness.

Past Health

Prenatal Status. How was this pregnancy spaced? Was it planned? What was the mother's attitude toward the pregnancy? What was the father's attitude? Was there medical supervision for the mother? At what month was the supervision started? What was the mother's health during pregnancy? Were there any complications (bleeding, excessive nausea and vomiting, unusual weight gain, high blood pressure, swelling of hands and feet, infections [rubella or STIs], falls)? During what month were diet and medications prescribed or taken during pregnancy (dose and duration)? Record the mother's use of alcohol, street drugs, or cigarettes and any X-ray studies taken during pregnancy.

Start with an open-ended question: "Tell me about your pregnancy." If she questions the relevancy of the statement, mention that these questions are important to gain a complete picture of the child's health.

Labour and Delivery. Parity of the mother, duration of the pregnancy, name of the hospital, course and duration of labour, use of anaesthesia, type of delivery (vertex, breech, Caesarean section), birth weight, Apgar scores, onset of breathing, any cyanosis, need for resuscitation, and use of special equipment or procedures.

Postnatal Status. Any problems in the nursery, length of hospital stay, neonatal jaundice, whether the baby was discharged with the mother, whether the baby was breast- or bottle-fed, weight gain, any feeding problems, "blue spells," colic, diarrhea, patterns of crying and sleeping, the mother's health postpartum, and the mother's reaction to the baby.

Childhood Illnesses. Age and any complications of measles, mumps, rubella, chicken pox, whooping cough, strep throat, and frequent ear infections. Also, any recent exposure to illness.

Serious Accidents or Injuries. Age of occurrence, extent of injury, how the child was treated, and complications of auto accidents, falls, head injuries, fractures, burns, and poisonings.

Serious or Chronic Illnesses. Age of onset, how the child was treated, and complications of meningitis or encephalitis; seizure disorders; asthma, pneumonia, and other chronic lung conditions; rheumatic fever; scarlet fever; diabetes; kidney problems; sickle-cell anemia; high blood pressure; and allergies.

Operations or Hospitalizations. Reason for care, age at admission, name of surgeon or healthcare professional, name of hospital, duration of stay, how child reacted to hospitalization, and any complications. (If child reacted poorly, he or she may be afraid now and will need special preparation for the examination that is to follow.)

Immunizations. Age when administered, date administered, and any reactions following immunizations. Appendix A on the Evolve Web site lists suggested immunization schedules.

Allergies. Any drugs, foods, contact agents, and environmental agents to which the child is allergic, and reaction to allergen. Note allergic reactions particularly common in childhood, such as allergic rhinitis, insect hypersensitivity, eczema, and urticaria.

Medications. Any prescription and over-the-counter medications (or vitamins) the child takes, including the dose, daily schedule, why the medication is given, and any problems.

Developmental History

Growth. Height and weight at birth and at 1, 2, 5, and 10 years, any periods of rapid growth or weight loss, and process of dentition (age of tooth eruption and pattern of loss).

Milestones. Age when child first held head erect, rolled over, sat alone, walked alone, cut his or her first tooth, said his or her first words with meaning, spoke in sentences, was toilet trained, tied shoes, dressed without help. Does the parent believe this development has been normal? How does this child's development compare with siblings or peers?

Current Development (Children 1 Month Through Preschool). Gross motor skills (rolls over, sits alone, walks alone, skips, climbs), fine motor skills (inspects hands, brings hands to mouth, pincer grasp, stacks blocks, feeds self, uses crayon to draw, uses scissors), language skills (vocalizes, first words with meaning, sentences, persistence of baby talk, speech problems), and personal–social skills (smiles, tracks movement with eyes to midline, past midline, attends to sound by turning head, recognizes own name). If the child is undergoing toilet training, indicate the method used, age at which bladder and bowel controlled, parents' attitude toward toilet training, and terms used for toileting.

School-Age Child. Gross motor skills (runs, jumps, climbs, rides bicycle, general coordination), fine motor skills (ties shoelace, uses scissors, writes name and numbers, draws pictures), and language skills (vocabulary, verbal ability, able to tell time, reading level).

Nutritional History

The amount of nutritional information needed depends on the child's age; the younger the child is, the more detailed and specific the data should be. For the infant, record whether breastfeeding or bottle-feeding is used. If the child is breastfed, record nursing frequency and duration, any supplements (vitamin, iron, fluoride, bottles), family support for nursing, and age and method of weaning. If the child is bottle-fed, record type of formula used, frequency and amount, any problems with feeding (spitting up, colic, diarrhea), supplements used, and any bottle propping. Record introduction of solid foods (age when the child began eating solids, which foods, whether foods are home or commercially made, amount given, child's reaction to new food, parent's reaction to feeding).

For preschool- and school-age children and adolescents, record the child's appetite, 24-hour diet recall (meals, snacks, amounts), vitamins taken, how much junk food is eaten, who eats with the child, food likes and dislikes, and parent's perception of child's nutrition.

A week-long diary of food intake may be more accurate than a spot 24-hour recall. Also, consider cultural practices in assessing child's diet.

Family History

As with the adult, diagram a family tree for the child, including siblings, parents, and grandparents. Give the age, health, or age and cause of death of each. Ask specifically for the family history of heart disease, high blood pressure, diabetes, blood disorders, cancer, sickle-cell anemia, arthritis, allergies, obesity, cystic fibrosis, alcoholism, mental illness, seizure disorder, kidney disease, intellectual disability, learning disabilities, birth defects, and sudden infant death. (When interviewing the mother, ask about the "child's father," not "your husband," in case of the separation of the child's biological parents.)

Review of Systems

General. Significant gain or loss of weight, failure to gain weight appropriate for age, frequent colds, ear infections, illnesses, energy level, fatigue, overactivity, and behaviour change (irritability, increased crying, nervousness).

Skin. Birthmarks, skin disease, pigment or colour change, mottling, change in mole, pruritus, rash, lesion, acne, easy bruising or petechiae, easy bleeding, and changes in hair or nails.

Head. Headache, head injury, dizziness.

Eyes. Strabismus, diplopia, pain, redness, discharge, cataracts, vision changes, reading problems. Is the child able to see the board at school? Does the child sit too close to the television?
Health Promotion. Use of eyeglasses, date of last vision screening.

Ears. Earaches, frequency of ear infections, myringotomy tubes in ears, discharge (characteristics), cerumen, ringing or crackling, and whether parent perceives any hearing problems.
Health Promotion. How does the child clean his or her ears?

Nose and Sinuses. Discharge and its characteristics, frequency of colds, nasal stuffiness, nosebleeds, and allergies.

Mouth and Throat. History of cleft lip or palate, frequency of sore throats, toothache, caries, sores in mouth or tongue, tonsils present, mouth breathing, difficulty chewing, difficulty swallowing, and hoarseness or voice change.
Health Promotion. Child's pattern of brushing teeth and last dental checkup.

Neck. Swollen or tender glands, limitation of movement, or stiffness.

Breast. For preadolescent and adolescent girls, when did they notice that their breasts were changing? What is the girl's self-perception of development? For older adolescents, does the girl perform breast self-examination? (See Chapter 17 for suggested phrasing of questions.)

Respiratory System. Croup or asthma, wheezing or noisy breathing, shortness of breath, chronic cough.

Cardiovascular System. Congenital heart problems, history of murmur, and cyanosis (what prompts this condition). Is there any limitation of activity, or can the child keep up with peers? Is there any dyspnea on exertion, palpitations, high blood pressure, or coldness in the extremities?

Gastrointestinal System. Abdominal pain, nausea and vomiting, history of ulcer, frequency of bowel movements, stool colour and characteristics, diarrhea, constipation or stool-holding, rectal bleeding, anal itching, history of pinworms, and use of laxatives.

Urinary System. Painful urination, polyuria or oliguria, narrowed stream, urine colour (cloudy, dark), history of urinary tract infection, whether toilet trained, when toilet training was planned, any problems, bedwetting (when the child started, frequency, associated with stress, how child feels about it).

Male Genital System. Penis or testicular pain, whether told if testes are descended, any sores or lesions, discharge, hernia or hydrocele, or swelling in scrotum during crying. For the preadolescent and adolescent boy, has he noticed any change in the penis and scrotum? Is the boy familiar with normal growth patterns, nocturnal emissions, and sex education? Screen for sexual abuse. (See Chapter 24 for suggested phrasing of questions.)

Female Genital System. Has the girl noted any genital itching, rash, vaginal discharge? For the preadolescent and adolescent girl, when did menstruation start? Was she prepared? Screen for sexual abuse. (See Chapter 26 for suggested phrasing of questions.)

Sexual Health. What is the child's attitude toward the opposite sex? Who provides sex education? How does the family deal with sex education, masturbation, dating patterns? Is the adolescent in a relationship involving intercourse? Does he or she have information on birth control and STIs? (See Chapters 24 and 26 for suggested phrasing of questions.)

Musculoskeletal System. In bones and joints: arthritis, joint pain, stiffness, swelling, limitation of movement, gait strength, and coordination. In muscles: pain, cramps, and weakness. In the back: pain, posture, spinal curvature, and any treatment.

Neurological System. Numbness and tingling. (Behaviour and cognitive issues are covered in the sections on development and interpersonal relationships.)

Hematological Systems. Excessive bruising, lymph node swelling, and exposure to toxic agents or radiation.

Endocrine System. History of diabetes or thyroid disease; excessive hunger, thirst, or urinating; abnormal hair distribution; and precocious or delayed puberty.

Functional Assessment (Including Activities of Daily Living)

Interpersonal Relationships. Within the family constellation, record the child's position in family; whether the child is adopted; who lives with the child; who is the primary caretaker; who is the caretaker if both parents work outside of the home; any support from relatives, neighbours, or friends; and the ethnic or cultural milieu.

Indicate family cohesion. Does the family enjoy activities as a unit? Has there been a recent family change or crisis (death, divorce, move)? Record information on child's self-image and level of independence. Does the child use a security blanket or toy? Is there any repetitive behaviour (bed-rocking, head-banging), pica, thumb-sucking, or nail-biting? Note method of discipline used. Indicate type used at home. How effective is it? Who disciplines the child? Is there any occurrence of negativism, temper tantrums, withdrawal, or aggressive behaviour?

Provide information on the child's friends: whether the child makes friends easily. How does the child get along with friends? Does he or she play with same-age or older or younger children?

Activity and Rest. Record the child's play activities. Indicate amount of active and quiet play, outdoor play, time watching television, and special hobbies or activities. Record sleep and rest. Indicate pattern and number of hours at night and during the day and the child's routine at bedtime. Is the child a sound sleeper, or is he or she wakeful? Does the child have nightmares, night terrors, or somnambulation? How does the parent respond? Does the child have naps during the day?

Record school attendance. Has the child had any experience with daycare or nursery school? In what grade is the child in school? Has the child ever skipped a grade or been held back? Does the child seem to like school? What is his or her school performance? Are the parent and child satisfied with the performance? Were days missed in school? Provide a reason for the absence. (These questions give an important index to child's functioning outside the home.)

Economic Status. Ask about the parent(s)' occupation. Indicate the number of hours each parent is away from home. Do parents perceive their income as adequate? What is the effect of illness on financial status?

Home Environment. Where does family live (house, apartment)? Is the size of the home adequate? Is there access to an outdoor play area? Does the child share a room, have his or her own bed, and have toys appropriate for his or her age?

Environmental Hazards. Inquire about home safety (precautions for poisons, medications, household products, presence of gates for stairways, and safe yard equipment). Provide information on the child's residence (adequate heating, ventilation, bathroom facilities), neighbourhood (residential or industrial, age of neighbours, safe play areas, playmates available, distance to school, amount of traffic, is area remote or congested and overcrowded, is crime a problem, presence of air or water pollution), and automobile (child safety seat, seatbelts).

Coping and Stress Management. Does the child have the ability to adapt to new situations? Record recent stressful experiences (death, divorce, move, loss of special friend). How does the child cope with stress? Has there been any recent change in behaviour or mood? Has counselling ever been sought?

Smoking and Drug Use. Has the child ever tried cigarette smoking? How much did he or she smoke? Has the child ever tried alcohol? How much alcohol did he or she drink weekly or daily? Has the child ever tried other drugs (marijuana, cocaine, amphetamines, barbiturates)?

Health Promotion. Who is the healthcare professional? When was the child's last checkup? Who is the dental care provider, and when was the last dental checkup? Provide date and result of screening for vision, hearing, urinalysis, phenylketonuria, hematocrit, tuberculosis skin test, sickle-cell trait, blood lead, and other tests specific to high-risk populations.

The Adolescent

This section presents a psychosocial review of symptoms intended to maximize communication with youth. The **HEEADSSS** method of interviewing focuses on assessment of the Home environment, Education and employment, Eating, peer-related Activities, Drugs, Sexuality, Suicide or depression, and Safety from injury and violence (Fig. 5-2). The tool minimizes adolescent stress because it moves from expected and less-threatening questions to those that are more personal. The tool presents the questions in three colours: green are considered essential to explore with every adolescent; blue are important for you to ask if time permits; red questions delve in more deeply if the situation demands it (Goldenring & Rosen, 2004). Interview the youth alone, while the parent waits outside and fills out past health questionnaires.

The HEEADSSS psychosocial interview for adolescents

Home
Who lives with you? Where do you live? Do you have your own room?
What are relationships like at home?
To whom are you closest at home?
To whom can you talk at home?
Is there anyone new at home? Has someone left recently?
Have you moved recently?
Have you ever had to live away from home? (Why?)
Have you ever run away? (Why?)
Is there any physical violence at home?

Education and employment
What are your favourite subjects at school? Your least favourite subjects?
How are your grades? Any recent changes? Any dramatic changes in the past?
Have you changed schools in the past few years?
What are your future education and employment plans and goals?
Are you working? Where? How much?
Tell me about your friends at school.
Is your school a safe place? (Why?)
Have you ever had to repeat a class? Have you ever had to repeat a grade?
Have you ever been suspended? Expelled? Have you ever considered dropping out?
How well do you get along with the people at school? Work?
Have your responsibilities at work increased?
Do you feel connected to your school? Do you feel as if you belong?
Are there adults at school you feel you could talk to about something important? (Who?)

Eating
What do you like and not like about your body?
Have there been any recent changes in your weight?
Have you dieted in the last year? How? How often?
Have you done anything else to try to manage your weight?
How much exercise do you get in an average day? Week?
What do you think would be a healthy diet? How does that compare to your current eating patterns?
Do you worry about your weight? How often?
Do you eat in front of the TV? Computer?
Does it ever seem as though your eating is out of control?
Have you ever made yourself throw up on purpose to control your weight?
Have you ever taken diet pills?
What would it be like if you gained (lost) 10 pounds?

Activities
What do you and your *friends* do for fun? (with whom, where, and when?)
What do you and your *family* do for fun? (with whom, where, and when?)
Do you participate in any sports or other activities?
Do you regularly attend a church group, club, or other organized activity?
Do you have any hobbies?
Do you read for fun? (What?)
How much TV do you watch in a week? How about video games?
What music do you like to listen to?

Drugs
Do any of your friends use tobacco? Alcohol? Other drugs?
Does anyone in your family use tobacco? Alcohol? Other drugs?
Do you use tobacco? Alcohol? Other drugs?
Is there any history of alcohol or drug problems in your family?
Do you ever drink or use drugs when you're alone?
(Assess frequency, intensity, patterns of use or abuse, and how youth obtains or pays for drugs, alcohol, or tobacco.)

Sexuality
Have you ever been in a romantic relationship?
Tell me about the people that you've dated. *OR* Tell me about your sex life.
Have any of your relationships ever been sexual relationships?
Are your sexual activities enjoyable?
What does the term "safer sex" mean to you?
Are you interested in boys? Girls? Both?
Have you ever been forced or pressured into doing something sexual that you didn't want to do?
Have you ever been touched sexually in a way that you didn't want?
Have you ever been raped, on a date or any other time?
How many sexual partners have you had altogether?
Have you ever been pregnant or worried that you might be pregnant? (females)
Have you ever impregnated someone or worried that that might have happened? (males)
What are you using for birth control? Are you satisfied with your method?
Do you use condoms every time you have intercourse?
Does anything ever get in the way of always using a condom?
Have you ever had an STIs or worried that you had an STI?

Suicide and depression
Do you feel sad or down more than usual? Do you find yourself crying more than usual?
Are you "bored" all the time?
Are you having trouble getting to sleep?
Have you thought a lot about hurting yourself or someone else?
Does it seem that you've lost interest in things that you used to really enjoy?
Do you find yourself spending less and less time with friends?
Would you rather just be by yourself most of the time?
Have you ever tried to kill yourself?
Have you ever had to hurt yourself (by cutting yourself, for example) to calm down or feel better?
Have you started using alcohol or drugs to help you relax, calm down, or feel better?

Safety (savagery)
Have you ever been seriously injured? (How?) How about anyone else you know?
Do you always wear a seatbelt in the car?
Have you ever ridden with a driver who was drunk or high? When? How often?
Do you use safety equipment for sports and other physical activities (e.g., helmets for biking or skateboarding)?
Is there any violence in your home? Does the violence ever get physical?
Is there a lot of violence at your school? In your neighbourhood? Among your friends?
Have you ever been physically or sexually abused? Have you ever been raped, on a date or at any other time? (If not asked previously)
Have you ever been in a car or motorcycle accident? (What happened?)
Have you ever been picked on or bullied? Is that still a problem?
Have you participated in physical fights in school or your neighbourhood? Are you still getting into fights?
Have you ever felt that you had to carry a knife, gun, or other weapon to protect yourself? Do you still feel that way?

Green = essential questions
Blue = as time permits
Red = optional or when situation requires

Fig. 5-2

The Older Adult

This health history for the older adult includes the same format as that described for the younger adult, as well as some additional questions. These questions address ways in which the ADLs may have been affected by normal aging processes or by the effects of chronic illness or disability. There is no specific age at which to ask these additional questions. Use them when it seems appropriate.

It is important for you to recognize positive health measures: what the person has been doing to help himself or herself stay well and to live to an older age. Older people have spent a lifetime with a traditional healthcare system that searches only for pathology and what is wrong with their health. It may be a pleasant surprise to have a health professional affirm the things that they are "doing right" and to note health strengths.

As you study the following, keep in mind the format for the "younger" adult. Only *additional* questions or a varying focus is addressed here.

Reason for Seeking Care

It may take time to figure out the reason that the older person has come in for an examination. An aging person may shrug off a symptom as evidence of growing old and may be unsure whether it is "worth mentioning." Also, some older people have a conservative philosophy toward their health status: "If it isn't broken, don't fix it." These people come for care only when something is blatantly wrong.

An older person may have many chronic problems, such as diabetes, hypertension, or constipation. It is challenging to filter out what brought the person in this time. The final statement should be the *person's* reason for seeking care, not your assumption of what the problem is.

Past Health

General Health. Health state over the last 5 years.

Accidents or Injuries, Serious or Chronic Illnesses, Hospitalizations, Operations. These areas may produce lengthy responses, and the person probably will not relate them in chronological order. Let the person talk freely; you can reorder the events later when you prepare the write-up. The amount of data included here can indicate the amount of stress the person has faced during his or her lifetime. This section of the history can be filled out at home or before the interview if the person's vision and writing ability are adequate. Then you can concentrate remaining time of the interview on reviewing pertinent data and on the present health of the person.

Last Examination. Most recent mammography, colonoscopy, and tonometry.

Obstetrical Status. It is *not* necessary to collect a detailed account of each pregnancy and delivery if the woman has passed menopause and has no gynecological symptoms. Merely record the number of pregnancies and the health of each newborn.

Current Medications. For each medication, record the name, purpose, and daily schedule. Does the person have a system in place to remember to take the medicine? Does medicine seem to work? Are there any side effects? If so, does the person feel like skipping medicine because of them? Also consider the following issues:

- Some older persons take a large number of drugs, prescribed by different physicians.
- The person may not know drug name or purpose. When this occurs, ask the person to bring in the drug to be identified.
- Is cost a problem? When the person is unable to afford a drug, he or she may decrease the dosage, take one pill instead of two, or not refill the empty bottle immediately.
- Is travelling to the pharmacy to refill a prescription a problem?
- Is the person taking any over-the-counter medications? Some people use a local pharmacist for self-treatment.
- Has the person ever shared medications with neighbours or friends? Some establish "lay referral" networks by comparing symptoms and thus medications.

Family History

Family history is not as useful in predicting which familial diseases the person may contract because most of those will have occurred at an earlier age. But these data are useful to assess which diseases or causes of death of relatives the person has experienced. Also it describes the person's existing social network.

Review of Systems

Remember that these are *additional* items to question for the older adult. Refer to the history for the younger adult for the basic list.

General. Present weight and what the person would like to weigh (gives idea of body image).

Skin. Change in sensation to pain, heat, or cold.

Eyes. Use of bifocal glasses, any trouble adjusting to far vision (problems with stairs).

Ears. Increased sensitivity to background noise and whether conversation sounds garbled or distorted.

Mouth. Use of dentures, when the person wears them (always, all day, only at meals, only at social occasions, or never), method of cleaning, any difficulty wearing the dentures (loose, pain, makes whistling or clicking noise), cracks at corners of the mouth.

Respiratory System. Shortness of breath and level of activity that produces it. Shortness of breath often is an early sign of cardiac dysfunction, but many older people dismiss it as "a cold" or getting "winded" because of old age.

Cardiovascular System. If chest pain occurs, the person may not feel it as intensely as a younger person. Instead, the older adult may feel dyspnea on exertion.

Peripheral Vascular System. Wears constrictive clothing, garters, or rolls stockings at knees. Any colour change at feet or ankles.

Urinary System. Urinary retention, incomplete emptying, straining to urinate, change in force of stream. If a weakened stream occurs, men may note the need to stand closer to the toilet. Women may note incontinence when coughing, laughing, or sneezing.

Sexual Health. Ask about any changes in sexual relationship the person has experienced. Note that for men it is normal for an erection to develop slowly. (See Chapter 24.) For women, note any comments about vaginal dryness or pain with intercourse. Note for all whether aspects of sex are satisfactory and whether adequate privacy exists for sexual relationship.

Musculoskeletal System. Gait change (balance, weakness, difficulty with steps, fear of falling), use of any assistive device (cane, walker). Any joint stiffness? During what part of the day does the stiffness occur? Does pain or stiffness occur with activity or rest?

Neurological System. Any problem with memory (recent or remote) or disorientation (time of day, in what settings)?

Functional Assessment (Including Activities of Daily Living)

Functional assessment measures how a person manages day-to-day activities. For older people, the meaning of health becomes those activities that they can or cannot do. The *impact* of a disease on their daily activities and overall quality of life (called the *disease burden*) is more important to older people than the actual disease diagnosis or pathology. Thus the functional assessment—because it emphasizes function—is very important in assessing older people.

Many functional assessment instruments are available that objectively measure a person's present functional status and monitor any changes over time. Most instruments measure the performance of specific tasks such as the ADLs and IADLs. The Comprehensive Older Person's Evaluation (Table 5-1) is particularly useful because it contains the basic ADL and IADL functional assessment as well as physical, social, psychological, demographic, financial, and legal issues.

Whether or not a standardized instrument is used, the following functional assessment questions are important additions to the older adult's health history.

Self-Concept, Self-Esteem. When the aging person was an adolescent, educational opportunities were not as available as they are today, nor were they equally available for women. The aging person may be sensitive about having achieved only the level of elementary school education or less.

Occupation. Past positions, volunteer activities, and community activities. Many people continue to work past the age of 65; they grew up with a strong work ethic and are proud to continue. If the person is retired, how has he or she adjusted to the change in role? It may mean loss of social role or social status, loss of personal relationships formed at work, and reduced income.

Activity and Mobility. How does the person spend a typical day in work, hobbies, and leisure activities? Is there any day this routine changes (e.g., Sunday visits from family)? Note that the person suffering from chronic illness or disability may have a self-care deficit, musculoskeletal changes, such as arthritis, and mental confusion.

List significant leisure activities, hobbies, sports, and community activities. Is there a community senior citizen centre available for nutrition, social network, and screening of health status?

What is the type, amount, and frequency of the exercise? Is a warm-up included? How does the body respond?

Sleep and Rest. Usual sleep pattern: feel rested during the day? Is energy sufficient to carry out daily activities? Need naps? Is there a problem with night wakenings (nocturia, shortness of breath, light sleep, insomnia [difficulty falling asleep, awakening during night, early morning wakening])? If no routine, tend to nap all afternoon? Does insomnia worsen with lack of a daily schedule?

Nutrition and Elimination. Record a 24-hour recall of the diet. Is this typical of most days? (Nutrition may vary greatly. Ask the person to keep a weekly log to bring in.) What are the meal patterns? Are there three full meals or five to six smaller meals per day? How many convenience foods and soft foods are used? Who prepares meals? Eat alone? Who shops for food? How are groceries transported home? Is the income adequate for groceries? Is there a problem preparing meals (adequate vision, motor deficit, adequate energy)? Are the appliances and water and utilities adequate for meal preparation? Is there any difficulty chewing or swallowing? What are the food preferences (aging persons often eat high amounts of carbohydrates because these foods are cheaper, easier to make, and easier to chew)?

Interpersonal Relationships and Resources. Who else is at home with the person? Live alone? Is this satisfactory? Have a pet? How close are family or friends? How often does the person see family or friends? If infrequent, is this experienced as a loss?

Does the person live with family, such as a spouse, children, or a sibling? Is this a satisfactory arrangement? What is the role in family for preparation of meals, housework, and other activities? Are there any conflicts?

On whom does the person depend for emotional support? For help with problems? Who meets affection needs?

Coping and Stress Management. Has there been a recent change in living conditions or social circumstances, such as loss of occupation, spouse, or friends; move from home; illness of self or family member; or decrease in income? How dealing with stress? If a loved one has died, how responding to the loss? "How do you feel about being 'alone' and having to take on unfamiliar responsibilities now?"

Environmental Hazards. Home safety: one floor or are there stairs, state of repair, is money adequate to maintain home, are there exits for fire, heating and utilities adequate, how long in the present home? Transportation: own automobile, last driver's test, consider self a safe driver, income adequate for maintenance, public transportation access, receive drives from community resources, friends? Neighbourhood: secure in personal safety at day or night; danger of loss of possessions; amount of noise and pollution; access to family and friends, grocery store, drug store, laundry, church, temple, mosque, health-care facilities?

| TABLE 5-1 | Comprehensive Older Person's Evaluation |

Name (print): _____   Date of Visit: _____

Chief complaint: _____

Today I will ask you about your overall health and function and will be using a questionnaire to help me obtain this information. The first few questions are to check your memory.

Preliminary Cognition Questionnaire: *Record if answer is correct with (+); if answer is incorrect, with (−). Record total number of errors.*

	(+, −)
1) What is the date today?	_____
2) What day of the week is it?	_____
3) What is the name of this place?	_____
4) What is your telephone number or room number? *(record answer: _____)* *If subject does not have phone, ask:* What is your street address?	_____
5) How old are you? *(record answer: _____)*	_____
6) When were you born? *(record answer from records if patient cannot answer: _____)*	_____
7) Who is the prime minister of Canada now?	_____
8) Who was the prime minister just before him?	_____
9) What was your mother's maiden name?	_____
10) Subtract 3 from 20 and keep subtracting from each new number you get, all the way down.	_____

Total errors   _____

If more than 4 errors, ask #11. If more than 6 errors, complete questionnaire from informant.

11) Do you think you would benefit from a legal guardian, someone who would be responsible for your legal and financial matters?
  Do you have a living will? Would you like one?
  a) No
  b) Has functioning legal guardian for sole purpose of managing money
    (describe: _____)
  c) Has legal guardian
  d) Yes

Demographic Section
1) Patient's ethnocultural background *(record: _____)*
2) Patient's gender *(circle)*   Male   Female
3) How far did you go in school?
  a) Postgraduate education
  b) 4-year degree
  c) College or technical school
  d) High school complete
  e) High school incomplete
  f) 0–8 years

Social Support Section: Now there are a few questions about your family and friends.
4) Are you married, widowed, separated, divorced, or have you never been married?
  a) Now married
  b) Widowed
  c) Separated
  d) Divorced
  e) Never married
5) Who lives with you? *(circle all responses)*
  a) Spouse
  b) Other relative or friend *(specify: _____)*
  c) Group living situation (nonhealth)
  d) Lives alone
  e) Nursing home, number of years

6) Have you talked to any friends or relatives by phone during the last week?
  a) Yes
  b) No
7) Are you satisfied by seeing your relatives and friends as often as you want to, or are you somewhat dissatisfied about how little you see them?
  a) Satisfied *(skip to #8)*
  b) No *(ask A)*
    A) Do you feel you would like to be involved in a senior citizens centre for social events, or perhaps meals?
      1) No
      2) Is involved *(describe: _____)*
      3) Yes
8) Is there someone who would take care of you for as long as you needed if you were sick or disabled?
  a) Yes *(skip to C)*
  b) No *(ask A)*
    A) Is there someone who would take care of you for a short time?
      1) Yes *(skip to C)*
      2) No *(ask B)*
    B) Is there someone who could help you now and then?
      1) Yes *(ask C)*
      2) No *(ask C)*
    C) Whom would we call in case of an emergency?
      (record name and telephone: _____
      _____)

Financial Section
9) Do you own, or are you buying, your own home?
  a) Yes *(skip to #10)*
  b) No *(ask A)*
    A) Do you feel you need assistance with housing?
      1) No
      2) Has subsidized or other housing assistance
      3) Yes *(describe: _____)*
    B) What type of housing did you have prior to coming here?
10) Are you covered by private medical insurance, Medicare, or some disability plan? *(circle all that apply)*
  a) Private insurance *(specify and skip to #11):)*
  b) Medicare
  c) Disability *(specify and ask A: _____)*
  d) None
  e) Other *(specify: _____)*
    A) Do you feel you need additional assistance with your medical bills?
      1) No
      2) Yes
11) Which of these statements best describes your financial situation?
  a) My bills are no problem to me *(skip to #12)*
  b) My expenses make it difficult to meet my bills *(ask A)*
  c) My expenses are so heavy that I cannot meet my bills *(ask A)*
    A) Do you feel that you need financial assistance such as: *(circle all that apply)*
      1) Assistance to obtain enough food
      2) Social assistance
      3) Assistance in paying your heating or electrical bills
      4) Other financial assistance *(describe: _____)*

Adapted with permission from Pearlman, R. (1987). Development of a functional assessment questionnaire for geriatric patients: COPE. *Journal of Chronic Diseases, 40*, 85S–94S. With permission from Elsevier.

TABLE 5-1	Comprehensive Older Person's Evaluation—cont'd

Psychological Health Section: The next few questions are about how you feel about your life in general. There are no right or wrong answers, only what best applies to you. Please answer yes or no to each question.

	Yes	No
12) Is your daily life full of things that keep you interested?	____	____
13) Have you, at times, very much wanted to leave home?	____	____
14) Does it seem that no one understands you?	____	____
15) Are you happy most of the time?	____	____
16) Do you feel weak all over much of the time?	____	____
17) Is your sleep fitful and disturbed?	____	____

18) Taking everything into consideration, how would you describe your satisfaction with your life in general at the present time—good, fair, or poor?
   a) Good
   b) Fair
   c) Poor

19) Do you feel you now need help with your mental health; for example, a counsellor or psychiatrist?
   a) No
   b) Has (specify: _____)
   c) Yes

Physical Health Section: The next few questions are about your health.

20) During the past month (30 days), how many days were you so sick that you couldn't do your usual activities, such as working around the house or visiting with friends?

21) Relative to other people your age, how would you rate your overall health at the present time: excellent, good, fair, poor, or very poor?
   a) Excellent (skip to #22)
   b) Very good (skip to #22)
   c) Good (ask A)
   d) Fair (ask A)
   e) Poor (ask A)
      A) Do you feel you need additional medical services such as a doctor, nurse, visiting nurse, or physical therapist? (circle all that apply)
         1) Doctor
         2) Nurse
         3) Visiting nurse
         4) Physical therapist
         5) None

22) Do you use an aid for walking, such as a wheelchair, walker, cane, or anything else? (circle aid usually used)
   a) Wheelchair
   b) Other (specify: _____)
   c) Visiting nurse
   d) Walker
   e) None

23) How much do your health troubles stand in the way of your doing things you want to do: not at all, a little, or a great deal?
   a) Not at all (skip to #24)
   b) A little (ask A)
   c) A great deal (ask A)
      A) Do you think you need assistance to do your daily activities; for example, do you need a live-in aide or choreworker?
         1) Live-in aide
         2) Choreworker
         3) Has aide, choreworker, or other assistance (describe: _____)
         4) None needed

24) Have you had, or do you currently have, any of the following health problems? If yes, place an "X" in appropriate box and describe; medical record information may be used to help complete this section.

	HX	CURRENT	DESCRIBE
a) Arthritis or rheumatism?			
b) Lung or breathing problem?			
c) Hypertension?			
d) Heart trouble?			
e) Phlebitis or poor circulation problems in arms or legs?			
f) Diabetes or low blood sugar?			
g) Digestive ulcers?			
h) Other digestive problem?			
i) Cancer?			
j) Anemia?			
k) Effects of stroke?			
l) Other neurological problem? (specify: _____)			
m) Thyroid or other glandular problem? (specify: _____)			
n) Skin disorders such as pressure sores, leg ulcers, burns?			
o) Speech problem?			
p) Hearing problem?			
q) Vision or eye problem?			
r) Kidney or bladder problems, or incontinence?			
s) A problem of falls?			
t) Problem with eating or your weight? (specify: _____)			
u) Problem with depression or your nerves? (specify: _____)			
v) Problem with your behaviour (specify: _____ _____)			
w) Problem with your sexual activity?			
x) Problem with alcohol?			
y) Problem with pain?			
z) Other health problems? (specify: _____)			

Immunizations: _____

25) What medications are you currently taking, or have been

Continued

TABLE 5-1 | **Comprehensive Older Person's Evaluation—cont'd**

taking, in the last month? (May I see your medication bottles?) *(If patient cannot list, ask categories a–r and note dosage and schedule, or obtain information from medical or pharmacy records and verify accuracy with the patient.)*

Allergies:

	Rx (DOSAGE AND SCHEDULE)
a) Arthritis medication	
b) Pain medication	
c) Blood pressure medication	
d) Water pills or pills for fluid	
e) Medication for your heart	
f) Medication for your lungs	
g) Blood thinners	
h) Medication for your circulation	
i) Insulin or diabetes medication	
j) Seizure medication	
k) Thyroid pills	
l) Steroids	
m) Hormones	
n) Antibiotics	
o) Medicine for nerves or depression	
p) Prescription sleeping pills	
q) Other prescription drugs	
r) Other nonprescription drugs	

26) Many people have problems remembering to take their medications, especially ones they need to take on a regular basis. How often do you forget to take your medications? Would you say you forget often, sometimes, rarely, or never?
   a) Never   c) Sometimes
   b) Rarely   d) Often

Activities of Daily Living: The next set of questions asks whether you need help with any of the following activities of daily living.

27) I would like to know whether you can do these activities without any help at all, or if you need assistance to do them. Do you need help to: *(If yes, describe, including patient needs.)*

	YES	NO	DESCRIBE (INCLUDE NEEDS)
a) Use the telephone?			
b) Get to places out of walking distance (using transportation)?			
c) Shop for clothes and food?			
d) Do your housework?			
e) Handle your money?			
f) Feed yourself?			
g) Dress and undress yourself?			
h) Take care of your appearance?			
i) Get in and out of bed?			
j) Take a bath or shower?			
k) Prepare your meals?			
l) Do you have any problem getting to the bathroom on time?			

28) During the past 6 months, have you had any help with such things as shopping, housework, bathing, dressing, and getting around?
   a) Yes *(specify: _____)*
   b) No

Signature of person completing the form:

_____

BIBLIOGRAPHY

Bennett, R. L., Steinhaus, K. A., Ulrich, S. B., O'Sullivan, C. K., Resta, R. G., Lochner-Doyle, D., et al. (1995). Recommendations for standardized human pedigree nomenclature. Pedigree Standardization Task Force of the National Society of Genetic Counselors. *American Journal of Human Genetics, 56*(3), 745–752.

Berry, T. A., & Shooner, K. A. (2004). Family history—The first genetic screen. *Nursing Practice, 29*(11), 14–25.

Canadian Institute for Health Information. (2005). *More than half of all alcohol-related severe injuries due to motor vehicle collisions.* Retrieved Feb 12, 2008, from, http://secure.cihi.ca/cihiweb/dispPage.jsp?cw_page=media_22jun2005_e

Dell, A. C., & Roberts, G. (2006). *Research update: Alcohol use and pregnancy: An important Canadian public health and social issue* (Catalogue No. HP10-5/2006E). Ottawa, ON: Health Canada.

Ewing, J. A. (1984). Detecting alcoholism: The CAGE questionnaire. *Journal of the American Medical Association, 252,* 1905–1907.

Goldenring, J. M., & Rosen, D. S. (2004). Getting into adolescent heads: An essential update. *Contemporary Pediatrics, 21*(1), 64–75.

Gordon, M. (2002). *Manual of nursing diagnosis* (10th ed.). St. Louis, MO: Mosby.

Granger, C. V., Ottenbacher, K. J., Baker, J. G., & Ashok, S. (1995). Reliability of a brief outpatient functional outcome assessment measure. *American Journal of Physical Medicine, 74,* 469–475.

Joint Commission. (2007). *Hospitals, language, and culture.* Retrieved September 8, 2007, from http://www.jointcommission.org/PatientSafety/HLC/

Lesser, J. M., Hughes, S. V., Jemelka, J. R., & Kumar, S. (2005). Challenges and strategies for taking a comprehensive history in the elderly. *Geriatrics, 60*(11), 22–25.

Mahoney, F. I., & Barthel, D. W. (1965). Functional evaluation: The Barthel Index. *Maryland State Medical Journal, 14,* 61–65.

National Alcohol Strategy. (2007). *Reducing alcohol-related harm in Canada: Toward a culture of moderation. Recommendations for a national alcohol strategy.* Ottawa, ON: National Alcohol Strategy Working Group.

Parve, J. (2004). Remove vaccination barriers for children 12 to 24 months. *Nurse Practitioner, 29*(4), 35–38.

Pearlman, R. (1987). Development of a functional assessment questionnaire for geriatric patients: The comprehensive older person's evaluation (COPE). *Journal of Chronic Disease, 40,* 85S–94S.

Post, S. G., Puchalski, C. M., & Larson, D. B. (2000). Physician and patient spirituality: professional boundaries, competency, and ethics. *Annals of Internal Medicine, 132,* 578–583.

Public Health Agency of Canada. (2006). *Canadian immunization guide* (7th ed.). Retrieved February 12, 2008, from http://www.phac-aspc.gc.ca/publicat/cig-gci/index-eng.php

Reece, S. M. (2006). The 3rd National Family history initiative: Thanksgiving 2006. *Nurse Practitioner, 31*(11), 57–59.

About.com, Inc., a part of *The New York Times Company. TWEAK Alcohol Screening Test.* (2007). Retrieved May 23, 2008, from http://alcoholism.about.com/od/tests/a/tweak.htm

Volk, R. J., Steinbauer, J. R., Cantor, S. B., & Holzer, C. E. (1997). The Alcohol Use Disorders Identification Test (AUDIT) as a screen for at-risk drinking in primary care patients of different racial/ethnic backgrounds. *Addiction 92,* 197–206.

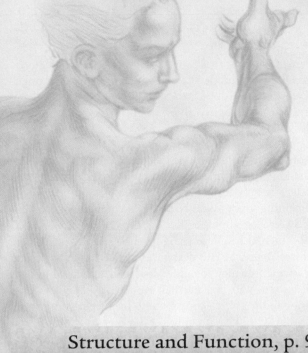

Mental Status Assessment

Written by **Carolyn Jarvis**, PhD, APN, CNP
Adapted by **Wendy Stanyon**, RN, Ed(D)

Structure and Function, p. 94

Defining Mental Status
Screening
Components of the Mental Status Examination

Objective Data, p. 96

Appearance
Behaviour
Cognitive Functions
Thought Processes and Perceptions
Supplemental Mental Status Examination

Documentation and Critical Thinking, p. 105

Abnormal Findings, p. 106

Abnormal Findings for Advanced Practice, p. 109

Electronic Resources

On Evolve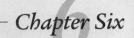

http://evolve.elsevier.com/Canada/Jarvis/examination/

- Interactive Case Studies
- Physical Examination Audio and Printable Summaries
- Bedside Assessment Summary Checklists
- Complete Physical Examination Form
- Nursing Diagnoses Boxes
- Health Promotion Guides
- Quick Assessments for 20 Common Conditions
- Multiple Choice Review Questions
- Chapter Objectives
- Appendices
- Weblinks

On the Companion CD

- Interactive Case Studies with Heart and Lung Sounds
- Health Promotion Guides
- Quick Assessments for 20 Common Conditions
- Head-to-Toe Physical Examination Video Clips

STRUCTURE AND FUNCTION

The World Health Organization (WHO) estimates that five of every 10 disabilities worldwide are mental health disorders. With one in five Canadians experiencing a mental health challenge during their lifetime, mental illness is not only a global health issue but also a major public health concern for this country.

At any given time 10.4% of Canadians are experiencing a mental illness (Health Canada, 2002). A variety of factors influence a person's mental health. Some are internal, some come from within the person's social network, and others are related to the individual's broader community. This "broader community" includes not only the healthcare and mental healthcare systems but also other sectors such as the economy, education, and housing. For example, according to Statistics Canada (2001), on any given night in 2001, more than 10,000 people in Canada were living in shelters. The Canadian Institute for Health Information conducted an extensive review of the literature related to mental health and homelessness. Its 2007 report, titled *Improving the Health of Canadians: Mental Health and Homelessness*, describes the pathways into homelessness. Clearly homelessness does not discriminate; it affects youth, men and women, one- and two-parent families, older adults, new immigrants, and Aboriginal people. No single circumstance influences an individual's mental health; rather, people are affected by a complex series of interacting factors. As such, strategies to improve the mental health of Canadians require active involvement from all community sectors.

In addition to internal, familial, and community influences, a person's mental health may be affected by larger social issues such as poverty, racism, and other forms of discrimination. As a culturally diverse country, Canada's population includes many immigrants as well as a large number of Aboriginal groups. People who are members of these groups often face unique challenges in terms of maintaining cultural, social, and economic integrity as important building blocks for mental health. Without adequate social resources or access to needed services, the stressors experienced by some ethnocultural and social groups in Canada can lead to increases in mental illnesses and suicide. For example, although there are great variations across communities, bands, and nations, the suicide rate among First Nations communities is twice as high as that of the general population, while the rate among Inuit is six to 11 times higher (Kirmayer et al., 2007; Public Health Agency of Canada [PHAC], 2006). These disturbingly high rates stem from the complex interplay of social determinants of health, intergenerational and historical traumas, and ongoing discrimination.

DEFINING MENTAL STATUS

Mental status is a person's emotional and cognitive functioning. Optimal functioning aims toward simultaneous life satisfaction in work, in caring relationships, and within the self. A variety of factors, including the physical environment and personal, social, cultural, and socioeconomic characteristics, can influence mental health, which is relative and ongoing. Everyone has "good" and "bad" days. Usually, mental status strikes a balance, allowing the person to function socially and occupationally.

The stress surrounding a traumatic life event (death of a loved one, serious illness) tips the balance, causing transient dysfunction. This is an expected response to a trauma. Mental status assessment during a traumatic life event can identify remaining strengths and can help the individual mobilize resources and use coping skills.

Good mental health is recognized as more than just the absence of illness. WHO describes mental health as a state of well-being in which the individual realizes his or her own abilities, copes with the normal stresses of life, works productively, and is able to contribute to his or her community (2007). PHAC (2006) broadly defines mental health as the capacity to feel, think, and behave in ways that enhance a person's ability to manage challenges and enjoy life. Characteristics indicative of mental health include finding enjoyment and balance in life, and demonstrating resilience, flexibility, and self-actualization (Canadian Mental Health Association, 2008). Some individuals are more mentally healthy than others, and a person's mental health can vary over time, depending on life circumstances.

A **mental illness** is a biological condition of the brain that causes alterations in thinking, mood, or behaviour (or any combination thereof) and is associated with significant distress and impaired daily functioning (PHAC, 2006). A complex interplay of many factors including genetics, biology, personality, socioeconomic status, and life events contribute to the development of a mental illness. Mental illness is not a single disease but a broad classification of many different disorders including disorders of thought, mood, or behaviour. The terms *mental illness* and *mental disorder* are often used interchangeably.

Mental illnesses are common and account for a large percentage of hospital stays every year. Mental illness also does not discriminate; anyone can be affected. Most Canadians, if they have not experienced a mental illness themselves, know someone who has been diagnosed with a mental illness.

Mental status assessment documents dysfunction and determines how that dysfunction affects self-care in everyday life. Mental status cannot be scrutinized directly as can heart sounds or the characteristics of the skin. Its functioning is inferred through an assessment of an individual's behaviours:

Consciousness: being aware of one's own existence, feelings, thoughts, and environment. This is the most elementary of mental status functions.

Language: using the voice to communicate one's thoughts and feelings. This is a basic tool of humans, and its loss has a heavy social impact on the individual.

Mood and affect: both of these elements deal with the prevailing feelings; **affect** is a temporary expression of feelings or state of mind, and **mood** is more durable, a prolonged display of feelings that colours the whole emotional life.

Orientation: the awareness of the objective world in relation to the self.

Attention: the power of concentration, the ability to focus on one specific thing without being distracted by many environmental stimuli.

Memory: the ability to lay down and store experiences and perceptions for later recall. *Recent* memory evokes day-to-day events; *remote* memory brings up years' worth of experiences.

Abstract reasoning: pondering a deeper meaning beyond the concrete and literal.

Thought process: the *way* a person thinks, the logical train of thought.

Thought content: *what* the person thinks—specific ideas, beliefs, the use of words.

Perceptions: an awareness of objects through the five senses.

 ## DEVELOPMENTAL CARE

Infants and Children

The maturation of emotional and cognitive functioning is described in detail in Chapter 2. It is difficult to separate and trace the development of just one aspect of mental status. All aspects are interdependent. For example, consciousness is rudimentary at birth because the cerebral cortex is not yet developed; the infant cannot distinguish the self from the mother's body. Consciousness gradually develops along with language, so that by 18 to 24 months the child learns that he or she is separate from objects in the environment and has words to express this. We also can trace language development: from the differentiated crying at 4 weeks, the cooing at 6 weeks, through one-word sentences at 1 year to multiword sentences at 2 years. Yet the concept of language as a social tool of communication occurs around 4 to 5 years of age, coincident with the child's readiness to co-operatively play with other children.

Attention gradually increases in span through preschool years so that, by school age, most children are able to sit and concentrate on their work for a period of time. Some children are late in developing concentration. School readiness coincides with the development of the thought process; around age 7, thinking becomes more logical and systematic, and the child is able to reason and understand. Abstract thinking, the ability to consider a hypothetical situation, usually develops between ages 12 and 15, although a few adolescents never achieve it.

The Aging Adult

The aging process leaves the parameters of mental status mostly intact. There is no decrease in general knowledge and little or no loss in vocabulary. Response time is slower than in youth; it takes a bit longer for the brain to process information and react to it. Thus performance on timed intelligence tests may be lower for the older adult—not because intelligence has declined, but because it takes longer to respond to the questions. The slower response time affects new learning; if a new presentation is rapidly paced, the older person does not have time to respond to it (Birren & Schaie, 2005).

Recent memory, which requires some processing (e.g., medication instructions, 24-hour diet recall, names of new acquaintances), is somewhat decreased with aging. Remote memory is not affected.

Age-related changes in sensory perception can affect mental status. For example, vision loss (as detailed in Chapter 14) may result in apathy, social isolation, and depression. Hearing changes are common in older adults (see the discussion of presbycusis in Chapter 15). Age-related hearing loss involves high sound frequencies. Consonants are high-frequency sounds, so older adults who have difficulty hearing them have problems with normal conversation. This problem produces frustration, suspicion, and social isolation, and also makes the person look confused.

The era of older adulthood contains more potential for loss than do earlier eras, such as loss of loved ones, loss of job status and prestige, loss of income, and the loss of an energetic and resilient body. The grief and despair surrounding these losses can affect mental status, and result in disorientation, disability, or depression.

SCREENING

In 2005 the Canadian Task Force on Preventative Health Care re-examined the literature on the benefits of screening for depression in primary care settings. After an extensive, systematic review, the task force concluded that there is fair evidence to support routine screening for depression in the general population in primary healthcare settings as a way of improving detection rates (MacMillan et al., 2005). In studies in which the screening process was linked to an integrated system of treatment and follow-up, there was improvement in patient outcomes. A number of screening tools exist; however, there is some evidence to suggest that asking two simple questions regarding mood and anhedonia—"Over the past 2 weeks, have you felt down, depressed, or hopeless?" and "Over the past 2 weeks, have you felt little interest or pleasure in doing things?"—may be as effective as more thorough assessment tools (MacMillan et al., 2005).

COMPONENTS OF THE MENTAL STATUS EXAMINATION

The full mental status examination is a systematic check of emotional and cognitive functioning. However, the steps described here rarely need to be taken in their entirety. Usually, you can assess mental status through the context of the health history interview. During that time, keep in mind the four main headings of mental status assessment:

Appearance, Behaviour, Cognition,
and Thought processes, or
A, B, C, T

Integrating the mental status examination into the health history interview is sufficient for most people. You will collect ample data to be able to assess mental health strengths and coping skills, and to screen for any dysfunction.

It is necessary to perform a full mental status examination when you discover any abnormality in affect or behaviour, and in the following situations:

- Family members concerned about a person's behavioural changes, such as memory loss, inappropriate social interaction.
- Brain lesions (trauma, tumour, brain attack [also known as cerebrovascular accident or stroke]). A mental status assessment documents any emotional or cognitive change associated with the lesion. Not recognizing these changes hinders care planning and creates problems with social readjustment.
- Aphasia (the impairment of language ability secondary to brain damage). A mental status examination assesses language dysfunction as well as any emotional problems associated with it, such as depression or agitation.
- Symptoms of psychiatric mental illness, especially with acute onset.

In every mental status examination, note these factors from the health history that could affect your interpretation of the findings:

- Any known illnesses or health problems, such as alcoholism or chronic renal disease.
- Current medications the side effects of which may cause confusion or depression.
- The usual educational and behavioural level—note that factor as the normal baseline, and do not expect performance on the mental status examination to exceed it.
- Responses to personal history questions, indicating current stress, social interaction patterns, sleep habits, drug and alcohol use.

In the following examination, the sequence of steps forms a *hierarchy* in which the most basic functions (consciousness, language) are assessed first. The first steps must be accurately assessed to ensure validity for the steps that follow. That is, if consciousness is clouded, then the person cannot be expected to have full attention and to co-operate with new learning. Or, if language is impaired, subsequent assessment of new learning or abstract reasoning (anything that requires language functioning) can give erroneous conclusions.

OBJECTIVE DATA

EQUIPMENT NEEDED
(Occasionally)
Pencil, paper, reading material

Normal Range of Findings	**Abnormal Findings**

APPEARANCE

Posture. *Posture* is erect and *position* is relaxed.

> Sitting on edge of chair or curled in bed, tense muscles, frowning, darting watchful eyes, restless pacing occur with anxiety and with hyperthyroidism. Sitting slumped in chair, slow walk and dragging feet occur with depression and some organic brain diseases.

Body Movements. *Body movements* are voluntary, deliberate, coordinated, and smooth and even.

> Restless, fidgety movements, or hyperkinetic appearance occurs with anxiety.
> Apathy and psychomotor slowing occur with depression and organic brain disease.
> Abnormal posturing and bizarre gestures occur with schizophrenia.
> Facial grimaces.

Dress. *Dress* is appropriate for setting, season, age, gender, and social group. Clothing fits and is put on appropriately.

> Inappropriate dress can occur with organic brain syndrome.
> Eccentric dress combination and bizarre makeup occur with schizophrenia or manic syndrome.

Normal Range of Findings	Abnormal Findings

Grooming and Hygiene. The person is clean and well groomed; hair is neat and clean; women have moderate or no makeup; men are shaved, or beard or mustache is well groomed. Nails are clean (though some jobs leave nails chronically dirty). Note: A dishevelled appearance in a previously well-groomed person is significant. Use care in interpreting clothing that is dishevelled, bizarre, or in poor repair, piercings, and tattoos, because these sometimes reflect the person's economic status or a deliberate fashion trend (especially among adolescents).

Unilateral neglect (total inattention to one side of body) occurs following some cerebrovascular accidents.

Inappropriate dress, poor hygiene, and lack of concern with appearance occur with depression and severe Alzheimer's disease. Meticulously dressed and groomed appearance and fastidious manner may occur with obsessive–compulsive disorders.

BEHAVIOUR

Level of Consciousness. The person is awake, alert, aware of stimuli from the environment and within the self, and responds appropriately to stimuli.

Lethargic, obtunded (Table 6-3 on p. 106).

Facial Expression. The look is appropriate to the situation and changes appropriately with the topic. There is comfortable eye contact unless precluded by cultural norm, e.g., for members of some Aboriginal cultures.

Flat, masklike expression occurs with parkinsonism and depression.

Speech. Judge the quality of speech by noting that the person makes laryngeal sounds effortlessly and shares conversation appropriately.

The pace of the conversation is moderate, and stream of talking is fluent.

Dysphonia is abnormal volume, pitch; (Table 6-4 on p. 107).
Monopolizes interview. Silent, secretive, or uncommunicative.
Slow, monotonous speech with parkinsonism, depression. Rapid-fire, pressured, and loud talking occur with manic syndrome.

Articulation (ability to form words) is clear and understandable.

Dysarthria is distorted speech (see Table 6-4, p. 107). Misuse of words; omits letters, syllables, or words; transposes words; occurs with aphasia. Circumlocution, or repetitious abnormal patterns: neologism, echolalia (Table 6-6 on p. 109).
Unduly long word-finding or failure in word search occurs with aphasia.

Word choice is effortless and appropriate to educational level. The person completes sentences, occasionally pausing to think.

Mood and Affect. Judge this by body language and facial expression, and by asking directly, "How do you feel today," or "How do you usually feel?" The mood should be appropriate to the person's place and condition and change appropriately with topics. The person is willing to co-operate with you.

See Table 6-5 on p. 108. Wide mood swings occur with manic syndrome. Altered mood states are apparent in schizophrenia. Heightened emotional activity or severely limited emotional responses.

COGNITIVE FUNCTIONS

Orientation. You can discern orientation through the course of the interview, or ask for it directly, using tact. "Some people have trouble keeping up with the dates while in the hospital. Do you know today's date?" Assess:

Time: day of week, date, year, season
Place: where person lives, present location, type of building, name of city and province
Person: own name, age, who examiner is, type of worker

Many hospitalized people normally have trouble with the exact date but are fully oriented on the remaining items.

Disorientation occurs with organic brain disorders, such as delirium and dementia. Orientation is usually lost in this order—first to time, then to place, and rarely to person.

Normal Range of Findings	Abnormal Findings
Attention Span. Check the person's ability to concentrate by noting whether he or she completes a thought without wandering. Note any distractibility or difficulty attending to you. Or, give a series of directions to follow and note the correct sequence of behaviours, such as, "Please take this glass of water with your left hand, drink from it, shift it to your right hand, and set it on the table." Note that attention span commonly is impaired in people who are anxious, fatigued, or drug intoxicated.	Digression from initial thought. Irrelevant replies to questions. Easily distracted; "stimulus bound," that is, any new stimulus quickly draws attention. Confusion, negativism.
Recent Memory. Assess recent memory in the context of the interview by the 24-hour diet recall or by asking the time the person arrived at the agency. Ask questions you can corroborate. This screens for the occasional person who confabulates or makes up answers to fill in the gaps of memory loss.	Recent memory deficit occurs with organic disorders, such as delirium, dementia, amnestic syndrome, or Korsakoff's syndrome in chronic alcoholism.
Remote Memory. In the context of the interview, ask the person verifiable past events; for example, ask to describe past health, the first job, birthday and anniversary dates, and historical events that are relevant for that person.	Remote memory is lost when cortical storage area for that memory is damaged, such as in Alzheimer's dementia or any disease that damages the cerebral cortex.

New Learning—The Four Unrelated Words Test. This tests the person's ability to lay down new memories. It is a highly sensitive and valid memory test. It requires more effort than does the recall of personal or historical events. It also avoids the danger of unverifiable material.

Say to the person, "I am going to say four words. I want you to remember them. In a few minutes I will ask you to recall them." To be sure that the person has understood, have the words repeated. Pick four words with semantic and phonetic diversity:

1. brown   1. fun
2. honesty   2. carrot
3. tulip   3. ankle
4. eyedropper 4. loyalty

After 5 minutes, ask for the recall of the four words. To test the duration of memory, ask for a recall at 10 minutes and at 30 minutes. The normal response for persons under 60 years is an accurate three- or four-word recall after a 5-, 10-, and 30-minute delay (Strub & Black, 2000).

> People with Alzheimer's dementia score a zero- or one-word recall. Impaired new learning ability also occurs with anxiety (due to inattention and distractibility) and depression (due to a lack of interest or motivation).

Additional Testing for Persons With Aphasia

Word Comprehension. Point to articles in the room, parts of the body, articles from pockets, and ask the person to name them.

Reading. Ask the person to read available print. Be aware that reading is related to educational level. Use caution that you are not just testing literacy.

Writing. Ask the person to make up and write a sentence. Note coherence, spelling, and parts of speech (the sentence should have a subject and verb).

> Aphasia is the loss of the ability to speak or write coherently, or to understand speech or writing, due to a brain attack (cerebral vascular accident or CVA). See Table 6-4 on p. 107.
>
> An awareness of a patient's reading and writing impairment is important in planning health teaching and rehabilitation.

Objective Data

Normal Range of Findings	Abnormal Findings

Higher Intellectual Function

Tests of higher intellectual functioning measure problem-solving and reasoning abilities. Results are closely related to the person's general intelligence and must be assessed considering educational and cultural backgrounds. These tests have been used to discriminate between organic brain disease and psychiatric disorders; errors on the tests indicate organic dysfunction.

Although they have been widely used, there is little evidence that most of these tests are valid in detecting organic brain disease. Furthermore, most of these tests have little relevance for daily clinical care. Thus, many time-honoured, standard tests of higher intellectual function are not discussed here, such as fund of general knowledge, digit span repetition, calculation, proverb interpretation and similarities to test abstract reasoning, or hypothetical situations to test judgement.

Judgement

A person exercises judgement when he or she can compare and evaluate the alternatives in a situation and reach an appropriate course of action. Rather than testing the person's response to a hypothetical situation (e.g., "What would you do if you found a stamped, addressed envelope lying on the sidewalk?"), you should be more interested in the person's judgement about daily or long-term life goals, the likelihood of acting in response to delusions or hallucinations, and the capacity for violent or suicidal behaviour.

To assess judgement in the context of the interview, note what the person says about job plans, social or family obligations, and plans for the future. Job and future plans should be realistic, considering the person's health situation. Also, ask the person to describe the rationale for personal health care, and how he or she decided about whether or not to comply with prescribed health regimens. The person's actions and decisions should be realistic.

Impaired judgement (unrealistic or impulsive decisions, wish fulfillment) occurs with intellectual disability, emotional dysfunction, schizophrenia, and organic brain disease.

THOUGHT PROCESSES AND PERCEPTIONS

Thought Processes. Ask yourself, "Does this person make sense? Can I follow what the person is saying?" The *way* a person thinks should be logical, goal directed, coherent, and relevant. The person should complete a thought.

Illogical, unrealistic thought processes. Digression from initial thought. Ideas run together. Evidence of blocking (person stops in middle of thought). See Table 6-6 on p. 109.

Thought Content. *What* the person says should be consistent and logical.

Obsessions, compulsions (Table 6-7 on p. 110).

Perceptions. The person should be consistently aware of reality. The perceptions should be congruent with yours. Ask the following questions:

- How do people treat you?
- Do other people talk about you?
- Do you feel like you are being watched, followed, or controlled?
- Is your imagination very active?
- Have you heard your name when alone?

Illusions, hallucinations (Table 6-8 on p. 110). Auditory and visual hallucinations occur with psychiatric and organic brain disease and with psychedelic drugs. Tactile hallucinations occur with alcohol withdrawal.

Normal Range of Findings

Abnormal Findings

Screen for Suicidal Thoughts. When the person expresses feelings of sadness, hopelessness, despair or grief, it is important to assess any possible risk of the person causing physical harm to himself or herself. Begin with more general questions. If you hear affirmative answers, continue with more specific questions:

- Have you ever felt so blue you thought of hurting yourself?
- Do you feel like hurting yourself now?
- Do you have a plan to hurt yourself?
- What would happen if you were dead?
- How would other people react if you were dead?

It is very difficult to question people about possible suicidal wishes, especially for beginning examiners. Examiners fear invading privacy and may have their own normal denial of death and suicide. However, the risk is far greater if you skip these questions when you have the slightest clue that they are appropriate. You may be the only healthcare professional to pick up clues of suicide risk. You are responsible for encouraging the person to talk about suicidal thoughts. Sometimes you cannot prevent a suicide when someone really wishes to kill himself or herself. However, for the people who are ambivalent, and they are the majority, you can buy time so the person can be helped to find an alternative. Share any concerns you have about a person's suicide ideation with a mental healthcare professional.

A precise suicide plan to take place in the next 24 to 48 hours using a lethal method constitutes high risk. Important clues and warning signs of suicide:
    Prior suicide attempts
    Depression, hopelessness
    Social withdrawal, running away
    Self-mutilation
    Hypersomnia or insomnia
    Slowed psychomotor activity
    Anorexia
    Verbal suicide messages (defeat, failure, worthlessness, loss, giving up, desire to kill self)
    Death themes in art, jokes, writing, behaviours
    Saying goodbye (giving away prized possessions)
    Additional content on mental disorders is listed in Table 6-9 on p. 111; Table 6-10 on p. 112; Table 6-11 on p. 113; Table 6-12 on p. 114; and Table 6-13 on p. 115.

SUPPLEMENTAL MENTAL STATUS EXAMINATION

The Folstein MiniMental State Examination (MMSE) is the most widely used cognitive screening test (Folstein et al., 1975; replicated by Depaulo et al., 1978; Table 6-1 on p. 101). A simplified scored form of the cognitive functions of the mental status examination, it is quick and easy, includes a standard set of only 11 questions, and requires only 5 to 10 minutes to administer. It is useful for both initial and serial measurements, so you can use it to demonstrate worsening or improvement of cognition over time and with treatment. It concentrates only on cognitive functioning, not mood or thought processes. It is a valid detector of organic disease; thus it is a good screening tool to detect dementia and delirium and to differentiate these from psychiatric mental illness.

In 1991 Molloy et al. proposed a Standardized MMSE (SMMSE). This version was developed to standardize administration methods, including the verbal instructions and questions to be given to patients, time limits, and scoring methods. Findings from the Molloy et al. (1991) research study comparing the SMMSE with the traditional MMSE indicated that the SMMSE was easier to administer and had an increased inter-rater reliability.

The maximum score on the test is 30; people with normal mental status average 27. Scores between 24 and 30 indicate no cognitive impairment.

Scores that occur with dementia and delirium are classified as follows: 18 to 23 = mild cognitive impairment; 0 to 7 = severe cognitive impairment.

TABLE 6-1	MiniMental State Examination

NAME OF SUBJECT _____   Age _____

NAME OF EXAMINER _____   Years of School Completed _____

Approach the patient with respect and encouragement.

Ask: Do you have any trouble with your memory?   ☐ Yes ☐ No   Date of Examination _____

May I ask you some questions about your memory?   ☐ Yes ☐ No

Score	Item

5 ( )   **TIME ORIENTATION**
Ask: What is the year _____ (1), season _____ (1),
month of the year _____ (1), date _____ (1),
day of the week _____ (1)?

5 ( )   **PLACE ORIENTATION**
Ask: Where are we now? What is the province _____ (1), city _____ (1),
part of the city _____ (1), building _____ (1),
floor of the building _____ (1)?

3 ( )   **REGISTRATION OF THREE WORDS**
Say: Listen carefully. I am going to say three words. You say them back after I stop.
Ready? Here they are . . . PONY (wait 1 second), QUARTER (wait 1 second), ORANGE (wait one second).
What were those words?
_____ (1)
_____ (1)
_____ (1)
Give 1 point for each correct answer, then repeat them until the patient learns all three.

5 ( )   **SERIAL 7s AS A TEST OF ATTENTION AND CALCULATION**
Ask: Subtract 7 from 100 and continue to subtract 7 from each subsequent remainder until I tell you to stop.
What is 100 take away 7? _____ (1)
Say: Keep Going. _____ (1), _____ (1),
_____ (1), _____ (1)

3 ( )   **RECALL OF THREE WORDS**
Ask: What were those three words I asked you to remember? Give one point for each correct answer.
_____ (1),
_____ (1),
_____ (1)

2 ( )   **NAMING**
Ask: What is this? (show pencil) _____ (1). What is this? (show watch) _____ (1).

1 ( )   **REPETITION**
Say: Now I am going to ask you to repeat what I say. Ready? No ifs, ands, or buts.
Now you say that. _____ (1)

3 ( )   **COMPREHENSION**
Say: Listen carefully because I am going to ask you to do something:
Take this paper in your left hand (1), fold it in half (1), and put it on the floor. (1)

1 ( )   **READING**
Say: Please read the following and do what it says, but do not say it aloud. (1)

Close your eyes

1 ( )   **WRITING**
Say: Please write a sentence. If patient does not respond, say: Write about the weather. (1)
_____

1 ( )   **DRAWING**
Say: Please copy this design.

TOTAL SCORE _____   Assess level of consciousness along a continuum

Alert   Drowsy   Stupor   Coma

	YES	NO		YES	NO	FUNCTION BY PROXY
Cooperative:	☐	☐	Deterioration from previous			Please record date when patient was last able to
Depressed:	☐	☐	level of functioning:	☐	☐	perform the following tasks.
Anxious:	☐	☐	Family History of Dementia:	☐	☐	Ask caregiver if patient independently handles:
Poor Vision:	☐	☐	Head Trauma:	☐	☐	
Poor Hearing:	☐	☐	Stroke:	☐	☐	
Native Language:	_____		Alcohol Abuse:	☐	☐	
			Thyroid Disease:	☐	☐	

	YES	NO	DATE
Money/Bills:	☐	☐	_____
Medication:	☐	☐	_____
Transportation:	☐	☐	_____
Telephone:	☐	☐	_____

From Folstein, M.F., Folstein, S.E., & McHugh, P.R. (1975). Mini-mental state. *Journal of Psychiatric Research, 12,* 189–198. Reprinted with permission. © 1975, 1998. Mini-Mental LLC.

Objective Data

Normal Range of Findings	Abnormal Findings

 DEVELOPMENTAL CARE

Infants and Children

The mental status assessment of infants and children covers behavioural, cognitive, and psychosocial development, and examines how the child is coping with his or her environment. Essentially, you will follow the same A-B-C-T guidelines as for the adult, with special consideration for developmental milestones. Your best examination "technique" arises from thorough knowledge of developmental milestones as described in Chapter 2. Abnormalities are often problems of *omission;* the child does not achieve a milestone you would expect.

The parent's health history, especially the sections on the developmental history and personal history, yields most of the mental status data.

In addition, the Nipissing District Developmental Screen (see Chapter 2) is a screening tool designed to help parents and caregivers monitor the growth and development of children from birth to 6 years of age. The following developmental areas are assessed: vision, hearing, communication, gross motor, fine motor, cognitive, social–emotional, and self-help skills.

The Pediatric Symptom Checklist (PSC; Table 6-2) is a brief screening questionnaire used to improve the recognition and treatment of psychosocial problems in school-aged children. It can be given to the parent when you take the history. Available in more than a dozen languages, the standard 35-item PSC form lists a broad range of emotional and behavioural concerns that reflect parents' impressions of their children's psychosocial functioning (Pagano et al., 2000).

For the adolescent, follow the same A-B-C-T guidelines as described for the adult.

The Aging Adult

It is important to conduct even a brief examination of all older people. Confusion is common in older adults and is easily misdiagnosed. Between one third and one half of older adults admitted to acute care medical and surgical services show varying degress of confusion. The chance of developing a cognitive impairment increases with the aging process. Approximately 16% of Canadians over the age of 65 will develop some impairment in cognition. For example, memory loss and degenerative brain disease such as Alzheimer's disease or another dementia will affect an additional 8% of the population. With one in three Canadians over the age of 85 being diagnosed with Alzheimer's disease or another dementia, the estimated cost to the healthcare system is $5.5 billion per year, which equates to $15 million a day. Beyond these financial costs to the system, there are also the personal costs to the individual living with dementia as well as the social costs for the family members and caregivers (Canadian Institutes of Health Research, 2007).

Check sensory status before assessing any aspect of mental status. Vision and hearing changes due to aging may alter alertness and leave the person looking confused. When older people cannot hear your questions, they may not perform up to their actual level of ability. One group of older people with psychiatric mental illness tested significantly better when they wore hearing aids (Kreeger et al., 1995).

Follow the same A-B-C-T guidelines as described for the younger adult with the *additional* considerations listed on page 104.

TABLE 6-2	Pediatric Symptom Checklist[1]

Emotional and physical health go together in children. Because parents are often the first to notice a problem with their child's behaviour, emotions, or learning, you may help your child get the best care possible by answering these questions. Please indicate which statement best describes your child.

		Never (0)	Sometimes (1)	Often (2)
1.	Complains of aches and pains	1.	_____	_____	_____
2.	Spends more time alone	2.	_____	_____	_____
3.	Tires easily, has little energy	3.	_____	_____	_____
4.	Fidgety, unable to sit still	4.	_____	_____	_____
5.	Has trouble with teacher	5.	_____	_____	_____
6.	Less interested in school	6.	_____	_____	_____
7.	Acts as if driven by a motor	7.	_____	_____	_____
8.	Daydreams too much	8.	_____	_____	_____
9.	Distracted easily	9.	_____	_____	_____
10.	Is afraid of new situations	10.	_____	_____	_____
11.	Feels sad, unhappy	11.	_____	_____	_____
12.	Is irritable, angry	12.	_____	_____	_____
13.	Feels hopeless	13.	_____	_____	_____
14.	Has trouble concentrating	14.	_____	_____	_____
15.	Less interested in friends	15.	_____	_____	_____
16.	Fights with other children	16.	_____	_____	_____
17.	Absent from school	17.	_____	_____	_____
18.	School grades dropping	18.	_____	_____	_____
19.	Is down on himself or herself	19.	_____	_____	_____
20.	Visits the doctor, who finds nothing wrong	20.	_____	_____	_____
21.	Has trouble sleeping	21.	_____	_____	_____
22.	Worries a lot	22.	_____	_____	_____
23.	Wants to be with you more than before	23.	_____	_____	_____
24.	Feels he or she is bad	24.	_____	_____	_____
25.	Takes unnecessary risks	25.	_____	_____	_____
26.	Gets hurt frequently	26.	_____	_____	_____
27.	Seems to be having less fun	27.	_____	_____	_____
28.	Acts younger than children his or her age	28.	_____	_____	_____
29.	Does not listen to rules	29.	_____	_____	_____
30.	Does not show feelings	30.	_____	_____	_____
31.	Does not understand other people's feelings	31.	_____	_____	_____
32.	Teases others	32.	_____	_____	_____
33.	Blames others for his or her troubles	33.	_____	_____	_____
34.	Takes things that do not belong to him or her	34.	_____	_____	_____
35.	Refuses to share	35.	_____	_____	_____

Does your child have any emotional or behavioural problems for which she/he needs help? _____ No   _____ Yes

Are there any services that you would like your child to receive for these problems? _____ No   _____ Yes

If yes, what type of services? _____

[1]Scoring is a point system: 0 = never; 1 = sometimes; 2 = often.
Item scores are summed, with a possible range of scores from 0 to 70. If one to three items are left blank by parents, they are simply ignored (score = 0). If four or more items are left blank, the questionnaire is considered invalid. For children age 6 or older, the cut-off score is 28 or higher (28 = impaired, 27 = not impaired).

Objective Data

Normal Range of Findings	Abnormal Findings

Behaviour

Level of Consciousness. In a hospital or extended care setting, the Glasgow Coma Scale (see Chapter 23) is a quantitative tool that is useful in testing consciousness in older adults who may be experiencing confusion. It gives a numerical value to the person's response in eye-opening, best verbal response, and best motor response. This system avoids ambiguity when numerous examiners care for the same person.

Cognitive Functions

Orientation. Many older adults experience social isolation, loss of structure without a job, a change in residence, or some short-term memory loss. These factors affect orientation, and this person may not provide the precise date or complete name of the clinic or setting. You may consider older adults oriented if they know *generally* where they are and the present period. That is, consider them oriented to time if the year and month are correctly stated. Orientation to place is accepted with the correct identification of the type of setting (e.g., the hospital) and the name of the town.

New Learning. In people of normal cognitive function, an age-related decline occurs in performance in the Four Unrelated Words Test described on p. 98. Persons in the eighth decade average two of four words recalled over 5 minutes. They will improve their performance at 10 and 30 minutes after being reminded by verbal cues (e.g., "one word was a colour; a common flower in Holland is _____").

People with Alzheimer's dementia do not improve their performance on subsequent trials.

Supplemental Mental Status Examination

Set Test. The Set Test was developed specifically for use with older adults. The original study tested people 65 to 85 years of age. It is a quantifiable test, designed to screen for dementia (Isaacs & Kennie, 1973). The test is easy to administer and takes less than 5 minutes. Ask the person to name 10 items in each of four categories or sets: fruits, animals, colours, and towns (FACT). Do not coach, prompt, or hurry the person. Each correct answer is one point. The maximum total score is 40. No one with a score over 25 has been found to have dementia. (Note: Since this is a verbal test, do not use it with persons with hearing impairments or aphasia.)

The Set Test is a more holistic approach to testing cognitive function. It assesses mental function as a whole instead of examining individual parts of cognitive function. That is, by asking the person to categorize, name, remember, and count the items in the test, you are really assessing this person's alertness, motivation, concentration, short-term memory, and problem-solving ability.

Set Test scores of less than 15 indicate dementia. Scores between 15 and 24 show less association with dementia and should be evaluated carefully.

Clock Test. Clock-drawing tests are a widely accepted cognitive screening tool. The person is asked to draw a clock face to depict a specific time, which requires a variety of cognitive functions, including long-term memory, auditory processing, visual–spatial acuity, concentration, numerical knowledge, and abstract thinking. The main advantages to this type of screening tool are the short time it takes to administer—approximately 2 minutes—and the fact that it can be used by individuals with little or no experience in cognitive assessment and minimal training in test administration. However, clock-drawing tests are not recommended for use as the sole screening tool for dementia as there are some notable limitations. With no single standard for administering or scoring the test, comparative studies have shown a definite variation in reliability, depending on the test method used. As well, the efficacy of these tests in detecting dementia is influenced by the severity of the cognitive impairment, and adverse performance effects resulting from limited education and advanced age have also been identified (Lorentz et al., 2002).

Summary Checklist: Mental Status Assessment

 For a PDA-downloadable version, go to http://evolve.elsevier.com/Canada/Jarvis/examination/.

1. **Appearance**
   Posture
   Body movements
   Dress
   Grooming and hygiene

2. **Behaviour**
   Level of consciousness
   Facial expression
   Speech (quality, pace, articulation, word choice)
   Mood and affect

3. **Cognitive functions**
   Orientation
   Attention span
   Recent and remote memory
   New learning—the Four Unrelated Words Test
   Judgement

4. **Thought processes**
   Thought content
   Perceptions
   Screen for suicidal thoughts (when indicated)

5. **Perform the MiniMental State Examination**

❖— DOCUMENTATION AND CRITICAL THINKING —❖

Sample Charting

Appearance: Person's posture is erect, with no involuntary body movements. Dress and grooming are appropriate for season and setting.

Behaviour: Person is alert, with appropriate facial expression and fluent, understandable speech. Affect and verbal responses are appropriate.

Cognitive functions: Oriented to time, person, place. Able to attend co-operatively with examiner. Recent and remote memory intact. Can recall four unrelated words at 5-, 10-, and 30-minute testing intervals. Future plans include returning to home and to local university once individual therapy is established and medication is adjusted.

Thought processes: Perceptions and thought processes are logical and coherent. No suicide ideation.

Score on MiniMental State Examination is 28.

Focused Assessment: Clinical Case Study

SUBJECTIVE

- Lola P. is a 79-year-old married woman, with a recent hospitalization for evaluation of increasing memory loss, confusion, and socially inappropriate behaviour. Her family reports that Mrs. P's hygiene and grooming have decreased; she eats very little and has lost weight, does not sleep through the night, has angry emotional outbursts that are unlike her former demeanour, and does not recognize her younger grandchildren. Her husband reports that she has drifted away from the stove while cooking, allowing food to burn on the stovetop. He has found her wandering through the house in the middle of the night, unsure of where she is. She used to "talk on the phone for hours" but now he has to push her into conversations.

OBJECTIVE

During this hospitalization, Mrs. P. has undergone a series of medical tests, including a negative lumbar puncture test, normal electroencephalogram (EEG), and a benign head computed tomography (CT) scan. Her physician now suggests a diagnosis of senile dementia of the Alzheimer's type (SDAT).

Appearance: Sitting quietly, somewhat slumped, picking on loose threads on her dress. Hooded, zippered sweatshirt top worn over dress. Hair is gathered in loose ponytail with stray wisps. No makeup.

Behaviour: Awake and gazing at hands and lap. Expression is flat and vacant. Will make eye contact when called by name, although gaze quickly shifts back to lap. Speech is a bit slow but articulate; some trouble with word choice.

Cognitive functions: Oriented to person and place. Can state the season, but not the day of the week or the year. Is not able to repeat the correct sequence of complex directions involving lifting and shifting glass of water to the other hand. Scores a one-word recall on the Four Unrelated Words Test. Cannot tell examiner how she would plan a grocery-shopping trip.

Thought processes: Experiences blocking in train of thought. Thought content is logical. Acts cranky and suspicious with family members. No suicide ideation.

MiniMental State Examination score is 17, and shows poor recall ability and marked difficulty with serial 7s.

Continued

ASSESSMENT

Chronic confusion
Impaired social interaction
Impaired memory
Wandering

Nursing Diagnoses Commonly Associated With Mental Health Disorders

All nursing diagnoses can be found on the Evolve Web site at **http://evolve.elsevier.com/Canada/Jarvis/examination/.**

 ABNORMAL FINDINGS

TABLE 6-3   Levels of Consciousness

The terms below are commonly used in clinical practice. They spread over a continuum from full alertness to deep coma. The terms are qualitative and therefore are not always reliable. (A *quantitative* tool that serves the same purpose and eliminates ambiguity is the Glasgow Coma Scale in Chapter 23.) These terms are widely accepted, however, and are useful as long as all co-workers agree on definitions and are consistent in their application. To increase clarity when using these terms, record also:

1. The level of stimulus used, ranging progressively from
   a. Name called in normal tone of voice
   b. Name called in loud voice
   c. Light touch on person's arm
   d. Vigorous shake of shoulder
   e. Pain applied

2. The person's response
   a. Amount and quality of movement
   b. Presence and coherence of speech
   c. Opening of eyes and making eye contact
3. What the person does on cessation of your stimulus

(1) Alert
Awake or readily aroused, oriented, fully aware of external and internal stimuli and responds appropriately, conducts meaningful interpersonal interactions.

(2) Lethargic (or Somnolent)
Not fully alert, drifts off to sleep when not stimulated, can be aroused to name when called in normal voice but looks drowsy, responds appropriately to questions or commands but thinking seems slow and fuzzy, inattentive, loses train of thought, spontaneous movements are decreased.

(3) Obtunded
(Transitional state between lethargy and stupor; some sources omit this level.)
Sleeps most of time, difficult to arouse—needs loud shout or vigorous shake, acts confused when is aroused, converses in monosyllables, speech may be mumbled and incoherent, requires constant stimulation for even marginal co-operation.

(4) Stupor or Semi-Coma
Spontaneously unconscious, responds only to persistent and vigorous shake or pain; has appropriate motor response (i.e., withdraws hand to avoid pain); otherwise can only groan, mumble, or move restlessly; reflex activity persists.

(5) Coma
Completely unconscious, no response to pain or to any external or internal stimuli (e.g., when suctioned, does not try to push the catheter away), light coma has some reflex activity but no purposeful movement, deep coma has no motor response.

Acute Confusional State (Delirium)
Clouding of consciousness (dulled cognition, impaired alertness); inattentive; incoherent conversation; impaired recent memory and confabulatory for recent events; often agitated and having visual hallucinations; disoriented, with confusion worse at night when environmental stimuli are decreased.

Adapted from Strub, R.L. & Black, F.W. (2000). *Mental status examination in neurology* (4th ed.). Philadelphia, PA: Davis, with permission.

Abnormal Findings

TABLE 6-4	Speech Disorders	
Condition	Disorder of	Description
Dysphonia	Voice	Difficulty or discomfort in talking, with abnormal pitch or volume, due to laryngeal disease. Voice sounds hoarse or whispered, but articulation and language are intact.
Dysarthria	Articulation	Distorted speech sounds; speech may sound unintelligible; basic language (word choice, grammar, comprehension) intact.
Aphasia	Language comprehension and production secondary to brain damage	True language disturbance, defect in word choice and grammar or defect in comprehension; defect is in *higher* integrative language processing.

Types of Aphasia

An earlier dichotomy classified aphasias as expressive (difficulty producing language) or receptive (difficulty understanding language). Since all people with aphasia have some difficulty with expression, beginning examiners tend to classify them all as expressive. The following system is more descriptive.

Condition	Description
Global aphasia	The most common and severe form. Spontaneous speech is absent or reduced to a few stereotyped words or sounds. Comprehension is absent or reduced to only the person's own name and a few select words. Repetition, reading, and writing are severely impaired. Prognosis for language recovery is poor. Caused by a large lesion that damages most of combined anterior and posterior language areas.
Broca's aphasia	Expressive aphasia. The person can understand language but cannot express him- or herself using language. This is characterized by nonfluent, dysarthric, and effortful speech. The speech is mostly nouns and verbs (high-content words) with few grammatic fillers, termed "agrammatic" or "telegraphic" speech. Repetition and reading aloud are severely impaired. Auditory and reading comprehensions are surprisingly intact. Lesion is in anterior language area called the *motor speech cortex* or *Broca's area*.
Wernicke's aphasia	Receptive aphasia. The linguistic opposite of Broca's aphasia. The person can hear sounds and words but cannot relate them to previous experiences. Speech is fluent, effortless, and well articulated but has many paraphasias (word substitutions that are malformed or wrong) and neologisms (made-up words) and often lacks substantive words. Speech can be totally incomprehensible. Often, there is a great urge to speak. Repetition, reading, and writing also are impaired. Lesion is in posterior language area called the *association auditory cortext* or *Wernicke's area*.

(For a discussion of other types of aphasia [e.g., conduction, anomic, transcortical, and so on], please consult a neurology text.)

Abnormal Findings

TABLE 6-5	Abnormalities of Mood and Affect	
Type of Mood or Affect	Definition	Clinical Example
Flat affect (blunted affect)	Lack of emotional response; no expression of feelings; voice monotonous and face immobile	Topic varies, expression does not
Depression	Sad, gloomy, dejected; symptoms may occur with rainy weather, after a holiday, or with an illness; if the situation is temporary, symptoms fade quickly	"I've got the blues."
Depersonalization (lack of ego boundaries)	Loss of identity, feels estranged, perplexed about own identity and meaning of existence	"I don't feel real." "I feel like I'm not really here."
Elation	Joy and optimism, overconfidence, increased motor activity, not necessarily pathological	"I'm feeling very happy."
Euphoria	Excessive well-being, unusually cheerful or elated, that is inappropriate considering physical and mental condition, implies a pathological mood	"I am high." "I feel like I'm flying." "I feel on top of the world."
Anxiety	Worried, uneasy, apprehensive from the anticipation of a danger whose source is unknown	"I feel nervous and high strung." "I worry all the time." "I can't seem to make up my mind."
Fear	Worried, uneasy, apprehensive; external danger is known and identified	Fear of flying in airplanes
Irritability	Annoyed, easily provoked, impatient	Person internalizes a feeling of tension, and a seemingly mild stimulus "sets him (or her) off"
Rage	Furious, loss of control	Person has expressed violent behaviour toward self or others
Ambivalence	The existence of opposing emotions toward an idea, object, person	A person feels love and hate toward another at the same time
Lability	Rapid shift of emotions	Person expresses euphoric, tearful, angry feelings in rapid succession
Inappropriate affect	Affect clearly discordant with the content of the person's speech	Laughs while discussing admission for liver biopsy

ABNORMAL FINDINGS
FOR ADVANCED PRACTICE

TABLE 6-6	Abnormalities of Thought Process	
Type of Process	Definition	Clinical Example
Blocking	Sudden interruption in train of thought, unable to complete sentence, seems related to strong emotion	"Forgot what I was going to say."
Confabulation	Fabricates events to fill in memory gaps	Mr. J gives detailed description of his long walk around the hospital although you know he remained in his room all afternoon.
Neologism	Coining a new word; invented word has no real meaning except for the person; may condense several words	"I'll have to turn on my thinkilator."
Circumlocution	Roundabout expression, substituting a phrase when cannot think of name of object	Says "the thing you open the door with" instead of "key."
Circumstantiality	Talks with excessive and unnecessary detail, delays reaching point; sentences have a meaningful connection but are irrelevant (this occurs normally in some people)	"When was my surgery? Well I was 28, I was living with my aunt, she's the one with psoriasis, she had it bad that year because of the heat, the heat was worse then than it was the summer of '92, . . . "
Loosening associations	Shifting from one topic to an unrelated topic; person seems unaware that topics are unconnected	"My boss is angry with me and it wasn't even my fault. *(pause)* I saw that movie, too, *Lassie.* I felt really bad about it. But she kept trying to land the airplane and she never knew what was going on."
Flight of ideas	Abrupt change, rapid skipping from topic to topic, practically continuous flow of accelerated speech; topics usually have recognizable associations or are plays on words	"Take this pill? The pill is blue. I feel blue. *(sings)* She wore blue velvet."
Word salad	Incoherent mixture of words, phrases, and sentences; illogical, disconnected, includes neologisms	"Beauty, red based five, pigeon, the street corner, sort of."
Perseveration	Persistent repeating of verbal or motor response, even with varied stimuli	"I'm going to lock the door, lock the door. I walk every day and I lock the door. I usually take the dog and I lock the door."
Echolalia	Imitation, repeats others' words or phrases, often with a mumbling, mocking, or mechanical tone	Nurse: "I want you to take your pill." Patient *(mocking):* "Take your pill. Take your pill."
Clanging	Word choice based on sound, not meaning, includes nonsense rhymes and puns	"My feet are cold. Cold, bold, told. The bell tolled for me."

TABLE 6-7	Abnormalities of Thought Content	
Type of Content	Definition	Clinical Example
Phobia	Strong, persistent, irrational fear of an object or situation; feels driven to avoid it	Cats, dogs, heights, enclosed spaces
Hypochondriasis	Morbid worrying about his or her own health, feels sick with no actual basis for that assumption	Preoccupied with the fear of having cancer; any symptom or physical sign means cancer
Obsession	Unwanted, persistent thoughts or impulses; logic will not purge them from consciousness; experienced as intrusive and senseless	Violence (parent having repeated impulse to kill a loved child); contamination (becoming infected by shaking hands)
Compulsion	Unwanted repetitive, purposeful act; driven to do it; behaviour thought to neutralize or prevent discomfort or some dreaded event	Hand washing, counting, checking and rechecking, touching
Delusions	Firm, fixed, false beliefs; irrational; person clings to delusion despite objective evidence to contrary	Grandiose—person believes he or she is God; famous, historical, or sports figure or other well-known person Persecution—"They are out to get me."

TABLE 6-8	Abnormalities of Perception	
Type of Perception	Definition	Clinical Example
Hallucination	Sensory perceptions for which there are no external stimuli; may strike any sense: visual, auditory, tactile, olfactory, gustatory	Visual: seeing an image (ghost) of a person who is not there; auditory: hearing voices or music
Illusion	*Mis*perception of an actual existing stimulus, by any sense	Folds of bedsheets appear to be animated

TABLE 6-9	Delirium, Dementia, and Amnestic Disorders[1]

Delirium

A. **Disturbance of consciousness** (i.e., reduced clarity of awareness of the environment) with reduced ability to focus, sustain, or shift attention

B. A **change in cognition** (such as memory deficit, disorientation, language disturbance) or the development of a perceptual disturbance

C. The disturbance **develops over a short period of time** (usually hours to days) and **tends to fluctuate** during the course of the day

Delirium may be due to a **general medical condition:** systemic infections, metabolic disorders (e.g., hypoxia, hypercarbia, hypoglycemia), fluid or electrolyte imbalances, liver or kidney disease, thiamine deficiency, postoperative states, hypertensive encephalopathy, or following seizures or head trauma.
Delirium also may be **substance induced** (i.e., due to a drug of abuse, a medication, or toxin exposure).

Dementia

A. The development of multiple cognitive deficits, manifested by memory impairment and one or more of 2. a, b, c, or d
   1. **Memory impairment** (impaired ability to learn new information or to recall previously learned information), and
   2. One (or more) of the following cognitive disturbances:
      a. Aphasia (language disturbance)
      b. Apraxia (impaired ability to carry out motor activities despite intact motor function)
      c. Agnosia (failure to recognize or identify objects despite intact sensory function)
      d. Disturbance in executive functioning (i.e., planning, organizing, sequencing, abstracting)

B. The cognitive deficits must be sufficiently severe to cause **impairment in occupational or social functioning** and must represent a decline from a previously higher level of functioning

Dementias have a common symptom presentation but are differentiated based on etiology, which includes senile dementia of the Alzheimer's type or SDAT (course is characterized by gradual onset and continuing cognitive decline); dementia due to cerebrovascular disease (characterized by focal neurological signs and symptoms, e.g., exaggeration of deep tendon reflexes, extensor plantar response, gait abnormalities, weakness of an extremity); human immunodeficiency virus disease; head trauma; Parkinson's disease, and others.

Amnestic Disorder

A. The development of **memory impairment** (inability to learn new information or to recall previously learned information) in the absence of other significant cognitive impairments

B. The memory disturbance causes significant **impairment in social or occupational functioning** and represents a significant decline from a previous level of functioning

This may be due to pathology (closed head trauma, penetrating projectile wounds, surgical intervention, hypoxia, infarction of the posterior cerebral artery, herpes simplex encephalitis), or it may be substance induced (e.g., alcohol-induced amnestic disorder due to thiamine deficiency associated with prolonged, heavy ingestion of alcohol).

[1]The terms *organic mental disorder* and *organic brain syndrome* are no longer used for these disorders. These diagnostic categories are meant to be illustrative, not inclusive. Please refer to the original source for additional details and for further categories.

TABLE 6-10	Substance Use Disorders

"Substances" refer to those agents taken nonmedically to alter mood or behaviour

Intoxication: ingestion of substance produces maladaptive behaviour changes due to effects on the central nervous system

Abuse: daily use needed to function, inability to stop, impaired social and occupational functioning, recurrent use when it is physically hazardous, substance-related legal problems

Dependence: physiological dependence on substance

Tolerance: requires increased amount of substance to produce same effect

Withdrawal: cessation of substance produces a syndrome of physiological symptoms

Substance	Intoxication	Withdrawal
Alcohol	**Appearance.** Unsteady gait, incoordination, nystagmus, flushed face **Behaviour.** Sedation, relief of anxiety, dulled concentration, impaired judgement, expansive, uninhibited behaviour, talkativeness, slurred speech, impaired memory, irritability, depression, emotional lability	**Uncomplicated.** (Shortly after cessation of drinking, peaks at second day, improves by fourth to fifth day.) Coarse tremor of hands, tongue, eyelids; anorexia; nausea and vomiting; malaise; autonomic hyperactivity (tachycardia, sweating, elevated blood pressure); headache; insomnia; anxiety; depression or irritability; transient hallucinations or illusions **Withdrawal delirium, "delirium tremens."** (Much less common than uncomplicated, occurs within 1 week of cessation.) Coarse, irregular tremor; marked autonomic hyperactivity (tachycardia, sweating); vivid hallucinations; delusions; agitated behaviour; fever
Sedatives, hypnotics	Similar to alcohol **Appearance.** Unsteady gait, incoordination **Behaviour.** Talkativeness, slurred speech, inattention, impaired memory, irritability, emotional lability, sexual aggressiveness, impaired judgement, impaired social or occupational functioning	Anxiety or irritability; nausea or vomiting; malaise; autonomic hyperactivity (tachycardia, sweating); orthostatic hypotension; coarse tremor of hands, tongue, and eyelids; marked insomnia; grand mal seizures
Nicotine	**Appearance.** Alerting, increased systolic blood pressure, increased heart rate, vasoconstriction **Behaviour.** Nausea, vomiting, indigestion (first use); loss of appetite, head rush, dizziness, jittery feeling, mild stimulant	Vasodilation, headaches; anger, irritability, frustration, anxiety, nervousness, awakening at night, difficulty concentrating, depression, hunger, impatience or restlessness
Cannabis (marijuana)	**Appearance.** Injected (reddened) conjunctivae, tachycardia, dry mouth, increased appetite, especially for "junk" food **Behaviour.** Euphoria, anxiety, slowed time perception, increased perceptions, impaired judgement, social withdrawal, suspiciousness or paranoid ideation	
Cocaine	**Appearance.** Pupillary dilation, tachycardia or bradycardia, elevated or lowered blood pressure, sweating, chills, nausea, vomiting, weight loss **Behaviour.** Euphoria, talkativeness, hypervigilance, pacing, psychomotor agitation, impaired social or occupational functioning, fighting, grandiosity, visual or tactile hallucinations	Dysphoric mood (anxiety, depression, irritability), fatigue, insomnia or hypersomnia, psychomotor agitation

Continued

Abnormal Findings

TABLE 6-10	Substance Use Disorders—cont'd	
Substance	Intoxication	Withdrawal
Amphetamines	Similar to cocaine **Appearance.** Pupillary dilation, tachycardia or bradycardia, elevated or lowered blood pressure, sweating or chills, nausea and vomiting, weight loss **Behaviour.** Elation, talkativeness, hypervigilance, psychomotor agitation, fighting, grandiosity, impaired judgement, impaired social and occupational functioning	Dysphoric mood (anxiety, depression, irritability), fatigue, insomnia or hypersomnia, psychomotor agitation
Opiates (morphine, heroin, meperidine)	**Appearance.** Pinpoint pupils, decreased blood pressure, pulse, respirations, and temperature **Behaviour.** Lethargy; somnolence; slurred speech; initial euphoria followed by apathy, dysphoria, and psychomotor retardation; inattention; impaired memory; impaired judgement; impaired social or occupational functioning	Dilated pupils, lacrimation, runny nose, tachycardia, fever, elevated blood pressure, piloerection, sweating, diarrhea, yawning, insomnia, restlessness, irritability, depression, nausea, vomiting, malaise, tremor, muscle and joint pains; symptoms are remarkably similar to clinical picture of influenza

TABLE 6-11	Schizophrenia[1]

A. Characteristic Symptoms

Two (or more) of the following, each present for a significant part of a 1-month period:
1. Delusions, that is, involving a phenomenon that the person's culture would regard as totally implausible, such as thought broadcasting, being controlled by a dead person
2. Hallucinations (auditory are more common), such as voices speaking directly to the person or commenting on his or her ongoing behaviour
3. Disorganized speech, such as frequent derailment or incoherence
4. Grossly disorganized or catatonic behaviour
5. Negative symptoms, that is, affective flattening, alogia (inability to speak), or avolition

B. Social/Occupational Dysfunction

One or more major areas of functioning such as work, interpersonal relations, or self-care are markedly below the level achieved prior to onset of the disturbance

C. Duration

Continuous signs persist for at least 6 months, including at least 1 month of symptoms from criterion A (i.e., active phase) and may include periods of prodromal or residual symptoms

[1]These diagnostic categories are meant to be illustrative, not inclusive. The reader is referred to the original source or a psychiatry textbook for further categories and schizophrenia subtypes, such as paranoid type, catatonic type, and disorganized type.

Abnormal Findings

| TABLE 6-12 | Mood Disorders[1] |

Major Depressive Episode
Characteristics

A. Five (or more) of the following symptoms are present during the same 2-week period and represent a change from previous functioning; at least one of the symptoms is either (1) depressed mood or (2) loss of interest or pleasure. Note: Do not include symptoms that are clearly caused by a general medical condition, or delusions or hallucinations.
  1. **Depressed mood** most of the day nearly every day, as indicated by either subjective report (e.g., feels sad or empty) or by observation by others (e.g., appears tearful)
     Note: In children and adolescents, can be irritable mood
  2. Markedly **diminished interest or pleasure** in all, or almost all, activities most of the day nearly every day
  3. Significant **weight loss** when not dieting, weight gain (e.g., a change of >5% body weight in a month), or decrease or increase in appetite nearly every day
     Note: In children, consider failure to make expected weight gains
  4. **Insomnia** or hypersomnia nearly every day
  5. **Psychomotor agitation** or retardation nearly every day
  6. **Fatigue** or loss of energy nearly every day
  7. Feelings of **worthlessness** or excessive or inappropriate guilt nearly every day
  8. **Diminished ability to think** or concentrate, or indecisiveness, nearly every day
  9. Recurrent **thoughts of death** (not just fear of dying), recurrent suicidal ideation without a specific plan, or a suicide attempt or a specific plan for committing suicide

B. The symptoms cause clinically significant distress or impairment in social, occupational, or other important areas of functioning.

C. The symptoms are not due to the direct physiological effects of a substance (e.g., drug of abuse, a medication) or a general medical condition (e.g., hypothyroidism) and are not better accounted for by bereavement, as with loss of a loved one (unless persist for longer than 2 months or are characterized by functional impairment, morbid preoccupation with worthlessness, suicidal ideation, psychotic symptoms, or psychomotor retardation).

Manic Episode
Characteristics

A. A distinct period of abnormally and **persistently elevated, expansive, or irritable mood,** lasting at least 1 week (or any duration if hospitalization is necessary).

B. During this period of mood disturbance, three (or more) of the following symptoms have persisted (four if the mood is only irritable):
  1. Inflated self-esteem or grandiosity
  2. Decreased need for sleep (e.g., feels rested after only 3 hours of sleep)
  3. More talkative than usual or pressure to keep talking
  4. Flight of ideas or subjective experience that thoughts are racing
  5. Distractibility (i.e., attention too easily drawn to unimportant or irrelevant external stimuli)
  6. Increase in goal-directed activity (either socially, at work or school, or sexually) or psychomotor agitation
  7. Excessive involvement in pleasurable activities that have a high potential for painful consequences (e.g., engaging in unrestrained buying sprees, sexual indiscretions, or foolish business investments)

C. The mood disturbance is sufficiently severe to cause marked impairment in occupational functioning or in usual social activities or relationships with others, or to necessitate hospitalization to prevent harm to self or others, or there are psychotic features.

D. The symptoms are not due to the direct physiological effects of a substance (e.g., a drug of abuse, a medication) or a general medical condition (e.g., hyperthyroidism).

Major depressive disorder is characterized by one or more major depressive episodes (i.e., at least 2 weeks of depressed mood or loss of interest accompanied by at least four additional symptoms of depression); **dysthymic disorder** is characterized by at least 2 years of depressed mood for more days than not, accompanied by additional depressive symptoms; **bipolar disorder** is characterized by one or more manic episodes usually accompanied by major depressive episodes.

Adapted from American Psychiatric Association. (2000). *Diagnostic and statistical manual of mental disorders,* (4th ed., Rev. ed.). Washington, DC: American Psychiatric Association. Reprinted with permission from the *Diagnostic and Statistical Manual of Mental Disorders* (4th ed., Rev. ed.). © 2000 American Psychiatric Association.

[1]These diagnostic categories are meant to be illustrative, not inclusive. The reader is referred to the original source or a psychiatry textbook for further categories, such as personality disorders or somatiform disorders.

Abnormal Findings

TABLE 6-13	Anxiety Disorders[1]

Panic Attack

A discrete period of **intense fear or discomfort,** in which four (or more) of the following symptoms develop abruptly and reach a peak within 10 minutes:
1. Palpitations, pounding heart, or accelerated heart rate
2. Sweating
3. Trembling or shaking
4. Sensations of shortness of breath or smothering
5. Feeling of choking
6. Chest pain or discomfort
7. Nausea or abdominal distress
8. Feeling dizzy, unsteady, lightheaded, or faint
9. Derealization (feelings of unreality) or depersonalization (being detached from oneself)
10. Fear of losing control or going crazy
11. Fear of dying
12. Paraesthesias (numbness or tingling sensations)
13. Chills or hot flashes

Agoraphobia

A. Anxiety about being in places or situations from which escape might be difficult (or embarrassing) or in which help may not be available in the event of having a panic attack or panic-like symptoms—agoraphobic fears typically involve being outside the home alone; being in a crowd or standing in a line; being on a bridge; and travelling in a bus, train, or automobile.
B. The situations are avoided (e.g., travel is restricted), are endured with marked distress or with anxiety about having a panic attack or panic-like symptoms, or the person requires the presence of a companion.

Panic Disorder

A. Both 1 and 2 occur:
　1. Recurrent unexpected panic attacks (see above)
　2. At least one of the attacks has been followed by 1 month (or more) of one (or more) of the following:
　　a. Persistent concern about having additional attacks
　　b. Worry about the implications of the attack or its consequences (e.g., losing control, having a heart attack, "going crazy")
　　c. A significant change in behaviour related to the attacks
B. Agoraphobia may be present or absent.

Specific Phobia

A. Marked and persistent fear that is excessive or unreasonable, cued by a specific object or situation (e.g., flying, heights, animals, receiving an injection, seeing blood).
B. Exposure to the phobic stimulus almost invariably provokes an immediate anxiety response, which may be a panic attack. Note: In children, the anxiety may be expressed by crying, tantrums, freezing, or clinging.
C. The person recognizes that the fear is excessive or unreasonable.
D. The phobic situation is avoided or is endured with intense anxiety or distress.
E. This interferes significantly with the person's normal routine, occupational (or academic) functioning, or social activities or relationships.

Social Phobia

A. A marked and persistent fear of one or more social or performance situations in which the person is exposed to unfamiliar people or to possible scrutiny by others; the individual fears that he or she will act in a way (or show anxiety symptoms) that will be humiliating or embarrassing.
B.–E.: The same as in specific phobia.

Continued

Abnormal Findings

TABLE 6-13	Anxiety Disorders[1]—cont'd

Obsessive–Compulsive Disorder

A. Person has either **obsessions:**
   1. Recurrent and persistent thoughts, impulses, or images that are experienced as intrusive and inappropriate and that cause marked anxiety or distress
   2. The thoughts, impulses, or images are not simply excessive worries about real-life problems
   3. The person attempts to ignore or suppress such thoughts, impulses, or images, or to neutralize them with some other thought or action
   4. The person recognizes that the obsessional thoughts are a product of his or her own mind (not imposed from without)

   or **compulsions:**

   1. Repetitive behaviours (e.g., hand washing, ordering, checking) or mental acts (e.g., praying, counting, repeating words silently) that the person feels driven to perform in response to an obsession, or according to rules that must be applied rigidly
   2. The behaviours or mental acts are aimed at preventing or reducing distress or at preventing some dreaded event or situation
B. At some point, the person has recognized that the obsessions or compulsions are excessive or unreasonable.
C. The obsessions or compulsions cause marked distress; are time consuming; or significantly interfere with the person's normal routine, occupational (or academic) functioning, or usual social activities or relationships.

Post-traumatic Stress Disorder

A. The person has been exposed to a traumatic event in which
   1. The person experienced, witnessed, or was confronted with the actual or threatened death or serious injury of self or others
   2. The person's response involved intense fear, helplessness, or horror
B. The traumatic event is persistently re-experienced by:
   1. Recurrent and intrusive distressing recollections of the event, including images, thoughts, or perceptions
   2. Recurrent distressing dreams of the event
   3. Acting or feeling as if the traumatic event were recurring
C. Persistent avoidance of stimuli associated with the trauma and numbing of general responsiveness (e.g., feeling of detachment or estrangement from others, unable to have loving feelings, sense of a foreshortened future)
D. Persistent symptoms of increased arousal:
   1. Difficulty falling or staying asleep   4. Hypervigilance
   2. Irritability or outbursts of anger   5. Exaggerated startle response
   3. Difficulty concentrating

Generalized Anxiety Disorder

A. Excessive anxiety and worry occurring more days than not for at least 6 months about a number of events or activities (such as work or school performance)
B. The person finds it difficult to control the worry
C. The anxiety and worry are associated with three (or more) of the following:
   1. Restlessness or feeling keyed up or on edge   4. Irritability
   2. Being easily fatigued   5. Muscle tension
   3. Difficulty concentrating or mind going blank   6. Sleep disturbance

Adapted from American Psychiatric Association. (2000). *Diagnostic and statistical manual of mental disorders,* (4th ed., Rev. ed.). Washington, DC: American Psychiatric Association. Reprinted with permission from the *Diagnostic and Statistical Manual of Mental Disorders* (4th ed., Rev. ed.). © 2000 American Psychiatric Association.
[1]These diagnostic categories are meant to be illustrative, not inclusive. The reader is referred to the original source or a psychiatry textbook for further details and categories of anxiety disorders.

BIBLIOGRAPHY

American Psychiatric Association. (2000). *Diagnostic and statistical manual of mental disorders* (4th ed., Rev. ed.). Washington, DC: Author.

Birren, J. E., & Schaie, K. W. (Eds.). (2005). *Handbook of the psychology of aging* (6th ed.). San Diego, CA: Academic Press.

Blackwell, J., & Niederhauser, C. (2003). Diagnose and manage autistic children. *Nurse Practitioner, 28*(6), 36–45.

Brown, E. L., Raue, P., Murphy, C. F., & Bruce, M. (2002). Assessing behavioral health using OASIS. Part 2: Cognitive impairment, problematic behaviors, and anxiety. *Home Healthcare Nurse, 20*(4), 236.

Canadian Institute for Health Information. (2007). *Improving the health of Canadians: Mental health and homelessness.* Ottawa, ON: Author.

Canadian Institutes of Health Research. (2007). *CIHR Institute of Aging strategic plan 2007–2012.* Ottawa, ON: Author.

Canadian Mental Health Association (CMHA). (2008). *Meaning of mental health.* Retrieved May 7, 2008, from http://www.cmha.ca/bins/content_page.asp?cid=2-267-1319&lang=1

Clark, B., & Halm, M. (2003). Postprocedural acute confusion in the elderly: Assessment tools can minimize this common condition. *American Journal of Nursing, 103*(5), 64UU–64AA3.

Cochran, H. (2003). Diagnose and treat primary insomnia. *Nurse Practitioner, 28*(9), 13–29.

Davis, B. (2004). Assessing adults with mental disorders in primary care. *Nurse Practitioner, 29*(5), 19–29.

De Nisco, S., Tiago, C., & Kravitz, C. (2005). Evaluation and treatment of pediatric ADHD. *Nurse Practitioner, 30*(8), 14–25.

Depaulo, J. R., Jr., & Folstein, M. F. (1978). Psychiatric disturbances in neurological patients: Detection, recognition and hospital course. *Annals of Neurology, 4*, 225–228.

Élie, M., Rousseau, F., Cole, M., Primeau, F., McCusker, J., & Bellavance, F. (2000). Prevalence and detection of delirium in elderly emergency department patients. *Canadian Medical Association Journal, 163*, 977–981.

Folstein, M. F., Folstein, S. E., & McHugh, P. R. (1975). "Mini-mental state": A practical method for grading the cognitive state of patients for the clinician. *Journal of Psychiatric Research, 12*, 189–198.

Garand, L., Mitchell, A., Dietrick, A., Hijjawi, J., & Pan, D. (2006). Suicide in older adults: Nursing assessment of suicide risk. *Issues in Mental Health Nursing, 29*, 355–370.

Gary, F. A. (2005). Stigma: Barrier to mental health care among ethnic minorities. *Issues in Mental Health Nursing, 26*, 979–999.

Guess, K. F. (2006). Posttraumatic stress disorder. *Nurse Practitioner, 31*(3), 26–35.

Harwood, G. A. (2005). Alcohol abuse: Screening in primary care. *Nurse Practitioner, 30*(2), 56–61.

Health Canada. (2002). *Report on mental illness in Canada.* Ottawa, ON: Author.

Helms, L. (2006). Prescribing SSRIs for adolescents with depression. *Nurse Practitioner, 31*(11), 46–51.

Isaacs, B., & Kennie, A. (1973). The set test as an aid to the detection of dementia in old people. *British Journal of Psychiatry, 123*, 467–470.

Kane, R. L., Ouslander, J. G., & Abrass, I. B. (2003). *Essentials of clinical geriatrics* (5th ed.). New York, NY: McGraw-Hill.

Kirmayer, L., Bass, G., Holton, T., Paul, K., Simpson, C., Tait, C. (2007). *Suicide among Aboriginal people in Canada.* Ottawa, ON: Aboriginal Healing Foundation.

Kreeger, J. L., Raulin, M. L., Grace, J., & Priest, B. L. (1995). Effect of hearing enhancement on mental status ratings in geriatric psychiatric patients. *American Journal of Psychiatry, 152*, 629–631.

Lee, K. A., & Ward, T. M. (2005). Critical components of a sleep assessment for clinical practice settings. *Issues Mental Health Nursing, 26*, 739–750.

Lemiengre, J., Nelis, T., Joosten, E., Braes, T., Foreman, M., Gastmans, C., et al. (2006). Detection of delirium by bedside nurses using the confusion assessment method. *Journal of the American Geriatric Society, 54*, 685–689.

Lorentz, W., Scanlan, J. M., & Borson, S. (2002). Brief screening tests for dementia. *Canadian Journal of Psychiatry, 47*, 723–733.

MacMillan, H. L., Patterson, C. J. S., & Wathen, C. N. (2005). Screening for depression in primary care: Recommendation statement from the Canadian Task Force on Preventive Health Care. *Canadian Medical Association Journal, 172*(1), 33–35.

Marshall, R. D., Turner, J. B., Lewis-Fernandez, R., Karestan, K., Yuval, N., Dohrenwend, B. P. (2006). Symptom patterns associated with chronic PTSD in male veterans. *Journal of Nervous and Mental Disease, 194*, 275–278.

Maynard, C. K. (2003a). Assess and manage somatization. *Nurse Practitioner, 28*(4), 20–31.

Maynard, C. K. (2003b). Differentiate depression from dementia. *Nurse Practitioner, 28*(3), 18–29.

Milano, C. (2006). Narcotics abuse in correctional facilities: Is pain medication being used inappropriately? *American Journal of Nursing, 106*(2), 22.

MacMillan, H.L., Patterson, C. J. S., & Wathen, C. N. (2005). Screening for depression in primary care: Recommendation statement from the Canadian Task Force on Preventive Health Care. *CMAJ, 172* (1), 33–35.

Molloy, D. W., Alemeyehu, E., & Roberts, R. (1991). Reliability of a standardized Mini-Mental State Examination compared with the traditional Mini-Mental State Examination. *American Journal of Psychiatry, 148*, 102–105.

Murphy, K. (2004). Recognizing depression in children. *Nurse Practitioner, 29*(9), 18–31.

Pagano, M. E., Cassidy, L. J., Little, M., Murphy, J. M., & Jellinek, M. (2000). Identifying psychosocial dysfunction in school-age children: The Pediatric Symptom Checklist as a self-report measure. *Psychology in the Schools, 37*(2), 91–106.

Pape, B., & Galipeault, J. P. (2002). *Mental health promotion for people with mental illness.* Ottawa, ON: Health Canada.

Public Health Agency of Canada. (2006). *The human face of mental health and mental illness in Canada.* Ottawa, ON: Minister of Public Works and Government Services Canada.

Spector, A. Z. (2006). Fatherhood and depression: A review of risks, factors, and clinical application. *Issues in Mental Health Nursing, 27*, 867–883.

Statistics Canada. (2001). *2001 census: Analysis series—Collective dwellings.* Ottawa, ON: Author.

Strub, R. L., & Black, F. W. (2000). *Mental status examination in neurology* (4th ed.). Philadelphia, PA: F.A. Davis.

Thayer, K. M., & Bruce, M. L. (2006). Recognition and management of major depression. *Nurse Practitioner, 31*(5), 12–25.

Torrisi, D., & McDaniel, H. (2003). Better outcomes for depressed patients. *Nurse Practitioner, 28*(8), 32–38.

Trossman, S. (2006). Rx for medical marijuana: promoting research on and acceptance of this treatment option for patients. *American Journal of Nursing, 106*(4), 77–79.

World Health Organization. (2007). *Mental health: Strengthening mental health promotion.* Geneva, Switzerland: Author.

World Health Organization. (2001). *The World Health report 2001—Mental health: New understanding, new hope.* Geneva, Switzerland: Author.

Web Sites of Interest

Aboriginal Healing Foundation—http://www.ahf.ca/

Alzheimer Society—http://www.alzheimer.ca/

Canadian Coalition for Seniors' Mental Health—http://www.ccsmh.ca/

Canadian Institute for Health Information—http://www.cihi.ca

Canadian Mental Health Association—http://www.cmha.ca/bins/index.asp

Centre for Addiction and Mental Health—http://www.camh.net/

Mental Health Commission of Canada—http://www.mentalhealth commission.ca/mhcc.html

Mental Health Glossary, Royal Ottawa Health Care Group—http://www.rohcg.on.ca/resources/glossary-e.cfm

Mood Disorder Society of Canada—http://www.mooddisorderscanada.ca/

National Eating Disorder Information Centre—http://www.nedic.ca/

Schizophrenia Society of Canada—http://www.schizophrenia.ca/

Seniors Mental Health Web site created to facilitate activities related to supporting seniors' mental health—http://www.seniorsmentalhealth.ca/index.html

Chapter Seven

Interpersonal Violence Assessment

Written by **Colleen Varcoe**, PhD, RN
Based on the original chapter by **Daniel J. Sheridan**, PhD, RN, CNS, FNE-A, FAAN,
and **Shawna S. Mudd**, MSN, CRNP

Interpersonal violence, including intimate partner violence, sexual assault, child abuse, and elder abuse, is a serious problem that healthcare professionals must recognize, assess, and respond to. In Canada, mandatory requirements for reporting child abuse exist but not for reporting other forms of violence. However, all forms of interpersonal violence have significant, long-lasting health consequences and require a meaningful response by healthcare professionals.

INTIMATE PARTNER VIOLENCE DEFINED

Intimate partner violence (IPV) encompasses spousal violence and violence committed by current or former dating partners (Johnson, 2006). **Spousal abuse** refers to physical or sexual violence, psychological violence, or financial abuse within current or former marital or common-law relationships, including same-sex spousal relationships. Behaviours used to dominate another person in the context of an intimate relationship may include physical or sexual assault and acts such as verbal abuse, imprisonment, humiliation, stalking, and denial of access to financial resources, shelter, or services (Tjaden et al., 2000). Gender is a key risk for IPV. "Men's and boys' experiences of violence are different than women's and girls' in important ways. While men are more likely to be injured by strangers in a public or social venue, women are in greater danger of experiencing violence from intimate partners in their own homes. Women are also at greater risk of sexual violence" (Johnson, 2006, p. 1). For women, IPV is acknowledged to be a *pattern of physical, sexual, or emotional violence (or all three) in the context of coercive control* (Cherniak et al., 2005; Tjaden et al., 2000).

SEXUAL ASSAULT DEFINED

Sexual assault usually occurs either within the context of a partner relationship or by a known assailant but may also be perpetrated by a stranger. The Canadian *Criminal Code* identifies both sexual assault and sexual touching as crimes. There are four levels of **sexual assault**: (1) sexual assault that is forced sexual activity without physical injury, (2) sexual assault with a weapon or verbal threats to a third party, (3) sexual assault causing bodily harm, and (4) aggravated sexual assault, which is forced sexual activity where the attacker seriously injures, wounds, maims, disfigures, or endangers life.

CHILD ABUSE AND NEGLECT DEFINED

In Canada, child abuse and exploitation are prohibited by the *Criminal Code* (Department of Justice Canada, 2007a). Most provinces and territories have child welfare laws that require the public, including healthcare professionals, to report suspected child abuse. The Department of Justice Canada defines **child abuse** as "the violence, mistreatment or neglect that a child or adolescent may experience while in the care of someone they either trust or depend on, such as a parent, sibling, other relative, caregiver or guardian. Abuse may take place anywhere and may occur, for example, within the child's home or that of someone known to the child. There are many different forms of abuse and a child may be subjected to more than one form" (2007a, p. 1). Child abuse and IPV against women often overlap, with estimates that children are also abused in up to 70% of families in which women are abused (Edleson, 1999; Folsom et al., 2003). Box 7-1 shows Department of Justice definitions consistent with those used in most provincial and territorial laws.

BOX 7-1 | Types of CHILD ABUSE

Physical abuse may consist of just one incident, or it may happen repeatedly. It involves deliberately using force against a child in such a way that the child is either injured or is at risk of being injured. Physical abuse includes beating, hitting, shaking, pushing, choking, biting, burning, kicking, and assaulting a child with a weapon. It also includes holding a child under water, or any other dangerous or harmful use of force or restraint. Female genital mutilation is another form of physical abuse.

Sexual abuse and exploitation involve using a child for sexual purposes. Examples of child sexual abuse include fondling, inviting a child to touch or be touched sexually, intercourse, rape, incest, sodomy, exhibitionism, and involving a child in prostitution or pornography.

Neglect is often chronic, and it usually involves repeated incidents. It involves failing to provide what a child needs for his or her physical, psychological, or emotional development and well-being. For example, neglect includes failing to provide a child with food, clothing, shelter, cleanliness, medical care, and protection from harm. Emotional neglect includes failing to provide a child with love, safety, and a sense of worth.

Emotional abuse involves harming a child's sense of self. It includes acts (or omissions) that result in, or place a child at risk of, serious behavioural, cognitive, emotional, or mental health problems. For example, emotional abuse may include verbal threats, social isolation, intimidation, exploitation, and routinely making unreasonable demands. It also includes terrorizing a child or exposing the child to family violence.

Abuse is a misuse of power and a violation of trust. Children who are being abused are usually in a position of dependence on the person who is abusing them. An abuser may use a number of different tactics to gain access to a child, exert power and control over the child, and prevent the child from telling anyone about the abuse or seeking support. The abuse may happen once or in a repeated and escalating pattern over a period of months or years, and may change form over time.

ELDER ABUSE AND NEGLECT DEFINED

Elder abuse and neglect are forms of IPV that continue into older adulthood or arise as persons become more vulnerable with age. As with any form of IPV, in older adults, too, it is gendered—that is, older women are at higher risk than men. The Department of Justice Canada (2007b) defines **elder abuse and neglect** as "violence, mistreatment or neglect that older adults living in either private residences or institutions may experience at the hands of their spouses, children, other family members, caregivers, service providers or other individuals in situations of power or trust" (p. 1). Elder abuse and neglect include violence in the home, violence in institutions, and even self-neglect (McDonald et al., 2000). Older adults who become frail and require medical or other health-related services may experience abuse involving failure to facilitate their access to medical or health services, failure to provide medical attention due to age, or conducting a procedure or treatment without the informed consent of the patient or the patient's recognized substitute decision maker. The Department of Justice (2007b) identifies many forms of elder abuse and neglect, including psychological, financial, physical, sexual, and spiritual abuses and neglect. Although age and gender can increase vulnerability, it is important to note that other factors, such as economic dependence, disabilities (e.g., intellectual and physical disabilities), and rural isolation also increase vulnerability to violence.

EFFECTS OF VIOLENCE ON HEALTH

IPV, child abuse, and elder abuse remain significant problems globally and in Canada, although all estimates are widely acknowledged to be underestimates. According to the most conservative estimates in the 2004 Canadian General Social Survey, 7% of women and 6% of men in current or previous spousal relationships reported having experienced some form of spousal violence during the previous 5 years, but violence against women tended to be much more severe (Statistics Canada, 2006). In the years between 1995 and 2004, men perpetrated 86% of one-time incidents, 94% of repeat (two to four) incidents, and 97% of chronic incidents. In that same time frame, the rate of spousal homicide against women was three to five times higher than the rate of male spousal homicide (Statistics Canada, 2006). Critiques of prevalence studies in Canada suggest that as many as 23% of women experience IPV each year (Clark et al., 2003).

Lifetime rates of physical assault by an intimate partner have been estimated at 25 to 30% in Canada and the United States (Johnson et al., 1995; Jones et al., 1999). Physical assault is often accompanied by sexual violence or emotional abuse, and many women experience IPV in more than one relationship over their lifetime (Johnson, 1996). The most detailed information on sexual assault is available from the 1993 National Violence Against Women Survey (Johnson, 1996). At that time, 39% of Canadian adult women reported having had at least one experience of sexual assault since the age of 16. In 2000, women made up the vast majority of victims of sexual assault (86%) and other types of sexual offences (78%) (Statistics Canada, 2001).

Estimates of child abuse are also difficult to make and often based on *reported* cases only. With data from child welfare authorities, the Canadian Incidence Study of Reported Child Abuse and Neglect estimated a rate of 21.52 investigations of child abuse per 1000 children (Public Health Agency of Canada, 2001). It is critical to note that the greatest proportion of reported and substantiated child abuse cases involved **neglect** (Table 7-1). Analyses of this report support the growing

TABLE 7-1	Investigations of Types of Child Maltreatment	
Types of Abuse	Percent of Investigations	Percent Substantiated
Physical abuse	31	34
Sexual abuse	10	38
Neglect	40	43
Emotional maltreatment	19	54

concern that insufficient attention has been paid to neglect in comparison with sexual abuse, in part because sexual abuse is a more sensational issue (McLean, 2001). Emphasis has been on risk assessment and urgent intervention for abuse but not on the more frequent cases of neglect. Because they found that 96% of substantiated cases did not involve severe physical harm (harm was severe enough to warrant medical attention in about 4% of substantiated cases), Trocmé et al. (2003) argued that assessment and investigation priorities need to be revised and to include consideration of long-term needs for housing, income, child care, and so on. Importantly, socioeconomic status has been consistently shown to be related to parenting effectiveness (Wekerle et al., 2007), also suggesting that healthcare professionals should assess for longer-term and broader social support.

The extent of elder abuse is also difficult to determine, but Statistics Canada reported that in the 1999 General Social Survey on Victimization, approximately 7% of the sample of >4000 adults over 65 years of age reported that they had experienced some form of emotional or financial abuse by an adult child, spouse, or caregiver in the 5 years prior to the survey, with the vast majority committed by spouses. Emotional abuse was more frequently reported (7%) than financial abuse (1%). The two most common forms of emotional abuse reported were snubbing or name-calling, and limiting contact with family and friends. Only a small proportion of older adults (1%) reported experiencing physical or sexual abuse. Almost 2% of older Canadians indicated that they had experienced more than one type of abuse (Canadian Centre for Justice Statistics, 2002).

All forms of violence have significant effects on health, and since individuals may experience multiple forms of violence and multiple incidences of violence, the health effects are likely to be cumulative. The health consequences of IPV are due not only to physical assault but also to sexual assault (Campbell et al., 1999a) and to emotional abuse (Carlson, 2005).

A persuasive body of knowledge accumulated in the past two decades has established that violent experiences have significant effects on women's health. The health consequences of IPV include:

- **Direct effects** of physical injuries, such as bruises and fractures (Muellman et al., 1996)
- **Chronic physical health problems,** such as chronic pain and arthritis; frequent headaches and migraines; visual problems; unexplained dizziness and fainting; sexually transmitted infections (STIs); unwanted pregnancies; gynecological symptoms; hypertension; viral infections such as colds and flu; peptic ulcers; and functional or irritable bowel disease (Campbell et al., 1997; Kendall-Tackett et al., 2003; Letourneau et al., 1999; Wuest et al., 2007)
- **Mental health problems,** including clinical depression; acute and chronic symptoms of anxiety; serious sleep disturbances; symptoms consistent with post-traumatic stress disorder (PTSD); substance abuse and dependence; and thoughts of suicide, which are significantly higher among women who have been abused than among those not abused (Campbell, 2002; Cascardi et al., 1999; Eby et al., 1995; Fischbach et al., 1997)

The most obvious healthcare problem for abused women is injury, with approximately 52% reporting they were injured seriously enough to need medical attention from an abusive incident (Bachman et al., 1995). Such injuries have particular patterns that can be recognized. Head and neck injuries and musculoskeletal injuries such as sprains and fractures are common (Bhandari et al., 2006).

Chronic health problems are less obviously linked to IPV but are very significant clinically. In many controlled investigations of women in a variety of healthcare settings, abused women have been found to have significantly more chronic health problems, including more neurological, gastrointestinal, and gynecological symptoms and chronic pain (Campbell, 2002; Campbell et al., 2001; Coker et al., 2000; Leserman et al., 1998; Letourneau et al., 1999; McCauley et al., 1995; Plichta, 1996; Wuest et al., 2007). Abused women also visit healthcare professionals more often than women not battered and incur higher healthcare costs (Coker et al., 2004; Rivara et al., 2007b; Schollenberger et al., 2003; Snow Jones et al., 2006; Wisner et al., 1999), with potential long-term costs both for themselves and employers (Reeves & O'Leary, 2007). In terms of mental health, abused women also experienced significantly more depression, suicidality (suicidal thoughts and attempts), and PTSD symptoms, as well as substance abuse (Golding, 1999). The forced sex that accompanies physical abuse in 40 to 45% of the cases contributes to a host of gynecological health problems including chronic pelvic pain, unintended pregnancy, STIs (including HIV), and urinary tract infections (Campbell and Soeken, 1999a; Letourneau et al., 1999; Maman et al., 2000). Abuse during pregnancy is also a significant health issue, with serious consequences for both the pregnant mother (e.g., antepartum hemorrhage, death, depression, substance abuse) and the infant (low birth weight, increased risk of child abuse) (Gazmararian et al., 2000; Janssen et al., 2003; Murphy et al., 2001).

Although more than 50% of abused women say they have been injured, only 25 to 30% say they have actually sought health care for one of the injuries (Du Mont et al., 2005; Plichta, 1996). Even so, the majority of abused women (80%) say they have been in a healthcare setting for some reason, either for regular checkups or for one of the chronic health problems described previously. Because many abused women may not be ready to seek help from a shelter or from the criminal justice system (Landenburger, 1998) or are reluctant to do so (Beaulaurier et al., 2007; Fugate et al., 2005), the healthcare system can be an extremely important early point of contact. By dealing effectively with abuse in its early stages, it is hoped that the pattern of violence can be stopped and chronic health problems avoided or minimized.

Professionals need to be alert for the conditions particularly associated with IPV, including gynecological problems (especially STIs, pelvic pain, and complaints of sexual dysfunction), chronic irritable bowel syndrome, back pain, depression, and the presenting symptoms of PTSD (especially problems sleeping and "panic" attacks or problems with "nerves"). When these problems occur, and especially when they persist, a thorough and repeated assessment of interpersonal violence is needed. In this case, an instrument such as the Women's Experience of Battering scale (Coker et al., 2000) might be used, or gentle indirect queries (e.g., "I am concerned about your health conditions; is there any chance that stress at home is contributing to these problems?") may be used. The health effects of violence on women and the associated social and economic costs also extend to the women's children (Bogat et al., 2006; Rivara et al., 2007b; Suh et al., 1990), in part due to witnessing abuse (Carlson, 2000; Knapp, 1998).

The health effects of elder abuse are not nearly as well studied. Complications from intentional injury can range from minor pain and discomfort to life-threatening injuries. Bleeding from intentional trauma can cause significant changes in circulatory homeostasis, leading to marked fluctuations in blood pressure and pulse, shock, and ultimately death. Localized infections can progress to generalized sepsis, even death, in older patients who are immunocompromised. The actual assault or the stress leading up to or following an assault can contribute to cardiac complications. All of the STIs and related complications that are sequelae of abuse in younger women are also present in older women who have been sexually assaulted. In addition, postmenopausal women have more friable vaginal mucosal tissue secondary to de-estrogenation, putting them at greater risk for STIs and vaginal trauma.

Abuse of older adults often is coupled with neglect. Neglect can manifest as symptoms of dehydration and malnutrition. Neglect can be intentional or nonintentional. Some family members or caregivers working with older persons consciously, and with malice, withhold food, water, medication, and appropriate necessities, often concurrently stealing the financial assets of the older, dependent person. This type of neglect is often, by definition, criminal in nature.

Some family members or caregivers working with an older person struggle with their own severe physical and cognitive health challenges. In spite of the caregiver's good intentions, the older patient may experience profound unintentional neglect. While unintentional neglect is usually not viewed as a crime, it must still be addressed. Self-neglect raises often unanswerable questions about one's right to live autonomously versus society's obligation to care for a person who is not able to care for herself or himself.

Older women face specific barriers to getting help. They may be more vulnerable because of economic dependence, physical and cognitive health challenges, and isolation. Services may not be appropriate to their needs when dealing with IPV. Leaving their partners may not be possible, but services and social expectations are not oriented to the fact that leaving poses special challenges to older women (Beaulaurier et al., 2007).

There are many possible long-term physical and psychological effects of child maltreatment. The immediate consequences can include a spectrum of physical injuries such as bruises, fractures, and lacerations, and can involve more severe injury such as head trauma. More severe forms of maltreatment can lead to death or long-term disability such as intellectual disability, blindness, and physical disability.

Child maltreatment can have effects on a child's development by disrupting the bond between child and caregiver (Hagele, 2005). Ongoing child maltreatment can lead to changes in brain structure and chemistry, which may lead to long-term physical, psychological, emotional, social, and cognitive dysfunctions in adulthood (Hagele, 2005). While physical harm occurs as a consequence of child abuse, other forms of abuse, which often co-occur, are also harmful. For example, an analysis of 554 youth found that verbal aggression was associated with moderate to large effects on psychiatric symptoms, comparable with the effects of witnessing intimate partner violence or nonfamilial sexual abuse, and larger than those associated with familial physical abuse (Teicher et al., 2006). Childhood abuse puts children at risk of depression and PTSD, of participating in harmful activities, of having difficulties in relationships, and of having negative beliefs and attitudes toward others. Each of these increases the likelihood of health problems, and they are closely related to each other (Kendall-Tackett, 2002). Child abuse is related to substance use, eating disorders, suicide, high-risk sexual behaviour, and sleep disorders. Child abuse may also increase vulnerability to later revictimization, and homelessness. The idea that people who are abused as children are more likely to abuse their children is popular, but evidence of this is inconclusive (Ozturk Ertem et al., 2000; Renner et al., 2006).

Canada's Department of Justice notes that

> there is no single, definitive cause of child abuse, and any child—regardless of age, gender, race, ethnicity, cultural identity, socioeconomic status, spirituality, sexual orientation, physical or mental abilities or personality—may be vulnerable to being abused. . . . Many experts believe that child abuse is linked to inequalities among people in our society and the power imbalance between adults and children. A child is usually in a position of dependence on his or her abuser, and has little or no power compared to the abuser. There is increasing understanding that a child's vulnerability to abuse may be increased by factors such as dislocation, colonization, racism, sexism, homophobia, poverty and social isolation. For example, in the past, many children sent to institutions experienced abuse [Fig.7-1]. Most of these children were from marginalized groups in our society including, among others, children with disabilities, children from racial and ethnic minorities, Aboriginal children and children living in poverty. There are also factors that may increase a child's vulnerability to being abused—or compound the effects of abuse. For example, a child's caregivers may experience barriers that prevent them from acquiring the necessary skills, resources and supports to prevent abuse, or they may lack access to the services and supports they need to address it. (Department of Justice Canada (2007a)

Although identifiable risk factors for child maltreatment exist, a study on missed cases of abusive head trauma conducted by Jenny et al. (1999) found several factors significant to missed injuries. They found that missed cases of abusive head injury occurred more often in White children than children in racialized groups, in children living with both parents, in younger children, and in children with less severe presenting

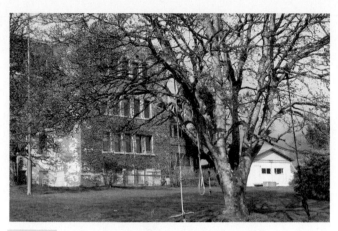

Fig. 7-1   For many generations, children from communities along the coast of British Columbia were taken from their families and sent to residential schools, including this one in Alert Bay, where they experienced multiple forms of abuse.

symptoms. These dynamics may reflect stereotypical thinking regarding who is abused. For example, in one Canadian study, nurses tended to anticipate IPV among poor and racialized people and to anticipate child abuse in Aboriginal families (Varcoe, 2001). Such attitudes may contribute to the fact that Aboriginal families are more often investigated because of neglect. Blackstock et al. (2004) analyzed the Canadian investigations of child abuse and found that at every decision point in the cases, Aboriginal children are over-represented: investigations were more likely to be substantiated, cases were more likely to be kept open for ongoing services, and children were more likely to be placed in out-of-home care.

HEALTHCARE PROFESSIONALS' RESPONSES TO INTIMATE PARTNER VIOLENCE

To date, the healthcare response to IPV has been inadequate at best. Research has consistently shown that healthcare professionals fail to identify when their patients are abused. The main recommendation for healthcare professionals has been to routinely screen for violence. However, evidence, to date, is inconclusive regarding whether this is effective (Coker, 2006). A systematic review of available literature published in English (Ramsey et al., 2002) found that of the studies that compared screening with no screening, most detected a greater proportion of abused women. However, detecting abuse does not necessarily lead to meaningful responses. Intervention studies used weak study designs and gave inconsistent results. No studies measured quality of life, mental health outcomes, or potential harm to women from screening programs. Ramsay et al. (2002) concluded that other than increased referral to outside agencies, little evidence exists that screening leads to changes in important outcomes such as decreased exposure to violence. Currently, in Canada, studies are under way to examine the effects of screening more broadly (http://www.fhs.mcmaster.ca/vaw/).

Some of the challenges to screening for abuse include the following:
- People who are experiencing violence may not identify their experiences as abuse.
- People who are experiencing violence may be ashamed or anticipate judgement by those caring for them.
- Privacy for disclosure may not be available in healthcare settings.
- Women may fear the responses from healthcare professionals, including acts that will increase their risks, such as those that increase danger for themselves or family members, or increase the risk of their children being apprehended.
- Healthcare professionals may ask screening questions more often of racialized or poor women, further perpetuating stereotypes of abuse and minimizing the abusive experiences of middle-class and Euro-Canadian women (Cory et al., 2007).

Even when the abuse is recognized, women's experiences with healthcare professionals tend to be negative (Bacchus et al., 2003; Gerbert et al., 1999; Humphreys et al., 2003; McCloskey et al., 2005). Research has shown that women often find professional responses to abuse unsympathetic, disempowering, victim-blaming, and focusing on physical consequences of violence rather than the wider effects and the context of women's lives (Gerbert et al., 1996; McMurray et al., 1994). Healthcare professionals often provide inappropriate or even harmful treatment (Plichta, 1991). A Canadian study of emergency department responses to violence against women showed that nurses' responses were shaped by stereotypical thinking about violence as primarily a problem of poor and racialized people, by judgements of the extent to which women "deserved" help, and by the patterns of practice that required nurses to process patients as quickly as possible (Varcoe, 2001). Healthcare professionals often lack knowledge about IPV, have attitudes and values that inhibit an effective response, and think they have no time to respond (Tower, 2007).

Assessing for IPV should be seen as part of a larger response to violence. The BC Women's Hospital Woman Abuse Response Team has developed the Safety and Health Enhancement (SHE) model (Fig. 7-2) (Cory et al., 2007), which guides healthcare professionals to develop more effective responses, beginning with effective policy and research driving the process rather than violence driving the process, as depicted in the Compounding Harms model (see Fig. 7-2). Key features of the approach include:
- **Putting safety first**—always beginning with attention to the patients' and your emotional, cultural, and physical safety
- **Making connections**—knowing and connecting with a range of resources and services so that you can facilitate access for patients
- **Offering more than band-aid solutions**—shifting from focusing on disclosure of abuse to being responsive to an individual's needs
- **Doing no harm**—ensuring that healthcare responses do not disempower, demean, or increase danger

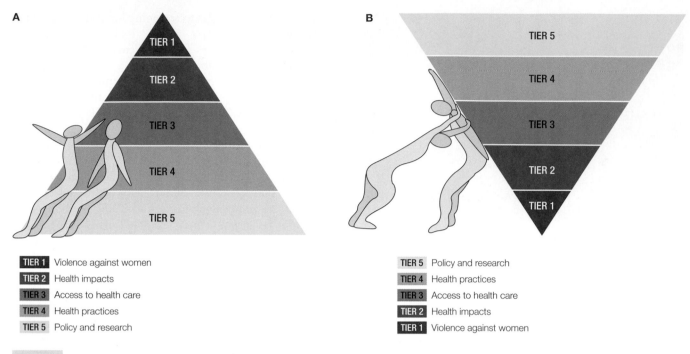

A

TIER 1
TIER 2
TIER 3
TIER 4
TIER 5

TIER 1 Violence against women
TIER 2 Health impacts
TIER 3 Access to health care
TIER 4 Health practices
TIER 5 Policy and research

B

TIER 5
TIER 4
TIER 3
TIER 2
TIER 1

TIER 5 Policy and research
TIER 4 Health practices
TIER 3 Access to health care
TIER 2 Health impacts
TIER 1 Violence against women

Fig. 7-2   **A**, Safety and Health Enhancement (SHE) model. **B**, Compounding Harms model.

- **Seeing the big picture**—keeping the wider context of women's lives in mind, and seeing violence as a widespread social problem rather than an individual aberration

Assessing for IPV

Even if it is not known whether screening is useful, healthcare professionals cannot ignore the problem of violence (Coker, 2006). Although the idea of screening may imply that healthcare professionals need to know a person's history of abuse to complete a good assessment or provide good care, this is not true. Further, research has found that women are prepared to disclose IPV to healthcare professionals when they feel confident and safe enough to do so (Bacchus et al., 2003; Gerbert et al., 1999). Healthcare professionals can:

- Assume that a majority of patients will have a history of abuse of some form
- Assume that any patient may be currently experiencing abuse
- Provide care that is appropriate for people who have histories of, or are experiencing, abuse, *regardless* of whether abuse has been disclosed

Based on awareness that abuse may be part of any patient's history, and using a relational approach as described in earlier chapters, assessment should routinely include:

- **Listening** in a nonjudgemental and accepting manner
- Having a **high index of suspicion** for abuse (MacMillan et al., 2003) when patients present with direct injuries consistent with abuse, chronic health problems associated with abuse (e.g., chronic pain), mental health problems consistent with abuse, or factors known to increase vulnerability (e.g., disabilities, economic dependence, isolation)
- **Assessing and intervening collaboratively**

Listening

Because women report that they feel judged and disbelieved by healthcare professionals, it is vital to begin by examining your own knowledge and beliefs about IPV. If a healthcare professional thinks that women should "just leave" or that they are responsible for the abuse they experience, these ideas will be conveyed to patients, discouraging them from seeking further help or from disclosure.

Listening nonjudgementally requires healthcare professionals to critically evaluate social judgements that are commonly made about women who are abused and to acquire sufficient knowledge to counter those negative judgements. Questions you might ask yourself are:

- What do I know about IPV? Who do I hold responsible for IPV? What do I think are the causes of IPV?
- What are my own personal experiences of violence, and how do they shape my understanding?
- What groups do I see as most vulnerable to IPV?
- How might my beliefs about IPV be conveyed to patients in ways that are judgemental or affirming?

Your practice environment also shapes your ability to listen effectively to and assess your patients. Hollingsworth et al. (2006) found that emergency nurses in Ontario who believed that assessing and responding to women who have experienced abuse is futile were less likely to engage in appropriate clinical practices, whereas those who had more positive beliefs about the benefits of assessing and responding to abuse were more likely to engage in appropriate clinical practices. In contrast to literature showing health professionals as unsympathetic and uninterested in providing care to women who have experienced abuse, they found that the nurses had relatively high levels of positive expectations regarding outcomes. Because *any* of your patients may have a history of abuse, it is critical to listen to *all* patients with that in mind and be confident that you can make a positive difference in their lives. This means using interpreters routinely with all patients who speak a different language from you. Questions to ask about your work environment include:

- How is "listening" to patients valued (by colleagues, managers, work expectations)? What time is available for listening?
- How much privacy is afforded when assessing patients?
- What is the workplace cultural norm with regard to attitudes toward patients (are you encouraged to see yourself as the expert?), women, and people who experience violence?
- How do these factors shape your practice? And how might you optimize the environment?

Your listening in a nonjudgemental manner can be very empowering for a woman who previously may have encountered disbelief, blame, or judgement from friends or professionals (Lempert, 1997; McMurray et al., 1994) and will contribute to building trust so that the woman may feel confident enough to disclose abuse. Both women who have experienced abuse and professionals with experience responding to abuse assert that validation of the woman's worth as a human being and abuse as undeserved are the most important aspects of an effective response and the foundation for a trusting relationship (Gerbert et al., 1999, 2000). Expressing interest in the conditions of women's lives beyond the immediate presenting health problem can be a way of conveying openness to women. For example, with any patient, simple questions such as, "How are your work and your home life affecting your health?" can convey interest and acceptance. Further, if the woman "hints" at or discloses abuse, conveying belief in her story by continuing to be nonjudgemental can also empower her. Sometimes women who are experiencing IPV will offer explanations for illnesses or injuries that downplay, overlook, or deny abuse—perhaps because of shame, fear of judgement, or fear of the consequences of disclosure, or because the woman has not connected her health problems to abuse. If done in a nonjudgemental, validating manner, openly indicating a possible connection to abuse can invite a direct conversation about IPV.

Anticipating Abuse

Based on the available statistics, about 50% of your female patients will have experienced at least one incident of physical or sexual assault in their lifetime. Because statistics suggest that about 7% of women currently in relationships have experienced violence in the past 5 years, violence will be a relevant issue to many. Some patients, however, are more vulnerable to abuse: those who are isolated, economically dependent on others, or dependent on others for care (e.g., those with disabilities). Further, as noted previously, specific injuries, such as fractures, bruises, and sprains, many chronic health challenges, and many mental health issues are associated with IPV. Thinking about IPV as a possible contributing factor is important in relation to diverse health issues ranging from substance abuse, to vaginal bleeding, to migraines. Given the high association of chronic pain with histories of abuse (Campbell, 2002; Kendall-Tackett et al., 2003; Walsh et al., 2007), you should have a high index of suspicion for abuse with any person experiencing chronic pain and

identify the factors related to abuse that are most relevant in your specific clinical area.

Assessing Collaboratively

Because research has repeatedly shown that women feel disempowered by healthcare professionals, which echoes their experiences of abuse, it is crucial to foster women's sense of control in decision making (Ford-Gilboe et al., 2005; Wuest et al., 2003), including helping them identify the risks and benefits of seeking help (Ford-Gilboe et al., 2006). When beginning most assessments, you will not know the women's abuse histories. Based on the relational approach introduced in Chapter 1 (Doane et al., 2005), a collaborative approach to assessment involves:

- Following the lead of women—conveying a willingness to listen and trustworthiness, allowing women to take the lead in disclosing (or not), and drawing on their knowledge to assess their levels of danger and options
- Listening to and for cues that might suggest abuse
- Self-observation—paying attention to how your assumptions and biases may shape your interactions and how you are reacting
- Pattern recognition—attending to patterns of physical symptoms (e.g. injuries, chronic pain) and health problems (e.g., substance abuse, sleep problems)
- Collaboratively developing knowledge—for example, helping women connect health problems to abuse, helping women evaluate their levels of danger
- Naming and supporting capacity—focusing on women's strengths and capacities

Assessment for abuse is much broader than screening. However, it may be useful to adapt questions designed for screening purposes in your assessments to follow the lead of the woman presenting with suggestions that her intimate relationships may be negatively impacting her health or with health problems or circumstances that warrant a high index of suspicion for abuse. For example, an 80-year-old woman presenting with tachycardia replied to the nurse's observation that her relationship did not seem to be helping her health, with the disclosure that "this [tachycardia] happens every time he gets like that." The nurse was able to clarify the woman's meaning, that the woman's husband battered her frequently.

Inquiring about a woman's relationships and their impact on her health should be included in the assessment of any woman (e.g., "How do the people in your life affect your health?"), as it will provide important information beyond what might be classified as violence or abuse.

Even when a woman describes abuse, she may downplay it, saying it is "only emotional" or "not that bad" or "we just fight a lot." More abuse may be revealed as you listen. This is not "denial" on the woman's part but rather the normal minimization that often accompanies trauma from violence.

It is appropriate for you to show that you are concerned and even distressed about the degree of violence. One message that needs to be conveyed during the assessment is that the abuse is not the woman's fault; this can be stated several times. Another important message is that you are concerned and that help is available. Still another is that several health problems can occur because of violence. In fact, in a survey of 265 abused women who accepted a referral to a social worker, 59% said it was because the medical provider expressed concern that their presenting health problem was related to IPV (McCaw et al., 2002).

Specific clinical contexts have assessment approaches that integrate attention to violence. For example, in the perinatal context, in contrast to the usual assumption that pregnancy is a positive event, it is important to approach all pregnant women with openness to the possibility that being in an abusive relationship may be one of her many challenges.

Humphreys et al. (2003) propose that when abuse is suspected or confirmed, appropriate clinical responses include:
- Assessing the woman's level of risk and developing a safety plan
- Conducting a thorough health assessment
- Identifying personal strengths and support systems
- Identifying appropriate goals with the woman in collaboration with other healthcare professionals

Assessment related to sexual assault should be based on the same principles as assessment for IPV. The emotional, cultural, and physical safety of the patient should come first, and a validating, nonjudgemental response is essential. It is important that the patient remain in control of care as much as possible, including the decision to call the police and to have forensic evidence collected. Sexual assault victims may be male or female, and assault may occur within the context of an intimate relationship (e.g., a spousal or dating relationship) or in a nonintimate relationship (with a client of a sex worker, or with others such as co-workers, employers, healthcare professionals, etc.). Assault by unknown assailants is much less common. McConkey et al. (2001) note that a survivor may seek treatment immediately or within days or weeks after the assault. Survivors may go to a primary care setting to receive treatment for prevention of pregnancy or STIs. Many survivors are embarrassed and fear being dismissed as undeserving of care, especially those who are victims of date rape, use alcohol or drugs, or for whom the assault is associated with sex work. In case of a known assailant, the survivor may be fearful of seeking treatment (McConkey et al., 2001).

HEALTHCARE PROFESSIONALS' RESPONSES TO ELDER AND VULNERABLE PERSON ABUSE AND NEGLECT

Assessing possible elder abuse and neglect can be more complicated than assessments for IPV. The older person can present for health care cognitively and physically intact or with multiple health, physical, and cognitive challenges. Assessment for IPV in the older woman is very similar to assessing for IPV among younger women if the patient is cognitively intact.

While some older women have been in abusive relationships for decades, others are experiencing for the first time physical and sexual violence from normally nonabusive partners who themselves may be afflicted with behaviour-altering neurological illnesses (Alzheimer's disease, organic brain syndromes). An older battered woman in a long-term abusive relationship may be trying to outlive her abuser, whereas the newly abused older woman may be reluctant to disclose abuse because of embarrassment, shame, and fears that her partner will be institutionalized. Assessment of physical abuse or neglect in the cognitively challenged person is much more complicated. Physical findings that are inconsistent with the history provided by the patient, family member, or caregiver are significant red flags for possible abuse and neglect.

HEALTHCARE PROFESSIONALS' RESPONSES TO CHILD ABUSE

In Canada, screening for child abuse is not recommended. Because of the high rate of false-positive screening test results and the potential for incorrectly labelling individuals as child abusers, the possible harms associated with screening outweigh the benefits (MacMillan, 2000). Although screening is not recommended, reporting suspected child abuse is mandatory in most provinces and territories, meaning that the identification of child abuse relies on careful assessment by healthcare professionals.

It is important that approaches to child abuse be similar to those recommended for IPV but modified (1) to take into account that children are even more vulnerable to family members, and (2) to accommodate the developmental stage of each child. Keep in mind that:
- Any child may be at risk of some form of abuse, regardless of the ethnicity or income of the family
- Neglect and emotional abuse are the most common forms of abuse and are harmful, so if you rely only on obvious indicators of physical abuse or look only for cues of sexual abuse, you may overlook significant damage
- Parents are not the only possible perpetrators of child abuse
- Many allegations of suspected child abuse are unsubstantiated
- While some situations warrant removal of children from their parents, this step also is stressful for children, and in most cases the children will remain in contact with their parents for life
- Assessments for child abuse are evaluations of parenting, and often focus uncritically on evaluating mothers against culturally specific dominant stereotypes of mothering even when the mother is not the perpetrator (Tanner et al., 2000)
- Ethically, as a healthcare professional, you are obligated to provide "good" care to all, including a child's parents
- While you must intervene and report suspected child abuse, your role as a healthcare professional is not to "rescue" the child at the expense of your relationship with the parents or of the relationship between the child and the parents

Again, your assumptions and beliefs will be conveyed to children and parents. It is crucial to reflect on your own ideas and experiences so that you can work toward the short- and long-term well-being of all parties. Assessment and intervention for suspected child abuse is possible without alienating the parents, regardless of whether the parents are suspected of perpetrating the abuse.

Assessing for Child Abuse

Assessing for child abuse means integrating awareness of the possibility of child abuse into every assessment. It is important to be alert for signs of physical abuse and intentional injury. However, it is crucial to carefully evaluate any physical injury within the context of a child's age and developmental stage. Is the injury that is being reported in line with the child's developmental level? For example, the explanation that a 3-week-old child was injured rolling off a bed is not developmentally plausible. Because the nurse may not be able to directly observe the child's motor and cognitive milestones during the history-taking, it is important to ask the caregivers directly. Is your child crawling, pulling up to stand, or walking? What other developmental issues are currently being faced at home: tantrums, potty training, and so on? It is also important to be aware of the possible indicators of neglect and emotional and sexual abuse, as these are much more challenging to determine. Tanner et al. (2000) recommend repeated observations of parenting and critical reflection on the part of professionals to take into account biases that arise from stereotypical and dominant assumptions in one's own cultural context. Horwath (2002) describes the Framework for the Assessment of Children in Need and Their Families, which can help professionals focus on broader issues rather than on dramatic situations of severe physical abuse. The framework features an assessment triangle with three interrelated systems or domains: the child's developmental needs, parenting capacity, and family and environmental factors (Fig. 7-3). The framework attends to the complexity of responding to child neglect, but Horwath cautions that the tensions among these domains must be taken into account to avoid losing focus on the child in question.

Responses to known child abuse are much more comprehensive than the well-publicized interventions of placing children in out-of-home care. There has been some evidence of the successful support of parents. For example, in Canada, two randomized controlled trials showed a reduction in the incidence of child abuse or outcomes related to physical abuse and neglect among first-time disadvantaged mothers and their infants who received a program of home visitation by nurses in the perinatal period extending through infancy (MacMillan, 2000).

Mandatory Reporting of Child Abuse

In Canada, provincial and territorial jurisdictions have the legislative responsibility for child and family services (child welfare). One exception is the federal responsibility for Aboriginal peoples with status under the *Indian Act* (Canada). Each province and territory has specific legislation providing protection for neglected and abused children. *Child Welfare in Canada* (Human Resources and Child Welfare Canada, 2000) outlines the roles and responsibilities of provincial and ter-

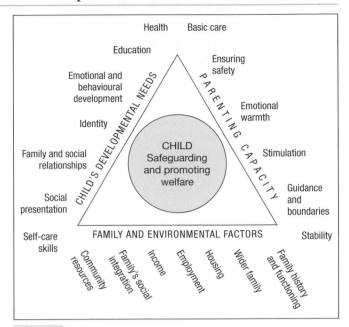

Fig. 7-3   Framework for the assessment of children in need and their families

ritorial child welfare authorities in the provision of child protection and preventive and support services. Most provinces and territories have legislation that makes it mandatory for the public, including healthcare professionals, to report child abuse. If you are working with children, you should review the specific requirements for the jurisdiction in which you are working by visiting the Human Resources and Social Development Canada Web site at http://www.hrsdc.gc.ca/en/cs/sp/sdc/socpol/publications/reports/2000-000033/page03.shtml.

If you suspect that a child is being maltreated, you should involve other members of the healthcare team. Most healthcare settings have access to social workers who are specifically trained in dealing with child abuse. They will often be the first point of contact for reporting suspected abuse.

HISTORY

It is important also to assess and document prior abuse, including prior IPV, childhood physical and sexual abuse, and prior rapes of all kinds (stranger, date, intimate partner). Cumulative trauma has been shown to be associated with more severe mental and physical health problems (Koss et al., 1994; McCauley et al., 1997). Also, determine the history of traumatic injuries, since these may have an impact on the current health condition. For instance, a woman may have experienced prior episodes of head trauma and strangulation, both of which may be related to chronic but subtle neurological symptoms and problems (Diaz-Olavarrieta et al., 1999). A mental status examination is also important, both for potential head trauma and neurological symptoms and for mental health problems. Pay particular attention to the most frequent mental health problems associated with violence: depression, suicidality, PTSD, substance abuse, and anxiety. Chapter 6 gives direction for conducting this part of the history.

If child abuse is suspected and if the child is verbal, a history should be obtained away from the caregivers through open-ended questions or spontaneous statements. It is important to remember that children may have suffered significant trauma but may respond only minimally to open-ended questions (Myers et al., 2002). Keeping the questions short and using age-appropriate language and familiar words can help to enrich the history-taking. Children older than 11 years of age can generally be expected to provide a history at the level of most adults (Myers et al., 2002).

The medical history is also an important part of your evaluation. Has the child had previous hospitalizations or injuries, or does he or she suffer from any chronic medical conditions? Does the child take any medication that may cause easy bruising? Does the child have a history of repeated visits to the hospital? Was there a delay in seeking care for anything other than a minor injury?

PHYSICAL EXAMINATION

Important components of the physical examination of the known survivor of IPV or elder abuse include a complete head-to-toe visual examination, especially if the patient is receiving healthcare services secondary to reported abuse. When the examination discovers physical findings, accurate use of medical terminology to describe injuries is essential (see Chapter 12). In Canada, it is controversial whether forensic evidence is supportive of women who experience IPV. For example, a study in British Columbia found that health records were inaccurate reflections of the woman's experience and were most often used to undermine the woman and her legal claims (Cory et al., 2003). However, there is some evidence that forensic examinations do lead to a higher probability of charges and conviction rates in sexual assault cases (Du Mont et al., 2000; McGregor et al., 2002).

There is no scientific evidence to support the accurate dating of injuries based on the colour of the contusion (Langlois & Greshman, 2001). However, a new bruise is usually red and will often develop a purple or purple-blue appearance 12 to 36 hours after blunt-force trauma. The colour of bruises (and ecchymoses) generally progresses from purple-blue to bluish green to greenish brown to brownish yellow before fading away.

Physical assessment following sexual assault can also include the collection of forensic evidence, that is, evidence that can be admitted in court. Such collection usually requires the expert skills of a specially trained sexual assault nurse examiner (SANE) or physician. The details of collection of such evidence are beyond the scope of this chapter.

Bruising is an important sign of elder abuse. There are multiple factors that can contribute to older adults bruising more readily or more severely than younger people. Medications and abnormal blood values related to their side effects, as well as underlying hematological disorders, can affect ease of bruising or the formation of ecchymosis. Common medications that increase risk for bruising or bleeding complications include, but are not limited to, the following: aspirin, ibuprofen, any of the nonsteroidal anti-inflammatory drugs, warfarin, heparin, valproic acid, prednisone, and clopidogrel. Vitamin supplements also may contribute to hematological complications (Doyle et al., 2001). Mosqueda et al. (2005) studied older adults who had accidental bruises and found that nearly 90% of their bruises were on their extremities and no accidental bruises were found on the neck, ears, genitalia, buttocks, or soles of the feet.

Any health evaluation for known or suspected elder abuse and neglect should include baseline laboratory tests, including, at a minimum, a complete blood count (CBC) with platelet level, basic blood chemistries (including BUN, creatinine, protein, and albumin), serum liver function tests, a coagulation panel, and a urinalysis (Geroff & Olshaker, 2001).

Physical Examination of Children

A visual inspection from head to toe is important in any physical examination of the child. Significant injuries can be hidden under clothing, diapers, socks, and long hair. The American Academy of Pediatrics (2002) defines significant trauma as any injury beyond temporary redness of the skin. Accidental bruising in healthy, active children is common, but the presence of bruises in babies has significance in evaluating for abuse. Children who are not yet walking with support—"cruising"—typically should not have bruises (Sugar et al., 1999). Bruising in infants who are not yet cruising, usually infants less than 9 months of age, should alert you to possible abusive mechanisms to the injury or an underlying medical illness.

Once children begin to walk, bruising, particularly on the bony prominences, is common (Sugar et al., 1999). Reece and Ludwig (2001) found that in children who were walking, 40 to 50% had bruises over the bony prominences of the front of their bodies. Sugar et al. (1999) found that bruising in "atypical" places such as the buttocks, hands, feet, and abdomen was exceedingly rare and should arouse concerns. Furthermore, any bruise that takes the shape of an object should be considered highly specific for abuse. Bruising found in nonmobile children should raise concerns about other injuries, including fractures and intracranial injury (Barber & Sibert, 2000).

The Canadian Paediatric Society has provided comprehensive guidelines to healthcare professionals regarding abusive head trauma (AHT), including what was previously known as "shaken baby syndrome." It advises that AHT should always be considered in infants without a definite diagnosis. Symptoms can include lethargy, decreased feeding, irritability, vomiting, respiratory distress, apnea, seizures, and an altered level of consciousness. The guidelines stress that the accompanying caregiver may not know the cause of the child's symptoms or may not give a complete and accurate history. The guidelines state that a full assessment for suspected AHT should be considered in infants and young children with:

- An acute or chronic injury that has inadequate, inconsistent, evolving, or no explanation
- A severe head injury allegedly the result of a short fall or minor trauma
- An unexplained symptomatic head injury in a child who was well when last seen
- Subdural hemorrhage, retinal hemorrhage, or rib, skull, or metaphyseal fractures

DOCUMENTATION

Documentation of intimate partner violence and elder abuse must include objective progress notes, written in unbiased language. Injury maps and photographic documentation may be useful. Examples of photographic documentation of patients of Dr. Dan Sheridan are included in this chapter (Figs. 7-4 through 7-6*).

Written documentation of histories of IPV and elder abuse need to be verbatim reports but within reason. It is clinically unrealistic to document verbatim every statement made by an abused patient. However, it is critical to document exceptionally poignant statements made by the victim that identify the reported perpetrator and severe threats of harm made by the reported perpetrator. Other aspects of the abuse history, including reports of past abusive incidents, can be paraphrased with the use of partial direct quotations.

When quoting or paraphrasing the history, you should not sanitize words reportedly heard by the victim. Verbatim documentation of the reported perpetrator's threats interlaced with curses and expletives can be extremely useful in future court proceedings. Also, be careful to use the exact terms an abused patient may use to describe sexual organs or sexually assaultive behaviours.

Photographic documentation in the medical record can be invaluable. Prior written consent to take photographs should be obtained from all cognitively intact, competent adults. Most healthcare facilities have standardized consent-to-photograph forms. If a patient is unconscious or cognitively impaired, taking photographs without consent is generally viewed as ethically sound, since it is a noninvasive, painless intervention that may help a suspected abuse victim.

When documenting the history and physical findings of child abuse and neglect, use the words of the child to describe how his or her injury occurred. Remember that the possibility arises that the abuser may be accompanying the child. If the child is nonverbal, use statements from caregivers. It is important to know your employer or institutional protocol for obtaining history in cases of suspected child maltreatment. Some protocols may delay a full interview until it can be conducted by a forensically trained interviewer.

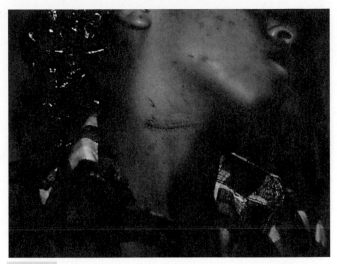

Fig. 7-4　Patterned, fingernail-like scratch abrasions to the left lateral neck from a manual strangulation mechanism of injury.

ASSESSING FOR RISK OF HOMICIDE

Women in both the United States and Canada have more often been killed by a husband, boyfriend, or ex-husband than by anyone else, and about three fourths of these women were abused by the man who subsequently killed them (Campbell et al., 2001; Statistics Canada, 2005). Statistics Canada (2005) reported that of 78 spouses killed in Canada in 2004, 62 were women killed by male spouses. In a study of intimate partner homicide of women in the United States, 42% of the women killed had been seen somewhere in the healthcare system (the emergency department in the majority of cases, but also in primary care, prenatal care, and other settings) for something in the year before she was killed (Sharps et al., 2001). These encounters were missed opportunities for healthcare professionals to identify IPV and intervene to decrease the danger.

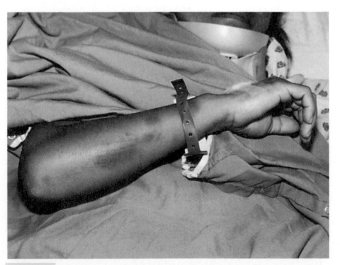

Fig. 7-5　Patterned, defensive-posture-like bruises to the right forearm.

---

*Many of these photos were first published in Sheridan, 2001. Reprinted here with the author's permission.

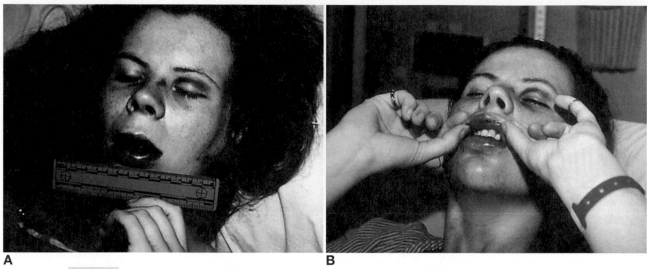

A   **B**

Fig. 7-6   Series of two photographs to illustrate how photographs can be used to demonstrate mechanisms of injuries. **A,** Victim has obvious facial trauma to her left eyelid, left lateral nose, and mouth. The left lateral nose contusion was caused by the nose piece of her glasses being forcefully pushed into her skin from a punch to the left eye. The patient's glasses absorbed much of the punch force and were broken (not shown). A second punch produced the mouth trauma. **B,** The force of the mouth punch caused the upper teeth to leave patterned contusion, abrasion, and minor laceration to the oral mucosa of the upper lip.

The same study found reliability and validity support for the Danger Assessment (DA), a 19-item yes/no instrument that has been used extensively by nurses in the healthcare system as well as advocates in other settings involving battered women (Campbell et al., 2001) (Fig. 7-7). The instrument starts with a calendar so that women can more accurately see for themselves how frequent and severe the violence has become over the past year. This is also an excellent tool for assessment of frequency and severity for the healthcare professional. Although there are no predetermined cutoff scores on the DA, the more yes answers there are, the more serious is the danger of the woman's situation. In the previously described multi-city study, abused women who were victims of homicide had an average score of 7.1 on the original 15-item DA. The DA is copyrighted, so users need to use it intact and are asked to communicate with the author if they are planning to use it for research purposes. It can also be downloaded from http://www.son.jhmi.edu.

CULTURAL AND SOCIAL CONSIDERATIONS

Violence is a widespread sociocultural problem, but in Western societies, there is a tendency to treat interpersonal violence as a problem of individuals. Rather than social prevention and intervention, efforts to deal with violence are targeted toward individuals, often leaving victims responsible for dealing with violence. Further, despite the fact that it is

well known that violence occurs across all societies and cultural groups, there is a tendency to associate violence with particular groups. To effectively deal with violence, healthcare professionals must take three steps. First, as argued in earlier chapters, healthcare professionals must work to evaluate how their own cultural values and beliefs and the dominant values operating in health care affect the care they provide. Second, healthcare professionals need to consider their own stereotypes and assumptions regarding IPV, sexual assault, child abuse and neglect, and elder abuse and neglect, and replace those stereotypes and assumptions with knowledge regarding all forms of violence. Third, healthcare professionals need to take into account how ideas about certain groups of people (e.g., stereotypes about some groups as being more violent or more likely to be abusive toward children) support discrimination in the provision of health care and deter people from seeking health care.

Rather than assessing how culture, narrowly defined as ethnicity, shapes experiences of violence, it is important to assess how culture in the broader sense shapes such experiences. For example, rather than focusing on particular ethnocultural groups, it is more useful to consider how racialization, gender, experiences of immigration, discrimination, language barriers, and inequitable access to employment and resources shape experiences of violence and access to social support in response to violence (Hyman et al., 2006; Jiwani, 2000; Martin et al., 1995; Varcoe, 2008).

DANGER ASSESSMENT
Jacquelyn C. Campbell, Ph.D., R.N.
Copyright 1985, 1988, 2001

Several risk factors have been associated with homicides (murders) of both batterers and battered women in research conducted after the murders have taken place. We cannot predict what will happen in your case, but we would like you to be aware of the danger of homicide in situations of severe battering and for you to see how many of the risk factors apply to your situation.

Using the calendar, please mark the approximate dates during the past year when you were beaten by your husband or partner. Write on that date how bad the incident was according to the following scale:

1. Slapping, pushing; no injuries and/or lasting pain
2. Punching, kicking; bruises, cuts, and/or continuing pain
3. "Beating up"; severe contusions, burns, broken bones
4. Threat to use weapon; head injury, internal injury, permanent injury
5. Use of weapon; wounds from weapon

(If **any** of the descriptions for the higher number apply, use the higher number.)

Mark **Yes** or **No** for each of the following. ("He" refers to your husband, partner, ex-husband, ex-partner, or whoever is currently physically hurting you.)

_____ 1. Has the physical violence increased in severity or frequency over the past year?
_____ 2. Has he ever used a weapon against you or threatened you with a weapon?
_____ 3. Does he ever try to choke you?
_____ 4. Does he own a gun?
_____ 5. Has he ever forced you to have sex when you did not wish to do so?
_____ 6. Does he use drugs? By drugs, I mean "uppers" or amphetamines, speed, angel dust, cocaine, "crack," street drugs or mixtures.
_____ 7. Does he threaten to kill you and/or do you believe he is capable of killing you?
_____ 8. Is he drunk every day or almost every day? (In terms of quantity of alcohol.)
_____ 9. Does he control most or all of your daily activities? For instance: does he tell you who you can be friends with, when you can see your family, how much money you can use, or when you can take the car? (If he tries, but you do not let him, check here: _____)
_____ 10. Have you ever been beaten by him while you were pregnant? (If you have never been pregnant by him, check here: _____)
_____ 11. Is he violently and constantly jealous of you? (For instance, does he say "If I can't have you, no one can"?)
_____ 12. Have you ever threatened or tried to commit suicide?
_____ 13. Has he ever threatened or tried to commit suicide?
_____ 14. Does he threaten to harm your children?
_____ 15. Do you have a child that is not his?
_____ 16. Is he unemployed?
_____ 17. Have you left him during the past year? (If you have *never* lived with him, check here: _____)
_____ 18. Do you currently have another (different) intimate partner?
_____ 19. Does he follow or spy on you, leave threatening notes, destroy your property, or call you when you don't want him to?

_____ Total "Yes" Answers

Thank you. Please talk to your nurse, advocate, or counsellor about what the Danger Assessment means in terms of your situation.

Fig. 7-7   Danger assessment.

BIBLIOGRAPHY

American Academy of Pediatrics. (1998). The role of the pediatrician in recognizing and intervening on behalf of abused women. *Pediatrics, 101*, 1091–1092.

Bacchus, L., Mezey, G., & Bewley, S. (2003). Experiences of seeking help from health professionals in a sample of women who experienced domestic violence. *Health and Social Care in the Community, 11*(1), 10–18.

Bachman, R., & Saltzman, L. E. (1995). *Violence against women: estimates from the redesigned survey.* Washington, DC: Bureau of Justice Statistics, National Institute of Justice.

Barber, M. A., & Sibert, J. R. (2000). Diagnosing physical child abuse: The way forward. *Post-Graduate Medical Journal, 76*, 743–749.

Beaulaurier, R., Seff, L., Newman, F., & Dunlop, B. (2007). External barriers to help seeking for older women who experience intimate partner violence. *Journal of Family Violence, 22*, 747–755.

Bhandari, M., Dosanjh, S., Tornetta, P., III, & Matthews, D. (2006). Musculoskeletal manifestations of physical abuse after intimate partner violence. *Journal of Trauma, 61*, 1473–1479.

Blackstock, C., Trocmé, N., & Bennett, M. (2004). Child maltreatment investigations among Aboriginal and non-Aboriginal families in Canada. *Violence Against Women, 10*, 901–916.

Bogat, G. A., DeJonghe, E., Levendosky, A. A., Davidson, W. S., & von Eye, A. (2006). Trauma symptoms among infants exposed to intimate partner violence. *Child Abuse and Neglect, 30*(2), 109–125.

Campbell, J., & Soeken, K. (1999a). Forced sex and intimate partner violence: Effects on women's health. *Violence against Women, 5*, 1017–1035.

Campbell, J., & Soeken, K. L. (1999b). Women's responses to battering: A test of the model. *Research in Nursing and Health, 22*, 49–58.

Campbell, J., Jones, A. S., Dienemann, J., Kub, J., Schollenberger, J., O'Campo, P., et al. (2002). Intimate partner violence and physical health consequences. *Archives of Internal Medicine, 162*, 1157–1163.

Campbell, J. C. (2002). Health consequences of intimate partner violence. *Lancet, 359*(9314), 1331–1336.

Campbell, J. C., & Lewandowski, L. (1997). Mental and psychical health effects of intimate partner violence on women and children. *Psychiatric Clinics of North America, 20*, 353–374.

Campbell, J. C., Sharps, P., & Glass, N. E. (2001). Risk assessment for intimate partner homicide. In G. F. Pinard & L. Pagani (Eds.), *Clinical assessment of dangerousness: Empirical contributions.* New York, NY: Cambridge University Press.

Campbell, R., Sefl, T., & Ahrens, C. E. (2003). The physical health consequences of rape: Assessing survivors' somatic symptoms in a racially diverse population. *Women's Studies Quarterly, 31*(1–2), 90–104.

Canadian Centre for Justice Statistics. (2002). *Family violence in Canada: A statistical profile.* Ottawa, ON: Statistics Canada.

Canadian Paediatric Society. (2007). *Position statements: Multidisciplinary guidelines on the identification, investigation and management of suspected abusive head trauma; Joint statement on shaken baby syndrome.* Retrieved June 5, 2008, from http://www.cps.ca/english/publications/YouthMaltreatment.htm

Carlson, B. (2000). Children exposed to intimate partner violence: Research findings and implications for intervention. *Trauma, Violence, and Abuse, 1*, 321–342.

Carlson, B. (2005). The most important things learned about violence and trauma in the past 20 years. *Journal of Interpersonal Violence, 20*, 119–126.

Cascardi, M., Daniel O'Leary, K., & Schlee, K. A. (1999). Co-occurrence and correlates of posttraumatic stress disorder and major depression in physically abused women. *Journal of Family Violence, 14*, 227–249.

Cherniak, D., Grant, L., Mason, R., Moore, B., & Pellizzari, R. (2005). Society of Obstetricians and Gynaecologists of Canada (SOGC) clinical practice guidelines: Intimate partner violence consensus statement. *Society of Obstetricians and Gynaecologists of Canada (SOGC) Clinical Practice Guidelines, 157.*

Clark, J. P., & Du Mont, J. (2003). Intimate partner violence and health: A critique of Canadian prevalence studies. *Revue Canadienne de Sante Publique, 94*(1), 52–58.

Coker, A., Smith, P. H., McKeown, R. E., & King, M. J. (2000). Frequency and correlates of intimate partner violence by type: Physical, sexual, and psychological battering. *American Journal of Public Health, 90*, 553–559.

Coker, A. L. (2006). Preventing intimate partner violence: How we will rise to this challenge. *American Journal of Preventive Medicine*, 528–529.

Coker, A. L., Fadden, M. K., Reeder, C. E., & Smith, P. H. (2004). Physical partner violence and medicaid utilization and expenditures. *Public Health Reports, 119*, 557–567.

Cory, J., & Dechief, L. (2007). *Safety and Health Enhancement (SHE) framework for women experiencing abuse.* Retrieved June 5, 2008, from http://www.bcwomens.ca/Services/HealthServices/WomanAbuseResponse/Resources.htm

Cory, J., Ruebesat, G., Hankivsky, O., & Dechief, L. (2003). *Reasonable doubt: The use of health records in criminal and civil cases of violence against women in relationships.* Retrieved June 5, 2008, from http://www.bcifv.org/resources/healthrecordsbrochure02.pdf

Department of Justice Canada. (2007a). *Child abuse fact sheet.* Retrieved June 5, 2008, from http://www.justice.gc.ca/en/ps/fm/childafs.html

Department of Justice Canada. (2007b). *Elder abuse fact sheet.* Retrieved June 5, 2008, from http://www.justice.gc.ca/en/ps/fm/adultsfs.html#head1

Diaz-Olavarrieta, C., Campbell, J., Garcia de la Cadena, C., Paz, F., & Villa, A. R. (1999). Domestic violence against patients with chronic neurologic disorders. *Archives of Neurology, 56*, 681–685.

Doane, G., & Varcoe, C. (2005). *Family nursing as relational inquiry: Developing health-promoting practice.* Philadelphia, PA: Lippincott, Williams & Wilkins.

Doyle, R. M., Harold, C., & Johnson, P. (Eds.). (2001). *Nursing herbal medicine handbook.* Springhouse, PA: Springhouse Corporation.

Du Mont, J., Forte, T., Cohen, M. M., Hyman, I., & Romans, S. (2005). Changing help-seeking rates for intimate partner violence in Canada. *Women and Health, 41*(1), 1–19.

Du Mont, J., McGregor, M. J., Myhr, T. L., & Miller, K.-L. (2000). Predicting legal outcomes from medicolegal findings: An examination of sexual assault in two jurisdictions. *Journal of Women's Health and Law, 1*, 219–233.

Eby, K. K., Campbell, J. C., Sullivan, C. M., & Davidson, W. S. (1995). Health effects of experiences of sexual violence for women with abusive partners. *Health Care for Women International, 16*, 563–576.

Edleson, J. L. (1999). The overlap between child maltreatment and woman battering. *Violence Against Women, 5*, 134–154.

Fischbach, R., & Herbert, B. (1997). Domestic violence and mental health: Correlates and conundrums within and across cultures. *Social Science and Medicine, 45*, 1161–1176.

Folsom, W. S., Christensen, M. L., Avery, L., & Moore, C. (2003). The co-occurrence of child abuse and domestic violence: an issue of service delivery for social service professionals. *Child and Adolescent Social Work Journal, 20*, 375–387.

Ford-Gilboe, M., Wuest, J., & Merritt-Gray, M. (2005). Strengthening capacity to limit intrusion: Theorizing family health promotion in the aftermath of woman abuse. *Qualitative Health Research, 15*, 477–501.

Ford-Gilboe, M., Wuest, J., Varcoe, C., & Merritt-Gray, M. (2006). Developing an evidence-based health advocacy intervention to support women who have left abusive partners. *Canadian Journal of Nursing Research, 38*(1), 147–167.

Fugate, M., Landis, L., Riordan, K., Naureckas, S., & Engel, B. (2005). Barriers to domestic violence help seeking: Implications for intervention. *Violence Against Women, 11*, 290–310.

Gazmararian, J. A., Petersen, R., Spitz, A. M., Goodwin, M. M., Saltzman, L. E., & Marks, J. S. (2000). Violence and reproductive health: Current knowledge and future research directions. *Maternal and Child Health Journal, 4*(2), 79–84.

Gerbert, B., Abercrombie, P., Caspers, N., Love, C., & Bronstone, A. (1999). How health care providers help battered women: The survivor's perspective. *Women and Health, 29,* 115–135.

Gerbert, B., Caspers, N., Bronstone, A., Moe, J., & Abercrombie, P. (1999). A qualitative analysis of how physicians with expertise in domestic violence approach the identification of victims. *Annals of Internal Medicine, 131,* 578–584.

Gerbert, B., Caspers, N., Milliken, N., Berlia, M., Bronstone, A., & Mof, J. (2000). Interventions that help victims of domestic violence. *Journal of Family Practice, 49,* 889.

Gerbert, B., Johnston, K., Caspers, N., Bleecker, T., Woods, A., & Rosenbaum, A. (1996). Experiences of battered women in health care settings: A qualitative study. *Women and Health, 24,* 1–17.

Geroff, A. J., & Olshaker, J. S. (2001). Elder abuse. In J. S. Olshaker, M. C. Jackson, & W. S. Smock (Eds.), *Forensic emergency medicine.* Philadelphia, PA: Lippincott Williams & Wilkins.

Golding, J. M. (1999). Intimate partner violence as a risk factor for mental disorders: A meta-analysis. *Journal of Family Violence, 14*(2), 99–132.

Hagele, D. M. (2005). The impact of maltreatment on the developing child. *NC Medical Journal, 66,* 356–359.

Hollingsworth, E., & Ford-Gilboe, M. (2006). Registered nurses' self-efficacy for assessing and responding to woman abuse in emergency department settings. *Canadian Journal of Nursing Research, 38*(4), 54–77.

Horwath, J. (2002). Maintaining a focus on the child? First impressions of the framework for the assessment of children in need and their families in cases of child neglect. *Child Abuse Review, 11*(4), 195–213.

Human Resources and Child Welfare Canada (2000). *Child welfare in Canada.* Retrieved June 5, 2008, from http://www.hrsdc.gc.ca/en/cs/sp/sdc/socpol/publications/reports/2000-000033/page00.shtml

Humphreys, C., & Thiara, R. (2003). Mental health and domestic violence: "I call it symptoms of abuse". *British Journal of Social Work, 33*(2), 209–226.

Humphreys, J., & Campbell, J. C. (2003). *Family violence in nursing practice.* New York, NY: Lippincott, Williams & Wilkins.

Hyman, I., Forte, T., Du Mont, J., Romans, S., & Cohen, M. (2006). The association between length of stay in Canada and intimate partner violence among immigrant women. *American Journal of Public Health, 96,* 654–659.

Janssen, P. A., Holt, V. L., Sugg, N. K., Emanuel, I., Critchlow, C. M., & Henderson, A. D. (2003). Intimate partner violence and adverse pregnancy outcomes: A population-based study. *American Journal of Obstetrics and Gynecology, 188,* 1341.

Jenny, C., Hymel, K. P., Ritzen, A., Reinert, S. E., & Hay, T. C. (1999). Analysis of missed cases of abusive head trauma. *Journal of the American Medical Association, 281,* 621–626.

Jiwani, Y. (2000). *Race, gender, violence and health care: Immigrant women of colour who have experienced violence and their encounters with the health care system.* Vancouver, BC: Feminist Research, Education, Development and Action.

Johnson, H. (1996). *Dangerous domains: Violence against women in Canada.* Scarborough, ON: International Thompson Publishing.

Johnson, H. (2006). *Measuring violence against women: Statistical trends.* Ottawa, ON: Statistics Canada.

Johnson, H., & Sacco, V. (1995). Researching violence against women: Statistics Canada's national survey. *Canadian Journal of Criminology, July,* 281–304.

Jones, A. S., Gielen, A. C., Campbell, J. C., Schollenberger, J., Dienemann, J. A., Kub, J., et al. (1999). Annual and lifetime prevalence of partner abuse in a sample of female HMO enrollees. *Women's Health Issues, 9,* 295–305.

Kendall-Tackett, K. (2002). The health effects of childhood abuse: four pathways by which abuse can influence health. *Child Abuse and Neglect, 26,* 715.

Kendall-Tackett, K., Marshall, R., & Ness, K. (2003). Chronic pain syndromes and violence against women. *Women and Therapy, 26,* 45–56.

Knapp, J. F. (1998). The impact of children witnessing violence. *Violence Among Children and Adolescents, 45,* 355–364.

Koss, M. P., Goodman, L. A., & Browne, A. (1994). *No safe haven: Male violence against women at home, at work, and in the community.* Washington, DC: American Psychological Association.

Landenburger, K. (1998). Exploration of women's identity: Clinical approaches with abused women. In J. Campbell (Ed.), *Empowering survivors of abuse: Health care for battered women and their children.* Newbury Park, CA: Sage.

Langlois, N. E. I., & Greshman, G. A. (2001). The aging of bruises: A review and study of the colour changes with time. *Forensic Science International, 50,* 227–238.

Lempert, L. B. (1997). The other side of help: Negative effects in the help-seeking processes of abused women. *Qualitative Sociology, 20,* 289–309.

Leserman, J., Li, D., Drossman, D. A., & Hu, Y. J. B. (1998). Selected symptoms associated with sexual and physical abuse among female patients with gastrointestinal disorders: The impact on subsequent health care visits. *Psychological Medicine, 28,* 417–425.

Letourneau, E., Holmes, M., & Chasedunn-Roark, J. (1999). Gynecologic health consequences to victims of interpersonal violence. *Women's Health Issues, 9*(2), 115–120.

MacMillan, H. L. (2000). Preventive health care, 2000 update: prevention of child maltreatment. *Canadian Medical Association Journal, 163,* 1451–1458.

MacMillan, H. L., & Wathen, C. N. (2003). Violence against women: Integrating the evidence into clinical practice. *Canadian Medical Association Journal, 169,* 570–571.

Maman, S., Campbell, J., Sweat, M., & Gielen, A. C. (2000). The intersection of HIV and violence: directions for future research and interventions. *Social Science and Medicine, 4,* 459–478.

Martin, D. L., & Mosher, J. E. (1995). Unkept promises: Experiences of immigrant women with the neo-criminalization of wife abuse. *Canadian Journal of Women and the Law, 8,* 3–44.

McCauley, J., Kern, D.E., Kolodner, K., Dill, L., Schroeder, A.F., DeChant, H. K., et al. (1995). The "battering syndrome": Prevalence and clinical characteristics of domestic violence in primary care internal medicine practices. *Annals of Internal Medicine, 123,* 737–746.

McCauley, J., Kern, D.E., Kolodner, K., Dill, L., Schroeder, A.F., DeChant, H. K., et al. (1997). Clinical characteristics of women with a history of childhood abuse: Unhealed wounds. *Journal of the American Medical Association, 277,* 1362–1368.

McCaw, B., Berman, W. H., Syme, S. L., & Hunkeler, E. F. (2002). Women referred for on-site domestic violence services in a managed care organization. *Women and Health, 35*(2/3), 23–40.

McCloskey, K., & Grigsby, N. (2005). The ubiquitous clinical problem of adult intimate partner violence: The need for routine assessment. *Professional Psychology: Research and Practice, 36,* 264–275.

McConkey, T. E., Sole, M. L., & Holcomb, L. (2001). Assessing the female sexual assault survivor. *Nurse Practitioner, 26*(7 Pt. 1), 28.

McDonald, L., & Collins, A. (2000). *Abuse and neglect of older adults: A discussion paper.* Ottawa, ON: Health Canada.

McGregor, M. J., Du Mont, J., & Myhr, T. L. (2002). Sexual assault forensic medical examination: Is evidence related to successful prosecution? *Annals of Emergency Medicine, 39,* 639–647.

McLean, C. (2001). Less sensational but more dangerous. *Report/Newsmagazine (National Edition), 28*(22), 44.

McMurray, A., & Moore, K. (1994). Domestic violence: Are we listening? Do we see? *Australian Journal of Advanced Nursing, 12*(1), 23–28.

Mosqueda, L., Burnight, K., & Liao, S. (2005). The life cycle of bruises in older adults. *Journal of the American Geriatrics Society, 53,* 1339–1343.

Muellman, R. L., Lenaghan, P. A., & Pakieser, R. A. (1996). Battered women: Injury locations and types. *Annals of Emergency Medicine, 28,* 468–492.

Murphy, C. C., Schei, B., Myhr, T. L., & Du Mont, J. (2001). Abuse: A risk factor for low birth weight? A systematic review and meta-analysis. *Canadian Medical Association Journal, 164*, 1567–1572.

Myers, J. E., Berliner, L., Briere, J., Hendrix, C. T., Jenny, C., & Reid, T. A. (2002). *The APSAC handbook on child maltreatment.* Thousand Oaks, CA: Sage Publications.

Ozturk Ertem, I., Leventhal, J. M., & Dobbs, S. (2000). Intergenerational continuity of child physical abuse: How good is the evidence? *Lancet, 356*(9232), 814.

Plichta, S. B. (1991). The effects of woman abuse on health care utilization and health status: A literature review. *Women's Health Issues, 2*(3), 154–163.

Plichta, S. B. (1996). Violence and abuse: Implications for women's health. In M. K. Falik & K. S. Collins (Eds.), *Women's health: The Commonwealth Fund survey.* Baltimore, MD: Johns Hopkins University Press.

Public Health Agency of Canada. (2001). *The Canadian incidence study of reported child abuse and neglect highlights.* Retrieved June 5, 2008, from http://www.phac-aspc.gc.ca/cm-vee/cishl01/

Ramsey, J., Richardson, J., Carter, Y. H., Davidson, L. L., & Feder, G. (2002). Should health professionals screen women for domestic violence? Systematic review. *British Medical Journal, 325*(7359), 314–318.

Reece, R. M., & Ludwig, S. (2001). *Child abuse: Medical diagnosis and management* (2nd ed.). Philadelphia, PA: Lippincott Williams & Wilkins.

Renner, L. M., & Slack, K. S. (2006). Intimate partner violence and child maltreatment: understanding intra- and intergenerational connections. *Child Abuse and Neglect, 30*, 599–617.

Reeves, C., & O'Leary-Kelly, A. M. (2007). The effects and costs of intimate partner violence for work organizations. *Journal of Interpersonal Violence, 22*, 327–344.

Rivara, F. P., Anderson, M. L., Fishman, P., Bonomi, A. E., Reid, R. J., Carrell, D., et al. (2007). Healthcare utilization and costs for women with a history of intimate partner violence. *American Journal of Preventive Medicine, 32*(2), 89–96.

Rivara, F. P., Anderson, M. L., Fishman, P., Bonomi, A. E., Reid, R. J., Carrell, D., et al. (2007). Intimate partner violence and health care costs and utilization for children living in the home. *Pediatrics, 120*, 1270–1277.

Schollenberger, J., Campbell, J., Sharps, P. W., O'Campo, P., Gielen, A.C., Dienemann, J., et al. (2003). African American HMO enrollees: Their experiences with partner abuse and its effect on their health and use of medical services. *Violence Against Women, 9*, 599–618.

Sharps, P., Koziol-Mclain, J., McFarlane, J., Sachs, C., & Xu, X. (2001). Opportunities for prevention of femicide by health care providers. *Preventive Medicine, 33*, 373–380.

Sheridan, D. J. (2001). Treating survivors of intimate partner abuse: forensic identification and documentation. In J. S. Olshaker, M. C. Jackson, & W. S. Smock (Eds.), *Forensic emergency medicine.* Philadelphia, PA: Lippincott Williams & Wilkins.

Snow-Jones, A., Dienemann, J., Schollenberger, J., Kub, J., O'Campo, P., Gielen, A. C., et al. (2006). Long-term costs of intimate partner violence in a sample of female HMO enrollees. *Women's Health Issues, 16*, 252–261.

Statistics Canada. (2001). *Family violence in Canada: A statistical profile 2001.* Ottawa, ON: Canadian Centre for Justice Statistics.

Statistics Canada. (2005). *Statistics Canada—The Daily. Homicides.* Retrieved June 5, 2008, from http://www.statcan.ca/Daily/English/051006/d051006b.htm

Statistics Canada. (2006). *Family violence in Canada: A statistical profile 2006.* Ottawa, ON: Canadian Centre for Justice Statistics.

Sugar, N. F., Taylor, J. A., & Feldman, K. W. (1999). Bruises in infants and toddlers: Those who don't cruise rarely bruise. *Archives of Pediatric and Adolescent Medicine, 153*, 399–403.

Suh, E. K., & Abel, E. M. (1990). The impact of spousal violence on the children of the abused. *Journal of Independent Social Work, 4*, 27–34.

Tanner, K., & Turney, D. (2000). The role of observation in the assessment of child neglect. *Child Abuse Review, 9*, 337–348.

Teicher, M. H., Samson, J. A., Polcari, A., & McGreenery, C. E. (2006). Sticks, stones, and hurtful words: relative effects of various forms of childhood maltreatment. *American Journal of Psychiatry, 163*, 993–1000.

Tjaden, P., & Thoennes, N. (2000). *Extent, nature and consequences of intimate partner violence: Findings from the National Violence Against Women survey. National Institute of Justice and the Centers for Disease Control and Prevention.* Washington, DC: U.S. Department of Justice, Office of Justice Programs, National Institute of Justice.

Tjaden, P., & Thoennes, N. (2000). *Full report of the prevalence, incidence, and consequences of violence against women* (NCJ-183781). Washington, DC: National Institute of Justice.

Tower, M. (2007). Intimate partner violence and the health care response: a postmodern critique. *Health Care for Women International, 28*, 438–452.

Trocmé, N., MacMillan, H., Fallon, B., & De Marco, R. (2003). Nature and severity of physical harm caused by child abuse and neglect: results from the Canadian Incidence Study. *Canadian Medical Association Journal, 169*, 911–915.

Varcoe, C. (1997). *Untying our hands: The social context of nursing in relation to violence against women.* Unpublished doctoral dissertation. Vancouver, BC: University of British Columbia.

Varcoe, C. (2001). Abuse obscured: an ethnographic account of emergency nursing in relation to violence against women. *Canadian Journal of Nursing Research, 32*(4), 95–115.

Varcoe, C. (2008). Inequality, violence and women's health. In B. S. Bolaria & H. Dickinson (Eds.), *Health, illness and health care in Canada* (4th ed.). Toronto, ON: Nelson.

Walsh, C. A., Jamieson, E., MacMillan, H., & Boyle, M. (2007). Child abuse and chronic pain in a community survey of women. *Journal of Interpersonal Violence, 22*, 1536–1554.

Wekerle, C., Wall, A.-M., Leung, E., & Trocmé, N. (2007). Cumulative stress and substantiated maltreatment: The importance of caregiver vulnerability and adult partner violence. *Child Abuse and Neglect, 31*, 427–443.

Wisner, C. L., Gilmer, T. P., Saltzman, L. E., & Zink, T. M. (1999). Intimate partner violence against women: Do victims cost health plans more? *Journal of Family Practice, 48*, 439–443.

Wuest, J., Ford-Gilboe, M., Merritt-Gray, M., & Berman, H. (2003). Intrusion: The central problem for health promotion among children and single mothers after leaving an abusive partner. *Qualitative Health Research, 13*, 597–622.

Wuest, J., Merritt-Gray, M., Lent, B., Varcoe, C., Conners, A. J., & Ford-Gilboe, M. (2007). Patterns of medication use among women survivors of intimate partner violence. *Canadian Journal of Public Health, 98*, 460–464.

Chapter Eight

Assessment Techniques and the Clinical Setting

Written by **Carolyn Jarvis**, PhD, APN, CNP
Adapted by **June MacDonald-Jenkins**, RN, BScN, MSc

CULTIVATING YOUR SENSES

SETTING

EQUIPMENT

A SAFER ENVIRONMENT

THE CLINICAL SETTING

Electronic Resources

On Evolve *evolve*

http://evolve.elsevier.com/Canada/Jarvis/examination/

- Interactive Case Studies
- Physical Examination Audio and Printable Summaries
- Bedside Assessment Summary Checklists
- Complete Physical Examination Form
- Nursing Diagnoses Boxes
- Health Promotion Guides
- Quick Assessments for 20 Common Conditions
- Multiple Choice Review Questions
- Chapter Objectives
- Appendices
- Weblinks

On the Companion CD

- Interactive Case Studies with Heart and Lung Sounds
- Health Promotion Guides
- Quick Assessments for 20 Common Conditions
- Head-to-Toe Physical Examination Video Clips

The health history described in the preceding chapters provides **subjective** data for health assessment, the individual's *own* perception of the health state. Unit 3 presents **objective** data, the signs perceived by the examiner through the physical examination.

The physical examination requires that the examiner develop technical skills and a knowledge base. The technical skills are the tools to gather data. You will relate those data to your knowledge base and to your previous experience. A sturdy knowledge base enables you to look *for,* rather than merely look *at.* Consider a statement by the eighteenth century German poet Göethe: "We see only what we know." To recognize a significant finding, you need to know what to look for.

CULTIVATING YOUR SENSES

You will use your senses—sight, smell, touch, and hearing—to gather data during the physical examination. You always have perceived the world through your senses, but now they will be focused in a new way. Applying your senses to assess each person's health state may seem awkward at first, but this will be polished with repetition and tutored practice. The skills requisite for the physical examination are **inspection, palpation, percussion,** and **auscultation.** The skills are performed one at a time and in this order.

Inspection

Inspection is concentrated watching. It is close, careful scrutiny, first of the individual as a whole and then of each body system. Inspection begins the moment you first meet the person and develop a "general survey." (Specific data to consider for the general survey are presented in the following chapter.) Then as you proceed through the examination, start the assessment of each body system with inspection.

Inspection always comes first. Initially you may feel embarrassed "staring" at the person without also "doing something." But do not be too eager to touch the person. A focused inspection takes time and yields a surprising amount of data. Train yourself not to rush through inspection by holding your hands behind your back.

Learn to use each person as his or her own control and compare the right and left sides of the body. The two sides are nearly symmetrical. Inspection requires good lighting, adequate exposure, and occasional use of certain instruments (otoscope, ophthalmoscope, penlight, nasal and vaginal specula) to enlarge your view.

Palpation

Palpation follows and often confirms points you noted during inspection. Palpation applies your sense of touch to assess these factors: texture, temperature, moisture, organ location and size, as well as any swelling, vibration or pulsation, rigidity or spasticity, crepitation, presence of lumps or masses, and presence of tenderness or pain. Different parts of the hands are best suited for assessing different factors:

- Fingertips—best for fine tactile discrimination, as of skin texture, swelling, pulsation, and determining presence of lumps
- A grasping action of the fingers and thumb—to detect the position, shape, and consistency of an organ or mass
- The dorsa (backs) of hands and fingers—best for determining temperature because the skin here is thinner than on the palms
- Base of fingers (metacarpophalangeal joints) or ulnar surface of the hand—best for vibration.

Your palpation technique should be slow and systematic. A person stiffens when touched suddenly, making it difficult for you to feel very much. Use a calm, gentle approach. Warm your hands by kneading them together or holding them under warm water. Identify any tender areas, and palpate them last.

Start with light palpation to detect surface characteristics and to accustom the person to being touched. Then perform deeper palpation, perhaps by helping the person use relaxation techniques such as imagery or deep breathing. Your sense of touch becomes blunted with heavy or continuous pressure. When deep palpation is needed (as for abdominal contents), intermittent pressure is better than one long continuous palpation. Avoid any situation in which deep palpation could cause internal injury or pain.

Bimanual palpation requires the use of both of your hands to envelop or capture certain body parts or organs—such as the kidneys, uterus, or adnexa—for more precise delimitation (see Chapters 21 and 26).

Percussion

Percussion is tapping the person's skin with short, sharp strokes to assess underlying structures. The strokes yield a palpable vibration and a characteristic sound that depicts the location, size, and density of the underlying organ. Why learn percussion when an X-ray study is so much more accurate? Because your percussing hands are always available, are easily portable, and give instant feedback. Percussion has the following uses:

- Mapping out the *location* and *size* of an organ by exploring where the percussion note changes between the borders of an organ and its neighbours
- Signalling the *density* (air, fluid, or solid) of a structure by a characteristic note
- Detecting an abnormal mass if it is fairly superficial; the percussion vibrations penetrate about 5 cm deep—a deeper mass would give no change in percussion
- Eliciting pain if the underlying structure is inflamed, as with sinus areas or over the kidney
- Eliciting a deep tendon reflex using the percussion hammer

Two methods of percussion can be used—*direct* (sometimes called immediate) and *indirect* (or mediate). In direct percussion the striking hand directly contacts the body wall. This produces a sound and is used in percussing the infant's thorax or the adult's sinus areas. *Indirect* percussion is used more often and involves both hands. The striking hand contacts the stationary hand fixed on the person's skin. This yields a sound and a subtle vibration. The procedure is as follows.

The Stationary Hand

Hyperextend the middle finger (sometimes called the pleximeter) and place its distal portion, the phalanx and distal interphalangeal joint, *firmly* against the person's skin. Avoid the person's ribs and scapulae. Percussing over a bone yields no data because it always sounds "dull." Lift the rest of the stationary hand up off the person's skin (Fig. 8-1). Otherwise the resting hand will dampen off the produced vibrations, just as a drummer uses the hand to halt a drum roll.

The Striking Hand

Use the middle finger of your dominant hand as the *striking finger* (sometimes called the plexor) (Fig. 8-2). Hold your forearm close to the skin surface, with your upper arm and shoulder steady. Scan your muscles to make sure they are steady but not rigid. The action is all in the wrist, and it *must* be relaxed. Spread your fingers, swish your wrist, and bounce your middle finger off the stationary one. Aim for just behind the nail bed or at the distal interphalangeal joint; the goal is to hit the portion of the finger that is pushing the hardest into the skin surface. Flex the striking finger so that its tip, not the finger pad, makes contact. It hits directly at right angles to the stationary finger.

Percuss two times in this location using even, staccato blows. Lift the striking finger off quickly; a resting finger damps off vibrations. Then move to a new body location and repeat, keeping your technique even. The force of the blow determines the loudness of the note. You do not need a very loud sound; use just enough force to achieve a clear note. The thickness of the person's body wall will be a factor. You will need a stronger percussion stroke for obese persons or those with very muscular body walls.

Percussion can be an awkward technique for beginning examiners. You may feel surprised and embarrassed if your striking finger misses your stationary hand completely. You may wince if the fingernail of your striking finger is too long and painfully gouges your stationary finger. As with all new skills, refinement follows practice. After a few weeks your hand placement becomes precise and feels natural, and your ears learn to perceive the subtle difference in percussion notes.

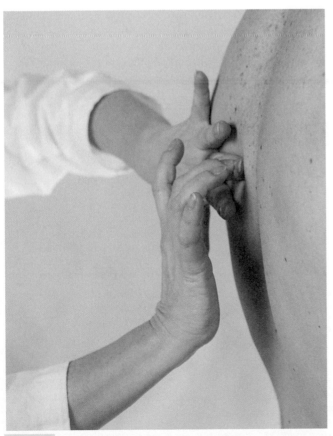

Fig. 8-1

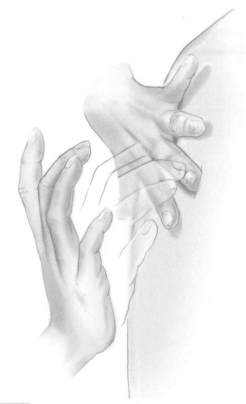

Fig. 8-2

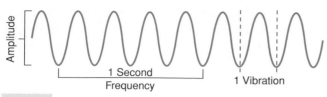

Fig. 8-3   Sound wave.

Production of Sound

All sound results from vibration of some structure (Fig. 8-3). Percussing over a body structure causes vibrations that produce characteristic waves and are heard as "notes" (Table 8-1). Each of the five percussion notes is differentiated by the following components:

1. **Amplitude** (or intensity), a loud or soft sound. The louder the sound, the greater the amplitude. Loudness depends on the force of the blow and the structure's ability to vibrate.
2. **Pitch** (or frequency), the number of vibrations per second, written as "cps," or cycles per second. More rapid vibrations produce a high-pitched tone; slower vibrations yield a low-pitched tone.
3. **Quality** (timbre), a subjective difference due to a sound's distinctive overtones. A pure tone is a sound of one frequency. Variations within a sound wave produce overtones. Overtones allow you to distinguish a C on a piano from a C on a violin.
4. **Duration,** the length of time the note lingers.

A basic principle is that a structure with relatively more air (such as the lungs) produces a louder, deeper, and longer sound because it vibrates freely, whereas a denser, more solid structure (such as the liver) gives a softer, higher, shorter sound because it does not vibrate as easily. Although Table 8-1 describes five "normal" percussion notes, variations occur in clinical practice. The "note" you hear depends on the nature of the underlying structure, as well as the thickness of the body wall and your correct technique. Do not learn these various notes just from written description. Practise on a willing partner.

Auscultation

Auscultation is listening to sounds produced by the body, such as the heart and blood vessels and the lungs and abdomen. Likely you already have heard certain body sounds with your ear alone—for example, the harsh gurgling of very congested breathing. However, most body sounds are very soft and must be channelled through a **stethoscope** for you to evaluate them. The stethoscope does not magnify sound but does block out extraneous room sounds. Of all the equipment you will use, the stethoscope quickly becomes a very personal instrument. Take time to learn its features and to fit one individually to yourself.

The fit and quality of the stethoscope are important. You cannot assess what you cannot hear through a poor instrument. The slope of the earpiece should point forward toward your nose. This matches the natural slope of your ear canal and efficiently blocks out environmental sound. If necessary, twist the earpieces to parallel the slope of your ear canals. The earpieces should fit snugly, but if they hurt, they are inserted too far. Adjust the tension and experiment with different rubber or plastic earplugs to achieve the most comfort. The tubing should be of thick material, with an internal diameter of 4 mm and about 36 to 46 cm long. Longer tubing may distort the sound.

TABLE 8-1	Characteristics of Percussion Notes				
	Amplitude	Pitch	Quality	Duration	Sample Location
Resonant	Medium-loud	Low	Clear, hollow	Moderate	Over normal lung tissue
Hyperresonant	Louder	Lower	Booming	Longer	Normal over child's lung Abnormal in the adult, over lungs with increased amount of air, as in emphysema
Tympany	Loud	High	Musical and drumlike (like the kettle drum)	Sustained longest	Over air-filled viscus, such as the stomach or the intestine
Dull	Soft	High	Muffled thud	Short	Relatively dense organ, as liver or spleen
Flat	Very soft	High	A dead stop of sound, absolute dullness	Very short	When no air is present, over thigh muscles, bone, or tumour

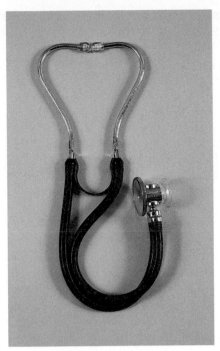

Fig. 8-4   Stethoscope diaphragm (left) and bell (right).

Choose a stethoscope with two end pieces—a diaphragm and a bell (Fig. 8-4). You will use the **diaphragm** most often because its flat edge is best for high-pitched sounds—breath, bowel, and normal heart sounds. (Since your stethoscope touches many people, clean the end pieces with an alcohol swab to eliminate a possible vector of infection.) Hold the diaphragm firmly against the person's skin—firm enough to leave a slight ring afterward. The **bell** end piece has a deep, hollow cup-like shape. It is best for soft, low-pitched sounds such as extra heart sounds or murmurs. Hold it lightly against the person's skin—just enough that it forms a perfect seal. Any harder causes the person's skin to act as a diaphragm, obliterating the low-pitched sounds.

Some newer stethoscopes have one end piece with a "tunable diaphragm." This enables you to listen to both low- and high-frequency sounds without rotation of the endpiece. For low-frequency sounds (traditional bell mode) hold the end piece very lightly on the skin; for high-frequency sounds (traditional diaphragm mode) press the end piece firmly on the skin.

Before you can evaluate body sounds, you must eliminate any confusing artifacts:

- Any extra room noise can produce a "roaring" in your stethoscope, so the room must be quiet.
- Keep the examination room warm. If the person starts shivering, the involuntary muscle contractions could drown out other sounds.
- Clean the stethoscope end piece with an alcohol wipe. Then warm it by rubbing it in your palm.
- The friction on the end piece from a man's hairy chest causes a crackling sound that mimics an abnormal breath

sound called *crackles*. To minimize this problem, wet the hair before auscultating the area.

- Never listen through a gown. Reach under a gown to listen, but take care that no clothing rubs on the stethoscope.
- Finally, avoid your own "artifact," such as breathing on the tubing, or the "thump" from bumping the tubing together.

Auscultation is a skill that beginning examiners are eager to learn, but one that is difficult to master. First you must learn the wide range of normal sounds. Once you can recognize normal sounds, you can distinguish the abnormal sounds and "extra" sounds. Be aware that in some body locations you may hear more than one sound; this can be confusing. You will need to listen selectively, to only one thing at a time. As you listen, ask yourself: What am I *actually hearing?* . . . What *should* I be hearing at this spot?

SETTING

The examination room should be warm and comfortable, quiet, private, and well lit. When possible, stop any distracting noises—such as humming machinery, radio or television, or people talking—that could make it difficult to hear body sounds. Your time with the individual should be secure from interruptions from other healthcare personnel. Lighting with natural daylight is best, although it is often not available; artificial light from two sources will suffice and will prevent shadows. A wall-mounted or gooseneck stand lamp is needed for high-intensity lighting.

Position the examination table so that both sides of the person are easily accessible (Fig. 8-5). The table should be at a height at which you can stand without stooping and should be equipped to raise the person's head up to 45 degrees. A roll-up stool is used for the sections of the examination for which you must be sitting. A bedside stand or table is needed to lay out all your equipment.

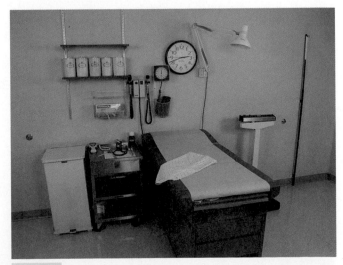

Fig. 8-5

EQUIPMENT

During the examination, you do not want to be searching for equipment or to have to leave the room to find an item. Have all your equipment at easy reach and laid out in an organized fashion (Fig. 8-6). The following items are usually needed for a screening physical examination:

- Platform scale with height attachment
- Skinfold calipers
- Sphygmomanometer
- Stethoscope with bell and diaphragm end pieces
- Thermometer
- Pulse oximeter (in hospital setting)
- Flashlight or penlight
- Otoscope/ophthalmoscope
- Tuning fork
- Nasal speculum (if a short, broad speculum is not included with the otoscope)
- Tongue depressor
- Pocket vision screener
- Skin-marking pen
- Flexible tape measure and ruler marked in centimetres
- Reflex hammer
- Sharp object (split tongue blade)
- Cotton balls
- Bivalve vaginal speculum
- Clean gloves
- Materials for cytological study
- Lubricant
- Fecal occult blood test materials

Most of the equipment is described as it comes into use throughout the text. However, consider these introductory comments on the otoscope and ophthalmoscope.

The **otoscope** funnels light into the ear canal and onto the tympanic membrane. The base serves both as the handle and the battery power source. To attach the head, press it down onto the male adaptor end of the base and turn clockwise until you feel a stop. To turn the light on, press the red button rheostat down and clockwise. (Always turn it off after use to increase the life of the bulb and battery.) Five specula, each a different size, are available to attach to the head (Fig. 8-7). (The short, broad speculum is for viewing the nares.) Choose

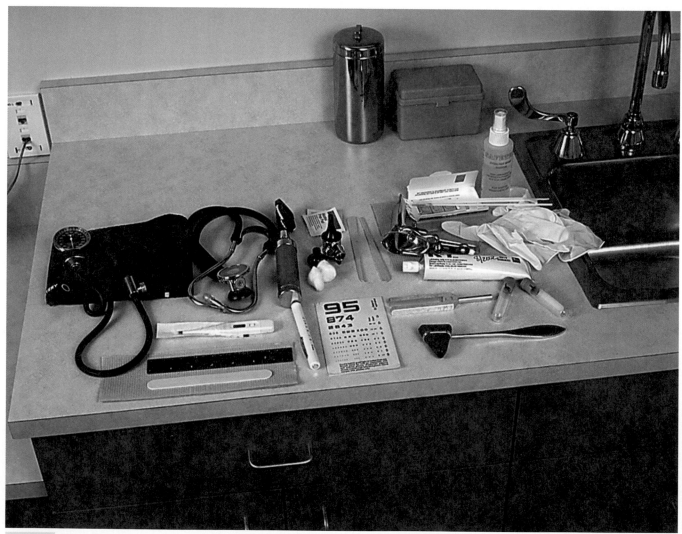

Fig. 8-6

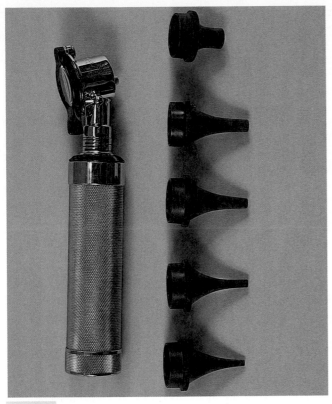

Fig. 8-7   Otoscope.

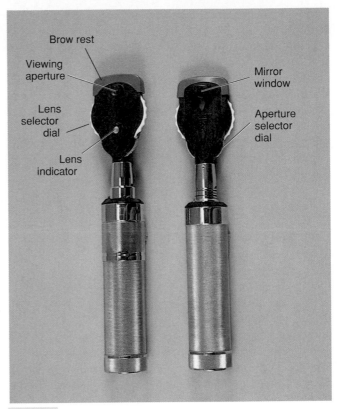

Fig. 8-8   Ophthalmoscope.

the largest one that will fit comfortably into the person's ear canal. See Chapter 15 for technique on use of the otoscope.

The **ophthalmoscope** illuminates the internal eye structures. Its system of lenses and mirrors enables you to look through the pupil at the fundus (background) of the eye, much like looking through a keyhole at a room beyond. The ophthalmoscope head attaches to the base male adaptor just as the otoscope head does (Fig. 8-8). The head has five different parts:

1. Viewing aperture, with five different apertures
2. Aperture selector dial on the front
3. Mirror window on the front
4. Lens selector dial
5. Lens indicator

Select the aperture to be used (Fig. 8-9).

○ Large (full spot) for dilated pupils

○ Small for undilated pupils

● Red-free filter — a green beam, used to examine the optic disc for hemorrhage (which looks black) and melanin deposits (which look grey)

⊕ Grid — to determine fixation pattern and to assess size and location of lesions on the fundus

▯ Slit — to examine the anterior portion of the eye and to assess elevation or depression of lesions on the fundus

Fig. 8-9

Rotating the lens selector dial brings the object into focus. The lens indicator shows a number, or *dioptre*, that indicates the value of the lens in position. The black numbers indicate a positive lens, from 0 to $+40$. The red numbers indicate a negative lens, from 0 to -20. The ophthalmoscope can compensate for myopia (nearsightedness) or hyperopia (farsightedness) in the examiner but will not correct for astigmatism. See Chapter 14 for details on how to hold the instrument and what to inspect.

The following equipment occasionally will be used, depending on the individual's needs: goniometer to measure joint range of motion, Doppler sonometer to augment pulse or blood pressure measurement, fetoscope for auscultating fetal heart tones, and pelvimeter to measure pelvic width.

For a child you also will need appropriate pediatric-sized end pieces for the stethoscope and otoscope specula, materials for developmental assessment, age-appropriate toys, and a nipple or pacifier for an infant.

A Clean Field

Do not let your stethoscope become a *staph*-oscope! Stethoscopes and other equipment that are frequently used on many patients can become a common vehicle for transmission of infection. Cleaning with an alcohol swab between patients is an effective control.

Designate a "clean" versus a "used" area for handling of your equipment. In a hospital setting, you may use the over-bed table for your clean surface and the bedside stand for the used equipment surface. In a clinic setting, use two separate areas of the pull-up table. Distinguish the clean area by one or two disposable paper towels. On the towels, place all the new, newly cleaned, or newly alcohol-swabbed equipment that you will use on this patient. Use alcohol swabs to clean all equipment that you carry from patient to patient (e.g., your stethoscope end pieces, the reflex hammer, ruler). As you proceed through the examination, pick up each piece of equipment from the clean area, and after use on the patient, relegate it to the used area, or (as in the case of tongue blades, gloves) throw it directly in the trash.

A SAFER ENVIRONMENT

In addition to monitoring the cleanliness of your equipment, take all steps to avoid any possible transmission of infection between patients or between patient and examiner. A **nosocomial** infection (an infection acquired during hospitalization) is a hazard because hospitals have sites that are possible reservoirs for virulent micro-organisms. Some of these micro-organisms have become resistant to antibiotics, such as methicillin-resistant *Staphylococcus aureus* (MRSA), vancomycin-resistant *Enterococcus* (VRE), or multidrug-resistant tuberculosis. Other micro-organisms include those for which there is currently no known cure, such as HIV.

The single most important step to decrease risk of micro-organism transmission is to wash your hands promptly and thoroughly. Ensure that you remove all jewellery prior to washing and that your hands are rinsed under running water;

lather the soap and rub your hands together, thoroughly covering all surfaces for 10 to 15 seconds (longer if hands appear visibly soiled). Rinse and dry thoroughly with a single-use towel or forced-air dryer. Ensure that you turn off the faucets without recontaminating your hands. Hospitals now have dispensers mounted on the wall outside every patient room. These dispensers contain a waterless, quick-drying, antiseptic solution for hand washing on entering and leaving the room.

Wear gloves when the potential exists for contact with any body fluids (e.g., blood, mucous membranes, body fluids, drainage, open skin lesions). Wearing gloves is *not* a protective substitute to washing hands, however, because gloves may have undetectable holes or may become torn during use, or hands may become contaminated as gloves are removed. Wear a gown, mask, and protective eyewear when the potential exists for any blood or body fluid spattering (e.g., suctioning, arterial puncture).

Health Canada's Laboratory Centre for Disease Control guidelines include the latest epidemiological information for decreasing transmission of bloodborne and other infections in hospitals. The guidelines include two tiers of precautions. **Routine Practices** (Table 8-2) are intended for use with *all* patients regardless of their risk or presumed infection status. Routine Practices are designed to reduce the risk of transmission of micro-organisms from both recognized and unrecognized sources, and they apply to (1) blood; (2) all body fluids, secretions, and excretions *except sweat,* whether or not they contain visible blood; (3) nonintact skin; and (4) mucous membranes.

TABLE 8-2	**Routine Practices for Use With All Patients**

A. **Wash hands** after touching blood, body fluids, secretions, excretions, and contaminated items, whether or not you are wearing gloves. Wash hands immediately after gloves are removed and between patient contacts. May need to wash hands between procedures on the same patient to prevent cross-contamination of different body sites.

B. **Wear clean gloves** when touching blood, body fluids, secretions, excretions, items contaminated with these, mucous membranes, and nonintact skin. Change gloves between tasks and procedures on the same patient after contact with material that may contain a high concentration of micro-organisms. Remove gloves promptly after use, before touching noncontaminated items, and before going to another patient, and wash hands immediately.

C. **Wear a mask and eye protection** to protect mucous membranes during procedures and patient care activities that are likely to generate splashes of blood, body fluids, secretions, and excretions.

D. **Wear a gown** (clean, nonsterile, appropriate to activity) to protect skin and prevent soiling of clothing during procedures and patient care activities that are likely to generate splashes of blood, body fluids, secretions, or excretions. Remove a soiled gown promptly and wash hands.

E. **Place in a private room** any patient who contaminates the environment or who does not or cannot assist in appropriate hygiene or environmental control. Some transmission-based precautions call for providing single accommodations or other negative-pressure enhanced environments for certain contact and airborne-transmitted pathogens.

F. **Take care with used patient care equipment,** soiled with blood, body fluids, secretions, and excretions; handle it in a manner that prevents skin and mucous membrane exposure, contamination of clothing, and transfer of micro-organisms to other patients and environments. Do not use the reusable equipment on another patient until it has been cleaned and reprocessed appropriately. Discard single-use items appropriately. Personal care supplies should never be shared between patients.

G. **Prevent injuries due to bloodborne pathogens** when using or handling needles, scalpels, and other sharp instruments. Never recap used needles, manipulate them using both hands, or direct the point of a needle toward any part of the body; rather, use either a one-handed "scoop" technique or an appropriate mechanical device. Do not remove used needles from disposable syringes by hand, or otherwise bend, break, or manipulate used needles by hand. Place used disposable syringes, needles, scalpel blades, and other sharp items in appropriate puncture-resistant containers. Use mouthpieces, resuscitation bags, or other ventilation devices instead of mouth-to-mouth resuscitation methods in areas where the need for resuscitation is predictable.

H. **Follow environmental control policies** for the routine care, cleaning, and disinfection of environmental surfaces, beds, bed rails, bedside equipment, and other frequently touched surfaces. Take care with used linen soiled with blood, body fluids, secretions, and excretions; handle, transport, and process this linen in a manner that prevents skin and mucous membrane exposure.

The second tier is **transmission-based precautions,** intended for use with patients with documented or suspected transmissible infections. They are designed *in addition to* Routine Practices to interrupt transmission in hospitals. Routes of transmission have been classified as contact (direct, indirect, and droplet), airborne, common vehicle (single contaminated source, such as food), and vectorborne. They may be combined for diseases that have multiple routes of transmission, such as varicella (chicken pox) (Appendices B-1 and B-2 on the Evolve Web site). Vectorborne transmission by insects of a pathogen such as West Nile virus has been reported in Canada.

THE CLINICAL SETTING

General Approach

Consider your emotional state and that of the person being examined. The patient is usually anxious due to the anticipation of being examined by a stranger and the unknown outcome of the examination. If anxiety can be reduced, the person will feel more comfortable and the data gathered will more closely describe the person's natural state. Anxiety can be reduced by an examiner who is confident and self-assured, as well as considerate and unhurried.

Usually, a beginning examiner feels anything *but* self-assured! Most worry about their technical skill, about missing something significant, or about forgetting a step. Many are embarrassed themselves about encountering a partially dressed individual. All these fears are natural and common. The best way to minimize them is with a lot of tutored practice on a healthy willing subject, usually a fellow student. You have to feel comfortable with your motor skills before you can absorb what you are actually seeing or hearing in a "real" patient. This comes with practice under the guidance of an experienced tutor, in an atmosphere in which it is acceptable to make mistakes and to ask questions. Your subject should "act like a patient" so that you can deal with the "real" situation while still in a safe setting. After you feel comfortable in the laboratory setting, accompany your tutor as he or she examines an actual patient so that you can observe an experienced examiner.

Hands On

With this preparation, it is possible to interact with your own patient in a confident manner. Begin by measuring the person's height, weight, blood pressure, temperature, pulse, and respirations (see Chapter 9). If needed, measure visual acuity at this time using the Snellen eye chart. All of these are familiar, relatively nonthreatening actions; they will gradually accustom the person to the examination. Then ask the person to change into an examining gown, leaving his or her underpants on. The person will feel more comfortable, and the underpants can easily be removed just before the genital examination. Unless your assistance is needed, leave the room as the person undresses. Keep in mind that some patients may not wish to disrobe fully or at all depending on ethnocultural considerations.

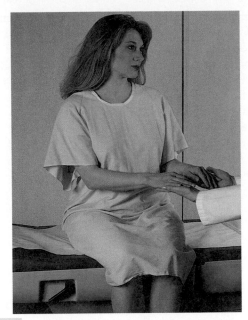

Fig. 8-10

As you re-enter the room, wash your hands in the person's presence. This indicates you are protective of this person and are starting fresh for him or her. Explain each step in the examination and how the person can co-operate. Encourage the person to ask questions. Keep your own movements slow, methodical, and deliberate.

Begin by touching the person's hands, checking skin colour, nail beds, and metacarpophalangeal joints (Fig. 8-10; see Chapters 12 and 22). Again, this is a less threatening way to ease a person into being touched. Most people are used to having relative strangers touch their hands.

As you proceed through the examination, avoid distractions and concentrate on one step at a time. The sequence of the steps may differ depending on the age of the person and your own preference. However, you should establish a system that works for you and stick to it to avoid omissions. Organize the steps so the person does not change positions too often. Although proper exposure is necessary, use additional drapes to maintain the person's privacy and to prevent chilling.

Do not hesitate to write out the examination sequence and refer to it as you proceed. The patient will accept this as quite natural if you explain you are making brief notations to ensure accuracy. Many agencies use a printed form. You will find that you will glance at the form less and less as you gain experience. Even with a form, you sometimes may forget a step in the examination. When you realize this, perform the manoeuvre in the next logical place in the sequence. (See Chapter 27 for the sequence of steps in the complete physical examination.)

As you proceed through the examination, occasionally offer some brief teaching about the person's body. For example, you might say, "This tapping on your back (percussion) is a little like playing different drums. The different notes I hear tell me where each organ starts and stops. You probably can hear the difference yourself from within your body." Or, "Everyone has two sounds for each heartbeat, something like this—lub-dup. Your own beats sound normal." Do not do this with every single step, or you will be hard pressed to make a comment when you do come across an abnormality. But some sharing of information builds rapport and increases the person's confidence in you as an examiner. It also gives the person a little more control in a situation in which it is easy to feel completely helpless.

At some point, you may want to linger in one location to concentrate on some complicated findings. To avoid causing anxiety, tell the person, "I always listen to heart sounds on a number of places on the chest. Just because I am listening a long time does not necessarily mean anything is wrong with you." And it follows that sometimes you *will* discover a finding that may be abnormal and you want another examiner to double-check. You need to give the person some information, yet you should not alarm the person unnecessarily. Say something like, "I do not have a complete assessment of your heart sounds. I want Ms. Wright to listen to you, too."

At the end of the examination, summarize your findings and share the necessary information with the person. Thank the person for the time spent. In a hospital setting, apprise the person of what is scheduled next. Before you leave a hospitalized person, lower the bed; make the person comfortable and safe; and return the bedside table, television, or any equipment to the way it was originally. In a clinic or home care setting, your assessment data provides the basis of information needed to develop a collaborative plan of care with your client.

❧ DEVELOPMENTAL CARE

Children are different from adults. Their difference in size is obvious. Their bodies grow in a predictable pattern that is assessed during the physical examination. However, their behaviour is also different. Behaviour grows and develops through predictable stages, just as the body does. Each examiner needs to know the expected emotional and cognitive features of these stages and to perform the physical examination based on developmental principles (Berk, 2007; Hockenberry et al., 2006).

With all children, the goal is to increase their comfort in the setting. This approach reveals their natural state as much as possible and will give them a more positive memory of healthcare professionals. Remember that a "routine" examination is anything but routine to children. You can increase their comfort by attending to the following developmental principles and approaches. The *order* of the developmental stages is more meaningful than the exact chronological age. Each child is an individual and will not fit exactly into one category. For example, if your efforts to "play games" with the preschooler are rebuffed, modify your approach to the security measures used with the toddler.

The Infant

Erik Erikson defines the major task of infancy as establishing trust. An infant is completely dependent on the parent for his or her basic needs. If these needs are met promptly and consistently, the infant feels secure and learns to trust others.

Position

- The parent always should be present to understand normal growth and development and for the child's feeling of security.
- Place the neonate or young infant flat on a padded examination table (Fig. 8-11). The infant also may be held against the parent's chest for some steps.
- Once the baby can sit without support (around 6 months), as much of the examination as possible should be performed while the infant is in the parent's lap.
- By 9 to 12 months, the infant is acutely aware of the surroundings. Anything outside the infant's range of vision is "lost," so the parent must be in full view.

Preparation

- Timing should be 1 to 2 hours after feeding, when the baby is not too drowsy or too hungry.
- Maintain a warm environment. A neonate may require an overhead radiant heater.
- An infant will not object to being nude. Have the parent remove outer clothing, but leave a diaper on a boy.
- An infant does not mind being touched, but make sure your hands and stethoscope end piece are warm.
- Use a soft, crooning voice during the examination; the baby responds more to the feeling in the tone of the voice than to what is actually said.
- An infant likes eye contact; lock eyes from time to time.

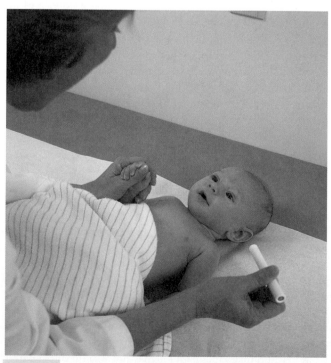

Fig. 8-11

- Smile; a baby prefers a smiling face to a frowning one. (Often beginning examiners are so absorbed in their technique that they look serious or stern.) Take time to play.
- Keep movements smooth and deliberate, not jerky.
- Use a pacifier for crying or during invasive steps.
- Offer brightly coloured toys for a distraction when the infant is fussy.
- Let an older baby touch the stethoscope or tongue blade.

Sequence

- Seize the opportunity with a sleeping baby to listen to heart, lung, and abdomen sounds first.
- Perform least distressing steps first. (See the sequence in Chapter 27.) Save the invasive steps of examination of the eye, ear, nose, and throat until last.
- Elicit the Moro or "startle" reflex at the end of the examination because it may cause the baby to cry.

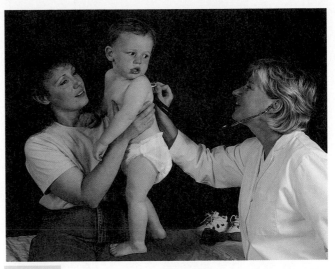

Fig. 8-12

The Toddler

The toddler is at Erikson's stage of developing autonomy. However, the need to explore the world and be independent is in conflict with the basic dependency on the parent. This often results in frustration and negativism. The toddler may be difficult to examine; do not take this personally. Since he or she is acutely aware of the new environment, the toddler may be frightened and cling to the parent. Also, the toddler has fear of invasive procedures and dislikes being restrained (Fig. 8-12).

Position

- The toddler should be sitting up on the parent's lap for all of the examination. When the toddler must be supine (as in the abdominal examination), move chairs to sit knee-to-knee with the parent. Have the toddler lie in the parent's lap with the toddler's legs in your lap.
- Enlist the aid of a co-operative parent to help position the toddler during invasive procedures. The child's legs can be captured between the parent's. The parent can encircle the child's head with one arm, holding it against the chest, and hold the child's arms with the other arm. (See Fig. 16-20.)

Preparation

- Children 1 or 2 years of age can understand symbols, so a security object, such as a special blanket or teddy bear, is helpful.
- Begin by greeting the child and the accompanying parent by name, but with a child 1 to 6 years old, focus more on the parent. By essentially "ignoring" the child at first, you allow the child to adjust gradually and to size you up from a safe distance. Then turn your attention gradually to the child, at first to a toy or object the child is holding, or perhaps to compliment a dress, the hair, or what a big girl or boy the child is. If the child is ready, you will note these signals: eye contact with you, smiling, talking with you, or accepting a toy or a piece of equipment.

- A 2-year-old child does not like to take off his or her clothes; have the parent undress the child one part at a time.
- Children 1 or 2 years of age like to say "No." Do not offer a choice when there really is none. Avoid saying, "May I listen to your heart now?" When the 1- or 2-year-old child says "No," and you go ahead and do it anyway, you lose trust. Instead, use clear firm instructions, in a tone that expects co-operation: "Now it is time for you to lie down so I can check your tummy."
- Also, 1- or 2-year-old children like to make choices. When possible, enhance autonomy by offering the *limited option:* "Shall I listen to your heart next, or your tummy?"
- Demonstrate the procedures on the parent (see Fig. 15-14).
- Praise the child when he or she is co-operative.

Sequence

- Collect some objective data during the history, which is a less stressful time. While you are focusing on the parent, note the child's gross motor and fine motor skills and gait.
- Begin with "games," such as cranial nerve testing.
- Start with nonthreatening areas. Save distressing procedures—such as examination of the head, ear, nose, or throat—for last.

The Preschool Child

The preschool child displays developing initiative. The preschooler takes on tasks independently and plans the task and sees it through. A child of this age is often co-operative, helpful, and easy to involve. However, children of this age have fantasies and may see illness as punishment for being "bad." The concept of body image is limited. The child fears any body injury or mutilation, so he or she will recoil from invasive procedures (e.g., tongue blade, rectal temperature, injection, and venipuncture).

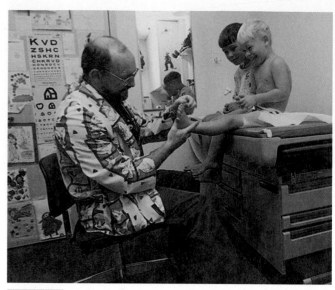

Fig. 8-13

Fig. 8-14

Position

- With a 3-year-old child, the parent should be present and may hold the child on his or her lap (Fig. 8-13).
- A 4- or 5-year-old child usually feels comfortable on the "Big Girl" or "Big Boy" (examining) table, with the parent present.

Preparation

- A preschooler can talk. Verbal communication becomes helpful now, but remember that the child's understanding is still limited. Use short, simple explanations.
- The preschooler is usually willing to undress. Leave underpants on until the genital examination.
- Talk to the child and explain the steps in the examination exactly.
- Do not allow a choice when there is none.
- As with the toddler, enhance the autonomy of the preschooler by offering choice when possible.
- Allow the child to play with equipment to reduce fears (Fig. 8-14).
- A preschooler likes to help; have the child hold the stethoscope for you.
- Use games. Have the child "blow out" the light on the penlight as you listen to the breath sounds or pretend to listen to the heart sounds of the child's teddy bear first. One technique that is absorbing to a preschooler is to trace their shape on the examining table paper (Hockenberry et al., 2006). You can comment on how big the child is, then fill in the outline with a heart or stomach and listen to the paper doll first. After the examination, the child can take the paper doll home as a souvenir.
- Use a slow, patient, deliberate approach. Do not rush.
- During the examination give the preschooler needed feedback and reassurance: "Your tummy feels just fine."
- Compliment the child on his or her co-operation.

Sequence

- Examine the thorax, abdomen, extremities, and genitalia first. Although the preschooler is usually co-operative, continue to assess head, eye, ear, nose, and throat last.

The School-Age Child

During the school-age period, the major task of the child is developing industry. The child is developing basic competency in school and in social networks and desires the approval of parents and teachers. When successful, the child has a feeling of accomplishment. During the examination, the child is co-operative and is interested in learning about the body. Language is more sophisticated now, but do not overestimate and treat the school-age child as a small adult. The child's level of understanding does not match that of his or her speech.

Position

- The school-age child should be sitting on the examination table.
- A 5-year-old child has a sense of modesty. If appropriate to the examination, let the older child (an 11- or 12-year-old child) decide whether parents or siblings should be present.

Preparation

- Break the ice with small talk about family, school, friends, music, or sports.
- The child should undress himself or herself, leave underpants on, and use a gown and drape.
- Demonstrate equipment—a school-age child is curious to know how equipment works.
- Comment on the body and how it works (Fig. 8-15). An 8- or 9-year-old child has some understanding of the body and is interested to learn more. It is rewarding to

see the child's eyes light up when he or she hears the heart sounds.

Sequence

- As with the adult, progress from head to toes.

The Adolescent

The major task of adolescence is developing a self-identity. This takes shape from various sets of values and different social roles (son or daughter, sibling, and student). In the end, each person needs to feel satisfied and comfortable with who he or she is. In the process, the adolescent is increasingly self-conscious and introspective. Peer group values and acceptance are important.

Position

- The adolescent should be sitting on the examination table.
- Examine the adolescent alone, without a parent or sibling present.

Preparation

- The body is changing rapidly. During the examination, the adolescent needs feedback that his or her own body is healthy and developing normally.
- The adolescent has a keen awareness of body image, often comparing himself or herself to peers. Apprise the adolescent of the wide variation among teenagers on the rate of growth and development (see Sex Maturity Ratings, Chapters 17, 24, and 26).
- Communicate with some care. Do not treat the teenager like a child, but do not overestimate and treat him or her like an adult either.

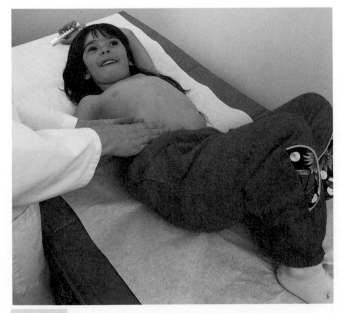

Fig. 8-15

- Since the person is idealistic at this age, the adolescent is ripe for health teaching. Positive attitudes developed now may last through adult life. Focus your teaching on ways adolescents can achieve their own wellness.

Sequence

- As with the adult, a head-to-toe approach is appropriate. Examine genitalia last, and do it quickly.

The Aging Adult

During later years, the tasks are developing the meaning of life and one's own existence and adjusting to changes in physical strength and health.

Position

- The older adult should be sitting on the examination table; a frail older adult may need to be supine.
- Arrange the sequence to allow as few position changes as possible.
- Allow rest periods when needed.

Preparation

- Adjust examination pace to meet the possible slowed pace of the older person. It is better to break the complete examination into a few visits than to rush through the examination and turn off the person.
- Use physical touch (unless there is a cultural contraindication). This is especially important with the aging person because other senses, such as vision and hearing, may be diminished.
- Do not mistake diminished vision or hearing for confusion. Confusion of sudden onset may signify a disease state. It is noted by short-term memory loss, diminished thought process, diminished attention span, and labile emotions (see Chapter 6).
- Be aware that the later years contain more of life's stress. Loss is inevitable, including changes in physical appearance of the face and body, declining energy level, loss of job through retirement, loss of financial security, loss of long-time home, and death of friends or spouse. How the person adapts to these losses significantly affects health assessment.

Sequence

- Use the head-to-toe approach as in the younger adult.

The Ill Person

For the person in some distress, alter the position during the examination. For example, a person with shortness of breath or ear pain may want to sit up, whereas a person with faintness or overwhelming fatigue may want to be supine. Initially it may be necessary just to examine the body areas appropriate to the problem, collecting a **mini-database.** You may return to finish a complete assessment after the initial distress is alleviated.

BIBLIOGRAPHY

Amella, E. J. (2004). Presentation of illness in older adults. *American Journal of Nursing, 104*(10), 40–52.

Berk, L. E. (2007). *Development through the lifespan* (4th ed.). Boston: Allyn and Bacon.

Garner, J. S. (1996). Hospital Infection Control Practices Advisory Committee: Guideline for isolation precautions in hospitals. *American Journal of Infection Control, 24,* 24–52.

Gewanter, B., Klein, R., & Jones, S. (2002). Antibiotic-resistant bacteria on the rise. *American Journal of Nursing, 102*(3), 116.

Health Canada. (1999). Infection control guidelines: Hand washing, cleaning, disinfection and sterilization in health care. *Canada Communicable Disease Report, 24S8,* 1–55.

Health Canada. (1999). Infection control guidelines: Routine practices and additional precautions for preventing the transmission of infection in health care. *Canada Communicable Disease Report, 25S4,* 1–148. Retrieved April 16, 2008, from http://www.phac-aspc.gc.ca/publicat/ccdr-rmtc/99pdf/cdr25s4e.pdf

Hockenberry, M., & Wilson, D. (2006). *Wong's nursing care of infants and children* (8th ed.). St Louis, MO: Mosby.

Markel, H. (2006). The stethoscope and the art of listening. *New England Journal of Medicine, 354,* 551–553.

O'Keefe, M. (2001). Revitalizing the art of auscultation. *Journal of Emergency Medical Services, 26*(5), 79–80.

Perkin, R. M., & Van Stralen, D. (2000). 20 things you may not know about pediatrics. *Journal of Emergency Medical Service, 25*(3), 38–49.

Romero, D. V., Treston, J., & O'Sullivan, A. L. (2006). Hand-to-hand preventing MRSA. *Nurse Practitioner, 31*(3), 16–25.

Romig, L. E. (2001). PREP for peds: Size-up & approach tips for pediatric calls. *Journal of Emergency Medical Service, 26*(5), 24–33.

Schuster, R. J., & Weber, M. L. (2003). Noise in the ambulatory health care setting: How loud is too loud? *Journal of Ambulatory Care Management, 26,* 243–249.

Shaner, H., & Botter, M. L. (2003). Pollution: Health care's unintended legacy. *American Journal of Nursing, 103*(3), 79–84.

Sheff, B. (2003). Multidrug-resistant microorganisms still making waves. *Nursing, 33*(11), 59–63.

Stone, J. T., Wyman, J. F., & Salisbury, S. A. (1998). *Clinical gerontological nursing: A guide to advanced practice* (2nd ed.). Philadelphia, PA: W.B. Saunders.

Thofern, U. A. R. (2000). Bacterial contamination of hospital physicians' stethoscopes. *Infection Control and Hospital Epidemiology, 21,* 558–559.

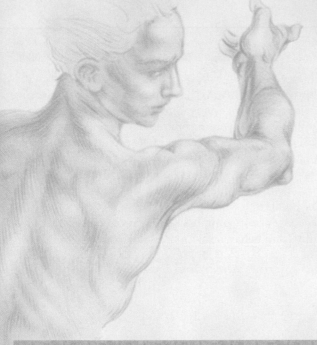

General Survey, Measurement, and Vital Signs

Written by **Carolyn Jarvis**, PhD, APN, CNP
Adapted by **June MacDonald-Jenkins**, RN, BScN, MSc

Electronic Resources

On Evolve *evolve*

http://evolve.elsevier.com/Canada/Jarvis/examination/

- Interactive Case Studies
- Physical Examination Audio and Printable Summaries
- Bedside Assessment Summary Checklists
- Complete Physical Examination Form
- Nursing Diagnoses Boxes
- Health Promotion Guides
- Quick Assessments for 20 Common Conditions
- Multiple Choice Review Questions
- Chapter Objectives
- Appendices
- Weblinks

On the Companion CD

- Interactive Case Studies with Heart and Lung Sounds
- Health Promotion Guides
- Quick Assessments for 20 Common Conditions
- Head-to-Toe Physical Examination Video Clips

OBJECTIVE DATA

The general survey is a study of the whole person, covering the general health state and any obvious physical characteristics. It is an introduction for the physical examination that will follow; it should give an overall impression, a "gestalt," of the person (see Sample Charting). Objective parameters are used to form the general survey, but these apply to the whole person, not just to one body system.

Launch a general survey at the moment you first encounter the person. What leaves an immediate impression? Does the person stand promptly as his or her name is called and walk easily to meet you? Or does the person look sick, rising slowly or with effort, with shoulders slumped and eyes without lustre or downcast? Is the hospitalized patient conversing with visitors, involved in reading or television, or lying perfectly still? Even as you introduce yourself and shake hands, you collect data. Does the person fully extend the arm, shake your hand firmly, make eye contact, or smile? Are the palms dry, or wet and clammy? As you proceed through the health history, the measurements, and the vital signs, note the following points that will add up to the general survey. Consider these four areas: **physical appearance, body structure, mobility,** and **behaviour.**

Normal Range of Findings	Abnormal Findings

THE GENERAL SURVEY

Physical Appearance

Age—The person appears his or her stated age.

Appears older than stated age, as with chronic illness, chronic alcoholism.

Sex—Sexual development is appropriate for gender and age.

Delayed or precocious puberty.

Level of consciousness—The person is alert and oriented, attends to your questions and responds appropriately.

Confused, drowsy, lethargic (see Table 6-3, p. 106).

Skin colour—Colour tone is even, pigmentation varying with genetic background, skin is intact with no obvious lesions.

Pallor, cyanosis, jaundice, erythema, any lesions (see Chapter 12).

Facial features—Facial features are symmetrical with movement.

Immobile, masklike, asymmetric, drooping (see Table 13-4, p. 294).

No signs of acute distress are present.

Respiratory signs—shortness of breath, wheezing.

Pain, indicated by facial grimace, holding body part.

Body Structure

Stature—The height appears within normal range for age, genetic heritage (see Measurement, p. 152).

Excessively short or tall (Table 9-6, p. 178).

Nutrition—The weight appears within normal range for height and body build; body fat distribution is even.

Cachectic, emaciated.

Simple obesity, with even fat distribution.

Centripetal (truncal) obesity—fat concentrated in face, neck, trunk, with thin extremities, as in Cushing's syndrome (hyperadrenalism) (see Table 9-6, p. 178).

Symmetry—Body parts look equal bilaterally and are in relative proportion to each other.

Unilateral atrophy or hypertrophy.

Asymmetrical location of a body part.

Posture—The person stands comfortably erect as appropriate for age. Note the normal "plumb line" through anterior ear, shoulder, hip, patella, ankle. Exceptions are the standing toddler who has a normally protuberant abdomen ("toddler lordosis") and the aging person who may be stooped with kyphosis.

Rigid spine and neck; moves as one unit (e.g., arthritis).

Stiff and tense, ready to spring from chair, fidgety movements.

Shoulders slumped; looks deflated (e.g., depression).

Position—The person sits comfortably in a chair or on the bed or examination table, arms relaxed at sides, head turned to examiner.

Tripod—leaning forward with arms braced on chair arms; occurs with chronic pulmonary disease.

Objective Data

Normal Range of Findings	Abnormal Findings

Sitting straight up and resists lying down (e.g., congestive heart failure).

Curled up in fetal position (e.g., acute abdominal pain).

Body build, contour—Proportions are
1. Arm span (fingertip to fingertip) equals height.
2. Body length from crown to pubis roughly equal to length from pubis to sole.
   Obvious physical deformities—note any congenital or acquired defects.

Elongated arm span, arm span greater than height (e.g., Marfan's syndrome hypogonadism) (see Table 9-6, p. 178).

Missing extremities or digits; webbed digits; shortened limb.

Mobility

Gait—Normally, the base is as wide as the shoulder width; foot placement is accurate; the walk is smooth, even, and well-balanced; and associated movements, such as symmetrical arm swing, are present.

Exceptionally wide base. Staggered, stumbling.

Shuffling, dragging, nonfunctional leg.

Limping with injury.

Propulsion—difficulty stopping (see Table 23-5, p. 703.

Range of motion—Note full mobility for each joint, and that movement is deliberate, accurate, smooth, and coordinated. (See Chapter 22 for information on more detailed testing of joint range of motion.)

No involuntary movement.

Limited joint range of motion.

Paralysis—absent movement.

Movement jerky, uncoordinated.

Tics, tremors, seizures (see Table 23-4, p. 701).

Behaviour

Facial expression—The person maintains eye contact (unless a cultural taboo exists), expressions are appropriate to the situation; e.g., thoughtful, serious, or smiling. (Note expressions both while the face is at rest and while the person is talking.)

Flat, depressed, angry, sad, anxious. However, note that anxiety is common in ill people. Also, some people smile when they are anxious.

Mood and affect—The person is comfortable and co-operative with the examiner and interacts pleasantly.

Hostile, distrustful, suspicious, crying.

Speech—Articulation (the ability to form words) is clear and understandable.

Dysarthria and dysphagia (see Table 6-4, p. 107). Speech defect, monotone, garbled speech.

The stream of talking is fluent, with an even pace.

The person conveys ideas clearly.

Word choice is appropriate to culture and education.

The person communicates in native language easily by himself or herself or with an interpreter.

Extremes of few words or of constant talking.

Dress—Clothing is appropriate to the climate, looks clean and fits the body, and is appropriate to the person's culture and age group; for example, Amish women may wear nineteenth century–style clothing, and Indian women may wear saris. Culturally determined dress should not be labelled as bizarre by Western standards or by adult expectations.

Trousers too large and held up by belt suggests weight loss, as does the addition of new holes in belt. If the belt is moved to a looser fit, it may indicate obesity or ascites.

Consistent wear of certain clothing may provide clues: long sleeves may conceal needle marks of drug abuse; broadbrimmed hats may reveal sun intolerance; Velcro fasteners instead of buttons may indicate chronic motor dysfunction.

Personal hygiene—The person appears clean and groomed appropriately for his or her age, occupation, and socioeconomic group. (Note that a wide variation of dress and hygiene is "normal.")

Hair is groomed, brushed. Women's makeup is appropriate for age and culture.

In a previously carefully groomed woman, unkempt hair and absent makeup may indicate malaise or illness.

Objective Data

Normal Range of Findings	Abnormal Findings

MEASUREMENT

Weight

Use a standardized *balance* or electronic standing scale. Instruct the person to remove his or her shoes and heavy outer clothing before standing on the scale. When a sequence of repeated weights is necessary, aim for approximately the same time of day and the same type of clothing worn each time. Record the weight in kilograms and in pounds.

Show the person how his or her own weight compares to the recommended range for height. Compare the person's current weight with that from the previous health visit. A recent weight loss may be explained by successful dieting. A weight gain usually reflects overabundant caloric intake, unhealthy eating habits, sedentary lifestyle, or fluid accumulation.

An unexplained weight loss may be a sign of a short-term illness (e.g., fever, infection, disease of the mouth or throat) or a chronic illness (endocrine disease, malignancy, mental health dysfunction).

Obesity is >120% ideal body weight and occasionally may be due to endocrine disorders, drug therapy (e.g., corticosteroids), or depression.

Height

Use a wall-mounted device or the measuring pole on the balance scale. Align the extended headpiece with the top of the head. The person should be shoeless, standing straight with gentle traction under the jaw, and looking straight ahead. Feet, shoulders, and buttocks should be in contact with the pole or the wall.

Body Mass Index

Body mass index (BMI) is a practical marker of optimal weight for height and an indicator of obesity or protein-calorie malnutrition (Fig. 9-1). It is calculated by:

$$BMI = \frac{Weight\ (in\ kilograms)}{Height\ (in\ metres)^2} \quad or \quad \frac{Weight\ (in\ pounds)}{Height\ (in\ inches)^2} \times 703$$

For a quick determination of BMI (kg/m^2), use a straightedge to help locate the point on the chart where height (cm or in) and weight (kg or lb) intersect (Fig. 9-1). Read the number on the dashed line closest to this point. For example, an individual who weighs 69 kg and is 173 cm tall has a BMI of approximately 23.

BMI interpretation for adults (World Health Organization (WHO, 2007):
   <18.5 Underweight
   18.5 to 24.9 Normal weight
   25.0 to 29.9 Overweight
   30.0 to 39.9 Obesity
   ≥40 Extreme obesity
BMI interpretation for children ages 2 to 20 years (CDC, 2000):
   85th to 95th percentile = risk for overweight

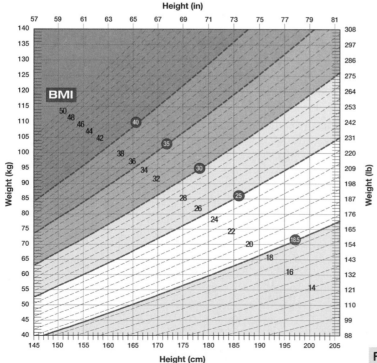

Fig. 9-1 Body mass index (BMI) nomogram.

Objective Data

Normal Range of Findings	Abnormal Findings

Waist-to-Hip Ratio

The waist-to-hip ratio assesses body fat distribution as an indicator of health risk. Obese persons with a greater proportion of fat in the upper body, especially in the abdomen, have android obesity; obese persons with most of their fat in the hips and thighs have gynoid obesity. The equation is:

$$\text{Waist-to-hip ratio} = \frac{\text{Waist circumference}}{\text{Hip circumference}}$$

where waist circumference is measured at the smallest circumference below the rib cage and above the iliac crest, and hip circumference is measured at the largest circumference of the buttocks. In addition, **waist circumference (WC)** alone can be used to predict greater health risk. Measure at the end of gentle expiration.

Health Canada guidelines for body weight classification in adults use BMI measurement and WC as indicators of health risk. This is in keeping with internationally adopted recommendations from WHO (2000), which are derived from population data. It is important to recognize that weight classification is only a component of a comprehensive health assessment. This classification system is not intended for use with those under 18 years of age or with pregnant or lactating women.

Abnormal Findings (right column):

A waist-to-hip ratio of 1.0 or > in men or 0.8 or > in women is indicative of android (upper body obesity) and an increased risk for obesity-related diseases and early mortality.

A WC >88 cm (35 in) in women and >102 cm (40 in) in men increases risk of cardiovascular and metabolic diseases.

VITAL SIGNS

Temperature

Cellular metabolism requires a stable core, or "deep body," temperature of a mean of 37.2°C (99°F). The body maintains a steady temperature through a thermostat, or feedback mechanism, regulated in the hypothalamus of the brain. The thermostat balances heat production (from metabolism, exercise, food digestion, external factors) with heat loss (through radiation, evaporation of sweat, convection, conduction).

The various routes of temperature measurement reflect the body's core temperature. The normal oral temperature in a resting person is 37°C (98.6°F), with a range of 35.8°C to 37.3°C (96.4°F to 99.1°F). The rectal temperature measures 0.4°C to 0.5°C (0.7°F to 1°F) higher.

The normal temperature is influenced by
- A diurnal cycle of 1° to 1.5°C (1°F to 1.5°F), with the trough occurring in the early morning hours and the peak occurring in late afternoon to early evening.
- The menstruation cycle in women. Progesterone secretion, occurring with ovulation at midcycle, causes a 0.5°F to 1.0°F rise in temperature that continues until menses.
- Exercise. Moderate to hard exercise increases body temperature.
- Age. Wider normal variations occur in the infant and young child due to less effective heat control mechanisms. In older adults, temperature is usually lower than in other age groups, with a mean of 36.2°C (97.2°F).

The **oral** temperature is accurate and convenient. The oral sublingual site has a rich blood supply (from the carotid arteries) that quickly responds to changes in inner core temperature.

Due to environmental concerns of mercury pollution from medical waste incinerators, mercury-containing oral thermometers and sphygmomanometers are being replaced with electronic equipment (Goldman et al., 2001). Shake a mercury-free glass thermometer down to 35.5°C (96°F) and place it at the base of the tongue in either of the posterior sublingual pockets—*not* in front

Abnormal Findings (right column):

The thermostatic function of the hypothalamus may become scrambled during illness or central nervous system disorders.

Hyperthermia, or fever, is caused by pyrogens secreted by toxic bacteria during infections or from tissue breakdown such as that following myocardial infarction, trauma, surgery, or malignancy. Neurological disorders (e.g., a cerebral vascular accident, cerebral edema, brain trauma, tumour, or surgery) also can reset the brain's thermostat at a higher level, resulting in heat production and conservation.

Hypothermia is usually due to accidental, prolonged exposure to cold. It also may be purposefully induced to lower the body's oxygen requirements during heart or peripheral vascular surgery, neurosurgery, amputation, or gastrointestinal hemorrhage.

Normal Range of Findings	**Abnormal Findings**

of the tongue. Instruct the person to keep his or her lips closed. Leave in place 3 to 4 minutes if the person is afebrile, and up to 8 minutes if febrile. (Take other vital signs during this time.) Wait 20 minutes prior to taking the temperature if the person has just taken hot or iced liquids and 2 minutes if he or she has just smoked, and 5 minutes if he or she has just chewed gum.

The **electronic thermometer** has the advantages of swift and accurate measurement (usually in 20 to 30 seconds) as well as safe, unbreakable, disposable probe covers. The instrument must be fully charged and correctly calibrated. Most children enjoy watching their temperature numbers advance on the box.

The **axillary** temperature is safe and accurate for infants and young children when the environment is reasonably controlled (see Developmental Care, p. 163).

Take a **rectal** temperature only when the other routes are not practical—for example, for comatose or confused persons, for persons in shock, or for those who cannot close the mouth because of breathing or oxygen tubes, wired mandible, or other facial dysfunction or if no tympanic membrane thermometer equipment is available. Wear gloves and insert a lubricated rectal probe cover on an electronic thermometer only 2 to 3 cm (1 in) into the adult rectum, directed toward the umbilicus. (For a glass thermometer, leave in place for $2\frac{1}{2}$ min). Disadvantages to the rectal route are patient discomfort and the time-consuming and disruptive nature of the activity.

The **tympanic membrane thermometer (TMT)** senses infrared emissions of the tympanic membrane (eardrum). The tympanic membrane shares the same vascular supply that perfuses the hypothalamus (the internal carotid artery); thus it is an accurate measurement of core temperature (Gilbert et al., 2002).

The tympanic membrane thermometer is a noninvasive, nontraumatic device that is extremely quick and efficient. The probe tip has the shape of an otoscope, the instrument used to inspect the ear. Gently place the covered probe tip in the person's ear canal (see Fig. 9-15 on p. 176). Do not force it and do not occlude the canal. Activate the device and you can read the temperature in 2 to 3 seconds.

There is minimal chance of cross-contamination with the tympanic thermometer because the ear canal is lined with skin and not mucous membrane. This thermometer is used with unconscious patients or with those who are unable or unwilling to co-operate with traditional techniques (i.e., those in critical care units, emergency departments, recovery areas, labour and delivery units). The tympanic thermometer has the advantages of speed, convenience, safety, reduced risk of injury and infection, and noninvasiveness.

In Canada Celsius is the official measurement system used for reporting body temperature. Some older adults remain more familiar with the Fahrenheit scale. Use this conversion:

$$\text{Degrees C} = \tfrac{5}{9}\,(\text{F} - 32)$$
$$\text{Degrees F} = (\tfrac{9}{5} \times \text{C}) + 32$$

Familiarize yourself with both scales. Note that it is far easier to learn to *think* in the Celsius scale than to take the time for paper-and-pencil conversions. Begin by memorizing these convenient equivalents:

$$104°\text{F} = 40°\text{C}; \quad 98.6°\text{F} = 37°\text{C}; \quad 95°\text{F} = 35°\text{C}$$

Objective Data

Normal Range of Findings	Abnormal Findings

Pulse

With every beat, the heart pumps an amount of blood—the **stroke volume**—into the aorta. This is about 70 ml in the adult. The force flares the arterial walls and generates a pressure wave, which is felt in the periphery as the **pulse.** Palpating the peripheral pulse gives the rate and rhythm of the heartbeat, as well as local data on the condition of the artery. The *radial* pulse is usually palpated while vital signs are measured.

Using the pads of your first three fingers, palpate the radial pulse at the flexor aspect of the wrist laterally along the radius bone (Fig. 9-2). Push until you feel the strongest pulsation. If the rhythm is regular, count the number of beats in 30 seconds and multiply by 2. Although the 15-second interval is frequently practised, any one-beat error in counting results in a recorded error of four beats per minute. The 30-second interval is the most accurate and efficient when heart rates are normal or rapid and when rhythms are regular. However, if the rhythm is irregular, count for a full minute. As you begin the counting interval, start your count with "zero" for the first pulse felt. The second pulse felt is "one," and so on. Assess the pulse, including (1) rate, (2) rhythm, (3) force, and (4) elasticity.

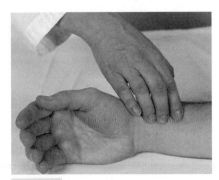

Fig. 9-2

Rate

In the resting adult, the normal heart rate range is 60 to 100 beats per minute (bpm). The rate normally varies with age, being more rapid in infancy and childhood and more moderate during adult and older years. The rate also varies with gender; after puberty, females have a slightly faster rate than males (Table 9-1).

In the adult, a heart rate less than 60 bpm is **bradycardia.** This occurs normally in the well-trained athlete whose heart muscle develops along with the skeletal muscles. The stronger, more efficient heart muscle pushes out a larger stroke volume with each beat, thus requiring fewer beats per minute to maintain a stable cardiac output. (Review the equation $CO = SV \times R$, or Cardiac output = Stroke volume × Rate, in Chapter 19.) A more rapid heart rate, over 100 bpm, is **tachycardia.** It occurs normally with anxiety or with increased exercise to match the body's demand for increased metabolism.

For descriptions of abnormal rates and rhythms, see Table 20-1, p. 547.

Tachycardia occurs with fever, sepsis, and following myocardial infarction.

| Normal Range of Findings | Abnormal Findings |

TABLE 9-1	Normal Resting Pulse Rates Across Age Groups	
Age	Average (Beats Per Minute)	Normal Limits
Newborn	120	70–190
1 yr	120	80–160
2 yr	110	80–130
4 yr	100	80–120
6 yr	100	75–115
8 yr	90	70–110
10 yr	90	70–110
12 yr		
Female	90	70–110
Male	85	65–105
14 yr		
Female	85	65–105
Male	80	60–100
16 yr		
Female	80	60–100
Male	75	55–95
18 yr		
Female	75	55–95
Male	70	50–90
Well-conditioned athlete	May be 50–60	50–100
Adult	74–76	60–100
Aging	74–76	60–100

Rhythm

The rhythm of the pulse normally has an even tempo. However, one irregularity that is commonly found in children and young adults is **sinus arrhythmia.** Here the heart rate varies with the respiratory cycle, speeding up at the peak of inspiration and slowing to normal with expiration. Inspiration momentarily causes a decreased stroke volume from the left side of the heart; to compensate, the heart rate increases. (See Chapter 19 for a full discussion on sinus arrhythmia.) If any other irregularities are felt, auscultate heart sounds for a more complete assessment (see Chapter 19).

Force

The force of the pulse shows the strength of the heart's stroke volume. A "weak, thready" pulse reflects a decreased stroke volume (e.g., as occurs with hemorrhagic shock). A "full, bounding" pulse denotes an increased stroke volume, as with anxiety, exercise, and some abnormal conditions. The pulse force is recorded using a three-point scale:

3+—Full, bounding
2+—Normal
1+—Weak, thready
0—Absent

Some agencies use a four-point scale; make sure your system is consistent with that used by the rest of your staff. Either scale is somewhat subjective. Experience will increase your clinical judgement.

Elasticity

With normal elasticity, the artery feels springy, straight, resilient.

Chapter 19 presents assessment of the precordium, including listening to the heart rate and rhythm as well as the quality of heart sounds. Chapter 20, on peripheral vascular assessment, presents further data on other pulse sites.

Objective Data

Normal Range of Findings	Abnormal Findings

Respirations

Normally, a person's breathing is relaxed, regular, automatic, and silent. Because most people are unaware of their breathing, do not mention that you will be counting the respirations, because sudden awareness may alter the normal pattern. Instead, maintain your position of counting the radial pulse and unobtrusively count the respirations. Count for 30 seconds or for a full minute if you suspect an abnormality. Avoid the 15-second interval. The result can vary by a factor of + or −4, which is significant with such a small number.

Note that respiratory rates presented in Table 9-2 normally are more rapid in infants and children. Also, a fairly constant ratio of pulse rate to respiratory rate exists, which is about 4:1. Normally, both pulse and respiratory rates rise as a response to exercise or anxiety. More detailed assessment on respiratory status is presented in Chapter 18.

TABLE 9-2	Normal Respiratory Rates
Age	Breaths Per Minute
Neonate	30–40
1 yr	20–40
2 yr	25–32
4 yr	23–30
6 yr	21–26
8 yr	20–26
10 yr	20–26
12 yr	18–22
14 yr	18–22
16 yr	12–20
18 yr	16–20
Adult	10–20

Blood Pressure

Blood pressure (BP) is the force of the blood pushing against the side of its container, the vessel wall. The strength of the push changes with the event in the cardiac cycle. The **systolic** pressure is the maximum pressure felt on the artery during left ventricular contraction, or systole. The **diastolic** pressure is the elastic recoil, or resting, pressure that the blood exerts constantly between each contraction. The **pulse pressure** is the difference between the systolic and diastolic and reflects the stroke volume (Fig. 9-3). The **mean arterial pressure (MAP)** is the pressure forcing blood into the tissues, averaged over the cardiac cycle. This is not an arithmetic average of systolic and diastolic pressures because diastole lasts longer. Rather, it is a value closer to diastolic pressure plus one third the pulse pressure.

The average BP in the young adult is 120/80 mm Hg, although this varies normally with many factors, such as:

- **Age.** Normally, a gradual rise occurs through childhood and into the adult years (see Fig. 9-18, p. 171).
- **Gender.** Before puberty, no difference exists between males and females. After puberty, females usually show a lower BP reading than do male counterparts. After menopause, BP in females is higher than in male counterparts.
- **Ethnocultural background.** In Canada, adults of African descent usually have a higher BP than do Euro-Canadians of the same age. The incidence of hypertension is twice as high in this group; reasons for the difference are not fully understood, but it appears to be due to genetics and environmental factors.

Normal Range of Findings	**Abnormal Findings**

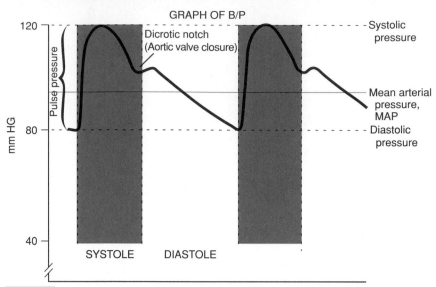

Fig. 9-3   A graph of B/P from systole through Diastole

- **Diurnal rhythm.** A daily cycle of a peak and a trough occurs: the BP climbs to a high in late afternoon or early evening and then declines to an early morning low.
- **Weight.** BP is higher in obese persons than in persons of normal weight of the same age (including adolescents).
- **Exercise.** Increasing activity yields a proportionate increase in BP. Within 5 minutes of terminating the exercise, the BP normally returns to baseline.
- **Emotions.** The BP momentarily rises with fear, anger, and pain as a result of stimulation of the sympathetic nervous system.
- **Stress.** The BP is elevated in persons feeling continual tension because of lifestyle, occupational stress, or life problems.

The level of **BP** is determined by five factors:

1. **Cardiac output.** If the heart pumps more blood into the container (i.e., the blood vessels), the pressure on the container walls increases (Fig. 9-4).
2. **Peripheral vascular resistance.** Peripheral vascular resistance is the opposition to blood flow through the arteries. When the container becomes smaller (e.g., in constricted vessels), the pressure needed to push the contents becomes greater.
3. **Volume of circulating blood.** Volume of circulating blood refers to how tightly the blood is packed into the arteries. Increasing the contents in the container increases the pressure.
4. **Viscosity.** The "thickness" of blood is determined by its formed elements, the blood cells. When the contents are thicker, the pressure increases.
5. **Elasticity of vessel walls.** When the container walls are stiff and rigid, the pressure needed to push the contents increases.

Blood pressure is measured with a stethoscope and an aneroid *sphygmomanometer*. The aneroid gauge is subject to drift; it must be recalibrated at least once each year and it must rest at zero.

The cuff consists of an inflatable rubber bladder inside a cloth cover. The width of the rubber bladder should equal 40% of the circumference of the person's arm. The length of the bladder should equal 80% of this circumference. When using an automated device, ensure you select the cuff size recommended by the manufacturer.

FACTORS CONTROLLING BLOOD PRESSURE

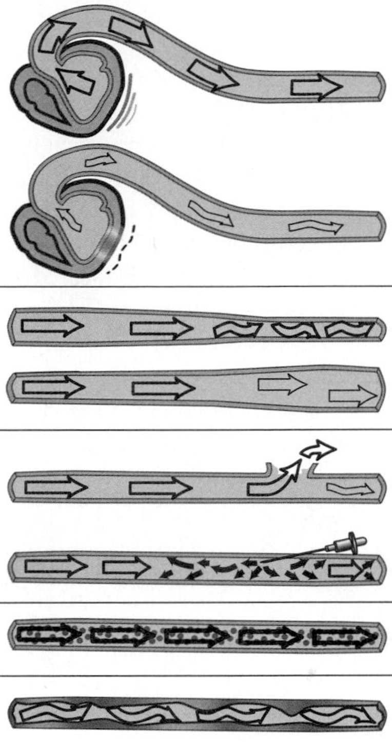

FACTOR	CONDITION		RESULT
Cardiac output	↑ with heavy exercise to meet body demand for increased metabolism		↑BP
	↓ with pump failure (weak pumping action after myocardial infarction, or in shock)		↓BP
Vascular resistance	↑ resistance (vasoconstriction)		↑BP
	↓ resistance (vasodilatation)		↓BP
Volume	↓ volume (hemorrhage)		↓BP
	↑ volume (increased sodium and water retention, intravenous fluid overload)		↑BP
Viscosity	↑ viscosity (increased hematocrit in polycythemia)		↑BP
Elasticity of arterial walls	↑ rigidity, hardening as in arteriosclerosis (heart pumping against greater resistance)		↑BP

Fig. 9-4

Illustration Copyright Pat Thomas, © 2006.

Normal Range of Findings

Available cuffs include six sizes that fit newborn infants to the extra-large adult, as well as tapered cuffs for the cone-shaped obese arm and thigh cuffs. Match the appropriate size cuff to the person's arm size and shape and not to the person's age (Fig. 9-5).

Abnormal Findings

The cuff size is important; using a cuff that is too narrow yields a falsely high BP because it takes extra pressure to compress the artery.

┌ Thigh cuff or large arm cuff

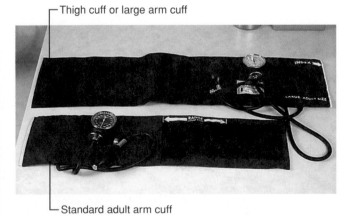

└ Standard adult arm cuff

Fig. 9-5

Arm Pressure

A comfortable, relaxed person yields a valid blood pressure. Many people are anxious at the beginning of an examination; allow at least a 5-minute rest before measuring the BP. Then take two or more BP measurements separated by 2 minutes.

Objective Data

Normal Range of Findings	Abnormal Findings

For each person, verify BP in both arms once, either on admission or for the first complete physical examination. It is not necessary to continue to check both arms for screening or monitoring. Occasionally a 5– to 10–mm Hg difference may occur in BP in the two arms (if values are different, use the higher value).

A difference in the two arms of more than 10 to 15 mm Hg may indicate arterial obstruction on the side with the lower reading.

The person may be sitting or lying, with the bare arm supported at heart level. (If used, place the mercury manometer so that it is vertical and at your eye level.) When the patient is sitting, the feet should be flat on the floor because BP has a false high measurement when legs are crossed versus uncrossed (Canadian Hypertension Education Program [CHEP], 2007).

Palpate the brachial artery, which is located just above the antecubital fossa, medial to the biceps tendon. With the cuff deflated, centre it about 2.5 cm (1 in) above the brachial artery and wrap it evenly.

Now palpate the brachial or the radial artery (Fig. 9-6). Inflate the cuff until the artery pulsation is obliterated and then 20 to 30 mm Hg beyond. This will avoid missing an **auscultatory gap,** which is a period when Korotkoff's sounds disappear during auscultation (Table 9-3).

An auscultatory gap occurs in about 5% of people, most often in hypertension caused by a noncompliant arterial system.

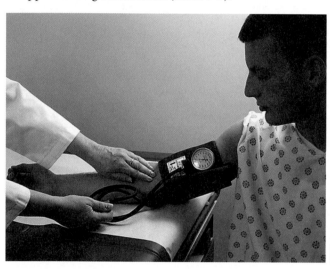

Fig. 9-6

Place the bell of the stethoscope over the site of the brachial artery, making a light but airtight seal (Fig. 9-7). The diaphragm end piece is usually adequate, but the bell is designed to pick up low-pitched sounds such as the sounds of a blood pressure reading.
So if you have a bell, use it.

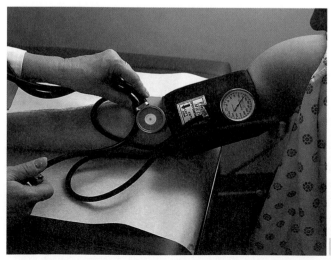

Fig. 9-7

Objective Data

TABLE 9-3	Korotkoff's Sounds		
Phase	Quality	Description	Rationale
Cuff correctly inflated	No sound		Cuff inflation compresses brachial artery. Cuff pressure exceeds heart's systolic pressure, occluding brachial artery blood flow.
I	Tapping	Soft, clear tapping, increasing in intensity	The **systolic** pressure. As the cuff pressure lowers to reach intraluminal systolic pressure, the artery opens, and blood first spurts into the brachial artery. Blood is at very high velocity because of small opening of artery and large pressure difference across opening. This creates turbulent flow, which is audible.
Auscultatory gap	No sound	Silence for 30–40 mm Hg during deflation, an abnormal finding	Sounds temporarily disappear during end of phase I, then reappear in phase II. Common with hypertension. If undetected, results in falsely low systolic or falsely high diastolic reading.
II	Swooshing	Softer murmur follows tapping	Turbulent blood flow through still partially occluded artery.
III	Knocking	Crisp, high-pitched sounds	Longer duration of blood flow through artery. Artery closes just briefly during late diastole.
IV	Abrupt muffling	Sound mutes to a low-pitched, cushioned murmur; blowing quality	Artery no longer closes in any part of cardiac cycle. Change in quality, not intensity.
V	Silence		Decreased velocity of blood flow. Streamlined blood flow is silent. The last audible sound (marking the disappearance of sounds) is **diastolic** pressure. The fifth Korotkoff sound is now used to define diastolic pressure in all age groups (Chobanian et al., 2003).

Brachial artery occluded by cuff, no blood flow

Artery intermittently compressed, blood spurts into artery

Cuff deflated, artery flows free

Auscultatory sound — Silence — I Clear tapping — IV Abrupt muffling — V Silence

Normal Range of Findings

Deflate the cuff slowly and evenly, about 2 mm Hg per heartbeat. Note the points at which you hear the first appearance of sound, the muffling of sound, and the final disappearance of sound. These are phases I, IV, and V of **Korotkoff's sounds,** which are the components of a BP reading first described by a Russian surgeon in 1905 (see Table 9-3).

Abnormal Findings

Objective Data

Normal Range of Findings

For all age groups, the fifth Korotkoff phase is now used to define diastolic pressure (CHEP, 2007). However, when a variance greater than 10 to 12 mm Hg exists between phases IV and V, record *both* phases along with the systolic reading (e.g., 142/98/80). Clear communication is important because the results significantly affect diagnosis and planning of care. Seated BPs are used to determine and monitor treatment decisions. Standing BPs are used to diagnose postural hypotension. See Table 9-4 for a list of common errors in blood pressure measurement.

Abnormal Findings

Hypotension, abnormally low BP; **hypertension**, abnormally high BP (see parameters in Table 9-6, on p. 178).

TABLE 9-4	Common Errors in Blood Pressure Measurement		
Common Error	**Result**	**Rationale**	
Taking blood pressure reading when person is anxious or angry or has just been active	Falsely high	Sympathetic nervous system stimulation	
Faulty arm position			
Above level of heart	Falsely low	Eliminates effect of hydrostatic pressure	
Below level of heart	Falsely high	Additional force of gravity added to brachial artery pressure	
Person supports own arm	Falsely high diastolic	Sustained isometric muscular contraction	
Faulty leg position (e.g., person's legs are crossed)	Falsely high systolic and diastolic	Translocation of blood volume from dependent legs to thoracic area	
Examiner's eyes are not level with meniscus of mercury column			
Looking up at meniscus	Falsely high	Parallax	
Looking down on meniscus	Falsely low		
Inaccurate cuff size (This is the most common error.)			
Cuff too narrow for extremity	Falsely high	Needs excessive pressure to occlude brachial artery	
Cuff wrap is too loose or uneven, or bladder balloons out of wrap	Falsely high	Needs excessive pressure to occlude brachial artery	
Failure to palpate radial artery while inflating			
Poor inflation of the cuff	Falsely low systolic	Miss initial systolic tapping or may tune in during *auscultatory gap* (tapping sounds disappear for 10–40 mm Hg and then return; common with hypertension)	
Both of these conditions can cause a falsely low systolic			
Overinflation of the cuff	Pain		
Pushing stethoscope too hard on brachial artery	Falsely low diastolic	Excessive pressure distorts artery and the sounds continue	
Deflating cuff			
Too quickly	Falsely low systolic or falsely high diastolic	Insufficient time to hear tapping	
Too slowly	Falsely high diastolic	Venous congestion in forearm makes sounds less audible	
Halting during descent and reinflating cuff to recheck systolic	Falsely high diastolic	Venous congestion in forearm	
Failure to wait 1–2 min before repeating entire reading	Falsely high diastolic	Venous congestion in forearm	
Any observer error			
Examiner's "subconscious bias"; a preconceived idea of what blood pressure reading *should* be due to person's age, race, sex, weight, history, or condition	Error anywhere		
Examiner's haste	Error anywhere		
Faulty technique			
Examiner's digit preference, "hears" more results that end in zero than would occur by chance alone (e.g., 130/80)			
Diminished hearing acuity			
Defective or inaccurately calibrated equipment			

Objective Data

Normal Range of Findings	Abnormal Findings

Orthostatic (or Postural) Vital Signs

Take serial measurements of pulse and blood pressure when you suspect volume depletion; when the person is known to have hypertension or is taking anti-hypertensive medications; or when the person reports fainting or syncope. Have the person rest supine for 2 or 3 minutes, take baseline readings of pulse and BP, and then repeat the measurements with the person sitting and then standing. For the person who is too weak or dizzy to stand, assess supine and then sitting with legs dangling. When the position is changed from supine to standing, normally a slight decrease (less than 10 mm Hg) in systolic pressure may occur.

Orthostatic hypotension, a drop in systolic pressure of more than 20 mm Hg, or orthostatic pulse increases of 20 bpm or more, occurs with a quick change to a standing position. These changes are due to abrupt peripheral vasodilatation without a compensatory increase in cardiac output. Orthostatic changes also occur with prolonged bedrest, older age, hypovolemia, and some drugs.

Record the BP by using even numbers. Also record the person's position, the arm used, and the cuff size, if different from the standard adult cuff. Record the pulse rate and rhythm, noting whether the pulse is regular.

Thigh Pressure

When BP measured at the arm is excessively high, particularly in adolescents and young adults, compare it with the thigh pressure to check for **coarctation** of the aorta (a congenital form of narrowing). Normally, the *thigh pressure is higher* than that in the arm. If possible, turn the person into the prone position on the abdomen. (If the person must remain in the supine position, bend the knee slightly.) Wrap a large cuff, 18 to 20 cm, around the lower third of the thigh, centered over the popliteal artery on the back of the knee. Auscultate the popliteal artery for the reading (Fig. 9-8). Normally, the systolic value is 10 to 40 mm Hg higher in the thigh than in the arm, and the diastolic pressure is the same.

With **coarctation of the aorta,** arm pressures are high. Thigh pressure is *lower* because the blood supply to the thigh is below the constriction.

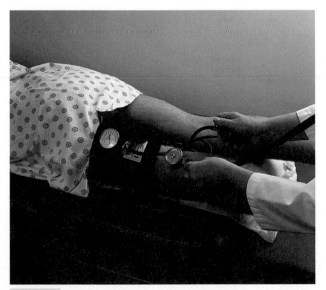

Fig. 9-8

🟣 DEVELOPMENTAL CARE

Infants and Children

General Survey

Physical appearance, body structure, mobility—Note the same basic elements as with the adult, with consideration to age and development.

Behaviour—Note the response to stimuli and level of alertness appropriate for age.

Objective Data

Objective Data

Normal Range of Findings	Abnormal Findings

Normal Range of Findings

Parental bonding—Note the child's interactions with parents, that parent and child show a mutual response and are warm and affectionate, appropriate to the child's condition. The parent provides appropriate physical care of child and promotes new learning.

Measurement

Weight. Weigh an infant on a platform-type balance scale (Fig. 9-9). To check calibration, set the weight at zero and observe the beam balance. Guard the baby so that he or she does not fall. Weigh to the nearest 10 g (½ oz) for infants and 100 g (¼ lb) for toddlers.

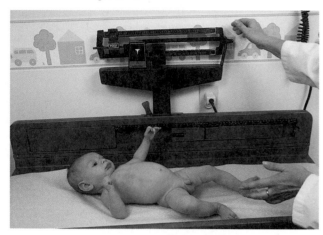

Fig. 9-9

By age 2 or 3 years, use the upright scale. Leave underpants on the child. Some young children are fearful of the rickety standing platform and may prefer sitting on the infant scale. Use the upright scale with preschoolers and school-age children, maintaining modesty with light clothing (Fig. 9-10).

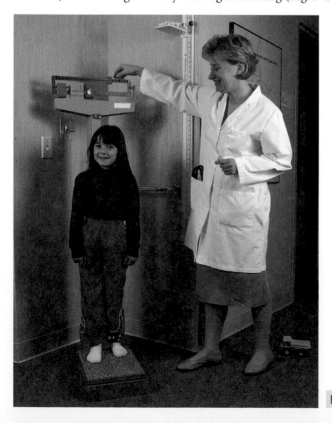

Fig. 9-10

Abnormal Findings

Some signs of child abuse are that the child avoids eye contact; the child exhibits no separation anxiety when you would expect it for age; the parent is disgusted by child's odour, sounds, drooling, or stools.

Deprivation of physical or emotional care (see Chapter 7).

Normal Range of Findings	Abnormal Findings

Length. Until age 2 years, measure the infant's body length supine by using a horizontal measuring board (Fig. 9-11). Hold the head in the midline. Because the infant normally has flexed legs, extend them momentarily by holding the knees together and pushing them down until the legs are flat on the table. Avoid using a tape measure along the infant's length because this is inaccurate.

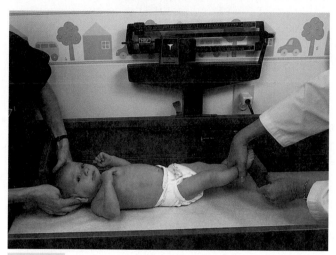

Fig. 9-11

For age 2 or 3 years, measure the child's height by standing the child against the pole on the platform scale or back against a flat ruler taped to the wall (Fig. 9-12). (Sometimes a child will stand more erect against the solid wall than against the narrow measuring pole on the scale.) Encourage the child to stand straight and tall and to look straight ahead without tilting the head. The shoulders, buttocks, and heels should touch the wall. Hold a book or flat board on the child's head at a right angle to the wall. Mark just under the book, noting the measure to the nearest 1 mm (⅛ in).

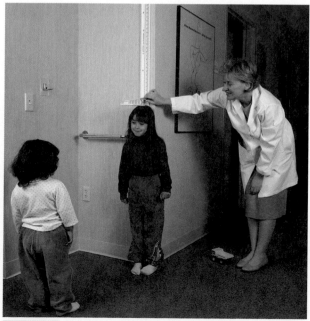

Fig. 9-12

Normal Range of Findings

Physical growth is perhaps the best index of a child's general health. The child's height and weight are recorded at every healthcare visit to determine normal growth patterns. The results are plotted on growth charts based on data from the National Center for Health Statistics (NCHS). Normal limits range from the 5th to the 95th percentile on standardized charts. (See Appendix D on the Evolve Web site for samples.) In 2006 WHO released a new set of child growth standards that better reflect the diversity of the global population. Based on height, weight, and BMI, these assessment tools minimize variations noted using the NCHS tools, which are based on norms established for Euro-American children. The WHO standards are being accepted globally as a more accurate measure of growth and development. (See the Evolve Web site for growth assessment forms for boys and girls.)

Healthy childhood growth is continuous but uneven, with rapid growth spurts occurring during infancy and adolescence. Results are more reliable when comparing numerous growth measures over a long time. These charts also compare the individual child's measurements against those of the general population.

Use your judgement and consider the genetic background of the small-for-age child. Explore the growth patterns of the parents and siblings. Studies have indicated that Canadian Crees have a higher prevalence of macrosomia (birth weight >90th percentile) than their non-Aboriginal counterparts (33% versus 11%). Even after controlling for gestational diabetes, which is known to contribute to higher birth weights, the rates remained significantly higher, indicating potential genetic differences in fetal growth (Rodrigues et al., 2000).

Head Circumference. Measure the infant's head circumference at birth and at each well-child visit up to age 2 years and then yearly up to 6 years (Fig. 9-13). Circle the tape around the head at the prominent frontal and occipital bones; the widest span is correct. Plot the measurement on standardized growth charts. Compare the infant's head size with that expected for age. A series of measurements is more valuable than a single figure to show the *rate* of head growth.

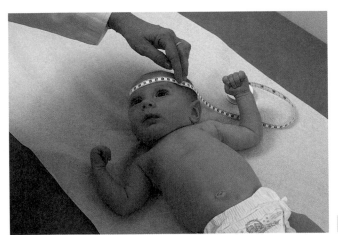

Fig. 9-13

The newborn's head measures about 32 to 38 cm (averaging around 34 cm) and is about 2 cm larger than the chest circumference. The chest grows at a faster rate than the cranium; at some time between 6 months and 2 years, both measurements are about the same, and after 2 years the chest circumference is greater than the head circumference.

Measurement of the chest circumference is valuable in a comparison with the head circumference, but not necessarily by itself. Encircle the tape around the chest at the nipple line. It should be snug, but not so tight that it leaves a mark (Fig. 9-14).

Abnormal Findings

Using NCHS charts

Further explore any growth measure that
- Falls below the 5th or above the 95th percentile with no genetic explanation
- Shows a wide percentile difference between height and weight—for example, a 10th-percentile height with a 95th-percentile weight
- Shows that growth has suddenly stopped when it had been steady
- Fails to show normal growth spurts during infancy and adolescence

Using WHO charts
- A child's score that is far from the median of 0, such as −3 or 3, indicates growth challenges.
- Z score lines indicate distance from the growth average.

Enlarged head circumference occurs with increased intracranial pressure (see Chapter 13).

Normal Range of Findings	Abnormal Findings

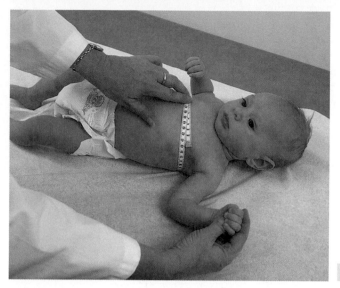

Fig. 9-14

Vital Signs

Measure vital signs with the same purpose and frequency as you would in an adult. With an *infant,* reverse the order of vital sign measurement to respiration, pulse, and temperature. Taking a rectal temperature may cause the infant to cry, which will increase the respiratory and pulse rate, thus masking the normal resting values. A *preschooler's* normal fear of body mutilation is increased with any invasive procedure. Whenever possible, avoid the rectal route and take a tympanic, inguinal, or axillary temperature. When this is not feasible, use the reverse order and measure the rectal temperature last. Promote the co-operation of the *school-age child* by explaining the procedure completely and encouraging the child to handle the equipment. Your approach to measuring vital signs with the *adolescent* is much the same as with the adult.

Temperature

Tympanic. Tympanic temperature (TMT) measurement is useful with toddlers who squirm at the restraint needed for the rectal route, and it is useful with preschoolers who are not yet able to co-operate for an oral temperature yet fear the disrobing and invasion of a rectal temperature. The TMT measurement is so rapid that it is usually over before the child realizes it (Fig. 9-15).

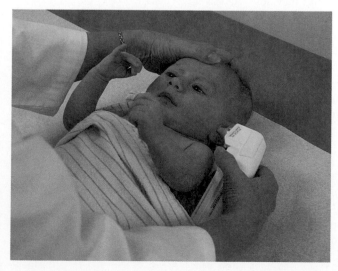

Fig. 9-15

Normal Range of Findings	Abnormal Findings

Objective Data

The data on TMT use with newborn infants and young children are conflicting. In a study of healthy neonates, Sganga et al. (2000) found that tympanic thermometers had a lack of correlation with other methods, making them a poor choice for healthy infants. In a study of infants aged 3 to 36 months in outpatient settings, Jean-Mary et al. (2002) found the TMT useful for noninvasive screening, but if the history or physical examination suggests a possible febrile illness, the rectal value should be used for clinical accuracy. However, Nimah et al. (2006) studied critically ill hospitalized children less than 7 years old and concluded the TMT measurements more accurately reflected core temperatures during febrile and nonfebrile states.

Inguinal. The inguinal route is safer than the rectal route. Its results may be closer to core temperature than the axillary site because the inguinal area has a rich supply of blood vessels, it lacks the brown fat tissue that interferes with axillary temperatures, and you can form a tight skin-to-skin seal (Cusson et al., 1997). Abduct the infant's leg and locate the femoral pulse. Place the bulb of the thermometer lateral to the pulse site, and adduct the leg to create a seal. (In a glass thermometer, a stable temperature will register in 3 to 5 minutes.)

Axillary. The axillary route is safer and more accessible than the rectal route; however, its accuracy and reliability have been questioned (Cusson et al., 1997). When cold receptors are stimulated, brown fat tissue in the area releases heat through chemical energy, which artificially raises skin temperature. Studies on preterm infants show only small differences between axillary and rectal temperature measurement, which may be because brown fat is not present until 34 weeks' gestation (Bliss-Holtz, 1995). When the axillary route is used, place the tip well into the axilla, and hold the child's arm close to the body. (In a glass thermometer, a stable axillary temperature will register by $5\frac{1}{2}$ minutes.)

Oral. Use the oral route when the child is old enough to keep the mouth closed. This is usually at age 5 or 6 years, although some 4-year-old children can co-operate. When available, use an electronic thermometer because it is unbreakable and it registers quickly.

Rectal. The Canadian Paediatric Society (2004) position statement on temperature measurement in infants and children articulates the pros and cons of all methods. It continues to recommend rectal temperature taking as the definitive technique in infants and children 5 years of age and younger. From birth to age 2 years, rectal is the definitive choice, followed by axillary when screening low-risk children. For children 2 to 5 years old, rectal remains the definitive route. For children older than 5 years of age, oral temperature is the primary method, followed by axillary and tympanic temperatures. An infant may be supine or side-lying, with the examiner's hand flexing the knees up onto the abdomen. (When supine, cover the boy's penis with a diaper.) An infant also may lie prone across the adult's lap. Separate the buttocks with one hand, and insert the lubricated electronic rectal probe *no farther than* 2.5 cm (1 in). Any deeper insertion risks rectal perforation because the colon curves posteriorly at 3 cm ($1\frac{1}{4}$ in). (In a glass thermometer, a temperature will register by 3 minutes.)

Normally, rectal temperatures measure higher in infants and young children than in adults, with an average of 37.8°C (100°F) at 18 months. Also, the temperature normally may be elevated in the late afternoon, after vigorous playing, or after eating.

Up to ages 6 to 8 years, children have higher fevers with illness than adults do. Even with minor infections, fevers may elevate to 39.5°C to 40.5°C (103°F to 105°F).

Pulse

Palpate or auscultate an apical rate with infants and toddlers. (See Chapter 19 for location of apex and technique.) In children older than 2 years, use the radial site. Count the pulse for a full minute to take into account normal irregularities, such as sinus arrhythmia. The heart rate normally fluctuates more with infants and children than with adults in response to exercise, emotion, and illness.

Normal Range of Findings	Abnormal Findings

Respirations

Watch the infant's abdomen for movement, because the infant's respirations are normally more diaphragmatic than thoracic (Fig. 9-16). Count a full minute because the pattern varies significantly from rapid breaths to short periods of apnea. Note the normal rate in Table 9-2 on page 157.

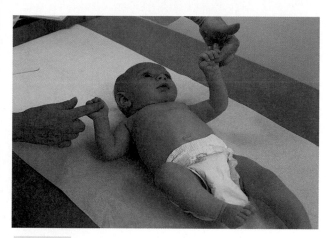

Fig. 9-16

Blood Pressure

In children aged 3 years and older and in younger children at risk, measure a routine BP at least annually. For accurate measurement in children, make some adjustment in the choice of equipment and technique. The most common error is to use the incorrect size cuff. The cuff width must cover two thirds of the upper arm, and the cuff bladder must completely encircle it.

Use a pediatric-sized end piece on the stethoscope to locate the sounds. If possible, allow a crying infant to become quiet for 5 to 10 minutes before measuring the BP; crying may elevate the systolic pressure by 30 to 50 mm Hg. Use the disappearance of sound (phase V Korotkoff) for the diastolic reading in children as well as adults. Note the new guidelines for normal BP values by age-groups *based on the child's height* (Appendices E-1 and E-2 on the Evolve Web site). In children, height is more strongly correlated with BP than is age. The new charts avoid the misclassification as normotensive or hypertensive of children who are at the extremes of normal growth (National High Blood Pressure Education Program [NHBPEP], 1996). That is, for children of the same age, BP classified as 90th and 95th percentiles is lower for very short children, whereas tall children are given a higher normal range.

Children under 3 years of age have such small arm vessels that it is difficult to hear Korotkoff's sounds with a stethoscope. Instead, use an electronic BP device that uses *oscillometry*, such as Dinamap, and gives a digital readout for systolic, diastolic, MAP and pulse. Or use a *Doppler* ultrasound device to amplify the sounds. This instrument is easy to use and can be used by one examiner. (Note the technique for using the Doppler device on p. 172.)

Further explore any blood pressure that is greater than the 95th percentile and refer for diagnostic evaluation. For the child whose BP falls in the 90 to 95th percentile and whose high BP cannot be explained by height or weight, monitor the BP every 6 months.

The Aging Adult

General Survey

Physical appearance—By the eighth and ninth decades, body contour is sharper, with more angular facial features, and body proportions are redistributed. (See measuring weight and height, p. 152.)

Posture—A general flexion occurs by the eight or ninth decade.

Objective Data

| Normal Range of Findings | Abnormal Findings |

Gait—Older adults often use a wider base to compensate for diminished balance, arms may be held out to help balance, and steps may be shorter or uneven.

Measurement

Weight. The older person appears sharper in contour with more prominent bony landmarks than are found in the younger adult. Body weight decreases during the 80s and 90s. This factor is more evident in males, perhaps because of greater muscle shrinkage. The distribution of fat also changes during the 80s and 90s. Even with good nutrition, subcutaneous fat is lost from the face and periphery (especially the forearms), whereas additional fat is deposited on the abdomen and hips (Fig. 9-17).

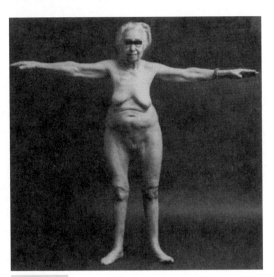

Fig. 9-17

Height. By the 80s and 90s, many people are shorter than they were in their 70s. This results from shortening in the spinal column due to thinning of the vertebral discs and shortening of the individual vertebrae, as well as slight flexion in the knees and hips and the postural changes of kyphosis. Because long bones do not shorten with age, the overall body proportion looks different—a shorter trunk with relatively long extremities (see Fig. 9-17).

Vital Signs

Temperature. Changes in the body's temperature regulatory mechanism leave the older adult less likely to have fever but at a greater risk for hypothermia. Thus the temperature is a less reliable index of the older person's true health state. Sweat gland activity is also diminished.

Pulse. The normal range of heart rate is 60 to 100 bpm, but the rhythm may be slightly irregular. The radial artery may feel stiff, rigid, and tortuous in an older person, although this condition does not necessarily imply vascular disease in the heart or brain. The increasingly rigid arterial wall needs a faster upstroke of blood, so the pulse is actually easier to palpate.

Respirations. Aging causes a decrease in vital capacity and a decreased inspiratory reserve volume. You may note a shallower inspiratory phase and an increased respiratory rate.

Blood Pressure. The aorta and major arteries tend to harden with age. As the heart pumps against a stiffer aorta, the systolic pressure increases, leading to a widened pulse pressure (see Fig. 9-18 for mean BP readings in apparently healthy persons from birth to older adult). With many older people, both the systolic and diastolic pressures increase, making it difficult to distinguish normal aging values from abnormal hypertension.

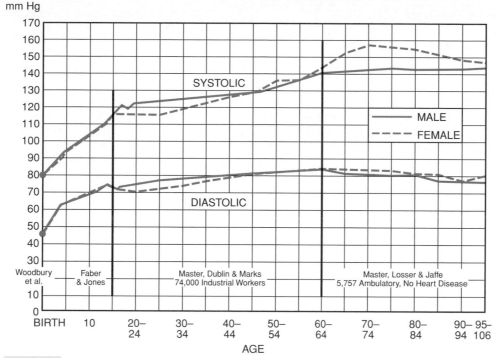

Fig. 9-18   Mean blood pressure readings in apparently healthy people, birth to older adult

Normal Range of Findings	Abnormal Findings

ADDITIONAL TECHNIQUES

Measurement of Oxygen Saturation

The **pulse oximeter** is a noninvasive method to assess arterial oxygen saturation (SpO$_2$). A sensor attached to the person's finger or earlobe has a diode that emits light and a detector that measures the relative amount of light absorbed by oxyhemoglobin (HbO$_2$) and unoxygenated (reduced) hemoglobin (Hb). The pulse oximeter compares the ratio of light emitted to light absorbed and converts this ratio into the percentage of oxygen saturation. Because it only measures light absorption of pulsatile flow, the result is arterial oxygen saturation. A healthy person with no lung disease and no anemia normally has an SpO$_2$ of 97 to 98%.

Select the appropriate pulse oximeter probe. The finger probe is spring loaded and feels like a clothespin attached to the finger but does not hurt (Fig. 9-19). At lower oxygen saturations, the earlobe probe is more accurate and is less affected by peripheral vasoconstriction (Grap, 2002).

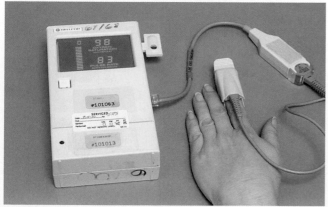

Fig. 9-19

The Doppler Technique

In many situations, pulse and BP measurement are enhanced by using an electronic device, the *Doppler ultrasonic flowmeter*. The Doppler technique works by a principle discovered in the nineteenth century by an Austrian physicist, Johannes Doppler. Sound varies in pitch in relation to the distance between the sound source and the listener; the pitch is higher when the distance is small, and the pitch lowers as the distance increases. Think of a railroad train speeding toward you; its train whistle sounds higher the closer it gets, and the pitch of the whistle lowers as the train moves away.

In this case, the sound source is the blood pumping through the artery in a rhythmic manner. A handheld transducer picks up changes in sound frequency and amplifies them as the blood flows and ebbs. The listener hears a whooshing pulsatile beat.

The Doppler technique is used to locate the peripheral pulse sites (see Chapter 20 for further discussion of this technique). For BP measurement, the Doppler technique will augment Korotkoff's sounds (Fig. 9-20). Through this technique, you can evaluate sounds that are hard to hear with a stethoscope, such as those in critically ill individuals with a low BP, in infants with small arms, and in obese persons in whom the sounds are muffled by layers of fat. Also, proper cuff placement is difficult on the obese person's cone-shaped upper arm. In this situation, you can place the cuff on the more even forearm and hold the Doppler probe over the radial artery. For either location, use the following procedure:

- Apply coupling gel to the transducer probe.
- Turn the Doppler flowmeter on.
- Touch the probe to the skin, holding the probe perpendicular to the artery.
- A pulsatile whooshing sound indicates location of the artery. You may need to rotate the probe, but maintain contact with the skin. Do not push the probe too hard or you will wipe out the pulse.
- Inflate the cuff until the sounds disappear; then proceed another 20 to 30 mm Hg beyond that point.
- Slowly deflate the cuff, noting the point at which the first whooshing sounds appear. This is the systolic pressure.
- It is difficult to hear the muffling of sounds or a reliable disappearance of sounds indicating the diastolic pressure (phases IV and V of Korotkoff's sounds). However, the systolic pressure alone gives valuable data on the level of tissue perfusion and on blood flow through patent vessels.

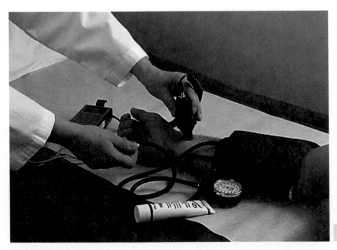

Fig. 9-20

Objective Data

Normal Range of Findings	Abnormal Findings

PROMOTING HEALTH AND SELF-CARE

As you measure height and weight and collect vital signs, it is a good time to begin a teaching plan to help the individual keep these physical signs within normal limits. CHEP considers the following **health behaviours** to be the foundation of hypertension control. Even if your patient is normotensive and has body weight in normal limits, the following recommendations will help keep blood pressure under control (CHEP, 2007):

- Lose weight, if you are more than 10% above ideal weight.
- Limit alcohol intake to no more than two drinks a day—a regular-sized bottle or can of beer, 45 mL (1.5 oz) of hard liquor, or 300 mL (10.5 oz) of wine.
- Get regular aerobic exercise (e.g., a 30- to 45-minute brisk walk) most days of the week.
- Cut sodium intake from the average 3100 mg/d to less than 1500 mg/d.
- Include the recommended daily allowances of potassium, calcium, and magnesium in your diet.
- Stop smoking.
- Reduce dietary saturated fat and cholesterol.

Canadians are so focused on the impact of dietary sodium on BP that in the fall of 2007, the minister of health announced a National Sodium Reduction Strategy (Blood Pressure Canada, 2007).

With over five million Canadians diagnosed with hypertension, CHEP recommends that the diagnosis of hypertension be expedited to ensure early intervention. See Fig. 9-21 for recommendations for management.

These recommendations establish a protocol for early detection, with patients being diagnosed within one to five visits. The practice of accepting self-administered/ home BP measurements (S/H BPMs) has sped up the process significantly. Ambulatory BP monitors (ABPM) are useful to determine readings outside the office setting for those with suspected office-induced hypertension.

Objective Data

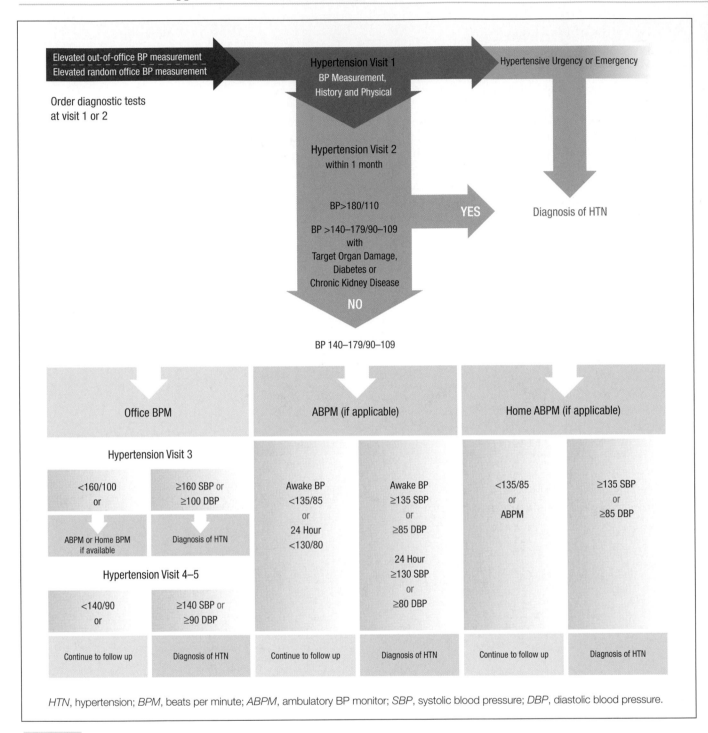

HTN, hypertension; *BPM*, beats per minute; *ABPM*, ambulatory BP monitor; *SBP*, systolic blood pressure; *DBP*, diastolic blood pressure.

Fig. 9-21   Canadian recommendations for the assessment of hypertensive patients.

DOCUMENTATION AND CRITICAL THINKING

Sample Charting

A.J. is a female 47-year-old African Canadian high-school principal, well nourished, well developed, appears stated age. She is alert, oriented, co-operative, with no signs of acute distress. Ht 163 cm (5'4"), Wt 57 kg (126 lbs), TPR 37°C-76-14, B/P 146/84 right arm, sitting.

Focused Assessment: Clinical Case Study*

Mrs. Grazia S. is a 76-year-old Hispanic female, retired secretary, in previous good health, who is brought to the emergency department by her 83-year-old husband. They have both been ill during the night with nausea, vomiting, abdominal pain, and diarrhea, which they attribute to eating "bad food" at a buffet-style restaurant the night before. Mr. S's condition has improved during the next day, but Mrs. S is worse, with severe vomiting, diarrhea, weakness, dizziness, and abdominal pain.

SUBJECTIVE

• Extreme fatigue. Weakness and dizziness occur whenever patient tries to sit or stand up: "Feels like I'm going to black out." Severe nausea and vomiting, thirsty but cannot keep anything down; even sips of water result in "dry heaves." Abdominal pain is moderate aching, intermittent. Diarrhea is watery brown stool, profuse during the night, somewhat diminished now.

OBJECTIVE

Vital signs: Temp 37.2°C (99° F), BP (supine) 102/64, pulse (supine) 70, regular rhythm, respirations 18.
Helped to seated, leg dangling position, vitals: BP 74/52, pulse 138, regular rhythm, respirations 20. Skin pale and moist (diaphoretic).
Reports lightheaded and dizzy in seated position. Returned to supine.
Respiratory: Breath sounds clear in all fields, no adventitious sounds.
Cardiovascular: Regular rate (70 bpm) and rhythm when supine, S_1 and S_2 are not accentuated or diminished, no extra sounds. All pulses present, 2+ and equal bilaterally. Carotids 2+ with no carotid bruit.
Abdomen: Bowel sounds hyperactive, skin pale and moist, abdomen soft and mildly tender to palpation. No enlargement of liver or spleen.
Neuro: Level of consciousness—alert and oriented; pupils equal, round, react to light and accommodation. Sensory status normal. Mild weakness in arms and legs. Gait and standing leg strength not tested due to inability to stand. Deep tendon reflexes 2+ and equal bilaterally. Babinski reflex → toes curl inward.

ASSESSMENT

Orthostatic hypotension, orthostatic pulse increase, and syncopal symptoms, R/T hypovolemia
Diarrhea, possibly R/T ingestion of contaminated food
Risk for hyperthermia, R/T dehydration and aging
Deficient fluid volume

Nursing Diagnoses Commonly Associated With Measurement or Vital Sign Disorders

All nursing diagnoses can be found on the Evolve Web site at **http://evolve.elsevier.com/Canada/Jarvis/examination/.**

*Please note that space does not allow for the inclusion of a detailed plan for each clinical case study in this text. Please consult the appropriate text for current treatment plan.

Documentation and Critical Thinking

ABNORMAL FINDINGS

TABLE 9-5 | **Abnormalities in Body Height and Proportion**

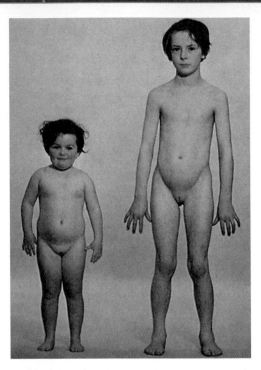

Hypopituitary Dwarfism

Deficiency in growth hormone in childhood results in retardation of growth below the 3rd percentile, delayed puberty, hypothyroidism, and adrenal insufficiency. The 9-year-old girl at left appears much younger than her chronological age, with infantile facial features and chubbiness. The age-matched girl at right shows increased height, more mature facies, and loss of infantile fat.

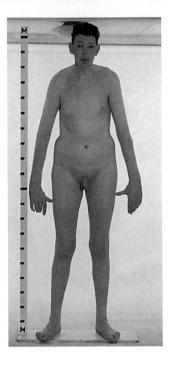

Gigantism

Excessive secretion of growth hormone by the anterior pituitary resulting in overgrowth of entire body. When this occurs during childhood, before closure of bone epiphyses in puberty, it causes increased height (here 2.09 m, or 6 ft 9 in), and weight and delayed sexual development.

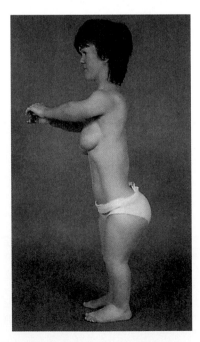

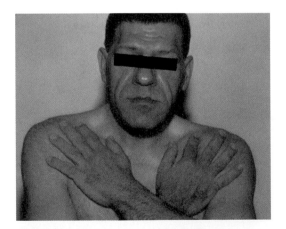

Acromegaly (Hyperpituitarism)

Excessive secretion of growth hormone in adulthood, after normal completion of body growth, causes overgrowth of bone in the face, head, hands, and feet, but no change in height. Internal organs also enlarge, which may result in cardiomegaly or hepatomegaly.

Reprinted from the Clinical Slide Collection on the Rheumatic Diseases, © 1991, 1995, 1997. Used by permission of the American College of Rheumatology.

Achondroplastic Dwarfism

Text continued on following page

TABLE 9-5 | **Abnormalities in Body Height and Proportion—cont'd**

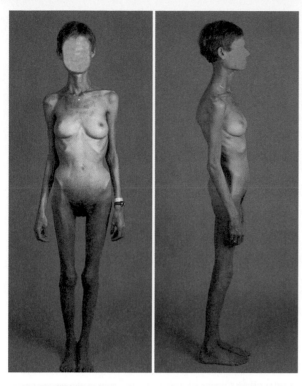

Anorexia Nervosa

A serious psychological disorder characterized by severe and life-threatening weight loss and amenorrhea in an otherwise-healthy adolescent or young adult. Behaviour is characterized by fanatic concern about weight, aversion to food, distorted body image (perceives self as fat despite skeletal appearance), starvation diets, frenetic exercise patterns, and striving for perfection.

Achondroplastic Dwarfism (see figure on previous page)

Congenital skeletal malformation caused by a genetic disorder in converting cartilage to bone. Characterized by relatively large head with frontal bossing and midplace hypoplasia, short stature, and short limbs, and often thoracic kyphosis, prominent lumbar lordosis, and abdominal protrusion. The mean adult height in men is about 131.5 cm (51.8 in) and in women about 125 cm (49.2 in).

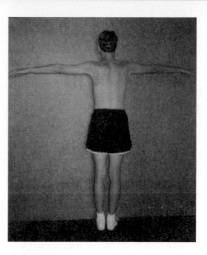

Marfan's Syndrome

Abraham Lincoln, Paganini, and Rachmaninoff are thought to have had this inherited connective tissue disorder, characterized by tall, thin stature (greater than 95th percentile), arachnodactyly (long, thin fingers), hyperextensible joints, arm span greater than height, pubis-to-sole measurement exceeding crown-to-pubis measurement, sternal deformity, high-arched narrow palate, and pes planus. Early morbidity and mortality occur as a result of cardiovascular complications such as mitral regurgitation and aortic dissection.

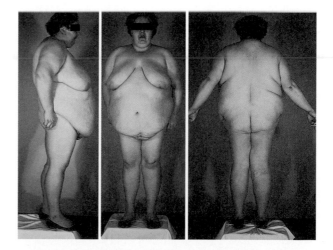

Endogenous Obesity—Cushing's Syndrome

Either administration of adrenocorticotropic hormone (ACTH) or excessive production of ACTH by the pituitary will stimulate the adrenal cortex to secrete excess cortisol. This causes Cushing's syndrome, characterized by weight gain and edema with central trunk and cervical obesity ("buffalo hump") and round plethoric face ("moon face"). Excessive catabolism causes muscle wasting; weakness; thin arms and legs; reduced height; and thin, fragile skin with purple abdominal striae, bruising, and acne. Note the obesity here is markedly different from *exogenous obesity* due to excessive caloric intake, in which body fat is evenly distributed and muscle strength is intact.

TABLE 9-6 | Abnormalities in Blood Pressure

Hypotension

In normotensive adults: <95/60
In hypertensive adults: < the person's average reading, but >95/60
In children: < expected value for age

Occurs With	Rationale
Acute myocardial infarction (MI)	Decreased cardiac output
Shock	Decreased cardiac output
Hemorrhage	Decrease in total blood volume
Vasodilatation	Decrease in peripheral vascular resistance
Addison's disease (hypofunction of adrenal glands)	Decrease in aldosterone production

Associated Symptoms and Signs

In conditions of decreased cardiac output, a low BP is accompanied by an increased pulse, dizziness, diaphoresis, confusion, and blurred vision. The skin feels cool and clammy because the superficial blood vessels constrict to shunt blood to the vital organs. An individual having an acute MI may also complain of crushing substernal chest pain, high epigastric pain, and shoulder or jaw pain.

Hypertension

Essential or Primary Hypertension

This occurs from no known cause but is responsible for about 95% of cases of hypertension in adults.

Classification and Follow-Up of Blood Pressure for Adults Age 18 and Older[1]

BP Classification	SBP (mm Hg)[1]		DBP (mm Hg)[1]	Lifestyle Modification	Initial Drug Therapy Without Compelling Indication	Initial Drug Therapy With Compelling Indication
Normal	<120	and	<80	Encourage		
Prehypertension	120–139	or	80–89	Yes	No antihypertensive drug indicated	Drug(s) for the compelling indications[3]
Stage 1 Hypertension	140–159	or	90–99	Yes	Thiazide-type diuretics for most. May consider ACEI, ARB, BB, CCB, or combination.	Drug(s) for the compelling indications.[3] Other antihypertensive drugs (diuretics, ACEI, ARB, BB, CCB) as needed.
Stage 2 Hypertension	≥160	or	≥100	Yes	Two-drug combination for most,[2] usually thiazide-type diuretic and ACEI, or ARB or BB or CCB.	Drug(s) for the compelling indications.[3] Other antihypertensive drugs (diuretics, ACEI, ARB, BB, CCB) as needed.

Data on classification of hypertension in adults adapted from the seventh report of the Joint National Committee on Prevention, Detection, Evaluation and Treatment of High Blood Pressure (JNC-7). Reprinted in *Journal of the American Medical Association,* 289, 2560–2572; and http://www.nhlbi.nih.gov/guidelines/hypertension.
DBP, diastolic blood pressure; *SBP,* systolic blood pressure.
Drug abbreviations: *ACEI,* angiotensin-converting enzyme inhibitor; *ARB,* angiotensin receptor blocker; *BB,* β-blocker; *CCB,* calcium channel blocker.
[1]Treatment determined by highest BP category.
[2]Initial combined therapy should be used cautiously in those at risk for orthostatic hypotension.
[3]Treat patients with chronic kidney disease or diabetes to BP goal of <130/80 mm Hg.

TABLE 9-6	Abnormalities in Blood Pressure—cont'd

Cardiovascular Risk Stratification in Patients With Hypertension

Major Risk Factors

Smoking
Dyslipidemia
Diabetes mellitus
Age >60 y
Gender (men and postmenopausal women)
Family history of cardiovascular disease: women <65 y
or men <55 y

Target Organ Damage/Clinical Cardiovascular Disease

Heart diseases
   Left ventricular atrophy
   Angina or prior myocardial infarction
   Prior coronary revascularization
   Heart failure
Stroke or transient ischemic attack
Nephropathy
Peripheral arterial disease
Retinopathy

Lifestyle Modifications for Hypertension Prevention and Management

- Lose weight if overweight
- Limit alcohol intake to no more than two drinks a day or less—a regular-sized bottle or can of beer, 45 mL (1.5 oz) of hard liquor, or 300 mL (10.5 oz) of wine.
- Increase aerobic physical activity (30–45 min most days of the week)
- Reduce sodium intake to no more than 1500 mg/d
- Maintain adequate intake of dietary potassium (approximately 90 mmol/L/d)
- Maintain adequate intake of dietary calcium and magnesium for general health
- Stop smoking and reduce intake of dietary saturated fat and cholesterol for overall cardiovascular health

Abnormal Findings

BIBLIOGRAPHY

Abraham, S. J., Clifford, L., & Najjar, M. F. (1976). Height and weight of adults 18–74 years of age in the United States. *Advancedata, 3*, 1–8.

Barr, G. D., Allen, C. M., & Shinefield, H. R. (1972). Height and weight of 7,500 children of three skin colors. *American Journal of Diseases of Children, 124*, 866–872.

Barton, S. J., Gaffney, R., Chase, T., Rayens, M. K., & Piyabanditkul, L. (2003). Pediatric temperature measurement and child/parent/nurse preference using three temperature measurement instruments. *Journal of Pediatric Nursing, 18*, 314–320.

Beevers, G., Lip, G. Y. H., & O'Brien, E. (2001). ADB of hypertension: Blood pressure measurement, II: Conventional sphygmomanometry: Technique of auscultatory blood pressure measurement. *British Medical Journal, 322*(7293), 1043–1047.

Blacher, J., Staessen, J. A., Girerd, X., Gasowski, J., Thijs, L., Liu, L., et al. (2000). Pulse pressure not mean pressure determines cardiovascular risk in older hypertensive patients. *Archives of Internal Medicine, 160*, 1085–1089.

Blazys, D. (2000). Orthostatic blood pressure. *Journal of Emergency Nursing, 26*, 479–480.

Bliss-Holtz, J. (1995). Methods of newborn infant temperature monitoring: A research review. *Issues in Comprehensive Pediatric Nursing, 18*, 287–298.

Blood Pressure Canada. (2007). First steps taken towards a national sodium reduction strategy. *Blood Pressure Canada News.* Retrieved on May 8, 2008, from http://hypertension.ca/bpc/first-steps-taken-towards-a-national-sodium-reduction-strategy/

Canadian Hypertension Society. (2005). Management of hypertension: A summary of new and important aspects of the 2005 Canadian Hypertension Education Program recommendations for the management of hypertension. *Canadian Nurse, 101*(5), 25.

Canadian Hypertension Education Program. (2007). *Hypertension. 2007 public recommendations.* Retrieved January 16, 2008, from http://hypertension.ca/bpc/wp-content/uploads/2007/11/chep2007march-locked.pdf

Canadian Paediatric Society. (2004). CPS position statement: Temperature measurement in paediatrics. *Paediatrics and Child Health, 9*, 171–180.

Canzanello, V. J., Jensen, P. L., & Schwartz, G. L. (2001). Are aneroid sphygmomanometers accurate in hospital and clinic settings? *Archives of Internal Medicine, 161*, 729–731.

Centers for Disease Control and Prevention. (2000). *Growth charts.* Atlanta, GA: National Center for Health Statistics in collaboration with the National Center for Chronic Disease Prevention and Health Promotion. Retrieved July 5, 2006, from http://www.cdc.gov/growth_charts

Chobanian, A. V., Bakris, G. L., Black, H. R., Cushman, W. C., Green, L. A., Izzo, J. L., Jr., et al. (2003). The seventh report of the Joint National Committee on Prevention, Detection, Evaluation and Treatment of High Blood Pressure: The JNC 7 report. *Journal of the American Medical Association, 289*, 2560–2572.

Craig, J. V., Lancaster, G. A., Taylor, S., Williamson, P. R., & Smyth, R. L. (2002). Infrared ear thermometry compared with rectal thermometry in children: A systematic review. *Lancet, 360*(9333), 603–609.

Cruickshank, J. K., Mzayek, F., & Liu, L. (2005). Origins of the "black/white" difference in blood pressure: Roles of birth weight, postnatal growth, early blood pressure, and adolescent body size. *Circulation, 111*, 1932–1937.

Cusson, R. M., Madonia, J. A., & Taekmen, J. B. (1997). The effect of environment on body site temperatures in full-term neonates. *Nursing Research, 46*, 202–207.

Fisher, A. A, Davis, M. W., Srikusalanukul, W., & Budge, M. M. (2005). Postprandial hypotension predicts all-cause mortality in older, low-level care residents. *Journal of the American Geriatric Society, 53,* 1313–1320.

Franklin, S. S. (2004). Pulse pressure as a risk factor. *Clinical and Experimental Hypertension, 26,* 645–652.

Gilbert, M., Barton, A. J., & Counsell, C. M. (2002). Comparison of oral and tympanic temperatures in adult surgical patients. *Applied Nursing Research, 15*(1), 42–47.

Giuliano, K. K., Giuliano, A. J., Scott, S. S., MacLachlan, E., Pysznik, E., Elliot, S., et al. (2000). Temperature measurement in critically ill adults: A comparison of tympanic and oral methods. *American Journal of Critical Care, 9,* 254–261.

Goldman, L. R., & Shannon, M. W. (2001). Technical report: Mercury in the environment: Implications for pediatricians. *Pediatrics, 108*(1), 197–205.

Grap, M. J. (2002). Pulse oximetry. *Critical Care Nurse, 22*(3), 69.

Health Canada. (2003). *Canadian guidelines for body weight classifications in adults* (Catalogue No. H49-179/2003E). Ottawa, ON: Author.

Hines, S. E. (2000). Performing a focused physical examination. *Patient Care, 34*(23), 76–106.

Hockenberry, M. J., & Wilson, D. (2007). *Wong's nursing care of infants and children* (8th ed.). St Louis, MO: Mosby.

Hwu, Y., Coates, V. E., & Lin, F. (2000). A study of the effectiveness of different measuring times and counting methods of human radial pulse rates. *Journal of Clinical Nursing, 9*(1), 146–152.

Jean-Mary, M. B., Dicanzio, J., Shaw, J., & Bernstein, H. H. (2002). Limited accuracy and reliability of infrared axillary and aural thermometers in a pediatric outpatient population. *Journal of Pediatrics, 141,* 671–676.

Kamienski, M. C. (2003). Reye syndrome. *American Journal of Nursing, 103*(7), 54–57.

Keele-Smith, R., & Price-Daniel, C. (2001). Effects of crossing legs on blood pressure measurement. *Clinical Nursing Research, 10*(3), 202–213.

Khorshid, L., Eşser, I., Zaybak, A., & Yapucu, Ü. (2004). Comparing mercury-in-glass, tympanic and disposable thermometers in measuring body temperature in healthy young people. *Journal of Clinical Nursing, 14,* 496–500.

Lanham, D. M., Walker, B., Klocke, E., & Jennings, M. (1999). Accuracy of tympanic temperature readings in children under 6 years of age. *Pediatric Nursing, 25*(1), 39–42.

Lipman, T. H., McGinley, A., & Hughes, J. (2006). Evaluation of the accuracy of height assessment of premenopausal and menopausal women. *Journal of Obstetric, Gynecologic, and Neonatal Nursing, 35,* 516–522.

Mitsnefes, M. M. (2006). Hypertension in children and adolescents. *Pediatric Clinics of North America, 53,* 493–512.

Moore, J. (2005). Hypertension: Catching the silent killer. *Nurse Practitioner, 30*(10), 16–35.

Morrison, R. E., & Lewis, J. B. (2004). Fever: Sorting out the potentially dangerous causes. *Consultant, 44,* 245–255.

National High Blood Pressure Education Program. (1996). Update on the 1987 task force report on high blood pressure in children and adolescents. *Pediatrics, 98,* 649–667.

Nimah, M. M., Bshesh, K., Callahan, J. D., & Jacobs, B. R. (2006). Infrared tympanic thermometry in comparison with other temperature measurement techniques in febrile children. *Pediatric Critical Care Medicine, 7*(1), 48–55.

O'Brien, E. (2000). Replacing the mercury sphygmomanometer: Requires clinicians to demand better automated devices. *British Medical Journal, 320*(7238), 815–816.

Overfield, T. (1995). *Biologic variation in health and illness: Race, age and sex differences* (2nd ed.). Menlo Park, CA: Addison Wesley.

Pesola, G. R., Pesola, H. R., Nelson, M. J., & Westfal, R. E. (2001). The normal difference in bilateral indirect blood pressure recordings in normotensive individuals. *American Journal of Emergency Medicine, 19*(1), 43–45.

Pickersgill, J., Fowler, H., Boothman, J., Thompson, K., Wilcock, S., & Tanner, J. (2003). Temperature taking: Children's preferences. *Pediatric Nursing, 15*(2), 22–25.

Robson, J. R. K., Larkin, F. A., Bursick, J. H., & Perri, K. P. (1975). Growth standards for infants and children: A cross-sectional study. *Pediatrics, 56,* 1014–1020.

Rodrigues, S., Robinson, E. J., Kramer, M. S., & Gray-MacDonald, K. (2000). High rates of infant macrosomia: A comparison of a Canadian native and non-native population. *Journal of Nutrition, 130,* 806–812.

Ryan-Krause, P. (2002). Identify and manage Marfan syndrome in children. *Nurse Practitioner, 27*(10), 26–36.

Sachse, D. (2001). Acromegaly. *American Journal of Nursing, 101*(11), 69–77.

Schell, K. A. (2006). Evidence-based practice: Noninvasive blood pressure measurement in children. *Pediatric Nursing, 32,* 263–267.

Schell, K., Lyons, D., Bradley, E., Bucher, L., Seckel, M., Wakai, S., et al. (2006). Clinical comparison of autonomic, noninvasive measurements of blood pressure in the forearm and upper arm with the patient supine or with the head of the bed raised 45 degrees: A follow-up study. *American Journal of Critical Care, 15,* 196–205.

Schrezenmaier, C., Gehrking, J. A., Hines, S. M., Low, P. A., Benrud-Larson, L. M., & Sandroni, P. (2005). Evaluation of orthostatic hypotension: Relationship of a new self-report instrument to laboratory-based measures. *Mayo Clinic Proceedings, 80,* 330–334.

Sganga, A., Wallace, R., Kiehl, E., Irving, T., & Witter, L. (2000). A comparison of four methods of normal newborn temperature measurement. *American Journal of Maternal Child Nursing, 25*(2), 66–79.

Sund-Levander, M., Grodzinsky, E., Loyd, D., & Wahren, L. K. (2004). Errors in body temperature assessment related to individual variation, measuring technique, and equipment. *International Journal of Nursing Practice, 10,* 216–223.

Todd, B. (2006). *Clostridium difficile*: Familiar pathogen, changing epidemiology. *American Journal of Nursing, 106*(5), 33–36.

U.S. Preventive Services Task Force. (2004). Screening for high blood pressure: Recommendations and rationale. *American Journal of Nursing, 104*(11), 82–87.

World Health Organization. (2000). *Obesity: Preventing and managing the global epidemic: Report of a WHO consultation on obesity.* Geneva, Switzerland: Author.

World Health Organization. (2006). *Training course on child growth assessment: Version 1.* Retrieved January 16, 2008, from http://www.who.int/childgrowth/training/Facilitator_Guide.pdf

World Health Organization. (2006). *BMI classification.* Retrieved January 16, 2008, from http://www.who.int/bmi/index.jsp?introPage=intro_3.html

Yarows, S. A., & Qian, K. (2001). Accuracy of aneroid sphygmomanometers in clinical usage. *Blood Pressure Monitoring, 6*(2), 101–106.

Pain Assessment: The Fifth Vital Sign

Written by **Carolyn Jarvis**, PhD, APN, CNP
Adapted by **Mona Sawhney**, RN, MN, ACNP

Electronic Resources

On Evolve **evolve**

http://evolve.elsevier.com/Canada/Jarvis/examination/

- Interactive Case Studies
- Physical Examination Audio and Printable Summaries
- Bedside Assessment Summary Checklists
- Complete Physical Examination Form
- Nursing Diagnoses Boxes
- Health Promotion Guides
- Quick Assessments for 20 Common Conditions
- Multiple Choice Review Questions
- Chapter Objectives
- Appendices
- Weblinks

On the Companion CD

- Interactive Case Studies with Heart and Lung Sounds
- Health Promotion Guides
- Quick Assessments for 20 Common Conditions
- Head-to-Toe Physical Examination Video Clips

— STRUCTURE AND FUNCTION —

NEUROANATOMICAL PATHWAY

Pain is a highly complex and subjective experience that originates from the central (CNS) or peripheral nervous system (PNS) or both. Specialized nerve endings called **nociceptors** are designed to detect painful sensations from the periphery and transmit them to the central nervous system. Nociceptors are located within the skin; connective tissue; muscle; and the thoracic, abdominal, and pelvic viscera. These nociceptors can be stimulated directly by trauma or injury or secondarily by chemical mediators that are released from the site of tissue damage.

Nociceptors carry the pain signal to the central nervous system by two primary sensory (or afferent) fibres: **Aδ and C fibres** (Fig. 10-1). Aδ fibres are myelinated and larger in diameter, and they transmit the pain signal rapidly to the CNS. Very localized, short-term, and sharp sensations result from Aδ fibre stimulation. In contrast, C fibres are unmyelinated and smaller, and they transmit the signal more slowly. Sensations are diffuse and aching, and they persist after the initial injury.

Peripheral sensory Aδ and C fibres enter the spinal cord by posterior nerve roots within the dorsal horn by the tract of Lissauer. The fibres synapse with **interneurons** located within a specified area of the cord called the **substantia gelatinosa.** A cross section shows that the grey matter of the spinal cord is divided into a series of consecutively numbered laminae (layers of nerve cells) (see Fig. 10-1). The substantia gelatinosa is lamina II, which receives sensory input from various areas of the body. The pain signals then cross over to the other side of the spinal cord and ascend to the brain by the **anterolateral spinothalamic tract.**

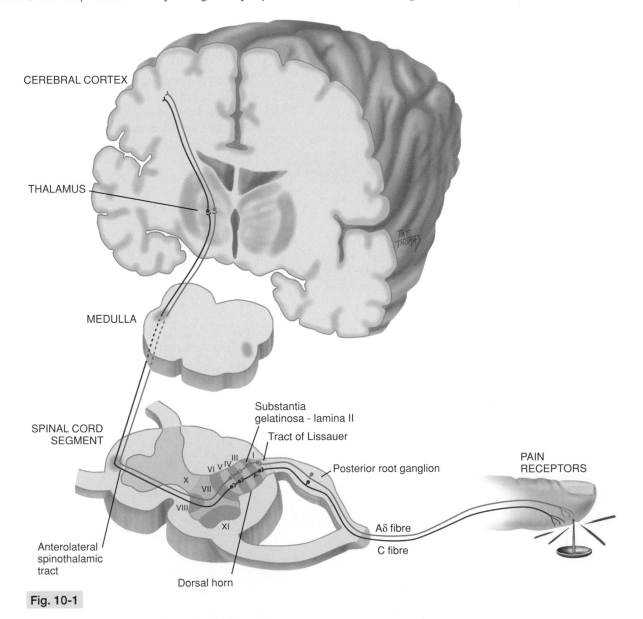

CEREBRAL CORTEX

THALAMUS

MEDULLA

SPINAL CORD SEGMENT

Substantia gelatinosa - lamina II

Tract of Lissauer

Posterior root ganglion

PAIN RECEPTORS

Aδ fibre

C fibre

Anterolateral spinothalamic tract

Dorsal horn

Fig. 10-1

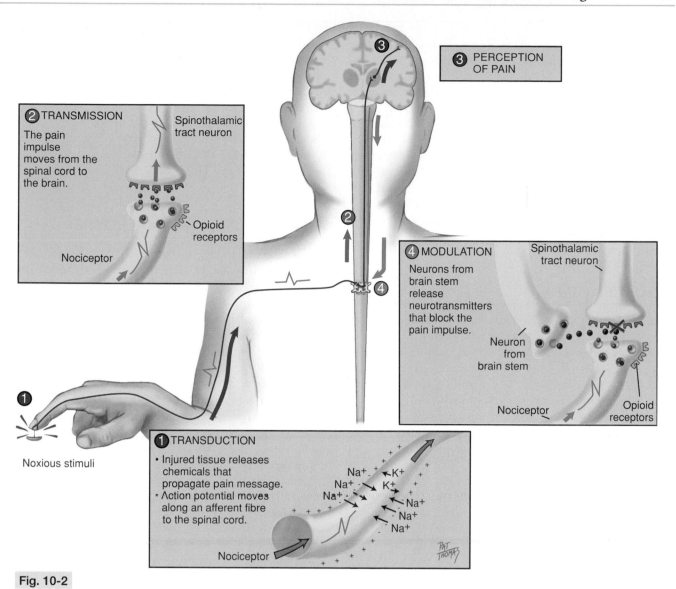

Fig. 10-2

NOCICEPTION

It is important to understand that pain occurs on a cellular level. Only then can you appreciate a patient's report of painful sensations that may develop after the initial site of injury heals. **Nociception** is the term used to describe how noxious stimuli are typically perceived as pain. Nociception can be divided into four phases: (1) transduction, (2) transmission, (3) perception, and (4) modulation (Fig. 10-2).

Initially, the first phase of **transduction** occurs when a noxious stimulus in the form of traumatic or chemical injury, burn, incision, or tumour takes place in the periphery. The periphery includes the skin, as well as somatic and visceral structures. These injured tissues then release a variety of chemicals, including substance P, histamine, prostaglandins, serotonin, and bradykinin. These chemicals are neurotransmitters that propagate a pain message, or action potential, along sensory afferent nerve fibres to the spinal cord. These nerve fibres terminate in the dorsal horn of the spinal cord. Because the initial afferent fibres stop in the dorsal horn, a second set of neurotransmitters carries the pain impulse across the synaptic cleft to the dorsal horn neurons. These neurotransmitters include substance P, glutamate, and adenosine triphosphate (ATP).

In the second phase, known as **transmission,** the pain impulse moves from the level of the spinal cord to the brain. Within the spinal cord, at the site of the synaptic cleft, are opioid receptors that can block this pain signalling with endogenous or exogenous opioids. However, if left uninterrupted, the pain impulse moves to the brain via various ascending fibres within the spinothalamic tract that terminate in the brain stem and thalamus. Once the pain impulse moves through the thalamus, the message is dispersed to higher cortical areas via mechanisms that are not clearly understood at this time.

The third phase, **perception,** indicates the conscious awareness of a painful sensation. Cortical structures such as the limbic system account for the emotional response to pain, and somatosensory areas can characterize the sensation. Only when the noxious stimuli are interpreted in these higher cortical structures can this sensation be identified as pain.

Lastly, the pain message is inhibited through the phase of **modulation.** Descending pathways from the brain stem to the spinal cord produce a third set of neurotransmitters that slows down or impedes the pain impulse, producing an analgesic effect. These neurotransmitters include serotonin; norepinephrine; neurotensin; γ-aminobutyric acid (GABA); and our own endogenous opioids, β-endorphins, enkephalins, and dynorphins.

SOURCES OF PAIN

Pain is based on its origin. Pain can be classified as nociceptive, neuropathic, or both. **Nociceptive** pain occurs due to tissue injury. This pain usually resolves as tissue healing takes place. It is well localized and often described as aching or throbbing. Nociceptive pain can be further classified as **somatic** or **visceral. Somatic** nociceptive pain can be superficial (superficial somatic or cutaneous pain) derived from skin surface and subcutaneous tissues or deep (deep somatic pain) derived from joints, tendons, muscles, or bone. **Visceral** pain originates from the larger interior organs (i.e., kidney, stomach, intestine, gallbladder, pancreas). The pain can stem from direct injury to the organ or from stretching of the organ from tumour, ischemia, distension, or severe contraction. Visceral pain can be constant or intermittent, and it may be poorly localized or referred to another area of the body. Examples of visceral pain include ureteral colic, acute appendicitis, and pancreatitis.

Neuropathic pain is defined as pain "initiated or caused by a primary lesion or dysfunction of the nervous system" (Merskey et al., 1994). It can be caused by injury to either the peripheral or central nervous system, or both. Neuropathic pain is a challenging problem because the pain can be severe and difficult to manage. Examples of neuropathic pain originating from the central nervous system include poststroke pain, pain related to multiple sclerosis, and pain due to spinal cord injury. Common causes of neuropathic pain from the peripheral nervous system include post-herpetic neuralgia, diabetic neuropathy, and myofascial pain. Neuropathic pain can be described as burning, shooting, or lancinating. The patient may have allodynia, which is pain in response to a normally nonpainful stimulus, or hyperalgesia, which is an increased pain response to a normally painful stimulus (Moulin et al., 2007).

Pain that is felt at a particular site but originates from another location is termed **referred pain.** Both sites are innervated by the same spinal nerve, and it is difficult for the brain to differentiate the point of origin. Referred pain may originate from visceral or somatic structures. Various structures maintain their same embryonic innervation. For example, an inflamed appendix in the right lower quadrant of the abdomen may have referred pain in the periumbilical area. It is useful to have knowledge of areas of referred pain for diagnostic purposes (see Table 21-2, p. 588).

TYPES OF PAIN (BY DURATION)

Pain can be classified by its duration. The duration can provide information on possible underlying mechanisms and treatment decisions. Pain is divided into acute or chronic categories. **Acute pain** is short term and self-limiting, often follows a predictable trajectory, and dissipates after an injury heals. Examples of causes of acute pain include surgery, trauma, and kidney stones. Acute pain in an individual serves a self-protective purpose; acute pain warns the individual of actual or potential tissue damage.

In contrast, **persistent pain** (or **chronic pain**) is defined as pain that has been present for 6 months or longer than the time of expected tissue healing (Jovey et al., 2003). Persistent pain can be categorized as malignant (cancer-related pain) or nonmalignant. It can last 5, 15, or 20 years and beyond. Malignant pain often parallels the pathology created by the tumour cells. The pain is induced by tissue necrosis or stretching of an organ by the growing tumour. The pain fluctuates within the course of the disease. Persistent nonmalignant pain is often associated with musculoskeletal conditions, such as arthritis, low back pain, or fibromyalgia. Research tells us that unrelieved acute pain can lead to persistent pain through a process called peripheral and central sensitization. Peripheral sensitization is the reduction of the pain threshold and an increased response of the peripheral end of the nociceptors. Central sensitization is an increase in excitability of neurons within the central nervous system (Kehlet et al., 2006).

Persistent pain does not stop when the injury heals. It continues after the predicted trajectory. Persistent pain outlasts its protective purpose, and the level of pain intensity does not correspond with the physical findings. Unfortunately, many patients with persistent pain are not believed and often are labelled as malingers, attention seekers, drug seekers, and so forth. Persistent pain originates from abnormal processing of pain fibres from peripheral or central sites. Because the pain is transmitted on a cellular level, current technology cannot reliably detect this process. Therefore, the most important and reliable indicator for pain is the patient's self-report.

DEVELOPMENTAL CARE

Infants

Infants have the same capacity for pain as adults. By 20 weeks' gestation, ascending fibres, neurotransmitters, and the cerebral cortex are developed and functioning to the extent that the fetus is capable of feeling pain (Anand, 1993). However, inhibitory neurotransmitters are in insufficient supply until birth at full term. Therefore, the preterm infant is rendered more sensitive to painful stimuli.

Preverbal infants are at high risk for undertreatment of pain because of persistent myths and beliefs that infants do not remember pain. In fact, new research indicates that repetitive and poorly controlled pain in infants (daily heel sticks, venipunctures) can result in lifelong adverse consequences such as neurodevelopmental problems, poor weight gain, learning disabilities, psychiatric disorders, and alcoholism (Anand, 2000).

The Aging Adult

No evidence exists to suggest that older individuals perceive pain to a lesser degree or that sensitivity is diminished. Although pain is a common experience among individuals 65 years of age and older, it is *not* a normal process of aging. Pain indicates pathology or injury. Pain should never be considered something to tolerate or accept in one's later years. Unfortunately, many clinicians and older adults wrongfully assume that pain should be expected in aging, which leads to less aggressive treatment. Older adults have additional fears about becoming dependent, undergoing invasive procedures, taking pain medications, and having a financial burden. The most common pain-producing conditions for aging adults include pathologies such as arthritis, osteoarthritis, osteoporosis, peripheral vascular disease, cancer, peripheral neuropathies, angina, and chronic constipation.

The somatosensory cortex is generally unaffected by dementia of the Alzheimer's type. Sensory discrimination is preserved in impaired but cognitively intact adults (Vreeling et al., 1995). Because the limbic system is affected by Alzheimer's disease, current research focuses on how the person interprets and reports these pain messages (Buffum et al., 2001).

Gender Differences

Gender differences are influenced by societal expectations, hormones, and genetic makeup. Traditionally, men have been raised to be more stoic about pain, and more affective or emotional displays of pain are accepted for women. Hormonal changes are found to have strong influences on pain sensitivity for women. Women are two to three times more likely to experience migraines during child-bearing years, are more sensitive to pain during the premenstrual period, and are six times more likely to have fibromyalgia (Fillingim, 2000). With recent findings from the Human Genome Project, genetic differences between both sexes may account for the differences in pain perception (Mogil, 2002). A pain gene exists, which helps to explain why some people feel more/less pain even with the same stimulus. Efforts are being made to tailor pharmacological agents to improve pain treatment based upon genetic sequencing.

CULTURAL AND SOCIAL CONSIDERATIONS

Please review the ethnocultural variations in Chapter 3. To enhance ethnocultural sensitivity, healthcare professionals need to work with patients and their families so that mutual goals are identified and the patients' understanding and beliefs about pain are taken into account (McCaffery et al., 1999).

The following are questions you can ask to assess an individual's beliefs about pain (Lasch, 2000):

- What do you call your pain? What name do you give it?
- Why do you think you have this pain?
- What does your pain mean for your body?
- How severe is it? Will it last a long or short time?
- Do you have any fears about your pain? If so, what do you fear most about your pain?
- What are the chief problems that your pain causes for you?
- What kind of treatment do you think you should receive? What are the most important results you hope to receive from treatment?
- What cultural remedies have you tried to help you with your pain?
- Have you seen a traditional healer for your pain? Do you want to?
- Who, if anyone, in your family do you talk to about your pain? What do they know? What do you want them to know?
- Do you have family and friends that help you because of your pain? If so, who helps you?

SUBJECTIVE DATA

Pain is defined as an "unpleasant sensory and emotional experience associated with actual or potential tissue damage or described in terms of such damage. Pain is always subjective" (American Pain Society, 1992, p. 250). "Pain is whatever the experiencing person says it is, existing whenever he says it does," (McCaffery, 1968, p. 95).

Since pain is a subjective experience, the self-report of pain is the most reliable indicator that an individual is experiencing pain. Complex physiological, genetic, and psychosocial factors contribute to the conversion of neurochemical activity to the pain experience, the individual's reaction to the painful sensation, and any related changes to an individual's mood and behaviour (Kehlet et al., 2006). With knowledge that pain occurs on a neurochemical level, the clinician cannot base the diagnosis of pain exclusively on physical examination findings, although these findings can lend support.

Examiner Asks	Rationale
INITIAL PAIN ASSESSMENT	
1. Where is your pain?	Pain may be localized or occurring in multiple sites.
2. When did your pain start?	Identifies onset and duration. This aids in identifying if the pain is acute or persistent (chronic)
3. What does your pain feel like? • Burning, stabbing, aching • Throbbing, firelike, squeezing • Cramping, sharp, itching, tingling • Shooting, crushing, sharp, dull	Identifies quality of pain and helps differentiate between nociceptive and neuropathic pain mechanisms. Neuropathic pain is described as burning, shooting, and tingling. Nociceptive pain originating from visceral sites is described as "aching" if localized and "cramping" if poorly localized, and from somatic sites it is described as "throbbing/aching."
4. How much pain do you have now? • How much pain do you have at rest? • How much pain do you have when moving?	Identifies intensity (refer to various intensity scales).
5. What makes your pain better or worse? (Include behavioural, pharmacological, nonpharmacological interventions)	Identifies alleviating and aggravating factors. Evaluates effectiveness of current treatment.
6. How does pain limit your function or activities?	Identifies degree of impairment and quality of life.
7. How do you usually behave when you are in pain? How would others know you are in pain?	Nonverbal behaviours are extremely variable, especially for persistent pain syndromes. Will aid in detection of pain and assessment.
8. What does this pain mean to you? Why do you think you are having pain?	Can identify myths, misconceptions, beliefs, such as, "I'm getting old"; "It's a punishment from God."

Subjective Data

PAIN ASSESSMENT TOOLS

Pain is multidimensional in scope, encompassing physical, affective, and functional domains. Various tools have been developed to capture unidimensional aspects (i.e., intensity) or multidimensional components. Select the pain assessment tool based on its purpose, time involved in administration, and the patient's ability to comprehend and complete the tool. First, teach patients how to use each tool, with practice sessions to strengthen the validity and reliability of the response. Enlarge the print when appropriate for individuals with impaired vision. The printed language should be translated to the native language of the patient if needed.

Validated comprehensive **pain assessment tools** are useful in assessing persistent pain conditions or complex acute pain problems. A few examples include the Initial Pain Assessment, The Brief Pain Inventory, and the McGill Questionnaire.

In the **Initial Pain Assessment** (McCaffery and Pasero, 1999 [not provided here]), the clinician asks the patient to answer eight questions concerning location, duration, quality, intensity, and aggravating/relieving factors. Further, the clinician adds questions about manner of expressing pain and the effects of pain that impairs one's quality of life.

The Brief Pain Inventory (Daut and Cleeland, 1982) asks the patient to rate the pain within the past 24 hours using graduated scales (0 to 10) with respect to its impact on areas such as mood, walking ability, and sleep (Fig. 10-3). **The Short-Form McGill Pain Questionnaire** (Melzack, 1987 [not provided here]) asks the patient to rank a list of descriptors in terms of their intensity and to give an overall intensity rating to his or her pain.

Pain rating scales are unidimensional and are intended to reflect pain intensity. They come in various forms. Pain rating scales can indicate a baseline intensity, track changes, and give some degree of evaluation to a treatment modality. **Numeric rating scales** ask the patient to choose a number that rates the level of pain, with 0 being no pain and the highest anchor 10 indicating the worst pain. It can be administered verbally or visually along a vertical or horizontal line (Fig. 10-4).

In general, older adults find the numeric rating scale too abstract and have difficulty responding, especially with a fluctuating chronic pain experience. An alternative is the simple **Descriptor Scale**, which lists words that describe different levels of pain intensity, such as *no pain, mild pain, moderate pain,* and *severe pain.* Older adults will often respond to scales in which words are used. Again, it is essential to teach the person how to use the scale to ensure accuracy.

INFANTS AND CHILDREN

Because infants are "preverbal and incapable of self-report," pain assessment is dependent upon behavioural and physiological cues. Refer to the Objective Data section. It is important to underscore the understanding that infants *do* feel pain.

Children 2 years of age can report pain and point to its location. They cannot rate pain intensity at this developmental level. It is helpful to ask the parent or caregiver what words their child uses to report pain (e.g., boo–boo, owie). Be aware that some children will try to be "grown up and brave" and often deny having pain in the presence of a stranger or if they are fearful of receiving a "shot." Rating scales can be introduced at 4 or 5 years of age. The Wong-Baker Scale is one example; the child is asked to choose a face that shows, "how much hurt you have now." The Faces Pain Scale—Revised (FPS-R) presents the child with drawings of facial expressions representing increasing levels of pain intensity. The child is asked to select the face that best represents his or her pain intensity, and the resulting score is the corresponding rank order of the expression chosen. The FPS-R is available in 31 languages (www.painsourcebook.ca). A sample of the FPS-R can be found in Appendix B.

Subjective Data

Brief Pain Inventory

Date: ___/___/___   Time: _____

Name: _____

      Last   First   Middle initial

1. Throughout our lives, most of us have had pain from time to time (such as minor headaches, sprains, and tooth-aches). Have you had pain other than these everyday kinds of pain today?
   1. Yes   2. No

2. On the diagram, shade in the areas where you feel pain. Put an X on the area that hurts the most.

Right   Left   Left   Right

3. Please rate your pain by circling the one number that best describes your pain at its **worst** in the past 24 hours.

0	1	2	3	4	5	6	7	8	9	10

   No pain   Pain as bad as you can imagine

4. Please rate your pain by circling the one number that best describes your pain at its **least** in the past 24 hours.

0	1	2	3	4	5	6	7	8	9	10

   No pain   Pain as bad as you can imagine

5. Please rate your pain by circling the one number that best describes your pain on the **average**.

0	1	2	3	4	5	6	7	8	9	10

   No pain   Pain as bad as you can imagine

6. Please rate your pain by circling the one number that tells how much pain you have **right now**.

0	1	2	3	4	5	6	7	8	9	10

   No pain   Pain as bad as you can imagine

7. What treatments or medications are you receiving for your pain?

   _____

8. In the past 24 hours, how much **relief** have pain treatments or medications provided? Please circle the one percentage that most shows how much relief you have received.

0%	10	20	30	40	50	60	70	80	90	100%

   No relief   Complete relief

9. Circle the one number that describes how, during the past 24 hours, pain has **interfered** with your:

   A: General activity

0	1	2	3	4	5	6	7	8	9	10

   Does not interfere   Completely interferes

   B: Mood

0	1	2	3	4	5	6	7	8	9	10

   Does not interfere   Completely interferes

   C: Walking ability

0	1	2	3	4	5	6	7	8	9	10

   Does not interfere   Completely interferes

   D: Normal work (includes both work outside the home and housework)

0	1	2	3	4	5	6	7	8	9	10

   Does not interfere   Completely interferes

   E: Relations with other people

0	1	2	3	4	5	6	7	8	9	10

   Does not interfere   Completely interferes

   F: Sleep

0	1	2	3	4	5	6	7	8	9	10

   Does not interfere   Completely interferes

   G: Enjoyment of life

0	1	2	3	4	5	6	7	8	9	10

   Does not interfere   Completely interferes

Fig. 10-3   Brief pain inventory

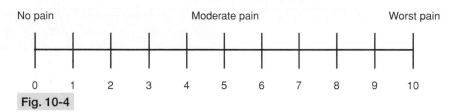

Fig. 10-4

OBJECTIVE DATA

PREPARATION

The physical examination process can help you understand the nature of the pain. Consider whether this is an acute or chronic condition. Recall that physical findings may not always support the patient's pain complaints, particularly for chronic pain syndromes. Pain should not be discounted when objective physical evidence is not found. Based on the patient's pain report, make every effort to reduce or eliminate the pain with appropriate analgesic and nonpharmacological interventions. According to the American Pain Society (1992), "In cases in which the cause of acute pain is uncertain, establishing a diagnosis is a priority, but symptomatic treatment of pain should be given while the investigation is proceeding. With occasional exceptions, (e.g., the *initial* examination of the patient with an acute condition of the abdomen), it is rarely justified to defer analgesia until a diagnosis is made. In fact, a comfortable patient is better able to cooperate with diagnostic procedures" (p. 3).

EQUIPMENT NEEDED

Tape measure to measure circumference of swollen joints or extremities
Tongue blade

Normal Range of Findings	Abnormal Findings
### THE JOINTS	
Note the size and contour of the joint. Measure circumference of the involved joint for comparison with baseline. Check active or passive range of motion (see complete technique, Chapter 22). Joint motion normally causes no tenderness, pain, or crepitation.	Swelling, inflammation, injury, deformity, diminished range of motion, increased pain on palpation. Crepitation is an audible and palpable crunching that accompanies movement.
### THE MUSCLES AND SKIN	
Inspect the skin and tissues for colour, swelling, and any masses or deformity.	Bruising, lesions, open wounds, tissue damage, atrophy, bulging, change in hair distribution.
To assess for changes in sensation, ask the person to close his or her eyes. Test the person's ability to perceive sensation by breaking a tongue blade in two lengthwise, lightly pressing the sharp and blunted ends on the skin in a random fashion, and asking to identify it as sharp or dull (see Fig. 23-23, p. 656). This test will help you identify location and extent of altered sensation.	Absent pain sensation (analgesia); increased pain sensation (hyperalgesia); or if a severe pain sensation is evoked with a stimulus that does not normally induce pain (e.g., the blunt end of the tongue blade; cotton ball; clothing) (allodynia).
### THE ABDOMEN	
Observe for contour and symmetry. Palpate for muscle guarding and organ size (see complete technique in Chapter 21). Note any areas of referred pain (see Table 21-2, p. 588).	Swelling, bulging, herniation, inflammation, organ enlargement.

Objective Data

Table 10-1 lists physiological changes resulting from poorly controlled pain.

NONVERBAL PAIN BEHAVIOURS

Individuals may be unable to verbalize the presence of pain for a variety of reasons. However, those individuals who are unable to report their pain are at high risk for the undertreatment of pain. This may be due to the lack of identification of the presence of pain.

Validated tools for the assessment of pain are available to healthcare professionals to assess pain in those who are unable to verbally communicate their pain. Individuals who are nonverbal but are cognitively intact may be able to indicate the intensity of their pain using a Numeric Rating Scale or the FPS-R, to write down a description of the quality of their pain, or to point to where their pain is located.

When the individual cannot verbally communicate the pain, you can assess pain using behavioural cues. Recall that individuals react to painful stimuli with a wide variety of behaviours. Behaviours are influenced by a wide variety of factors, including the nature of the pain (acute versus persistent), age, and cultural and gender expectations.

Behaviours that may indicate that an individual is experiencing pain include rocking, negative vocalizations, frowning, grimacing, noisy breathing, irritability, agitation, rubbing a painful area, and bracing. Other less apparent indicators that an individual is experiencing pain include flat affect, decreased interaction, decreased intake, and an altered sleep pattern. Sleeping is one behaviour in response to pain as self-distraction. Unfortunately, healthcare professionals may inadvertently interpret this behaviour as the absence of pain and not follow up with an appropriate pain management intervention.

Acute Pain Behaviours

Because acute pain involves autonomic responses and has a protective purpose, individuals experiencing moderate to intense levels of pain *may* exhibit the following behaviours: guarding, grimacing, vocalizations such as moaning, agitation, restlessness, stillness, diaphoresis, or change in vital signs. These behaviours should not be used exclusively to rule out or confirm the presence of pain as pulse and blood pressure can be altered by a fluid volume, medications, and blood loss.

Persistent (Chronic) Pain Behaviours

Persons with persistent pain often live with the experience for months and years. One cannot function physiologically and go on with life in a repetitive state of grimacing, diaphoresis, guarding, and so on. The person adapts over time, and clinicians cannot look for or anticipate the same acute pain behaviours in order to confirm a pain diagnosis.

Persons with persistent pain typically try to give little indication that they are in pain and therefore are at higher risk for underdetection. Whenever possible, it is best to ask the person how he or she behaves when in pain. Chronic pain behaviours, such as being with other people, movement, exercise, prayer, sleeping, or inactivity, underscore the more subtle, less anticipated ways in which persons behave when they are experiencing chronic pain.

TABLE 10-1	Physiological Changes from Poorly Controlled Pain
Pain is not a benign symptom. Poorly controlled acute and chronic pain have a negative impact on physiological systems.	
Physiological System	**Acute Pain Responses**
Cardiac	Tachycardia
	Elevated blood pressure
	Increased myocardial oxygen demand
	Increased cardiac output
Pulmonary	Hypoventilation
	Hypoxia
	Decreased cough
	Atelectasis
Gastrointestinal	Nausea
	Vomiting
	Ileus
Renal	Oliguria
	Urinary retention
Musculoskeletal	Spasm
	Joint stiffness
Endocrine	Increased adrenergic activity
Central nervous system	Fear
	Anxiety
	Fatigue
Immune	Impaired cellular immunity
	Impaired wound healing
Poorly controlled persistent pain	Depression
	Isolation
	Limited mobility and function
	Confusion
	Family distress
	Diminished quality of life

The Unconscious Individual

Individuals who are unconscious due to physiological reasons or medications to sedate them may experience pain. Assessment of pain in these individuals is particularly challenging. Behavioural and observational tools can be helpful in identifying pain in these individuals. The Critical-Care Pain Observation Tool (CPOT) was developed to assess pain in patients in the intensive care unit, but it may be helpful in assessing pain in any unconscious adult. Behaviours assessed include facial expression, body movement, muscle tension, negative vocalizations, and compliance with a ventilator (Table 10-2). The individual can receive a score between 0 and 8, with a higher score being more indicative of pain.

♥ DEVELOPMENTAL CARE

Infants

Pain in neonates and infants can be assessed and managed effectively using reliable, valid, and clinically sensitive assessment tools. Pain measures that include more than one

TABLE 10-2	The Critical-Care Pain Observation Tool		
Indicator	Description	Score	
Facial expression	No muscular tension observed	Relaxed, neutral	0
	Presence of frowning, brow lowering, orbit tightening, and levator contraction	Tense	1
	All of the above facial movements plus eyelid tightly closed	Grimacing	2
Body movements	Does not move at all (does not necessarily mean absence of pain)	Absence of movements	0
	Slow, cautious movements, touching or rubbing the pain site, seeking attention through movements	Protection	1
	Pulling tube, attempting to sit up, moving limbs/thrashing, not following commands, striking at staff, trying to climb out of bed	Restlessness	2
Muscle tension			
Evaluation by passive flexion and extension of upper extremities	No resistance to passive movements	Relaxed	0
	Resistance to passive movements	Tense, rigid	1
	Strong resistance to passive movements, inability to complete them	Very tense or rigid	2
Compliance with the ventilator (intubated patients)	Alarms not activated, easy ventilation	Tolerating ventilator or movement	0
	Alarms stop spontaneously	Coughing but tolerating	1
	Asynchrony: blocking ventilation, alarms frequently activated	Fighting ventilator	2
OR			
Vocalization (extubated patients)	Talking in normal tone or no sound	Talking in normal tone or no sound	0
	Sighing, moaning	Sighing, moaning	1
	Crying out, sobbing	Crying out, sobbing	2
Total, range			0–8

assessment approach within a given instrument are used for measuring pain in neonates and infants. Most measures include both behavioural and physiological indicators, and some also include contextual factors, such as the gestational age or behavioural sleep/wake state of the infant. There are several published measures that combine behavioural and physiological indicators for assessing pain in infants with varying degrees of established reliability and validity, such as the Neonatal Pain, Agitation, and Sedation Scale (NPASS) and the Premature Infant Pain Profile (PIPP). The PIPP has been the most rigorously validated of these measures.

PIPP is a behavioural measure of pain for premature infants (Table 10-3). It was developed at the Universities of Toronto and McGill in Canada. Indicators of pain that are assessed include gestational age; behavioural state before painful stimulus; and change in heart rate, change in oxygen saturation, brow bulge, eye squeeze, and nasolabial furrow during painful stimulus.

Because the sympathetic nervous system is engaged particularly in acute episodes of pain, physiological changes take place that may indicate the presence of pain. These include sweating, increases in blood pressure and heart rate, vomiting, nausea, and changes in oxygen saturation. However, like in the adult, these physiological changes cannot be used exclusively to confirm or deny pain because of other factors such as stress, medications, and fluid changes.

Note that these measures target acute pain. No biological markers have been identified for long-term chronic pain in infants or children. Therefore, evaluate the whole individual. Look for changes in temperament, expression, and activity. If a procedure or disease process is known to induce pain in adults (e.g., circumcision, surgery, sickle cell disease, cancer), it *will* induce pain in the infant or child.

The Aging Adult

Although pain should not be considered a "normal" part of aging, it is prevalent. When the older adult reports a history of conditions such as osteoarthritis, peripheral vascular disease, cancer, osteoporosis, angina, or chronic constipation, be alert and anticipate a pain problem. Older adults will often deny having pain for fear of dependency, further testing or invasive procedures, cost, and fear of taking pain killers and becoming dependent. During the interview you must establish an empathic and caring rapport to gain trust.

When you look for behavioural cues, look at changes in functional status. Observe for changes in dressing, walking, toileting, or involvement in activities. A slowness and rigidity may develop, and fatigue may occur. Look for a sudden onset of acute confusion, which may indicate poorly controlled pain. However, you will need to rule out other competing explanations such as infection or adverse reaction from medications.

Objective Data

TABLE 10-3	PIPP: Premature Infant Pain Profile[1]					
Process	Indicator	0	1	2	3	Score
Chart Observe infant 15 s	Gestational age Behavioural state	36 wk and more Active/awake Eyes open Facial movements	32–35 wk, 6 d Quiet/awake Eyes open No facial movements	28–31 wk, 6 d Active/sleep Eyes closed Facial movements	<28 weeks Quiet/sleep Eyes closed No facial movements	
Observe baseline Heart rate ___ Oxygen saturation ___						
Observe infant 30 s	Heart rate Max ____ Oxygen saturation Min _____ Brow bulge	0–4 beats/min increase 0–2.4% decrease None 0–9% of time	5–14 beats/min increase 2.5–4.9% decrease Minimum 10–39% of time	15–24 beats/min increase 5.0–7.4% decrease Moderate 40–69% of time	25 beats/min increase 7.5% or more decrease Maximum 70% of time or more	
	Eye squeeze	None 0–9% of time	Minimum 10–39% of time	Moderate 40–69% of time	Maximum 70% of time or more	
	Nasolabial furrow	None 0–9% of time	Minimum 10–39% of time	Moderate 40–69% of time	Maximum 70% of time or more Total score	

[1]Scoring instructions include scoring gestational age before examining the infant, the behavioural state before the potentially painful event by observing the infant for 15 s, recording the baseline heart rate and oxygen saturation, and observing the infant for 30 s immediately following the painful event. Score physiological and facial changes seen during this time and record immediately. The maximum score is 21, and the higher the score, the more intense is the pain behaviour.

❖ — DOCUMENTATION AND CRITICAL THINKING — ❖

Sample Charting

SUBJECTIVE

Starting within the past 2 weeks, states having severe epigastric pain within a half hour of eating greasy fatty foods. Pain is stabbing and squeezing in nature with radiation to right shoulder blade. Rates pain as a 10 on a scale of 0 to 10. Nausea accompanies pain. Takes antacids, with minimal relief. Pain diminishes after bringing knees to chest and "not moving" for a 1-hour period.

OBJECTIVE

Patient diaphoretic, grimacing, and having difficulty concentrating. Breathless during history. Arms guarding upper abdominal area. Abdomen distended. Severe tenderness noted on light right upper quadrant and epigastric palpation. Bowel sounds hyperactive in all four quadrants.

ASSESSMENT

Acute episodic visceral pain

Focused Assessment: Clinical Case Study 1

R.M. is a 20-year-old male diagnosed with sickle cell crisis. Admitted to the emergency department.

SUBJECTIVE

- Within the past 48 hours, R.M. reports increasing pain in upper and lower extremity joints and swelling of right knee. States having "stomach flu" 1 week before with periods of vomiting and diarrhea. Pain is aching and constant in nature. Rates pain as 10+ on a scale of 0 to 10. Reports difficulty walking and climbing stairs. Taking ibuprofen, two tablets every 4 hours, and using ice packs, with no relief.

OBJECTIVE

Requiring assistance to sit on examination table. Unable to bear weight on right leg. Affect flat, clenches jaw during position changes. Tenderness localized in elbow, wrist, finger, and knee joints. Diminished range of motion in wrists and knees (right knee 36 cm, left knee 30 cm diameter). Right knee warm and boggy to touch.

ASSESSMENT

Acute nociceptive pain

Focused Assessment: Clinical Case Study 2

A.G. is an 85-year-old female with a 20-year history of osteoarthritis.

SUBJECTIVE

- A.G. reports increased pain and stiffness in her neck, arms, and lower back for the past month. Denies radiation of pain. Denies tingling or numbness in upper or lower extremities.
- Having difficulty getting in and out of bathtub and dressing herself. Describes pain as aching, with good and bad days. Becomes frustrated when asked to rate her pain intensity. Replies, "I don't know what number to give; it hurts a lot, on and off." Takes acetaminophen extra strength, two tablets, when the pain "really gets the best of me," with some degree of relief. Does not take part in "field trips" offered by assisted living facility because she "hurts too much."

OBJECTIVE

Localized tenderness noted upon palpation to C3 and C4; unable to flex neck to chest. Crepitus noted in both shoulder joints. No swelling noted. Muscle strength 1+ and equal for upper extremities. Lumbar area tender to moderate palpation. Rubs lower back frequently; limited flexion at the waist. Gait slow and unsteady. Facial expression stoic.

ASSESSMENT

Persistent (chronic) pain

ABNORMAL FINDINGS
FOR ADVANCED PRACTICE

Abnormal Findings

COMPLEX REGIONAL PAIN SYNDROME

Complex regional pain syndrome (CRPS) is a chronic progressive nerve condition, characterized by burning pain, swelling, stiffness, and discoloration of the affected extremity. It affects both men and women, usually around 40 to 60 years old, and occurs weeks to months after a nerve injury (e.g., carpal tunnel syndrome, broken leg, cerebral lesions). Pathophysiology involves a complex interaction of sensory, motor, and autonomic nerves, as well as the immune system. The nerve injury may modify the usual pain pathway, causing a neuropathic "wind-up" or "short-circuit" mechanism.

A key feature is that a typically innocuous stimulus (e.g., a light brush of a cotton ball or clothing) can create a severe, intense painful response. Other subjective data include burning pain often disproportionate to the degree of injury and joint pain during movement. Objective data include swelling, disappearance of skin wrinkles, cool skin temperature, discoloration, brittle nails, and finally atrophic changes (pale, dry, shiny skin, and muscle atrophy). Treatment is beyond the scope of this text but initially includes oral medication to decrease symptoms and physical therapy to regain limb function.

BIBLIOGRAPHY

American Pain Society. (1992). *Principles of analgesic use in the treatment of acute and cancer pain* (3rd ed.). Glenview, IL: Author.

Anand, K. J. S. (1993). The applied physiology of pain. In K. J. S. Anand & R. J. McGrath (Eds.), *Pain in neonates*. Amsterdam, The Netherlands: Elsevier.

Anand, K. J. S. (2000). Effects of perinatal pain and stress. *Progress in Brain Research, 122*, 117–119.

Arnstein, P. (2006). Placebo: No relief for Ms. Mahoney's pain. *American Journal of Nursing, 106*(2), 54–66.

Banasik, J. L. (2005). Pain. In L. E. Copstead-Kirkhorn & J. L. Banasik, J.L. (Eds.), *Pathophysiology: Biological and behavioral perspectives* (3rd ed.). Philadelphia, PA: W.B. Saunders.

Beyer, J. E. (1983). *The oucher: A user's manual and technical report.* Evanston, IL: Judson.

Buffum, M. D., Miaskowski, C., Sands, L., & Brod, M. (2001). A pilot study of the relationship between discomfort and agitation in patients with dementia. *Geriatric Nursing, 22*(2), 80–85.

Curtis, S., Kolytolo, C., & Broome, M. E. (2004). Somatosensory function and pain. In C. M. Porth (Ed.), *Pathophysiology: Concepts of altered health states* (7th ed.). Philadelphia, PA: Lippincott.

D'Arcy, Y. (2005a). Field guide to pain. Part 1. Screening for pain in primary care. *Nurse Practitioner, 30*(9), 46–48.

D'Arcy, Y. (2005b). Field guide to pain. Part 2. Developing a plan of care. *Nurse Practitioner, 30*(10), 60–62.

D'Arcy, Y. (2005c). Field guide to pain. Part 3. Care after a pain management referral. *Nurse Practitioner, 30*(11), 62–64.

Daut, R. L., & Cleeland, C. S. (1982). The prevalence and severity of pain in cancer. *Cancer, 50*, 1913–1918.

Ezenwa, M. O., Ameringer, S., Ward, S., & Serlin, R. C. (2006). Racial and ethnic disparities in pain management in the United States. *Journal of Nursing Scholarship, 38*, 225–233.

Fillingim, R. B. (2000). *Sex, gender and pain.* Seattle, WA: IASP Press.

Gelians, C., et al. (2006). Validation of the critical care observation tool in adult patients. *American Journal of Critical Care, 15*, 420–427.

Hockenberry, M. J., Wilson, D., & Winkelstein, M. L. (2005). *Wong's essentials of pediatric nursing* (7th ed.). St. Louis: Mosby.

International Association for the Study of Pain. (1995). Pain measurement in children. *Pain Clinical Updates, 1*(3), 2.

Jovey, R. D., Ennis, J., Gardner-Nix, J., Goldman, B., Hays, H., & Lynch, M. (2003). Use of opioid analgesics for the treatment of chronic non-cancer pain. A consensus statement and guidelines from the Canadian Pain Society. *Pain Research and Management, 8*(Suppl.A), 3A–14A.

Kehlet, H., Jensen, T. S., & Woolf, C. J. (2006). Persistent postsurgical pain: risk factors and prevention. *Lancet. 367*(9522):1618–1625.

Krechel, S. W., & Bildner, J. (1995). CRIES: A new neonatal postoperative pain measurement score. Initial testing of validity and reliability. *Paediatric Anaesthesiology, 5*(1), 53–61.

Kwekkeboom, K. L., & Gretarsdottir, E. (2006). Systematic review of relaxation interventions for pain. *Journal of Nursing Scholarship, 38*, 269–277.

Lasch, K. E. (2000). Culture, pain, and culturally sensitive pain care. *Pain Management Nursing, 1*(3 Suppl. 1), 16–22.

McCaffery, M. (1968). *Nursing practice theories related to cognition, bodily pain, and man-environment interactions.* Los Angeles, CA: UCLA, Students' Store.

McCaffery, M., & Pasero, C. (1999). *Pain: Clinical manual* (2nd ed.). St Louis, MO: Mosby.

Melzack, R. (1987). The short-form McGill Pain Questionnaire. *Pain, 30*, 191–197.

Mendell, J. R., & Sahenk, Z. (2003). Painful sensory neuropathy. *New England Journal of Medicine, 348*, 1243–1255.

Merskey, H., Bogduk, N. (Eds.). (1994). *Classification of chronic pain: Descriptors of chronic pain syndromes and definitions of pain terms* (2nd ed, pp. 209–214). Seattle, WA: IASP Press.

Mogil, J. S. (2002). Pain genetics: Pre- and post-genomic findings. *International Association for the Study of Pain Technical Corner Newsletter, 2*, 3–6.

Moulin, D. E., Clark, A. J., Gilron, I., Ware, M. A., Watson, C. P. N., Sessle, B. J., et al. (2007). Pharmacological management of chronic neuropathic pain—Consensus statement and guidelines from the Canadian Pain Society. *Pain Research and Management, 12*(1), 13–21.

Pasero, C., & McCaffery, M. (2005). No self-report means no pain-intensity rating. *American Journal of Nursing, 105*(10), 50–53.

Polomano, R. C., & Farrar, J. T. (2006). Pain and neuropathy in cancer survivors. *American Journal of Nursing, 106*(3), 39–47.

Reyes, S. (2003). Nursing assessment of infant pain. *Perinatal and Neonatal Nursing, 17*, 291–303.

Solano, J. P., Gomes, B., & Higginson, I. J. (2006). A comparison of symptom prevalence in far advanced cancer, AIDS, heart disease, chronic obstructive pulmonary disease and renal disease. *Journal of Pain Symptom Management, 31*(1), 58–69.

Stevens, B., Johnston, C., et al. (1996). Premature Infant Pain Profile: Development and initial validation. *Clinical Journal of Pain, 12*(1), 13–22.

Turk, D. C., & Melzack, R. (Eds.). (1992). *Handbook of pain assessment.* New York, NY: Guilford Press.

Vreeling, F. W., Houx, P. J., Jolles, J., & Verhey, F. R. (1995). Primitive reflexes in Alzheimer's disease and vascular dementia. *Journal of Geriatric Psychiatry and Neurology, 8*, 111–117.

Nutritional Assessment

Written by **Joyce K. Keithley**, DNSc, RN, FAAN
Adapted by **Ellen Vogel**, PhD, RD, FDC, and **Christina Vaillancourt**, RD, CDE

Electronic Resources

On Evolve *evolve*

http://evolve.elsevier.com/Canada/Jarvis/examination/
- Interactive Case Studies
- Physical Examination Audio and Printable Summaries
- Bedside Assessment Summary Checklists
- Complete Physical Examination Form
- Nursing Diagnoses Boxes
- Health Promotion Guides
- Quick Assessments for 20 Common Conditions
- Multiple Choice Review Questions
- Chapter Objectives
- Appendices
- Weblinks

On the Companion CD

- Interactive Case Studies with Heart and Lung Sounds
- Health Promotion Guides
- Quick Assessments for 20 Common Conditions
- Head-to-Toe Physical Examination Video Clips

STRUCTURE AND FUNCTION

DEFINING NUTRITIONAL STATUS

Nutritional status refers to the degree of balance between nutrient intake and nutrient requirements. This balance is affected by many factors, including income (personal buying power); education; social support networks; physical environment; and the requisite knowledge, skills, and time to purchase and prepare healthy food. Raine (2005) offers an overview and synthesis of the determinants of healthy eating in Canada in supplement format. Two articles included in the supplement examine the determinants of healthy eating in two life-stage groups, namely, children and youth (Taylor et al., 2005), and in Canada's Aboriginal populations (Willows, 2005).

Optimal nutritional status is achieved when sufficient nutrients are consumed to support day-to-day body needs and any increased metabolic demands due to growth, pregnancy, or illness. Persons having optimal nutritional status are more active, have fewer physical illnesses, and live longer than those who are malnourished.

Undernutrition occurs when nutritional reserves are depleted or when nutrient intake is inadequate to meet day-to-day needs or additional metabolic demands. Vulnerable groups—infants, children, pregnant women, recent immigrants, persons with low incomes, hospitalized people, and older adults—are at risk for impaired growth and development, lowered resistance to infection and disease, delayed wound healing, longer hospital stays, and higher healthcare costs.

Overnutrition is caused by the consumption of nutrients—especially calories, sodium, and fat—in excess of body needs. A major nutritional problem today, overnutrition can lead to obesity and is a risk factor for heart disease, type 2 diabetes, hypertension, stroke, gallbladder disease, sleep apnea, certain cancers, and osteoarthritis (NHLBI, 2006). Overall, 23.1% of Canadian adults, an estimated 5.5 million, were obese (body mass index [BMI] >30.0) when heights and weights were measured in the 2004 Canadian Community Health Survey. Another 36.1% (an estimated 8.6 million Canadians) were categorized as being overweight (BMI 25.0–29.9). Together these data suggest that over half (59.2%) of Canadians, aged 18 and older, were either overweight or obese (Statistics Canada, 2005a).

In Canada, the proportion of children and adolescents who are overweight or obese has increased significantly in recent years. For children, the term overweight is defined as a BMI in the ≥95th percentile based on age- and gender-specific BMI charts. In 2004, 8% of Canadian children and adolescents were obese and 18% were overweight, compared with only 3% who were obese and 12% who were overweight in 1978–1979. Being overweight during childhood and adolescence is associated with an increased risk for being overweight during adulthood (NHLBI, 2006).

DEVELOPMENTAL CARE

Infants and Children

The time from birth to 4 months of age is the most rapid period of growth in the life cycle. Although infants lose weight during the first few days of life, birth weight is usually regained by the seventh to tenth day after birth. Thereafter, infants double their birth weight by 4 months and triple it by 1 year of age. Breastfeeding is recommended for full-term infants for the first year of life because breast milk is ideally formulated to promote normal infant growth and development and natural immunity. Although relatively few contraindications to breastfeeding exist, women who are human immunodeficiency virus (HIV) positive should not breastfeed, since HIV can be transmitted through breast milk. The number of pounds gained by infants during the second year is approximately the birth weight.

Infants increase their length by 50% during the first year of life and double it by 4 years of age. Brain size also increases very rapidly during infancy and childhood. By age 2 years, the brain has reached 50% of its adult size; by age 4, 75%; and by age 8, 100%. For this reason, infants and children younger than 2 should not drink skim or low-fat milk or be placed on low-fat diets—fat (calories and essential fatty acids) is mandatory for proper growth and central nervous system development.

Adolescence

Following a period of slow growth in late childhood, adolescence is characterized by rapid physical growth and endocrine and hormonal changes. Caloric and protein requirements increase to meet this demand, and because of bone growth and increasing muscle mass (and, in girls, the onset of menarche), calcium and iron requirements also increase. Typically, these increased requirements cannot be met by three meals per day; therefore, nutritious snacks play an important role in achieving adequate nutrient intake.

In general, adolescent boys grow taller and have less body fat than adolescent girls. The percentage of body fat increases in females to about 25% and decreases in males (replaced by muscle mass) to about 12%. Typically, girls double their body weight between the ages of 8 and 14; boys double their body weight between the ages of 10 and 17 years.

Pregnancy and Lactation

To support the synthesis of maternal and fetal tissues, sufficient calories, protein, vitamins, and minerals must be consumed. The recommended weight gain is 11.5 to 16 kg (25 to 35 lb) for women of normal weight, 12.5 to 18 kg (28 to 40 lb) for women who are underweight, and 7 to 11 kg (15 to 24 lb) for women who are overweight. See Appendix F on the Evolve

Web site for the increased requirements associated with pregnant and lactating women. Appendix G on the Evolve Web site gives recommended weight gain guidelines based on body mass index, and illustrates degrees of desirable weight gain during pregnancy, as recommended by the Subcommittee on Nutritional Status and Weight Gain During Pregnancy (National Academy of Sciences, 1990).

Adulthood

During adulthood, growth and nutrient needs stabilize. Most adults are in relatively good health. However, lifestyle factors such as cigarette smoking, stress, lack of exercise, excessive alcohol intake, and diets high in saturated fat, cholesterol, salt, and sugar and low in fibre are contributing factors for the development of hypertension, obesity, atherosclerosis, cancer, osteoporosis, and diabetes mellitus. The adult years, therefore, are an important time for education, preserving health and preventing or delaying the onset of chronic disease.

The Aging Adult

As people age, a number of changes occur that make them prone to undernutrition or overnutrition. Poor physical or mental health, social isolation, alcoholism, limited functional ability, poverty, and polypharmacy are the major risk factors for malnutrition in older adults (Furman, 2006).

Normal physiological changes in older adults that directly affect nutritional status include poor dentition, decreased visual acuity, decreased saliva production, slowed gastrointestinal motility, decreased gastrointestinal absorption, and diminished olfactory and taste sensitivity. Important features that have an impact on nutritional requirements in the older years are a decrease in energy requirements due to loss of lean body mass, the most metabolically active tissue, and an increase in fat mass.

Socioeconomic conditions also frequently have a significant effect on the nutritional status of the older adult. The decline in the number of extended families and the increased mobility of families reduce available support systems. Access to facilities for meal preparation, having a suitable eating environment, access to grocery stores, physical limitations, limited income, and social isolation are frequent problems and can obviously interfere with the acquisition of a balanced diet. Medications must also be considered, because older adults frequently take multiple medications that have a potential for interaction both with nutrients and with one another.

🌐 CULTURAL AND SOCIAL CONSIDERATIONS

Food security is described as the condition in which all people, at all times, have access to nutritious, safe, personally acceptable, and culturally appropriate foods, produced in ways that are environmentally sound and socially just (Fairholm, 1999). In Canada, income-related *food insecurity* is increasingly acknowledged as a key social determinant of health. Recent data indicated that in 2004 over 2.7 million Canadians (9.2% of the population) were food insecure at some point in the previous year as a result of financial challenges they faced (Health Canada, 2004). The prevalence of household food insecurity was higher in certain groups, including lone-parent families with one or more young children, those receiving social assistance, and Aboriginal people living off-reserve. Isolated communities in Canada are particularly vulnerable to food insecurity as a result of decreased availability and accessibility to food. Surveys reported a high prevalence of food insecurity (40 to 83%) in isolated Aboriginal communities (Indian Affairs and Northern Development, 2003, 2004).

Because foods and eating customs are culturally distinct, each person has a unique cultural heritage that may affect nutritional status. Immigrants commonly maintain traditional eating customs long after the language and manner of dress of an adopted country become routine (especially for holidays and observance of religious customs). Occupation, class, religion, gender, and health awareness also have a great bearing on eating practices.

The changing cultural profile in Canada encourages the availability of a variety of ethnically diverse foods and cuisines. This aspect of the Canadian eating environment is reflected in updated nutrition education resources, including *Eating Well with Canada's Food Guide* (Health Canada, 2007) (see Appendix D).

An example of a new resource designed to complement Canada's Food Guide is *Eating Well with Canada's Food Guide—First Nations, Inuit and Métis,* a food guide tailored to reflect the traditions and food choices of those population groups (Health Canada, 2007b). This guide includes both traditional and store-bought foods that are generally available, affordable, and accessible to Aboriginal peoples across Canada. It is anticipated that other adaptations of Canada's Food Guide will soon be available from Health Canada for use by specific ethnic groups.

Newly arriving immigrants and refugees may be at risk for undernutrition for a variety of reasons. In some situations they come from countries with limited food supplies caused by poverty, poor sanitation, war, or political strife. General

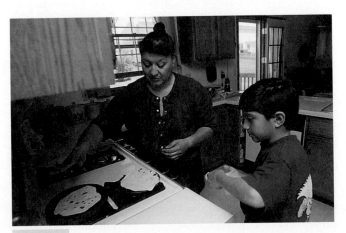

Fig. 11-1

undernutrition, hypertension, diarrhea, lactose intolerance, osteomalacia (soft bones), scurvy, and dental caries are among the more common nutrition-related problems of new immigrants from developing countries.

When immigrants and refugees arrive in Canada, a series of other factors also contribute to their nutritional problems. They find themselves in a new country with a completely new language, culture, and society. They are faced with unfamiliar foods, food storage requirements and facilities, food preparation requirements, and food-buying habits. Many familiar foods are difficult or impossible to obtain. Low income may also limit their access to familiar foods. When traditional food habits are disrupted by a new culture, borderline deficiencies or adverse nutritional consequences may result.

Because rapid changes in eating patterns and customs are occurring in all countries, what are considered customs today may not be considered traditional in a few years. The best way to learn about the eating patterns of people is to talk with them, eat with them, and ask about their dietary customs. It is important to keep in mind that recent immigrant groups, such as the Southeast Asians, are often shorter and weigh less than their Western counterparts, so standard tables of weight for age, height for age, and weight for height may not be appropriate to evaluate growth and development of immigrant children. At present no reliable standards to evaluate every immigrant group exist.

The cultural factors that must be considered when assessing nutritional status are the cultural definition of food, frequency and number of meals eaten away from home, form and content of ceremonial meals, amount and types of foods eaten, and regularity of food consumption. Because inaccuracies may occur, the 24-hour dietary recalls or 3-day food records used traditionally for assessment may be inadequate when dealing with people from culturally diverse backgrounds. Standard dietary handbooks may fail to provide culture-specific diet information because nutritional content and exchange tables are generally based on Western diets. Another source of error may originate from cultural patterns of eating. For example, many low-income ethnic groups eat sparingly or moderately during the week (i.e., simple rice or bean dishes), whereas weekend meals are markedly more elaborate (i.e., meats, fruits, vegetables, and sweets are added).

Although you may assume that "food" is a universal concept, you should ask the person to clarify what is meant by the term. For example, certain Latin American groups do not consider chili peppers—an important source of vitamins A and C—to be food and thus fail to list them as vegetables on daily food records. Among Vietnamese refugees, the dietary intake of calcium may appear inadequate, particularly with the low consumption of dairy products common among members of this group. Daily soups prepared by soaking bones in acidified broth or pickled or sweet and sour meats such as pork ribs (vinegar leaches calcium from the bones and makes it available to the body) are, however, commonly consumed, thus providing adequate quantities of calcium to meet daily requirements. Tofu is also a good source of calcium if calcium salts are used to precipitate the curd. In Middle Eastern countries, yogurt and feta cheese are the major dietary sources of calcium since milk is not commonly consumed by adults. The reason for this is lactose intolerance, a condition commonly found in people of non-European descent.

Food itself is only one part of eating. In some cultures, social contacts during meals are restricted to members of the immediate or extended family. For example, in some Middle Eastern cultures, men and women eat meals separately, or women may be permitted to eat with their husbands, but not with other males. Among some Hispanic groups, the male breadwinner is served first, then women and children. Etiquette during meals, the use of hands, type of eating utensils (e.g., chopsticks, special flatware), and protocols governing the order in which foods are consumed during a meal all vary cross-culturally.

Dietary Practices of Selected Cultural Groups

It is necessary to avoid **cultural stereotyping,** the tendency to view individuals of common cultural backgrounds similarly and according to a preconceived notion of how they "ought" to behave. For example, despite widely held stereotypes, we know that some Chinese people do not like rice, some Italians do not like spaghetti, some Irish do not like corned beef and cabbage, and so forth. Aggregate dietary preferences among people from certain cultural groups, however, can be described (e.g., characteristic ethnic dishes, methods of food preparation). Refer to topic-specific nutrition texts for detailed information about culture-specific diets and the nutritional value of ethnic foods.

Cultural food preferences are often interrelated with religious dietary beliefs and practices. Many religious groups use foods as symbols in celebrations and rituals. Knowing the person's religious practices related to food enables you to suggest improvements or modifications that do not conflict with dietary laws. Table 11-1 summarizes dietary practices for selected religious groups.

Other issues to consider when assessing nutritional status are fasting and other religious observations that may limit a person's food or liquid intake during specified times (e.g., many Catholics fast and abstain from meat on Ash Wednesday and the Fridays of Lent. People of Islamic faith fast from dawn to sunset during the month of Ramadan in the Islamic calendar and eat only twice a day—before dawn and after sunset. People of Jewish faith observe a 24-hour fast on Yom Kippur).

Kosher is the term that refers to the dietary laws of observant members of Jewish faith; mixing milk and meat products and the prohibition of eating pig meats and crustaceans are examples of the many rules within the system. Halal is the term that refers to the Islamic dietary laws (here, too, the prohibition of pig meat is one of many dietary laws).

PURPOSES AND COMPONENTS OF NUTRITIONAL ASSESSMENT

Nutritional status can be determined by the application of nutritional assessment techniques. In general, these techniques are noninvasive, inexpensive, and easy to perform.

The purposes of nutritional assessment are to (1) identify individuals who are malnourished or are at risk of developing malnutrition, (2) provide data for designing a nutrition plan of care that will prevent or minimize the development of malnutrition, and (3) establish baseline data for evaluating the efficacy of nutritional care.

Nutrition screening, the first step in assessing nutritional status, may be completed in any setting (e.g., clinic, home, hospital, long-term care facilities). Based on easily obtained data, nutrition screening is a quick and easy way to identify individuals at nutrition risk, such as those who have experienced weight loss, inadequate food intake, or recent illness. Parameters used for nutrition screening typically include weight and weight history, conditions associated with increased nutritional risk, diet information, and routine laboratory data. A variety of valid tools are available for screening different populations. For example, the Admission Nutrition Screening Tool (Kovacevich et al., 1997) was validated for use by nurses in hospitalized patients (Table 11-2), and the Nutrition Screening Initiative form (Fig. 11-2) was designed and validated in the outpatient, geriatric population (Dwyer, 1991).

Individuals identified at nutritional risk during screening should undergo a **comprehensive nutritional assessment,** which includes dietary history and clinical information,

TABLE 11-1	**Religious Dietary Practices**
Religious Group	**Food Restrictions**
Buddhism	All meat
Catholicism	Meat by some denominations on Ash Wednesday, Good Friday, and other holy days
	Alcoholic beverages by some denominations
Hinduism	Beef, pork, and some fowl
	Alcohol
	Garlic and onions by some
	Red-coloured foods (e.g., tomatoes) by some
Islam	All pork and pork products
	Meat not slaughtered according to ritual
	Alcoholic beverages and products containing alcohol (e.g., vanilla extract), coffee, and tea
	Food and beverages before sunset during Ramadan
Mormon	Alcoholic beverages
	Caffeinated beverages (e.g., coffee, tea, pop) and medicines containing caffeine, stimulants, or alcohol (e.g., Anacin, NoDoz, Nyquil)
	Food and beverages on first Sunday of each month
Orthodox Judaism	All pork and pork products
	Meat not slaughtered according to ritual
	All shellfish (e.g., crab, lobster, shrimp, oysters)
	Dairy products and meat at the same meal
	Leavened bread and cake during Passover
	Food and beverages on Yom Kippur
Seventh-Day Adventist	All pork and pork products
	Shellfish
	Meat, dairy products, and eggs by some
	Alcoholic beverages, coffee, and tea
	Highly seasoned foods

TABLE 11-2	**Admission Nutrition Screening Tool**

A. DIAGNOSIS

If the patient has at least ONE of the following diagnoses, circle and proceed to section E to consider the patient AT NUTRITIONAL RISK and stop here.
- Anorexia nervosa or bulimia nervosa
- Malabsorption (celiac sprue, ulcerative colitis, Crohn's disease, short bowel syndrome)
- Multiple trauma (closed head injury, penetrating trauma, multiple fractures)
- Decubitus ulcers
- Major gastrointestinal surgery within the past year
- Cachexia (temporal wasting, muscle wasting, cancer, cardiac)
- Coma
- Diabetes
- End-stage liver disease
- End-stage renal disease
- Nonhealing wounds

B. NUTRITION INTAKE HISTORY

If the patient has at least ONE of the following symptoms, circle and proceed to section E to consider the patient AT NUTRITIONAL RISK and stop here.
- Diarrhea (>500 mL × 2 days)
- Vomiting (>5 days)
- Reduced intake (<½ normal intake for >5 days)

C. AVERAGE BODY WEIGHT STANDARDS (BMI)

Determine the patient's current BMI by measuring their height and weight and compare it to the WHO standards for average weight (see pp. 152 and 207).
If their BMI is <18.5, proceed to section E to consider the patient AT NUTRITIONAL RISK and stop here.

D. WEIGHT HISTORY

Any recent unplanned weight loss? No___ Yes___ Amount (kg or lb)_____
If yes, within the past _____weeks or _____months
Current weight (kg or lb) _____
Usual weight (kg or lb) _____
Height (cm, ft, in) _____
Find percentage of weight loss:

$$\frac{\text{Usual wt} - \text{Current wt}}{\text{Usual wt}} \times 100 = \text{\_\_\_\_ \% wt loss}$$

Compare the % wt loss with the chart values and circle appropriate value

Length of Time	Significant (%)	Severe (%)
1 week	1–2	>2
2–3 weeks	2–3	>3
1 month	4–5	>5
3 months	7–8	>8
5+ months	10	>10

If the patient has experienced a significant or severe weight loss, proceed to section E and consider the patient AT NUTRITIONAL RISK

E. NURSE ASSESSMENT

Using the above criteria, what is this patient's nutritional risk? (circle one)

LOW NUTRITIONAL RISK   AT NUTRITIONAL RISK

Adapted from Kovacevich, D.S., et al. (1997). Nutrition risk classification: a valid and reproducible tool for nurses. *Nutrition in Clinical Practice, 12,* 20–25. Used with permission.

The warning signs of poor nutritional health are often overlooked. Use this checklist to find out if you or someone you know is at nutritional risk.

Read the statements below. Circle the number in the yes column for those that apply to you or someone you know. For each yes answer, score the number in the box. Total your nutritional score.

DETERMINE YOUR NUTRITIONAL HEALTH

	YES
I have an illness or condition that made me change the kind and/or amount of food I eat.	2
I eat fewer than 2 meals per day.	3
I eat few fruits or vegetables, or milk products.	2
I have 3 or more drinks of beer, liquor, or wine almost every day.	2
I have tooth or mouth problems that make it hard for me to eat.	2
I don't always have enough money to buy the food I need.	4
I eat alone most of the time.	1
I take 3 or more different prescribed or over-the-counter drugs a day.	1
Without wanting to, I have lost or gained 4.5 kg in the last 6 months.	2
I am not always physically able to shop, cook, and/or feed myself.	2
TOTAL	

Total Your Nutritional Score. If it's —

0-2 Good! Recheck your nutritional score in 6 months.

3-5 You are at moderate nutritional risk. See what can be done to improve your eating habits and lifestyle. Your office on aging, senior nutrition program, senior citizens centre, or health department can help. Recheck your nutritional score in 3 months.

6 or more You are at high nutritional risk. Bring this checklist the next time you see your doctor, dietitian, or other qualified health or social service professional. Talk with them about any problems you may have. Ask for help to improve your nutritional health.

These materials developed and distributed by the Nutrition Screening Initiative, a project of:

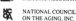

AMERICAN ACADEMY OF FAMILY PHYSICIANS

THE AMERICAN DIETETIC ASSOCIATION

NATIONAL COUNCIL ON THE AGING, INC.

Remember that warning signs suggest risk, but do not represent diagnosis of any condition.

Fig. 11-2

physical examination for clinical signs, anthropometric measures, and laboratory tests. The skills needed to collect the clinical and dietary history and to perform the physical examination are described in the Subjective Data and Objective Data sections that follow. Table 11-3 is an example of a Subjective Global Assessment form for compiling comprehensive nutritional assessment data.

Various methods for collecting current dietary intake information are available—24-hour recall, food frequency questionnaire, and food diary. Documentation of nutritional intake for hospitalized patients can best be achieved through calorie counts of nutrients consumed or infused.

The easiest and most popular method of obtaining information about dietary intake is the **24-hour recall.** The individual or family member completes a questionnaire or is interviewed and asked to recall everything eaten within the last 24 hours. However, several significant sources of error may occur when this method is used: (1) the individual or family member may not be able to recall the type or amount of food eaten; (2) intake within the last 24 hours may be atypical of usual intake; (3) the individual or family member may alter the truth for a variety of reasons; and (4) snack items and use of gravies, sauces, and condiments may be under-reported.

To counter some of the difficulties inherent in the 24-hour recall method, a **food frequency questionnaire** may also be completed. With this tool, information is collected on how

---

TABLE 11-3	Features of Subjective Global Assessment (SGA)

(Select appropriate category with a checkmark, or enter numerical value where indicated by "#".)

A. HISTORY

1. Weight change
   Overall loss in past 6 mo: amount = # _____ kg; % loss = # _____
   Change in past 2 wk: ____ increase, ____ no change, ____ decrease
2. Dietary intake change (relative to normal)
   ____ No change
   ____ Change ____ duration = # _____ weeks
   ____ Type: ____ suboptimal solid diet ____ full liquid diet ____ hypocaloric liquids ____ starvation
3. Gastrointestinal symptoms (that persisted for >2 wk)
   ____ none ____ nausea ____ vomiting
   ____ diarrhea ____ anorexia
4. Functional capacity
   ____ No dysfunction (e.g., full capacity)
   ____ Dysfunction ____ duration = # _____ wk
   ____ Type: ____ working suboptimally ____ ambulatory ____ bedridden
5. Disease and its relation to nutritional requirements
   Primary diagnosis (specify)
   Metabolic demand (stress): ____ no stress ____ low stress ____ moderate stress ____ high stress

B. PHYSICAL (for each trait specify 0 = normal, 1+ = mild, 2+ = moderate, 3+ = severe)

\# ____ loss of subcutaneous fat (triceps, chest)
\# ____ muscle wasting (quadriceps, deltoids)
\# ____ ankle edema
\# ____ sacral edema
\# ____ ascites

C. SGA RATING (select one)

____ A = Well nourished
____ B = Moderately malnourished (or suspected of being malnourished)
____ C = Severely malnourished

Reprinted with permission from Detsky, A.J., McLaughlin, J.R., Baker, J.P., Johnston, N., Whittaker, S., Mendelson, R.A., et al. (1987). What is subjective global assessment of nutritional status? *Journal of Parenteral and Enteral Nutrition, 11*(1), 9.

many times per day, week, or month the individual eats particular foods. Drawbacks to the use of the food frequency questionnaire are (1) it does not quantify amount of intake, and (2) like the 24-hour recall, it relies on the individual's or family member's memory of how often a food was eaten.

Food diaries or records require asking the individual or family member to write down everything consumed for a certain period of time. Three days—two weekdays and one weekend day—are customarily used. A food diary is most complete and accurate if the individual is instructed to record information immediately after eating. Potential problems with the food diary include (1) noncompliance, (2) inaccurate recording, (3) atypical intake on the recording days, and (4) conscious alteration of diet during the recording period.

Direct observation of the feeding and eating process can lead to detection of problems not readily identified through standard nutrition interviews. For example, observing the typical feeding techniques used by a parent or caregiver and

the interaction between the individual and caregiver can be of value when assessing failure to thrive in children or unintentional weight loss in older adults.

Eating Well With Canada's Food Guide (Health Canada, 2007a) and the Daily Reference Intakes (DRIs) are two guides commonly used to determine the adequacy or inadequacy of a diet. Refer to Canada's Food Guide (Fig. 11-3 or Appendix D or online at http://www.hc-sc.gc.ca/fn-an/food-guide-aliment/index_e.html) for additional information and for the interactive tools (My Food Guide) that allow you and your patients to personalize the information found in the guide. The DRIs are recommended amounts of nutrients to prevent deficiencies and reduce the risk of chronic diseases. In addition to recommending adequate intakes, the DRIs also specify upper limits of nutrients to avoid toxicity. With increased use of dietary supplements, the risk for nutrient toxicities is on the rise. Refer to nutrition texts for examples of the DRIs.

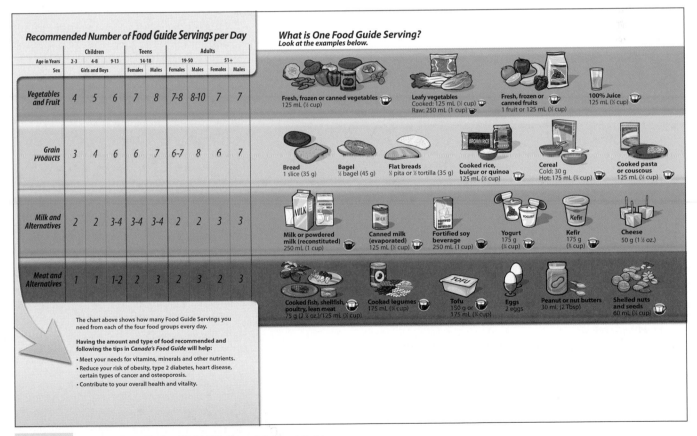

Fig. 11-3   Extract from *Eating Well With Canada's Food Guide*

SUBJECTIVE DATA

1. Eating patterns
2. Usual weight
3. Changes in appetite, taste, smell, chewing, swallowing
4. Recent surgery, trauma, burns, infection
5. Chronic illnesses
6. Nausea, vomiting, diarrhea, constipation
7. Food allergies or intolerances
8. Medications or nutritional supplements, or both
9. Self-care behaviours
10. Alcohol or illegal drug use
11. Exercise and activity patterns
12. Family history

Examiner Asks	Rationale
1. Eating patterns. • Number of meals and snacks per day? • Kind and amount of food eaten? • Fad, special, or alternative diets? • Where is food eaten? • Food preferences and dislikes? • Religious or cultural restrictions? • Able to feed self?	Most individuals are knowledgeable about, or interested in, the foods they consume. If misconceptions are present, begin gradual instruction to correct. Ethnicity and religious beliefs, or feeding difficulties, may affect intake of certain foods. Many alternative diets are not supported by scientific safety or efficacy data.
2. Usual weight. What is your usual weight? • 20% below or above desirable weight? • Recent weight change? • How much lost or gained? • Over what time period? • Reason for loss or gain?	Persons who have had a recent, unintentional weight loss or who are obese are at nutritional risk. Underweight individuals are vulnerable because their fuel reserves may be depleted. Excess weight is associated with a number of health problems, ranging from hypertension to cancer. Protein and calorie needs are often overlooked in acutely ill obese persons.
3. Changes in appetite, taste, smell, chewing, swallowing. • Type of change? • When did change occur?	Poor appetite, taste and smell alterations, as well as chewing and swallowing difficulties interfere with adequate nutrient intake and increase the likelihood of nutritional risk.
4. Recent surgery, trauma, burns, infection. • When? • Type? • How treated? • Conditions that increase nutrient loss (e.g., draining wounds, effusions, blood loss, dialysis)?	Persons who have had recent surgery, trauma, sepsis, or conditions causing nutrient losses may have caloric and nutrient needs that are two or three times greater than normal.
5. Chronic illnesses. • Type? • When diagnosed? • How treated? • Dietary modifications? • Recent cancer chemotherapy or radiation therapy?	Individuals with chronic illnesses that affect nutrient use (e.g., diabetes mellitus, pancreatitis, or malabsorption) or those receiving cancer treatment are twice as likely to have nutritional deficits.
6. Nausea, vomiting, diarrhea, constipation. Any problems? • Due to? • How long?	Gastrointestinal symptoms such as nausea, vomiting, diarrhea, or constipation may interfere with nutrient intake or absorption.

Examiner Asks	Rationale

7. Food allergies or intolerances.
- Any problematic foods?
- Type of reaction?
- How long?

Food allergies, especially peanut allergies, are on the rise and represent a major health concern. Refer to published guidelines for more information on the management of food allergies.

Intolerances may result in nutrient deficiencies (e.g., diarrhea after milk ingestion).

8. Medications and nutritional supplements.
- Prescription medications?
- Nonprescription?
- Use over a 24-hour period?

- Type of vitamin or mineral supplement? Amount? Duration of use?
- Herbal and botanical products? Specific type and brand and where obtained? How often used? Who recommended? How does it help you? Any problems?

Analgesics, antacids, anticonvulsants, antibiotics, diuretics, laxatives, antineoplastic drugs, steroids, and oral contraceptives are among the drugs that can interact with nutrients, impairing their digestion, absorption, metabolism, or utilization.

Vitamin and mineral supplements may cause harmful side effects if taken in large amounts.

Use of herbal and botanical supplements is commonly not reported, so ask about intake and discuss proper use and potential adverse effects. Refer to Natural Health Products Directorate (NHPD) Web site in reference list.

9. Self-care behaviours.
- Meal preparation facilities?
- Transportation for travel to market?
- Adequate income for food purchase?
- Who prepares meals and does shopping?
- Environment during mealtimes?

Socioeconomic factors may interfere with ingestion of adequate amounts of food or with usual diet.

10. Alcohol or illegal drug use.
- When was last drink of alcohol?
- Amount taken that episode?
- Amount alcohol each day? Each week?
- Duration of use?
- (Repeat questions for each drug used.)

These agents are often substituted for nutritious foods and increase requirements for some nutrients. Also, pregnant women who smoke, drink alcohol, or use illegal drugs give birth to a disproportionate number of infants with low birth weights, failure to thrive, and other serious complications.

11. Exercise and activity patterns.
- Amount?
- Type?

Caloric and nutrient needs rise with increased activity and exercise, especially competitive sports and manual labour. Inactive or sedentary lifestyles often lead to excess weight gain.

12. Family history. Family or personal history of heart disease, osteoporosis, cancer, gout, gastrointestinal disorders, obesity, or diabetes?
- Effect of each on eating patterns?
- Effect on activity patterns?

Long-term nutritional deficiencies or excesses may first become manifest as disease, such as these common examples during the adult years. Early identification of nutritional alterations permits dietary and activity modifications to occur promptly—at a time when the body can recover more fully.

Subjective Data

|

Subjective Data

Additional History for Infants and Children

Dietary histories of infants and children are generally obtained from the child's parents, guardian, babysitter, or daycare centre. Usually, the person responsible for food preparation is able to provide a fairly accurate dietary history. Having the caregivers keep a thorough daily food diary and occasionally requesting 24-hour recalls during clinic visits are the most commonly employed techniques for this population group.

1. Gestational nutrition.
- Maternal history of alcohol or illegal drug use?
- Any diet-related complications during gestation?
- Infant's birth weight?
- Any evidence of delayed physical or mental growth?

Low birth weight (<2500 g) is a major factor in infant morbidity and mortality. Poor gestational nutrition, low maternal weight gain, and maternal alcohol and drug use—all factors in low birth weight—can lead to birth defects and delayed growth and development.

2. Infant breastfed or bottle-fed.
- Type, frequency, amount, and duration of feeding?
- Any difficulties encountered?
- Timing and method of weaning?

Well-nourished infants have appropriate physical and social growth and development. Inexperienced mothers may have problems with breastfeeding or bottle-feeding or have questions about whether the infant is receiving adequate amounts of food.

3. Child's willingness to eat what you prepare.
- Any special likes or dislikes?
- How much will child eat?
- How do you control non-nutritious snack foods?
- How do you avoid food aspiration?

The preschool period is one of increasing growth. Lifelong food habits form. Use of small portions, finger foods, simple meals, and nutritious snacks are strategies to improve dietary intake. Avoid foods likely to be aspirated (e.g., hot dogs, nuts, grapes, round candies, popcorn).

Additional History for the Adolescent

1. Your present weight.
- What would you like to weigh?
- How do you feel about your present weight?
- On any special diet to lose weight?
- On other diets to lose weight? If so, were they successful?
- Constantly think about "feeling fat"?
- Intentionally vomit or use laxatives or diuretics after eating?

Obesity, particularly in girls, may precipitate fad dieting and malnutrition. Because of adolescents' increased body awareness and self-consciousness, they are prone to eating disorders (anorexia nervosa or bulimia), conditions in which the real or perceived body image does not compare favourably to an ideal image found in advertisements or pictures of fashion models.

2. Use of anabolic steroids or other agents to increase muscle size and physical performance?
- When?
- How much?
- Any problems?

Once confined to male professional athletes, the use of anabolic steroids and other performance-enhancing agents now extends to junior-high, high-school, and college males and females. Adverse effects include personality disorders (aggressiveness), and liver and other organ damage.

Examiner Asks	Rationale

* Use of caffeinated, energy boosting drinks? When? Type? Duration?

Energy boosting drinks like Red Bull may contain large amounts of caffeine, other stimulants, or herbal products. Side effects include dehydration, dangerously high blood pressure and heart rate, and sleep problems.

3. What snacks or fast foods do you like to eat?
* When?
* How much?

An accurate dietary history may be difficult because of between-meal snacks and meals eaten on the run. These often are omitted or forgotten during the interview or in a food diary.

4. Age first started menstruating.
* What is your menstrual flow like?

Menarche is usually delayed if malnutrition is present. Likewise, amenorrhea or scant menstrual flow is associated with nutritional deficiency.

Additional History for the Pregnant Female

1. How many times have you been pregnant?
* When?
* Any problems encountered during previous pregnancies?
* Problems this pregnancy?

A multiparous mother with pregnancies occurring less than 1 year apart has an increased chance of depleted nutritional reserves. Note previous complications of pregnancy (excessive vomiting, anemia, or gestational diabetes). Slower gastrointestinal motility and pressure from the fetus may cause constipation, hemorrhoids, and indigestion. A past history of a low-birth-weight infant suggests past nutritional problems. Giving birth to an infant weighing 4500 g (10 lb) or more may signal *latent* diabetes in the mother.

2. What foods do you prefer when pregnant?
* What foods do you avoid?
* Crave any particular foods?

The expectant mother is vulnerable to familial, cultural, and traditional influences for food choices. Cravings for, or aversions to, particular foods are common; evaluate for their potential contribution to, or interference with, dietary intake.

Additional History for the Aging Adult

1. How does your diet differ from when you were in your 40s and 50s?
* Why?
* What factors affect the way you eat?

Note any physiological or psychological changes of aging or socioeconomic changes that affect nutritional status.

2. Review the "Determine Your Nutritional Health" checklist (see Fig. 11-2, p. 200)

The Nutritional Screening Initiative (White et al., 1991) is a three-step approach for nutrition screening of the older person. The nutrition checklist in Figure 11-2 identifies major risk factors and indicators of poor nutritional status. Persons identified at risk should undergo level 1 and/or level 2 screening depending on whether they are at moderate or high risk of poor nutritional status. (See sample forms in Jarvis, C. *Laboratory Manual for Physical Examination and Health Assessment, First Canadian Edition.*)

OBJECTIVE DATA

CLINICAL SIGNS

Observation of an individual's general appearance—obese, cachectic (fat and muscle wasting), or edematous—can provide clues to overall nutritional status. More specific clinical signs and symptoms suggestive of nutritional deficiencies can be detected through a physical examination. Because clinical signs are late manifestations of malnutrition, only in areas in which rapid turnover of epithelial tissue occurs—skin, hair, mouth, lips, and eyes—are the nutritional deficiencies readily detectable. These signs may also be non-nutritional in origin. Therefore, laboratory testing is required to make an accurate diagnosis. Laboratory tests for assessment of nutritional status are reviewed later in this chapter. Clinical signs of various nutritional deficiencies are summarized in Table 11-4 and are depicted in the section on abnormalities at the end of this chapter (see Table 11-6).

EQUIPMENT NEEDED

Lange or Harpenden skinfold calipers
Ross insertion tape or other measurement tape
Anthropometer
Pen or pencil
Nutritional assessment data form

TABLE 11-4	Clinical Signs of Malnutrition		
Area of Examination	Normal Appearance	Signs Associated With Malnutrition	Nutrient Deficiency
Skin	Smooth, no signs of rashes, bruises, flaking	Dry, flaking, scaly	Vitamin A, vitamin B complex, linoleic acid
		Petechiae/ecchymoses	Vitamins C and K
		Follicular hyperkeratosis (dry, bumpy skin)	Vitamin A, linoleic acid
		Cracks in skin, lesions on the hands, legs, face, or neck	Niacin, tryptophan
		Pellagrous dermatosis (hyperpigmentation of skin exposed to sunlight)	Niacin
		Nasolabial seborrhea	Riboflavin, vitamin B_6
		Acneiform forehead rash	Vitamin B_6
		Eczema	Linoleic acid
		Xanthomas (excessive deposits of cholesterol)	Excessive serum levels of LDLs or VLDLs
Hair	Shiny, firm, does not fall out easily, healthy scalp	Dull, dry, sparse	Protein, zinc, linoleic acid
		Colour changes	Copper or protein
		Corkscrew hair	Copper
Eyes	Corneas are clear, shiny; membranes are pink and moist; no sores at corners of eyelids	Foamy plaques (Bitot's spots)	Vitamin A
		Dryness (xerophthalmia)	Vitamin A
		Softening (keratomalacia)	Vitamin A
		Pale conjunctivae	Iron, vitamins B_6, B_{12}
		Red conjunctivae	Riboflavin
		Blepharitis	B complex, biotin
Lips	Smooth, not chapped or swollen	Cheilosis (vertical cracks in lips)	Riboflavin, niacin
		Angular stomatitis (red cracks at sides of mouth)	Riboflavin, niacin, iron, vitamin B_6
Tongue	Red in appearance; not swollen or smooth, no lesions	Glossitis (beefy red)	Vitamin B complex
		Pale	Iron
		Papillary atrophy	Niacin
		Papillary hypertrophy	Multiple nutrients
		Magenta or purplish colour	Riboflavin
Gums	Reddish-pink, firm, no swelling or bleeding	Bleeding	Vitamin C
Nails	Smooth, pink	Brittle, ridged, or spoon shaped (koilonychia)	Iron
		Splinter hemorrhages	Vitamin C
Musculoskeletal	Erect posture, no malformations, good muscle tone, can walk or run without pain	Pain in calves, thighs	Thiamine
		Osteomalacia	Vitamin D, calcium
		Rickets	Vitamin D, calcium
		Joint pain	Vitamin C
		Muscle wasting	Protein, carbohydrate, fat
Neurological	Normal reflexes, appropriate affect	Peripheral neuropathy	Thiamine, vitamin B_6
		Hyporeflexia	Thiamine
		Disorientation or irritability	Vitamin B_{12}

Normal Range of Findings	Abnormal Findings

ANTHROPOMORPHIC MEASURES

Anthropometry is the measurement and evaluation of growth, development, and body composition. The most commonly used anthropometric measures are height, weight, waist-hip ratio, and waist circumference. Measurement of height, weight, and head circumference is described in Chapter 9.

Derived Weight Measures

Two derived weight measures are used to depict changes in body weight.

The **percent usual body weight** is calculated as follows:

$$\text{Percent usual body weight} = \frac{\text{Current weight}}{\text{Usual weight}} \times 100$$

Recent weight change is calculated using the following formula:

$$\text{Weight change} = \frac{\text{Usual weight} - \text{Current weight}}{\text{Usual weight}} \times 100$$

Body Mass Index

BMI provides a practical marker of optimal weight for height and an indicator of obesity or protein-calorie malnutrition (see Appendix C on the Evolve Web site). It is calculated by:

$$\text{BMI} = \frac{\text{Weight (in kilograms)}}{\text{Height (in metres)}^2}$$

$$\text{or} \quad \frac{\text{Weight (in pounds)}}{\text{Height (in inches)}^2} \times 703$$

Waist-to-Hip Ratio

The waist-to-hip ratio assesses body fat distribution as an indicator of health risk. Obese persons with a greater proportion of fat in the upper body, especially in the abdomen, have android obesity; obese persons with most of their fat in the hips and thighs have gynoid obesity. The equation is:

$$\text{Waist-to-hip ratio} = \frac{\text{Waist circumference}}{\text{Hip circumference}}$$

where waist circumference is measured in inches at the smallest circumference below the rib cage and above the umbilicus, and hip circumference is measured in inches at the largest circumference of the buttocks. In addition, **waist circumference (WC)** alone can be used to predict greater health risk.

A current weight of 85 to 95% of usual body weight indicates mild malnutrition; 75 to 84%, moderate malnutrition; and <75%, severe malnutrition.

An unintentional loss of >5% of body weight over 1 month, >7.5% of body weight over 3 months, or >10% of body weight over 6 months is clinically significant.

BMI interpretation for adults (Health Canada, 2003b):
- <18.5 — Underweight
- 18.5 to 24.9 — Normal weight
- 25.0 to 29.9 — Overweight
- 30.0 to 39.9 — Obesity
- ≥40 — Extreme obesity

BMI interpretation for children ages 2 to 20 years (CDC, 2000):
85th to 95th percentile = risk for overweight
See Appendix D on the Evolve Web site for CDC growth charts.

A waist-to-hip ratio of 1.0 or more in men or 0.8 or more in women is indicative of android (upper body obesity) and increasing risk for obesity-related diseases and early mortality.

A WC >89 cm (35 in) inches in women and >102 cm (40 in) in men increases risk of cardiovascular and metabolic diseases.

Normal Range of Findings	Abnormal Findings

 DEVELOPMENTAL CARE

Infants, Children, and Adolescents

Weight. During infancy, childhood, and adolescence, height and weight should be measured at regular intervals, because longitudinal growth is one of the best indices of nutritional status over time. See Chapter 9 for techniques.

Skinfold Thickness. Determination of skinfold thickness and body mass index may be useful in evaluating childhood and teenage overnutrition.

An estimated 8% of children and adolescents were obese, and 18% were overweight in Canada in 2004.

The Pregnant Female

Weight. Measure weight monthly up to 30 weeks' gestation, then every 2 weeks until the last month of pregnancy, when weight should be measured weekly. Appendix G on the Evolve Web site illustrates approximate weight gain considered normal for each week of pregnancy.

Consider the expectant mother at nutritional risk if her weight is 10% or more below ideal or 20% or more above the norm for her height and age group.

The Aging Adult

Height. With age, height declines in both men and women very slowly from the early 30s, leading to an average 2.9-cm loss in men and 4.9-cm loss in women (Gabriella & Sinclair, 1997; Rueben et al., 1995). Height measures may not be accurate in individuals confined to a bed or wheelchair or those over 60 years of age (because of osteoporotic changes). Therefore, arm span, which is correlated with height, may be a better measure for older people.

Other Measurements. Mid-upper arm circumference (MAC) and TSF measures may not be accurate and are difficult to obtain in older adults (because of sagging skin, changes in fat distribution, and declining muscle mass). (See Frisancho [1984] for data on weight and TSF thickness by height in US men and women age 55 to 74 years.) Body mass index and waist-to-hip ratio are better indicators of obesity in this age group.

LABORATORY STUDIES

Routine laboratory tests are objective, can detect preclinical nutritional deficiencies, and can be used to confirm subjective findings. Use caution, however, when interpreting test results that may be outside normal ranges, because they do not always reflect a nutritional problem and because standards for aging adults have not yet been firmly established.

The best routinely performed laboratory indicators of nutritional status are hemoglobin, hematocrit, cholesterol, triglycerides, total lymphocyte count, and serum albumin. Glucose, low- and high-density lipoproteins, prealbumin, transferrin, and total protein levels also provide meaningful information.

Hemoglobin. The hemoglobin determination is used to detect iron deficiency anemia. Normal values are as follows: **infants,** 1 to 3 days—145 to 225 g/L; 2 months—90 to 140 g/L; **children,** 6 to 12 years—115 to 155 g/L; **adults,** males—135 to 180 g/L; females—120 to 160 g/L.

Increased hemoglobin levels suggest hemoconcentration due to polycythemia vera or dehydration.

Decreased hemoglobin levels may indicate anemia, recent hemorrhage, or hemodilution caused by fluid retention.

A low value indicates insufficient hemoglobin formation; thus hematocrit and hemoglobin values should be interpreted together.

Hematocrit. Hematocrit, a measure of cell volume, is also an indicator of iron status. Normal values are as follows: **infants,** 1 to 3 days—0.44 to 0.72; 2 months—0.28 to 0.42; **children,** 6 to 12 years—0.35 to 0.45; **adults,** males—0.4 to 0.54; females—0.38 to 0.47.

Normal Range of Findings	Abnormal Findings

Cholesterol. Total cholesterol is measured to evaluate fat metabolism and to assess the risk of cardiovascular disease. Normal cholesterol concentration is <5.2 mmol/L.

Coronary artery disease risk steadily increases as serum cholesterol rises. Serum cholesterol levels of 5.2 to 6.2 mmol/L (borderline high) are associated with moderate risk and >6.2 mmol/L or more (high) with high risk of coronary artery disease, heart attack, brain attack, and peripheral vascular disease.

Triglycerides. Serum triglycerides (TGs) are used to screen for hyperlipidemia and to determine the risk of coronary artery disease. Normal range is <.69 mmol/L.

Serum TG levels are also associated with coronary artery disease and are categorized as *borderline,* 2.26 to 4.50 mmol/L, or *high,* >4.5 mmol/L.

Total Lymphocyte Count. The most commonly used tests of immune function are total lymphocyte count (TLC) and skin testing, also called delayed cutaneous hypersensitivity testing. TLC is an important indicator of visceral protein status and therefore of cellular immune function.

The TLC is derived from the white blood cell count (WBC) and the differential count:

$$TLC = WBC \times \frac{\text{Number of lymphocytes in differential}}{100 \text{ cells}}$$

where TLC is calculated in cells per cubic millimetre.

Normal values for all age categories are between 1000 and 4000 cells/mm^3.

Non-nutritional factors that affect TLC include hypoalbuminemia, metabolic stress (e.g., major surgery, trauma, sepsis), infection, cancer, and chronic diseases.

Lymphopenia is a decrease in circulating lymphocytes.

Lymphocytosis is an increase in circulating lymphocytes.

Skin Testing. Adequate immunity can also be demonstrated by a positive reaction to multiple skin test antigens. In these tests of immune function, at least six antigens are injected intradermally in the forearm area, and the response (redness and induration) is noted at 24 and 48 hours. A 5-mm or greater response to more than one antigen is generally considered to be a positive reaction (i.e., indicative of adequate immunity).

Commonly used antigens include *Candida,* tetanus toxoid, diphtheria toxoid, *Streptococcus,* old tuberculin, proteus, and trichophyton.

A response of <5 mm indicates anergy or immunoincompetence. Anergy occurs with malnutrition, hepatic failure, infection, and immunosuppressive drugs (e.g., chemotherapy agents, steroids).

Lymphopenia and the lack of a positive response to skin test antigens increase risk of infection and sepsis.

Serum Proteins. Serum albumin is another common measurement of visceral protein status. Because of its relatively long half-life (17 to 20 days) and large body pool (4.0 to 5.0 g/kg), albumin is not an early indicator of protein malnutrition.

Normal serum albumin concentration in infants and children older than 6 months and adults ranges from 35 to 50 g/L.

Levels of **serum transferrin,** an iron-transport protein, can be measured directly or by an indirect measurement of total iron-binding capacity. Serum transferrin, with a half-life of 8 to 10 days, may be a more sensitive indicator of visceral protein status than albumin.

The normal values for serum transferrin are 1.90 to 3.35 g/L.

Low serum albumin levels occur with protein–calorie malnutrition, altered hydration status, and decreased liver function.

A serum albumin level of 28 to 35 g/L represents moderate visceral protein depletion, and <28 g/L denotes severe depletion (Chernecky & Berger, 2008).

Levels of 1.5 to 1.7 g/L suggest mild protein deficiency; 1.0 to 1.5 g/L, moderate deficiency; and levels less than 1.0 g/L, severe deficiency (Lee & Nieman, 2003). Because many clinical conditions can alter serum albumin and transferrin levels, consider the person's history in conjunction with these values for accurate interpretation.

Prealbumin, or thyroxine-binding prealbumin, serves as a transport protein for thyroxine (T_4) and retinol-binding protein. With a shorter half-life (48 hours) than either albumin or transferrin, prealbumin is sensitive to acute changes in protein status and sudden demands on protein synthesis. Normal prealbumin levels range from 1.5 to 2.5 g/L.

Prealbumin levels are elevated in renal disease and reduced by surgery, trauma, burns, and infection. Prealbumin levels of 1.0 to 1.5 g/L indicate mild depletion; .5 to 1.0 g/L, moderate depletion; and less than .5 g/L, severe depletion.

Normal Range of Findings	Abnormal Findings

C-reactive protein (CRP), a plasma protein marker of inflammatory status produced by the liver, is used to monitor metabolic stress (e.g., trauma, surgery, burns) and as an indicator of when to begin nutritional support in critically ill patients. CRP is generally not detectable in the blood of healthy individuals.

Detectable levels of CRP are associated with increased risk of atherosclerosis and may be seen in other inflammatory conditions, such as infections, rheumatoid arthritis, or tuberculosis. The use of oral contraceptives and the effects of pregnancy during the last 4 to 5 months may also produce detectable CRP levels.

Nitrogen Balance. Nitrogen balance is also used as an index of protein nutritional status. Nitrogen is released with the catabolism of amino acids and is excreted in the urine as urea. Nitrogen balance therefore indicates whether the person is anabolic (positive nitrogen balance) or catabolic (negative nitrogen balance).

Nitrogen balance is estimated by a formula based on urine urea nitrogen (UUN) excreted during the previous 24 hours:

$$\text{Nitrogen} = \text{Nitrogen intake} - \text{Nitrogen excretion}$$
$$= \text{Protein intake}/6.25 - (24\text{-hour UUN} + 4)$$

where

Nitrogen balance is determined in grams
24-hour UNN = urinary urea nitrogen, measured in grams
4 = nonurea nitrogen losses via feces, skin, sweat, and lungs, measured in grams

In response to stress and increased protein demand, the body rapidly mobilizes its protein compartments, which results in increased production of urea and excretion of urea in the urine. With infection, an estimated loss of 9 to 11 g/d of UUN can be expected. In patients with major burns, 12 to 18 g/d of urea nitrogen may be expected in the urine (Blackburn et al., 1977).

Creatinine-Height Index. The creatinine-height index (CHI) is a method of estimating the amount of skeletal muscle mass. Creatinine is derived from the breakdown of creatine, an energy-containing complex found in muscle. Creatinine is excreted unchanged in the urine at a constant rate in proportion to the amount of body muscle.

Creatinine height index is calculated by first measuring urinary creatinine using a carefully collected 24-hour urine specimen. This value is then compared with ideal urinary creatinine levels from a creatinine-for-height-standard table, by means of the following equation:

$$\text{CHI} = \frac{\text{Actual 24-hour urine creatinine}}{\text{Ideal 24-hour urine creatinine for height}} \times 100$$

The person's CHI is then compared with a CHI standard table to determine the degree of skeletal muscle depletion.

The validities of CHI and nitrogen balance studies are dependent on the accuracy of the 24-hour urine collection. Failure to obtain an accurate sample and abnormal renal function result in underestimation of creatinine and nitrogen losses.

Assuming an accurate 24-hour urine specimen, a CHI of 60 to 80% of standard indicates a moderate deficit in body mass. A value of <60% indicates a severe deficit in body muscle mass (Blackburn et al., 1977). Stress, fever, and trauma can increase urinary creatinine excretion.

☙ DEVELOPMENTAL CARE

In infancy and childhood, laboratory tests are performed only when undernutrition is suspected or if the child has acute or chronic illnesses that affect nutritional status.

During adolescence, unless overt disease is suspected, laboratory evaluation of hemoglobin and hematocrit levels and urinalysis for glucose and protein levels are adequate.

In pregnancy, hemoglobin and hematocrit values can be used to detect deficiencies of protein, folacin, vitamin B$_{12}$, and iron. Urine is frequently tested for glucose and protein (albumin), which can signal diabetes, pre-eclampsia, and renal disease.

In older adulthood, all serum and urine data must be interpreted with an understanding of declining renal efficiency and a tendency for aging adults to be overhydrated or underhydrated.

Normal Range of Findings

Abnormal Findings

 CULTURAL AND SOCIAL CONSIDERATIONS

Biocultural Variations in Laboratory Studies

Biocultural variations occur with some laboratory tests, such as *hemoglobin*. The normal *hemoglobin level* for individuals of African descent is 1 g lower than levels for other groups, a factor that should be considered in the treatment of anemia.

Sickle-cell anemia is a *hemoglobin*-related, genetic health problem. It is a genetically inherited trait that may have emerged as a result of an adaptation to fight malaria in Africa. Sickle-cell anemia occurs in individuals of African descent and causes the normal red blood cell to assume a sickle shape. Sickle-cell anemia comprises the following blood characteristics:

1. The presence of two hemoglobin S genes (Hb SS)
2. The presence of the hemoglobin S gene with another abnormal hemoglobin gene (Hb SC, Hb SD, etc.)
3. The presence of the hemoglobin S gene with a different abnormality in hemoglobin synthesis

Some people (carriers) have the sickle-cell trait (HbSS, HbSC, or others), but do not experience symptoms of the syndrome. A similar phenomenon is found among people from China and Italy (Spector, 2004).

SERIAL ASSESSMENT

To monitor nutritional status in malnourished individuals or in individuals at risk for malnutrition, serial measurements of nutritional assessment parameters are made at routine intervals. At a minimum, weight and dietary intake should be evaluated weekly. Because the other nutritional assessment parameters change more slowly, data on these indicators may be collected biweekly or monthly.

Health Promotion

The keys to a healthy diet are (a) eat a variety of foods from all the basic food groups to ensure nutrient adequacy; (b) consume the recommended amounts of fruits and vegetables, whole grains, and fat-free or low-fat milk products or equivalents; (c) limit intake of foods high in saturated or trans fats, added sugars, starch, cholesterol, salt, and alcohol; (d) match calorie intake with calories expended; (e) engage in 30 to 60 minutes of moderate physical activity most days; and (f) follow food safety guidelines for handling, preparing, and storing foods.

Canada's *Physical Activity Guide* is designed to help individuals at specific life stages (i.e., older adults, children, youth) make wise choices about physical activity. Research indicated that the majority of Canadians were unaware that insufficient physical activity is a serious risk factor for premature death and chronic disease and disability (Health Canada, 2003a). According to Health Canada, two thirds of Canadians are currently inactive (Health Canada, 2003a).

Approaches to weight loss for those who are overweight and obese must be tailored to the individual, reflect cultural sensitivity, and take into consideration the patient's readiness to lose weight and his or her healthcare and self-care beliefs. Weight loss programs that recommend less than 1000 to 1200 calories per day may not provide adequate nutrients. Regardless of macronutrient composition, any diet that reduces calorie intake or advocates 1400 to 1500 calories per day results in weight loss. In other words, it is not eating too much of any particular nutrient, such as carbohydrate or fat, that makes us gain weight, but rather the overall number of calories ingested. The cardinal features of a successful long-term weight loss plan for adults 19 years and over are (a) getting regular physical exercise; (b) eating a low-calorie (≈1400 to 1500 kcal/d), low-fat (20 to 35% of total calories) diet; and (c) monitoring daily food intake (e.g., food diary, portion size) and body weight.

Based on the findings of the nutritional assessment, the type of malnutrition can be diagnosed. The four major types of malnutrition are obesity, marasmus, kwashiorkor, and a marasmus-kwashiorkor mix (Table 11-6, p. 215). Each type of malnutrition has characteristic clinical and laboratory findings and a distinct cause.

Objective Data

Summary Checklist: Nutritional Assessment

 For a PDA-downloadable version, go to http://evolve.elsevier.com/Canada/Jarvis/examination/.

1. Obtain a **health history** relevant to nutritional status
2. Elicit **dietary history,** if indicated
3. **Inspect** skin, hair, eyes, oral cavity, nails, and musculoskeletal and neurological systems for clinical signs and symptoms suggestive of nutritional deficiencies
4. **Measure** height, weight, and other anthropometric parameters, as indicated
5. Review relevant **laboratory tests**
6. Offer **health promotion** teaching

❧— DOCUMENTATION AND CRITICAL THINKING —❧

Sample Charting

SUBJECTIVE

No history of diseases or surgery that would alter intake or requirements; no recent weight changes; no appetite changes. Socioeconomic history is noncontributory. Does not smoke; drink alcohol; or use illegal, prescription, or over-the-counter drugs. No food allergies. Sedentary lifestyle; plays golf once per week.

OBJECTIVE

Dietary intake is adequate to meet protein and energy needs. No clinical signs of nutrient deficiencies. Height, weight, and screening laboratory tests within normal ranges.

Focused Assessment: Clinical Case Study 1

R.G. is a 33-year-old gay male diagnosed as HIV seropositive 5 years ago.

SUBJECTIVE

- He presents to the Infectious Disease Clinic with a 2-week history of diarrhea and anorexia, and a weight loss of 17 kg. Daily caloric intake averages 1000 kcal (usual intake is 2000 kcal). Describes diarrhea as "runny" and occurring 4 to 6 times a day.

OBJECTIVE

Inspection: Slightly raised patches resembling milk curds present in mouth and throat. General appearance is pale and cachectic.

Anthropometric: Height is 166.4 cm (64.9 in). Current weight is 50.9 kg (112 lb); usual and ideal body weight is 68 kg (150 lb). TSF measures 8.5 mm (normal value is 12.5 mm).

Laboratory: Serum albumin (18.6 g/L) and total lymphocyte count (1000/mm^3) are well below normal ranges. Stool is of watery consistency; stool analysis reveals *Cryptosporidium* infection.

ASSESSMENT

- Imbalanced nutrition: less than body requirements R/T anorexia, fever, diarrhea, and oral *Candida albicans*
- Protein–calorie malnutrition (marasmus)

Focused Assessment: Clinical Case Study 2

E.F. is an 87-year-old widow who lives alone in her own home. She has enjoyed good health all of her life.

SUBJECTIVE

- During the past year, she has experienced declining memory and no longer cooks or drives. Relies on children to take her grocery shopping and to prepare occasional meals. Income adequate. Describes her appetite as excellent. Spends her days watching television and reading. Experiences occasional constipation. Eats a well-balanced diet and enjoys high-carbohydrate foods such as cookies, candy, and doughnuts because they are easy to chew. Caloric intake is 1800 kcal/d.

OBJECTIVE

Inspection: No clinical signs of nutrient deficiencies.
Anthropometric: Height is 160 cm (62 in). Current weight is 56.8 kg (125 lb); usual weight is 56.8 kg (125 lb), and ideal weight is 56.4 kg (124 lb).
Laboratory: Hemoglobin, hematocrit, and albumin values within normal limits.

ASSESSMENT

- Normal nutriture
- Constipation related to inactivity and diet high in refined carbohydrates

Nursing Diagnoses Commonly Associated With Nutrition

All nursing diagnoses can be found on the Evolve Web site at **http://evolve.elsevier.com/Canada/Jarvis/examination/.**

◄ ABNORMAL FINDINGS ►

TABLE 11-5 | Classification of Malnutrition

Type/Etiology	Clinical Features	Anthropometric Measures	Laboratory Findings
Obesity due to caloric excess, refers to weights more than 20% above ideal body weight. Persons who are 100% or more above ideal body weight are categorized as morbidly obese. The causes of being overweight and obese are complex and multifaceted; genetic, social, cultural, pathological, psychological, and physiological factors have all been implicated. Regardless of the cause of obesity, the underlying problem is usually an imbalance of caloric intake and caloric expenditure. In most cases, a small caloric surplus over a long period of time results in the extra pounds. Although visceral protein levels and immunocompetence are generally normal in the obese individual, anthropometric measures are above normal.	Obese appearance	Weight >120% standard for height Body mass index >30 TSF >10% standard Waist-to-hip ratio >1.0 (men) or >0.8 (women)	Serum cholesterol 2.0 g/L Serum triglycerides >2.5 g/L

Continued

TABLE 11-5 | Classification of Malnutrition—cont'd

Type/Etiology	Clinical Features	Anthropometric Measures	Laboratory Findings
Marasmus (protein–calorie malnutrition) is due to inadequate intake of protein and calories or prolonged starvation. Anorexia, bowel obstruction, cancer cachexia, and chronic illness are among the clinical conditions leading to marasmus. Marasmus is characterized by decreased anthropometric measures—weight loss and subcutaneous fat and muscle wasting. Visceral protein levels may remain within normal ranges.	Starved appearance 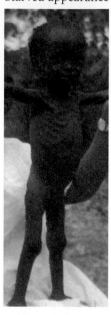	Weight ≤80% standard for height TSF <90% standard Mid-upper arm muscle circumference (MAMC) ≤90% standard	Creatinine-height index (CHI) <80% standard
Kwashiorkor (protein malnutrition) is due to diets that may be high in calories but that contain little or no protein, e.g., low-protein liquid diets, fad diets, and long-term use of dextrose-containing intravenous fluids. Individuals with kwashiorkor, in contrast to those with marasmus, have decreased visceral protein levels and depressed immune function but generally have adequate anthropometric measures. These individuals may therefore appear well nourished or even obese.	Well-nourished appearance Edematous	Weight ≥100% standard for height TSF ≥100% standard	Serum albumin <35 g/L Serum transferrinn <1.5 g/L Lymphocytes <1500 mm Anergy
Marasmus and kwashiorkor mix is due to prolonged inadequate intake of protein and calories (e.g., severe starvation, severe catabolic states). This condition combines elements of both marasmus and kwashiorkor. Nutritional assessment findings include muscle, fat, and visceral protein wasting, along with immune incompetence. Individuals with a marasmus-kwashiorkor mix are usually those who have undergone acute catabolic stress, such as major surgery, trauma, or burns, in combination with prolonged starvation. Without nutritional support, this type of malnutrition is associated with the highest risk of morbidity and mortality.	Emaciated appearance	Weight ≤70% standard TSF ≤80% standard MAMC ≤60% standard	Serum albumin <28 g/L Serum transferrin <1.0 g/L Lymphocytes <900 mm Anergy CHI 60% standard

TABLE 11-6 | Abnormalities Due to Nutritional Deficiencies

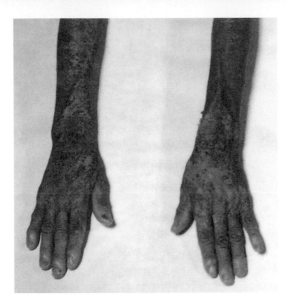

Pellagra

Pigmented keratotic scaling lesions resulting from a deficiency of niacin. These lesions are especially prominent in areas exposed to the sun, such as hands, forearms, neck, and legs.

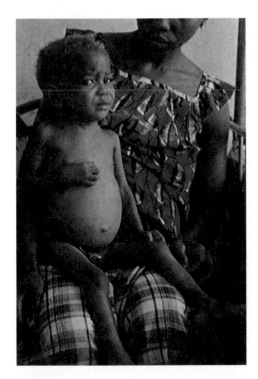

Kwashiorkor

Occurs in children and adults whose diets contain mostly carbohydrate and little or no protein and are under stress (growth, parasitic or viral infections, major surgery, trauma, or burns). Accompanying signs include generalized edema, scaling areas of decreased pigmentation, and decreased hair pigmentation.

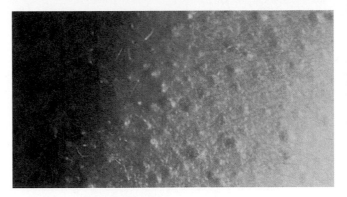

Follicular Hyperkeratosis

Dry, bumpy skin associated with vitamin A or linoleic acid (essential fatty acid) deficiency, or both. Linoleic acid deficiency may also result in eczematous skin, especially in infants.

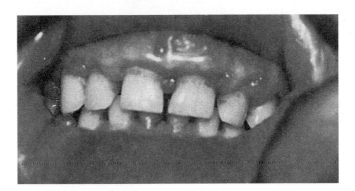

Scorbutic Gums

Deficiency of vitamin C. Gums are swollen, ulcerated, and bleeding due to vitamin C–induced defects in oral epithelial basement membrane and periodontal collagen fibre synthesis.

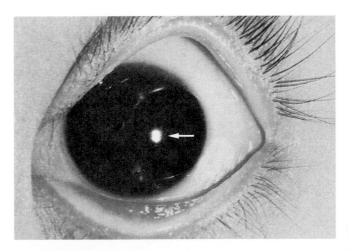

Bitot's Spots

Foamy plaques of the cornea that are a sign of vitamin A deficiency. Severe depletion may result in conjunctival xerosis (drying) and progress to corneal ulceration, and finally destruction of the eye (keratomalacia).

Continued

TABLE 11-6	Abnormalities Due to Nutritional Deficiencies—cont'd

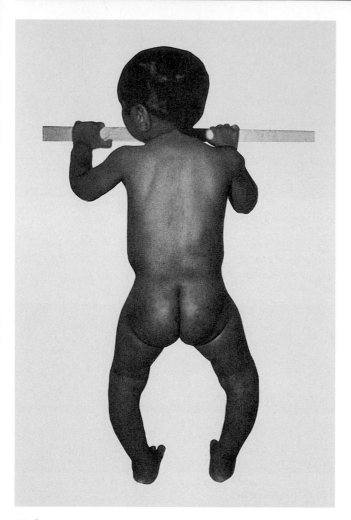

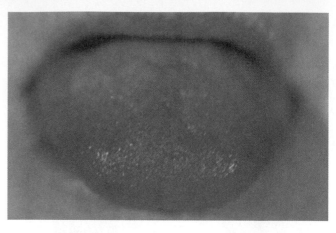

Magenta Tongue

"Magenta tongue" is a sign of riboflavin deficiency. In contrast, a pale tongue is probably attributable to iron deficiency; a beefy red-coloured tongue is caused by vitamin B complex deficiency.

Rickets

Sign of vitamin D and calcium deficiencies in children (disorders of cartilage cell growth, enlargement of epiphyseal growth plates) and adults (osteomalacia).

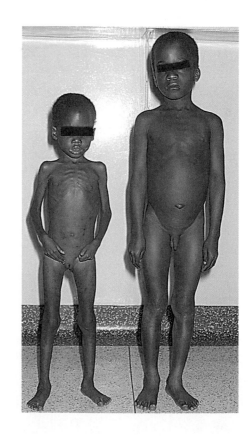

HIV Infection Discordant Twins ▶

A 4½-year-old girl infected with human immunodeficiency virus (HIV) with her uninfected twin brother. The girl has been sickly since shortly after birth and suffers from HIV-associated malnutrition.

ABNORMAL FINDINGS
FOR ADVANCED PRACTICE

TABLE 11-7 | **Metabolic Syndrome (MetS)**

A lack of consensus exists regarding operational definitions of metabolic syndrome. In 1998 the World Health Organization proposed a unifying definition that includes identification of the presence of insulin resistance. More recently the United States Expert Panel on Detection, Evaluation, and Treatment of High Blood Cholesterol in Adults (Adult Treatment Panel III [ATP III]) provided an operational definition based on three or more criteria that does not require a measure of insulin resistance (Table 11-8). Data from the Third National Health and Nutrition Survey, which employed the ATP III criteria, found that the overall prevalence of metabolic syndrome in the United States was approximately 20 to 25%.

TABLE 11-8	**Clinical Identification of Metabolic Syndrome Using NCEP ATP III Criteria**
Risk Factor	Defining Level[1]
FPG	≥6.1 mmol/L
BP	≥130/85 mm Hg
TGs	≥1.7 mmol/L
HDL-C	
Men	<1.0 mmol/L
Women	<1.3 mmol/L
Abdominal obesity	
Men	>102 cm
Women	>88 cm

[1]A diagnosis of metabolic syndrome is made when 3 or more of the risk determinants are present.
NCEP APT III, National Cholesterol Education Program Adult Treatment Panel III; *FPG*, fasting plasma glucose; *BP*, blood pressure; *HDL-C*, high-density lipoprotein cholesterol; *TG*, triglyceride.

Abnormal Findings

BIBLIOGRAPHY

Adult Treatment Panel III. (2001). Executive summary of the third report of the National Cholesterol Education Program (NCEP) Expert Panel on Detection, Evaluation, and Treatment of High Blood Cholesterol in Adults. *Journal of the American Medical Association, 285,* 2486–2497.

American Academy of Family Physicians, the American Dietetic Association, and National Council on Aging. (1994). *Nutrition interventions manual for professionals caring for older Americans.* Washington, DC: Nutrition Screening Initiative.

Blackburn, G. L., Bistrian, B. R., Maini, B. S., Schlamm, H. T., & Smith, M. F. (1977). Nutritional and metabolic assessment of the hospitalized patient. *Journal of Parenteral and Enteral Nutrition, 1*(1), 11–22.

Bolanowski, M., & Nilsson, B. E. (2001). Assessment of human body composition using dual-energy x-ray absorptiometry and bioelectrical impedance analysis. *Medical Science Monitor, 7,* 1029–1033.

Centers for Disease Control and Prevention. (2000). *Growth charts.* Retrieved July 5, 2006, from http://www.cdc.gov/growth_charts

Centers for Disease Control and Prevention. (2006). *Overweight and obesity: obesity trends.* Retrieved July 5, 2006, from http://www.cdc.gov/nccdphp/dnpa/obesity/trend/index.htm

Chernecky, C. C., & Berger, B. J. (2008). *Laboratory tests and diagnostic procedures* (5th ed.). St Louis, MO: Saunders.

Detsky, A. S., McLaughlin, J. R., Baker, J. P., Johnston, N., Whittaker, S., Mendelson, R. A., et al. (1987). What is subjective global assessment of nutritional status? *Journal of Parenteral and Enteral Nutrition, 11*(1), 8–14.

DiMaria-Ghalili, R. A., & Amella, E. (2005). Nutrition in older adults: Intervention and assessment can help curb the growing threat of malnutrition. *American Journal of Nursing, 105*(3), 40–49.

Dwyer, J. T. (1991). *Screening older Americans' nutritional health: Current practices and future possibilities* [Monograph]. Washington, DC: Nutrition Screening Initiative.

Fairholm, J. (1999). *Urban agriculture and food security initiatives in Canada: A survey of Canadian non-governmental organizations.* Ottawa, ON: International Development Research Centre.

Fischbacn, F. (2003). *A manual of laboratory and diagnostic tests* (7th ed.). Philadelphia, PA: Lippincott Williams & Wilkins.

Ford, E. S., Giles, W. H., & Dietz, W. H. (2002). Prevalence of the metabolic syndrome among U.S. adults: findings from the National Health and Nutrition Examination Survey. *Journal of the American Medical Association, 287,* 356–359.

Fraser, C. G. (2001). *Biological variation: from principles to practice.* Washington, DC: AAAC Press.

Frisancho, A. R. (1984). New standards of weight and body composition by frame size and height for assessment of nutritional status of adults and the elderly. *American Journal of Clinical Nutrition, 40,* 808–819.

Frisancho, A. R. (1990). *Anthropometric standards for the assessment of growth and nutritional status.* Ann Arbor, MI: University of Michigan Press.

Frisancho, A. R., & Flegel, P. N. (1983). Elbow breadth as a measure of frame size for U.S. males and females. *American Journal of Clinical Nutrition, 31,* 311–314.

Furman, E. F. (2006). Undernutrition in older adults across the continuum of care: Nutritional assessment, barriers, and interventions. *Journal of Gerontological Nursing, 32*(1), 22–27.

Gabriella, S. E., & Sinclair, A. J. (1997). Diagnosing undernutrition in elderly people. *Reviews in Clinical Gerontology, 7,* 367–371.

Health Canada. (2003a). *Canada's physical activity guide to healthy active living.* Retrieved June 5, 2008, from http://www.phac-aspc.gc.ca/pau-uap/paguide/intro.html

Health Canada. (2003b). *Canadian guidelines for body weight classification in adults.* Retrieved June 5, 2008, from http://www.hc-sc.gc.ca/fn-an/nutrition/weights-poids/guide-ld-adult/qa-qr-prof_e.html

Health Canada. (2004). *Canadian community health survey. Cycle 2.2, nutrition.* Retrieved June 5, 2008, from http://www.hc-sc.gc.ca/fn-an/surveill/nutrition/commun/income_food_sec-sec_alim_e.html

Health Canada. (2007a). *Eating well with Canada's food guide.* Retrieved June 5, 2008, from http://www.hc-sc.gc.ca/fn-an/food-guide-aliment/index_e.html

Health Canada. (2007b). *Eating well with Canada's food guide—First Nations, Inuit and Métis.* Retrieved June 5, 2008, from http://www.hc-sc.gc.ca/fn-an/pubs/fnim-pnim/index_e.html

Indian Affairs and Northern Development. (2003). *Nutrition and food security in Kugaaruk, Nunavut: Baseline survey for food mail pilot project.* Ottawa, ON: Indian Affairs and Northern Development.

Indian Affairs and Northern Development. (2004a). *Nutrition and food security in Fort Severn, Ontario: Baseline survey for the pilot food mail project.* Ottawa, ON: Indian Affairs and Northern Development.

Indian Affairs and Northern Development. (2004b). *Nutrition and food security in Kangiqsujuaq, Nunavik: Baseline survey for the food mail pilot project.* Ottawa, ON: Indian Affairs and Northern Development.

Ishida, D. N. (2001). Making inroads on cancer prevention and control with Asian Americans. *Seminars in Oncology Nursing, 17,* 220–228.

Jackson, R. T. (1990). Separate hemoglobin standards for blacks and whites: A critical review of the case for separate and unequal hemoglobin standards. *Medical Hypotheses, 32,* 181–189.

Kovacevich, D. S., Boney, A. R., Braunschweig, C. L., Perez, A., & Stevens, M. (1997). Nutrition risk classification: a valid and reproducible tool for nurses. *Nutrition in Clinical Practice, 12,* 20–25.

Lee, R. D., & Nieman, D. C. (2003). *Nutritional assessment* (3rd ed.). New York, NY: McGraw-Hill.

National Academy of Sciences. (1990). *Nutrition during pregnancy.* Washington, DC: National Academy Press.

National Academy of Sciences. (1991). *Nutrition during lactation.* Washington, DC: National Academy Press.

National Digestive Disease Clearing House. (2006). *Home page.* Retrieved August 10, 2006, from http://digestive.niddk.nih.gov/index.htm

National Heart, Lung, and Blood Institute, National Institutes of Health, Department of Health and Human Services. (2006). *Obesity education initiative.* Retrieved July 5, 2006, from http://www.nhlbi.nih.gov/about/oei/index.htm

National Institutes of Health. (2000). *The practical guide: identification, evaluation, and treatment of overweight and obesity in adults* [Monograph]. Washington, DC: NHLBI Obesity Education Initiative.

Ogden, C. L., Carroll, M. D., Curtin, L. R., McDowell, M. A., Tabak, C. J., & Flegal, K. M. (2006). Prevalence of overweight and obesity in the United States, 1999–2004. *Journal of the American Medical Association, 295,* 1549–1555.

Pesce-Hammond, K., & Wessel, J. (2005). Nutrition assessment and decision making. In R. Merritt (Ed.), *The A.S.P.E.N. nutrition support practice manual* (2nd ed., pp. 3–26). Silver Spring, MD: The American Society for Parenteral and Enteral Nutrition.

Raine, K. (2005). Determinants of healthy eating in Canada: An overview and synthesis. *Canadian Journal of Public Health, 96,* S8–S15.

Reuben, D. B., Greendale, G. A., & Harrison, G. G. (1995). Nutrition screening in older persons. *Journal of the American Geriatric Society, 43,* 415–425.

Smith, S. C., Jr., Allen, J., Blair, S. N., Bonow, R. O., Brass, L. M., Fonarow, G.C., et al. (2006). AHA/ACC guideline for secondary prevention for patients with coronary and other atherosclerotic vascular disease: 2006 update. *Circulation, 113,* 2363–2372.

Spector, R. E. (2004). *Cultural diversity in health and illness* (6th ed.). Upper Saddle River, NJ: Pearson Prentice Hall.

Statistics Canada. (2005a). *Measured obesity, adult obesity in Canada: Measured height and weight, 2004, no. 1* (Catalogue No. 82-620).

Retrieved June 5, 2008, from http://www.statcan.ca/english/research/82-620-MIE/2005001/articles/adults/aobesity.htm

Statistics Canada. (2005b). *Measured obesity, overweight Canadian children and adolescents, 2004, no. 1* (Catalogue No. 82-620). Retrieved June 5, 2008, from www.statcan.ca/english/research/82-620-MIE/2005001/articles/child/cobesity.htm

Subcommittee on Nutritional Status and Weight Gain during Pregnancy, Food and Nutrition Board, National Academy of Sciences. (1990). *Nutrition during pregnancy. Parts I and II*. Washington, DC: National Academy Press.

Taylor, J. P., Evers, S., & McKenna, M. (2005). Determinants of healthy eating in children and youth. *Canadian Journal of Public Health, 96*, S20–S27.

U.S. Department of Agriculture. Center for Nutrition Policy and Promotion. (2005). *MyPyramid*. Retrieved April 12, 2006, from http://www.mypyramid.gov

U.S. Department of Agriculture and Department of Health and Human Services. (2005). *Dietary guidelines for Americans 2005*. Retrieved April 12, 2006, from http://www.health.gov/dietaryguidelines

Weiss, R., Dziura, J., Burgert, T. S., Tamborlane, W. V., Taksali, S. E., Yeckel, C. W., et al. (2004). Obesity and the metabolic syndrome in children and adolescents. *New England Journal of Medicine, 350*, 2362–2374.

White, J. V., Ham, R. J., & Lipschitz, D. A. (1991). *Nutrition screening initiative: Toward a common view* [Monograph]. Washington, DC: Nutrition Screening Initiative.

Willows, N. D. (2005). Determinants of healthy eating in Aboriginal peoples in Canada: the current state of knowledge and research gaps. *Canadian Journal of Public Health, 96*, S32–S37.

Xu, Y., & Whitmer, K. (2006). C-reactive protein and cardiovascular disease in people with diabetes. *American Journal of Nursing, 106*(8), 66–72.

Skin, Hair, and Nails

Written by **Carolyn Jarvis**, PhD, APN, CNP
Adapted by **June MacDonald-Jenkins**, RN, BScN, MSc

Electronic Resources

On Evolve *evolve*

http://evolve.elsevier.com/Canada/Jarvis/examination/

- Interactive Case Studies
- Physical Examination Audio and Printable Summaries
- Bedside Assessment Summary Checklists
- Complete Physical Examination Form
- Nursing Diagnoses Boxes
- Health Promotion Guides
- Quick Assessments for 20 Common Conditions
- Multiple Choice Review Questions
- Chapter Objectives
- Appendices
- Weblinks

On the Companion CD

- Interactive Case Studies with Heart and Lung Sounds
- Health Promotion Guides
- Quick Assessments for 20 Common Conditions
- Head-to-Toe Physical Examination Video Clips

STRUCTURE AND FUNCTION

Think of the skin as the body's largest organ system—it covers 1.86 square metres of surface area in the average adult. The skin is the sentry that guards the body from environmental stresses (e.g., trauma, pathogens, dirt) and adapts it to other environmental influences (e.g., heat, cold).

SKIN

The skin has two layers—the outer highly differentiated *epidermis* and the inner supportive *dermis* (Fig. 12-1). Beneath these layers is a third layer, the *subcutaneous* layer of adipose tissue.

Epidermis

The *epidermis* is thin but tough. Its cells are bound tightly together into sheets that form a rugged protective barrier. It is stratified into several zones. The inner **stratum germinativum,** or basal cell layer, forms new skin cells. Their major ingredient is the tough, fibrous protein *keratin*. The melanocytes interspersed along this layer produce the pigment *melanin,* which gives brown tones to the skin and hair. All people have the same number of melanocytes; however, the amount of melanin they produce varies with genetic, hormonal, and environmental influences.

From the basal layer the new cells migrate up and flatten into the **stratum corneum.** This outer horny cell layer consists of dead keratinized cells that are interwoven and closely packed. The cells are constantly being shed, or desquamated, and are replaced with new cells from below. The epidermis is completely replaced every 4 weeks. In fact, each person sheds about half a kilogram of skin each year.

The epidermis is uniformly thin except on the surfaces that are exposed to friction, such as the palms and the soles. On these surfaces, skin is thicker because of work and weight-bearing. The epidermis is avascular; it is nourished by blood vessels in the dermis below.

Skin colour is derived from three sources: (1) mainly from the brown pigment melanin, (2) also from the yellow-orange tones of the pigment carotene, and (3) from the red-purple tones in the underlying vascular bed. All people have skin of varying shades of brown, yellow, and red; the relative proportion of these shades affects the prevailing colour. Skin colour is further modified by the thickness of the skin and by the presence of edema.

Dermis

The *dermis* is the inner supportive layer consisting mostly of connective tissue, or *collagen.* This is the tough, fibrous

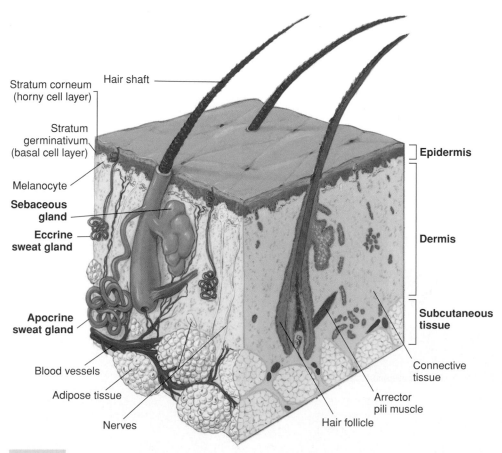

Stratum corneum (horny cell layer)
Hair shaft
Stratum germinativum (basal cell layer)
Melanocyte
Sebaceous gland
Eccrine sweat gland
Apocrine sweat gland
Blood vessels
Adipose tissue
Nerves
Epidermis
Dermis
Subcutaneous tissue
Connective tissue
Arrector pili muscle
Hair follicle

Fig. 12-1

protein that enables the skin to resist tearing. The dermis also has resilient elastic tissue that allows the skin to stretch with body movements. The nerves, sensory receptors, blood vessels, and lymphatics lie in the dermis. Also, appendages from the epidermis—such as the hair follicles, sebaceous glands, and sweat glands—are embedded in the dermis.

Subcutaneous Layer

The *subcutaneous layer* is adipose tissue, which is made up of lobules of fat cells. The subcutaneous tissue stores fat for energy, provides insulation for temperature control, and aids in protection by its soft cushioning effect. Also, the loose subcutaneous layer gives skin its increased mobility over structures underneath.

EPIDERMAL APPENDAGES

Epidermal appendages are formed by a tubular invagination of the epidermis down into the underlying dermis.

Hair

Hair is *vestigial* for humans; it no longer is needed for protection from cold or trauma. However, hair is highly significant in most cultures for its cosmetic and psychological meaning (see Cultural and Social Considerations).

Hairs are threads of keratin. The hair *shaft* is the visible projecting part, and the *root* is below the surface embedded in the follicle. At the root the *bulb matrix* is the expanded area where new cells are produced at a high rate. Hair growth is cyclical, with active and resting phases. Each follicle functions independently so that while some hairs are resting, others are growing. Around the hair follicle are the muscular *arrector pili,* which contract and elevate the hair so that it resembles "goose flesh" during exposure to cold or in emotional states.

People have two types of hair. Fine, faint **vellus hair** covers most of the body (except the palms and soles, the dorsa of the distal parts of the fingers, the umbilicus, the glans penis, and inside the labia). The other type is **terminal hair,** the darker thicker hair that grows on the scalp and eyebrows and, after puberty, on the axillae, pubic area, and the face and chest in the male.

Sebaceous Glands

Sebaceous glands produce a protective lipid substance, *sebum,* which is secreted through the hair follicles. Sebum oils and lubricates the skin and hair and forms an emulsion with water that retards water loss from the skin. (Dry skin results from loss of water, not directly from loss of oil.) Sebaceous glands are everywhere except on the palms and soles. They are most abundant in the scalp, forehead, face, and chin.

Sweat Glands

There are two types of sweat glands. The **eccrine** glands are coiled tubules that open directly onto the skin surface and produce a dilute saline solution called *sweat.* The evaporation of sweat reduces body temperature. Eccrine glands are widely distributed through the body and are mature in the 2-month-old infant.

The **apocrine** glands produce a thick, milky secretion and open into the hair follicles. They are located mainly in the axillae, anogenital area, nipples, and navel and are vestigial in humans. They become active during puberty, and secretion occurs with emotional and sexual stimulation. Bacterial flora residing on the skin surface react with apocrine sweat to produce a characteristic musky body odour. The functioning of apocrine glands decreases in the aging adult.

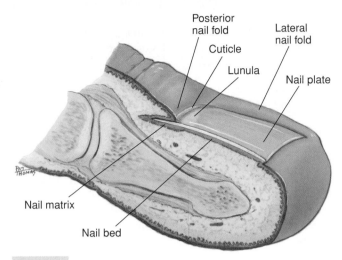

Fig. 12-2

Nails

The nails are hard plates of keratin on the dorsal edges of the fingers and toes (Fig. 12-2). The nail plate is clear, with fine longitudinal ridges that become prominent in aging. Nails take their pink colour from the underlying nail bed of highly vascular epithelial cells. The lunula is the white opaque semi-lunar area at the proximal end of the nail. It lies over the nail matrix where new keratinized cells are formed. The nail folds overlap the posterior and lateral borders. The cuticle works like a gasket to cover and protect the nail matrix.

FUNCTION OF THE SKIN

The skin is a waterproof, highly resilient covering that has protective and adaptive properties:

- **Protection.** Skin minimizes injury from physical, chemical, thermal, and light wave sources.
- **Prevents penetration.** Skin is a barrier that stops invasion of micro-organisms and loss of water and electrolytes from within the body.
- **Perception.** Skin is a vast sensory surface holding the neurosensory end-organs for touch, pain, temperature, and pressure.
- **Temperature regulation.** Skin allows heat dissipation through sweat glands and heat storage through subcutaneous insulation.
- **Identification.** People identify one another by unique combinations of facial characteristics, hair, skin colour, and even fingerprints. Self-image is often enhanced or deterred by the way society's standards of beauty measure up to each person's perceived characteristics.

- **Communication.** Emotions are expressed in the sign language of the face and in the body posture. Vascular mechanisms such as blushing or blanching also signal emotional states.
- **Wound repair.** Skin allows cell replacement of surface wounds.
- **Absorption and excretion.** Skin allows limited excretion of some metabolic wastes, byproducts of cellular decomposition such as minerals, sugars, amino acids, cholesterol, uric acid, and urea.
- **Production of vitamin D.** The skin is the surface on which ultraviolet light converts cholesterol into vitamin D.

 ## DEVELOPMENTAL CARE

Infants and Children

The hair follicles develop in the fetus at 3 months' gestation; by midgestation most of the skin is covered with **lanugo,** the fine downy hair of the newborn infant. In the first few months after birth, this is replaced by fine vellus hair. Terminal hair on the scalp, if present at birth, tends to be soft and to suffer a patchy loss, especially at the temples and occiput. Also present at birth is **vernix caseosa,** the thick, cheesy substance made up of sebum and shed epithelial cells.

The newborn's skin is similar in structure to the adult's, but many of its functions are not fully developed. The newborn's skin is thin, smooth, and elastic and is relatively more permeable than that of the adult, so the infant is at greater risk for fluid loss. Sebum, which holds water in the skin, is present for the first few weeks of life, producing milia and cradle cap in some babies. Then sebaceous glands decrease in size and production and do not resume functioning until puberty. Temperature regulation is ineffective. Eccrine sweat glands do not secrete in response to heat until the first few months of life and then only minimally throughout childhood. The skin cannot protect much against cold because it cannot contract and shiver and because the subcutaneous layer is inefficient. Also, the pigment system is inefficient at birth.

As the child grows, the epidermis thickens, toughens, and darkens and the skin becomes better lubricated. Hair growth accelerates. At puberty, secretion from apocrine sweat glands increases in response to heat and emotional stimuli, producing body odour. Sebaceous glands become more active—the skin looks oily, and acne develops. Subcutaneous fat deposits increase, especially in females.

Secondary sex characteristics that appear during adolescence are evident in the integument (i.e., skin). In the female the diameter of the areola enlarges and darkens, and breast tissue develops. Coarse pubic hair develops in males and females, then axillary hair, and then coarse facial hair in males.

The Pregnant Female

The change in hormone levels results in increased pigment in the areolae and nipples, vulva, and sometimes in the midline of the abdomen (**linea nigra**) or in the face (**chloasma**). Hyperestrogenemia probably also causes the common vascular spiders and palmar erythema. Connective tissue develops increased fragility, resulting in **striae gravidarum,** which may develop in the skin of the abdomen, breasts, or thighs. Metabolism is increased in pregnancy; as a way to dissipate heat, the peripheral vasculature dilates, and the sweat and sebaceous glands increase secretion. Fat deposits are laid down, particularly in the buttocks and hips, as maternal reserves for the nursing baby.

The Aging Adult

The skin is a mirror that reflects aging changes that proceed in *all* our organ systems; it just happens to be the one organ we can view directly. The aging process carries a slow atrophy of skin structures. The aging skin loses its elasticity; it folds and sags. By the 70s to 80s, it looks parchment thin, lax, dry, and wrinkled.

The epidermis's outer layer, the *stratum corneum,* thins and flattens. This allows chemicals easier access into the body. Wrinkling occurs because the underlying dermis also thins and flattens. A loss of elastin, collagen, and subcutaneous fat occurs as well as a reduction in muscle tone. The loss of collagen increases the risk for shearing, tearing injuries.

Sweat glands and sebaceous glands decrease in number and function, leaving dry skin. Decreased response of the sweat glands to thermoregulatory demand also puts the older person at greater risk for heat stroke. The vascularity of the skin diminishes while the vascular fragility increases; a minor trauma may produce dark red discoloured areas, or **senile purpura.**

Sun exposure and, to a somewhat lesser extent, cigarette smoking further accentuate aging changes in the skin. Coarse wrinkling, decreased elasticity, atrophy, speckled and uneven colouring, more pigment changes, and a yellowed leathery texture occur. Chronic sun damage is even more prominent in pale or light-skinned persons.

An accumulation of factors place the aging person at risk for skin disease and breakdown: the thinning of the skin, the decrease in vascularity and nutrients, the loss of protective cushioning of the subcutaneous layer, a lifetime of environmental trauma to skin, the social changes of aging (e.g., less nutrition, limited financial resources), the increasingly sedentary lifestyle, and the chance of immobility. When skin breakdown does occur, subsequent cell replacement is slower, and wound healing is delayed.

In the aging hair matrix, the number of functioning melanocytes decreases, so the hair looks grey or white and feels thin and fine. A person's genetic script determines the onset of greying and the number of grey hairs. Hair distribution changes. Males may have a symmetrical W-shaped balding in the frontal areas. Some testosterone is present in both males and females; as it decreases with age, axillary and pubic hair decrease. As the female's estrogen also decreases, testosterone is unopposed and the female may have some bristly facial hairs. Nails grow more slowly. Their surface is lusterless and is characterized by longitudinal ridges resulting from local trauma at the nail matrix.

Because the aging changes in the skin and hair can be viewed directly, they carry profound a psychological impact. For many people, self-esteem is linked to a youthful appearance. This view is compounded by media advertising in Western society. Although sagging and wrinkling skin and graying and thinning hair are normal processes of aging, they can prompt a loss of self-esteem for many adults.

CULTURAL AND SOCIAL CONSIDERATIONS

Awareness of normal biocultural differences and the ability to recognize the unique clinical manifestations of disease are especially important for darkly pigmented people. As described earlier, melanin is responsible for the various colors and tones of skin observed among people from culturally diverse backgrounds. Melanin protects the skin against harmful ultraviolet rays, a genetic advantage accounting for the lower incidence of skin cancer among darkly pigmented individuals of African, Indian, or Aboriginal descent. The incidence of melanoma is 20 times higher among individuals of lighter skin pigment versus their darker counterparts.

Areas of the skin affected by hormones and, in some cases, differing for culturally diverse people, are the sexual skin areas, such as the nipples, areola, scrotum, and labia majora. In general, these areas are darker than other parts of the skin in both adults and children, especially among individuals of African or Asian descent.

The apocrine and eccrine sweat glands are important for fluid balance and for thermoregulation. When apocrine gland secretions are contaminated by normal skin flora, odor results.

Inuit people have made an interesting environmental adaptation; they sweat less than Euro-Canadians on their trunks and extremities but more on their faces. This adaptation allows for temperature regulation without causing perspiration and dampness of their clothes, which would decrease their ability to insulate against severe cold weather and would pose a serious threat to their survival.

Alcohol flush syndrome, mistakenly called Asian flush previously, is a condition characterized by a genetic disposition that can cause a range of symptoms such as redness and flushing of the face, heat sensation, splotchy redness of the neck, and accelerated intoxication in the presence of ingested alcohol. It is found in approximately 90% of individuals of Aboriginal descent and 50% of those of Asian descent.

These unpleasant side effects sometimes prevent further drinking that may lead to further inebriation, but the symptoms can lead to a misassumption that the people affected are more easily inebriated than others.

Perhaps one of the most obvious and widely variable racial differences occurs with the hair. The hair of people of African descent varies widely in texture. It is very fragile and ranges from long and straight to short, spiralled, thick, and kinky. The hair and scalp have a natural tendency to be dry and require daily combing, gentle brushing, and the application of oil. Hair care products designed to specifically care for kinky hair should be available in clinical settings. In comparison, people of Asian descent generally have straight, silky hair.

Hair condition is significant in diagnosing and treating certain disease states. For example, hair texture becomes dry, brittle, and lustreless with inadequate nutrition. The hair of children of African descent with severe malnutrition (e.g., marasmus) frequently changes not only in texture but in colour. The child's hair often becomes less kinky and assumes a copper-red colour.

Subjective Data

SUBJECTIVE DATA

1. Previous history of skin disease (allergies, hives, psoriasis, eczema)
2. Change in pigmentation
3. Change in mole (size or colour)
4. Excessive dryness or moisture
5. Pruritus
6. Excessive bruising
7. Rash or lesion
8. Medications
9. Hair loss
10. Change in nails
11. Environmental or occupational hazards
12. Self-care behaviours

Examiner Asks	Rationale
1. Previous history of skin disease. Any previous skin disease or problem? • How was this treated? • Any family history of allergies or allergic skin problem? • Any known allergies to drugs, plants, animals? • Any birthmarks, tattoos?	Significant familial predisposition: allergies, hay fever, psoriasis, atopic dermatitis (eczema), acne. Identify offending allergen. Use of nonsterile equipment to apply tattoos increases risk of hepatitis C.
2. Change in pigmentation. Any **change in skin colour** or **pigmentation**?	Hypopigmentation—loss of pigmentation; hyperpigmentation—increase in colour.

Subjective Data

Examiner Asks	Rationale
• A generalized colour change (all over), or localized?	Generalized change suggests systemic illness: pallor, jaundice, cyanosis.
3. Change in mole. Any **change in a mole:** colour, size, shape, sudden appearance of tenderness, bleeding, itching? • Any "sores" that do not heal?	Signs suggest neoplasm in pigmented nevus. Person may be unaware of change in nevus on back or buttocks that he or she cannot see.
4. Excessive dryness or moisture. Any change in the feel of your skin: temperature, **moisture,** texture? • Any excess **dryness?** Is this seasonal or constant?	Seborrhea—oily. Xerosis—dry.
5. Pruritus. Any skin itching? Is this mild (prickling, tingling) or intense (intolerable)? • Does it awaken you from sleep? • Where is the itching? When did it start? • Any other skin pain or soreness? Where?	Pruritus is the most common of skin symptoms; occurs with dry skin, aging, drug reactions, allergy, obstructive jaundice, uremia, lice. Presence or absence of pruritus may be significant for diagnosis. Scratching may cause excoriation of primary lesion.
6. Excessive bruising. Any excess **bruising?** Where on the body? • How did this happen? • How long have you had it?	Multiple cuts and bruises, bruises in various stages of healing, bruises above knees and elbows, and illogical explanation—consider the possibility of abuse. Frequent falls may be due to dizziness of neurological or cardiovascular origin. Also, frequent minor trauma may be a side effect of alcoholism or other drug abuse.
7. Rash or lesion. Any skin **rash** or **lesion?** • Onset. When did you first notice it? • Location. Where did it start? • Where did it spread? • Character or quality. Describe the colour. • Is it raised or flat? Any crust, odour? Does it feel tender, warm? • Duration. How long have you had it? • Setting. Anyone at home or work with a similar rash? Have you been camping, acquired a new pet, tried a new food, drug? Does the rash seem to come with stress? • Alleviating and aggravating factors. What home care have you tried? Bath, lotions, heat? Do they help, or make it worse? • Associated symptoms. Any itching, fever? • What do you think rash or lesion means? • Coping strategies. How has rash or lesion affected your self-care, hygiene, ability to function at work, at home, and socially? • Any new or increased stress in your life?	Rashes are a common cause of seeking health care. A careful history is important; it may be an accurate predictor of the type of lesion you will see in the examination and its cause. Identify the primary site—it may give clue to cause. Migration pattern, evolution. Identify new or relevant exposure, any household or social contacts with similar symptoms. Myriad over-the-counter remedies are available. Many people try them and seek professional help only when they do not see improvement. Assess person's perception of cause: fear of cancer, illnesses borne by ticks, or sexually transmitted infections. Assess effectiveness of coping strategies. Chronic skin diseases may increase risk of loss of self-esteem, social isolation, and anxiety. Stress can exacerbate chronic skin illness.

Examiner Asks	Rationale
8. Medications. What **medications** do you take? • Prescription and over-the-counter? • Recent change?	Drugs may produce allergic skin eruption: aspirin, antibiotics, barbiturates, some tonics. Drugs may increase sunlight sensitivity and give burn response: sulfonamides, thiazide diuretics, oral hypoglycemic agents, and tetracycline. Drugs can cause hyperpigmentation: antimalarials, antineoplastic agents, hormones, metals, tetracycline.
• How long on medication?	Even after a long time on medication, a person may develop sensitivity.
9. Hair loss. Any recent **hair loss?** • A gradual or sudden onset? Symmetrical? Associated with fever, illness, increased stress?	Alopecia is a significant loss. A full head of hair equates with vitality in many cultures. If treated as a trivial problem, the person may seek alternative, unproven methods of treatment.
• Any unusual hair growth? • Any recent change in texture, appearance?	Hirsutism is shaggy or excessive hair.
10. Change in nails. Any **change in nails:** shape, colour, brittleness? Do you tend to bite or chew nails?	
11. Environmental or occupational hazards. Any **environmental** or **occupational** hazards? • Any hazard-related problems with your occupation, such as dyes, toxic chemicals, radiation? • How about hobbies? Do you perform any household or furniture repair work? • How much sun exposure do you get from outdoor work, leisure activities, sunbathing, tanning salons?	Majority of skin neoplasms result from occupational or environmental agents. People at risk include outdoor sports enthusiasts, farmers, sailors, outdoor workers; also creosote workers, roofers, coal workers. Unprotected sun exposure accelerates aging and produces lesions. At more risk: light-skinned people, those over 40 years old, and those regularly in sun.
• Recently been bitten by insect: bee, tick, mosquito? • Any recent exposure to plants, animals in yard work, camping?	Identify contactants that produce lesions or contact dermatitis. Tell people with chronic recurrent urticaria (hives) to keep diary of meals and environment to identify precipitating factors.
12. Self-care behaviours. What do you do to care for your skin, hair, nails? What cosmetics, soaps, chemicals do you use? • Clip cuticles on nails, use adhesive for false fingernails?	Assess **self-care** and influence on self-concept—may be important with this society's media stress on high norms of beauty. Many over-the-counter remedies are costly and exacerbate skin problems.
• If you have allergies, how do you control your environment to minimize exposure? • Do you perform a skin self-examination? • Do you use sunscreen? What number SPF?	

Additional History for Infants and Children

1. Does the child have any birthmarks?

2. Was there any change in skin colour as a newborn?
• Any jaundice? Which day after birth?
• Any cyanosis? What were the circumstances?

Examiner Asks	Rationale
3. Have you noted any rash or sores? What seems to bring it on? • Have you introduced a new food or formula? When? Does your child eat chocolate, cow's milk, eggs?	Generalized rash—consider allergic reaction to new food. Irritability and general fussiness may indicate the presence of pruritus.
4. Does the child have any diaper rash? How do you care for this? How do you wash diapers? How often do you change diapers? How do you clean skin?	Occlusive diapers or infrequent changing may cause rash. Infant may be allergic to certain detergent or to disposable wipes.

5. Does the child have any burns or bruises?
  • Where?
  • How did it happen?
	A careful history is important to distinguish expected childhood bumps and bruises from any lesion that may indicate child abuse or neglect: cigarette burns; excessive bruising, especially above knees or elbows; linear whip marks. With abuse the history often will not coincide with the physical appearance and location of lesion.

6. Has the child had any exposure to contagious skin conditions: scabies, impetigo, lice? Or to communicable diseases: measles, chicken pox, scarlet fever? Or to toxic plants: poison ivy? • Are the child's vaccinations up to date?	
7. Does the child have any habits or habitual movements, such as nail-biting, twisting hair, rubbing head on mattress?	
8. What steps are taken to protect the child from sun exposure? What about sunscreens and sunblocks? How do you treat a sunburn?	Excessive sun exposure, especially severe or blistering sunburns in childhood, increases risk for melanoma in later life (Roebuck & Siegel, 2006).

Additional History for the Adolescent

1. Have you noticed any skin problems such as pimples, blackheads?
  • How long have you had them?
  • How do you treat this?
  • How do you feel about it?
	About 70% of teens will have acne, and the psychological effect often is more significant than the physical effect. Self-treatment is common. Many myths surround the cause of acne. Cause is unknown; acne is not caused by poor diet, oily complexion, or contagion.

Additional History for the Aging Adult

1. What changes have you noticed in your skin in the last few years?	Assess impact of aging on self-concept. Normal aging changes may cause distress. Many changes attributed to aging are due to chronic sun damage. Most skin cancers appear in aging people, although sun damage often begins decades earlier.
2. Any delay in wound healing? • Any skin itching?	Pruritus is very common with aging. Consider side effects of medicine or systemic disease (e.g., liver or kidney disease, cancer, lymphoma), but senile pruritus is usually due to dry skin (xerosis).

Examiner Asks	Rationale
	Exacerbated by too-frequent bathing or use of soap. Scratching with dirty, jagged fingernails produces excoriations.
3. Any other skin pain?	Some diseases, such as herpes zoster (shingles), produce more intense sensations of pain, itching in aging people. Other diseases (e.g., diabetes) may reduce pain sensation in extremities. Also, some aging people tolerate chronic pain as "part of growing old," and hesitate to "complain."
4. Any change in feet, toenails? Any bunions? Is it possible to wear shoes?	Some aging people cannot reach down to their feet to give self-care.
5. Do you experience frequent falls?	Multiple bruises, trauma from falls.
6. Any history of diabetes, peripheral vascular disease?	Risk for skin lesions in feet or ankles.
7. What do you do to care for your skin?	Application of bland lotions is important to retain moisture in aging skin. Dermatitis may ensue from certain cosmetics, creams, ointments, and dyes applied to achieve a youthful appearance. Aging skin has a delayed inflammatory response when exposed to irritants. If the person is not alerted by warning signs (e.g., pruritus, redness), exposure may continue and dermatitis may ensue.

OBJECTIVE DATA

PREPARATION

Try to control external variables that may influence skin colour and confuse your findings, both in light-skinned and in dark-skinned persons (Table 12-1).

Learn to consciously attend to skin characteristics. The danger is one of omission. You grow so accustomed to seeing the skin that you are likely to ignore it as you assess the organ systems underneath. Yet the skin holds information about the body's circulation, nutritional status, and signs of systemic diseases as well as topical data on the integument itself.

Know the person's normal skin colouring. Baseline knowledge is important to assess colour or pigment changes. If this is the first time you are examining the person, ask about his or her usual skin colour and about any self-monitoring practices.

The Complete Physical Examination. Although it is presented alone in this chapter, skin assessment is integrated throughout the complete examination; it is not a separate step. At the beginning of the examination, assessing the person's hands and fingernails is a nonthreatening way to accustom him or her to your touch. Most people are used to having relative strangers shake their hands or touch their arms. As you move through the examination, scrutinize the outer skin surface first before you concentrate on the underlying structures. Separate intertriginous areas (areas with skinfolds) such as under large breasts, obese abdomen, and the groin and inspect them thoroughly. These areas are dark, warm, and moist and provide the perfect conditions for irritation or infection. Last, always remove the person's socks and inspect the feet, toenails, and the area between the toes.

EQUIPMENT NEEDED

Strong direct lighting (natural daylight is ideal to evaluate skin characteristics but is usually not available in the clinical area)

Small centimetre ruler

Penlight

Gloves

Needed for special procedures:

Wood's light (filtered ultraviolet light)

Magnifying glass, for minute lesions

Materials for laboratory tests: potassium hydroxide (KOH), glass slide

TABLE 12-1	External Variables Influencing Skin Colour				
Variable			Causes		Misleading Outcome
Emotions					
Fear, anger	→		Peripheral vasoconstriction	→	False pallor
Embarrassment	→		Flushing in face and neck	→	False erythema
Environment					
Hot room	→		Vasodilatation	→	False erythema
Chilly or air-conditioned room	→		Vasoconstriction	→	False pallor, coolness
Cigarette smoking	→		Vasoconstriction	→	False pallor
Physical					
Prolonged elevation	→		Decreased arterial perfusion	→	Pallor, coolness
Dependent position	→		Venous pooling	→	Redness, warmth, distended veins
Immobilization, prolonged inactivity	→		Slowed circulation	→	Pallor coolness, nail beds pale, prolonged capillary filling time

In a hospitalized setting, a more formalized tool may be used to determine factors that may result in putting the patient at risk for skin tears or breakdown. One such scale that is commonly used is the Braden Risk Assessment Scale™. Primarily used in the community and hospital settings, it is an efficient measurement tool to assist in objective skin risk assessment. For the complete scale, please see Appendix A.

The Regional Examination. At times, an individual seeks health care because of a skin change, and your assessment will be focused on the skin alone. Ask the person to remove his or her clothing and assess the skin as one entity. Stand back at first to get an overall impression; this helps reveal distribution patterns. Then inspect lesions carefully. With a skin rash, check all areas of the body because there are some locations the person cannot see. You cannot rely on the history alone that the rash is limited to one location. Inspect mucous membranes, too, because some disorders have characteristic lesions here.

The skills used are inspection and palpation because some skin changes have accompanying signs that can be felt.

Normal Range of Findings	Abnormal Findings

INSPECT AND PALPATE THE SKIN

Colour

General Pigmentation. Observe the skin tone. Normally it is consistent with genetic background and varies from pinkish tan to ruddy dark tan or from light to dark brown and may have yellow or olive overtones. Dark-skinned people normally have areas of lighter pigmentation on the palms, nail beds, and lips (Fig. 12-3, *A*).

An acquired condition is **vitiligo**, the complete absence of melanin pigment in patchy areas of white or light skin on the face, neck, hands, feet, body folds, and around orifices (Fig. 12-3, *B*). Vitiligo can occur in all people, although dark-skinned people are more severely affected and potentially suffer a greater threat to their body image.

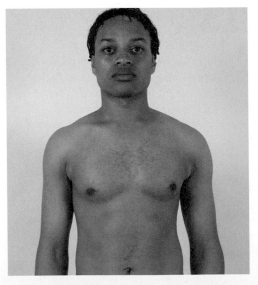

Fig. 12-3A

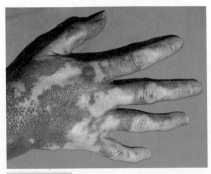

Fig. 12-3B   Vitiligo.

Normal Range of Findings

General pigmentation is darker in sun-exposed areas. Common (benign) pigmented areas also occur:

- **Freckles** (ephelides)—small, flat macules of brown melanin pigment that occur on sun-exposed skin (Fig. 12-4, *A*).
- **Mole** (nevus)—a proliferation of melanocytes, tan to brown colour, flat or raised. Acquired nevi are characterized by their symmetry, small size (6 mm or less), smooth borders, and single uniform pigmentation. The **junctional nevus** (Fig. 12-4, *B*) is macular only and occurs in children and adolescents. In young adults it progresses to the **compound nevi** (Fig. 12-4, *C*) that are macular and papular. The intradermal nevus (mainly in older age) has nevus cells in only the dermis.
- **Birthmarks**—may be tan to brown in colour.

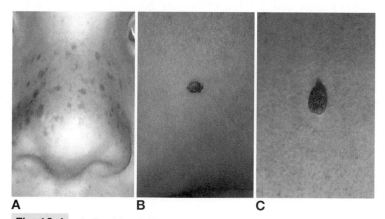

Fig. 12-4   A, Freckles. B, Junctional nevus. C, Compound nevus.

Widespread Colour Change. Note any colour change over the entire body skin, such as pallor (white), erythema (red), cyanosis (blue), and jaundice (yellow). Note whether the colour change is transient and expected or if it is due to pathology.

In dark-skinned people the amount of normal pigment may mask colour changes. Lips and nail beds show some colour change, but they vary with the person's skin colour and may not always be accurate signs. The more reliable sites are those with the least pigmentation, such as under the tongue, the buccal mucosa, the palpebral conjunctiva, and the sclera. See Table 12-2 on pp. 248 and 249 for specific clues to assessment.

Pallor. When the red-pink tones from the oxygenated hemoglobin in the blood are lost, the skin takes on the colour of connective tissue (collagen), which is mostly white. Pallor is common in acute high-stress states, such as anxiety or fear, because of the powerful peripheral vasoconstriction from sympathetic nervous system stimulation. The skin also looks pale with vasoconstriction from exposure to cold and cigarette smoking and in the presence of edema.

Look for pallor in dark-skinned people by the absence of the underlying red tones that normally give brown or black skin its lustre. The brown-skinned individual demonstrates pallor with a more yellowish brown colour, and the black-skinned person will appear ashen or grey. Generalized pallor can be observed in the mucous membranes, lips, and nail beds. The palpebral conjunctiva and nail beds are preferred sites for assessing the pallor of anemia. When inspecting the conjunctiva, lower the lid sufficiently to visualize the conjunctiva near the *outer* canthus as well as the inner canthus. The coloration is often lighter near the inner canthus.

Abnormal Findings

Danger signs: abnormal characteristics of pigmented lesions are summarized in the mnemonic **ABCDE:**

Asymmetry (*not* regularly round or oval, two halves of lesion do not look the same)

Border irregularity (notching, scalloping, ragged edges or poorly defined margins)

Colour variation (areas of brown, tan, black, blue, red, white, or combination)

Diameter greater than 6 mm (i.e., the size of a pencil eraser), although early melanomas may be diagnosed at a smaller size (Oliviero, 2002).

Elevation and Enlargement

Additional symptoms: change in mole's size, a new pigmented lesion, and development of itching, burning, or bleeding in a mole. Any of these signs should raise suspicion of malignant melanoma and warrant referral.

Ashen-grey colour in dark skin or marked pallor in Whites occurs with anemia, shock, arterial insufficiency (see Table 12-2, p. 248).

The pallor of impending shock is accompanied by other subtle manifestations, such as increasing pulse rate, oliguria, apprehension, and restlessness.

Anemias, particularly chronic iron deficiency anemia, may show "spoon" nails, with a concave shape. A lemon yellow tint of the face and slightly yellow sclera accompany pernicious anemia, also indicated by neurological deficits and a red, painful tongue. Fatigue, exertional dyspnea, rapid pulse, dizziness, and impaired mental function accompany most severe anemias.

Normal Range of Findings	Abnormal Findings

Erythema. Erythema is an intense redness of the skin from excess blood (hyperemia) in the dilated superficial capillaries. This sign is *expected* with fever, local inflammation, or with emotional reactions such as blushing in vascular flush areas (cheeks, neck, and upper chest).

Erythema occurs with polycythemia, venous stasis, carbon monoxide poisoning, and the extravascular presence of red blood cells (petechiae, ecchymosis, hematoma) (see Table 12-2, p. 248, and Table 12-7, 256).

When erythema is associated with fever or localized inflammation, it is characterized by increased skin temperature from the increased rate of blood flow through the blood vessels. Because you cannot see inflammation in dark-skinned persons, it is often necessary to palpate the skin for increased warmth, taut or tightly pulled surfaces that may be indicative of edema, and hardening of deep tissues or blood vessels.

Cyanosis. This is a bluish, mottled discoloration that signifies decreased perfusion; the tissues are not adequately perfused with oxygenated blood. Be aware that cyanosis can be a nonspecific sign. A person who is anemic could have hypoxemia without ever looking blue because not enough hemoglobin is present (either oxygenated or reduced) to colour the skin. On the other hand, a person with polycythemia (an increase in the number of red blood cells) looks ruddy blue at all times and may not necessarily be hypoxemic. This person just is unable to fully oxygenate the massive numbers of red blood cells. Last, do not confuse cyanosis with the common and normal bluish tone on the lips of dark-skinned persons of Mediterranean origin.

Cyanosis indicates hypoxemia and occurs with shock, heart failure, chronic bronchitis, and congenital heart disease.

Cyanosis is difficult to observe in a person with dark pigmentation (see Table 12-2, p. 248). Given that most conditions causing cyanosis also cause decreased oxygenation of the brain, other clinical signs—such as changes in level of consciousness and signs of respiratory distress—will be evident.

Jaundice. Jaundice is exhibited by a yellow colour, indicating rising amounts of bilirubin in the blood. Except for physiological jaundice in the newborn (p. 240), jaundice does not occur normally. Jaundice is *first* noted in the junction of the hard and soft palates in the mouth and in the sclera. But do not confuse scleral jaundice with the normal yellow subconjunctival fatty deposits that are common in the outer sclera of dark-skinned persons. The scleral yellow of jaundice extends up to the edge of the iris.

Jaundice occurs with hepatitis, cirrhosis, sickle-cell disease, transfusion reaction, and hemolytic disease of the newborn.

As levels of serum bilirubin rise, jaundice is evident in the skin over the rest of the body. This is best assessed in direct natural daylight. Common calluses on palms and soles often look yellow—do not interpret these as jaundice.

Light or clay-coloured stools and dark golden urine often accompany jaundice in both light- and dark-skinned people.

Temperature

Note the temperature of your own hands. Then use the backs (dorsa) of your hands to palpate the person and check bilaterally. The skin should be warm, and the temperature should be equal bilaterally; warmth suggests normal circulatory status. Hands and feet may be slightly cooler in a cool environment.

Hypothermia. Generalized coolness may be induced, such as in hypothermia used for surgery or high fever. Localized coolness is expected with an immobilized extremity, as when a limb is in a cast or with an intravenous infusion.

General hypothermia accompanies central circulatory problem such as shock.

Localized hypothermia occurs in peripheral arterial insufficiency and Raynaud's disease.

Hyperthermia. Generalized hyperthermia occurs with an increased metabolic rate, such as in fever or after heavy exercise. A localized area feels hyperthermic with trauma, infection, or sunburn.

Hyperthyroidism has an increased metabolic rate, causing warm, moist skin.

Moisture

Perspiration appears normally on the face, hands, axilla, and skinfolds in response to activity, a warm environment, or anxiety. **Diaphoresis,** or profuse perspiration, accompanies an increased metabolic rate, such as occurs in heavy activity or fever.

Diaphoresis occurs with thyrotoxicosis and with stimulation of the nervous system with anxiety or pain.

Normal Range of Findings	Abnormal Findings

Look for **dehydration** in the oral mucous membranes. Normally there is none, and the mucous membranes look smooth and moist. Be aware that dark skin may normally look dry and flaky, but this does not necessarily indicate systemic dehydration.

With dehydration, mucous membranes look dry and the lips look parched and cracked. With extreme dryness the skin is fissured, resembling cracks in a dry lake bed.

Texture

Normal skin feels smooth and firm, with an even surface.

Hyperthyroidism—skin feels smoother and softer, like velvet.
Hypothyroidism—skin feels rough, dry, and flaky.

Thickness

The epidermis is uniformly thin over most of the body, although thickened callus areas are normal on palms and soles. A callus is a circumscribed overgrowth of epidermis and is an adaptation to excessive pressure from the friction of work and weight bearing.

Very thin, shiny skin (atrophic) occurs with arterial insufficiency.

Edema

Edema is fluid accumulating in the intercellular spaces; it is not present normally. To check for edema, imprint your thumbs firmly against the ankle malleolus or the tibia. Normally the skin surface stays smooth. If your pressure leaves a dent in the skin, "pitting" edema is present. Its presence is graded on a four-point scale:

1+ Mild pitting, slight indentation, no perceptible swelling of the leg
2+ Moderate pitting, indentation subsides rapidly
3+ Deep pitting, indentation remains for a short time, leg looks swollen
4+ Very deep pitting, indentation lasts a long time, leg is very swollen

This scale is somewhat subjective; outcomes vary among examiners (see further content on grading scale in Chapter 20).

Edema masks normal skin colour and obscures pathological conditions such as jaundice or cyanosis because the fluid lies between the surface and the pigmented and vascular layers. It makes dark skin look lighter.

Edema is most evident in dependent parts of the body (feet, ankles, and sacral areas), where the skin looks puffy and tight. Edema makes the hair follicles more prominent, so you note a pig-skin or orange peel look (called *peau d'orange*).
Unilateral edema—consider a local or peripheral cause.
Bilateral edema or edema that is generalized over the whole body *(anasarca)*—consider a central problem such as heart failure or kidney failure.

Mobility and Turgor

Pinch up a large fold of skin on the anterior chest under the clavicle (Fig. 12-5). Mobility is the skin's ease of rising, and turgor is its ability to return to place promptly when released. This reflects the elasticity of the skin.

Mobility is decreased when edema is present.
Poor turgor is evident in severe dehydration or extreme weight loss; the pinched skin recedes slowly or "tents" and stands by itself.
Scleroderma, literally "hard skin," is a chronic connective tissue disorder associated with decreased mobility (see Table 13-4, p. 294).

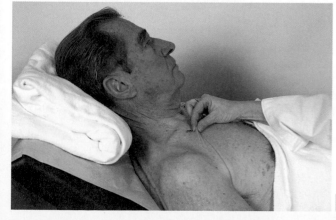

Fig. 12-5

Objective Data

Vascularity or Bruising

Cherry (senile) angiomas are small (1 to 5 mm), smooth, slightly raised bright red dots that commonly appear on the trunk in all adults over 30 years old (Fig. 12-6). They normally increase in size and number with aging and are not significant.

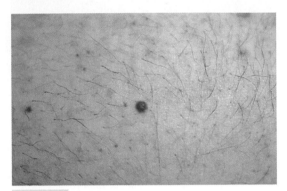

Fig. 12-6   Cherry angioma.

Any bruising (ecchymosis) should be consistent with the expected trauma of life. There are normally no venous dilatations or varicosities.

Document the presence of any tattoos (a permanent skin design from indelible pigment) on the person's chart. Advise the person that the use of tattoo needles and tattoo parlour equipment of doubtful sterility increases the risk of hepatitis C.

Multiple bruises at different stages of healing and excessive bruises above knees or elbows should raise concern about physical abuse (see Table 12-6, p. 255).

Needle marks or tracks from intravenous injection of street drugs may be visible on the antecubital fossae, forearms, or any available vein.

Lesions

If any lesions are present, note the:
1. Colour.
2. Elevation: flat, raised, or pedunculated.
3. Pattern or shape: the grouping or distinctness of each lesion, for example, annular, grouped, confluent, linear. The pattern may be characteristic of a certain disease.
4. Size, in centimetres: Use a ruler to measure. Avoid household descriptions such as "quarter size" or "pea size."
5. Location and distribution on body: Is it generalized or localized to area of a specific irritant; around jewellery, watchband, around eyes?
6. Any exudate. Note its colour and any odour.

Palpate lesions. Wear a glove if you anticipate contact with blood, mucosa, any body fluid, or skin lesion. Roll a nodule between the thumb and index finger to assess depth. Gently scrape a scale to see if it comes off. Note the nature of its base or if it bleeds when the scale comes off. Note the surrounding skin temperature. However, the erythema associated with rashes is not always accompanied by noticeable increases in skin temperature.

Does the lesion blanch with pressure or stretch? Stretching the area of skin between your thumb and index finger decreases (blanches) the normal underlying red tones, thus providing more contrast and brightening the macules. Red macules from dilated blood vessels *will* blanch momentarily, whereas those from extravasated blood (petechiae) do not. Blanching also helps identify a macular rash in dark-skinned people.

Lesions are traumatic or pathological changes in previously normal structures. When a lesion develops on previously unaltered skin, it is **primary.** However, when a lesion changes over time or changes because of a factor such as scratching or infection, it is **secondary.** Study Table 12-3, p. 249, for the shapes and Tables 12-4 and 12-5, pp. 251 and 253, for the characteristics of primary and secondary skin lesions. The terms used (*macule, papule,* etc.) are helpful to describe any lesion you encounter.

Note the pattern and characteristics of common skin lesions (see Table 12-9, p. 260) and malignant skin lesions (Table 12-10, p. 262), and lesions associated with acquired immune deficiency syndrome (AIDS) (Table 12-11, p. 263).

Objective Data

Normal Range of Findings	Abnormal Findings

Use a magnifier and light for closer inspection of the lesion (Fig. 12-7). Use a Wood's light (i.e., an ultraviolet light filtered through a special glass) to detect fluorescing lesions. With the room darkened, shine the Wood's light on the area.

Lesions with blue-green fluorescence indicate fungal infection, such as tinea capitis (scalp ringworm).

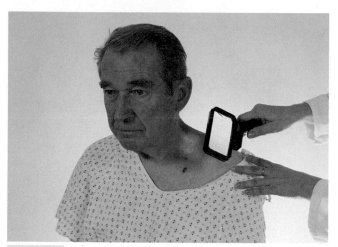

Fig. 12-7

Potassium Hydroxide Preparation. Microscopic examination of skin scrapings helps diagnose superficial fungal infections. Use a sharp sterile blade and lightly scrape the scale from the edge of a scaling lesion. Place on a clean slide. Add a drop of 10 to 20% KOH to dissolve nonfungal skin debris; send to the laboratory.

INSPECT AND PALPATE THE HAIR

Colour

Hair colour comes from melanin production and may vary from pale blonde to total black. Greying begins as early as the third decade of life because of reduced melanin production in the follicles. Genetic factors affect the age of onset of greying.

Texture

Scalp hair may be fine or thick and may look straight, curly, or kinky. It should look shiny, although this characteristic may be lost with the use of some beauty products such as dyes, rinses, or permanents.

Note dull, coarse, or brittle scalp hair.
Grey, scaly, well-defined areas with broken hairs accompany tinea capitis, a ringworm infection found mostly in school-age children (see Table 12-13, p. 265).

Distribution

Fine vellus hair coats the body, whereas coarser terminal hairs grow at the eyebrows, eyelashes, and scalp. During puberty, distribution conforms to normal male and female patterns. At first, coarse curly hairs develop in the pubic area, then in the axillae, and last in the facial area in boys. In the genital area the female pattern is an inverted triangle; the male pattern is an upright triangle with pubic hair extending up to the umbilicus. In individuals of Asian descent, body hair may be diminished.

Genital hair absent or with abnormal configuration suggests endocrine abnormalities.
Hirsutism—excess body hair. In females, this forms a male pattern of hair distribution on the face and chest and indicates endocrine abnormalities (see Table 12-13, p. 265).

Objective Data

Normal Range of Findings	Abnormal Findings

Objective Data

Lesions

Separate the hair into sections and lift it, observing the scalp. With a history of itching, inspect the hair behind the ears and in the occipital area as well. All areas should be clean and free of any lesions or pest inhabitants. Many people normally have seborrhea (dandruff), which is indicated by loose white flakes.

Head or pubic lice. Distinguish dandruff from nits (eggs) of lice, which are oval, adherent to hair shaft, and cause intense itching (see Table 12-13, p. 265).

INSPECT AND PALPATE THE NAILS

Shape and Contour

The nail surface is normally slightly curved or flat, and the posterior and lateral nail folds are smooth and rounded. Nail edges are smooth, rounded, and clean, suggesting adequate self-care.

Jagged nails, bitten to the quick, or traumatized nail folds from chronic nervous picking suggest nervous habits.

Chronically dirty nails suggest poor self-care or some occupations in which it is impossible to keep them clean.

The Profile Sign. View the index finger at its profile and note the angle of the nail base; it should be about 160 degrees (Fig. 12-8). The nail base is firm to palpation. Curved nails are a variation of normal with a convex profile. They may look like clubbed nails, but notice that the angle between nail base and nail is normal (i.e., 160 degrees or less).

Clubbing of nails occurs with congenital chronic cyanotic heart disease and with emphysema and chronic bronchitis.

In early clubbing, the angle straightens out to 180 degrees and the nail base feels spongy to palpation.

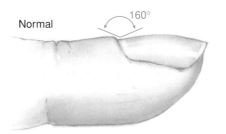 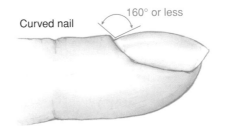 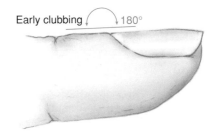

Normal 160°   Curved nail 160° or less   Early clubbing 180°

Fig. 12-8

Consistency

The surface is smooth and regular, not brittle or splitting.

Pits, transverse grooves, or lines may indicate a nutrient deficiency or may accompany acute illness in which nail growth is disturbed (see Table 12-14, p. 267).

Nail thickness is uniform.

Nails are thickened and ridged with arterial insufficiency.

The nail is firmly adherent to the nail bed, and the nail base is firm to palpation.

A spongy nail base accompanies clubbing.

Normal Range of Findings	Abnormal Findings

Colour

The translucent nail plate is a window to the even, pink nail bed underneath.

Dark-skinned people may have brown-black pigmented areas or linear bands or streaks along the nail edge (Fig. 12-9). All people normally may have white hairline linear markings from trauma or picking at the cuticle (Fig. 12-10). Note any abnormal marking in the nail beds.

Cyanosis or marked pallor.

Brown linear streaks (especially sudden appearance) are abnormal in light-skinned people and may indicate melanoma.

Splinter hemorrhages, transverse ridges, or Beau's lines (see Table 12-14, p. 267).

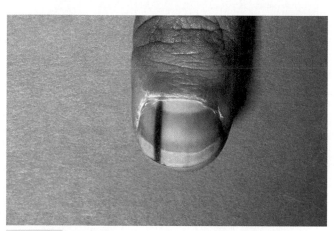

Fig. 12-9   Linear pigmentation.

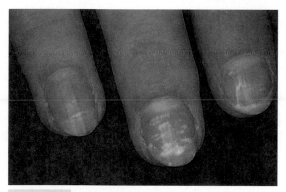

Fig. 12-10   Leukonychia striata.

Capillary Refill. Depress the nail edge to blanch and then release, noting the return of colour. Normally, colour return is instant, or at least within a few seconds in a cold environment. This indicates the status of the peripheral circulation. A sluggish colour return takes longer than 1 or 2 seconds.

Inspect the toenails. Separate the toes and note the smooth skin in between.

Cyanotic nail beds or sluggish colour return: consider cardiovascular or respiratory dysfunction.

PROMOTING HEALTH AND SELF-CARE

Teach Skin Self-Examination

Teach all adults to examine their skin once a month, using the ABCDE rule (see p. 231) to raise warning signals of any suspicious lesions. Use a well-lighted room that has a full-length mirror. It helps to have a small handheld mirror. Ask a relative to search skin areas difficult to see (e.g., behind ears, back of neck, back). Follow the sequence outlined in Figure 12-11 and report any suspicious lesions promptly to a physician or nurse.

Objective Data

Objective Data

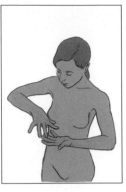

1. Undress completely. Check forearms, palms, space between fingers. Turn over hands and study the backs.

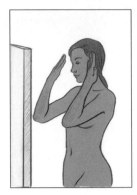

2. Face mirror; bend arms at elbow. Study arms in mirror.

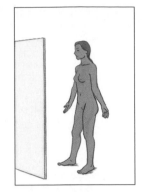

3. Face mirror and study entire front of body. Start at face, neck, torso, working down to lower legs.

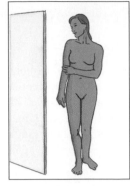

4. Pivot to right side facing mirror. Study sides of upper arms, working down to ankles. Repeat with left side.

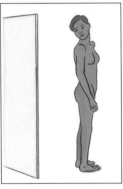

5. With back to mirror, study buttocks, thighs, lower legs.

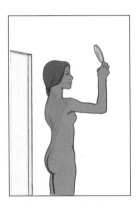

6. Use the hand-held mirror to study upper back.

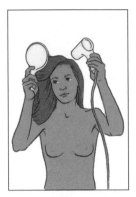

7. Use the hand-held mirror to study scalp, lifting the hair. A blow-dryer on a cool setting helps to lift hair.

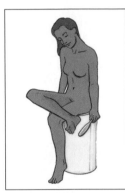

8. Sit on chair or bed. Study insides of each leg and soles of feet. Use the small mirror to help.

Fig. 12-11   Skin self-examination.

Normal Range of Findings	Abnormal Findings

🌸 DEVELOPMENTAL CARE

Infants

Skin Colour—General Pigmentation. Newborns of African descent initially have lighter-toned skin than their parents because of a pigment function that is not yet in full production. Their full melanotic colour is evident in the nail beds and scrotal folds. The **mongolian spot** is a common variation of hyperpigmentation in newborns of Aboriginal, African, East Indian, or Hispanic descent (Fig. 12-12). It is a blue-black to purple macular area at the sacrum or buttocks, but sometimes it occurs on the abdomen, thighs, shoulders, or arms. It is due to deep dermal melanocytes. It gradually fades during the first year. By adulthood these spots are lighter but are frequently still visible. Mongolian spots are present in 90% of individuals of African descent and 80% of individuals of Asian or Aboriginal descent. If you are unfamiliar with mongolian spots, be careful not to confuse them with bruises. Recognition of this normal variation is particularly important when dealing with children who might be erroneously identified as victims of child abuse.

Bruising is a common soft tissue injury that follows a rapid, traumatic, or breech birth.

Normal Range of Findings	Abnormal Findings

Multiple bruises in various stages of healing, or pattern injury, suggest child abuse (see Table 12-6, p. 255).

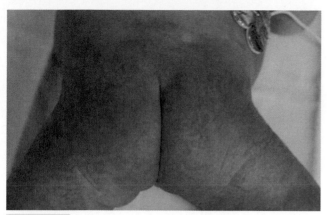

Fig. 12-12   Mongolian spot.

The **café au lait spot** is a large round or oval patch of light brown pigmentation (hence, the name "coffee with milk"), which is usually present at birth (Fig. 12-13). Most often these patches are normal.

Six or more café au lait macules, each more than 1.5 cm in diameter, are diagnostic of neurofibromatosis, an inherited neurocutaneous disease.

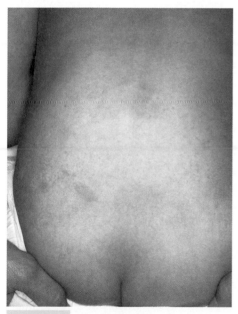

Fig. 12-13   Café au lait spot.

Skin Colour Change.   Three erythematous states are common variations in the neonate:
1. The newborn's skin has a beefy-red flush for the first 24 hours because of vasomotor instability; then the colour fades to its normal colour.
2. Another finding, the **harlequin colour change,** occurs when the baby is in a side-lying position. The lower half of the body turns red and the upper half blanches with a distinct demarcation line down the midline. The cause is unknown, and its occurrence is transient.
3. Finally, **erythema toxicum** is a common rash that appears in the first 3 to 4 days of life. Sometimes called the "flea bite" rash or newborn rash, it consists of tiny, punctate, red macules and papules on the cheeks, trunk, chest, back, and buttocks (Fig. 12-14). The cause is unknown; no treatment is needed.

Normal Range of Findings

Abnormal Findings

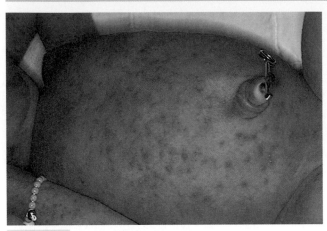

Fig. 12-14 Erythema toxicum.

Two temporary cyanotic conditions may occur:

1. A newborn may have **acrocyanosis,** a bluish colour around the lips, hands and fingernails, and feet and toenails. This may last for a few hours and disappear with warming.
2. **Cutis marmorata** is a transient mottling in the trunk and extremities in response to cooler room temperatures (Fig. 12-15). It forms a reticulated red or blue pattern over the skin.

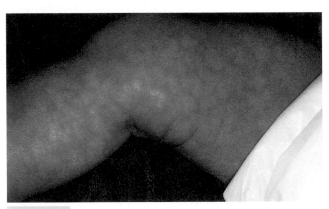

Fig. 12-15 Cutis marmorata.

Physiological jaundice is a common variation in about half of all newborns. A yellowing of the skin, sclera, and mucous membranes develops after the third or fourth day of life because of the increased numbers of red blood cells that hemolyze after birth. The hemoglobin in the red blood cells is metabolized by the liver and spleen; its pigment is converted into bilirubin.

Carotenemia also produces a yellow-orange colour in light-skinned persons but no yellowing in the sclera or mucous membranes. It comes from ingesting large amounts of foods containing carotene, a vitamin A precursor. Carotene-rich foods are popular as prepared infant foods, and the absorption of carotene is enhanced by mashing, pureeing, and cooking. The colour is best seen on the palms and soles, the forehead, tip of the nose and nasolabial folds, the chin, behind the ears, and over the knuckles; it fades to normal colour within 2 to 6 weeks of withdrawing carotene-rich foods from the diet.

Moisture. The vernix caseosa is the moist, white, cream cheese–like substance that covers part of the skin in all newborns. Perspiration is present after 1 month of age.

Persistent generalized cyanosis indicates distress, such as cyanotic congenital heart disease.

Persistent or pronounced cutis marmorata occurs with Down syndrome or prematurity.

Green-brown discoloration of the skin, nails, and cord occurs with passing of meconium in utero, indicating fetal distress.

Jaundice on the first day of life may indicate hemolytic disease. Jaundice after 2 weeks of age may indicate biliary tract obstruction.

Green-tinged vernix occurs with meconium staining.

In children, excessive sweating may accompany hypoglycemia, heart disease, or hyperthyroidism.

Normal Range of Findings	Abnormal Findings

Texture. A common variation occurring in the infant is **milia** (Fig. 12-16). Milia are tiny while papules on the cheeks, forehead, and across the nose and chin caused by sebum that occludes the opening of the follicles. Tell parents not to squeeze the lesions; milia resolve spontaneously within a few weeks.

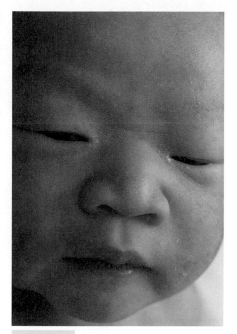

Fig. 12-16 Milia.

Thickness. In the neonate, the epidermis is normally thin, but you will also note well-defined areas of subcutaneous fat. The baby's skin dimples over joints, but there is no break in the skin. Check for any defect or break in the skin, especially over the length of the spine.

Mobility and Turgor. Test mobility and turgor over the abdomen in an infant.

Vascularity or Bruising. Some vascular markings are common birthmarks in the newborn. A **storkbite** (salmon patch) is a flat, irregularly shaped red or pink patch found on the forehead, eyelid, or upper lip but most commonly at the back of the neck (nuchal area) (Fig. 12-17). It is present at birth and usually fades during the first year.

Lack of subcutaneous fat occurs in prematurity and malnutrition.

A red sacrococcygeal dimple occurs with a pilonidal cyst or sinus (see Table 25-2, p. 750).

Poor turgor, or "tenting," indicates dehydration or malnutrition.

Port-wine stain, strawberry mark (immature hemangioma), cavernous hemangioma (see Table 12-7, 256).

Bruising may suggest abuse (see Table 12-6, 255).

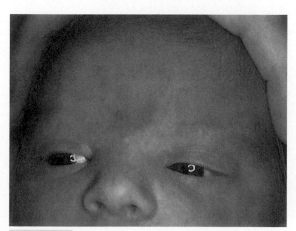

Fig. 12-17 Storkbite.

Objective Data

Normal Range of Findings	Abnormal Findings

Hair. A newborn's skin is covered with fine downy lanugo (Fig. 12-18), especially in a preterm infant. Dark-skinned newborns have more lanugo than lighter-skinned newborns. Scalp hair may be lost in the few weeks after birth, especially at the temples and occiput. It grows back slowly.

Scaly crusted scalp occurs with seborrheic dermatitis (cradle cap [see Table 12-13, p. 265]).

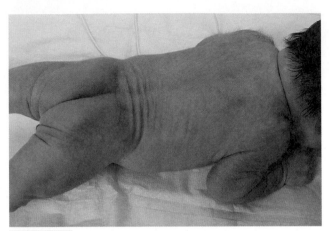

Fig. 12-18   Lanugo.

Nails. A newborn's nail beds may be blue (cyanotic) for the first few hours of life; then they turn pink.

Adolescents

The increase in sebaceous gland activity creates increased oiliness and **acne.** Acne is the most common skin problem of adolescence. Almost all teens have some acne, even if it is the milder form of open comedones (blackheads) (Fig. 12-19, *A*) and closed comedones (whiteheads). Severe acne includes papules, pustules, and nodules (Fig. 12-19, *B*). Acne lesions usually appear on the face and sometimes on the chest, back, and shoulders. Acne may appear in children as early as 7 to 8 years of age; then the lesions increase in number and severity and peak at 14 to 16 years in girls and at 16 to 19 years in boys.

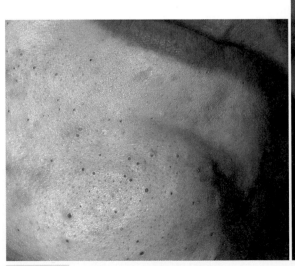
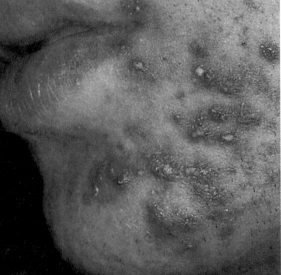

Fig. 12-19   A, Open comedones. B, Acne.

Normal Range of Findings	Abnormal Findings

The Pregnant Female

Striae are jagged linear "stretch marks" of silver to pink colour that appear during the second trimester on the abdomen, breasts, and sometimes thighs. They occur in one half of all pregnancies. They fade after delivery but do not disappear. Another skin change on the abdomen is the **linea nigra,** a brownish black line down the midline (see Fig. 29-3). **Chloasma** is an irregular brown patch of hyperpigmentation on the face. It may occur with pregnancy or in women taking oral contraceptive pills. Chloasma disappears after delivery or stopping the pills. **Vascular spiders** occur in two thirds of all pregnancies, primarily in Euro-Canadians. These lesions have tiny red centres with radiating branches and occur on the face, neck, upper chest, and arms.

The Aging Adult

Skin Colour and Pigmentation. Common variations of hyperpigmentation are senile lentigines and keratoses.

Senile Lentigines. Commonly called liver spots, these are small, flat, brown macules (Fig. 12-20). These circumscribed areas are clusters of melanocytes that appear after extensive sun exposure. They appear on the forearms and dorsa of the hands. They are not malignant and require no treatment.

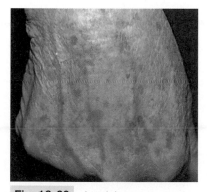

Fig. 12-20   Lentigines.

Keratoses. These lesions are raised, thickened areas of pigmentation that look crusted, scaly, and warty. One type, **seborrheic keratosis,** looks dark, greasy, and "stuck on" (Fig. 12-21). They develop mostly on the trunk but also on the face and hands and on unexposed as well as on sun-exposed areas. They do not become cancerous.

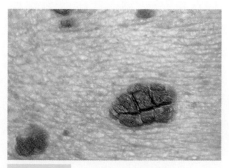

Fig. 12-21   Seborrheic keratosis.

Objective Data

Normal Range of Findings	**Abnormal Findings**

Another type, **actinic (senile** or **solar) keratosis,** is less common (Fig. 12-22). These lesions are red-tan scaly plaques that increase over the years to become raised and roughened. They may have a silvery white scale adherent to the plaque. They occur on sun-exposed surfaces and are directly related to sun exposure. They are premalignant and may develop into squamous cell carcinoma.

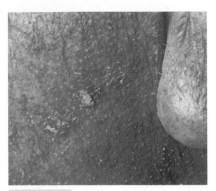

Fig. 12-22   Actinic keratosis.

Moisture. Dry skin (xerosis) is common in the aging person because of a decline in the size, number, and output of the sweat glands and sebaceous glands. The skin itches and looks flaky and loose.

Texture. Common variations occurring in the aging adult are **acrochordons,** or "skin tags," which are overgrowths of normal skin that form a stalk and are polyplike (Fig. 12-23). They occur frequently on eyelids, cheeks and neck, and axillae and trunk.

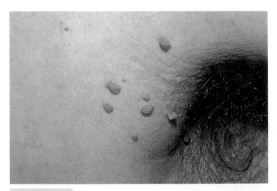

Fig. 12-23   Skin tags

Sebaceous hyperplasia consists of raised yellow papules with a central depression. They are more common in men, occurring over the forehead, nose, or cheeks. They have a pebbly look (Fig. 12-24).

Normal Range of Findings

Abnormal Findings

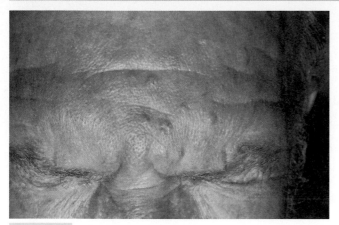

Fig. 12-24   Sebaceous hyperplasia.

Thickness. With aging, the skin looks as thin as parchment and the subcutaneous fat diminishes. Thinner skin is evident over the dorsa of the hands, forearms, lower legs, dorsa of feet, and over bony prominences. The skin may feel thicker over the abdomen and chest.

Mobility and Turgor. The turgor is decreased (less elasticity), and the skin recedes slowly or "tents" and stands by itself (Fig. 12-25).

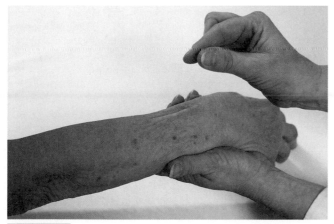

Fig. 12-25

Hair. With aging, the hair growth decreases, and the amount decreases in the axillae and pubic areas. After menopause, women may develop bristly hairs on the chin or upper lip resulting from unopposed androgens. In men, coarse terminal hairs develop in the ears, nose, and eyebrows, although the beard is unchanged. Male-pattern balding, or alopecia, is a genetic trait. It is usually a gradual receding of the anterior hairline in a symmetrical W shape. In men and women, scalp hair gradually turns grey because of the decrease in melanocyte function.

Nails. With aging, the nail growth rate decreases, and local injuries in the nail matrix may produce longitudinal ridges. The surface may be brittle or peeling and sometimes yellowed. Toenails also are thickened and may grow misshapen, almost grotesque. The thickening may be a process of aging or it may be due to chronic peripheral vascular disease.

Fungal infections are common in aging, with thickened crumbling toenails and erythematous scaling on contiguous skin surfaces.

Objective Data

Summary Checklist: Skin, Hair, and Nails Examination

For a PDA-downloadable version, go to http://evolve.elsevier.com/Canada/Jarvis/examination.

1. **Inspect the skin**
   Colour
   General pigmentation
   Areas of hypopigmentation or
     hyperpigmentation
   Abnormal colour changes
2. **Palpate the skin**
   Temperature
   Moisture
   Texture

Thickness
Edema
Mobility and turgor
Hygiene
Vascularity or bruising
3. **Note any lesions**
   Colour
   Shape and configuration
   Size
   Location and distribution on body

4. **Inspect and palpate the hair**
   Texture
   Distribution
   Any scalp lesions
5. **Inspect and palpate the nails**
   Shape and contour
   Consistency
   Colour
6. **Teach skin self-examination**

Promoting Health: Artificial Tanning and Skin Cancer Risk

The Dangers of Tanning Salons

We know that prolonged sun exposure can lead to skin cancer, yet why is it that we do not realize the potential dangers of tanning booths? The skin examination is an opportunity for healthcare professionals to educate the public about the dangers of excessive ultraviolet (UV) exposure. As you examine an individual's skin, take the time to ask about the use of tanning salons. Ask about solar exposure and outdoor sun-protective precautions as well.

The popularity of indoor tanning salons appears to be growing, despite public health warnings and increasing evidence of the dangers of artificial UV radiation. The Canadian Cancer Society has identified risk factors for the development of skin cancer with prolonged exposure to UV rays. Individuals most at risk are those who have a history of skin cancer, are under the age of 18, are fair skinned, have freckles or moles, have a family history of skin cancer, or are using medications that increase their sensitivity to UV rays.

There are many documented adverse effects of sunbeds, including acute sunburn, suppression of cutaneous DNA repair and immune functioning, ocular disorders, and increased risk of skin cancer, specifically squamous/basal cell carcinoma and melanoma. Health Canada has stated that the use of sunbeds and sunlamps is known to be a human carcinogen. In addition, the World Health Organization has publically recognized the dangers of sunbed use and declared that, worldwide, no person under the age of 18 years should use a sunbed. Yet, despite these warnings, the tanning industry appears to have convinced the public that indoor tanning is healthy, emphasizing that tanning produces a psychological sense of well-being and can even induce vitamin D production. Further, they claim that getting a tan before you go out into the sun can actually prevent sunburn, a known risk factor for skin cancer. "Pretanning" before a vacation or outdoor sun exposure is a particularly dangerous practice because not only does it lead to extra UV exposure, but it also appears to lead to decreased use of subsequent outdoor sun-protective precautions. At best, artificial "pretans" only offer the protection equal to a sunscreen with an SPF 2 to 3, well under the minimal protective recommendation of SPF 15.

Although Health Canada regulates manufacturers of indoor tanning equipment and limits the amount of UV radiation that can be emitted, it does not regulate the proportion of UVB emitted. Most tanning salons promote their devices emitting UVA light, which is thought to be "safer" than UVB light; however, UVB light usage is increasing as it intensifies tanning results. Further, the amount of UVA light received in a tanning salon may be two to three times more than the UVA light we receive from the sun and is a known risk factor for melanoma. Women who use tanning beds more than once a month are 55% more likely to have malignant melanoma. In addition, people who use tanning booths are 2.5 times more likely to have squamous cell carcinoma and 1.5 times more likely to have basal cell carcinoma.

Although one of the sources of vitamin D is exposure to UV light, an adequate level of vitamin D is typically attained through incidental exposure to the sun and normal dietary intake of vitamin D. Sources of vitamin D that do not carry an increased risk of skin cancer include vitamin D supplements or food sources supplemented with vitamin D.

Many individuals feel that tanning gives you a "healthy glow"; on the contrary, the long-term use of tanning can lead to something more frightening and deadly.

Levine, J.A. et al. (2005). The indoor UV tanning industry: A review of skin cancer risk, health benefit claims, and regulation, Journal of the American Academy of Dermatology, 53(6), 1038–1044.
Canadian Cancer Society: www.cancer.ca
Health Canada: www.healthcanada.ca

Objective Data

❧—— DOCUMENTATION AND CRITICAL THINKING ——❧

Sample Charting

SUBJECTIVE

No history of skin disease; no present change in pigmentation or in nevi; no pruritus, bruising, rash, or lesions. On no medications. No work-related skin hazards. Uses sunblock cream when outdoors.

OBJECTIVE

Skin: Colour tan-pink, even pigmentation, with no nevi. Warm to touch, dry, smooth, and even. Turgor good, no lesions.
Hair: Even distribution, thick texture, no lesions or pest inhabitants.
Nails: No clubbing or deformities. Nail beds pink with prompt capillary refill.

ASSESSMENT

Warm, dry intact skin.

Focused Assessment: Clinical Case Study

Ethan E. is a 3-year-old male presenting with his mother, who seeks health care because of Ethan's fever, fatigue, and rash of 3 days' duration.

SUBJECTIVE

- 2 weeks PTA (prior to arrival)—Ethan was playing with a child who was subsequently diagnosed as having chicken pox.
- 3 days PTA—mother reports fever 37.7°C to 38.3°C and fatigue, irritability. That evening noted "tiny blisters" on chest and back.
- 1 day PTA—blisters on chest changed to white with scab on top. New eruption of blisters on shoulders, thighs, face. Intense itching and scratching.

OBJECTIVE

Temp 38.0°C, P 110, R 24
Skin: Generalized vesiculopustular rash covering face, trunk, upper arms, and thighs. Small vesicles on face, pustules and red-honey-coloured crusts on trunk. Otherwise skin is warm and dry, turgor good.
Ears: Tympanic membranes pearl grey with landmarks intact. No discharge.
Mouth and throat: Mucosa dark pink, no lesions. Tonsils 1+, no exudate. No lymphadenopathy.
Heart: S_1, S_2 normal, not accentuated or diminished, no murmurs or extra sounds.
Lungs: Hyperresonant to percussion. Breath sounds clear, no adventitious sounds.

ASSESSMENT

Varicella
Impaired skin integrity R/T infection and scratching

Documentation
and Critical Thinking

ABNORMAL FINDINGS

TABLE 12-2	Detecting Colour Changes in Light and Dark Skin	
	Note Appearance	
Etiology	**Light Skin**	**Dark Skin**
Pallor		
Anemia—decreased hematocrit Shock—decreased perfusion, vasoconstriction	Generalized pallor	Brown skin appears yellow-brown, dull; black skin appears ashen grey, dull; skin loses its healthy glow—check areas with least pigmentation, such as conjunctivae, mucous membranes
Local arterial insufficiency	Marked localized pallor (e.g., lower extremities, especially when elevated)	Ashen grey, dull; cool to palpitation
Albinism—total absence of pigment melanin throughout the integument	Whitish pink	Tan, cream, white
Vitiligo—patchy depigmentation from destruction of melanocytes	Patchy milky white spots, often symmetrical bilaterally	Same
Cyanosis		
Increased amount of unoxygenated hemoglobin Central—chronic heart and lung disease cause arterial desaturation	Dusky blue	Dark but dull, lifeless; only severe cyanosis is apparent in skin—check conjunctivae, oral mucosa, nail beds
Peripheral—exposure to cold, anxiety	Nail beds dusky	
Erythema		
Hyperemia—increased blood flow through engorged arterioles, such as in inflammation, fever, alcohol intake, blushing	Red, bright pink	Purplish tinge, but difficult to see; palpate for increased warmth with inflammation, taut skin, and hardening of deep tissues
Polycythemia—increased red blood cells, capillary stasis	Ruddy blue in face, oral mucosa, conjunctiva, hands and feet	Well concealed by pigment—check for redness in lips
Carbon monoxide poisoning	Bright cherry red in face and upper torso	Cherry-red colour in nail beds, lips, and oral mucosa
Venous stasis—decreased blood flow from area, engorged venules	Dusky rubour of dependent extremities; a prelude to necrosis with pressure sore	Easily masked; use palpation for warmth or edema
Jaundice		
Increased serum bilirubin, more than 2 to 3 mg/100 mL from liver inflammation or hemolytic disease, such as after severe burns, some infections	Yellow in sclera, hard palate, mucous membranes, then over skin	Check sclera for yellow near limbus; do not mistake normal yellowish fatty deposits in the periphery under the eyelids for jaundice—jaundice best noted in junction of hard and soft palate and also palms
Carotenemia—increased serum carotene from ingestion of large amounts of carotene-rich foods	Yellow-orange in forehead, palms and soles, nasolabial folds, but no yellowing in sclera or mucous membranes	Yellow-orange tinge in palms and soles
Uremia—renal failure causes retained urochrome pigments in the blood	Orange-green or grey overlying pallor of anemia; may also have ecchymoses and purpura	Easily masked; rely on laboratory and clinical findings

Continued

TABLE 12-2	Detecting Colour Changes in Light and Dark Skin—cont'd	
	Note Appearance	
Etiology	Light Skin	Dark Skin
Brown-Tan		
Addison's disease—cortisol deficiency stimulates increased melanin production	Bronzed appearance, an "eternal tan," most apparent around nipples, perineum, genitalia, and pressure points (inner thighs, buttocks, elbow, axillae)	Easily masked; rely on laboratory and clinical findings
Café au lait spots—caused by increased melanin pigment in basal cell layer	Tan to light brown, irregularly shaped, oval patch with well-defined borders	

TABLE 12-3	Common Shapes and Configurations of Lesions

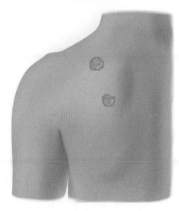

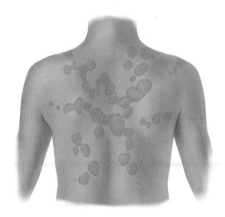

ANNULAR, or circular, begins in centre and spreads to periphery (e.g., tinea corporis or ringworm, tinea versicolor, pityriasis rosea).

CONFLUENT, lesions run together (e.g., urticaria [hives]).

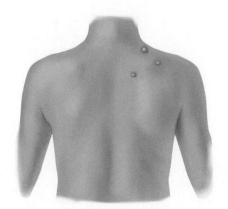

◀ **DISCRETE,** distinct, individual lesions that remain separate (e.g., molluscum).

| TABLE 12-3 | Common Shapes and Configurations of Lesions—cont'd |

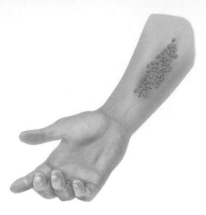

GROUPED, clusters of lesions (e.g., vesicles of contact dermatitis).

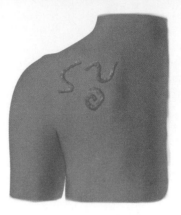

GYRATE, twisted, coiled spiral, snakelike.

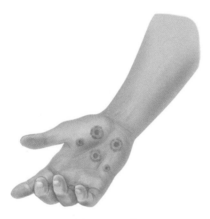

TARGET, or iris, resembles iris of eye, concentric rings of colour in the lesions (e.g., erythema multiforme).

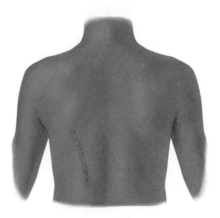

LINEAR, a scratch, streak, line, or stripe.

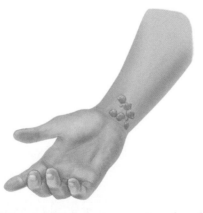

POLYCYCLIC, annular lesions grow together (e.g., lichen planus, psoriasis).

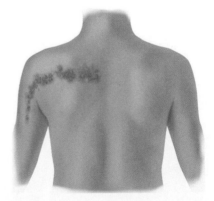

ZOSTERIFORM, linear arrangement along a nerve route (e.g., herpes zoster).

TABLE 12-4 | Primary Skin Lesions[1]

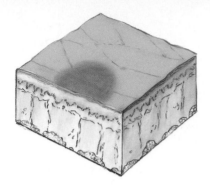

Macule

Solely a colour change, flat and circumscribed, of less than 1 cm. Examples: freckles, flat nevi, hypopigmentation, petechiae, measles, scarlet fever.

Patch

Macules that are larger than 1 cm. Examples: mongolian spot, vitiligo, café au lait spot, chloasma, measles rash.

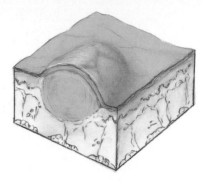

Papule

Something you can feel (i.e., solid, elevated, circumscribed, less than 1 cm diameter) caused by superficial thickening in the epidermis. Examples: elevated nevus (mole), lichen planus, molluscum, wart (verruca).

Plaque

Papules coalesce to form surface elevation wider than 1 cm. A plateaulike, disc-shaped lesion. Examples: psoriasis, lichen planus.

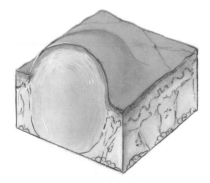

Nodule ▲

Solid, elevated, hard or soft, larger than 1 cm. May extend deeper into dermis than papule. Examples: xanthoma, fibroma, intradermal nevi.

Tumour

Larger than a few centimetres in diameter, firm or soft, deeper into dermis; may be benign or malignant, although "tumour" implies "cancer" to most people. Examples: lipoma, hemangioma.

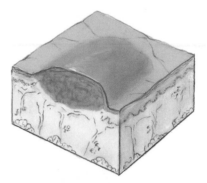

Wheal ▲

Superficial, raised, transient, and erythematous; slightly irregular shape due to edema (fluid held diffusely in the tissues). Examples: mosquito bite, allergic reaction, dermographism.

[1]The immediate result of a specific causative factor; primary lesions develop on previously unaltered skin.

TABLE 12-4 | **Primary Skin Lesions—cont'd**

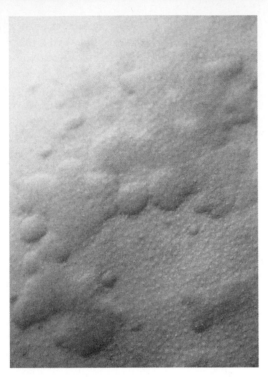

Urticaria (Hives)

Wheals coalesce to form extensive reaction, intensely pruritic.

Reprinted by permission of the publisher from Fireman, P. (1995). Atlas of allergies *(2nd ed.). Mosby.*

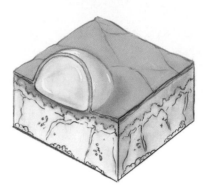

Vesicle

Elevated cavity containing free fluid, up to 1 cm; a "blister." Clear serum flows if wall is ruptured. Examples: herpes simplex, early varicella (chicken pox), herpes zoster (shingles), contact dermatitis.

Bulla

Larger than 1 cm diameter; usually single chambered (unilocular); superficial in epidermis; it is thin walled, so it ruptures easily. Examples: friction blister, pemphigus, burns, contact dermatitis.

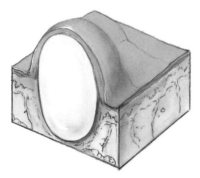

Cyst

Encapsulated fluid-filled cavity in dermis or subcutaneous layer, tensely elevating skin. Examples: sebaceous cyst, wen.

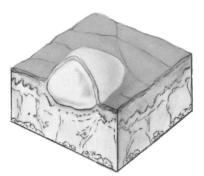

Pustule

Turbid fluid (pus) in the cavity. Circumscribed and elevated. Examples: impetigo, acne.

TABLE 12-5 | Secondary Skin Lesions[1]

DEBRIS ON SKIN SURFACE

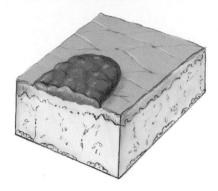

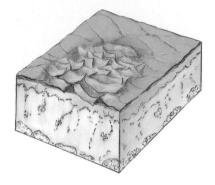

Crust

The thickened, dried-out exudate left when vesicles/pustules burst or dry up. Colour can be red-brown, honey, or yellow, depending on the fluid's ingredients (blood, serum, pus). Examples: impetigo (dry, honey-coloured), weeping eczematous dermatitis, scab after abrasion.

Scale

Compact, desiccated flakes of skin, dry or greasy, silvery or white, from shedding of dead excess keratin cells. Examples: after scarlet fever or drug reaction (laminated sheets), psoriasis (silver, micalike), seborrheic dermatitis (yellow, greasy), eczema, ichthyosis (large, adherent, laminated), dry skin.

BREAK IN CONTINUITY OF SURFACE

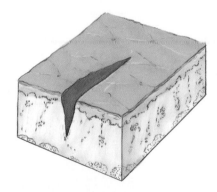

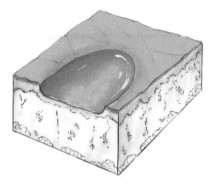

Fissure

Linear crack with abrupt edges, extends into dermis, dry or moist. Examples: cheilosis—at corners of mouth due to excess moisture; athlete's foot.

Erosion

Scooped-out but shallow depression. Superficial; epidermis lost; moist but no bleeding; heals without scar because erosion does not extend into dermis.

---

[1]Resulting from a change in a primary lesion from the passage of time; an evolutionary change.
Note: Combinations of primary and secondary lesions may coexist in the same person. Such combined designations may be termed papulosquamous, maculopapular, vesiculopustular, or papulovesicular.

TABLE 12-5 | Secondary Skin Lesions—cont'd

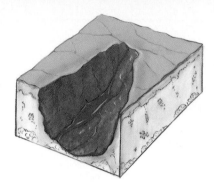

Ulcer

Deeper depression extending into dermis, irregular shape; may bleed; leaves scar when heals. Examples: stasis ulcer, pressure sore, chancre.

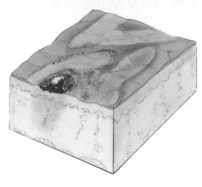

Excoriation

Self-inflicted abrasion; superficial; sometimes crusted; scratches from intense itching. Examples: insect bites, scabies, dermatitis, varicella.

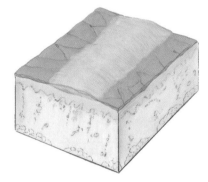

Scar

After a skin lesion is repaired, normal tissue is lost and replaced with connective tissue (collagen). This is a permanent fibrotic change. Examples: healed area of surgery or injury, acne.

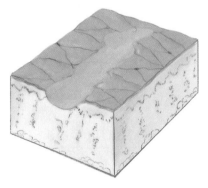

Atrophic Scar

Resulting skin level depressed with loss of tissue; a thinning of the epidermis. Example: striae.

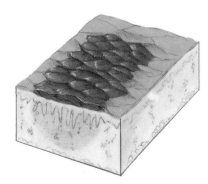

Lichenification

Prolonged intense scratching eventually thickens the skin and produces tightly packed sets of papules; looks like surface of moss (or lichen).

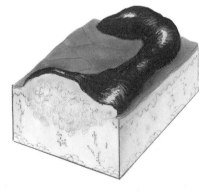

Keloid

A hypertrophic scar. The resulting skin level is elevated by excess scar tissue, which is invasive beyond the site of original injury. May increase long after healing occurs. Looks smooth, rubbery, "clawlike," and has a higher incidence among individuals of African descent.

TABLE 12-6	Lesions Caused by Trauma or Abuse

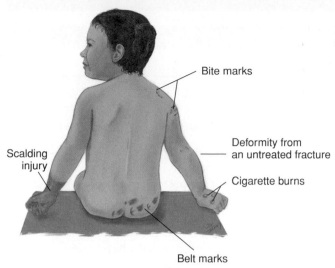

Bite marks

Deformity from
an untreated fracture

Cigarette burns

Scalding
injury

Belt marks

◄ Pattern Injury

Pattern injury is a bruise or wound whose shape suggests the instrument or weapon that caused it (e.g., belt buckle, broomstick, burning cigarette, pinch marks, bite marks, or scalding hot liquid). Inflicted scalding-water immersion burns usually have a clear border, like a glove or sock, indicating that body part was held under water intentionally. Deformity results from an untreated fracture because the bone heals out of alignment.

These physical signs suggest child abuse, together with a history that does not match the severity or type of injury, and indicate an impaired or dysfunctional parent–child relationship.

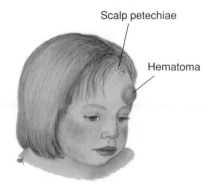

Scalp petechiae

Hematoma

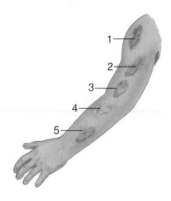

1
2
3
4
5

Hematoma

A hematoma is a bruise you can feel. It elevates the skin and is seen as swelling. Multiple petechiae and purpura may occur on the face when prolonged vigorous crying or coughing raises venous pressure.

Contusion (Bruise)

A large patch of capillary bleeding into tissues. Colour in light-skinned person is usually (1) red-blue or purple immediately after or within 24 hours of trauma→(2) blue to purple→(3) blue-green→(4) yellow→(5) brown→complete disappearance. A recent bruise in dark-skinned person is deep, dark purple. Note that it is *not* possible to date the age of a bruise from its colour.

Pressure on a bruise will *not* cause it to blanch. A bruise usually occurs from trauma; also from bleeding disorders and liver dysfunction.

ABNORMAL FINDINGS
FOR ADVANCED PRACTICE

TABLE 12-7	Vascular Lesions

HEMANGIOMAS

Caused by a benign proliferation of blood vessels in the dermis.

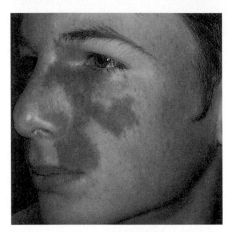

◀ Port-Wine Stain (Nevus Flammeus)

A large, flat macular patch covering the scalp or face, frequently along the distribution of cranial nerve V. The colour is dark red, bluish, or purplish and intensifies with crying, exertion, or exposure to heat or cold. The marking consists of mature capillaries. It is present at birth and usually does not fade. The use of yellow light lasers now makes photoablation of the lesion possible, with minimal adverse effects.

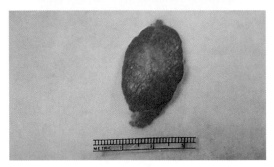

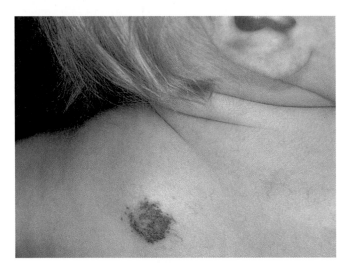

Strawberry Mark (Immature Hemangioma)

A raised bright red area with well-defined borders about 2 to 3 cm in diameter. It does not blanch with pressure. It consists of immature capillaries, is present at birth or develops in the first few months, and usually disappears by age 5 to 7 years. Requires no treatment, although parental and peer pressure may prompt treatment.

Cavernous Hemangioma (Mature)

A reddish blue, irregularly shaped, solid and spongy mass of blood vessels. It may be present at birth, may enlarge during the first 10 to 15 months, and will not involute spontaneously.

TELANGIECTASES

Caused by vascular dilatation; permanently enlarged and dilated blood vessels that are visible on the skin surface. Examples are as follows.

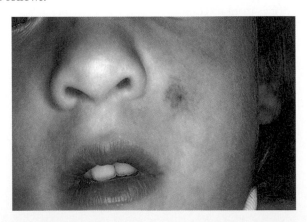

◀ Spider or Star Angioma

A fiery red, star-shaped marking with a solid circular centre. Capillary radiations extend from the central arterial body. With pressure, note a central pulsating body and blanching of extended legs. Develops on face, neck, or chest; may be associated with pregnancy, chronic liver disease, or estrogen therapy, or may be normal.

Continued

TABLE 12-7 | **Vascular Lesions—cont'd**

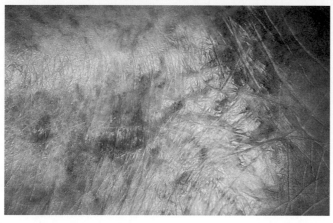

◀ **Venous Lake**

A blue-purple dilatation of venules and capillaries in a star-shaped, linear, or flaring pattern. Pressure causes them to empty or disappear. Located on the legs near varicose veins and also on the face, lips, ears, and chest.

PURPURIC LESIONS

Caused by blood flowing out of breaks in the vessels. Red blood cells and blood pigments are deposited in the tissues (extravascular). Difficult to see in dark-skinned people.

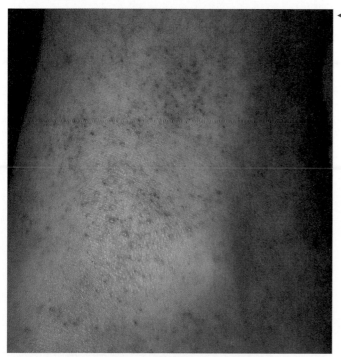

◀ **Petechiae**

Tiny punctate hemorrhages, 1 to 3 mm, round and discrete, dark red, purple, or brown. Caused by bleeding from superficial capillaries; will not blanch. May indicate abnormal clotting factors. In dark-skinned people, petechiae are best visualized in the areas of lighter melanization (e.g., the abdomen, buttocks, and volar surface of the forearm). When the skin is black or very dark brown, petechiae cannot be seen in the skin.

Most of the diseases that cause bleeding and microembolism formation—such as thrombocytopenia, subacute bacterial endocarditis, and other septicemias—are characterized by petechiae in the mucous membranes as well as on the skin. Thus you should inspect for petechiae in the mouth, particularly the buccal mucosa, and in the conjunctivae.

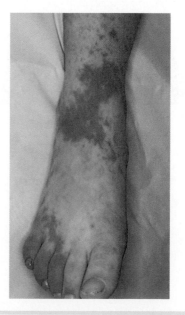

Purpura ▶

Confluent and extensive patch of petechiae and ecchymoses, >3 mm flat, red to purple, macular hemorrhage. Seen in generalized disorders such as thrombocytopenia and scurvy. Also occurs in old age as blood leaks from capillaries in response to minor trauma and diffuses through dermis.

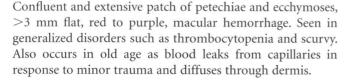

TABLE 12-8	Common Skin Lesions in Children

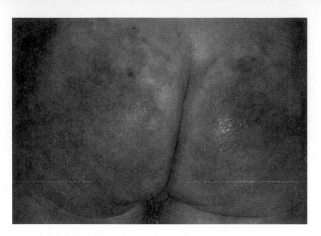

Diaper Dermatitis

Red, moist maculopapular patch with poorly defined borders in diaper area, extending along inguinal and gluteal folds. History of infrequent diaper changes or occlusive coverings. Inflammatory disease caused by skin irritation from ammonia, heat, moisture, occlusive diapers.

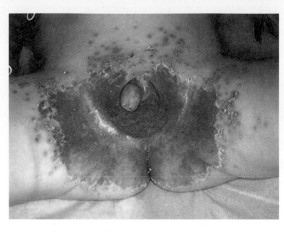

Intertrigo (Candidiasis)

Scalding red, moist patches with sharply demarcated borders, some loose scales. Usually in genital area extending along inguinal and gluteal folds. Aggravated by urine, feces, heat, and moisture, the *Candida* fungus infects the superficial skin layers.

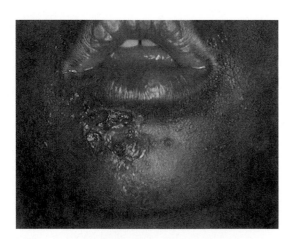

Impetigo

Moist, thin-roofed vesicles with thin, erythematous base. Rupture to form thick, honey-coloured crusts. Contagious bacterial infection of skin; most common in infants and children.

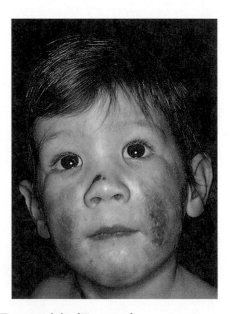

Atopic Dermatitis (Eczema)

Erythematous papules and vesicles, with weeping, oozing, and crusts. Lesions usually on scalp, forehead, cheeks, forearms and wrists, elbows, backs of knees. Paroxysmal and severe pruritus. Family history of allergies.

Continued

TABLE 12-8   Common Skin Lesions in Children—cont'd

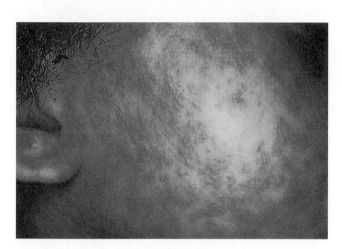

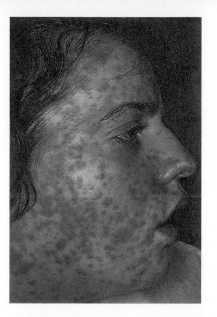

Measles (Rubeola) in Dark Skin

Measles (Rubeola) in Light Skin

Red-purple maculopapular blotchy rash in dark skin (on left) and in light skin (on right) appears on third or fourth day of illness. Rash appears first behind ears and spreads over face, then over neck, trunk, arms, and legs; looks "coppery" and does not blanch. Also characterized by Koplik's spots in mouth—bluish white, red-based elevations of 1 to 3 mm.

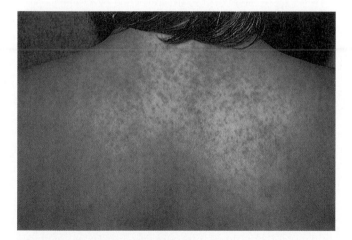

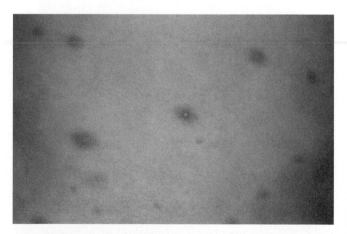

German Measles (Rubella)

Pink papular rash (similar to measles but paler) first appears on face, then spreads. Distinguished from measles by presence of neck lymphadenopathy and absence of Koplik's spots.

Chicken Pox (Varicella)

Small tight vesicles first appear on trunk, then spread to face, arms, and legs (not palms or soles). Shiny vesicles on an erythematous base are commonly described as the "dewdrop on a rose petal." Vesicles erupt in succeeding crops over several days, then become pustules, and then crusts. Intensely pruritic.

TABLE 12-9	Common Skin Lesions

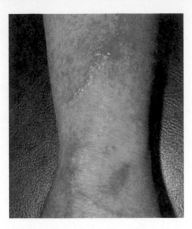

Primary Contact Dermatitis

Local inflammatory reaction to an irritant in the environment or an allergy. Characteristic location of lesions often gives clue. Often erythema shows first, followed by swelling, wheals (or urticaria), or maculopapular vesicles, scales. Frequently accompanied by intense pruritus. Example here: poison ivy.

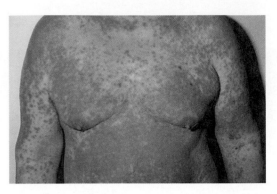

Allergic Drug Reaction

Erythematous and symmetrical rash, usually generalized. Some drugs produce urticarial rash or vesicles and bullae. History of drug ingestion.

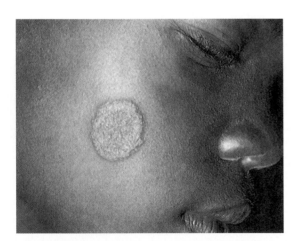

Tinea Corporis (Ringworm of the Body)

Scales—hyperpigmented in white-skinned individuals, depigmented in dark-skinned individuals—on chest, abdomen, back of arms forming multiple circular lesions with clear centres.

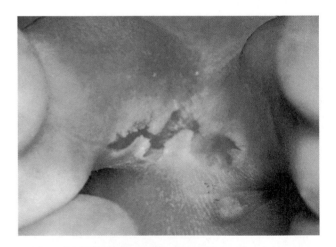

Tinea Pedis (Ringworm of the Foot)

"Athlete's foot," a fungal infection, first appears as small vesicles between toes, sides of feet, soles. Then grows scaly and hard. Found in chronically warm, moist feet: children after gymnasium activities, athletes, aging adults who cannot dry their feet well.

Continued

TABLE 12-9 | Common Skin Lesions—cont'd

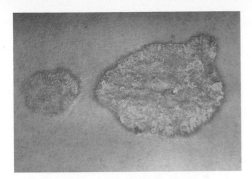

Psoriasis

Scaly erythematous patch, with silvery scales on top. Usually on scalp, outside of elbows and knees, low back, and anogenital area.

Tinea Versicolor

Fine, scaling, round patches of pink, tan, or white that do not tan in sunlight (hence the name), caused by a superficial fungal infection. Usual distribution is on neck, trunk, and upper arms—a short-sleeved turtleneck sweater area. Most common in otherwise-healthy young adults.

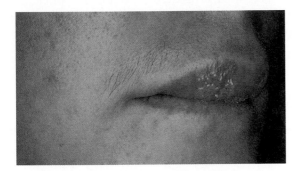

Labial Herpes Simplex (Cold Sores)

Herpes simplex virus (HSV) infection has a prodrome of skin tingling and sensitivity. Lesion then erupts with tight vesicles followed by pustules and then produces acute gingivostomatitis with many shallow, painful ulcers. Common location is upper lip; also in oral mucosa and tongue.

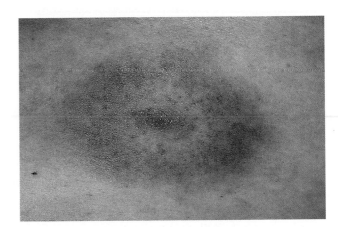

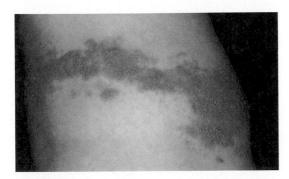

Herpes Zoster (Shingles)

Small grouped vesicles emerge along route of cutaneous sensory nerve, then pustules, then crusts. Caused by the varicella zoster virus (VZV), a reactivation of the dormant virus of chicken pox. Acute appearance, almost always unilateral, does not cross midline. Commonly on trunk, but can be anywhere. If on ophthalmic branch of cranial nerve V, it poses risk to eye. Most common in adults more than 50 years old. Pain is often severe and long lasting in aging adults, called *postherpetic neuralgia*.

Erythema Migrans of Lyme Disease

Lyme disease (LD) is not fatal, but may have serious arthritic, cardiac, or neurological sequelae. It is caused by a spirochete bacterium carried by the black or dark brown deer tick. Deer ticks are common in Canada and are carried across the country from endemic areas in the United States and Canada by migrating birds. Due to the tick's 2-year life cycle, individuals can become infected all year long (Ogden et al., 2006). The first stage (early localized LD) has the distinctive bull's-eye, red macular or papular rash (shown above) in 50% of cases. The rash radiates from the site of the tick bite (5 cm or larger), with some central clearing, and is usually located in axilla, midriff, inquina, or behind knee, with regional lymphadenopathy. Rash fades in 4 weeks; untreated individual then may have disseminated disease with fatigue, anorexia, fever, chills, joint or muscle aches. Antibiotic treatment shortens symptoms and decreases risk of sequelae.

| TABLE 12-10 | Malignant Skin Lesions |

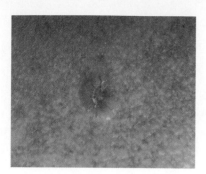

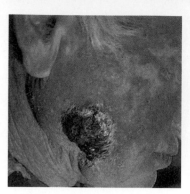

Basal Cell Carcinoma

Usually starts as a skin-coloured papule (may be deeply pigmented) with a translucent top and overlying telangiectasia. Then develops rounded pearly borders with central red ulcer, or looks like large open pore with central yellowing. One of the most common forms of skin cancer. It progresses slowly and rarely causes death.

Squamous Cell Carcinoma

Erythematous scaly patch with sharp margins, 1 cm or more. Develops central ulcer and surrounding erythema. Usually on hands or head, areas exposed to solar radiation. As common as basal cell carcinoma in Canada; progresses slowly and is usually easily removed by surgery.

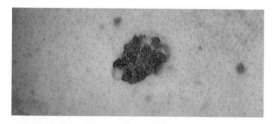

Malignant Melanoma

Half these lesions arise from pre-existing nevi. Usually brown; can be tan, black, pink-red, purple, or mixed pigmentation. Often irregular or notched borders. May have scaling, flaking, oozing texture. Common locations are on the trunk and back in men and women, on the legs in women, and on the palms, soles of feet, and the nails in those of African descent. Melanoma represents only 1 to 2% of all skin cancers, yet is the most fatal; 20% of all Canadians diagnosed with melanoma will die. Occurs earlier in life and progresses rapidly.

TABLE 12-11   Skin Lesions Associated With Acquired Immune Deficiency Syndrome

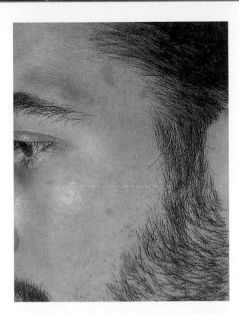

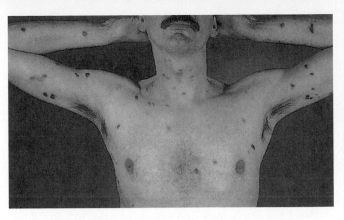

2. Epidemic Kaposi's Sarcoma: Plaque Stage ▲

Evolving lesions develop into raised papules or thickened plaques. These are oval and vary in colour from red to brown.

1. Epidemic Kaposi's Sarcoma: Patch Stage

An aggressive form of Kaposi's sarcoma is one of the diseases that characterizes AIDS. Here, multiple patch-stage early lesions are faint pink on the temple and beard area. They easily could be mistaken for bruises or nevi and be ignored.

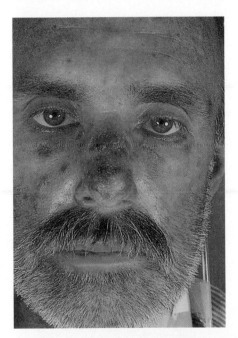

3. Epidemic Kaposi's Sarcoma: Advanced Disease

Advanced-stage, widely disseminated lesions involving skin, mucous membranes, and visceral organs. Here, violet-coloured tumours cover the nose and face, and a tiny cherry-red tumour nodule is on the inner canthus of the right eye.

TABLE 12-12 | **Infectious Disease as a Biological Weapon**

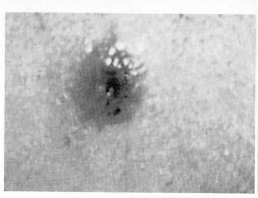
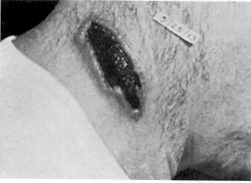

Anthrax

Cutaneous anthrax is caused by *Bacillus anthracis* (an encapsulated, spore-forming bacteria) when it comes in contact with a pre-existing lesion or broken skin, usually on the head, neck, or extremities. After 3 days, a red, raised, pruritic papule appears, followed by a round ulcer with surrounding vesicles a few days later (forearm lesion on left). Area edema and tender lymphadenopathy are common. A tough, painless, black scab, or *eschar*, forms in a few weeks (neck lesion on right), which loosens and falls off in another few weeks. Antibiotics decrease the risk of systemic disease.

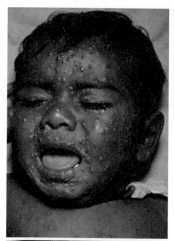

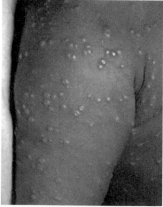

◄ **Smallpox (Variola Major)**

Smallpox is a viral infection with no known treatment, which was declared eradicated worldwide in 1980 by the World Health Organization, and routine vaccination stopped.

Disease is spread by direct contact or inhalation of respiratory droplets. After exposure and an incubation period of 10 to 12 days, the person develops flu-like symptoms of malaise, fever, myalgia, headache, vomiting; then a maculopapular rash appears, first on the oral mucosa, face and arms, later on the trunk. Lesions are uniform in appearance and become vesicular, then pustular and umbilicated (as opposed to chicken pox lesions, which are in various stages, more superficial, and are more numerous on the trunk). In a few weeks, the lesions form crusts and drop away leaving pitted scars. The present treatment is supportive only, and mortality rate is 30 to 40%.

TABLE 12-13   Abnormal Conditions of Hair

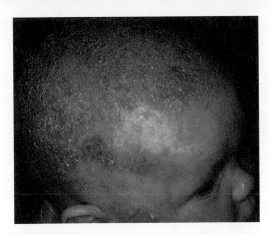

Seborrheic Dermatitis (Cradle Cap)

Thick, yellow to white, greasy, adherent scales with mild erythema on scalp and forehead; very common in early infancy. Resembles eczema lesions except cradle cap is distinguished by absence of pruritus, "greasy" yellow-pink lesions, and negative family history of allergy.

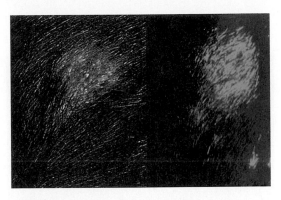

Tinea Capitis (Scalp Ringworm)

Rounded patchy hair loss on scalp, leaving broken-off hairs, pustules, and scales on skin. Caused by fungal infection; lesions may fluoresce blue-green under Wood's light. Usually seen in children and farmers; highly contagious; routes of transmission include other people, domestic animals, and soil.

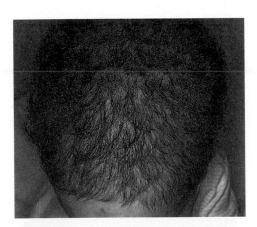

Toxic Alopecia

Patchy, asymmetric balding that accompanies severe illness or use of chemotherapy where growing hairs are lost and resting hairs are spared. Regrowth occurs after illness or discontinuation of toxin.

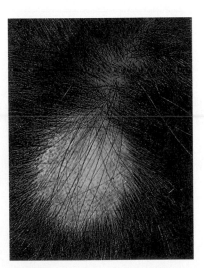

Alopecia Areata

Sudden appearance of a sharply circumscribed, round or oval balding patch, usually with smooth, soft, hairless skin underneath. Unknown cause; when limited to a few patches, person usually has complete regrowth.

TABLE 12-13 | **Abnormal Conditions of Hair—cont'd**

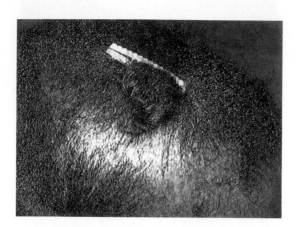

Traumatic Alopecia: Traction Alopecia

Linear or oval patch of hair loss along hairline, a part, or with scattered distribution; caused by trauma from hair rollers, tight braiding, tight ponytail, barrettes.

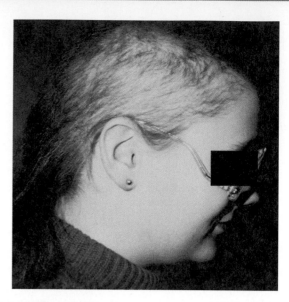

Trichotillomania

Traumatic self-induced hair loss usually the result of compulsive twisting or plucking. Forms irregularly shaped patch, with broken-off, stublike hairs of varying lengths; person is never completely bald. Occurs as child rubs or twists area absently while falling asleep, reading, or watching television. In adults it can be a serious problem and is usually a sign of a personality disorder.

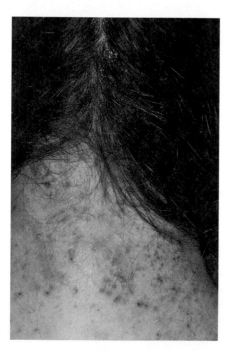

Pediculosis Capitis (Head Lice)

History includes intense itching of the scalp, especially the occiput. The nits (eggs) of lice are easier to see in the occipital area and around the ears, appearing as 2- to 3-mm oval translucent bodies, adherent to the hair shafts. Common among school-age children. Over-the-counter pediculicide shampoos are available; however, nit removal by daily combing of wet hair with a fine-tooth metal comb is especially important.

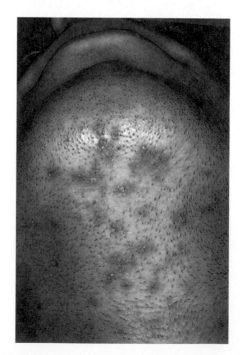

Folliculitis

Superficial infection of hair follicles. Multiple pustules, "whiteheads," with hair visible at centre and erythematous base. Usually on arms, legs, face, and buttocks.

Continued

TABLE 12-13 | Abnormal Conditions of Hair—cont'd

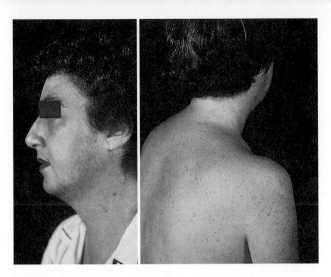

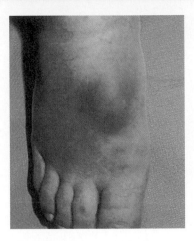

Hirsutism

Excess body hair in females forming a male sexual pattern (upper lip, face, chest, abdomen, arms, legs); caused by endocrine or metabolic dysfunction; occasionally idiopathic.

Furuncle and Abscess

Red, swollen, hard, tender, pus-filled lesion caused by acute localized bacterial (usually staphylococcal) infection; usually on back of neck, buttocks, occasionally on wrists or ankles. Furuncles are due to infected hair follicles, whereas abscesses are due to traumatic introduction of bacteria into the skin. Abscesses are usually larger and deeper than furuncles.

TABLE 12-14 | Abnormal Conditions of the Nails

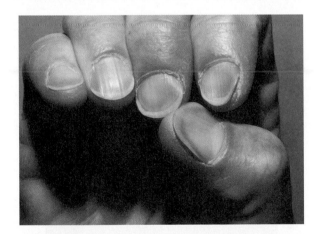

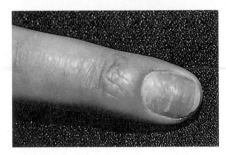

Paronychia

Red, swollen, tender inflammation of the nail folds. Acute paronychia is usually a bacterial infection; chronic paronychia is most often a fungal infection from a break in the cuticle in those who perform "wet" work.

Koilonychia (Spoon Nails)

Thin, depressed nails with lateral edges tilted up, forming a concave profile. May be congenital or a hereditary trait; if all nails are involved, may be due to iron deficiency anemia.

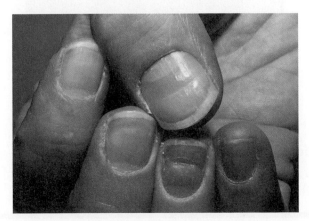

Beau's Line ▶

Transverse furrow or groove. A depression across the nail that extends down to the nail bed. Occurs with any trauma that temporarily impairs nail formation, such as acute illness, toxic reaction, or local trauma. Dent appears first at the cuticle and moves forward as nail grows.

TABLE 12-14	Abnormal Conditions of the Nails—cont'd

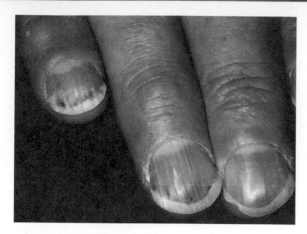

Splinter Hemorrhages

Red-brown linear streaks, embolic lesions, occur with subacute bacterial endocarditis; also may occur with minor trauma.

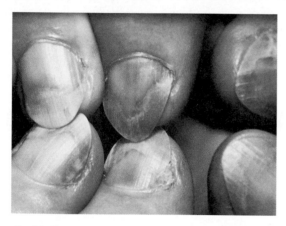

Onycholysis

This is a slow, persistent fungal infection of fingernails and, more often, toenails, common in older adults. Fungus causes change in colour (green where nail plate separates from bed), texture, thickness, with nail crumbling or breaking, and loosening of the nail plate, usually beginning at the distal edge and progressing proximally.

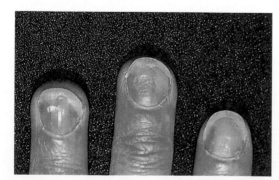

Pitting

Sharply defined pitting and crumbling of the nails with distal detachment often occurs with psoriasis.

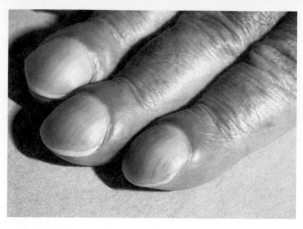

Late Clubbing

Proximal edge of nail elevates; angle is greater than 180 degrees. Distal phalanx looks rounder and wider. Seen with chronic obstructive pulmonary disease and congenital heart disease with cyanosis. Occurs first in thumb and index finger.

Reprinted from the Clinical Slide Collection on the Rheumatic Diseases, © 1991, 1995, 1997. Used by permission of the American College of Rheumatology.

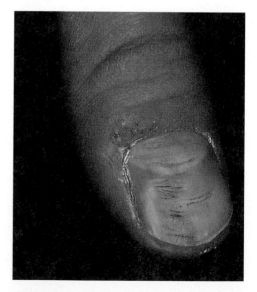

Habit-Tic Dystrophy

Depression down middle of nail or multiple horizontal ridges, caused by continuous picking of cuticle by another finger of same hand, which causes injury to nail base and nail matrix.

BIBLIOGRAPHY

Anderson, R. B., & Holman, J. R. (2006). Moles and melanoma: Clues to early detection. *Consultant, 46,* 1474–1481.

Bratton, R., & Corey, G. (2005). Tick-borne disease. *American Family Physician, 71,* 2323–2330.

Brook, I. (2005). Management of human and animal bite wounds: An overview. *Advances in Skin and Wound Care, 18,* 197–203.

Canadian Cancer Society. (2007). *SunSense guidelines.* Retrieved January, 26, 2008, from http://www.cancer.ca/ccs/internet/standard/0,3182,3172_13247__langId-en,00.html

Canadian Cancer Society/National Cancer Institute of Canada. (2007). *Canadian cancer statistics 2007.* Retrieved January 26, 2008, from http://www.cancer.ca/vgn/images/portal/cit_86751114/36/15/1816216925cw_2007stats_en.pdf

Dixon, T. C., & Guillemin, J. (1999). Anthrax. *New England Journal of Medicine, 341,* 815–825.

Emond, R. T., Welsby, P., & Rowland, H. (2003). *Colour atlas of infectious diseases* (4th ed.). St Louis, MO: Mosby.

Friedman-Kien, A. E. (1996). *Color atlas of AIDS* (2nd ed.). Philadelphia, PA: W.B. Saunders.

Gibson, W. (2006a). Rashes and fever in children: Sorting out the potentially dangerous, part 1. *Consultant, 46*(1), 49–60.

Gibson, W. (2006b). Rashes and fever in children: Sorting out the potentially dangerous, part 2. *Consultant, 46*(1), 83–88.

Gill, S. (2006). An overview of atopic eczema in children: A significant disease. *British Journal of Nursing, 15,* 494–499.

Godyn, J. J, Reyes, L., Siderits, R., & Hazra, A. (2005). Cutaneous anthrax: Conservative or surgical treatment? *Advances in Skin and Wound Care, 18,* 146–150.

Habif, T. P., Campbell, J. I., Chapman, M. S., Dinulos, J. G. H., & Zug, K. A. (2005). *Skin disease: Diagnosis and treatment* (2nd ed.). St. Louis, MO: Mosby.

Halpern, A., Phelan, D., & Oliveria, S. (2005). Skin self-examinations. *Dermatology Nursing, 17,* 109–114.

Hampton, T. (2005). Skin cancer's ranks rise: Immunosuppression to blame. *Journal of the American Medical Association, 294,* 1476–1480.

Health Canada. (2005). *Guidelines for tanning salon owners, operators and users: A guideline published in collaboration with federal, provincial and territorial radiation protection committee.* Retrieved January 26, 2008, from http://www.hc-sc.gc.ca/ahc-asc/alt_formats/hecs-sesc/pdf/psp-psp/ccrpb-bpcrpcc/guidelines_tanning_salon_owners_operators_users.pdf

Health Canada. (2006). *Preventing skin cancer.* Retrieved January 26, 2008, from http://www.hc-sc.gc.ca/iyh-vsv/alt_formats/cmcd-dcmc/pdf/skincancer_e.pdf

Holzberg, M. (2006). Common nail disorders. *Dermatology Clinics, 24,* 349–354.

James, W. (2005). Acne. *New England Journal of Medicine, 352,* 1463–1472.

Joslin, N. (2004). Early identification key to scleroderma treatment. *Nurse Practitioner, 29*(7), 24–41.

Karnath, B. (2005). Easy bruising and bleeding in the adult patient: a sign of underlying disease. *Hospital Physician, 41*(1), 35–39.

Lazovich, D., Forster, J., Sorensen, G., Emmons, K., Stryker, J., Demierre M. F., et al. (2004). Characteristics associated with use or intention to use indoor tanning among adolescents. *Archives of Pediatric and Adolescent Medicine, 158,* 918–924.

Luba, M., Bangs, S. A., Mohler, A. M., & Stulberg, D. L. (2003). Common benign skin tumors. *American Family Physician, 67,* 729–738.

Maguire-Eisen, M. (2003). Risk assessment and early detection of skin cancers. *Seminars in Oncology Nursing, 19*(1), 43–51.

Marks, J. G., & Miller, J. (2006). *Lookingbill and Marks' principles of dermatology* (4th ed.). Philadelphia, PA: W.B. Saunders.

Massey, D. (2006). The value and role of skin and nail assessment in the critically ill. *Nursing Critical Care, 11*(2), 80–85.

Mayer, B. W., & Burns, P. (2000). Differential diagnosis of abuse injuries in infants and young children. *Nurse Practitioner, 25*(10), 15–37.

Nadelman, R. (2006). Tick-borne diseases: A focus on Lyme disease. *Infections in Medicine, 23,* 267–272, 279–280.

Ogden, N., Trudel, L., Artsob, H., et al. (2006). *Ixodes scapularis* ticks collected by passive surveillance in Canada: Analysis of geographic distribution and infection with Lyme borreliosis agent *Borrelia burgdorferi. Journal of Medical Entomology, 43,* 600–609.

Oliviero, M. C. (2002). How to diagnose malignant melanoma. *Nurse Practitioner, 27*(2), 26–37.

Ollstein, R. (2004). Skin lesions in the elderly: Precancer and cancer. *Care Management Journal, 5,* 107–111.

Persell, D. J., Arangie, P., Young, C., Stokes, E. N., Payne, W. C., Skorga, P., et al. (2001). Preparing for bioterrorism: Category A agents. *Nurse Practitioner, 26*(12), 12–29.

Phelan, D. L., Oliveria, S. C. D., & Halpern, A. C. (2005). Patient experiences with photo books in monthly skin self-examinations. *Dermatology Nursing, 17,* 109–114.

Powell, F. (2005). Rosacea. *New England Journal of Medicine, 352,* 793–803.

Reilly, C. M., & Deason, D. (2002). Smallpox. *American Journal of Nursing, 102*(2), 51–55.

Roebuck, H. (2005). Face up to rosacea. *Nurse Practitioner, 30*(9), 24–35.

Roebuck, H., & Siegel, M. (2006). The ABCs of melanoma recognition. *Nurse Practitioner, 31*(6), 11–13.

Simmerman, J. M. (2002). Advances in DNA vaccines. *Nurse Practitioner, 27*(1), 53–61.

Specter, M. (2005, May 23). Higher risk: Crystal meth, the Internet, and dangerous choices about AIDS. *New Yorker,* 38–45.

Spector, R. E. (2004). *Cultural diversity in health and illness.* Upper Saddle River, NJ: Prentice Hall.

Sullivan, J. R., & Shear, N. H. (2002). Drug eruptions and other adverse drug effects in aged skin. *Clinics in Geriatric Medicine, 18*(1), 21–42.

Talbot, L., & Curtis, L. (1996). The challenges of assessing skin indicators in people of color. *Home Healthcare Nurse, 14,* 167–171.

Trent, J., & Kirsner, R. (2004). Cutaneous manifestations of HIV: A primer. *Advances in Skin and Wound Care, 17,* 116–129.

Tuchman, M., & Weinberg, J. (2006). Why everyone's skin needs to be examined. *Clinical Advisor, 9*(2), 33–34, 37–38.

U.S. Preventive Services Task Force. (2004). Counseling to prevent skin cancer: Recommendations and rationale. *American Journal of Nursing, 104*(4), 87–91.

Wakabayshi, I. (2005). Sensitivity of circulatory response to alcohol influences the relationship between alcohol consumption and blood pressure in Orientals. *Blood Pressure, 14,* 238–244.

Head, Face, and Neck, Including Regional Lymphatics

Written by **Carolyn Jarvis**, PhD, APN, CNP
Adapted by **June MacDonald-Jenkins**, RN, BScN, MSc

Electronic Resources

On Evolve *evolve*

**http://evolve.elsevier.com/Canada/Jarvis/
examination/**

- Interactive Case Studies
- Physical Examination Audio and
  Printable Summaries
- Bedside Assessment Summary Checklists
- Complete Physical Examination Form
- Nursing Diagnoses Boxes
- Health Promotion Guides
- Quick Assessments for 20 Common
  Conditions
- Multiple Choice Review Questions
- Chapter Objectives
- Appendices
- Weblinks

On the Companion CD

- Interactive Case Studies with Heart and
  Lung Sounds
- Health Promotion Guides
- Quick Assessments for 20 Common
  Conditions
- Head-to-Toe Physical Examination
  Video Clips

STRUCTURE AND FUNCTION

THE HEAD

The **skull** is a rigid bony box that protects the brain and special sense organs, and it includes the bones of the cranium and the face (Fig. 13-1). Note the location of these **cranial bones:** frontal, parietal, occipital, and temporal. Use these names to describe any of your findings in the corresponding areas.

The adjacent cranial bones unite at meshed immovable joints called the **sutures.** The bones are not firmly joined at birth; this allows for the mobility and change in shape needed for the birth process. The sutures gradually ossify during early childhood. The **coronal** suture *crowns* the head from ear to ear at the union of the frontal and parietal bones. The **sagittal** suture *separates* the head lengthwise between the two parietal bones. The **lambdoid** suture separates the parietal bones crosswise from the occipital bone.

The 14 **facial bones** also articulate at sutures (note the nasal bone, zygomatic bone, and maxilla), except for the mandible (the lower jaw). It moves up, down, and sideways from the temporomandibular joints, which are anterior to the ears.

The cranium is supported by the cervical vertebra: C1, the "atlas"; C2, the "axis"; and down to C7. The C7 vertebra has a long spinous process that is palpable when the head is flexed. Feel this useful landmark, the **vertebra prominens,** on your own neck.

The human **face** has myriad appearances and a large array of facial expressions that reflect mood. The expressions are formed by the facial muscles (Fig. 13-2), which are mediated by cranial nerve VII, the facial nerve. Facial muscle function is symmetrical bilaterally, except for an occasional quirk or wry expression.

Facial structures also are symmetrical; the eyebrows, eyes, ears, nose, and mouth appear about the same on both sides. The palpebral fissures—the openings between the eyelids— are equal bilaterally. Also, the nasolabial folds, the creases extending from the nose to each corner of the mouth, should look symmetrical. Facial sensations of pain or touch are mediated by the three sensory branches of cranial nerve V, the trigeminal nerve. (Testing for sensory function is described in Chapter 23.)

Two pairs of **salivary glands** are accessible to examination on the face (Fig. 13-3). The **parotid** glands are in the cheeks over the mandible, anterior to and below the ear. They are the largest of the salivary glands but are not normally palpable. The **submandibular** glands are beneath the mandible at the angle of the jaw. A third pair, the **sublingual** glands, lie in the floor of the mouth. (Salivary gland function follows in Chapter 16.) The **temporal artery** lies superior to the temporalis muscle, and its pulsation is palpable anterior to the ear.

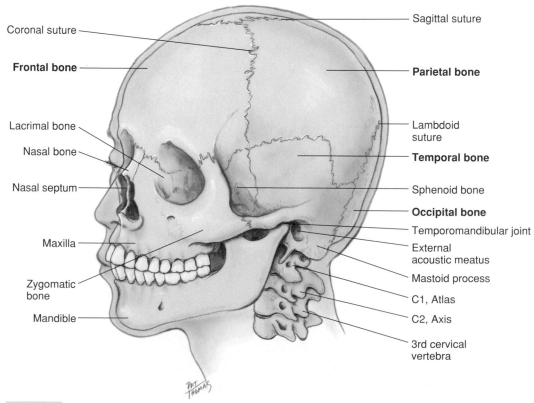

Coronal suture

Frontal bone

Lacrimal bone

Nasal bone

Nasal septum

Maxilla

Zygomatic bone

Mandible

Sagittal suture

Parietal bone

Lambdoid suture

Temporal bone

Sphenoid bone

Occipital bone

Temporomandibular joint

External acoustic meatus

Mastoid process

C1, Atlas

C2, Axis

3rd cervical vertebra

Fig. 13-1

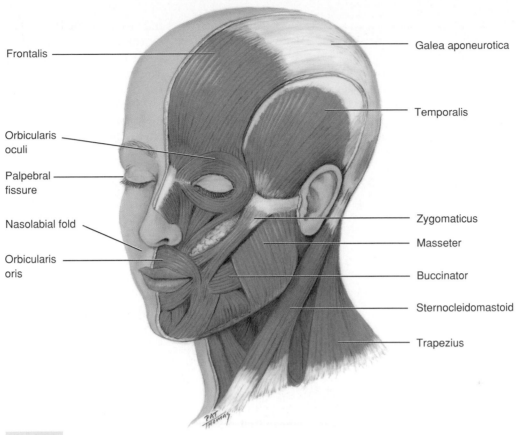

Frontalis

Galea aponeurotica

Temporalis

Orbicularis oculi

Palpebral fissure

Zygomaticus

Nasolabial fold

Masseter

Orbicularis oris

Buccinator

Sternocleidomastoid

Trapezius

Fig. 13-2   Facial muscles.

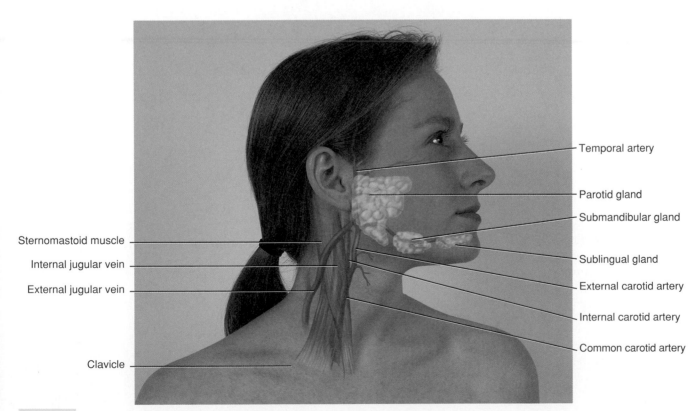

Temporal artery

Parotid gland

Submandibular gland

Sternomastoid muscle

Sublingual gland

Internal jugular vein

External jugular vein

External carotid artery

Internal carotid artery

Common carotid artery

Clavicle

Fig. 13-3

THE NECK

The **neck** is delimited by the base of the skull and inferior border of the mandible above, and by the manubrium sterni, the clavicle, the first rib, and the first thoracic vertebra below. Think of the neck as a *conduit* for the passage of many structures, which are lying in close proximity: vessels, muscles, nerves, lymphatics, and viscera of the respiratory and digestive systems. Blood vessels include the common and internal carotid arteries and their associated veins. The internal carotid branches off the common carotid and runs inward and upward to supply the brain; the external carotid supplies the face, salivary glands, and superficial temporal area. The carotid artery and internal jugular vein lie beneath the sternomastoid muscle. The external jugular vein runs diagonally across the sternomastoid muscle. (Assessment of the neck vessels is discussed in Chapter 19.)

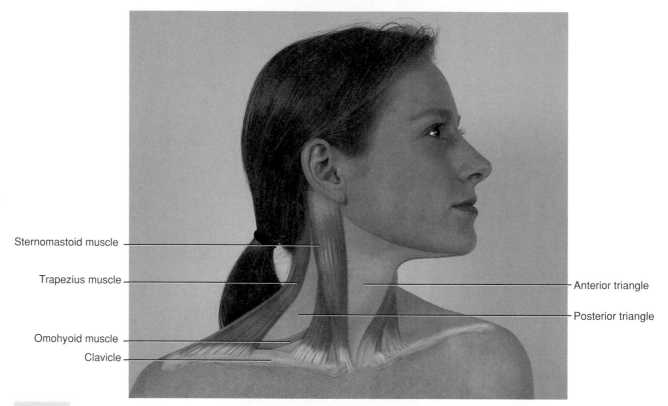

Sternomastoid muscle

Trapezius muscle

Omohyoid muscle

Clavicle

Anterior triangle

Posterior triangle

Fig. 13-4

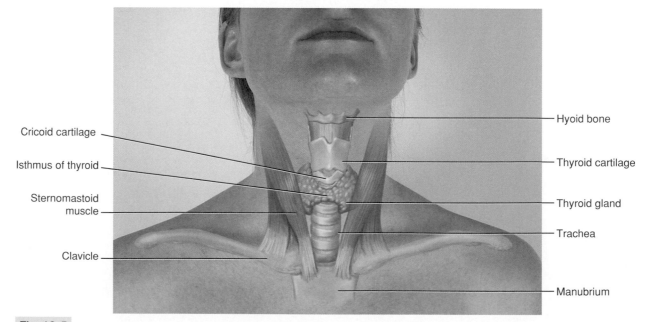

Cricoid cartilage

Isthmus of thyroid

Sternomastoid muscle

Clavicle

Hyoid bone

Thyroid cartilage

Thyroid gland

Trachea

Manubrium

Fig. 13-5

The major **neck muscles** are the **sternomastoid** and the **trapezius** (Fig. 13-4); they are innervated by cranial nerve XI, the spinal accessory. The sternomastoid muscle arises from the sternum and the medial part of the clavicle and extends diagonally across the neck to the mastoid process behind the ear. It accomplishes head rotation and head flexion. The two trapezius muscles form a trapezoid shape on the upper back. Each arises from the occipital bone and the vertebrae and extends fanning out to the scapula and clavicle. The trapezius muscles move the shoulders and extend and turn the head.

The sternomastoid muscle divides each side of the neck into two triangles. The **anterior triangle** lies in front, between the sternomastoid and the midline of the body, with its base up along the lower border of the mandible and its apex down at the suprasternal notch. The **posterior triangle** is behind the sternomastoid muscle, with the trapezius muscle on the other side and with its base along the clavicle below. It contains the posterior belly of the omohyoid muscle. These triangles are helpful guidelines when describing findings in the neck.

The **thyroid gland** is an important endocrine gland with a rich blood supply. It straddles the trachea in the middle of the neck (Fig. 13-5). This highly vascular endocrine gland synthesizes and secretes thyroxine (T_4) and triiodothyronine (T_3), hormones that stimulate the rate of cellular metabolism. The gland has two lobes, both conical in shape, each curving posteriorly between the trachea and the sternomastoid muscle. The lobes are connected in the middle by a thin isthmus lying over the second and third tracheal rings. (Sometimes a third lobe, the pyramidal lobe, is present. It is cone shaped,

usually on the left, and extends up toward the hyoid bone from the isthmus or from the neighbouring lobe.)

Just above the thyroid isthmus, within about 1 cm, is the **cricoid** cartilage or upper tracheal ring. The **thyroid** cartilage is above that, with a small palpable notch in its upper edge. This is the prominent "Adam's apple" in males. The highest is the **hyoid** bone, palpated high in the neck at the level of the floor of the mouth.

LYMPHATICS

The lymphatic system is discussed more fully in Chapter 20, p. 531. However, the head and neck have a rich supply of **lymph nodes** (Fig. 13-6). Although sources differ as to their nomenclature, one commonly used system is given here. Note that their labels correspond to adjacent structures.

- *Preauricular,* in front of the ear
- *Posterior auricular* (mastoid), superficial to the mastoid process
- *Occipital,* at the base of the skull
- *Submental,* midline, behind the tip of the mandible
- *Submandibular,* halfway between the angle and the tip of the mandible
- *Tonsillar,* under the angle of the mandible
- *Superficial cervical,* overlying the sternomastoid muscle
- *Deep cervical,* deep under the sternomastoid muscle
- *Posterior cervical,* in the posterior triangle along the edge of the trapezius muscle
- *Supraclavicular,* just above and behind the clavicle, at the sternomastoid muscle

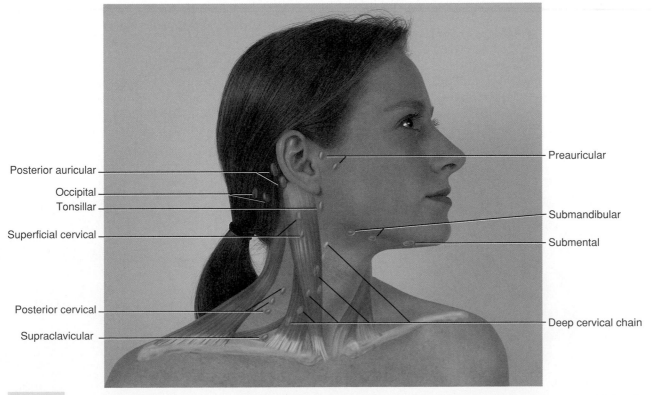

Posterior auricular

Occipital

Tonsillar

Superficial cervical

Posterior cervical

Supraclavicular

Preauricular

Submandibular

Submental

Deep cervical chain

Fig. 13-6

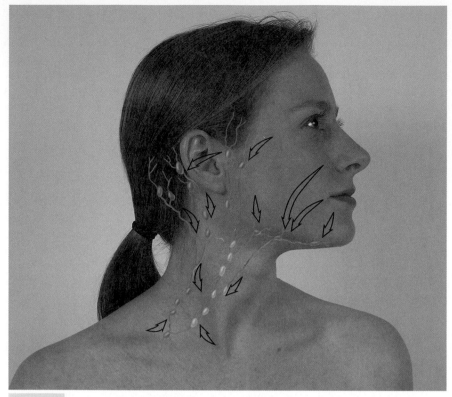

Fig. 13-7

You also should be familiar with the direction of the drainage patterns of the lymph nodes (Fig. 13-7). When nodes are abnormal, check the area they drain for the source of the problem. Explore the area proximal (upstream) to the location of the abnormal node.

The lymphatic system is an extensive vessel system, which is separate from the cardiovascular system and is phylogenetically older. The lymphatics are a major part of the immune system, whose job it is to detect and eliminate foreign substances from the body. The vessels allow the flow of clear, watery fluid (lymph) from the tissue spaces into the circulation. Lymph nodes are small, oval clusters of lymphatic tissue that are set at intervals along the lymph vessels like beads on a string. The nodes filter the lymph and engulf

pathogens, preventing potentially harmful substances from entering the circulation. Nodes are located throughout the body but are accessible to examination only in four areas: head and neck, arms, axillae, and inguinal region. The greatest supply is in the head and neck.

 DEVELOPMENTAL CARE

Infants and Children

The bones of the neonatal skull are separated by sutures and by **fontanelles,** the spaces where the sutures intersect (Fig. 13-8). These membrane-covered "soft spots" allow for growth of the brain during the first year. They gradually ossify; the

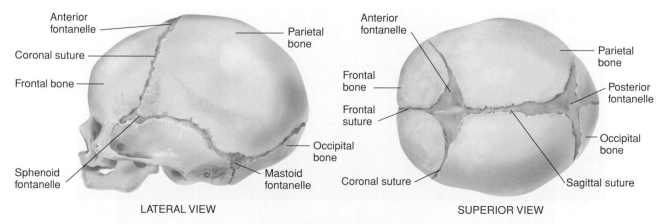

LATERAL VIEW

SUPERIOR VIEW

BONES OF THE NEONATAL SKULL

Fig. 13-8

© Pat Thomas, 2006.

triangle-shaped posterior fontanelle is closed by 1 to 2 months, and the diamond-shaped anterior fontanelle closes between 9 months and 2 years.

During the fetal period, head growth predominates. Head size is greater than chest circumference at birth. The head size grows during childhood, reaching 90% of its final size when the child is 6 years old. But during infancy, trunk growth predominates so that head size changes in proportion to body height. Facial bones grow at varying rates, especially nasal and jaw bones. In the toddler, the mandible and maxilla are small and the nasal bridge is low, so the whole face seems small compared with the skull.

Lymphoid tissue is well developed at birth and grows to adult size when the child is 6 years old. The child's lymphatic tissue continues to grow rapidly until age 10 or 11 years, actually exceeding its adult size before puberty. Then the lymphatic tissue slowly atrophies.

The appearance of acne in adolescence was discussed in the previous chapter. Facial hair also appears on boys at this time—first on the upper lip, then on cheeks and lower lip, and last on the chin. A noticeable enlargement of the thyroid cartilage occurs, and with it, the voice deepens.

The Pregnant Female

The thyroid gland enlarges slightly during pregnancy as a result of hyperplasia of the tissue and increased vascularity.

The Aging Adult

The facial bones and orbits appear more prominent, and the facial skin sags as a result of decreased elasticity, decreased subcutaneous fat, and decreased moisture in the skin. The lower face may look smaller if teeth have been lost.

SUBJECTIVE DATA

1. Headache	3. Dizziness	5. Lumps or swelling
2. Head injury	4. Neck pain, limitation of motion	6. History of head or neck surgery

Examiner Asks	Rationale
1. Headache. Any unusually frequent or unusually severe **headaches?** • Onset. When did *this kind* of headache start? • Gradual, over hours, or a day? • Or, suddenly, over minutes, or less than 1 hour? • Ever had *this kind* of headache before? • Location. Where do you feel it: frontal, temporal, behind your eyes, like a band around the head, in the sinus area, or in the occipital area? • Is pain localized on one side, or all over? • Character. Throbbing (pounding, shooting) or aching (viselike, constant pressure, dull)? • Is it mild, moderate, or severe? • Course and duration. What time of day do the headaches occur: morning, evening, awaken you from sleep? How long do they last? Hours, days? Have you noted any daily headaches, or several within a time period?	This is a more meaningful question than, "Do you ever have headaches?" because most people have had at least one headache. Because many conditions have a headache as a symptom, a detailed history is important. A red flag is a severe headache in an adult or child who has never had it before. Tension headaches tend to be occipital, frontal, or with bandlike tightness; migraines (vascular) tend to be supraorbital, retro-orbital, or frontotemporal; cluster headaches (vascular) produce pain around the eye, temple, forehead, cheek. Unilateral or bilateral (e.g., with cluster headaches pain is always unilateral and always on the same side of the head). Character is typically viselike with tension headache, throbbing with migraine or temporal arteritis. Quantity is often severe with migraine, or excruciating with cluster headache. Migraines occur about two per month, each lasting 1 to 3 days; one to two cluster headaches occur per day, each lasting $\frac{1}{2}$ to 2 hours for 1 or 2 months; then complete remission may last for months or years.

Examiner Asks	Rationale

- Precipitating factors. What brings it on: activity or exercise, work environment, emotional upset, anxiety, alcohol? (Also note signs of depression.)

- Associated factors. Any relation to other symptoms: any nausea and vomiting? (Note which came first, headache or nausea.) Any vision changes, pain with bright lights, neck pain or stiffness, fever, weakness, moodiness, stomach problems?

- Do you have any other illness?

- Do you take any medications?

- What makes it worse: movement, coughing, straining, exercise?
- Pattern. Any family history of headache?
  What is the frequency of your headaches: once a week? Are your headaches occurring closer together?
  Are they getting worse? Or are they getting better?
  (For females) When do they occur in relation to your menstrual periods?
- Effort to treat. What seems to help: going to sleep, medications, positions, rubbing the area?

- Coping strategies. How have these headaches affected your self-care, or your ability to function at work, home, and socially?

2. **Head injury.** Any **head injury** or blow to your head?
   - Onset. When? Please describe exactly what happened.
   - Setting: any hazardous conditions? Were you wearing a helmet or hard hat?
   - How about yourself just before injury: dizzy, lightheaded, had a blackout, had a seizure?
     Lost consciousness and then fell? (Note which came first.)
     Knocked unconscious? Or did you fall and lose consciousness a few minutes later?
   - Any history of illness (e.g., heart trouble, diabetes, epilepsy)?
   - Location. Exactly where did you hit your head?
   - Duration. How long were you unconscious?
     Any symptoms afterward—headache, vomiting, projectile vomiting?
     Any change in level of consciousness since injury: dazed or sleepy?

- Associated symptoms. Any pain in the head or the neck, vision change, discharge from ear or nose—is it bloody or watery? Are you able to move all extremities? Any tremors, staggered walk, numbness and tingling?
- Pattern. Symptoms became worse, better, unchanged since injury?
- Effort to treat. Emergency department or hospitalized? Any medications?

Rationale

Alcohol ingestion and daytime napping typically precipitate cluster headaches, whereas alcohol, letdown after stress, menstruation, and eating chocolate or cheese precipitate migraines.

Nausea, vomiting, and visual disturbances are associated with migraines; eye reddening and tearing, eyelid drooping, rhinorrhea, and nasal congestion are associated with cluster headaches; anxiety and stress are associated with tension headaches; nuchal rigidity and fever are associated with meningitis or encephalitis.

Hypertension, fever, hypothyroidism, and vasculitis produce headaches.

Oral contraceptives, bronchodilators, alcohol, nitrates, carbon monoxide inhalation produce headaches.

Migraines are associated with family history of migraine.

With migraines, people lie down to feel better, whereas with cluster headaches they need to move—even to pace the floor—to feel better.

Loss of consciousness *before* a fall may have a cardiovascular cause (e.g., heart block).

A change in level of consciousness is of prime importance in evaluating a neurological deficit.

Examiner Asks	Rationale

3. Dizziness. Experienced any **dizziness?**
(Determine exactly what the person means by dizziness.) Was it a feeling of lightheadedness or of falling? Or was it a spinning sensation?

Dizziness is a lightheaded, swimming sensation, feeling of falling. True *vertigo* is true rotational spinning from neurological disease (labyrinthine–vestibular apparatus, vestibular nuclei in brain stem).

When vertigo is *objective,* the perception is that the room spins. When vertigo is *subjective,* the perception is that the person spins.

- Onset. Abrupt or gradual? After a change in position, such as sudden standing?
- Associated factors. Any nausea and vomiting, pallor, immobility, decreased hearing acuity, or tinnitus along with the dizziness?

4. Neck pain, limitation of motion. Any **neck pain?**
- Onset. How did the pain start: injury, automobile accident, after lifting, from a fall? Or with fever? Or did it have a gradual onset?

Acute onset of stiffness with headache and fever occurs with meningeal inflammation.

- Location. Does pain radiate? To the shoulders, arms?
- Associated symptoms. Any **limitations to range of motion,** numbness or tingling in shoulders, arms, or hands?
- Precipitating factors. What movements cause pain? Do you need to lift or bend at work or home?
  Does stress seem to bring it on?
- Coping strategies. Able to do your work, to sleep?

Pain creates a vicious circle. Tension increases pain and disability, which produces more anxiety.

5. Lumps or swelling. Any **lumps or swelling** in the neck?
Any recent infection? Any tenderness?
For a lump that persists, how long have you had it? Has it changed in size?

Tenderness suggests acute infection.

A persistent lump arouses suspicion of malignancy. For those more than 40 years old, suspect malignancy until proven otherwise.

- Any history of prior irradiation of head, neck, upper chest?

Increased risk for salivary and thyroid tumours.

- Any difficulty swallowing?
- Do you smoke? For how long? How many packs a day? Do you chew tobacco?
- When was your last alcoholic drink? How much alcohol do you drink a day?
- Ever had a thyroid problem? Overfunctioning or underfunctioning? How was it treated: surgery, irradiation, any medication?

Dysphagia.

Smoking and chewing tobacco increase risk of oral and respiratory cancers.

Smoking and large alcohol consumption together increase the risk of cancer.

6. History of head or neck surgery. Ever had **surgery of the head or neck?**
For what condition? When did the surgery occur? How do you feel about results?

Surgery for head and neck cancer often is disfiguring and increases risk of body image disturbance.

Additional History for Infants and Children

1. Did the mother use alcohol or street drugs during pregnancy? How often? How much was used per episode?

Alcohol increases the risk of fetal alcohol syndrome, which includes distinctive facial features (see Table 13-3, p. 293). Cocaine use causes neurological, developmental, and emotional problems.

Examiner Asks	Rationale
2. Was delivery vaginal or by Caesarean section? Any difficulty? Use of forceps?	Forceps may increase the risk of caput succedaneum, cephalhematoma, and Bell's palsy.
3. What were you told about the baby's growth? Was it on schedule? Did the head seem to grow and fontanelles close on schedule? At what age (in months) did the baby achieve head control?	
Additional History for the Aging Adult	
1. If dizziness is a problem, how does this affect your daily activities? Are you able to drive safely, manoeuvre about the house safely?	Assess self-care. Assess potential for injury.
2. If neck pain is a problem, how does this affect your daily activities? Are you able to drive, perform at work, do housework, sleep, look down when using stairs?	

OBJECTIVE DATA

Normal Range of Findings	Abnormal Findings
THE HEAD	
INSPECT AND PALPATE THE SKULL	
Size and Shape	
Note the general size and shape. **Normocephalic** is the term that denotes a round symmetrical skull that is appropriately related to body size. Be aware that "normal" includes a wide range of sizes.	Deformities: microcephaly, abnormally small head; macrocephaly, abnormally large head (hydrocephaly, acromegaly, Paget's disease); see Table 13-1, p. 291.
To assess shape, place your fingers in the person's hair and palpate the scalp. The skull normally feels symmetrical and smooth. The cranial bones that have normal protrusions are the forehead, the lateral edge of each parietal bone, the occipital bone, and the mastoid process behind each ear. There is no tenderness to palpation.	Note lumps, depressions, or abnormal protrusions.
Temporal Area	
Palpate the temporal artery above the zygomatic (cheek) bone between the eye and top of the ear.	The artery looks more tortuous and feels hardened and tender with temporal arteritis.
The temporomandibular joint is just below the temporal artery and anterior to the tragus. Palpate the joint as the person opens the mouth, and note normally smooth movement with no limitation or tenderness.	Crepitation, limited range of motion (ROM), or tenderness.

Normal Range of Findings	Abnormal Findings

INSPECT THE FACE

Facial Structures

Inspect the face, noting the facial expression and its appropriateness to behaviour or reported mood. Anxiety is common in the hospitalized or ill person.

Although the shape of facial structures may vary somewhat among races, they always should be symmetrical. Note symmetry of eyebrows, palpebral fissures, nasolabial folds, and sides of the mouth.

Note any abnormal facial structures (coarse facial features, exophthalmos, changes in skin colour or pigmentation), or any abnormal swelling. Also note any involuntary movements (tics) in the facial muscles. Normally none occur.

Abnormal Findings:

Hostility or embarrassment.

Tense, rigid muscles may indicate anxiety or pain; a flat affect may indicate depression; excessive smiling may be inappropriate.

Marked asymmetry with central brain lesion (e.g., brain attack) or with peripheral cranial nerve VII damage (Bell's palsy). See Table 13-4, p. 294.

Edema in the face occurs first around the eyes (periorbital) and the cheeks, where the subcutaneous tissue is relatively loose.

Note grinding of jaws, tics, fasciculations, or excessive blinking.

THE NECK

INSPECT AND PALPATE THE NECK

Symmetry

Head position is centred in the midline, and the accessory neck muscles should be symmetrical. The head should be held erect and still.

Abnormal Findings:

Head tilt occurs with muscle spasm. Rigid head and neck occur with arthritis.

Range of Motion

Note any limitation of movement during active motion. Ask the person to touch the chin to the chest, turn the head to the right and left, try to touch each ear to the shoulder (without elevating shoulders), and to extend the head backward. When the neck is supple, motion is smooth and controlled.

Test muscle strength and the status of cranial nerve XI by trying to resist the person's movements with your hands as the person shrugs the shoulders and turns the head to each side.

As the person moves the head, note enlargement of the salivary glands and lymph glands. Normally no enlargement is present. Note a swollen parotid gland when the head is extended; look for swelling below the angle of the jaw. Also, note thyroid gland enlargement. Normally none is present.

Also note any obvious pulsations. The carotid artery runs medial to the sternomastoid muscle, and it creates a brisk localized pulsation just below the angle of the jaw. Normally, there are no other pulsations while the person is in the sitting position (see Chapter 19).

Abnormal Findings:

Note pain at any particular movement.

Note ratchety or limited movement from cervical arthritis or inflammation of neck muscles. The arthritic neck is rigid; the person turns at the shoulders rather than at the neck.

Thyroid enlargement may be a unilateral lump, or it may be diffuse and look like a doughnut lying across the lower neck (see Table 13-2, p. 292).

Lymph Nodes

Using a gentle circular motion of your fingerpads, palpate the lymph nodes (Fig. 13-9). (Normally, the salivary glands are not palpable. When symptoms warrant, check for parotid tenderness by palpating in a line from the outer corner of the

Abnormal Findings:

The parotid is swollen with mumps (see Table 13-2, p. 292).

Normal Range of Findings	**Abnormal Findings**

eye to the lobule of the ear.) Beginning with the preauricular lymph nodes in front of the ear, palpate the 10 groups of lymph nodes in a routine order. Many nodes are closely packed, so you must be systematic and thorough in your examination. Once you establish your sequence, do not vary or you may miss some small nodes.

Parotid enlargement has been found with acquired immune deficiency syndrome (AIDS).

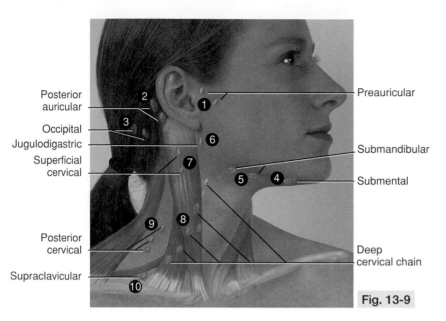

Posterior auricular
Occipital
Jugulodigastric
Superficial cervical
Posterior cervical
Supraclavicular

Preauricular
Submandibular
Submental
Deep cervical chain

Fig. 13-9

Use gentle pressure because strong pressure could push the nodes into the neck muscles. It is usually most efficient to palpate with both hands, comparing the two sides symmetrically. However, the submental gland under the tip of the chin is easier to explore with one hand. When you palpate with one hand, use your other hand to position the person's head. For the deep cervical chain, tip the person's head toward the side being examined to relax the ipsilateral muscle (Fig. 13-10). Then you can press your fingers under the muscle. Search for the supraclavicular node by having the person hunch the shoulders and elbows forward (Fig. 13-11); this relaxes the skin. The inferior belly of the omohyoid muscle crosses the posterior triangle here; do not mistake it for a lymph node.

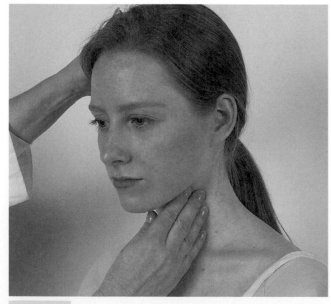

Fig. 13-10

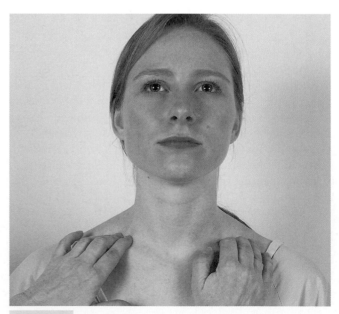

Fig. 13-11

Normal Range of Findings

If any nodes are palpable, note their location, size, shape, delimitation (discrete or matted together), mobility, consistency, and tenderness. Cervical nodes often are palpable in healthy persons, although this palpability decreases with age (Fig. 13-12). Normal nodes feel movable, discrete, soft, and nontender.

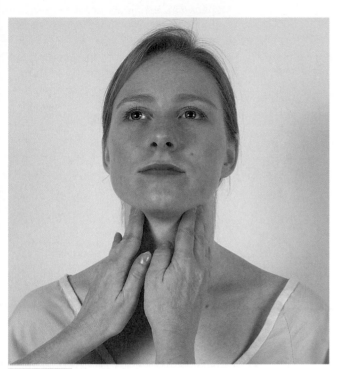

Fig. 13-12

If nodes are enlarged or tender, check the area they drain for the source of the problem. For example, those in the upper cervical or submandibular area often relate to inflammation or a neoplasm in the head and neck. Follow up on or refer your findings. An enlarged lymph node, particularly when you cannot find the source of the problem, deserves prompt attention.

Abnormal Findings

Lymphadenopathy is enlargement of the lymph nodes (>1 cm) from infection, allergy, or neoplasm.

The following criteria are common clues but are not definitive in all circumstances:

- Acute infection—nodes are bilateral, enlarged, warm, tender, and firm but freely movable.
- Chronic inflammation (e.g., in tuberculosis, the nodes are clumped).
- Cancerous nodes are hard, unilateral, nontender, and fixed.
- Nodes with human immunodeficiency virus (HIV) infection are enlarged, firm, nontender, and mobile. Occipital node enlargement is common with HIV infection.
- A single, enlarged, nontender, hard, left supraclavicular node (Virchow's node) may indicate a neoplasm in the thorax or abdomen.
- Painless, rubbery, discrete nodes that gradually appear occur with Hodgkin's lymphoma.

Normal Range of Findings	Abnormal Findings

Trachea

Normally, the trachea is midline; palpate for any tracheal shift. Place your index finger on the trachea in the sternal notch, and slip it off to each side (Fig. 13-13). The space should be symmetrical on both sides. Note any deviation from the midline.

Conditions of tracheal shift:
- The trachea is *pushed to the unaffected* (or healthy) side with an aortic aneurysm, a tumour, unilateral thyroid lobe enlargement, and pneumothorax.
- The trachea is *pulled toward the affected* (diseased) side with large atelectasis, pleural adhesions, or fibrosis.
- Tracheal tug is a rhythmic downward pull that is synchronous with systole and that occurs with aortic arch aneurysm.

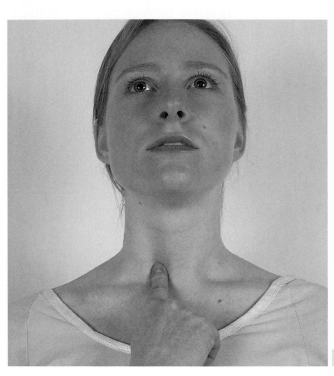

Fig. 13-13

Thyroid Gland

The thyroid gland is difficult to palpate; arrange your setting to maximize your likelihood of success. Position a standing lamp to shine tangentially across the neck to highlight any possible swelling. Supply the person with a glass of water, and first inspect the neck as the person takes a sip and swallows. Thyroid tissue moves up with a swallow.

Posterior Approach. To palpate, move behind the person (Fig. 13-14). Ask the person to sit up very straight and then to bend the head slightly forward and to the right. This will relax the neck muscles. Use the fingers of your left hand to push the trachea slightly to the right.

Look for diffused enlargement or a nodular lump.

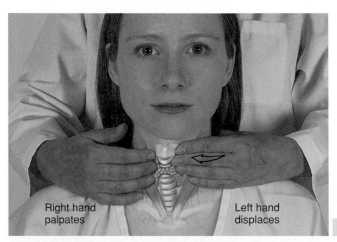

Right hand palpates   Left hand displaces

Fig. 13-14

Normal Range of Findings	Abnormal Findings

Then curve your right fingers between the trachea and the sternomastoid muscle, retracting it slightly, and ask the person to take a sip of water. The thyroid moves up under your fingers with the trachea and larynx as the person swallows. Reverse the procedure for the left side.

Usually you cannot palpate the normal adult thyroid. If the person has a long, thin neck, you sometimes will feel the isthmus over the tracheal rings. The lateral lobes usually are not palpable; check them for enlargement, consistency, symmetry, and the presence of nodules.

Abnormalities: enlarged lobes that are easily palpated before swallowing, or are tender to palpation; or the presence of nodules or lumps. See Table 13-2, p. 292.

Anterior Approach. This is an alternate method of palpating the thyroid, but it is more awkward to perform, especially for a beginning examiner. Stand facing the person. Ask him or her to tip the head forward and to the right. Use your right thumb to displace the trachea slightly to the person's right. Hook your left thumb and fingers around the sternomastoid muscle. Feel for lobe enlargement as the person swallows (Fig. 13-15).

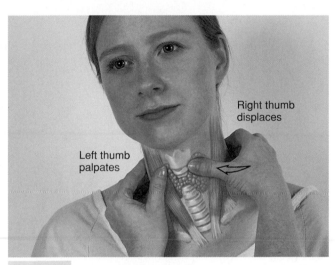

Right thumb displaces

Left thumb palpates

Fig. 13-15

Auscultate the Thyroid

If the thyroid gland is enlarged, auscultate it for the presence of a **bruit.** This is a soft, pulsatile, whooshing, blowing sound heard best with the bell of the stethoscope. The bruit is not present normally.

A bruit occurs with accelerated or turbulent blood flow, indicating hyperplasia of the thyroid (e.g., hyperthyroidism).

 DEVELOPMENTAL CARE

Infants and Children

Skull

Measure an infant's **head size** with measuring tape at each visit up to age 2 years, then yearly up to age 6 years. (Measurement of head circumference is presented in detail in Chapter 9.)

The newborn's head measures about 32 to 38 cm (average around 34 cm), and is 2 cm larger than chest circumference. At age 2 years, both measurements are the same. During childhood the chest circumference grows to exceed head circumference by 5 to 7 cm.

Note an abnormal increase in head size or failure to grow.

Microcephalic—head size below norms for age.

Macrocephalic—an enlarged head for age, or rapidly increasing in size (e.g., hydrocephalus [increased cerebrospinal fluid]).

Objective Data

Normal Range of Findings	Abnormal Findings

Normal Range of Findings

Observe the infant's head from all angles, not just the front. The contour should be symmetrical. Some racial variation occurs in normal head shapes; children of Nordic descent tend to have long heads, whereas those of Asian descent have broad heads.

Two common variations in the newborn cause the shape of the skull to look markedly asymmetrical: A **caput succedaneum** is edematous swelling and ecchymosis of the presenting part of the head caused by birth trauma (Fig. 13-16). It feels soft, and it may extend across suture lines. It gradually resolves during the first few days of life and needs no treatment.

Abnormal Findings

Frontal bulges, or "bossing," occur with prematurity or rickets.

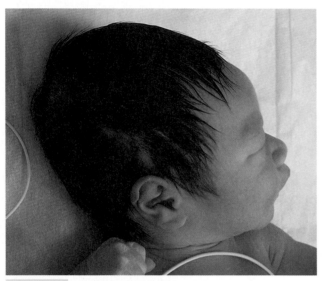

Fig. 13-16 Caput succedaneum.

A **cephalhematoma** is a subperiosteal hemorrhage, which is also a result of birth trauma (Fig. 13-17). It is soft, fluctuant, and well defined over one cranial bone because the periosteum (i.e., the covering over each bone) holds the bleeding in place. It appears several hours after birth and gradually increases in size. No discoloration is present, but it looks bizarre, so parents need reassurance that it will be reabsorbed during the first few weeks of life without treatment. Rarely, a large hematoma may persist to 3 months.

An infant with cephalhematoma is at greater risk for jaundice as the red blood cells within the hematoma are broken down and reabsorbed.

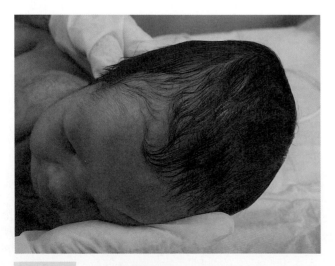

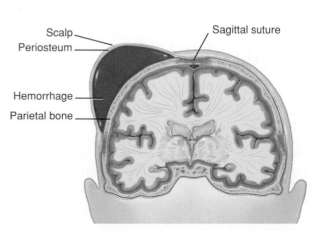

Scalp
Periosteum

Sagittal suture

Hemorrhage
Parietal bone

Fig. 13-17 Cephalhematoma.

Normal Range of Findings	Abnormal Findings

As you palpate the newborn's head, the suture lines feel like ridges. By 5 to 6 months, they are smooth and not palpable.

A newborn's head may feel asymmetrical and the involved ridges more prominent due to *moulding* of the cranial bones during engagement and passage through the birth canal. Moulding is overriding of the cranial bones; usually, the parietal bone overrides the frontal or occipital bone. Reassure parents that this lasts only a few days or a week. Babies delivered by Caesarean section are noted for their evenly round heads. Also, some asymmetry may occur if an infant continually sleeps in one position; this is a flattening of the dependent cranial bone, usually the occiput.

Gently palpate the skull and **fontanelles** while the infant is calm and somewhat in a sitting position (crying, lying down, or vomiting may cause the anterior fontanelle to look full and bulging). The skull should feel smooth and fused except at the fontanelles. The fontanelles feel firm, slightly concave, and well defined against the edges of the cranial bones. You may see slight arterial pulsations in the anterior fontanelle.

The posterior fontanelle may not be palpable at birth. If it is, it measures 1 cm and closes by 1 to 2 months. The anterior fontanelle may be small at birth and enlarges to 2.5 cm by 2.5 cm. A large diameter of 4 to 5 cm occasionally may be normal under 6 months. A small fontanelle usually is normal. The anterior fontanelle closes between 9 months and 2 years. Early closure may be insignificant if head growth proceeds normally.

Note the infant's **head posture** and **head control.** The infant can turn the head side to side by 2 weeks and shows the **tonic neck reflex** when supine and the head is turned to one side (extension of same arm and leg, flexion of opposite arm and leg). The tonic neck reflex disappears between 3 and 4 months, and then the head is maintained in the midline. Head control is achieved by 4 months, when the baby can hold the head erect and steady when pulled to a vertical position. (See Chapter 22 and Chapter 23 for further details on the musculoskeletal and neurological systems.)

Face

Check **facial features** for symmetry, appearance, and presence of swelling. Note symmetry of wrinkling when the infant cries or smiles (e.g., both sides of the lips rise and both sides of forehead wrinkle). Children love to comply when you ask them to "make a face." Normally, no swelling is evident. Parotid gland enlargement is seen best when the child sits and looks up at the ceiling; the swelling appears below the angle of the jaw.

Neck

An infant's neck looks short; it lengthens during the first 3 to 4 years. You can see the neck better by supporting the infant's shoulders and tilting the head back a little. This positioning also facilitates palpation of the trachea, which is buried deep in the neck. Feel for the row of cartilaginous rings in the midline or just slightly to the right of the midline.

Assess muscle development with gentle passive ROM. Cradle the infant's head with your hands and turn it side to side, and test forward flexion, extension, and rotation. Note any resistance to movement, especially flexion. Ask a child to actively move through the ROM, as you would an adult.

During infancy, cervical lymph nodes are not palpable normally. But a child's lymph nodes are—they feel more prominent than an adult's until after puberty,

Abnormal Findings (right column):

Sutures palpable when the child is older than 6 months.

Marked asymmetry, as in *craniosynostosis,* a severe deformity caused by premature closure of the sutures. Premature closing of the suture results in a long, narrow head.

Flattening also occurs in children with rickets.

A true tense or bulging fontanelle occurs with acute increased intracranial pressure.

Depressed and sunken fontanelles occur with dehydration or malnutrition.

Marked pulsations occur with increased intracranial pressure.

Delayed closure or larger-than-normal fontanelle size occurs with hydrocephalus, Down syndrome, hypothyroidism, or rickets.

A small fontanelle is a sign of microcephaly, as is early closure.

Tonic neck reflex beyond 5 months may indicate brain damage.

In children, head tilt occurs with habit spasm, poor vision, and brain tumour.

Head lag after 4 months may indicate intellectual or motor disability.

Unilateral immobility indicates nerve damage (central or peripheral) (e.g., note angle of mouth droop on paralyzed side).

Some facies are characteristic of congenital abnormalities or chronic allergy. See Tables 13-3 and 13-4, pp. 293 and 294.

A short neck or webbing (loose fanlike folds) may indicate congenital abnormality (e.g., Down or Turner's syndrome), or it may occur alone.

Head tilt and limited ROM occur with torticollis (wryneck), or from sternomastoid muscle injury during birth or a congenital defect.

Resistance to flexion (nuchal rigidity) and pain on flexion indicate meningeal irritation or meningitis.

Cervical nodes >1 cm are considered enlarged.

Normal Range of Findings	**Abnormal Findings**

when lymphoid tissue begins to atrophy. Palpable nodes less than 3 mm are normal. They may be up to 1 cm in size in the cervical and inguinal areas but are discrete, move easily, and are nontender. Children have a higher incidence of infection, so you will expect a greater incidence of inflammatory adenopathy. No other mass should occur in the neck.

The thyroid gland is difficult to palpate in an infant because of the short, thick neck. The child's thyroid may be palpable normally.

Special Procedures

Palpation. *Craniotabes* is a softening of the skull's outer layer. With a newborn, pressure along the suture of the parietal and occipital bones above the ear produces a snapping sensation because of the pliable skull bone. It is like indenting a Ping-Pong ball and feeling it snap back. Do not attempt this unless craniotabes is suspected because of other abnormal findings, and even then avoid excessive pressure. Craniotabes may be normal, especially with premature infants.

Percussion. With an infant, you may directly percuss with your plexor finger against the head surface. This yields a resonant or "cracked pot" sound, which is normal before closure of the fontanelles.

Auscultation. Bruits are common in the skull in children under 4 or 5 years of age or in children with anemia. They are systolic or continuous and are heard over the temporal area.

Transillumination. Use this procedure if you suspect an abnormal head size or an intracranial lesion. In a completely darkened room, hold a rubber-collared flashlight firmly against the infant's skull. You need a tight fit against the head. Explore all regions of the head: frontal, both sides, occiput (Fig. 13-18). A small ring of light around the flashlight is normal (less than 2 cm in the frontal area, less than 1 cm in the occipital area). But you should not see a larger halo around the rubber collar.

Abnormal Findings:

Thyroglossal duct cyst—cystic lump high up in midline, freely movable, and rises up when swallowing.

Supraclavicular nodes enlarge with Hodgkin's disease.

Craniotabes may occur with rickets, hydrocephaly, or congenital syphilis.

The sound occurs with hydrocephalus from separation of cranial sutures (Macewen's sign).

After 5 years of age, bruits indicate increased intracranial pressure, aneurysm, or arteriovenous shunt.

Presence of a halo of light through the skull indicates a loss or thinning of cerebral cortex. If the cortex is absent, the entire cranium lights up (Fig. 13-19).

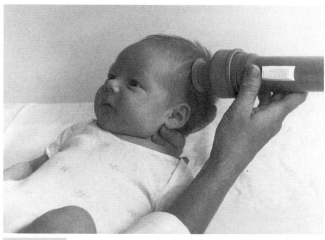

Fig. 13-18

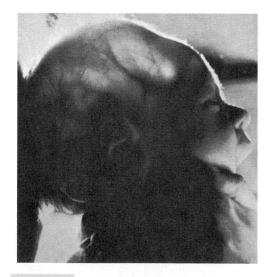

Fig. 13-19   Hydranencephaly.

The Pregnant Female

During the second trimester, chloasma may show on the face. This is a blotchy, hyperpigmented area over the cheeks and forehead that fades after delivery. The thyroid gland may be palpable normally during pregnancy.

The Aging Adult

The temporal arteries may look twisted and prominent. In some aging adults, a mild rhythmic tremor of the head may be normal. **Senile tremors** are benign and include head nodding (as if saying yes or no) and tongue protrusion. If some teeth have been lost, the lower face looks unusually small, with the mouth sunken in.

Normal Range of Findings	Abnormal Findings
The neck may show an increased cervical concave (or inward) curve when the head and jaw are extended forward to compensate for kyphosis of the spine. During the examination, direct the aging person to perform ROM slowly; he or she may experience dizziness with side movements. An aging person may have prolapse of the submandibular glands, which could be mistaken for a tumour. But drooping submandibular glands will feel soft and be present bilaterally.	

Summary Checklist: Head, Face, and Neck, Including Regional Lymphatics Examination

For a PDA-downloadable version, go to http://evolve.elsevier.com/Canada/Jarvis/examination/.

1. **Inspect and palpate the skull**
   General size and contour
   Note any deformities, lumps, tenderness
   Palpate temporal artery, temporomandibular joint

2. **Inspect the face**
   Facial expression
   Symmetry of movement (cranial nerve VII)
   Any involuntary movements, edema, lesions

3. **Inspect and palpate the neck**
   Active ROM
   Enlargement of salivary glands, lymph nodes, thyroid gland
   Position of the trachea

4. **Auscultate the thyroid** (if enlarged) for bruit

Promoting Health: Brain Injury Prevention

Use Your Head. Wear a Helmet.

In Canada, helmet use is legislated provincially. Safe Kids Canada is currently advocating that all provinces adopt the U.S. Consumer Product Safety Commission (CPSP) recommendations in regard to helmet safety standards. Bicycle helmet laws in Canada do not specify the CPSC standard, so there is a potential for cyclists to be in violation of the helmet law in their province.

When buying a new bicycle helmet in Canada, look for the CSA, ASTM, or CPSC standard. The CPSC standard is comparable to the CSA standard. For guidelines and information about which helmet to choose for activities to prevent brain and head injury, go to www.safekidscanada.ca or call 1-888 SAFE TIPS. Also ensure you are aware of individual provincial helmet legislation. The 2007 report titled *Reaching for the Top: A report by the advisor on healthy children and youth* stated that a pan-Canadian 5-year National Injury Prevention Strategy, which will include new national helmet legislation, will be implemented by December 2008. Ensure that you are using the most up-to-date legislated policy to guide your decision making. For more information about CPSC standards, go to www.cpsc.gov.

In general, all helmets are designed to absorb the impact energy in a collision or fall, protecting the brain from injury and trauma. However, all helmets are not created equal. Each type of helmet is specifically designed to protect the head and brain from the specific type(s) of impact that can take place in the particular sport or activity for which it is intended.

Wearing a properly fitted and safe bicycle helmet can reduce an individual's risk of head injury by 85% and reduce the risk of brain injury by 88%. A helmet needs to be comfortable, snug, and secured. It should not move in any direction when adjusted properly and the chinstrap needs to be securely buckled. A proper fit is as important as wearing the correct helmet. This is particularly important for children. It is important to select a helmet that fits now, not a helmet that a child will grow into.

Children and adults should wear a sport- or activity-specific helmet when participating in the following sports or recreational activities:

- Alpine skiing and snowboarding
- ATV riding
- Baseball
- Bicycling
- Football
- Go-karting
- Horseback riding
- Ice hockey
- Lacrosse
- Roller and in-line skating
- Rock climbing
- Scooter riding
- Skateboarding
- Snowmobiling
- Softball

Although a helmet has not yet been specifically designed for either ice-skating or sledding, wearing a bicycle, skateboard, or ski helmet may be preferable to wearing no helmet at all.

There are also certain activities for which an individual, especially a child, should not wear a helmet. For example, playing on playgrounds or climbing. In these situations, a helmet's chinstrap might get caught and pose a risk of strangulation. Further, the helmet itself may also pose an entrapment hazard or risk.

Leitch, K. (2007). *Reaching for the top: A report by the advisor on healthy children and youth*. Ottawa, ON: Health Canada.
Safe Kids Canada. (2005). Position statement on bicycle helmet legislation. Retrieved June 5, 2008, from http://www.sickkids.ca/SKCForPartners/custom/BikeLegislationPositionStatement.pdf
U.S. Consumer Product Safety Commission. (2006). *Which helmet for which activity?* Retrieved from http://www.cpsc.gov.

Objective Data

❧ — DOCUMENTATION AND CRITICAL THINKING — ❧

Sample Charting

SUBJECTIVE

Denies any unusually frequent or severe headache; no history of head injury, dizziness, or syncope; no neck pain, limitation of motion, nodules, or swelling.

OBJECTIVE

Head: Normocephalic, no lumps, no lesions, no tenderness.
Face: Symmetric, or drooping, no weakness, no involuntary movements.
Neck: Supple with full ROM, no pain. Symmetric, no lymphadenopathy or masses. Trachea midline, thyroid not palpable. No bruits.

ASSESSMENT

Normocephalic symmetric head and neck.

Focused Assessment: Clinical Case Study

Mara is a 19-year-old single female college student with a history of good health and no chronic illnesses; she enters the outpatient clinic today stating, "I think I've had a stroke!"

SUBJECTIVE

- 1 day PTA: first noticed at dinner at college cafeteria when joking with friends, started to stick out tongue and roll tongue and could not do it, right side of tongue was not working. Mara left room to look in mirror and became scared; when smiled, noticed right side was not working. Tried to pucker lips, could not. Could not whistle, could not raise eyebrow: "I looked like a Vulcan." No other movement disorder below neck. Mild pain behind right ear with buzzing in ear. Able to sleep last night, but roommate said Mara's right eyelid did not close completely during sleep.
- Today: still no movement on complete right side of face. Feeling self-conscious in class and during conversations with friends. Now has taste aversion, fluids with high water content taste especially bitter. No hearing loss.

OBJECTIVE

T 37°C, P 64, R 14, B/P 108/78.

Forehead appears smooth and immobile on right, unable to wrinkle right side. Unable to close right eye, Bell's phenomenon present with attempts to close (right eyeball rolls upward), right palpebral fissure appears wider. No corneal reflex on right. Unable to whistle or puff right cheek. Absent nasolabial fold on right. Mouth droops on right, sags on right when tries to smile. Slight drooling. Left side of face responds appropriately to all these movements. Superficial sensation intact.

Rest of musculoskeletal system intact: able to hold balance while standing, able to walk, walk heel-to-toe, do knee bend on each knee. Arm strength and range of motion intact.

ASSESSMENT

Right-sided facial paralysis, consistent with Bell's palsy
Disturbed body image R/T effects of loss of facial function
Risk for deficient fluid volume R/T taste aversion and dietary alteration
Risk for sensory deficit, visual impairment, R/T effects of neurological impairment

Nursing Diagnoses Commonly Associated With Head and Neck Disorders

All nursing diagnoses can be found on the Evolve Web site at **http://evolve.elsevier.com/Canada/Jarvis/examination/.**

ABNORMAL FINDINGS

TABLE 13-1	Abnormalities in Head Size and Contour

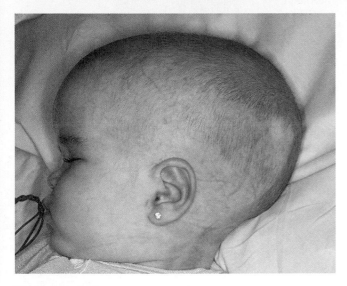

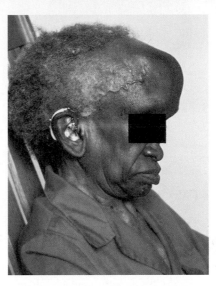

Hydrocephalus

Obstruction of drainage of cerebrospinal fluid results in excessive accumulation, increasing intracranial pressure, and enlargement of the head. The face looks small compared with the enlarged cranium. The increasing pressure also produces dilated scalp veins, frontal bossing, and downcast or "setting sun" eyes (sclera visible above iris). The cranial bones thin, sutures separate, and percussion yields a "cracked pot" sound (Macewen's sign).

Paget's Disease of Bone (Osteitis Deformans)

A localized bone disease of unknown etiology that softens, thickens, and deforms bone. It affects 3% of adults over age 40 years and 8–15% over the age of 75 years. Symptoms occur a decade earlier in men. The disease is characterized by bowed long bones, sudden fractures, frontal bossing, and enlarging skull bones that form an acorn-shaped cranium. Enlarging skull bones press on cranial nerves, causing symptoms of headache, vertigo, tinnitus, progressive deafness, and optic atrophy and compression of the spinal cord.

Reprinted from the Clinical Slide Collection on the Rheumatic Diseases. © 1991, 1995, 1997. Used by permission of the American College of Rheumatology.

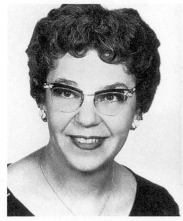
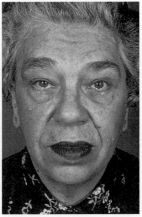

◀ Acromegaly

Excessive secretion of growth hormone from the pituitary after puberty creates an enlarged skull and thickened cranial bones. Note the elongated head, massive face, prominent nose and lower jaw, heavy eyebrow ridge, and coarse facial features, especially when compared with the same woman's face on the left pictured several years before she had a pituitary tumour.

TABLE 13-2	Swellings on the Head or Neck

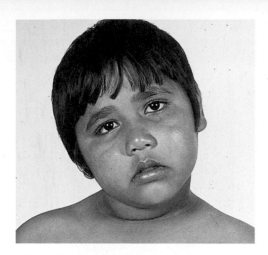

Torticollis (Wryneck)

A shortening or excessive contraction of the sternocleidomastoid muscle in the neck; it may be caused by an idiopathic, genetic, or acquired secondary injury that results in a lateral head tilt and chin rotation to the opposite side. Congenital torticollis may be caused by intrauterine malpositioning or by prenatal injury of the muscles or blood supply in the neck. You will feel a firm, discrete, nontender mass midmuscle on the involved side. This requires treatment, or the muscle becomes fibrotic and permanently shortened with permanent limitation of ROM, asymmetry of head and face, and visual problems from a nonhorizontal position of the eyes.

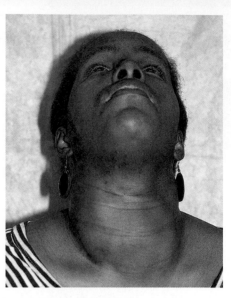

Thyroid—Multiple Nodules

Multiple nodules usually indicate inflammation or a multinodular goitre rather than a neoplasm. However, suspect any rapidly enlarging or firm nodule.

Thyroid—Single Nodule (not illustrated)

Most solitary nodules are benign, although a solitary nodule poses a greater risk of malignancy than do multiple nodules and poses a greater risk in a young person. Suspect any painless, rapidly growing nodule, especially the appearance of a single nodule in a young person. Cancerous nodules tend to be hard and are fixed to surrounding structures.

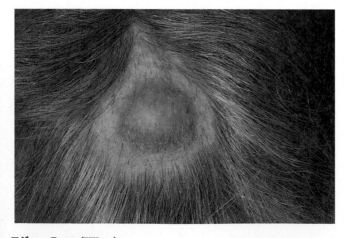

Pilar Cyst (Wen)

Smooth, firm, fluctuant swelling on the scalp. Tense pressure of the contents causes overlying skin to be shiny and taut. It is a benign growth.

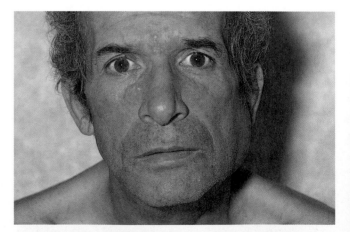

Parotid Gland Enlargement

Rapid painful inflammation of the parotid occurs with mumps. Parotid swelling also occurs with blockage of a duct, abscess, or tumour. Note swelling anterior to lower ear lobe. Stensen duct obstruction can occur in aging adults dehydrated from diuretics or anticholinergics.

TABLE 13-3   Pediatric Facial Abnormalities

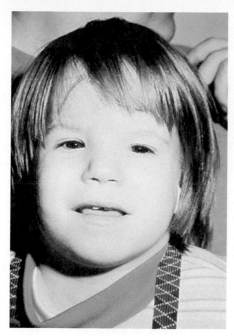

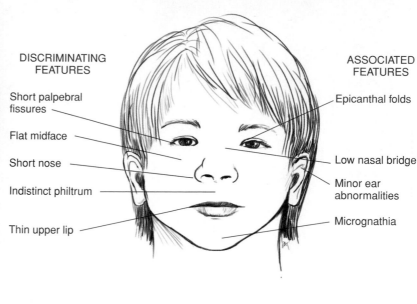

DISCRIMINATING
FEATURES

Short palpebral fissures

Flat midface

Short nose

Indistinct philtrum

Thin upper lip

ASSOCIATED
FEATURES

Epicanthal folds

Low nasal bridge

Minor ear abnormalities

Micrognathia

© Pat Thomas, 2006.

Fetal Alcohol Syndrome

A pregnant woman who abuses alcohol is at great risk of producing a baby with a wide range of growth and developmental abnormalities. Facial malformations may be recognizable at birth. Characteristic facies include narrow palpebral fissures, epicanthal folds, and midfacial hypoplasia.

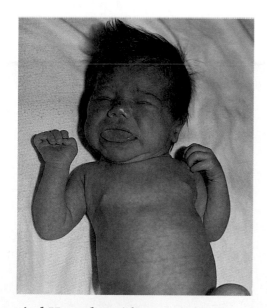

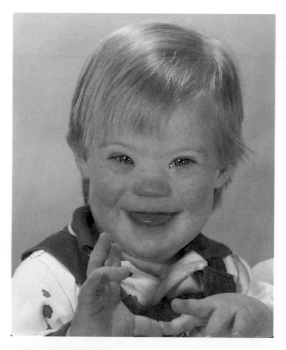

Congenital Hypothyroidism

Thyroid deficiency at an early age produces impaired growth and neurological deficit. Without neonatal screening, characteristic facies develop by 3 to 6 months of age: low hairline, hirsute forehead, swollen eyelids, narrow palpebral fissures, widely spaced eyes, depressed nasal bridge, puffy face, thick tongue protruding through an open mouth, and a dull expression. Head size is normal, but the anterior and posterior fontanelles are wide open.

Down Syndrome

Chromosomal aberration (trisomy 21). Head and face characteristics may include upslanting eyes with inner epicanthal folds, flat nasal bridge, small broad flat nose, protruding thick tongue, ear dysplasia, short broad neck with webbing, and small hands with single palmar crease.

TABLE 13-3	Pediatric Facial Abnormalities—cont'd

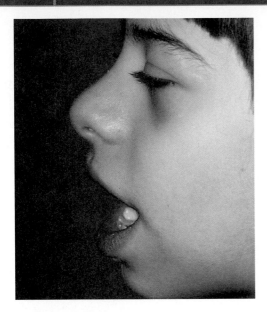

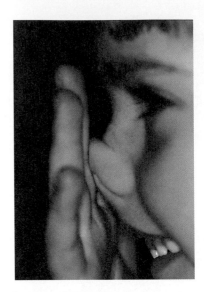

Atopic (Allergic) Facies

Children with chronic allergies such as atopic dermatitis often develop characteristic facial features. These include exhausted face, blue shadows below the eyes ("allergic shiners") from sluggish venous return, a double or single crease on the lower eyelids (Morgan's lines), central facial pallor, and open-mouth breathing (allergic gaping). The open-mouth breathing can lead to malocclusion of the teeth and malformed jaw because the child's bones are still forming.

Allergic Salute and Crease

The transverse line on the nose is also a feature of chronic allergies. It is formed when the child chronically uses the hand to push the nose up and back (the "allergic salute") to relieve itching and to free swollen turbinates, which allows air passage.

TABLE 13-4	Abnormal Facial Appearances With Chronic Illnesses

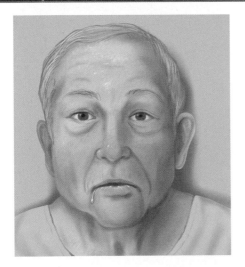

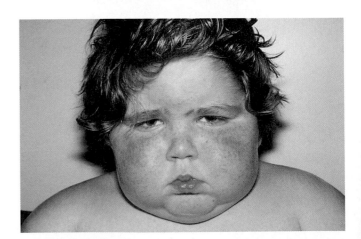

Parkinson's Syndrome

A deficiency of the neurotransmitter dopamine and degeneration of the basal ganglia in the brain. The immobility of features produces a face that is flat and expressionless, "masklike," with elevated eyebrows, staring gaze, oily skin, and drooling.

Cushing's Syndrome

With excessive secretion of adrenocorticotropic hormone (ACTH) and chronic steroid use, the person develops a plethoric, rounded, moonlike face, prominent jowls, red cheeks, hirsutism on the upper lip, lower cheeks, and chin, and acneiform rash on the chest.

Continued

TABLE 13-4 | **Abnormal Facial Appearances With Chronic Illnesses—cont'd**

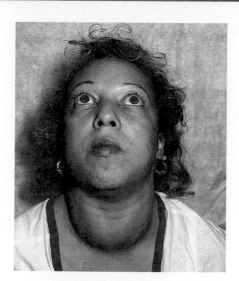

Hyperthyroidism

Goitre is an increase in the size of the thyroid gland and occurs with hyperthyroidism, Hashimoto's thyroiditis, and hypothyroidism. Graves' disease (shown here) is the most common cause of hyperthyroidism, manifested by goitre and exophthalmos (bulging eyeballs). Symptoms include nervousness, fatigue, weight loss, muscle cramps, and heat intolerance; signs include tachycardia, shortness of breath, excessive sweating, fine muscle tremor, thin silky hair and skin, infrequent blinking, and a staring appearance.

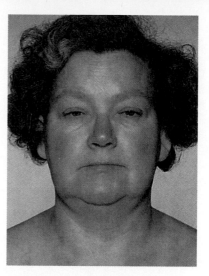

Myxedema (Hypothyroidism)

A deficiency of thyroid hormone, when severe, causes a nonpitting edema or myxedema. Note puffy edematous face, especially around eyes (periorbital edema), coarse facial features, dry skin, and dry coarse hair and eyebrows.

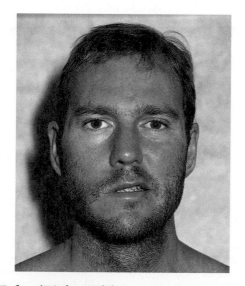

Bell's Palsy (Right Side)

A **lower motor neuron** lesion (**peripheral**), producing cranial nerve VII paralysis, which is almost always unilateral. It has a rapid onset, and the majority of cases are thought to be caused by herpes simplex virus (HSV). Note complete paralysis of one half of the face; person cannot wrinkle forehead, raise eyebrow, close eye, whistle, or show teeth on the right side. Former Canadian Prime Minister Jean Chrétien acquired Bell's palsy in his youth.

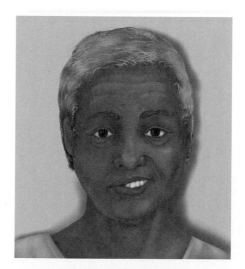

Brain Attack or Cerebrovascular Accident

An **upper motor neuron** lesion (**central**). A "stroke" is an acute neurological deficit caused by an obstruction of a cerebral vessel, as in atherosclerosis, or a rupture in a cerebral vessel. Note paralysis of lower facial muscles, but also note that the upper half of face is not affected because of the intact nerve from the unaffected hemisphere. The person is still able to wrinkle the forehead and close the eyes.

TABLE 13-4	Abnormal Facial Appearances With Chronic Illnesses—cont'd

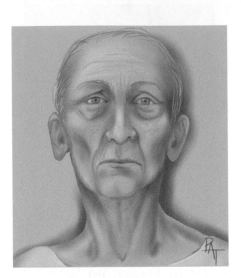

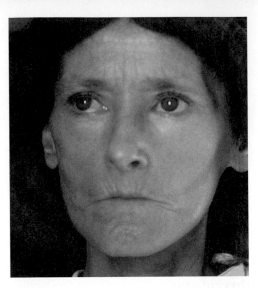

Cachectic Appearance

Accompanies chronic wasting diseases (such as cancer), dehydration, and starvation. Features include sunken eyes; hollow cheeks; and exhausted, defeated expression.

Scleroderma

Literally "hard skin," this rare connective tissue disease is characterized by chronic hardening and shrinking degenerative changes in the skin, blood vessels, synovium, and skeletal muscles. Changes can occur in skin, heart, esophagus, kidney, lung. Characteristic facies: hard, shiny skin on forehead and cheeks; thin, pursed lips with radial furrowing; absent skinfolds; muscle atrophy on face and neck; absence of expression.

Reprinted from the Clinical Slide Collection on the Rheumatic Diseases, © 1991, 1995, 1997. Used by permission of the American College of Rheumatology.

Abnormal Findings (side margin)

BIBLIOGRAPHY

Brown, J., & Skarin, A. (2004). Clinical mimics of lymphoma. *Oncologist, 9,* 406–416.

Fleener, V., & Holloway, B. (2004). Migraines: Not just an adult problem. *Nurse Practitioner, 29*(11), 27–40.

Herman, M. J. (2006). Torticollis in infants and children: common and unusual causes. *Instructor Course Lectures, 55,* 647–653.

Joslin, N. (2004). Early identification key to scleroderma treatment. *Nurse Practitioner, 29*(7), 24–41.

Kaniecki, R. (2003). Headache assessment and management. *Journal of the American Medical Association, 289,* 1430–1433.

Leitch, K. (2007). *Reaching for the top: A report by the advisor on healthy children and youth.* Ottawa: Health Canada.

Maizels, M. (2004). The patient with daily headaches. *American Family Physician, 70,* 2299–2306, 2313–2314.

Malchiodi, L. (2002). Thyroid storm. *American Journal of Nursing, 102*(5), 33–35.

Merritt, L. (2005). Part 2. Physical assessment of the infant with cleft lip and/or palate. *Advances in Neonatal Care, 5,* 125–134.

Mongini, F., Deregibus, A., Raviola, F., & Mongini, T. (2003). Confirmation of the distinction between chronic migraine and chronic tension-type headache by the McGill Pain Questionnaire. *Headache, 43,* 867–877.

Prisco, M. K. (2000). Evaluating neck masses. *Nurse Practitioner, 25*(4), 30–51.

Roodman, G. (2003). Recent developments in Paget's disease. *Advanced Studies in Medicine, 3,* 286–292.

Ruckenstein, M. (2006). The dizzy patient: How you can help. *Consultant, 46,* 145–152.

Ruoff, G. (2005). Chronic daily headache: Understanding and treatment. *Consultant, 45,* 871–886.

Safe Kids Canada. (2005). *Safe Kids Canada position statement on bicycle helmet legislation.* Retrieved from http://www.sickkids.ca/SKCForPartners/custom/BikeLegislationPositionStatement.pdf

Safe Kids Canada. (2007). *Helmets.* Retrieved February 1, 2008, from http://www.sickkids.ca/SKCForParents/section.asp?s=Safety+Information+by+Topic&sID=10774&ss=&ssID=&sss=Bike+Helmets&sssID=14486

Santiago-Rosado, L. (2005). Syncope: Step-by-step through the workup. *Consultant, 45,* 759–768.

Seidman-Riple, J., & Huang, J. (1994). Monograph series on aging-related diseases: VII. Paget's disease (osteitis deformans). *Chronic Diseases in Canada, 16*(2). Retrieved February 4, 2008, from http://www.phac-aspc.gc.ca/publicat/cdic-mcc/16-2/b_e.html

Simmons Holcomb, S. (2003a). Detecting thyroid disease, part 1. *Nursing, 33*(8), 32cc1–32cc4.

Simmons Holcomb, S. (2003b). Detecting thyroid disease, part 2. *Nursing, 33*(9), 32cc1–32cc4.

Sweet, J. (2004). A numb chin: It could be the first symptom of a malignancy. *Archives Internal Medicine, 164,* 1347–1348.

Weeks, B. (2005). Graves' disease: The importance of early diagnosis. *Nurse Practitioner, 30*(11), 34–47.

Eyes

Written by **Carolyn Jarvis**, PhD, APN, CNP
Adapted by **Annette J. Browne**, PhD, RN

Electronic Resources ——————⤎

On Evolve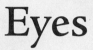

http://evolve.elsevier.com/Canada/Jarvis/examination/

- Interactive Case Studies
- Physical Examination Audio and Printable Summaries
- Bedside Assessment Summary Checklists
- Complete Physical Examination Form
- Nursing Diagnoses Boxes
- Health Promotion Guides
- Quick Assessments for 20 Common Conditions
- Multiple Choice Review Questions
- Chapter Objectives
- Appendices
- Weblinks

On the Companion CD

- Interactive Case Studies with Heart and Lung Sounds
- Health Promotion Guides
- Quick Assessments for 20 Common Conditions
- Head-to-Toe Physical Examination Video Clips

⤌ ——————————————⤎

Structure and Function

STRUCTURE AND FUNCTION

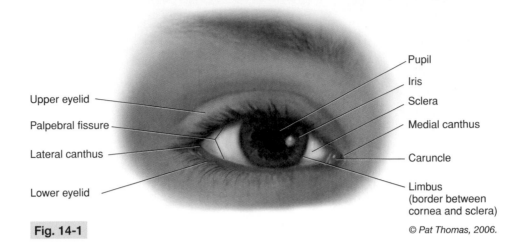

Upper eyelid

Palpebral fissure

Lateral canthus

Lower eyelid

Pupil

Iris

Sclera

Medial canthus

Caruncle

Limbus
(border between
cornea and sclera)

© Pat Thomas, 2006.

Fig. 14-1

EXTERNAL ANATOMY

The eye is the sensory organ of vision. Humans are very visual beings. More than half the neocortex is involved with processing visual information (Wehenmeyer & Gallman, 2002).

Because this sense is so important to humans, the eye is well protected by the bony orbital cavity, which is surrounded with a cushion of fat. The **eyelids** are like two movable shades that further protect the eye from injury, strong light, and dust. The upper eyelid is the larger and more mobile one. The eyelashes are short hairs in double or triple rows that curve outward from the lid margins, filtering out dust and dirt.

The **palpebral fissure** is the elliptical open space between the eyelids (Fig. 14-1). When closed, the lid margins approximate completely. When open, the upper lid covers part of the iris. The lower lid margin is just at the **limbus,** the border between the cornea and sclera. The **canthus** is the corner of the eye, the angle where the lids meet. At the inner canthus the **caruncle** is a small fleshy mass containing sebaceous glands.

Within the upper lid, **tarsal plates** are strips of connective tissue that give it shape (Fig. 14-2). The tarsal plates contain the **meibomian glands,** modified sebaceous glands that secrete an oily lubricating material onto the lids. This stops the tears from overflowing and helps to form an airtight seal when the lids are closed.

The exposed part of the eye has a transparent protective covering, the **conjunctiva.** The conjunctiva is a thin mucous membrane folded like an envelope between the eyelids and the eyeball. The *palpebral* conjunctiva lines the lids and is clear, with many small blood vessels. It forms a deep recess and then folds back over the eye. The *bulbar* conjunctiva overlays the eyeball, with the white sclera showing through. At the limbus the conjunctiva merges with the cornea. The cornea covers and protects the iris and pupil.

The **lacrimal apparatus** provides constant irrigation to keep the conjunctiva and cornea moist and lubricated (Fig. 14-3). The lacrimal gland, in the upper outer corner over the

eye, secretes tears. The tears wash across the eye and are drawn up evenly as the lid blinks. The tears drain into the **puncta,** visible on the upper and lower lids at the inner canthus. The tears then drain into the nasolacrimal sac, through the centimetre-long nasolacrimal duct, and empty into the inferior meatus inside the nose. A tiny fold of mucous membrane prevents air from being forced up the nasolacrimal duct when the nose is blown.

Extraocular Muscles. Six muscles attach the eyeball to its orbit (Fig. 14-4) and serve to direct the eye to points of the

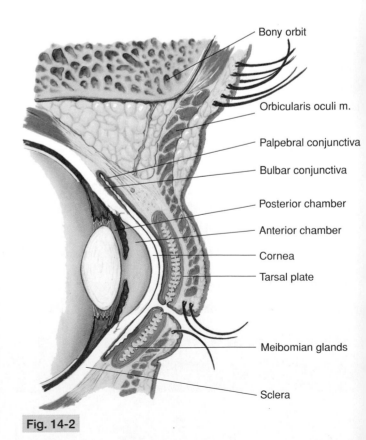

Bony orbit

Orbicularis oculi m.

Palpebral conjunctiva

Bulbar conjunctiva

Posterior chamber

Anterior chamber

Cornea

Tarsal plate

Meibomian glands

Sclera

Fig. 14-2

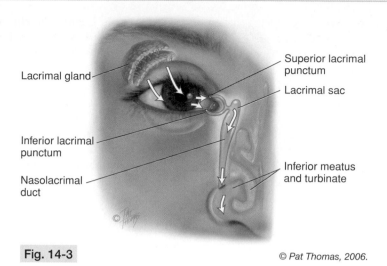

Fig. 14-3   © Pat Thomas, 2006.

person's interest. These extraocular muscles give the eye both straight and rotary movements. The four straight, or *rectus,* muscles are the superior, inferior, lateral, and medial rectus muscles. The two slanting, or *oblique,* muscles are the superior and inferior muscles.

Each muscle is coordinated, or yoked, with one in the other eye. This ensures that when the two eyes move, their axes always remain parallel (called *conjugate movement*). Parallel axes are important because the human brain can tolerate seeing only one image. Although some animals can perceive

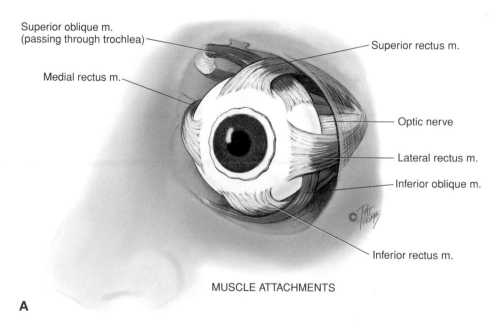

MUSCLE ATTACHMENTS

A

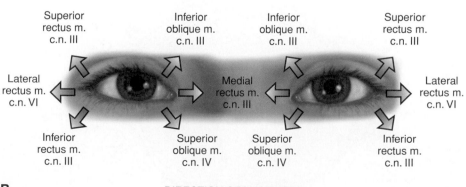

B

Fig. 14-4   DIRECTION OF MOVEMENT

© Pat Thomas, 2006.

two different pictures through each eye, human beings have a binocular, single-image visual system. This occurs because our eyes move as a pair. For example, the two yoked muscles that allow looking to the far right are the right lateral rectus and the left medial rectus.

Movement of the **extraocular muscles** (see Fig. 14-4) is stimulated by three **cranial nerves.** Cranial nerve VI, the abducens nerve, innervates the lateral rectus muscle (which abducts the eye); cranial nerve IV, the trochlear nerve, innervates the superior oblique muscle; and cranial nerve III, the oculomotor nerve, innervates all the rest—the superior, inferior, and medial rectus and the inferior oblique muscles. Note that the superior oblique muscle is located on the superior aspect of the eyeball, but when it contracts, it enables the person to look downward and inward.

INTERNAL ANATOMY

The eye is a sphere composed of three concentric coats: (1) the outer fibrous **sclera,** (2) the middle vascular **choroid,** and (3) the inner nervous **retina** (Fig. 14-5). Inside the retina is the transparent vitreous body. The only parts accessible to examination are the sclera anteriorly and the retina through the ophthalmoscope.

The Outer Layer. The **sclera** is a tough, protective, white covering. It is continuous anteriorly with the smooth, transparent cornea, which covers the iris and pupil. The cornea is part of the refracting media of the eye, bending incoming light rays so that they will be focused on the inner retina.

The **cornea** is very sensitive to touch; contact with a wisp of cotton stimulates a blink in both eyes, called the *corneal reflex.* The trigeminal nerve (cranial nerve V) carries the afferent sensation into the brain, and the facial nerve (cranial nerve VII) carries the efferent message that stimulates the blink.

The Middle Layer. The **choroid** has dark pigmentation to prevent light from reflecting internally and is heavily vascularized to deliver blood to the retina. Anteriorly, the choroid is continuous with the ciliary body and the iris. The muscles of the ciliary body control the thickness of the lens. The iris functions as a diaphragm, varying the opening at its centre, the pupil. This controls the amount of light admitted into the retina. The muscle fibres of the iris contract the pupil in bright light and to accommodate for near vision, and dilate the pupil when the light is dim and for far vision. The colour of the iris varies from person to person.

The **pupil** is round and regular. Its size is determined by a balance between the parasympathetic and sympathetic chains of the autonomic nervous system. Stimulation of the parasympathetic branch, through cranial nerve III, causes constriction of the pupil. Stimulation of the sympathetic branch dilates the pupil and elevates the eyelid. As mentioned earlier, the pupil size also reacts to the amount of ambient light and to accommodation, or focusing an object on the retina.

The **lens** is a biconvex disc located just posterior to the pupil. The transparent lens serves as a refracting medium, keeping a viewed object in continual focus on the retina. Its thickness is controlled by the ciliary body; the lens bulges for focusing on near objects and flattens for far objects.

The **anterior chamber** is posterior to the cornea and in front of the iris and lens. The **posterior chamber** lies behind the iris to the sides of the lens. These contain the clear, watery aqueous humor that is produced continually by the ciliary body. The continuous flow of fluid serves to deliver nutrients to the surrounding tissues and to drain metabolic wastes. Intraocular pressure is determined by a balance between the amount of aqueous humor produced and resistance to its outflow at the angle of the anterior chamber.

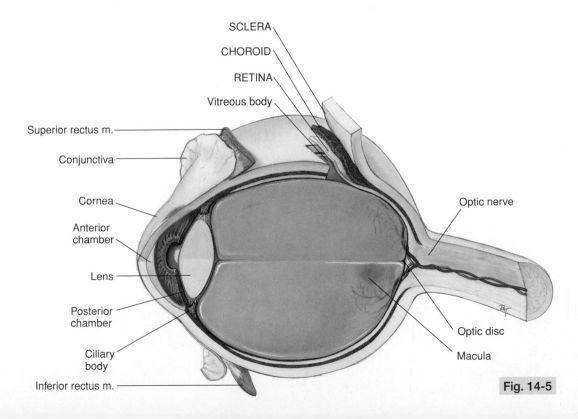

SCLERA
CHOROID
RETINA
Vitreous body
Superior rectus m.
Conjunctiva
Cornea
Anterior chamber
Lens
Posterior chamber
Ciliary body
Inferior rectus m.
Optic nerve
Optic disc
Macula

Fig. 14-5

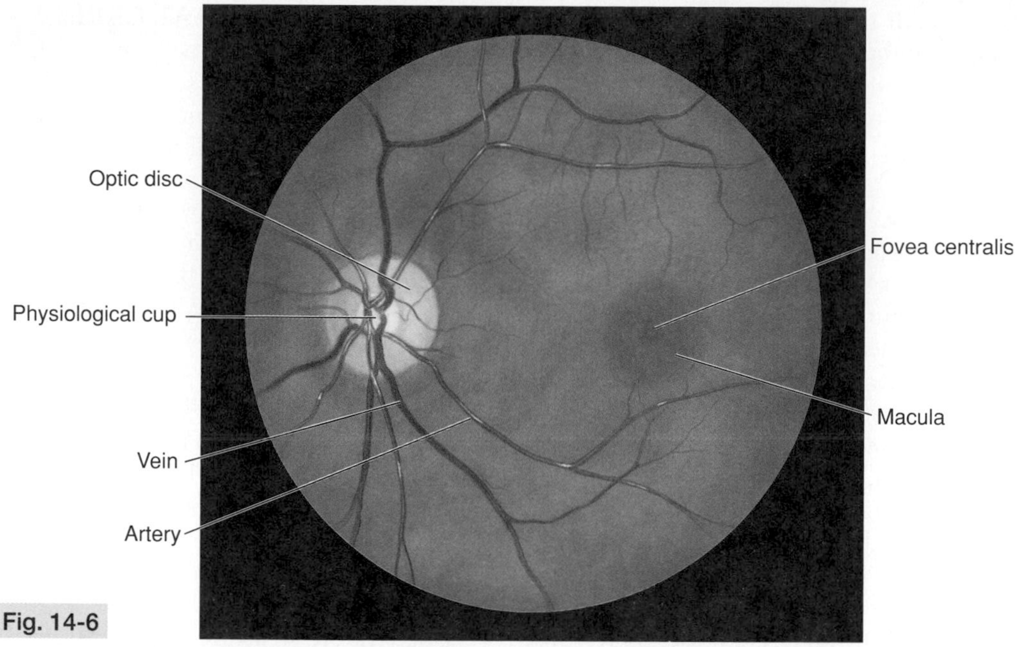

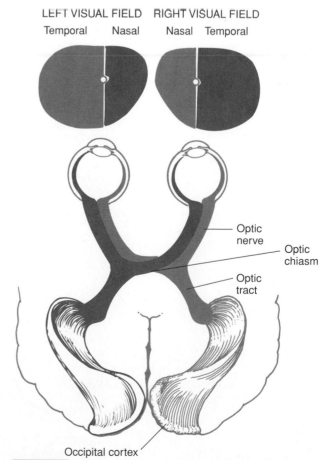

Optic disc

Physiological cup

Vein

Artery

Fovea centralis

Macula

Fig. 14-6

The Inner Layer. The **retina** is the visual receptive layer of the eye in which light waves are changed into nerve impulses. The retina surrounds the soft gelatinous vitreous humor. The retinal structures viewed through the ophthalmoscope are the optic disc, the retinal vessels, the general background, and the macula (Fig. 14-6).

The **optic disc** (or optic papilla) is the area in which fibres from the retina converge to form the optic nerve. Located toward the nasal side of the retina, it has these characteristics: a colour that varies from creamy yellow-orange to pink; a round or oval shape; margins that are distinct and sharply demarcated, especially on the temporal side; and a physiological cup, the smaller circular area inside the disc where the blood vessels exit and enter.

The **retinal vessels** normally include a paired artery and vein extending to each quadrant, growing progressively smaller in calibre as they reach the periphery. The arteries appear brighter red and narrower than the veins, and the arteries have a thin sliver of light on them (the arterial light reflex). The general background of the fundus varies in colour, depending on the person's skin colour. The **macula** is located on the temporal side of the fundus. It is a slightly darker pigmented region surrounding the **fovea centralis,** the area of sharpest and keenest vision. The macula receives and transduces light from the centre of the visual field.

VISUAL PATHWAYS AND VISUAL FIELDS

Objects reflect light. The light rays are refracted through the transparent media (cornea, aqueous humor, lens, and vitreous body) and strike the retina. The retina transforms the light stimulus into nerve impulses that are conducted through the optic nerve and the optic tract to the visual cortex of the occipital lobe.

The image formed on the retina is upside down and reversed from its actual appearance in the outside world (Fig. 14-7). That is, an object in the upper temporal visual field of the right eye reflects its image onto the lower nasal area of the retina. All retinal fibres collect to form the optic nerve, but they maintain this same spatial arrangement, with nasal fibres running medially and temporal fibres running laterally.

At the optic chiasm, nasal fibres (from both temporal visual fields) cross over. The left optic tract now has fibres

LEFT VISUAL FIELD   RIGHT VISUAL FIELD
Temporal   Nasal   Nasal   Temporal

Optic nerve

Optic chiasm

Optic tract

Occipital cortex

Fig. 14-7   Visual pathways (viewed from above).

Structure and Function

from the left half of each retina, and the right optic tract contains fibres only from the right. Thus the right side of the brain looks at the left side of the world.

VISUAL REFLEXES

Pupillary Light Reflex. The pupillary light reflex is the normal constriction of the pupils when bright light shines on the retina (Fig. 14-8). It is a subcortical reflex arc (i.e., a person has no conscious control over it); the afferent link is cranial nerve II, the optic nerve, and the efferent path is cranial III, the oculomotor nerve. When one eye is exposed to bright light, a *direct light reflex* occurs (constriction of that pupil) as well as a *consensual light reflex* (simultaneous constriction of the other pupil). This happens because the optic nerve carries the sensory afferent message in and then synapses with both sides of the brain. For example, consider the light reflex in a person who is blind in one eye. Stimulation of the normal eye produces both a direct and a consensual light reflex. Stimulation of the blind eye causes no response because the sensory afferent in cranial nerve II is destroyed.

Fixation. This is a reflex direction of the eye toward an object attracting a person's attention. The image is fixed in the centre of the visual field, the fovea centralis. This consists of very rapid ocular movements to put the target back on the fovea, and somewhat slower (smooth pursuit) movements to track the target and keep its image on the fovea. These ocular movements are impaired by drugs, alcohol, fatigue, and inattention.

Accommodation. This is adaptation of the eye for near vision. It is accomplished by increasing the curvature of the lens through movement of the ciliary muscles. Although the lens cannot be observed directly, the components of accommodation that can be observed are convergence (motion toward) of the axes of the eyeballs and pupillary constriction.

🏵 DEVELOPMENTAL CARE

Infants and Children

At birth, eye function is limited, but it matures fully during the early years. Peripheral vision is intact in the newborn infant. The macula, the area of keenest vision, is absent at birth but is developing by 4 months and is mature by 8 months. Eye movements may be poorly coordinated at birth. By 3 to 4 months of age, the infant establishes binocularity and can fixate on a single image with both eyes simultaneously. Most neonates (80%) are born farsighted; this gradually decreases after 7 to 8 years of age.

In structure, the eyeball reaches adult size by 8 years. At birth, the iris shows little pigmentation, and the pupils are small. The lens is nearly spherical at birth, becoming flatter throughout life. Its consistency changes from that of soft plastic at birth to rigid glass in old age.

The Aging Adult

Changes in eye structure contribute greatly to the distinct facial changes of the aging person. The skin loses its elasticity, causing wrinkling and drooping; fat tissues and muscles atrophy; and the external eye structures appear as on p. 324. Lacrimal glands involute, causing decreased tear production and a feeling of dryness and burning.

On the globe itself, the cornea may show an infiltration of degenerative lipid material around the limbus (see discussion of *arcus senilis,* p. 325). Pupil size decreases. The lens loses elasticity, becoming hard and glasslike. This glasslike quality decreases the lens's ability to change shape to accommodate for near vision; this condition is termed **presbyopia.** The average age at which people experience presbyopia is 40 years (Kaiser et al., 2003). By 70 years of age, the normally transparent fibres of the lens begin to thicken and yellow. This is nuclear sclerosis, or the beginning of a senile cataract.

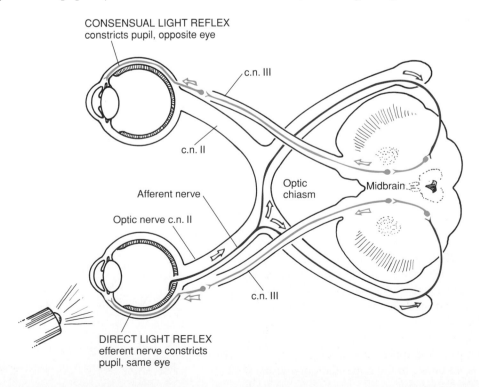

CONSENSUAL LIGHT REFLEX
constricts pupil, opposite eye

c.n. III

c.n. II

Afferent nerve

Optic nerve c.n. II

Optic chiasm

Midbrain

c.n. III

DIRECT LIGHT REFLEX
efferent nerve constricts
pupil, same eye

Fig. 14-8

Inside the globe, floaters appear in the vitreous as a result of debris that can accumulate because vitreous humor is not continuously renewed as aqueous humor is. Visual acuity may diminish gradually after 50 years of age, and even more so after 70 years. Near vision is commonly affected because of the decreased power of accommodation in the lens (presbyopia). As early as the fourth decade, a person may have blurred vision and difficulty reading. Also, the aging person needs more light to see because of a decreased adaptation to darkness, and this condition may affect the function of night driving.

The prevalence of age-related vision loss is increasing dramatically, with one in every nine Canadians over age 65 living with significant vision loss (Canadian National Institute for the Blind [CNIB], 2004). In the aging population the most common causes of decreased visual functioning are:

1. Macular degeneration, or the breakdown of cells in the macula of the retina.   Loss of central vision, the area of clearest vision, is the most common cause of blindness. Age-related macular degeneration (AMD) is the leading cause of blindness in Canada and remains the single most common cause of legal blindness in people over age 65 (Clinical Practice Guideline Expert Committee [CPGEC], 2007). In 2004, it was estimated that 2.1 million Canadians between the ages of 43 and 75 were affected by AMD (CNIB, 2004). It affects 28% of those aged 75 to 85 years, with women affected more often than men (Kane et al., 2003). With this, the person is unable to read fine print, sew, or do fine work and may have difficulty distinguishing faces. Depending on how much the lifestyle is oriented around activities requiring close work, loss of central vision may cause great distress. Peripheral vision is not affected, so the person can manage self-care and will not become completely disabled.

2. Cataract formation, or lens opacity, resulting from a clumping of proteins in the lens.   Some cataract formation should be expected by age 70 years. Cataracts represent the second most common cause of correctable visual impairment after the correction of refractive error (CPGEC, 2007). Advancing age remains the most common risk factor, with progression typically extending over a long period of time. Other common risk factors include diabetes mellitus, certain medications (steroids), diabetes, history of ocular trauma, and previous intraocular inflammation or surgery (CNIB, 2004). The prevalence of cataract is over 50% in those aged 70 to 79, and almost 100% in the 90+ age group.

3. Glaucoma, or increased intraocular pressure.   The age-adjusted rate for people over age 60 is 6 to 8% (Einarson et al., 2006). Chronic open-angle glaucoma is the most common type; it involves a gradual loss of peripheral vision.

4. Diabetic retinopathy.   This remains the leading cause of visual impairment in people under age 65 (CPGEC, 2007). This risk is highest in patients who present with concurrent proteinuria. Patients who are diabetic should be referred regularly for screening for diabetic retinopathy by an ophthalmologist (Canadian Diabetes Association, 2003).

To summarize, the number of partially sighted people is rising largely because of the increasing proportion of older adults in the population. The term *partially sighted* refers to those patients whose vision is outside normal limits (<20/60) and who cannot have improvement in their vision through medical or surgical means (Canadian Ophthalmological Society, 2008). In Canada, a visual acuity worse than 20/50 disqualifies people from obtaining a driver's licence or restricts their driving to daytime only, as do some visual field deficits (CNIB, 2008). Legal blindness is corrected vision that is 20/200 or worse, and peripheral vision <20 degrees.

The Canadian Ophthalmological Society's screening recommendations for adults are listed below (CPGEC, 2007, p. 43):

1. **Screening intervals in the asymptomatic low-risk patient**
   - Age 19 to 40 years: at least every 10 years
   - Age 41 to 55 years: at least every 5 years
   - Age 56 to 65 years: at least every 3 years
   - Age >65 years: at least every 2 years

2. **Screening in symptomatic patients**
   Any patient noting changes in visual acuity, visual field, colour vision, or physical changes to the eye should be assessed as soon as possible.

3. **Screening intervals in high-risk patients**
   Patients at higher risk of visual impairment (e.g., those with diabetes, cataract, macular degeneration, or glaucoma [or suspected glaucoma], or a family history of these conditions) should be assessed more frequently and thoroughly.
   - Age >40 years: at least every 3 years
   - Age >50 years: at least every 2 years
   - Age >60 years: at least annually

CULTURAL AND SOCIAL CONSIDERATIONS

Variability exists in the colour of the iris and in retinal pigmentation, with darker irides having darker retinas behind them. Individuals with light retinas generally have better night vision but can have pain in an environment that has too much light.

Research from the USA shows that primary open-angle glaucoma affects Black people three to six times more often than White people and is three to six times more likely to cause blindness in Blacks than in Whites (Kaiser et al., 2003). Reasons for this are not known.

Based on data from large-scale US studies, patients with a predisposition to visual deficits include those who wear glasses or contact lenses, have diabetes, are Black, or have a strong family history of glaucoma, AMD, or retinal detachment (CPGEC, 2007). In Canada, outreach efforts are particularly needed among Aboriginal people, whose incidence of diabetes is much higher (three to five times) than that of the general population (First Nations and Inuit Health, 2007). About one in four Aboriginal people report a problem with vision, compared with one in 10 in the general population (CNIB, 2004).

Canadians between the ages 19 and 64 must rely on private (third-party) insurance or out-of-pocket payment to see an eye specialist for routine vision screening (CPGEC, 2007). People who cannot afford vision testing or corrective lenses need to be referred to agencies that can provide that service free of charge or at a reduced cost.

SUBJECTIVE DATA

1. Vision difficulty (decreased acuity, blurring, blind spots)
2. Pain
3. Strabismus, diplopia
4. Redness, swelling
5. Watering, discharge
6. History of ocular problems
7. Glaucoma
8. Use of glasses or contact lenses
9. Self-care behaviours

Examiner Asks	Rationale
1. Vision difficulty (decreased acuity, blurring, blind spots). Any **difficulty seeing** or any blurring? Come on suddenly, or progress slowly? In one eye or both? • Constant, or does it come and go? • Do objects appear out of focus, or does it feel like a clouding over objects? Does it feel like "greyness" of vision? • Do spots move in front of your eyes? One or many? In one or both eyes? • Any halos/rainbows around objects? Or rings around lights? • Any blind spot? Does it move as you shift your gaze? Any loss of peripheral vision? • Any night blindness?	Floaters are common with myopia or after middle age as a result of condensed vitreous fibres. Usually not significant, but acute onset of floaters ("shade" or "cobwebs") may occur with retinal detachment. Halos around lights occur with acute narrow-angle glaucoma. **Scotoma,** a blind spot in the visual field surrounded by an area of normal or decreased vision, occurs with glaucoma, with optic nerve and visual pathway disorders. Night blindness occurs with optic atrophy, glaucoma, or vitamin A deficiency.
2. Pain. Any **eye pain?** Please describe. • Come on suddenly? • Quality—a burning or itching? • Or sharp, stabbing pain or pain with bright light? • A foreign body sensation? Or deep aching? Or headache in brow area?	*Sudden onset* of eye symptoms (pain, floaters, blind spot, loss of peripheral vision) may be an emergency. Refer immediately. Quality is valuable diagnostic indicator. **Photophobia** is inability to tolerate light. Note: Some common eye diseases cause no pain (e.g., refractive errors, cataract, glaucoma).
3. Strabismus, diplopia. Any history of crossed eyes? Now or in the past? Does this occur with eye fatigue? • Ever see double? Constant, or does it come and go? In one eye or both?	Strabismus is a deviation in the anteroposterior axis of the eye. **Diplopia** is the perception of two images of a single object.
4. Redness, swelling. Any **redness** or **swelling** in the eyes? • Any infections? Now or in the past? When do these occur? In a particular time of year? Are they seasonal?	
5. Watering, discharge. Any **watering** or excessive tearing? • Any **discharge?** Any matter in the eyes? Is it hard to open your eyes in the morning? What colour is the discharge? • How do you remove matter from eyes?	Lacrimation (tearing) and epiphora (excessive tearing) are due to irritants or obstruction in drainage of tears. Purulent discharge is thick and yellow. Crusts form at night. Assess hygiene practices and knowledge of cross-contamination.
6. History of ocular problems. Any **history** of injury or surgery to eye? Or any history of allergies?	Allergens may cause irritation of conjunctiva or cornea (e.g., makeup, contact lens solution).

Examiner Asks	Rationale
7. Glaucoma. Ever been tested for **glaucoma?** Results? • Any family history of glaucoma?	Glaucoma is characterized by increased intraocular pressure.
8. Use of glasses or contact lenses. Do you wear **glasses** or **contact lenses?** How do they work for you? • Last time your prescription was checked? Was it changed? • If you wear contact lenses, are there any problems such as pain, photophobia, watering, or swelling? • How do you care for contacts? How long do you wear them? How do you clean them? Do you remove them for certain activities?	Assess self-care behaviours.
9. Self-care behaviours. Last vision test? Who tested it? • Ever tested for colour vision? • Any environmental conditions at home or at work that may affect your eyes? For example, flying sparks, metal bits, smoke, dust, chemical fumes? If so, do you wear goggles to protect your eyes?	Self-care behaviours for eyes and vision. Work-related eye disease (e.g., an auto mechanic with a foreign body from metal working or radiation damage from welding).
10. What medications are you taking? Systemic or topical? Do you take any medication specifically for the eyes?	Some medications have ocular side effects; for example, prednisone may cause cataracts or increased intraocular pressure.
11. If you have experienced a vision loss, how do you cope? Do you have books with large print, books on audio tape, Braille? • Do you maintain living environment the same? • Do you sometimes fear complete loss of vision?	A constant spatial layout eases navigation through the home.

Additional History for Infants and Children

1. Any vaginal infections in the mother at time of delivery?	Genital herpes and gonorrheal vaginitis have ocular sequelae for the newborn.
2. Considering age of child, which developmental milestones of vision have you (parent) noted?	The parent is most often the one to detect vision problems.
3. Does the child have routine vision testing at school?	
4. Are you (parent) aware of safety measures to protect child's eyes from trauma? Do you inspect toys? • Have you taught the child safe care of sharp objects and how to carry and how to use them?	

Additional History for the Aging Adult

1. Have you noticed any visual difficulty with climbing stairs or driving? Any problem with night vision?	Any loss of depth perception or central vision.
2. When was the last time you were tested for glaucoma? • Any aching pain around eyes? Any loss of peripheral vision? • If you have glaucoma, how do you manage your eyedrops?	Compliance may be a problem if symptoms are absent. Assess ability to administer eyedrops.
3. Is there a history of cataracts? Any loss or progressive blurring of vision?	

Subjective Data

Examiner Asks	Rationale
4. Do your eyes ever feel dry? Burn? What do you do for this?	Decreased tear production may occur with aging.
5. Any decrease in usual activities, such as reading or sewing?	Macular degeneration causes a loss in central vision acuity.

❧ OBJECTIVE DATA ❧

PREPARATION

Position the person standing for vision screening; then sitting up with the head at your eye level.

EQUIPMENT NEEDED

Snellen eye chart
Handheld visual screener
Opaque card or occluder
Penlight
Applicator stick
Ophthalmoscope

Normal Range of Findings	Abnormal Findings

TEST CENTRAL VISUAL ACUITY

Snellen Eye Chart

The Snellen alphabet chart is the most commonly used and accurate measure of visual acuity. It has lines of letters arranged in decreasing size.

Place the Snellen alphabet chart in a well-lit spot at eye level. Position the person on a mark exactly 20 feet (6.1 m) from the chart. Hand the person an opaque card with which to shield one eye at a time during the test; inadvertent peeking may result when shielding the eye with the person's own fingers (Fig. 14-9). If the person wears glasses or contact lenses, leave them on. Remove only reading glasses because they will blur distance vision. Ask the person to read through the chart to the smallest line of letters possible. Encourage the person to try the next smallest line also. (Note: Use a Snellen picture chart for people who cannot read letters. See p. 321.)

Note hesitancy, squinting, leaning forward, misreading letters.

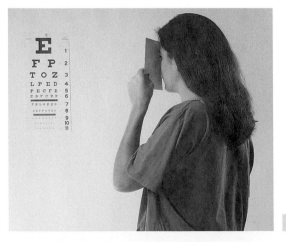

Fig. 14-9

Record the result using the numerical fraction at the end of the last successful line read. Indicate whether the person missed any letters or if corrective lenses were worn—for example, "O.D.* 20/30-1, with glasses."

*O.D., oculus dexter, or right eye.

Normal Range of Findings	Abnormal Findings

Normal visual acuity is 20/20. Contrary to some people's impression, the numerical fraction is *not* a percentage of normal vision. Instead, the top number (numerator) indicates the distance the person is standing from the chart, and the denominator gives the distance at which a normal eye could have read that particular line. Thus "20/20" means, "You can read at 20 ft (6.1 m) what the normal eye could have read at 20 ft."

The larger the denominator, the poorer the vision. If vision is poorer than 20/30, refer to an ophthalmologist or optometrist. Impaired vision may be due to refractive error, opacity in the media (cornea, lens, vitreous), or disorder in the retina or optic pathway.

If the person is unable to see even the largest letters, shorten the distance to the chart until it is seen and record that distance (e.g., "10/200"). If visual acuity is even lower, assess whether the person can count your fingers when they are spread in front of the eyes or distinguish light perception from your penlight.

Near Vision

For people over 40 years of age or for those who report increasing difficulty reading, test near vision with a handheld vision screener with various sizes of print (e.g., a Jaeger card) (Fig. 14-10). Hold the card in good light about 14 inches (35 cm) from the eye—this distance equals the print size on the chart used at 20 feet (6.1 m). Test each eye separately, with glasses on. A normal result is "14/14" in each eye, reading without hesitancy and without moving the card closer or farther away. When no vision screening card is available, ask the person to read from a magazine or newspaper.

Presbyopia, the decrease in power of accommodation with aging, is suggested when the person moves the card farther away.

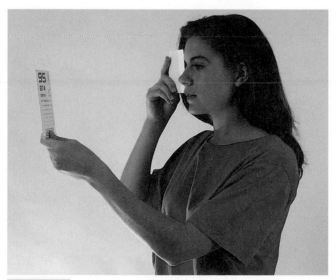

Fig. 14-10

Normal Range of Findings	Abnormal Findings

TEST VISUAL FIELDS

Confrontation Test

This is a gross measure of peripheral vision. It compares the person's peripheral vision with your own, assuming yours is normal (Fig. 14-11). Position yourself at eye level with the person, about 60 cm away. Direct the person to cover one eye with an opaque card, and with the other eye to look straight at you. Cover your own eye opposite to the person's covered one. You are testing the uncovered eye. Hold a pencil or your flicking finger as a target midline between you and the other person, and slowly advance it in from the periphery in several directions.

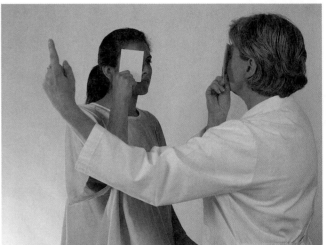

Fig. 14-11

Ask the person to say "now" as the target is first seen; this should be just as you see the object also. (This works with all but the temporal visual field, with which you would need a 2 m arm to avoid being seen initially! With the temporal direction, start the object somewhat behind the person.) Estimate the angle between the anteroposterior axis of the eye and the peripheral axis where the object is first seen. Normal results are about 50 degrees upward, 90 degrees temporal, 70 degrees down, and 60 degrees nasal (Fig. 14-12).

If the person is unable to see the object as examiner does, the test suggests peripheral field loss. Refer to an optometrist for more precise testing using a tangent screen (see Table 14-5 on p. 335).

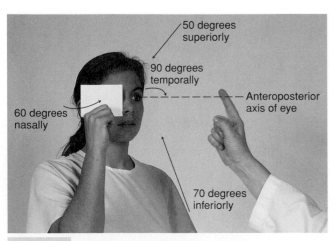

Fig. 14-12   Range of peripheral vision.

Normal Range of Findings	Abnormal Findings

INSPECT EXTRAOCULAR MUSCLE FUNCTION

Corneal Light Reflex (The Hirschberg Test)

Assess the parallel alignment of the eye axes by shining a light toward the person's eyes. Direct the person to stare straight ahead as you hold the light about 30 cm away. Note the reflection of the light on the corneas; it should be in exactly the same spot on each eye. See the bright white dots in Fig. 14-29 for symmetry of the corneal light reflex.

Asymmetry of the light reflex indicates deviation in alignment from eye muscle weakness or paralysis. If you see this, perform the cover test.

Cover Test

The cover test detects small degrees of deviated alignment by interrupting the fusion reflex that normally keeps the two eyes parallel. Ask the person to stare straight ahead at your nose even though the gaze may be interrupted. With an opaque card, cover one eye. As it is covered, note the uncovered eye. A normal response is a steady fixed gaze (Fig. 14-13, *A*).

Meanwhile, the macular image has been suppressed on the covered eye. If muscle weakness exists, the covered eye will drift into a relaxed position.

Now uncover the eye and observe it for movement. It should stare straight ahead (Fig. 14-13, *B*). If it jumps to re-establish fixation, eye muscle weakness exists. Repeat with the other eye.

If the eye jumps to fixate on the designated point, it was out of alignment before.

A **phoria** is a mild weakness noted only when fusion is blocked. **Tropia** is more severe—a constant misalignment of the eyes (see Table 14-1, p. 330).

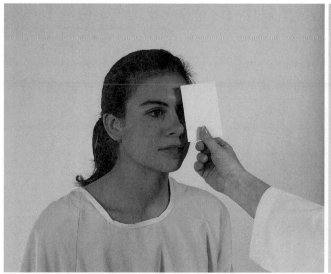
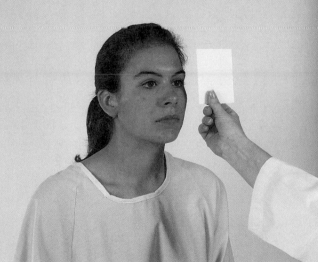

A   **B**

Fig. 14-13

Diagnostic Positions Test

Leading the eyes through the six cardinal positions of gaze will elicit any muscle weakness during movement (Fig. 14-14). Ask the person to hold the head steady and to follow the movement of your finger, pen, or penlight only with the eyes. Hold the target back about 30 cm so the person can focus on it comfortably, and move it to each of the six positions, hold it momentarily, then back to centre. Progress clockwise. A normal response is parallel tracking of the object with both eyes.

Eye movement is not parallel. Failure to follow in a certain direction indicates weakness of an extraocular muscle (EOM) or dysfunction of cranial nerve innervating it.

Normal Range of Findings	Abnormal Findings

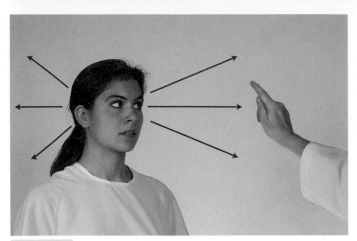

Fig. 14-14   Diagnostic Positions Test

In addition to parallel movement, note any **nystagmus,** a fine oscillating movement best seen around the iris. Mild nystagmus at extreme lateral gaze is normal; nystagmus at any other position is not.

Finally, note that the upper eyelid continues to overlap the superior part of the iris, even during downward movement. You should not see a white rim of sclera between the lid and the iris. If noted, this is termed "lid lag."

INSPECT EXTERNAL OCULAR STRUCTURES

Begin with the most external points, and logically work your way inward.

General

Already you will have noted the person's ability to move around the room, with vision functioning well enough to avoid obstacles and to respond to your directions. Also note the facial expression; a relaxed expression accompanies adequate vision.

Eyebrows

Normally the eyebrows are present bilaterally, move symmetrically as the facial expression changes, and have no scaling or lesions.

Eyelids and Lashes

The upper lids normally overlap the superior part of the iris, and approximate completely with the lower lids when closed. The skin is intact without redness, swelling, discharge, or lesions.

The palpebral fissures are horizontal in non-Asians, whereas Asians normally have an upward slant.

Note that the eyelashes are evenly distributed along the lid margins and curve outward.

Nystagmus occurs with disease of the semicircular canals in the ears, a paretic eye muscle, multiple sclerosis, or brain lesions.

Lid lag occurs with hyperthyroidism.

Groping with hands.

Squinting or craning forward.

Absent lateral third of brow with hypothyroidism.
Unequal or absent movement with nerve damage.
Scaling with seborrhea.

Lid lag with hyperthyroidism.
Incomplete closure creates risk for corneal damage.
Ptosis, drooping of upper lid.
Periorbital edema, lesions (see Tables 14-2 and 14-3 on pp. 331 to 333).
Ectropion and entropion (see Table 14-2, p. 331).

Normal Range of Findings	Abnormal Findings

Eyeballs

The eyeballs are aligned normally in their sockets with no protrusion or sunken appearance. Some people of African descent normally may have a slight protrusion of the eyeball beyond the supraorbital ridge.

Exophthalmos (protruding eyes) and enophthalmos (sunken eyes) (see Table 14-2, p. 331).

Conjunctiva and Sclera

Ask the person to look up. Using your thumbs, slide the lower lids down along the bony orbital rim. Take care not to push against the eyeball. Inspect the exposed area (Fig. 14-15). The eyeball looks moist and glossy. Numerous small blood vessels normally show through the transparent conjunctiva. Otherwise, the conjunctivae are clear and show the normal colour of the structure below—pink over the lower lids and white over the sclera. Note any colour change, swelling, or lesions.

General reddening (see Table 14-6, p. 336).

Cyanosis of the lower lids.

Pallor near the outer canthus of the lower lid may indicate anemia (the inner canthus normally contains less pigmentation).

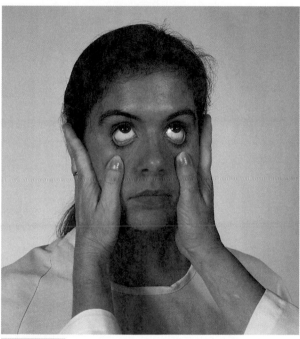

Fig. 14-15

The sclera is china white, although people with dark skin occasionally have a grey-blue or "muddy" colour to the sclera. Also in dark-skinned people, you normally may see small brown macules (like freckles) on the sclera, which should not be confused with foreign bodies or petechiae. Last, some people with dark skin may have yellowish fatty deposits beneath the lids away from the cornea. Do not confuse these yellow spots with the overall scleral yellowing that accompanies jaundice.

Scleral icterus is an even yellowing of the sclera extending up to the cornea, indicating jaundice.

Tenderness, foreign body, discharge, or lesions.

Eversion of the Upper Lid

This manoeuvre is not part of the normal examination, but it is useful when you must inspect the conjunctiva of the upper lid, as with eye pain or suspicion of a foreign body. Most people are apprehensive of any eye manipulation. Enhance their co-operation by using a calm and gentle, yet deliberate, approach.

Normal Range of Findings	Abnormal Findings

1. Ask the person to keep both eyes open and look down. This relaxes the eyelid, whereas closing it would tense the orbicularis muscle.
2. Slide the upper lid up along the bony orbit to lift up the eyelashes.
3. Grasp the lashes between your thumb and forefinger and gently pull down and outward.
4. With your other hand, place the tip of an applicator stick on the upper lid above the level of the internal tarsal plates (Fig. 14-16).

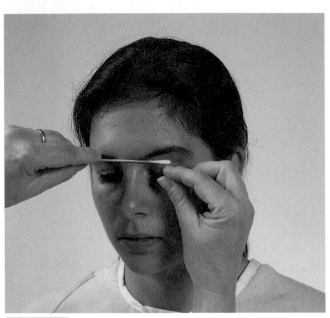

Fig. 14-16

5. Gently push down with the stick as you lift the lashes up. This uses the edge of the tarsal plate as a fulcrum and flips the lid inside out. Take special care not to push in on the eyeball.
6. Secure the everted position by holding the lashes against the bony orbital rim (Fig. 14-17).

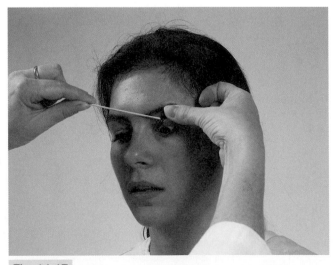

Fig. 14-17

Objective Data

Normal Range of Findings	Abnormal Findings

7. Inspect for any colour change, swelling, lesion, or foreign body.
8. To return to normal position, gently pull the lashes outward as the person looks up.

Lacrimal Apparatus

Ask the person to look down. With your thumbs, slide the outer part of the upper lid up along the bony orbit to expose under the lid. Inspect for any redness or swelling.

Normally, the puncta drain the tears into the lacrimal sac. Presence of excessive tearing may indicate blockage of the nasolacrimal duct. Check this by pressing the index finger against the sac, just inside the lower orbital rim, not against the side of the nose (Fig. 14-18). Pressure will slightly evert the lower lid, but there should be no other response to pressure.

Swelling of the lacrimal gland may show as a visible bulge in the outer part of the upper lid.

Puncta red, swollen, tender to pressure.
Watch for any regurgitation of fluid out of the puncta, which confirms duct blockage.

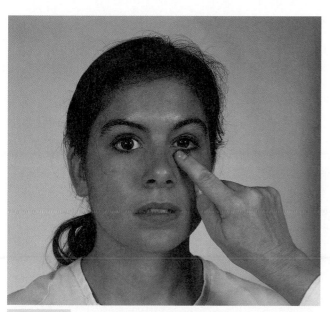

Fig. 14-18

INSPECT ANTERIOR EYEBALL STRUCTURES

Cornea and Lens

Shine a light from the side across the cornea, and check for smoothness and clarity. This oblique view highlights any abnormal irregularities in the corneal surface. There should be no opacities (cloudiness) in the cornea, the anterior chamber, or the lens behind the pupil. Do not confuse an **arcus senilis** with an opacity. The arcus senilis is a normal finding in aging persons and is illustrated on p. 325.

A corneal abrasion causes irregular ridges in reflected light, producing a shattered look to light rays (see Table 14-7, p. 337).

Iris and Pupil

The iris normally appears flat, with a round regular shape and even coloration. Note the size, shape, and equality of the pupils. Normally the pupils appear round, regular, and of equal size in both eyes. In the adult, resting size is from 3 to 5 mm. A small number of people (5%) normally have pupils of two different sizes, which is termed **anisocoria**.

Irregular shape.
Although they may be normal, all unequally sized pupils call for a consideration of central nervous system injury.

Normal Range of Findings	Abnormal Findings
To test the **pupillary light reflex,** darken the room and ask the person to gaze into the distance. (This dilates the pupils.) Advance a light in from the side* and note the response. Normally you will see (1) constriction of the same-sided pupil (a *direct light reflex*), and (2) simultaneous constriction of the other pupil (a *consensual light reflex*).	Dilated pupils. Dilated and fixed pupils. Constricted pupils. Unequal or no response to light (see Table 14-4, p. 334).

In the acute care setting, gauge the pupil size in millimetres, both before and after the light reflex. Recording the pupil size in millimetres is more accurate when many nurses and physicians care for the same person or when small changes may be significant signs of increasing intracranial pressure. Normally, the resting size is 3, 4, or 5 mm and decreases equally in response to light. A normal response is designated by:

$$R\frac{3}{1} = \frac{3}{1}L$$

This indicates that both pupils measure 3 mm in the resting state and that both constrict to 1 mm in response to light. A graduated scale printed on a handheld vision screener or taped onto a tongue blade facilitates your measurement (see Fig. 23-58 in Chapter 23).

Test for **accommodation** by asking the person to focus on a distant object (Fig. 14-19). This process dilates the pupils. Then have the person shift the gaze to a near object, such as your finger held about 7 to 8 cm from the nose. A normal response includes (1) pupillary constriction, and (2) convergence of the axes of the eyes.

Absence of constriction or convergence.
Asymmetrical response.

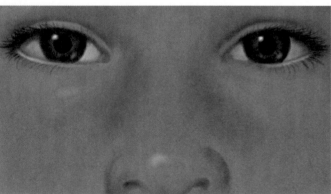
Far vision—pupils dilate

Fig. 14-19

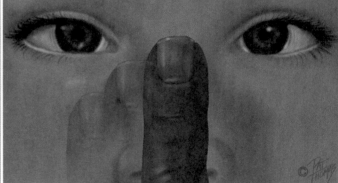
Near vision—pupils constrict

© Pat Thomas, 2006.

Record the normal response to all these manoeuvres as PERRLA, or **P**upils **E**qual, **R**ound, **R**eact to **L**ight, and **A**ccommodation.

INSPECT THE OCULAR FUNDUS

The ophthalmoscope enlarges your view of the eye so that you can inspect the **media** (anterior chamber, lens, vitreous) and the **ocular fundus** (the internal surface of the retina). It accomplishes this by directing a beam of light through the pupil to illuminate the inner structures. Thus, using the ophthalmoscope is like peering through a keyhole (the pupil) into an interesting room beyond.

*Always advance the light in from the *side* to test the light reflex. If you advance from the front, the pupils will constrict to accommodate for near vision. Thus, you do not know what the pure response to the light would have been.

Normal Range of Findings	Abnormal Findings

The ophthalmoscope should function as an appendage of your own eye. This takes some practice. Practise holding the instrument and focusing at objects around the room before you approach a "real" person. Hold the ophthalmoscope right up to your eye, braced firmly against the cheek and brow. Extend your index finger onto the lens selector dial so that you can refocus as needed during the procedure without taking your head away from the ophthalmoscope to look. Now look about the room, moving your head and the instrument together as one unit. Keep both your eyes open; just view the field through the ophthalmoscope.

Recall that the ophthalmoscope contains a set of lenses that control the focus (Fig. 14-20). The unit of strength of each lens is the *dioptre*. The black numbers indicate a positive dioptre; they focus on objects nearer in space to the ophthalmoscope. The red numbers show a negative dioptre and are for focusing on objects farther away.

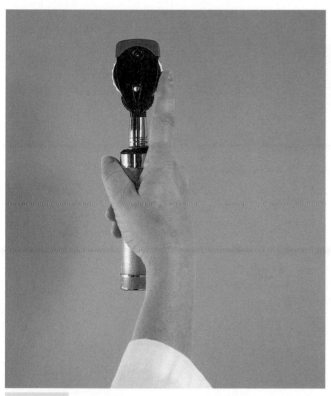

Fig. 14-20

To examine a person, darken the room to help dilate the pupils. (Dilating eyedrops are not needed during a screening examination. When indicated, they dilate the pupils for a wider look at the fundus background and macular area. Eyedrops are used only when glaucoma can be completely ruled out because dilating the pupils in the presence of glaucoma can precipitate an acute episode.) Remove your own eyeglasses and the other person's as they obstruct close movement; you can compensate for their correction by using the dioptre setting. Contact lenses may be left in; they pose no problem as long as they are clean.

Select the large round aperture with the white light for the routine examination. If the pupils are small, use the smaller white light. (Although the instrument has other shape and coloured apertures, these are rarely used in a screening examination.) The light must have maximum brightness; replace old or dim batteries.

Normal Range of Findings	Abnormal Findings

Tell the person, "Please keep looking at that light switch (or mark) on the wall across the room, even though my head will get in the way." Staring at a distant fixed object helps to dilate the pupils and to hold the retinal structures still.

Match sides with the person. That is, hold the ophthalmoscope in your *right* hand up to your *right* eye to view the person's *right* eye. You must do this to avoid bumping noses during the procedure. Place your free hand on the person's shoulder or forehead (Fig. 14-21, *A*). This helps orient you in space, because once you have the ophthalmoscope in position, you only have a very narrow range of vision. Also, your thumb can anchor the upper lid and help prevent blinking.

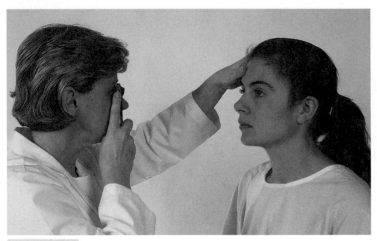

Fig. 14-21A

Begin about 25 cm away from the person at an angle about 15 degrees lateral to the person's line of vision. Note the red glow filling the person's pupil. This is the **red reflex,** caused by the reflection of your ophthalmoscope light off the inner retina. Keep sight of the red reflex, and steadily move closer to the eye. If you lose the red reflex, the light has wandered off the pupil and onto the iris or sclera. Adjust your angle to find it again.

As you advance, adjust the lens to +6 and note any opacities in the media. These appear as dark shadows or black dots interrupting the red reflex. Normally, none are present.

Cataracts appear as opaque black areas against the red reflex (see Table 14-8, p. 338).

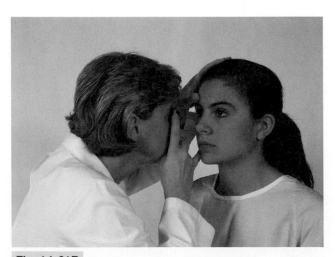

Fig. 14-21B

Normal Range of Findings	Abnormal Findings

Progress toward the person until your foreheads almost touch (Fig. 14-21, *B*). Adjust the dioptre setting to bring the ocular fundus into sharp focus. If you and the person have normal vision, this should be at 0. Moving the dioptres compensates for nearsightedness or farsightedness. Use the red lenses for nearsighted eyes and the black for farsighted eyes (Fig. 14-22).

NORMAL EYE

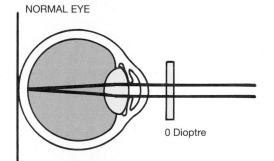

0 Dioptre

The person's eye and your eye are normal. The 0 dioptre (clear glass) will focus sharply on the retina.

MYOPIA (nearsightedness)

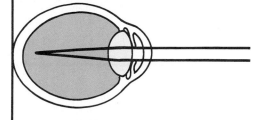

In myopia, the globe is longer than normal, and light rays focus in *front* of the retina.

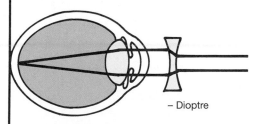

– Dioptre

Compensate for myopia in yourself or the other person by using a negative diptre (red number or concave lens). This corrects the focal point onto the retina.

HYPEROPIA (farsightedness)

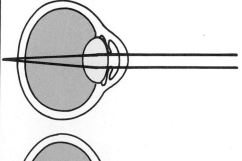

In hyperopia, the globe is shorter than normal. Light rays would focus behind the retina (if they could pass through).

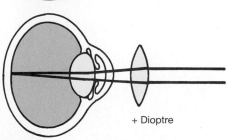

+ Dioptre

Compensate for hyperopia by using a positive dioptre (black number or convex lens). This blends the light rays so the focal point is on the retina.

Fig. 14-22

Objective Data

Normal Range of Findings	Abnormal Findings

Moving in on the 15-degree lateral line should bring your view just to the optic disc. If the disc is not in sight, track a blood vessel as it grows larger and it will lead you to the disc. Systematically inspect the structures in the ocular fundus: (1) optic disc, (2) retinal vessels, (3) general background, and (4) macula (Fig. 14-23). (Note the illustration here shows a large area of the fundus. Your actual view through the ophthalmoscope is much smaller—slightly larger than one disc diameter.)

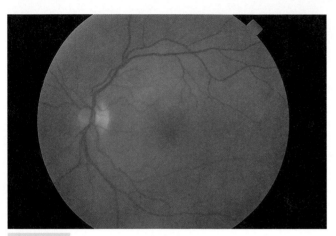

Fig. 14-23   Normal ocular fundus.

Optic Disc

The most prominent landmark is the optic disc, located on the nasal side of the retina. Explore these characteristics:

1.	**Colour**	Creamy yellow-orange to pink.
2.	**Shape**	Round or oval.
3.	**Margins**	Distinct and sharply demarcated, although the nasal edge may be slightly fuzzy.
4.	**Cup–disc ratio**	Distinctness varies. When visible, physiological cup is a brighter yellow-white than rest of the disc. Its width is not more than one half the disc diameter.

Two normal variations may occur around the disc margins. A **scleral crescent** is a grey-white new moon shape (Fig. 14-24). It occurs when pigmentation is absent in the choroid layer and you are looking directly at the sclera. A **pigment crescent** is black; it is due to accumulation of pigment in the choroid.

Abnormal Findings (right column):

Pallor. Hyperemia.
Irregularity.
Blurred margins.

Cup extending to the disc border (see Table 14-9, p. 338).

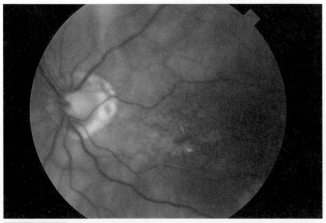

Fig. 14-24   Scleral crescent.

Normal Range of Findings	Abnormal Findings

The diameter of the disc, or DD, is a standard of measure for other fundus structures (Fig. 14-25). To describe a finding, note its clock-face position as well as its relationship to the disc in size and distance (e.g., ". . . at 5:00, 3 DD from the disc").

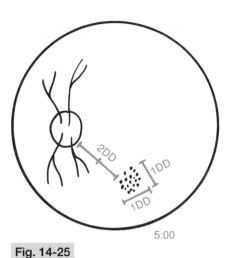

2DD
1DD
1DD
5:00

Fig. 14-25

Retinal Vessels

This is the only place in the body where you can view blood vessels directly. Many systemic diseases that affect the vascular system show signs in the retinal vessels. Follow a paired artery and vein out to the periphery in the four quadrants (see Fig. 14-23), noting these points:

1. **Number**	A paired artery and vein pass through each quadrant. Vessels look straighter at the nasal side.	Absence of major vessels.
2. **Colour**	Arteries are brighter red than are veins. Also, they have the arterial light reflex, with a thin stripe of light down the middle.	
3. **A:V ratio**	The ratio comparing the artery-to-vein width is 2:3 or 4:5.	Arteries too constricted. Veins dilated.
4. **Calibre**	Arteries and veins show a regular decrease in calibre as they extend to periphery.	Focal constriction. Neovascularization.
5. **A-V (arteriovenous) crossing**	An artery and vein may cross paths. This is not significant if within 2 DD of disc and if no sign of interruption in blood flow is seen. There should be no indenting or displacing of vessel.	Crossings more than 2 DD away from disc. Nicking or pinching of underlying vessel. Vessel engorged peripheral to crossing (see Table 14-10, p. 339).
6. **Tortuosity**	Mild vessel twisting when present in both eyes is usually congenital and not significant.	Extreme tortuosity or marked asymmetry in two eyes.
7. **Pulsations**	Present in veins near disc as their drainage meets the intermittent pressure of arterial systole. (Often hard to see.)	Absent pulsations.

General Background of the Fundus

The colour normally varies from light red to dark brown-red, generally corresponding with the person's skin colour. Your view of the fundus should be clear; no lesions should obstruct the retinal structures.

Abnormal lesions: hemorrhages, exudates, microaneurysms.

Normal Range of Findings	Abnormal Findings

Macula

The macula is 1 DD in size and located 2 DD temporal to the disc. Inspect this area last in the funduscopic examination. A bright light on this area of central vision causes some watering and discomfort and pupillary constriction. Note that the normal colour of the area is somewhat darker than the rest of the fundus but is even and homogeneous. Clumped pigment may occur with aging.

Clumped pigment occurs with trauma or retinal detachment.

Within the macula, you may note the foveal light reflex. This is a tiny white glistening dot reflecting your ophthalmoscope's light.

Hemorrhage or exudate in the macula occurs with senile macular degeneration.

 DEVELOPMENTAL CARE

Infants and Children

The eye examination is often deferred at birth because of transient edema of the lids from birth trauma or from the instillation of silver nitrate at birth. The eyes should be examined within a few days and at every well child visit thereafter.

Visual Acuity. The child's age determines the screening measures used. With a newborn, test visual reflexes and attending behaviours. Test **light perception** using the blink reflex; the neonate blinks in response to bright light (Fig. 14-26). Also, the pupillary light reflex shows that the pupils constrict in response to light. These reflexes indicate that the lower portion of the visual apparatus is intact. But you cannot infer that the infant can *see;* that requires later observation to show that the brain has received images and can interpret them.

Absent blinking.
Absent pupillary light reflex, especially after 3 weeks, indicates blindness.

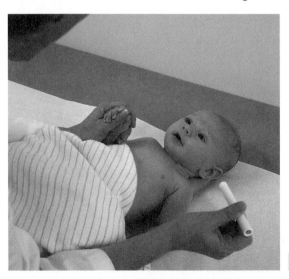

Fig. 14-26

As you introduce an object to the infant's line of vision, note these attending behaviours:

Birth to 2 weeks—Refusal to reopen eyes after exposure to bright light; increasing alertness to object; infant may fixate on an object.
By 2 to 4 weeks—Infant can fixate on an object.
By 1 month—Infant can fixate on and follow a light or bright toy.
By 3 to 4 months—Infant can fixate, follow, and reach for the toy.
By 6 to 10 months—Infant can fixate and follow the toy in all directions.

The Allen test (picture cards) screens children from 30 to 35 months of age and is even reliable with co-operative toddlers as young as 2 years of age. The test contains seven cards of familiar objects (birthday cake, teddy bear, tree, house, car, telephone, and horse and rider). First, show the pictures up close to the child to make sure the child can identify them. Then, present each picture at a distance of 4.5 m. Results are normal if the child can name three of seven cards within three to five trials.

Normal Range of Findings

Use a picture chart or the Snellen E chart for the preschooler from 3 to 6 years of age. The E chart shows the capital letter E in varying sizes pointing in different directions. The child points his or her fingers in the direction the "table legs" are pointing. By 7 to 8 years of age when the child is familiar with reading letters, begin to use the standard Snellen alphabet chart. Normally a child achieves 20/20 acuity by 6 to 7 years of age (Fig. 14-27).

The Canadian Paediatric Society (2007) recommends periodic screening for infants, children, and youth as outlined below:

A. Newborn to 3 months
- A complete examination of the skin and external eye structures as well as the conjunctiva, cornea, iris, and pupils is an integral part of the physical examination of all newborns, infants, and children.
- The red reflex should be inspected for lenticular opacities (cataracts) and signs of posterior eye disease (retinoblastoma).
- Failure of visualization or abnormalities of the red reflex are indications for referral to an ophthalmologist.
- Corneal light reflex should be tested to detect ocular misalignment.

B. Six to 12 months
- Conduct examination as above.
- Ocular alignment should again be observed to detect strabismus. The corneal light reflex should be central and the cover–uncover test normal.
- Fixation and following are observed.

C. Three to 5 years
- Conduct examination as above.
- Visual acuity testing with an optotype test (e.g., E acuity card or Allen chart) should be completed.
- A child with visual acuity <20/30 should be referred to an ophthalmologist.

D. Six to 18 years
- Visual acuity should be assessed every 2 years until age 10 years, then every 3 years thereafter (e.g., Snellen chart).

Abnormal Findings

The U.S.National Society for Prevention of Blindness states these criteria for referral:

1. Age 3 years—vision 20/50 or less in either eye.
2. Age 4 years and over—20/40 or less in either eye.
3. Difference between two eyes is one line or more.
4. Child shows other signs of vision impairment, regardless of acuity.

Screen two separate times before referral.

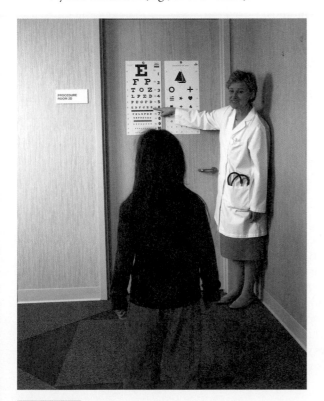

Fig. 14-27

Normal Range of Findings	Abnormal Findings

Visual Fields. Assess peripheral vision with the confrontation test in children older than 3 years when the preschooler is able to stay in position. As with the adult, the child should see the moving target at the same time your normal eyes do. Often a young child forgets to say "now" or "stop" as the moving object is seen. Rather, note the instant the child's eyes deviate or head shifts position to gaze at the moving object. Match this nearly automatic response with your own sighting.

Colour Vision. Colour blindness is an inherited recessive X-linked trait affecting about 8% of Euro-Canadian males. It is less common in males of African or First Nations descent, and it is rare in females. "Colour deficient" is a more accurate term because the condition is relative and not disabling. Often, it is just a social inconvenience, although it may affect the person's ability to discern traffic lights, or it may affect school performance in which colour is a learning tool.

Test only boys for colour vision, once between the ages of 4 and 8 years. Use Ishihara's test, a series of polychromatic cards. Each card has a pattern of dots printed against a background of many coloured dots. Ask the child to identify each pattern. A boy with normal colour vision can see each pattern. A colour blind person cannot see the letter against the field colour.

Extraocular Muscle Function. Testing for **strabismus** (squint, crossed eye) is an important screening measure during early childhood. Strabismus causes disconjugate vision because one eye deviates off the fixation point. To avoid diplopia or unclear images, the brain begins to suppress data from the weak eye (a suppression scotoma). Then visual acuity in this otherwise-normal eye begins to deteriorate from disuse. Early recognition and treatment are essential to restore binocular vision. Diagnosis after 6 years of age has a poor prognosis. Test misalignment by the corneal light reflex and the cover test.

Check the **corneal light reflex** by shining a light toward the child's eyes. The light should be reflected at exactly the same spot in the two corneas (see Fig. 14-29). Some asymmetry (where one light falls off centre) under 6 months of age is normal.

Perform the **cover test** on all children as described on p. 309. Some examiners omit the opaque card and place a hand on the child's head. The examiner's thumb extends down and blocks vision over the eye without actually touching the eye. One can use a familiar character puppet to attract the child's attention. The normal results are the same as those listed in the adult section.

Function of the extraocular muscles during movement can be assessed during the early weeks by the child's gaze following a brightly coloured toy as a target. An older infant can sit on the parent's lap as you move the toy in all directions. After 2 years of age, direct the child's gaze through the six cardinal positions of gaze. You may stabilize the child's chin with your hand to prevent him or her from moving the entire head.

External Eye Structures. Inspect the ocular structures as described in the earlier section. A neonate usually holds the eyes tightly shut. Do not attempt to pry them open; that just increases contraction of the orbicularis oculi muscle. Hold the newborn supine and gently lower the head; the eyes will open. Also, the eyes will open when you hold the infant at arm's length and slowly turn the infant in one direction (Fig. 14-28). In addition to inspecting the ocular structures, this also tests the vestibular function reflex. That is, the baby's eyes will look in the direction the body is being turned. When the turning stops, the eyes will shift to the opposite direction after a few quick beats of nystagmus. Also termed "doll's eyes," this reflex disappears by 2 months of age.

Untreated strabismus can lead to permanent visual damage. The resulting loss of vision from disuse is amblyopia ex anopsia.

Asymmetry in the corneal light reflex after 6 months is abnormal and must be referred.

Objective Data

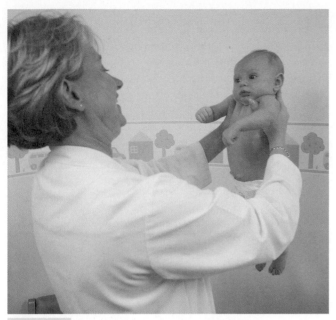

Fig. 14-28

Normal Range of Findings

Eyelids and Lashes. Normally the upper lids overlie the superior part of the iris. In newborns, the *setting-sun sign* is common. The eyes appear to deviate down, and you see a white rim of sclera over the iris. It may show as you rapidly change the neonate from a sitting to a supine position.

Many infants have an *epicanthal fold,* an excess skinfold extending over the inner corner of the eye, partly or totally overlapping the inner canthus. It occurs frequently in Asian children and in 20% of people of European descent. In non-Asians it disappears as the child grows, usually by 10 years of age. While they are present, epicanthal folds give a false appearance of misalignment, termed **pseudostrabismus** (Fig. 14-29). Yet the corneal light reflex is normal.

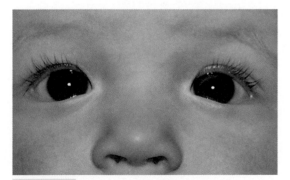

Fig. 14-29   Pseudostrabismus.

Asian infants normally have an upward slant of the palpebral fissures. Entropion, a turning inward of the eyelid, is found normally in some Asian children. If the lashes do not abrade the corneas, it is not significant.

Abnormal Findings

The setting-sun sign also occurs with hydrocephalus as the globes protrude.

Blank sunken eyes accompany malnutrition, dehydration, and a severe illness.

An upward lateral slope together with epicanthal folds and hypertelorism (large spacing between eyes) occurs with Down syndrome.

Objective Data

Objective Data

Normal Range of Findings

Conjunctiva and Sclera. A newborn may have a transient chemical conjunctivitis from the instillation of silver nitrate. This appears within 1 hour and lasts not more than 24 hours after birth. The sclera should be white and clear, although it may have a blue tint as a result of thinness at birth. The lacrimal glands are not functional at birth.

Iris and Pupils. The iris normally is blue or slate grey in light-skinned newborns and brown in dark-skinned infants. By 6 to 9 months, the permanent colour is differentiated. Brushfield's spots, or white specks around the edge of the iris, occasionally may be normal.

A searching nystagmus is common just after birth. The pupils are small but constrict to light.

The Ocular Fundus. The amount of data gathered during the funduscopic examination depends on the infant's ability to hold the eyes still and on your ability to glean as much data as possible in a brief period of time.

A complete funduscopic examination is difficult to perform on an infant, but at least check the red reflex when the infant fixates at the bright light for a few seconds. Note any interruption.

Perform a funduscopic examination on an infant between 2 and 6 months of age. Position the infant (up to 18 months) supine on the table. The fundus appears pale, and the vessels are not fully developed. There is no foveal light reflection because the macula area will not be mature until 1 year.

Inspect the fundus of the young child and school-age child as described in the preceding section on the adult. Allow the child to handle the equipment. Explain why you are darkening the room and that you will leave a small light on. Assure the child that the procedure will not hurt. Direct the young child to look at an appealing picture, or perhaps at a toy or an animal, during the examination.

The Aging Adult

Visual Acuity. Perform the same examination as described in the adult section. Central acuity may decrease, particularly after 70 years of age. Peripheral vision may be diminished.

Ocular Structures. The eyebrows may show a loss of the outer one third to one half of hair because of a decrease in hair follicles. The remaining brow hair is coarse (Fig. 14-30). As a result of atrophy of elastic tissues, the skin around the eyes may show wrinkles or crow's feet. The upper lid may be so elongated as to rest on the lashes, resulting in pseudoptosis.

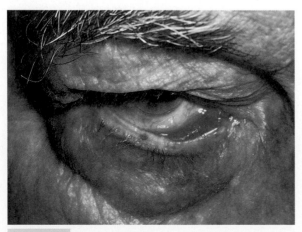

Fig. 14-30   Pseudoptosis.

Abnormal Findings

Ophthalmia neonatorum (conjunctivitis of the newborn) is a purulent discharge caused by a chemical irritant or a bacterial or viral agent from the birth canal.

Absence of iris colour occurs with albinism.

Brushfield's spots usually suggest Down syndrome.

Constant nystagmus, prolonged setting-sun sign, marked strabismus, and slow lateral movements suggest vision loss.

An interruption in the red reflex indicates an opacity in the cornea or lens. An absent red reflex occurs with congenital cataracts or retinal disorders.

Papilledema is rare in the infant because the fontanelles and open sutures will absorb any increased intracranial pressure if it occurs.

Normal Range of Findings

The eyes may appear sunken from atrophy of the orbital fat. Also, the orbital fat may herniate, causing bulging at the lower lids and inner third of the upper lids.

The lacrimal apparatus may decrease tear production, causing the eyes to look dry and lustreless and the person to report a burning sensation. **Pinguecu-lae** commonly show on the sclera (Fig. 14-31). These yellowish elevated nodules occur due to a thickening of the bulbar conjunctiva from prolonged exposure to sun, wind, and dust. Pingueculae appear at the 3:00 and 9:00 positions—first on the nasal side, then on the temporal side.

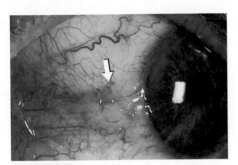

Fig. 14-31   Pinguecula.

The cornea may look cloudy with age. **Arcus senilis** is commonly seen around the cornea (Fig. 14-32). This is a grey-white arc or circle around the limbus; it is due to deposition of lipid material. As more lipid accumulates, the cornea may look thickened and raised, but the arcus has no effect on vision.

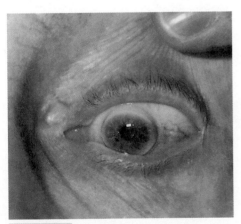

Fig. 14-32   Arcus senilis.

Xanthelasma are soft, raised yellow plaques occurring on the lids at the inner canthus (Fig. 14-33). They commonly occur around the fifth decade of life and more frequently in women. They occur with both high and normal blood levels of cholesterol and have no pathological significance.

Abnormal Findings

Ectropion (lower lid dropping away) and entropion (lower lid turning in) (see Table 14-2, p. 331).

Distinguish pinguecula from the abnormal **pterygium**, also an opacity on the bulbar conjunctiva, but one that grows over the cornea (see Table 14-7, p. 337).

Objective Data

Normal Range of Findings	**Abnormal Findings**

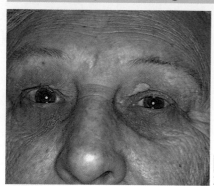

Fig. 14-33
Xanthelasma.

Pupils are small in old age, and the pupillary light reflex may be slowed. The lens loses transparency and looks opaque.

The Ocular Fundus. Retinal structures generally have less shine. The blood vessels look paler, narrower, and attenuated. Arterioles appear paler and straighter, with a narrower light reflex. More arteriovenous crossing defects occur.

A normal development on the retinal surface is **drusen,** or benign degenerative hyaline deposits (Fig. 14-34). They are small, round, yellow dots that are scattered haphazardly on the retina. Although they do not occur in a pattern, they are usually symmetrically placed in the two eyes. They have no effect on vision.

Drusen are easily confused with the abnormal finding *hard exudates,* which occur with a more circular or linear pattern (see Table 14-10, p. 339). Also, drusen in the macular area occur with macular degeneration.

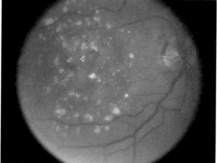

Fig. 14-34
Drusen.

Summary Checklist: Eye Examination

 For a PDA-downloadable version, go to http://evolve.elsevier.com/Canada/Jarvis/examination/.

1. **Test visual acuity**
   Snellen eye chart
   Near vision (those older than 40 years or those having difficulty reading)
2. **Test visual fields**—confrontation test
3. **Inspect extraocular muscle function**
   Corneal light reflex (Hirschberg's test)
   Cover test
   Diagnostic positions test

4. **Inspect external eye structures**
   General
   Eyebrows
   Eyelids and lashes
   Eyeball alignment
   Conjunctiva and sclera
   Lacrimal apparatus
5. **Inspect anterior eyeball structures**
   Cornea and lens
   Iris and pupil
      Size, shape, and equality
      Pupillary light reflex
      Accommodation

6. **Inspect the ocular fundus**
   Optic disc (colour, shape, margins, cup–disc ratio)
   Retinal vessels (number, colour, artery–vein [A:V] ratio, calibre, arteriovenous crossings, tortuosity, pulsations)
   General background (colour, integrity)
   Macula

Promoting Health: Screening for Glaucoma

Preventing Glaucoma

Glaucoma is the second leading cause of preventable blindness in Canada. Glaucoma is a condition in which the optic nerve is damaged, usually as a result of increasing pressure within the eye. The risk of glaucoma increases with age, but it can occur in anyone in any age group. Glaucoma is not curable, and an individual's vision, once lost, cannot be regained. However, with medication or surgery, it is possible to halt further loss of vision. Screening for glaucoma is the first step in early diagnosis and intervention. Primary open-angle glaucoma causes such insidious damage to the optic nerve and vision that few people have early awareness of the condition (CPGEC, 2007). As a result, only half of patients are diagnosed in developed countries such as Canada. However, it is an ideal disorder for screening because it is asymptomatic, typically progresses slowly, and can be effectively treated.

The prevalence of open-angle glaucoma is 60% greater in women than in men, between the ages of 70 and 79 (CNIB, 2004). Over age 80, almost 300% more women than men have open-angle glaucoma. In the United States, glaucoma-related vision compromise was reported as three times more prevalent in people of African or Hispanic descent (CPGEC, 2007). Increasing age and family history are major risk factors. Healthcare professionals should encourage regular eye examinations, especially for those with known risk factors. Risk factors for glaucoma include:

1. Being over 60 years of age
2. Being of African descent
3. Being a woman
4. Increased intraocular pressure (IOP) above 21 mm Hg
5. Family history of glaucoma
6. Steroid use
7. Decreased central corneal thickness less than 0.5 mm
8. Hypertension
9. Eye injury
10. Severe myopia (nearsightedness)
11. Diabetes
12. Use of certain other medications, including antihypertensives, antihistamines, anticholinergics, and antidepressants

There are two main types of glaucoma. To understand the difference, it is helpful to review the basic structure of the eye. The anterior and posterior chambers of the eye are filled with a fluid called aqueous humor. This fluid is produced in the posterior chamber and then passes into the anterior chamber through the pupil. The fluid moves out of the eye and into the bloodstream through a drainage area located in front of the iris. This drainage area is located in the angle formed between the iris and the point at which the iris appears to meet the inside of the cornea. If the flow of aqueous humor is blocked, intraocular pressure increases. This pressure eventually damages the optic nerve and results in a permanent loss of vision because, in the retina, neurons are not regenerated once they are lost.

Open-angle glaucoma is the most common type of glaucoma, accounting for more than 90% of all cases. With open-angle glaucoma, the angle between the iris and the cornea is open, but the fluid is slow to drain, creating a buildup of pressure. There are virtually no symptoms. Vision loss begins with the peripheral vision, which often goes unnoticed because individuals learn to compensate intuitively by turning their heads. As the condition progresses, individuals have a decreasing field of peripheral vision until eventually they may not be able to see anything on either side. This is referred to as tunnel vision.

Closed-angle glaucoma occurs when the space between the cornea and iris is narrower than normal. Anything that causes the pupil to dilate, such as dim light, eye drops, or certain medications, can block the drainage of fluid. Aging and injury also contribute to and can block the drainage of fluid. Closed-angle glaucoma causes sudden attacks of increased pressure that result in blurred vision, sensitivity to light, nausea, and halos around lights. The affected individuals must be treated immediately.

Regular comprehensive eye examinations are extremely important because glaucoma does not have symptoms in its early stages. These examinations should include:

1. Visual acuity testing
2. Visual field testing
3. Dilated eye examination
4. Tonometry to measure the pressure inside the eye

Screening with simple IOP testing and optic nerve examination tend to underestimate the prevalence of glaucoma (CPGEC, 2007). While visual field testing typically reveals damage, it is usually at a more advanced stage than the very early stage ideal for diagnosis and treatment. Other testing provided by ophthalmologists include frequency-doubling technology perimetry to demonstrate early damage to visual function, tomography to measure IOP, and laser imaging to assess the nerve fibre layer (Einarson et al., 2006).

Although individuals who wear glasses appear to have more regular eye examinations, healthcare professionals need to remind all individuals of the risk for glaucoma and the need for regular comprehensive eye examinations.

Fleming, C. et al. (2005). Screening for primary open-angle glaucoma in the primary care setting: An update from the United States Preventive Services Task Force, *Annals of Family Medicine, 3,* 167–172.

Salmon, J.F. Screening for chronic glaucoma, *Journal of Medical Screening,13,* 1–3.

Clinical Practice Guideline Expert Committee. (2007). Canadian Ophthalmological Society evidence-based clinical practice guidelines for the periodic eye examination in adults in Canada. *Canadian Journal of Ophthalmology, 42,* 39–45.

Documentation and Critical Thinking

❧— DOCUMENTATION AND CRITICAL THINKING —❧

Sample Charting

SUBJECTIVE

Vision reported good with no recent change. No eye pain, no inflammation, no discharge, no lesions. Wears no corrective lenses, vision last tested 1 year PTA, test for glaucoma at that time was normal.

OBJECTIVE

Snellen chart—O.D. 20/20, O.S. 20/20 −1. Fields normal by confrontation. Corneal light reflex symmetrical bilaterally. Diagnostic positions test shows EOMs intact. Brows and lashes present. No ptosis. Conjunctiva clear. Sclera white. No lesions. PERRLA.

Fundi: Red reflex present bilaterally. Discs flat with sharp margins. Vessels present in all quadrants without crossing defects. Retinal background has even colour with no hemorrhages or exudates. Macula has even colour.

ASSESSMENT

Healthy vision function
Healthy eye structures

Focused Assessment: Clinical Case Study 1

Emma K. is a 34-year-old married, female homemaker brought to the emergency department by police after a reported domestic quarrel.

SUBJECTIVE

• States husband struck her on the face and eyes with his fists about 1 hour PTA. "I ruined the dinner again. I can't do anything right." Pain in left cheek and both eyes felt immediately and continues. Alarmed at "bright red blood on eyeball." No bleeding from eye area or cheek. Vision intact just after trauma. Now reports difficulty opening lids.

OBJECTIVE

Sitting quietly and hunched over, hands over eyes. Voice tired and flat. L cheek swollen and discoloured, no laceration. Lids edematous and discoloured both eyes. No skin laceration. L lid swollen almost shut. L eye—round 1-mm bright red patch over lateral aspect of globe at 3:00 position. No active bleeding out of eye, iris intact, anterior chamber clear. R eye—conjunctiva clear, sclera white, cornea and iris intact, anterior chamber clear. PERRLA. Pupils R 4/1 = 4/1 L. Vision 14/14 both eyes by Jaeger card.

ASSESSMENT

Ecchymoses L cheek and both eyes
Subconjunctival hemorrhage L eye
Pain R/T inflammation
Chronic low self-esteem R/T effects of domestic violence

Focused Assessment: Clinical Case Study 2

Sam T. is a 63-year-old married, male postal carrier admitted to the medical centre for surgery for suspected brain tumour. After postanaesthesia recovery, Sam T. is admitted to the neurology ICU, awake, lethargic with slowed but correct verbal responses, oriented × 3, moving all four extremities, vital signs stable. Pupils R 4/2 = 4/2 L with sluggish response. Assessments are made q15 min.

SUBJECTIVE

• No response now to verbal stimuli.

OBJECTIVE

Semicomatose—no response to verbal stimuli, does withdraw R arm and leg purposefully to painful stimuli. No movement L arm or leg. Pupils R 5/5 ≠ L 4/2. Vitals remain stable as noted on graphic sheet.

ASSESSMENT

Unilateral dilated and fixed R pupil
Clouding of consciousness
Focal motor deficit—no movement L side
Ineffective tissue perfusion R/T interruption of cerebral flow

Focused Assessment: Clinical Case Study 3

Trung Q. is a 4-year-old male born in Southeast Asia who arrived in this country 1 month PTA. Lives with parents, two siblings. Speaks only native language; here with uncle, who acts as interpreter.

SUBJECTIVE

• Seeks care because RN in church sponsoring family noted "crossed eyes." Uncle states vision seemed normal to parents. Plays with toys and manipulates small objects without difficulty. Identifies objects in picture books; does not read.

OBJECTIVE

With uncle interpreting directions for test to Trung, vision by Snellen E chart—O.D. 20/30, O.S. 20/50 −1. Fields seem intact by confrontation—jerks head to gaze at object entering field.
EOMs: Asymmetrical corneal light reflex with outward deviation L eye. Cover test—as R eye covered, L eye jerks to fixate, R eye steady when uncovered. As L eye covered, R eye holds steady gaze, L eye jerks to fixate as uncovered. Diagnostic positions—able to gaze in six positions, although L eye obviously misaligned at extreme medial gaze.
Eye structures: Brows and lashes present and normal bilaterally. Upward palpebral slant, epicanthal folds bilaterally—consistent with shape of eyes. Conjunctiva clear, sclera white, iris intact, PERRLA.
Fundi: Discs flat with sharp margins. Observed vessels normal. Unable to see in all four quadrants or to see macular area.

ASSESSMENT

L exotropia
Abnormal vision in L eye
Disturbed visual sensory perception R/T effects of neurological impairment.

Focused Assessment: Clinical Case Study 4

Vera K. is an 87-year-old widowed, African Canadian, female homemaker living independently who is admitted to hospital for observation and adjustment of digitalis medication. Cardiac status has been stable during hospital stay.

SUBJECTIVE

• Reports desire to monitor own medication at home but fears problems because of blurred vision. First noted distant vision blurred 5 years ago but near vision seemed to improve at that time: "I started to read better without my glasses!" Since then, blurring of distant vision has increased, near vision now blurred also.
• Able to navigate home environment without difficulty. Fixes simple meals with cold foods. Receives hot meal from "Meals on Wheels" at lunch. Enjoys TV, though it looks somewhat blurred. Unable to write letters, sew, or read paper, which she regrets.

OBJECTIVE

Vision by Jaeger card O.D. 20/200, O.S. 20/400 −1, with glasses on. Fields intact by confrontation. EOMs intact. Brow hair absent lateral third. Upper lids have folds of redundant skin but lids do not droop. Lower lids and lashes intact. Xanthelasma present both inner canthi. Conjunctiva clear, sclera white, iris intact, L pupil looks cloudy, PERRLA, pupils R 3/2 = 3/2 L.
Fundi: Red reflex has central dark spot both eyes. Discs flat, with sharp margins. Observed vessels normal. Unable to see in all four quadrants or macular area because of small pupils.

ASSESSMENT

Central opacity, both eyes
Central visual acuity deficit, both eyes
Deficient diversional activity R/T poor vision

Nursing Diagnoses Commonly Associated With the Eye and Visual Disorders

All nursing diagnoses can be found on the Evolve Web site at **http://evolve.elsevier.com/Canada/Jarvis/examination/**.

ABNORMAL FINDINGS

TABLE 14-1	Extraocular Muscle Dysfunction

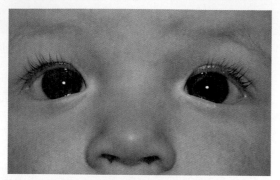

A, Pseudostrabismus.

◀ **Symmetrical Corneal Light Reflex**

A. **Pseudostrabismus** has the appearance of strabismus because of epicanthic fold but is normal for a young child.

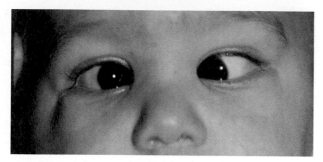

B, Left esotropia.

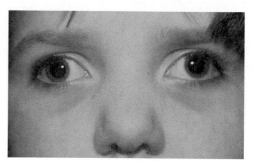

C, Exotropia.

Asymmetrical Corneal Light Reflex

Strabismus is true disparity of the eye axes. This constant misalignment is also termed *tropia* and is likely to cause amblyopia.
B. Esotropia—inward turn of the eye.
C. Exotropia—outward turning of the eyes.

Cover Test

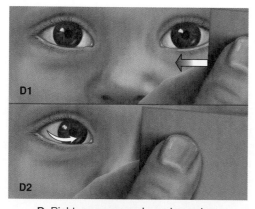

D, Right, or uncovered eye, is weaker.

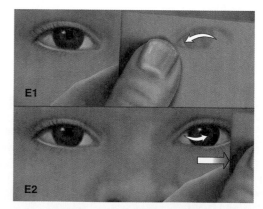

E, Left, or covered eye, is weaker.

D. Uncovered eye—If it jumps to fixate on designated point, it was out of alignment before (i.e., when you cover the stronger eye [D1], the weaker eye now tries to fixate [D2]).

Phoria—mild weakness, apparent only with the cover test and less likely to cause amblyopia than a tropia but still possible.

E. Covered eye—If this is the weaker eye, once macular image is suppressed it will drift to relaxed position (E1).

As eye is uncovered—If it jumps to re-establish fixation (E2), weakness exists.

Esophoria—nasal (inward) drift.
Exophoria—temporal (outward) drift.

| TABLE 14-1 | Extraocular Muscle Dysfunction—cont'd |

Diagnostic Positions Test

(Paralysis apparent during movement through six cardinal positions of gaze.)

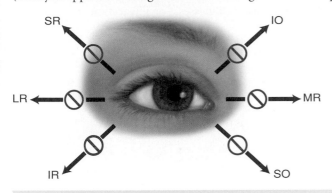

If eye will not turn:	Indicates paralysis in:	or cranial nerve
Straight nasal	Medial rectus	III
Up and nasal	Inferior oblique	III
Up and temporal	Superior rectus	III
Straight temporal	Lateral rectus	VI
Down and temporal	Inferior rectus	III
Down and nasal	Superior oblique	IV

| TABLE 14-2 | Abnormalities in the Eyelids |

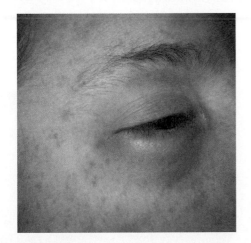

Periorbital Edema

Lids are swollen and puffy. Lid tissues are loosely connected, so excess fluid is easily apparent. This occurs with local infections; crying; and systemic conditions such as congestive heart failure, renal failure, allergy, hypothyroidism (myxedema).

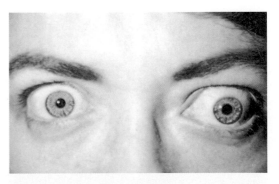

Exophthalmos (Protruding Eyes)

Exophthalmos is a forward displacement of the eyeballs and widened palpebral fissures. Note "lid lag," the upper lid rests well above the limbus, and white sclera is visible. Acquired bilateral exophthalmos is associated with thyrotoxicosis.

Continued

TABLE 14-2	Abnormalities in the Eyelids—cont'd

Enophthalmos (Sunken Eyes) (not illustrated)

A look of narrowed palpebral fissures shows with enophthalmos, in which the eyeballs are recessed. Bilateral enophthalmos is caused by loss of fat in the orbits and occurs with dehydration and chronic wasting illnesses. For illustration, see "Cachetic Appearance" in Table 13-4, p. 294.

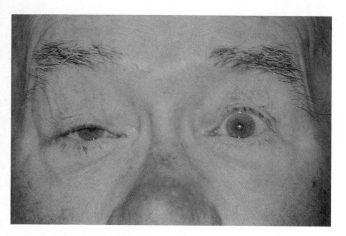

Ptosis (Drooping Upper Lid)

Ptosis occurs from neuromuscular weakness (e.g., myasthenia gravis with bilateral fatigue as the day progresses), oculomotor cranial nerve III damage, or sympathetic nerve damage (e.g., Horner's syndrome). It is a positional defect that gives the person a sleepy appearance and impairs vision.

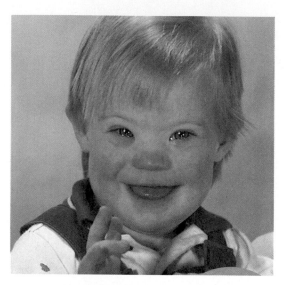

Upward Palpebral Slant

Although normal in many children, when combined with epicanthal folds, hypertelorism (large spacing between the eyes), and Brushfield's spots (light-coloured areas in outer iris), indicates Down syndrome.

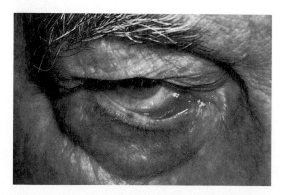

Ectropion

The lower lid is loose and rolling out, does not approximate to eyeball. Puncta cannot siphon tears effectively, so excess tearing results. The eyes feel dry and itchy because the tears do not drain correctly over the corner and toward the medial canthus. Exposed palpebral conjunctiva increases risk for inflammation. Occurs in aging as a result of atrophy of elastic and fibrous tissues but may result from trauma.

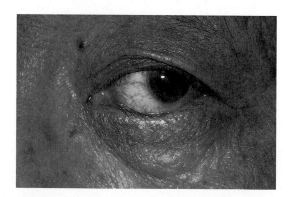

Entropion

The lower lid rolls in because of spasm of lids or scar tissue contracting. Constant rubbing of lashes may irritate cornea. The person feels a "foreign body" sensation.

TABLE 14-3   Lesions on the Eyelids

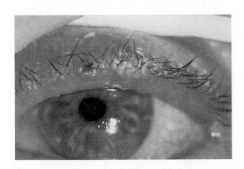

Blepharitis (Inflammation of the Eyelids)

Red, scaly, greasy flakes and thickened, crusted lid margins occur with staphylococcal infection or seborrheic dermatitis of the lid edge. Symptoms include burning, itching, tearing, foreign body sensation, and some pain.

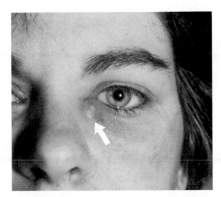

Chalazion

A beady nodule protruding on the lid, chalazion is an infection or retention cyst of a meibomian gland. It is a nontender, firm, discrete swelling with freely movable skin overlying the nodule. If it becomes inflamed, it points inside and not on lid margin (in contrast with stye).

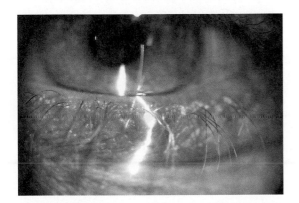

Hordeolum (Stye)

Hordeolum is a localized staphylococcal infection of the hair follicles at the lid margin. It is painful, red, and swollen—a pustule at the lid margin. Rubbing the eyes can cause cross-contamination and development of another stye.

Dacryocystitis (Inflammation of the Lacrimal Sac)

Dacryocystitis is infection and blockage of sac and duct. Pain, warmth, redness, and swelling occur below the inner canthus toward nose. Tearing is present. Pressure on sac yields purulent discharge from puncta.

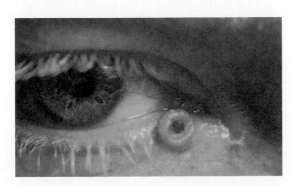

◄ **Basal Cell Carcinoma**

Carcinoma is rare, but it occurs most often on the lower lid and medial canthus. It looks like a papule with an ulcerated centre. Note the rolled-out pearly edges. It should be referred for removal though metastasis is rare.

Dacryoadenitis (Inflammation of the Lacrimal Gland) (not illustrated)

Dacryoadenitis is an infection of the lacrimal gland. Pain, swelling, and redness occur in the outer third of upper lid. It occurs with mumps, measles, and infectious mononucleosis, or from trauma.

Abnormal Findings

TABLE 14-4 | **Abnormalities in the Pupil**

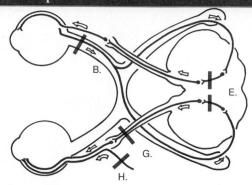

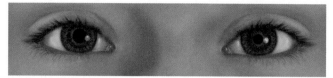

A. Unequal Pupil Size—Anisocoria

Although this exists normally in 5% of the population, consider central nervous system disease.

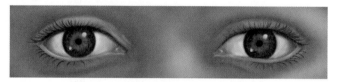

C. Constricted and Fixed Pupils—Miosis

Miosis occurs with the use of pilocarpine drops for glaucoma treatment, the use of narcotics, with iritis, and with damage of pons in the brain.

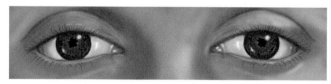

E. Argyll Robertson Pupil

No reaction to light, pupil does constrict with accommodation. Small and irregular bilaterally. Argyll Robertson pupil occurs with central nervous system syphilis, brain tumour, meningitis, and chronic alcoholism.

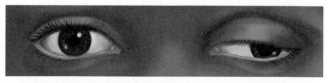

G. Cranial Nerve III Damage

Unilateral dilated pupil with no reaction to light or accommodation, occurs with oculomotor nerve damage. Ptosis may also be present, with eye deviating down and laterally.

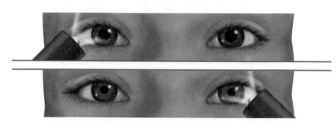

B. Monocular Blindness

When light is directed to the blind eye, no response occurs in either eye. When light is directed to normal eye, both pupils constrict (direct and consensual response to light) as long as the oculomotor nerve is intact.

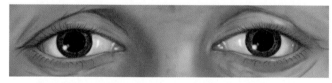

D. Dilated and Fixed Pupils—Mydriasis

Enlarged pupils occur with stimulation of the sympathetic nervous system, reaction to sympathomimetic drugs, use of dilating drops, acute glaucoma, past or recent trauma. Also, they herald central nervous system injury, circulatory arrest, or deep anaesthesia.

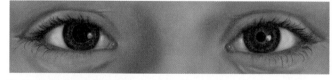

F. Tonic Pupil (Adie's Pupil)

Sluggish reaction to light and accommodation. Tonic pupil is usually unilateral, a large regular pupil that does react, but sluggishly after long latent time. No pathological significance.

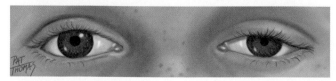

H. Horner Syndrome

Unilateral, small, regular pupil does react to light and accommodation. Occurs with Horner syndrome, a lesion of the sympathetic nerve. Also, note ptosis and absence of sweat (anhidrosis) on same side.

ABNORMAL FINDINGS
FOR ADVANCED PRACTICE

TABLE 14-5 | **Visual Field Loss**

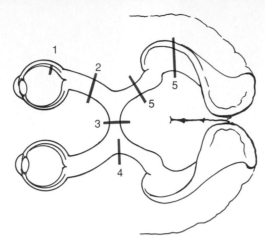

1. Retinal damage
   - Macula—central blind area (e.g., in diabetes):

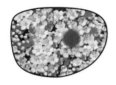

   - Localized damage—blind spot (scotoma) corresponding to particular area:

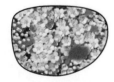

   - Increasing intraocular pressure—decrease in peripheral vision (e.g., glaucoma). Starts with paracentral scotoma in early stage:

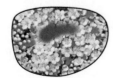

   - Retinal detachment. Person has shadow or diminished vision in one quadrant or one half of visual field:

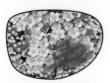

2. Lesion in globe or optic nerve. Injury here yields one blind eye, or unilateral blindness:

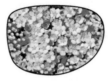

3. Lesion at optic chiasm (e.g., pituitary tumour). Injury to crossing fibres only yields a loss of nasal part of each retina and a loss of both temporal visual fields. Bi-temporal (heteronymous) hemianopsia:

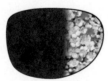

4. Lesion of outer uncrossed fibres at optic chiasm (e.g., aneurysm of left internal carotid artery exerts pressure on uncrossed fibres). Injury yields left nasal hemianopsia:

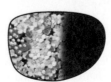

5. Lesion R optic tract or R optic radiation. Visual field loss in R nasal and L temporal fields. Loss of same half visual field in both eyes is homonymous hemianopsia:

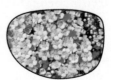

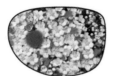
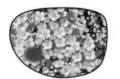
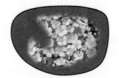
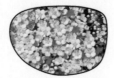
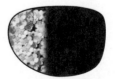
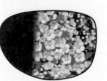
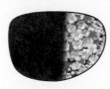

TABLE 14-6	**Vascular Disorders of the External Eye**

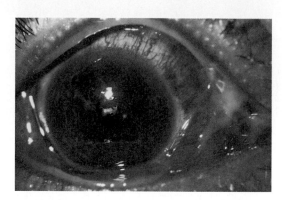

Conjunctivitis

Infection of the conjunctiva, "pink eye," has red, beefy-looking vessels at periphery but usually clearer around iris (although here it is severe). This is common from bacterial or viral infection, allergy, or chemical irritation. Purulent discharge accompanies bacterial infection. Preauricular lymph node is often swollen and painful, with a history of upper respiratory infection. Symptoms include itching, burning, foreign body sensation, and eyelids stuck together on awakening.

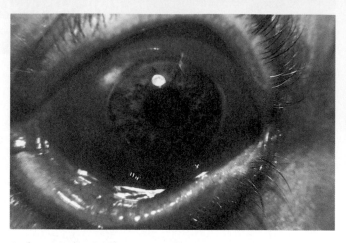

Subconjunctival Hemorrhage

A red patch on the sclera, subconjunctival hemorrhage looks alarming but is usually not serious. The red patch has clear edges, although here it is extensive. It occurs from increased intraocular pressure from coughing, sneezing, weight lifting, labour during childbirth, straining at stool, or trauma.

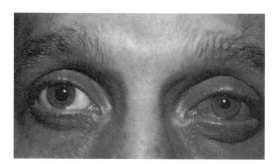

Iritis (Circumcorneal Redness)

Deep dull red halo around the iris and cornea. Note redness around iris, in contrast with conjunctivitis, in which the redness is more prominent at the periphery. Pupil shape may be irregular from swelling of iris. Person also has marked photophobia, constricted pupil, blurred vision, and throbbing pain. Warrants immediate referral.

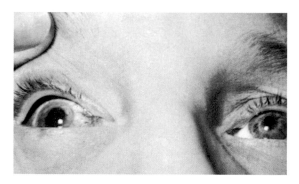

Acute Glaucoma

Acute, narrow-angle glaucoma shows a circumcorneal redness around the iris, with a dilated pupil. Pupil is oval, dilated; cornea looks "steamy"; and anterior chamber is shallow. Acute glaucoma occurs with sudden increase in intraocular pressure from blocked outflow from anterior chamber. The person experiences a sudden clouding of vision, sudden eye pain, and halos around lights. This requires emergency treatment to avoid permanent vision loss.

Abnormal Findings

TABLE 14-7 | **Abnormalities on the Cornea and Iris**

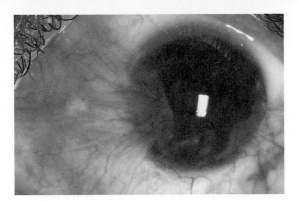

Pterygium

A triangular opaque wing of bulbar conjunctiva overgrows toward the centre of the cornea. It looks membranous, translucent, and yellow to white, usually invades from nasal side, and it may obstruct vision as it covers pupil. Occurs usually from chronic exposure to hot, dry, sandy climate, which stimulates the growth of a pinguecula (p. 325) into a pterygium.

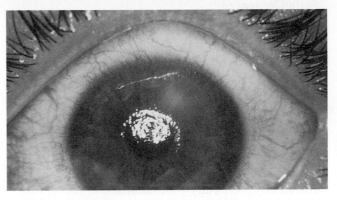

Corneal Abrasion

This is the most common result of a blunt eye injury, but irregular ridges usually visible only when fluorescein stain reveals yellow-green branching. Top layer of corneal epithelium removed, from scratches or poorly fitting or overworn contact lenses. Because the area is rich in nerve endings, the person feels intense pain, a foreign body sensation, and lacrimation, redness, and photophobia.

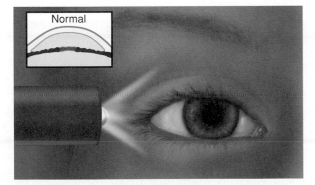

Normal Anterior Chamber (for Contrast)

A light directed across the eye from the temporal side illuminates the entire iris evenly because the normal iris is flat and creates no shadow.

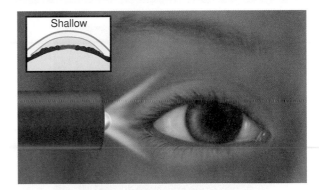

Shallow Anterior Chamber

The iris is pushed anteriorly because of increased intraocular pressure. Because direct light is received from the temporal side, only the temporal part of iris is illuminated; the nasal side is shadowed, the "shadow sign." This may be a sign of acute angle closure glaucoma; the iris looks bulging because aqueous humor cannot circulate.

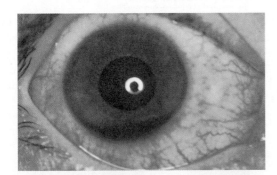

Hyphema

Blood in anterior chamber is a serious result of blunt trauma (a fist or a baseball) or spontaneous hemorrhage. Suspect scleral rupture or major intraocular trauma. Note that gravity settles blood.

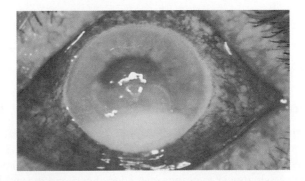

Hypopyon

Purulent matter in anterior chamber occurs with iritis and with inflammation in the anterior chamber.

TABLE 14-8	Opacities in the Lens

Senile Cataracts

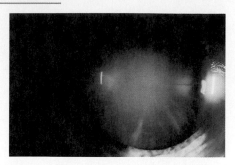

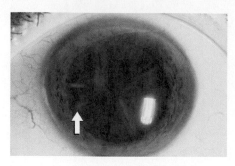

Central Grey Opacity—Nuclear Cataract

Nuclear cataract shows as an opaque grey surrounded by black background as it forms in the centre of lens nucleus. Through the ophthalmoscope, it looks like a black centre against the red reflex. It begins after age 40 years and develops slowly, gradually obstructing vision.

Star-Shaped Opacity—Cortical Cataract

Cortical cataract shows as asymmetrical, radial, white spokes with black centre. Through ophthalmoscope, black spokes are evident against the red reflex. This forms in outer cortex of lens, progressing faster than nuclear cataract.

TABLE 14-9	Abnormalities in the Optic Disc

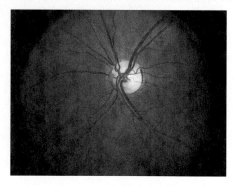

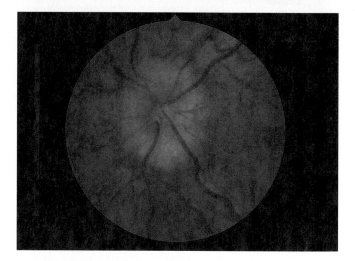

Optic Atrophy (Disc Pallor)

Optic atrophy is a white or grey colour of the disc as a result of partial or complete death of the optic nerve. This results in decreased visual acuity, decreased colour vision, and decreased contrast sensitivity.

Papilledema (Choked Disc)

Increased intracranial pressure causes venous stasis in the globe, showing redness, congestion, and elevation of the disc; blurred margins; hemorrhages; and absent venous pulsations. This is a serious sign of intracranial pressure, usually caused by a space-occupying mass (e.g., a brain tumour) or hematoma). Visual acuity is not affected.

Excessive Cup–Disc Ratio   ▶

With primary, open-angle glaucoma, the increased intraocular pressure decreases blood supply to retinal structures. The physiological cup enlarges to more than half of the disc diameter, vessels appear to plunge over edge of cup, and the vessels are displaced nasally. This is asymptomatic, although the person may have decreased vision or visual field defects in the late stages of glaucoma.

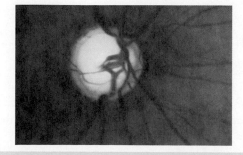

TABLE 14-10 | Abnormalities in Retinal Vessels and Background

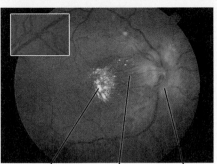

Macular star   Retinal folds   Disc edema

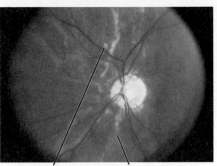

Elschnig spots   Siegrist streaks

Arteriovenous Crossing (Nicking)

Arteriovenous crossing with interruption of blood flow. When vein is occluded, it dilates distal to crossing. This person also has disc edema and hard exudates in a macular star pattern that occur with acutely elevated (malignant) hypertension. With hypertension, the arteriole wall thickens and becomes opaque so that no blood is seen inside it (silverwire arteries).

Narrowed (Attenuated) Arteries

This is a generalized decrease in diameter. The light reflex also narrows. It occurs with severe hypertension (shown here) and with occlusion of central retinal artery and retinitis pigmentosa.

Vessel Nicking

Nicking is a localized narrowing in vein caused by arteriole crossing. It is seen with hypertension and arteriosclerosis.

Diabetic Retinopathy

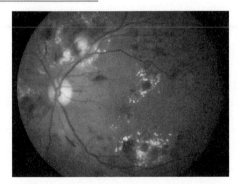

◄ Microaneurysms

Microaneurysms are round punctate red dots that are localized dilatations of a small vessel. Their edges are smooth and discrete. The vessel itself is too small to view with the ophthalmoscope; only the isolated red dots are seen. This occurs with diabetes.

Intraretinal Hemorrhages

Dot-shaped hemorrhages are deep intraretinal hemorrhages that look splattered on. They may be distinguished from microaneurysms by the blurred irregular edges. Flame-shaped hemorrhages are superficial retinal hemorrhages that look linear and spindle shaped. They occur with hypertension.

Exudates

Soft exudates or "cotton wool" areas look like fluffy grey-white cumulus clouds. They are arteriolar microinfarctions that envelop and obscure the vessels. They occur with diabetes, hypertension, subacute bacterial endocarditis, lupus, and papilledema of any cause. Hard exudates are numerous small yellow-white spots, having distinct edges and a smooth, solid-looking surface. They often form a circular pattern, clustered around a venous microinfarction. They also may form a linear or star pattern. (This is in contrast with drusen, which have a scattered haphazard location [see Fig. 14-34, p. 326].)

BIBLIOGRAPHY

Altersitz, K. (2006). Women's eye health series examine ocular complications, systemic disease. *Ocular Surgery News, 24*, 85.

Bakes, K., & Cadnapaphornchai, L. (2005). Clinical assessment of vision loss. *Emergency Medicine, 37*, 14–24.

Bal, S., & Hollingworth, G. (2005). 10-minute consultation: Red eye. *British Medical Journal, 331*, 438.

Bielory, L. (2006). Allergic diseases of the eye. *Medical Clinics of North America, 90*, 129–148.

Boyd-Monk, H. (2005). Bringing common eye emergencies into focus. *Nursing, 35*, 46–51.

Brown, G. (Ed.). (2005). Retinal, vitreous and macular disorders. *Current Opinion in Ophthalmology, 16*, 139–229.

Canadian Diabetes Association Clinical Practice Guidelines Expert Committee. (2003). Canadian Diabetes Association 2003 clinical practice guidelines for the prevention and management of diabetes in Canada. *Canadian Journal of Diabetes, 27*(Suppl. 2), S76–S80.

Canadian National Institute for the Blind. (2004). *A clear vision: Solutions to Canada's vision loss crisis*. Toronto: Canterbury Communications.

Canadian National Institute for the Blind. (2008). *Glossary of terms related to AMD*. Retrieved April 11, 2008, from http://www.cnib.ca/en/your-eyes/eye-conditions/amd/resources/glossary/Default.aspx

Canadian Ophthalmological Society. (2008). *Position statement. Low vision*. Retrieved April 11, 2008, from http://www.eyesite.ca/english/program-and-services/policy-statements-guidelines/low-vision.htm

Canadian Paediatric Society. (2007). *Position statement. Vision screening in infants, children and youth*. Retrieved April 11, 2008, from http://www.cps.ca/English/statements/CP/cp98-01.htm

Clinical Practice Guideline Expert Committee. (2007). Canadian Ophthalmological Society evidence-based clinical practice guidelines for the periodic eye examination in adults in Canada. *Canadian Journal of Ophthalmology, 42*, 39–45.

Einarson, T., Vicente, C., Machado, M., Covert, D., Trope, G., et al. (2006). Screening for glaucoma in Canada: A systematic review of the literature. *Canadian Journal of Ophthalmology, 41*, 709–721.

First Nations and Inuit Health. (2007). *Diabetes initiative*. Retrieved February 11, 2008, from http://www.hc-sc.gc.ca/fnih-spni/diseases-maladies/diabete/index_e.html

Gillett, P., & Goldblum, K. (2004). Ophthalmic patient assessment. *Journal of the American Society of Ophthalmic Registered Nurses, 29*, 23–28.

Groopman, J. (2003, September 29). The bionic eye: Can scientists use electronic implants to help the blind see? *New Yorker*, 48–54, 67–68.

Halle, C. (2002). Achieve new vision screening objectives. *Nurse Practitioner, 27*, 15–37.

Hammersmith, K. (Ed.). (2005). Corneal and external disorders. *Current Opinion in Ophthalmology, 16*, 231–250.

Helzner, E. P., Cauley, J. A., Pratt, S. R., Wisniewski, S. R., Zmuda, J. M., Talbott, E. O., et al. (2005). Race and sex differences in age-related hearing loss: The Health, Aging and Body Composition Study. *Journal of the American Geriatric Society, 53*, 2119–2127.

Houde, S. C. (2001). Age-related vision loss in the older adult. *Clinical Excellence for Nurse Practitioners, 5*, 185–196.

Hoyt, K., & Haley, R. (2005). Innovations in advanced practice: Assessment and management of eye emergencies. *Topics in Emergency Medicine, 27*, 101–117.

Kaiser, P. K., Friedman, N. J., & Pineda, R. (2003). *The Massachusetts Eye and Ear Infirmary illustrated manual of ophthalmology* (2nd ed.). Philadelphia: W.B. Saunders.

Kane, R. T., Ouslander, J. G., & Abrass, I. B. (2003). *Essentials of clinical geriatrics* (5th ed.). New York: McGraw-Hill.

Kerns, B., & Mason, J. (2004). Red eye: A guide through the differential diagnosis. *Emergency Medicine, 36*, 31, 35–36, 38.

Khaw, P., Shah, P., & Elkington, A. (2004). ABC of eyes: Injury to the eye. *British Medical Journal, 328*, 36–38.

McLaughlin, C., & Levin, A. (2006). The red reflex. *Pediatric Emergency Care, 22*, 137–140.

Miller, N., & Newman, N. (2004). The eye in neurological disease. *Lancet, 364*, 2045–2054.

Opstelten, W., & Zaal, M. (2005). Managing ophthalmic herpes zoster in primary care. *British Medical Journal, 331*, 147–151.

Watkinson, S. (2005). Visual impairment in older people. *Nursing Standard, 19*, 45–52.

Watkinson, S., & Graham, S. (2005). Visual impairment in children. *Nursing Standard, 19*, 58–65.

Wehenmeyer, J., & Gallman, E. (2002). *Neuroscience curriculum* (25th ed.). Urbana-Champaign: University of Illinois.

Whiteside, M., Wallhagen, M., & Pettengill, E. (2006). Sensory impairment in older adults: Part 2: Vision loss. *American Journal of Nursing, 106*, 52–62.

Wong, T. Y, Rosamond, W., Chang, P. P., Couper, D. J., Sharrett, A. R., Hubbard, L. D., et al. (2005). Retinopathy and risk of congestive heart failure. *Journal of the American Medical Association, 293*, 63–69.

World Health Organization. (2007). *Vision 2020. The right to sight. Global initiative for the elimination of avoidable blindness: Action plan 2006–2011*. Geneva, Switzerland: Author.

Web Sites of Interest

Canadian National Institute for the Blind—http://www.cnib.ca/

Canadian Ophthalmological Society—http://www.eyesite.ca/english/program-and-services/policy-statements-guidelines/index.htm

Canadian Paediatric Society: Vision Screening in Children—http://www.cps.ca/english/statements/CP/cp98-01.htm

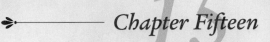

Chapter Fifteen

Ears

Written by **Carolyn Jarvis**, PhD, APN, CNP
Adapted by **June MacDonald-Jenkins**, RN, BScN, MSc

Electronic Resources

On Evolve *evolve*

http://evolve.elsevier.com/Canada/Jarvis/examination/

- Interactive Case Studies
- Physical Examination Audio and Printable Summaries
- Bedside Assessment Summary Checklists
- Complete Physical Examination Form
- Nursing Diagnoses Boxes
- Health Promotion Guides
- Quick Assessments for 20 Common Conditions
- Multiple Choice Review Questions
- Chapter Objectives
- Appendices
- Weblinks

On the Companion CD

- Interactive Case Studies with Heart and Lung Sounds
- Health Promotion Guides
- Quick Assessments for 20 Common Conditions
- Head-to-Toe Physical Examination Video Clips

STRUCTURE AND FUNCTION

The ear is the sensory organ for hearing and maintaining equilibrium. The ear has three parts: the external, middle, and inner ears. The external ear is called the **auricle** or **pinna** and consists of movable cartilage and skin (Fig. 15-1). Note the landmarks of the auricle and use these terms to describe your findings. The mastoid process, the bony prominence behind the lobule, is not part of the ear but is an important landmark.

EXTERNAL EAR

The external ear has a characteristic shape and serves to funnel sound waves into its opening, the **external auditory canal** (Fig. 15-2). The canal is a cul-de-sac 2.5 to 3 cm long in the adult and terminates at the eardrum, or tympanic membrane. The canal is lined with glands that secrete cerumen, a yellow waxy material that lubricates and protects the ear. The wax forms a sticky barrier that helps keep foreign bodies from entering and reaching the sensitive tympanic membrane. Cerumen migrates out to the meatus by the movements of chewing and talking.

The outer one third of the canal is cartilage; the inner two thirds consists of bone covered by thin sensitive skin. The canal has a slight S-curve in the adult. The outer one third curves up and toward the back of the head, whereas the inner two thirds angle down and forward toward the nose.

The **tympanic membrane (TM),** or **eardrum,** separates the external and middle ears and is tilted obliquely to the ear canal, facing downward and somewhat forward. It is a translucent membrane with a pearly grey colour and a prominent cone of light in the anteroinferior quadrant, which is the reflection of the otoscope light (Fig. 15-3). The drum is oval and slightly concave, pulled in at its centre by one of the middle ear ossicles, the **malleus.** The parts of the malleus show through the translucent drum; these are the **umbo,** the **manubrium** (handle), and the **short process.** The small, slack, superior section of the tympanic membrane is called the **pars flaccida.** The remainder of the drum, which is thicker and more taut, is the **pars tensa.** The **annulus** is the outer fibrous rim of the drum.

Lymphatic drainage of the external ear flows to the parotid, mastoid, and superficial cervical nodes.

MIDDLE EAR

The middle ear is a tiny air-filled cavity inside the temporal bone (see Fig. 15-2). It contains tiny ear bones, or auditory ossicles: the **malleus, incus,** and **stapes.** Several openings into the middle ear are present. Its opening to the outer ear is covered by the tympanic membrane. The openings to the inner ear are the oval window at the end of the stapes and the round window. Another opening is the **eustachian tube,** which connects the middle ear with the nasopharynx and allows passage of air. The tube is normally closed, but it opens with swallowing or yawning.

The middle ear has three functions: (1) it conducts sound vibrations from the outer ear to the central hearing apparatus in the inner ear, (2) it protects the inner ear by reducing the amplitude of loud sounds, and (3) its eustachian tube allows equalization of air pressure on each side of the tympanic membrane so that the membrane does not rupture (e.g., during altitude changes in an airplane).

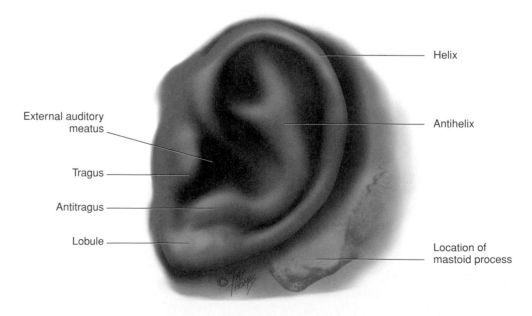

Helix

Antihelix

External auditory meatus

Tragus

Antitragus

Lobule

Location of mastoid process

AURICLE, OR PINNA

Fig. 15-1

© Pat Thomas, 2006.

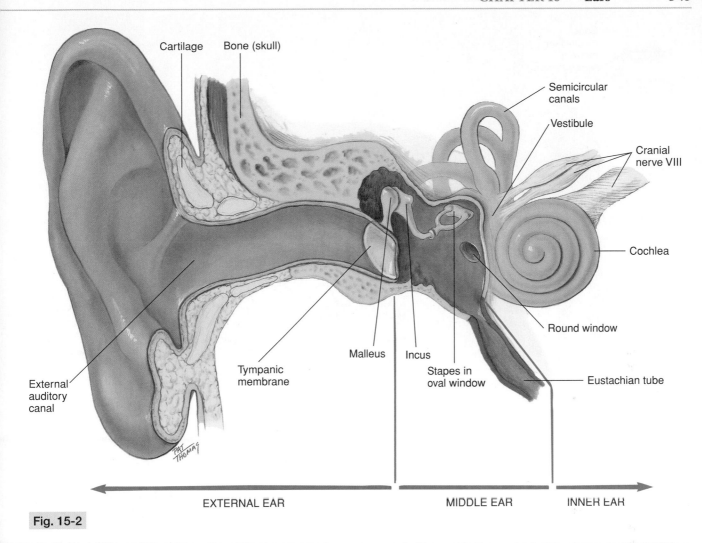

Cartilage   Bone (skull)

Semicircular canals

Vestibule

Cranial nerve VIII

Cochlea

Round window

Malleus   Incus

Stapes in oval window

Eustachian tube

External auditory canal

Tympanic membrane

EXTERNAL EAR   **MIDDLE EAR**   **INNER EAR**

Fig. 15-2

INNER EAR

The inner ear contains the **bony labyrinth,** which holds the sensory organs for equilibrium and hearing. Within the bony labyrinth, the **vestibule** and the **semicircular canals** comprise the vestibular apparatus, and the **cochlea** (Latin for "snail shell") contains the central hearing apparatus. Although the inner ear is not accessible to direct examination, its functions can be assessed.

HEARING

Concerning the function of hearing, the auditory system can be divided into three levels: peripheral, brainstem, and cerebral cortex. At the peripheral level, the ear transmits sound and converts its vibrations into electrical impulses, which can be analyzed by the brain. For example, you hear an alarm bell ringing in the hall. Its sound waves travel instantly to your ears. The *amplitude* is how loud the alarm is; its *frequency* is the pitch (in this case, high) or the number of cycles per second. The sound waves produce vibrations on your tympanic membrane. These vibrations are carried by the middle ear ossicles to your oval window. Then the sound waves travel through your cochlea, which is coiled like a snail's shell, and are dissipated against the round window. Along the way, the **basilar membrane** vibrates at a point specific to the frequency of the sound. In this case, the alarm's high frequency stimulates the basilar membrane at its base near the stapes (Fig. 15-4). The numerous fibres along the basilar membrane are the receptor hair cells of the **organ of Corti,** the sensory

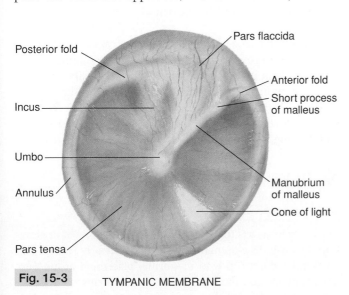

Posterior fold

Pars flaccida

Anterior fold

Short process of malleus

Incus

Umbo

Manubrium of malleus

Annulus

Cone of light

Pars tensa

Fig. 15-3   TYMPANIC MEMBRANE

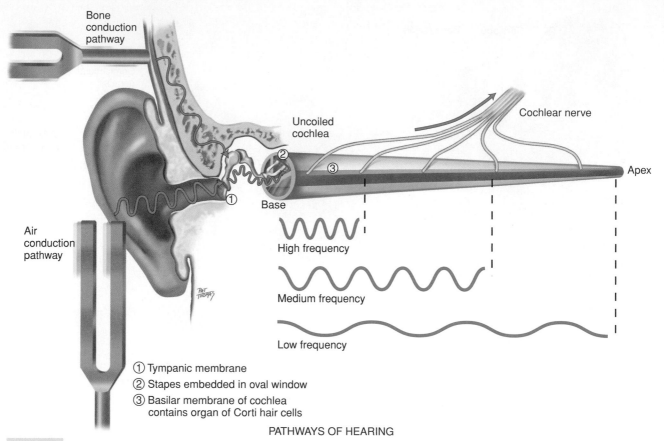

① Tympanic membrane
② Stapes embedded in oval window
③ Basilar membrane of cochlea contains organ of Corti hair cells

PATHWAYS OF HEARING

Fig. 15-4

organ of hearing. As the hair cells bend, they mediate the vibrations into electric impulses. The electrical impulses are conducted by the auditory portion of cranial nerve VIII to the brainstem.

The function at the brainstem level is *binaural interaction,* which permits locating the direction of a sound in space as well as identifying the sound. How does this work? Each ear is actually one half of the total sensory organ. The ears are located on each side of a movable head. The cranial nerve VIII from each ear sends signals to both sides of the brainstem. Areas in the brainstem are sensitive to differences in intensity and timing of the messages from the two ears, depending on the way the head is turned.

Finally, the function of the cortex is to interpret the meaning of the sound and begin the appropriate response. All this happens in the split second it takes you to react to the alarm.

Pathways of Hearing. The normal pathway of hearing is air conduction (AC), described above; it is the most efficient. An alternate route of hearing is by bone conduction (BC). Here, the bones of the skull vibrate. These vibrations are transmitted directly to the inner ear and to cranial nerve VIII.

Hearing Loss. Anything that obstructs the transmission of sound impairs hearing. A **conductive** hearing loss involves a mechanical dysfunction of the external or middle ear. It is a partial loss because the person is able to hear if the sound amplitude is increased enough to reach normal nerve elements in the inner ear. Conductive hearing loss may be caused by impacted cerumen, foreign bodies, a perforated tympanic membrane, pus or serum in the middle ear, or otosclerosis (a decrease in mobility of the ossicles).

Sensorineural (or perceptive) loss signifies pathology of the inner ear, cranial nerve VIII, or the auditory areas of the cerebral cortex. A simple increase in amplitude may not enable the person to understand words. Sensorineural hearing loss may be caused by *presbycusis,* a gradual nerve degeneration that occurs with aging, and by ototoxic drugs, which affect the hair cells in the cochlea. A **mixed loss** is a combination of conductive and sensorineural types in the same ear.

Equilibrium. The labyrinth in the inner ear constantly feeds information to your brain about your body's position in space. It works like a plumb line to determine verticality or depth. The ear's plumb lines register the angle of your head in relation to gravity. If the labyrinth ever becomes inflamed, it feeds the wrong information to the brain, creating a staggering gait and a strong, spinning, whirling sensation called *vertigo.*

❧ DEVELOPMENTAL CARE

Infants and Children

The inner ear starts to develop early in the fifth week of gestation. In early development the ear is posteriorly rotated and low set; later it ascends to its normal placement around eye level. If maternal rubella infection occurs during the first trimester, it can damage the organ of Corti and impair hearing.

The infant's eustachian tube is relatively shorter and wider and its position is more horizontal than the adult's, so it is easier for pathogens from the nasopharynx to migrate through to the middle ear (Fig. 15-5). The lumen is surrounded by lymphoid tissue, which increases during childhood; thus, the lumen is easily occluded. These factors place the infant at greater risk for middle ear infections than the adult.

The infant's and the young child's external auditory canal is shorter and has a slope opposite to that of the adult's (see Fig. 15-17 on p. 358).

The Adult

Otosclerosis is a common cause of conductive hearing loss in young adults between the ages of 20 and 40 years. It is a gradual hardening that causes the foot plate of the stapes to become fixed in the oval window, impeding the transmission of sound and causing progressive deafness.

The Aging Adult

In the aging person, cilia lining the ear canal become coarse and stiff. This may cause decreased hearing because it impedes sound waves travelling toward the tympanic membrane. It also causes cerumen to accumulate and oxidize, which greatly reduces hearing. The cerumen itself is drier because of atrophy of the apocrine glands. Also, a life history of frequent ear infections may result in scarring on the drum.

Impacted cerumen is a common but reversible cause of hearing loss in older people. After removal of cerumen, most people have significantly improved hearing ability. We can improve the hearing health of older people by routinely performing otoscopic examinations and by performing ear canal irrigations when impacted cerumen occurs.

A person living in a noise-polluted area (e.g., near an airport or a busy highway) has a greater risk of hearing loss. But **presbycusis** is a type of hearing loss that occurs with aging, even in people living in a quiet environment. It is a gradual

sensorineural loss caused by nerve degeneration in the inner ear or auditory nerve. More than 50% of all Canadians over the age of 65 have hearing loss. The person first notices a high-frequency tone loss; it is harder to hear consonants (high-pitched components of speech) than vowels. This makes words sound garbled. The ability to localize sound is impaired also. This communication dysfunction is accentuated when unfavourable background noise is present (e.g., with music, with dishes clattering, or at a large noisy party).

Canadian experts recommend that we have our hearing tested every 3 years starting at age 2, or prior if language skills are not developing. Individuals who listen to very loud music, work with high levels of industrial noise, or are over the age of 65 years should see an audiologist annually. There is significant evidence mounting that neonatal hearing screening should be implemented as routine practice (Durieux-Smith et al., 2008). In the absence of universal screening policies, all high-risk births should be screened. Local audiologists can test hearing and may refer patients to other healthcare professionals based upon their findings.

CULTURAL AND SOCIAL CONSIDERATIONS

Otitis media, or OM (middle ear infection), occurs because of obstruction of the eustachian tube or passage of nasopharyngeal secretions into the middle ear. Otitis media is one of the most common illnesses in children. The incidence and severity increase in children of Aboriginal descent. Acute otitis media rates are significantly higher in Aboriginal than in other North American populations (Dallaire et al., 2006).

The incidence of OM is also increased in premature infants, in those with Down syndrome, and in babies fed by bottle in a supine position. In the supine position the effects of gravity and sucking tend to draw the nasopharyngeal contents directly into the middle ear. Urge the parent to hold the baby partly upright against the arm while feeding. Do not prop the bottle or let the baby take a bottle to bed. Encouraging breastfeeding helps prevent this problem.

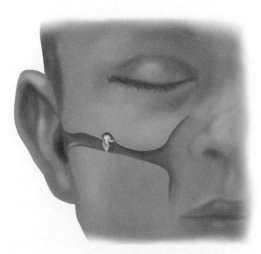

INFANT
Horizontal eustachian tube

Fig. 15-5

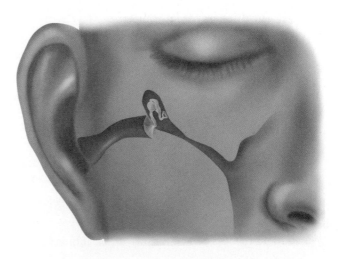

ADULT
Sloped eustachian tube

The most important side effect of acute OM is the persistence of fluid in the middle ear after treatment. This middle ear effusion can impair hearing, placing the child at risk for delayed cognitive development.

Cerumen is genetically determined and comes in two major types: (1) dry cerumen, which is grey, flaky, and frequently forms a thin mass in the ear canal, and (2) wet cerumen, which is honey brown to dark brown and moist. Individuals of Asian or Aboriginal descent have >80% frequency of dry cerumen, whereas individuals of African or Euro-Canadian descent have >97% frequency of wet cerumen (Overfield, 1995). The presence and composition of cerumen are not related to poor hygiene. Take caution to avoid mistaking the flaky, dry cerumen for eczematous lesions.

Almost 25% of all Canadians report some level of hearing loss, although about 10% of those identify themselves as "culturally deaf," "oral deaf," "deafened," or "hard of hearing." Hearing loss is the third most prevalent chronic condition in older adults. The Canadian Hearing Society (2007) has created a position statement regarding the social and ethical dilemmas faced by Canadians with hearing loss (see http://www.chs.ca).

SUBJECTIVE DATA

1. Earache
2. Infections
3. Discharge
4. Hearing loss
5. Environmental noise
6. Tinnitus
7. Vertigo
8. Self-care behaviours

Examiner Asks	Rationale
1. Earache. Any **earache** or other pain in ears? • Location—feel close to the surface or deep in the head? • Does it hurt when you push on the ear? • Character—dull, aching or sharp, stabbing? Constant or come and go? Is it affected by changing position of head? Ever had this kind of pain before? • Any accompanying cold symptoms or sore throat? Any problems with sinuses or teeth? • Ever been hit on the ear or on the side of the head, or had any sport injury? Ever had any trauma from a foreign body? • What have you tried to relieve pain?	**Otalgia** may be directly due to ear disease or may be referred pain from a problem in teeth or oropharynx. A virus/bacterium from upper respiratory infection (URI) may migrate up eustachian tube to involve middle ear. Trauma may rupture the TM. Assess effect of coping strategies.
2. Infections. Any ear **infections?** As an adult, or in childhood? • How frequent were they? How were they treated?	A history of chronic ear problems suggests possible sequelae.
3. Discharge. Any **discharge** from your ears? • Does it look like pus, or is it bloody? • Any odour to the discharge? • Any relationship between the discharge and the ear pain?	Discharge (otorrhea) suggests infection in canal or a perforated eardrum. For example: *External otitis*—purulent, sanguineous, or watery discharge. *Acute otitis media with perforation*—purulent discharge. *Cholesteatoma*—dirty yellow or grey discharge, foul odour. Typically with perforation—ear pain occurs first, stops with a popping sensation, then drainage occurs.
4. Hearing loss. Ever had any trouble hearing? • Onset—Did the loss come on slowly or all at once? • Character—Has all your hearing decreased, or just on hearing certain sounds?	Presbycusis has gradual onset over years, whereas a traumatic hearing loss is often sudden. Refer any sudden loss in one or both ears *not* associated with URI.

Examiner Asks	Rationale
• In what situations do you notice the loss: conversations, using the telephone, watching television, at a party?	Loss is apparent when competition from background noise is present, as at a party.
• Do people seem to shout at you?	*Recruitment*—a marked loss when sound is at low intensity, but sound actually becomes painful when repeated in a loud voice.
• Do ordinary sounds seem hollow, as if you are hearing in a barrel or under water? • Recently travelled by airplane? • Any family history of hearing loss? • Effort to treat—Any hearing aid or other device? Anything to help hearing?	Character of hearing loss when cerumen expands and becomes impacted, as after swimming or showering.
• Coping strategies—How does the loss affect your daily life? Any job problem? Feel embarrassed? Frustrated? How do your family, friends react?	Hearing loss can cause social isolation and can lessen pleasure of leisure activities.

Note to examiner: During history, note these clues from normal conversation that indicate possible hearing loss:

1. Lip reading or watching your face and lips closely rather than your eyes
2. Frowning or straining forward to hear
3. Posturing of head to catch sounds with better ear
4. Misunderstanding your questions or frequently asking you to repeat
5. Acting irritable or showing startle reflex when you raise your voice (recruitment)
6. Speech sounds garbled, possibly vowel sounds distorted
7. Inappropriately loud voice
8. Flat, monotonous tone of voice

Examiner Asks	Rationale
5. Environmental noise. Any loud noises at home or on the job? For example, do you live in a noise-polluted area, near an airport or busy traffic area? Now or in the past?	Old trauma to hearing initially goes unnoticed but results in further decibel loss in later years.
• Are you near other noises such as heavy machinery, loud persistent music, gunshots while hunting? • Coping strategies—Any steps to protect your ears, such as headphones or ear plugs?	
6. Tinnitus. Ever felt ringing, crackling, or buzzing in your ears? When did this occur?	Tinnitus originates within the person; it accompanies some hearing or ear disorders.
• Seem louder at night?	Tinnitus seems louder with no competition from environment noise.
• Are you taking any medications?	Many medications have ototoxic sequelae: aspirin, aminoglycosides (streptomycin, gentamicin, kanamycin, neomycin), ethacrynic acid, furosemide, indomethacin, naproxen, quinine, vancomycin and local anaesthetic.
7. Vertigo. Ever felt **vertigo,** that is, the room spinning around or yourself spinning? (Vertigo is a true twirling motion.)	True rotational spinning occurs with dysfunction of labyrinth. **Objective vertigo**—feels like room spins. **Subjective vertigo**—person feels like he or she spins.
• Ever felt dizzy, like you are not quite steady, like falling or losing your balance? Giddy, lightheaded?	Distinguish true vertigo from dizziness or lightheadedness.

Subjective Data

Examiner Asks	Rationale
8. Self-care behaviours. How do you clean your ears?	Assess potential trauma from invasive instruments. Cotton-tipped applicators can impact cerumen, causing hearing loss.
• Last time you had your hearing checked? • If a hearing loss was noted, did you obtain a hearing aid? How long have you had it? Do you wear it? How does it work? Any trouble with upkeep, cleaning, changing batteries?	Prescribe frequency of hearing assessment according to person's age or risk factors.

Additional History for Infants and Children

Examiner Asks	Rationale
1. Ear Infections. At what age was the child's first episode? How many ear infections in the last 6 months? How many total? How were these treated? • Has the child had any surgery, such as insertion of ear tubes or removal of tonsils?	A first episode that occurs in the first 3 months of life increases risk of recurrent OM. Recurrent OM is three episodes in past 3 months or four within past year (Carlson, 2005).
• Are the infections increasing in frequency, in severity, or staying the same? • Does anyone in the home smoke cigarettes?	
• Does your child receive child care outside your home? In a daycare centre or someone else's home? How many children in the group?	Passive and gestational smoke are risk factors for OM (Lieu et al., 2007). Bottle feeding (as opposed to breast-feeding) and attendance at group daycare are also risk factors for OM.
2. Does the child seem to be hearing well? • Have you noticed that the infant startles with loud noise? Did the infant babble around 6 months? Does he or she talk? At what age did talking start? Was the speech intelligible? • Ever had the child's hearing tested? If there was a hearing loss, did it follow any diseases in the child, or in the mother during pregnancy? (Note: It is important to catch any problem early, because a child with hearing loss is at risk for delayed speech and social development, and learning deficit.)	Children at risk for hearing deficit include those exposed to maternal rubella, syphilis, cytomegalovirus, toxoplasmosis, or to maternal ototoxic drugs in utero; premature infants; low-birth-weight infants; trauma or hypoxia at birth; and infants with congenital liver or kidney disease. In children the incidence of meningitis, measles, mumps, OM, and any illness with persistent high fever may increase risk of hearing deficit.
3. Does the child tend to put objects in the ears? Is the older child or adolescent active in contact sports?	These children are at increased risk for trauma.

OBJECTIVE DATA

PREPARATION

Position the adult sitting up straight with his or her head at your eye level. Occasionally the ear canal is partially filled with cerumen, which obstructs your view of the TM. If the eardrum is intact and no current infection is present, a preferred method of cleaning the adult canal is to soften the cerumen with a warmed solution of mineral oil and hydrogen peroxide. Then the canal is irrigated with warm water (body temperature) with a bulb syringe or a low-pulsatile dental irrigator (WaterPik). Direct fluid to the posterior wall. Leave space around the irrigator tip for water to escape. Do not irrigate if the history or the examination suggests perforation or infection.

EQUIPMENT NEEDED

Otoscope with bright light (fresh batteries give off white—not yellow—light)
Pneumatic bulb attachment, sometimes used with infant or young child
Tuning forks in 512 and 1024 Hz

Normal Range of Findings	Abnormal Findings

INSPECT AND PALPATE THE EXTERNAL EAR

Size and Shape

The ears are of equal size bilaterally with no swelling or thickening. Ears of unusual size and shape may be a normal familial trait with no clinical significance.

Microtia—ears smaller than 4 cm vertically.
Macrotia—ears larger than 10 cm vertically.
Edema.

Skin Condition

The skin colour is consistent with the person's facial skin colour. The skin is intact, with no lumps or lesions. On some people you may note **Darwin's tubercle,** a small painless nodule at the helix. This is a congenital variation and is not significant (Table 15-2, p. 361).

Reddened, excessively warm skin indicates inflammation (Table 15-1, p. 360).
Crusts and scaling occur with otitis externa, eczema, contact dermatitis, seborrhea.
Enlarged tender lymph nodes in the region indicate inflammation of the pinna or mastoid process.
Red-blue discoloration indicates frostbite.
Tophi, sebaceous cyst, chondrodermatitis, keloid, carcinoma (see Table 15-2, p. 361).

Tenderness

Move the pinna and push on the tragus. They should feel firm, and movement should produce no pain. Palpating the mastoid process should also produce no pain.

Pain with movement occurs with otitis externa and furuncle.
Pain at the mastoid process may indicate mastoiditis or lymphadenitis of the posterior auricular node.

The External Auditory Meatus

Note the size of the opening to direct your choice of speculum for the otoscope. No swelling, redness, or discharge should be present.

Atresia—absence or closure of the ear canal.
A sticky yellow discharge accompanies otitis externa or may indicate OM if the drum has ruptured.

Some cerumen is usually present. The colour varies from grey-yellow to light brown and black, and the texture varies from moist and waxy to dry and desiccated. A large amount of cerumen obscures visualization of the canal and drum.

Impacted cerumen is a common cause of conductive hearing loss.

INSPECT WITH THE OTOSCOPE

As you inspect the external ear, note the size of the auditory meatus. Then choose the largest speculum that will fit comfortably in the ear canal and attach it to the otoscope. Tilt the person's head slightly away from you toward the opposite shoulder. This method brings the obliquely sloping eardrum into better view.

Objective Data

Normal Range of Findings	Abnormal Findings

Pull the pinna up and back on an adult or older child; this helps straighten the S-shape of the canal (Fig. 15-6). (Pull the pinna down on an infant and a child under 3 years of age [Fig. 15-17, p. 356]). Hold the pinna gently but firmly. Do not release traction on the ear until you have finished the examination and the otoscope is removed.

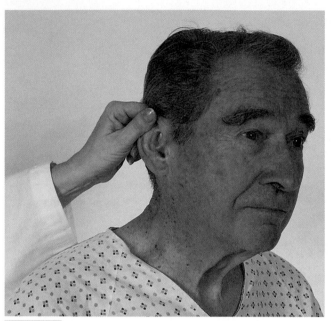

Fig. 15-6

Hold the otoscope "upside down" along your fingers and have the dorsa (back) of your hand along the person's cheek braced to steady the otoscope (Fig. 15-7). This position may feel awkward to you at first. It soon will feel natural and you will find it useful in preventing forceful insertion. Also, your stabilizing hand acts as a protecting lever if the person suddenly moves the head.

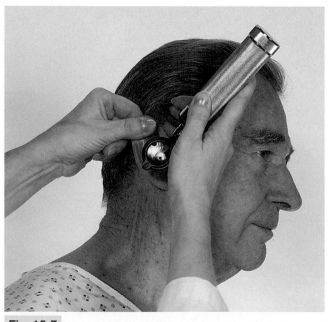

Fig. 15-7

Normal Range of Findings	Abnormal Findings

Insert the speculum slowly and carefully along the axis of the canal. Watch the insertion; then put your eye up to the otoscope. Avoid touching the inner "bony" section of the canal wall, which is covered by a thin epithelial layer and is sensitive to pain. Sometimes you cannot see anything but canal wall. If so, try to reposition the person's head, apply more traction on the pinna, and reangle the otoscope to look forward toward the person's nose.

Once it is in place, you may need to rotate the otoscope slightly to visualize all the eardrum; do this gently. Lastly, perform the otoscopic examination before you test hearing; ear canals with impacted cerumen give the erroneous impression of pathological hearing loss.

The External Canal

Note any redness and swelling, lesions, foreign bodies, or discharge. If any discharge is present, note the colour and odour. (Also, clean any discharge from the speculum before examining the other ear to avoid contamination with possibly infectious material.) For a person with a hearing aid, note any irritation on the canal wall from poorly fitting ear moulds.

Redness and swelling occur with otitis externa; canal may be completely closed with swelling.

Purulent otorrhea suggests otitis externa or OM if the drum has ruptured.

Frank blood or clear, watery drainage (cerebrospinal fluid [CSF]) after trauma suggests basal skull fracture and warrants immediate referral. CSF feels oily and is positive for glucose on TesTape.

Foreign body, polyp, furuncle, exostosis (Table 15-3, p. 363).

The Tympanic Membrane

Colour and Characteristics. Systematically explore the TM's landmarks (Fig. 15-8). The normal eardrum is shiny and translucent, with a pearl-grey colour. The cone-shaped light reflex is prominent in the anteroinferior quadrant (at 5:00 in the right drum and 7:00 in the left drum). This is the reflection of your otoscope light. Sections of the malleus are visible through the translucent drum: the umbo, manubrium, and short process. (Infrequently, you also may see the incus behind the drum; it shows as a whitish haze in the upper posterior area.) At the periphery the annulus looks whiter and denser.

Yellow-amber drum colour occurs with OM with effusion (serous).

Red colour occurs with acute OM.

Absent or distorted landmarks.

Air/fluid level or air bubbles behind drum indicate OM with effusion (Tables 15-4, p. 365, and 15-5, p. 366).

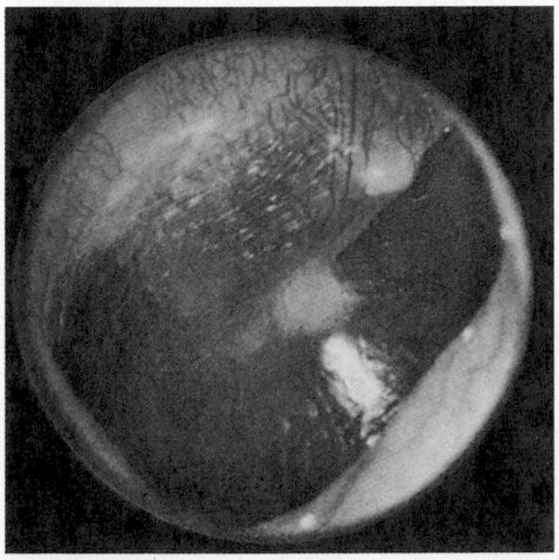

Fig. 15-8   Normal tympanic membrane *(right).*

Normal Range of Findings	**Abnormal Findings**

Position. The eardrum is flat, slightly pulled in at the centre, and flutters when the person performs the Valsalva manoeuvre or holds the nose and swallows (insufflation). You may elicit these manoeuvres to assess drum mobility. Avoid them with an aging person because they may disrupt equilibrium. Also avoid middle ear insufflation in a person with upper respiratory infection because it could propel infectious matter into the middle ear.

Integrity of Membrane. Inspect the eardrum and the entire circumference of the annulus for perforations. The normal TM is intact. Some adults may show scarring, which is a dense white patch on the drum. This is a sequela of repeated ear infections.

Retracted drum resulting from vacuum in middle ear with obstructed eustachian tube.

Bulging drum from increased pressure in OM.

Drum hypomobility is an early sign of OM (see Table 15-5, p. 366).

Perforation shows as a dark oval area or as a larger opening on the drum.

Vesicles on drum (see Table 15-5, p. 366).

TEST HEARING ACUITY

Your screening for a hearing deficit begins during the history; how well does the person hear conversational speech? An audiometer gives a precise quantitative measure of hearing by assessing the person's ability to hear sounds of varying frequency. Because this equipment usually is not available in the clinical setting, you may use alternate screening measures. These are "crude" tests. They are nonquantitative; they are useful to document the *presence* of hearing loss but do not measure the degree of loss. Refer any abnormal findings for more accurate measures with pure tone audiometry.

Whispered Voice Test

Test one ear at a time while masking hearing in the other ear to prevent sound transmission around the head. This is done by placing one finger on the tragus and rapidly pushing it in and out of the auditory meatus. Shield your lips so the person cannot compensate for a hearing loss (consciously or unconsciously) by lip reading or using the "good" ear. With your head 30 to 60 cm from the person's ear, exhale and whisper slowly some two-syllable words, such as Tuesday, armchair, baseball, and fourteen. Normally, the person repeats each word correctly after you say it.

The person is unable to hear whispered words. A whisper is a high-frequency sound and is used to detect high-tone loss.

Tuning Fork Tests

Tuning fork tests measure hearing by air conduction (AC) or by bone conduction (BC), in which the sound vibrates through the cranial bones to the inner ear. The AC route through the ear canal and middle ear is usually the more sensitive route. To activate the tuning fork, hold it by the stem and strike the tines softly on the back of your hand (Fig. 15-9). Also, grasping the tines with the thumb and index finger and stroking upward will cause the tuning fork to vibrate. This decreases the incidence of making the tone too loud.

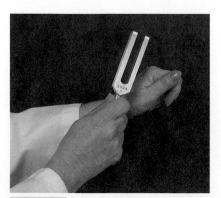

Fig. 15-9

Normal Range of Findings	Abnormal Findings

The **Weber test** is valuable when a person reports hearing better with one ear than the other. Place a vibrating tuning fork in the midline of the person's skull and ask whether the tone sounds the same in both ears or better in one (Fig. 15-10). The person should hear the tone by BC through the skull, and it should sound equally loud in both ears.

Sound lateralizes to one ear with a conductive or a sensorineural loss (Table 15-6, p. 368).

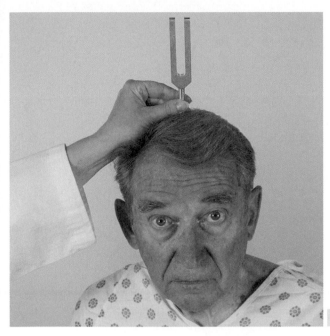

Fig. 15-10

The **Rinne test** compares AC and BC sound (Fig. 15-11). Place the stem of the vibrating tuning fork on the person's mastoid process and ask him or her to signal when the sound goes away. Quickly invert the fork so the vibrating end is near the ear canal; the person should still hear a sound (Fig. 15-12). Normally the sound is heard twice as long by AC (next to ear canal) as by BC (through the mastoid process). A normal response is a positive Rinne test, or "AC > BC." Repeat with the other ear.

Ratio of AC to BC is altered with hearing loss (see Table 15-6, p. 368).

Sound is heard longer by BC with a conductive loss.

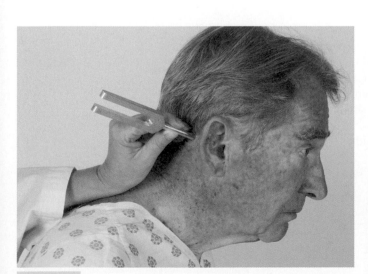

Fig. 15-11

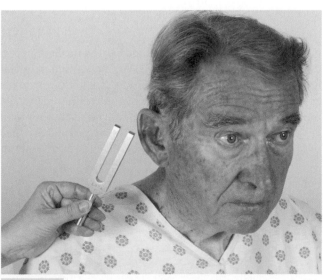

Fig. 15-12

Objective Data

Normal Range of Findings	Abnormal Findings

THE VESTIBULAR APPARATUS

The **Romberg test** assesses the ability of the vestibular apparatus in the inner ear to help maintain standing balance. Because the Romberg test also assesses intactness of the cerebellum and proprioception, it is discussed in Chapter 23 (see Fig. 23-17, p. 670).

❦ DEVELOPMENTAL CARE

Infants and Young Children

Examination of the external ear of an infant or young child is similar to that described for the adult, with the addition of examination of position and alignment on head. Note the ear position. The top of the pinna should match an imaginary line extending from the corner of the eye to the occiput. Also, the ear should be positioned within 10 degrees of vertical (Fig. 15-13).

Low-set ears or deviation in alignment may indicate intellectual disability or a genitourinary malformation.

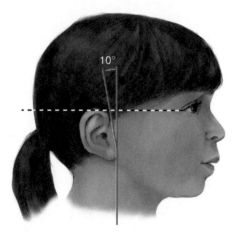

Normal alignment

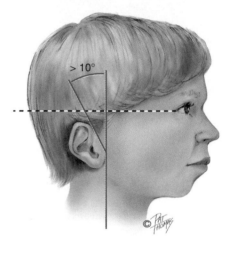

Low-set ears and deviation in alignment

© Pat Thomas, 2006.

Fig. 15-13

Otoscopic Examination. In addition to its place in the complete examination, eardrum assessment is mandatory for any infant or child requiring care for illness or fever. For the infant or young child, it is best to perform the otoscopic examination toward the end of the complete examination. Many young children protest vigorously during this procedure no matter how well you prepare, and it is difficult to re-establish co-operation afterward. Save the otoscopic examination until last. Then the parent can hold and comfort the child.

Normal Range of Findings	**Abnormal Findings**

To help prepare the child, let the child hold your funny-looking "flashlight." You may wish to have the child look in the parent's ear as you hold the otoscope (Fig. 15-14).

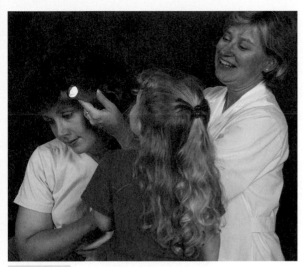

Fig. 15-14

Positioning of the child is important. You need a clear view of the canal. Avoid harsh restraint, but you must protect the eardrum from injury in case of sudden head movement. Enlist the aid of a co-operative parent. Prop an infant upright against the parent's chest or shoulder, with the parent's arm around the upper part of the head (Fig. 15-15). A toddler can be held in the parent's lap or may lie on the examining table with his or her arms secured (Fig. 15-16). In each case, the child's head is stabilized to avoid movement against the otoscope.

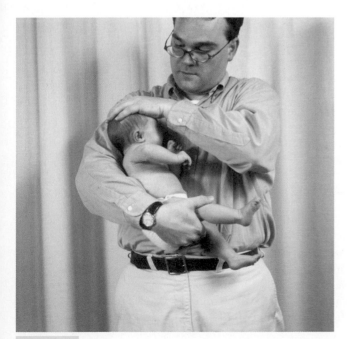

Fig. 15-15

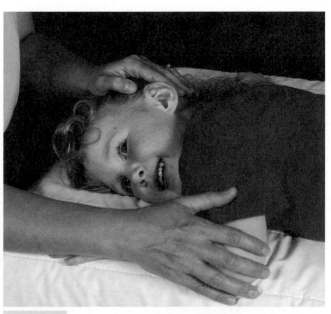

Fig. 15-16

Objective Data

Normal Range of Findings	**Abnormal Findings**

Remember to pull the pinna straight down on an infant or a child under 3 years old. This method will match the slope of the ear canal (Fig. 15-17).

ADULT

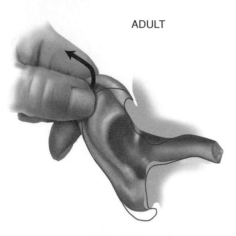

Adult—Pull
pinna up and back

YOUNG CHILD

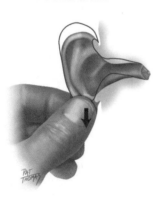

Infant or child under 3—Pull
pinna straight down   **Fig. 15-17**

At birth the patency of the ear canal is determined, but the otoscopic examination is not performed because the canal is filled with amniotic fluid and vernix caseosa. After a few days the TM is examined. During the first few days, the TM often looks thickened and opaque. It may look infected and have a mild redness from increased vascularity. The eardrum also looks infected in infants after crying.

The position of the eardrum is more horizontal in the neonate, making it more difficult to see completely and harder to differentiate from the canal wall. By 1 month of age, the drum is in the oblique (more vertical) position as in the older child, and examination is a bit easier.

When examining an infant or young child, a pneumatic bulb attachment enables you to direct a light puff of air toward the drum to assess vibratility (Fig. 15-18). For a secure seal, choose the largest speculum that will fit in the ear canal without causing pain. A rubber tip on the end of the speculum gives a better seal. Give a small pump to the bulb (positive pressure), then release the bulb (negative pressure). Normally the TM moves inward with a slight puff and outward with a slight release.

Tympanic membranes can turn pink from the child or infant crying. Use of the pneumatic bulb is the most reliable way to detect OM as there is little to no movement of the tympanic membrane.

Normal Range of Findings	Abnormal Findings

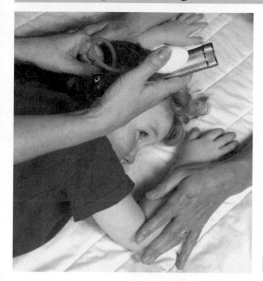

Fig. 15-18

An abnormal response is no movement. Drum hypomobility indicates effusion or a high vacuum in the middle ear. For the newborn's first 6 weeks, drum immobility is the best indicator of middle ear infection.

Normally the TM is intact. In a child being treated for chronic OM, you may note the presence of a tympanostomy tube in the central part of the eardrum. This is inserted surgically to equalize pressure and drain secretions. Finally, although the condition is not normal, it is not uncommon to note a foreign body in a child's canal, such as a small stone or a bead.

Chronic OM relieved by tympanostomy tubes (see Table 15-5, p. 366).

Foreign body (see Table 15-3, p. 363).

Test Hearing Acuity. Use the developmental milestones mentioned in this section to assess hearing in an infant. Also, attend to the parents' concern over the infant's inability to hear; their assessment is usually well founded.

The room should be silent and the baby contented. Make a loud sudden noise (hand clap or squeeze toy) out of the baby's peripheral range of vision of about 30 cm. You may need to repeat a few times, but you should note these responses:

- Newborn—startle (Moro) reflex, acoustic blink reflex
- 3 to 4 months—acoustic blink reflex, infant stops movement and appears to "listen," halts sucking, quiets if crying, cries if quiet
- 6 to 8 months—infant turns head to localize sound, responds to own name
- Preschool and school-age child—child must be screened with audiometry

Absence of alerting behaviour may indicate congenital deafness.

Failure to localize sound.
No intelligible speech by 2 years of age.

Note that a young child may be unaware of a hearing loss because the child does not know how one "ought" to hear. Note these behavioural manifestations of hearing loss:
1. The child is inattentive in casual conversation.
2. The child reacts more to movement and facial expression than to sound.
3. The child's facial expression is strained or puzzled.
4. The child frequently asks to have statements repeated.
5. The child confuses words that sound alike.
6. The child has an accompanying speech problem: speech is monotonous or garbled; the child mispronounces or omits sounds.
7. The child appears shy and withdrawn and "lives in a world of his or her own."
8. The child frequently complains of earaches.
9. The child hears better at times when the environment is more conducive to hearing.

The Aging Adult

An aging adult may have pendulous earlobes with linear wrinkling because of loss of elasticity of the pinna. Coarse, wiry hairs may be present at the opening of the ear canal. During otoscopy the eardrum normally may be whiter, more opaque, and duller than in the younger adult. It also may look thickened.

Objective Data

Normal Range of Findings	Abnormal Findings

A high-tone frequency hearing loss is apparent for those affected with presbycusis, the hearing loss that occurs with aging. This condition is revealed in difficulty hearing whispered words in the voice test and in difficulty hearing consonants during conversational speech. The aging adult feels that "people are mumbling" and feels isolated in family or friendship groups.

Summary Checklist: Ear Examination

 For a PDA-downloadable version, go to http://evolve.elsevier.com/Canada/Jarvis/examination/.

1. **Inspect external ear**
   Size and shape of auricle
   Position and alignment on head
   Note skin condition—colour, lumps, lesions
   Check movement of auricle and tragus for tenderness
   Evaluate external auditory meatus—note size, swelling, redness, discharge, cerumen, lesions, foreign bodies

2. **Otoscopic examination**
   External canal
   Cerumen, discharge, foreign bodies, lesions
   Redness or swelling of canal wall

3. **Inspect tympanic membrane**
   Colour and characteristics

   Note position (flat, bulging, retracted)
   Integrity of membrane

4. **Test hearing acuity**
   Note behavioural response to conversational speech
   Voice test
   Tuning fork tests—Weber and Rinne

Promoting Health

Use of Digital Music Players: Earbuds and Hearing Loss

Can you hear me now?

Today, there is growing concern about the potential for hearing loss in young people using digital music players and earbud headphones. Unlike earphones, which are placed over the ear, earbuds are placed directly in the ear canal, resulting in the sound being placed closer to the eardrum. Further, because the sound is digital, there is virtually no distortion, no matter how loud one turns up the volume. And probably most significant, because digital music players can hold thousands of songs and can play for hours without recharging, users tend to listen continuously for hours at a time.

Hearing loss occurs slowly and often goes unnoticed until it is quite extensive, so early prevention is the key. The risk of hearing loss increases as sound is played louder and for longer durations. For this reason, current research proposes the 60–60 rule. The 60–60 rule recommends that individuals use their digital music players and earbuds for no more than 60 minutes a day at levels below 60% of maximum volume. Many experts are suggesting that digital music players be designed to prevent the playing of music above 90 dB, about 60% of the maximum volume (≈120 dB) of the typical digital music player today. Simply put, it means dialling down the volume to a "6" or lower and taking a break at least every hour. Other ways to avoid hearing loss include using larger headphones that rest over the ear opening or noise-cancelling headphones that eliminate background noise so that listeners do not have to increase the volume as high. It is often difficult to explain this to young people who abound with youthful optimism and tend not to worry about future damage. However, listening with earbuds boosts sound signals by as much as 6 to 9 dB, about the difference between the sound of a vacuum cleaner and a motorcycle.

The decibel scale is logarithmic. In other words, 40 dB is 100 times as intense as 20 dB. Normal conversation takes place around 60 dB, whereas a chainsaw typically records at 100 dB and a rock concert at 120 dB. Government minimum safety standards in Canada dictate that 85 dB for 8 hours daily is considered the limit for occupational exposure to noise. Adopted by several provinces across the country, these standards exist to protect workers from hearing loss in the workplace. As the decibel level increases, exposure time needs to be cut significantly.

Although we know not to look into the sun because its intense rays will do damage to our eyes, we do not seem to realize that blasting our ears with intense sound is going to do damage, too. There is a certain irony when you see young people donning sunglasses and earbuds.

BIBLIOGRAPHY

Britt, R.R. (2006). *Sound science: HealthSciTech (2006): Retrieved May 26, 2008, from http://www.livescience.com/humanbiology/060104_earbuds.html*

Health Canada. (2006). *Hearing loss and leisure noise. Retrieved February 5, 2008, from http://www.hc-sc.gc.ca/iyh-vsv/environ/leisure-loisirs_e.html#is*

Keizer, G. (2005). *Eh? iPod earbuds can cause hearing loss: InformationWeek: Business innovation powered by technology (2005): Retrieved from http://www.informationweek.com/shared/printable ArticleSrc.jhtml?artcleID5175006733*

Portnuff, C.D.F., & Fligor, B.J. (2006, October). *Sound output levels of the iPod and other MP3 players: Is there potential risk to hearing? Presented at NIHL in Children Conference, Cincinnati, OH: Retrieved May 26, 2008, from http://www.hearingconservation.org/docs/virtualPressRoom/portnuff.htm*

Selvin, J. (2005). *Play it loud and you may pay for it: 4 Hearing Loss Retrieved May 26, 2008, from http://www.4hearingloss.com/archives/2005/09/play_it_loud_an.html*

Objective Data *(side tab)*

DOCUMENTATION AND CRITICAL THINKING

Sample Charting

SUBJECTIVE

States hearing is good, no earaches, infections, discharge, hearing loss, tinnitus, or vertigo.

OBJECTIVE

Pinna: Skin intact with no masses, lesions, tenderness, or discharge.
Otoscope: External canals are clear with no redness, swelling, lesions, foreign body, or discharge. Both tympanic membranes are pearly grey, with light reflex and landmarks intact, no perforations.
Hearing: Whispered words heard bilaterally. Weber test—tone heard midline without lateralization. Rinne test: AC > BC and = bilaterally.

ASSESSMENT

Healthy ear structures
Hearing accurate

Focused Assessment: Clinical Case Study

Jamal K. is a 9-month-old infant of African descent who is brought to the clinic by his mother because he "feels hot and was up crying all night."
History: Jamal is the third child of Mr. and Mrs. K. Mrs. K. received regular prenatal care. Jamal was born at 37 weeks' gestation; labour and delivery were uncomplicated. Jamal weighed 3200 g at birth, and was discharged 2 days after delivery. Jamal has been bottle-fed, with solids introduced at 5 months. Well-baby care has been regular; immunizations are up to date. Jamal has had two prior episodes of otitis media, no other illnesses.
Social History: Jamal lives with his family in a two-bedroom apartment over their grocery store and shares a bedroom with a 4-year-old brother and a 2-year-old brother. Mr. K. works full time in their grocery store; Mrs. K. provides child care in her own home for her children and for her sister's two young children. Both parents smoke cigarettes, one to two packs per day.

SUBJECTIVE

- 1 day PTA—Mrs. K. put Jamal down for nap with a bottle of juice, as is usual. Jamal woke up in the middle of the nap crying furiously. Quieted somewhat when held upright but still fussy. Took juice from bottle, refused solid baby food. Temperature 38°C rectally. Crying and fussy all night. Mrs. K. has given no medications to Jamal.

OBJECTIVE

Vital signs: Temp 38.4°C (tympanic), pulse 152, resp 36, Wt. 9.2 kg, Ht. 74 cm.
General: Alert, active, crying, and fussy. Developmentally appropriate for age.
Skin: Warm and dry, no rashes or lesions.
Head: Anterior fontanelle flat, 1 × 1.5 cm, posterior fontanelle closed.
Eyes: No exudate, conjunctivae clear, sclerae white, red reflex present bilaterally.
Ears: Both tympanic membranes dull red and bulging, no light reflex, no mobility on pneumatic otoscopy.
Mouth/throat: Oral mucosa pink, no lesions or exudate, tonsils 1+.
Neck: Supple, no lymphadenopathy.
Heart: Regular rate and rhythm, no murmurs.
Lungs: Breath sounds clear and equal bilaterally, unlaboured.
Abdomen: Bowel sounds present, abdomen soft, nontender.

ASSESSMENT

Acute otitis media, both ears
Pain R/T inflammation in TMs
Risk for ear infection injury R/T supine bottle-feeding, group child care, second-hand smoke
Deficient knowledge (parents) R/T lack of exposure to risk factors for otitis media

ABNORMAL FINDINGS

TABLE 15-1	Abnormalities of the External Ear

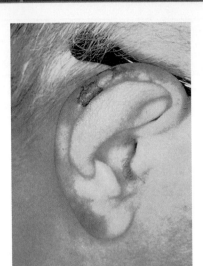

Frostbite

Reddish blue discoloration and swelling of auricle after exposure to extreme cold. Vesicles or bullae may develop, the person feels pain and tenderness, and ear necrosis may ensue.

Reprinted from the Clinical Slide Collection on the Rheumatic Diseases, © 1991, 1995, 1997. Used by permission of the American College of Rheumatology.

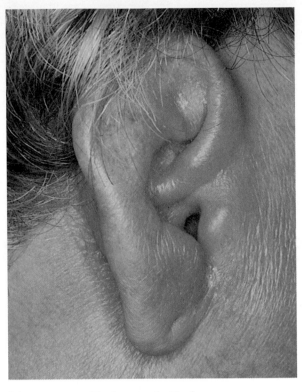

Otitis Externa (Swimmer's Ear)

An infection of the outer ear, with severe pain on movement of the pinna and tragus, redness and swelling of pinna and canal, scanty purulent discharge, scaling, itching, fever, and enlarged tender regional lymph nodes. Hearing is normal or slightly diminished. More common in hot humid weather. Swimming causes canal to become waterlogged and swell; skinfolds are set up for infection. Prevent by using rubbing alcohol or 2% acetic acid eardrops after every swim.

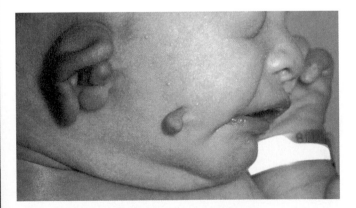

Branchial Remnant and Ear Deformity

A facial remnant or leftover of the embryological branchial arch usually appears as a skin tag, in this case one containing cartilage. They occur most often in the preauricular area, in front of the tragus. When bilateral, there is increased risk of renal anomalies.

Cerebrospinal Fluid Otorrhea (not illustrated)

Skull fracture of temporal bone causes cerebrospinal fluid to leak from ear canal and pool in concha when the person is supine. Cerebrospinal fluid feels oily and tests positive for glucose.

| TABLE 15-2 | **Lumps and Lesions on the External Ear** |

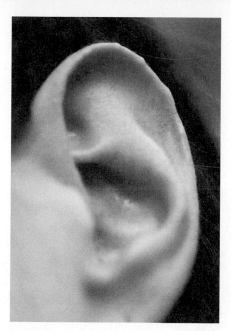

Darwin's Tubercle

Small painless nodule at the helix. It is a congenital variation and is not significant. Do not mistake it for a tophus.

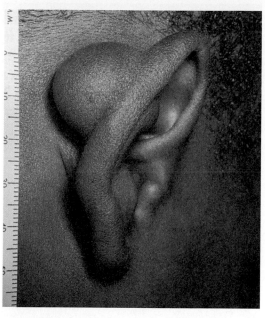

Sebaceous Cyst

Location is commonly behind lobule, in the postauricular fold. A nodule with central black punctum indicates blocked sebaceous gland. It is filled with waxy sebaceous material and is painful if it becomes infected. Often are multiple.

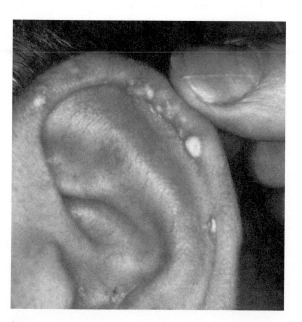

Tophi

Small, whitish yellow, hard, nontender nodules in or near helix or antihelix; contain greasy, chalky material of uric acid crystals and are a sign of gout.

Reprinted from the Clinical Slide Collection on the Rheumatic Diseases, © 1991, 1995, 1997. Used by permission of the American College of Rheumatology.

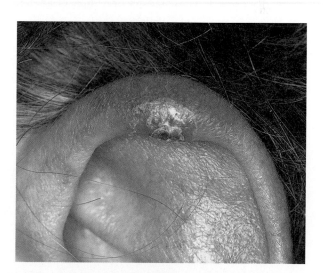

Chondrodermatitis Nodularis Helicus

Painful nodules develop on the rim of the helix (where there is no cushioning subcutaneous tissue) as a result of repetitive mechanical pressure or environmental trauma (sunlight). They are small, indurated, dull red, poorly defined, and very painful.

TABLE 15-2 | Lumps and Lesions on the External Ear—cont'd

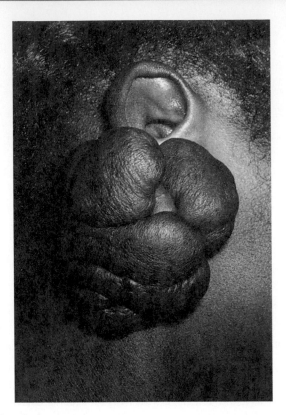

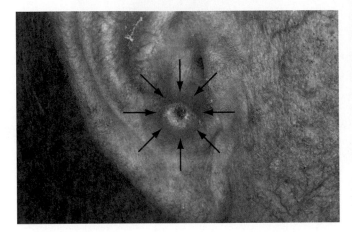

Keloid

Overgrowth of scar tissue, which invades original site of trauma. It is more common in dark-skinned people, although it also occurs in individuals with light skin. In the ear it is most common at lobule at the site of a pierced ear. Overgrowth shown here is unusually large.

Carcinoma

Ulcerated crusted nodule with indurated base that fails to heal. Bleeds intermittently. Must refer for biopsy. Usually occurs on the superior rim of the pinna, which has the most sun exposure. May occur also in ear canal and show chronic discharge that is either serosanguineous or bloody.

ABNORMAL FINDINGS
FOR ADVANCED PRACTICE

TABLE 15-3	Abnormalities in the Ear Canal

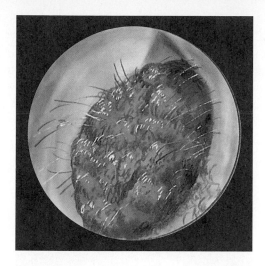

◀ **Excessive Cerumen**

Excessive cerumen is produced or is impacted because of narrow tortuous canal or poor cleaning method. May show as round ball partially obscuring drum or totally occluding canal. Even when canal is 90 to 95% blocked, hearing stays normal. But when last 5 to 10% is totally occluded (when cerumen expands after swimming or showering), person has ear fullness and sudden hearing loss.

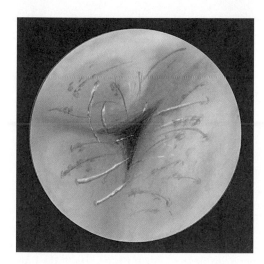

◀ **Otitis Externa**

Severe swelling of canal, inflammation, tenderness. Here canal lumen is narrowed to one fourth of normal size. (See complete description in Table 15-1, p. 360.)

TABLE 15-3   Abnormalities in the Ear Canal—cont'd

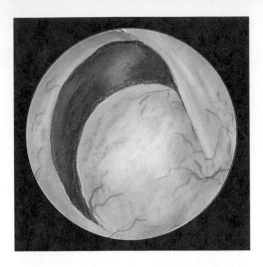

◀ **Osteoma**

Single, stony hard, rounded nodule that obscures the drum; nontender; overlying skin appears normal. Attached to inner third, the bony part, of canal. Benign, but refer for removal.

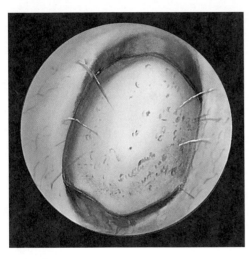

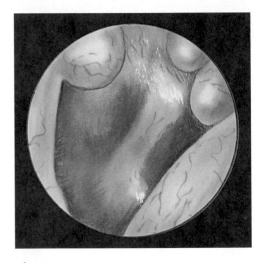

Foreign Body

Usually it is children who place a foreign body in the ear (here, a stone completely occludes the canal), which is later noted on routine examination. Common objects are beans, corn, breakfast cereals, jewellery beads, small stones, sponge rubber. Cotton is most common in adults and becomes impacted from cotton-tipped applicators. A trapped live insect is uncommon but makes the person especially frantic.

Exostosis

More common than osteoma. Small, bony hard, rounded nodules of hypertrophic bone, covered with normal epithelium. They arise near the drum but usually do not obstruct the view of the drum. They are usually multiple and bilateral. They may occur more frequently in cold-water swimmers. The condition needs no treatment, although it may cause accumulation of cerumen, which blocks the canal.

Continued

TABLE 15-3 | **Abnormalities in the Ear Canal—cont'd**

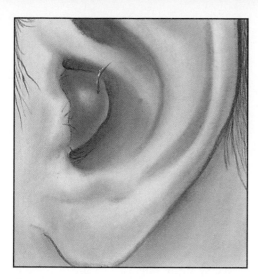

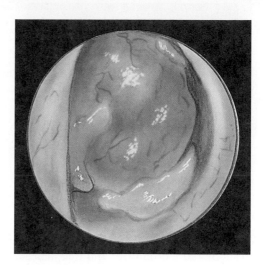

Furuncle

Exquisitely painful, reddened, infected hair follicle. Here, it occurs on the tragus but also may be on cartilaginous part of ear canal. Regional lymphadenopathy often accompanies a furuncle.

Polyp

Arises in canal from granulomatous or mucosal tissue; redder than surrounding skin and bleeds easily; bathed in foul purulent discharge; indicates chronic ear disease. Benign, but refer for excision.

TABLE 15-4 | **Abnormal Findings Seen on Otoscopy**

Appearance of Eardrum	Indicates	Suggested Condition
Yellow-amber colour	Serum or pus	Serous otitis media or chronic otitis media
Prominent landmarks	Retraction of drum	Negative pressure in middle ear from an obstructed eustachian tube
Air/fluid level or air bubbles	Serous fluid	Serous otitis media
Absent or distorted light reflex	Bulging of eardrum	Acute otitis media
Bright red colour	Infection in middle ear	Acute purulent otitis media
Blue or dark red colour	Blood behind drum	Trauma, skull fracture
Dark oval areas	Perforation	Drum rupture
White dense areas	Scarring	Sequelae of infections
Diminished or absent landmarks	Thickened drum	Chronic otitis media
Black or white dots on drum or canal	Colony of growth	Fungal infection

From Sherman, J.L. & Fields, S.K. (1998). *Guide to patient evaluation* (5th ed.) New York, NY: 1988, Medical Examination Publishing. Reprinted by permission of Elsevier, Inc.

Abnormal Findings

TABLE 15-5 | Abnormalities of the Tympanic Membrane

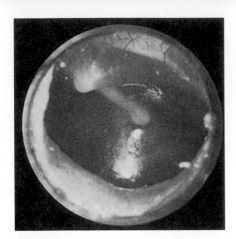

Retracted Drum

Landmarks look more prominent and well defined. Malleus handle looks shorter and more horizontal than normal. Short process is very prominent. Light reflex is absent or distorted. The drum is dull and lustreless and does not move. These signs indicate negative pressure and middle ear vacuum from obstructed eustachian tube and serous otitis media.

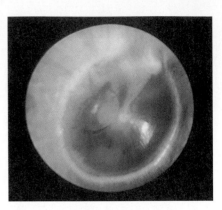

Otitis Media With Effusion (OME)

An amber-yellow drum suggests serum in middle ear that transudates to relieve negative pressure from the blocked eustachian tube. You may note an air/fluid level with fine black dividing line or air bubbles visible behind drum. Symptoms are feeling of fullness, transient hearing loss, popping sound with swallowing. Also called serous otitis media, glue ear.

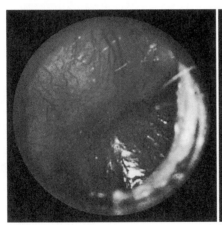

Early stage. Later stage.

Acute (Purulent) Otitis Media (above)

This results when the middle ear fluid is infected. An absent light reflex from increasing middle ear pressure is an early sign. Redness and bulging are first noted in superior part of drum (pars flaccida), along with earache and fever. Then fiery redness and bulging of entire drum occurs; deep throbbing pain; fever; transient hearing loss. Pneumatic otoscopy reveals drum hypomobility.

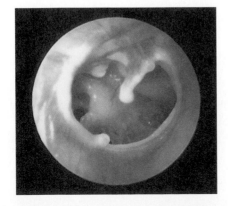

◀ Perforation

If the acute otitis media is not treated, the drum may rupture from increased pressure. Perforations also occur from trauma (e.g., a slap on the ear). Usually the perforation appears as a round or oval darkened area on the drum, but in this photo the perforation is very large. *Central* perforations occur in the pars tensa. *Marginal* perforations occur at the annulus. Marginal perforations are called *attic perforations* when they occur in superior part of the drum, the pars flaccida.

Continued

TABLE 15-5 | **Abnormalities of the Tympanic Membrane—cont'd**

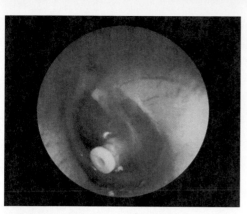

Insertion of Tympanostomy Tubes

Polyethylene tubes are inserted surgically into the eardrum to relieve middle ear pressure and promote drainage of chronic or recurrent middle ear infections. Number of acute infections tends to decrease because of improved aeration. Tubes extrude spontaneously in 12 to 18 months.

Reprinted from Fireman, P. (1995). Atlas of allergies, (2nd ed., p. 182), by permission of the publisher, Mosby.

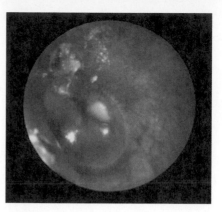

Cholesteatoma

An overgrowth of epidermal tissue in the middle ear or temporal bone may result over the years after a marginal tympanic membrane perforation. It has a pearly white, cheesy appearance. Growth of cholesteatoma can erode bone and produce hearing loss. Early signs include otorrhea, unilateral conductive hearing loss, tinnitus.

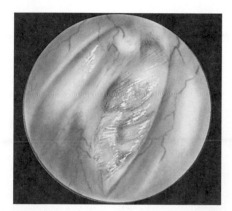

Scarred Drum

Dense white patches on the eardrum are sequelae of repeated ear infections. They do not necessarily affect hearing.

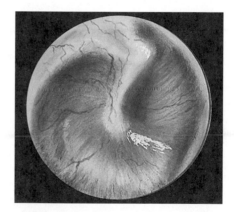

Blue Drum (Hemotympanum)

This indicates blood in the middle ear, as in trauma resulting in skull fracture.

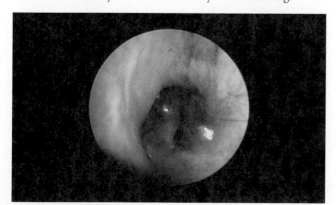

Bullous Myringitis

Small vesicles containing blood on the drum; accompany *Mycoplasma* pneumonia and virus infections. May have blood-tinged discharge and severe otalgia.

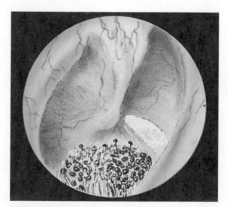

Fungal Infection (Otomycosis)

Colony of black or white dots on drum or canal wall suggests a yeast or fungal infection.

TABLE 15-6 | **Tuning Fork Tests**

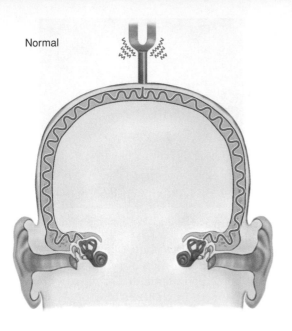

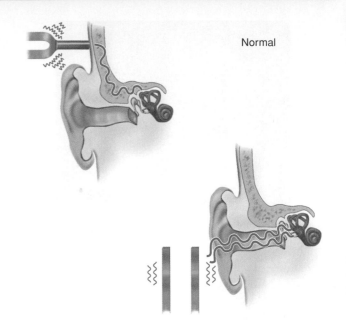

Weber Test

Normal—Sound is equally loud in both ears; sound does not lateralize.

Rinne Test

Normal—Sound is heard twice as long by air conduction (AC) as by bone conduction (BC); a "positive" Rinne, or AC > BC.

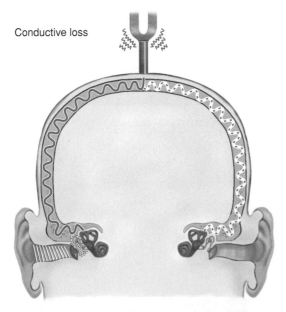

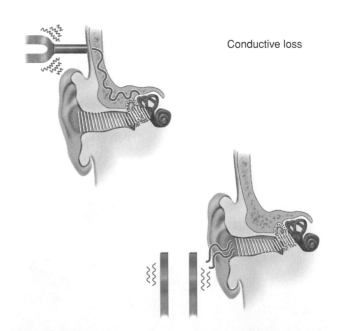

Conductive loss—Sound lateralizes to "poorer" ear from background room noise, which masks hearing in normal ear. "Poorer" ear (the one with conductive loss) is not distracted by background noise, thus has a better chance to hear bone-conducted sound. Examples: transient conductive loss with serous or purulent otitis media.

Conductive loss—Person hears as long by bone conduction (AC = BC) or even longer (AC < BC), a "negative" finding on the Rinne test.

Continued

TABLE 15-6	Tuning Fork Tests—cont'd

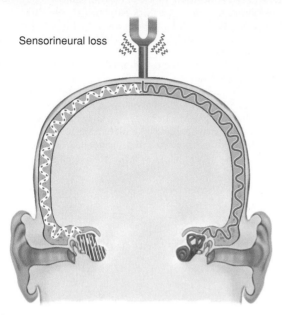

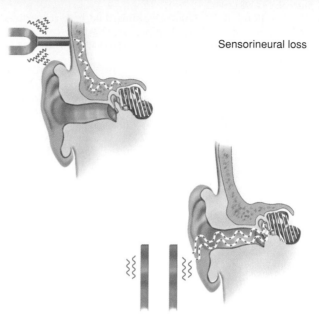

Weber Test

Sensorineural loss—Sound lateralizes to "better" ear or unaffected ear. "Poor" ear (the one with nerve loss) is unable to perceive the sound.

Rinne Test

Sensorineural loss—Normal ratio of AC > BC is intact but is reduced overall. That is, person hears poorly both ways.

Abnormal Findings

BIBLIOGRAPHY

American Academy of Pediatrics, Subcommittee on Management of Acute Otitis Media. (2004). Diagnosis and management of acute otitis media. *Pediatrics, 113,* 1451–1465.

Bagai, A., Thavendiranathan, P., & Detsky, A. (2006). Does this patient have hearing impairment? *Journal of the American Medical Association, 29,* 416–428.

Bernius, M., & Perlin, D. (2006). Pediatric ear, nose and throat emergencies. *Pediatric Clinics of North America, 53,* 195–214.

Block, S. (2005). Diagnosing acute otitis media: It's what you see, not what you hear. *Contemporary Pediatrics, 22,* 3–8.

Canadian Hearing Society. (2007). *The Canadian Hearing Society position paper on discrimination and audism.* Retrieved April 18, 2008, at http://www.chs.ca/info/publicaffairs/pdf/CHSPositionOnDiscrimination.pdf

Carlson, L. (2005). Otitis media: New information on an old disease. *Nurse Practitioner, 30,* 31–43.

Chantry, C., Howard, C., & Auinger, P. (2006). Full breastfeeding duration and associated decrease in respiratory tract infection in US children. *Pediatrics, 117,* 425–432.

Dallaire, F., Dewailly, E., Vézina, C., Bruneau S., & Ayotte P. (2006). Portrait of outpatient visits and hospitalizations for acute infections in Nunavik preschool children. *Canadian Journal of Public Health, 97,* 362–368.

Devaney, K. O., Boschman, C. R., Willard, S. C., Ferlito, A., & Rinaldo, A. (2005). Tumours of the external ear and temporal bone. *Lancet Oncology, 6,* 411–420.

Durieux-Smith, A., Fitzpatrick, E., & Whitingham, J. (2008). Universal newborn hearing screening: A question of evidence. *International Journal of Audiology, 47*(1), 1–10.

Gates, G., & Mills, J. (2005). Presbycusis. *Lancet, 366,* 1111–1120.

Health Canada. (2006). *Hearing loss and leisure noise.* Retrieved February 5, 2008, from http://www.hc-sc.gc.ca/iyh-vsv/environ/leisure-loisirs_e.html#is

Helzner, E. P., Cauley, J. A., Pratt, S. R., Wisniewski, S. R., Zmuda, J. M., Talbott, E. O., et al. (2005). Race and sex differences in age-related hearing loss: The Health, Aging, and Body Composition Study. *Journal of the American Geriatric Society, 53,* 2119–2127.

Holcomb, S. (2004). New guidelines improve treatment of otitis media. *Nurse Practitioner, 29,* 6–13.

Kane, R. L., Ouslander, J. G., & Abrass, I. E. (2003). *Essentials of clinical geriatrics* (5th ed.). New York, NY: McGraw-Hill.

Levy, B., Slade, M., & Gill, T. (2006). Hearing decline predicted by elders' stereotypes. *Journal of Gerontology, 61,* 82–87.

Lieu, J., & Feinstein, A. (2007). Effect of gestational and passive smoke exposure on ear infections in children. *Archives of Pediatric and Adolescent Medicine, 156,* 147–154.

Moore, A. (2006). The otoscope. *Journal of the American Medical Association, 295,* 2115–2116.

National Center for Health Statistics. (2006). *Health, United States, 2005 with chartbook on trends in the health of Americans* (DHHS Publication No. 2005-1232). Hyattsville, MD: Author.

Overfield, T. (1995). *Biologic variation in health and illness: Race, age, and sex differences* (2nd ed.). New York, NY: CRC Press.

Rash, E. (2004). Recognize cholesteatomas early. *Nurse Practitioner, 29,* 24–29.

Rothman, R., Owens, T., & Simel, D. (2003). Does this child have acute otitis media? *Journal of the American Medical Association, 290,* 1633–1640.

Sangster, J. F, Grace, T. M., & Seewald, R. C. (1991). Hearing loss in elderly patients in family practice. *Canadian Medical Association Journal, 144,* 981–984.

Singh, A., & Bond, B. L. (2006). Does this child have acute otitis media? *Annals of Emergency Medicine, 47,* 113–116.

Spilman, L. (2002). Examination of the external ear. *Advances in Neonatal Care, 2,* 72–80.

Terris, M. H., Magit, A. E., & Davidson, T. E. (1995). Otitis media with effusion in infants and children. *Postgraduate Medicine, 97,* 137–151.

U.S. Preventive Services Task Force. (2002). Newborn hearing screening: Recommendations and rationale. *American Journal of Nursing, 102,* 83–89.

Urkin, J., Gazala, E., & Bar-David, Y. (2004). Cleaning earwax: Why you shouldn't play it by ear. *Contemporary Pediatrics, 21,* 73–80.

Valtonen, H., Tuomilehto, H., Qvarnberg, Y., & Nuutinen, J. (2005). A 14-year prospective follow-up study of children treated early in life with tympanostomy tubes, 2: Hearing outcomes. *Archives of Otolaryngology—Head and Neck Surgery, 131,* 299–303.

Wallhagen, M., Pettengill, E., & Whiteside, M. (2006). Sensory impairment in older adults, part 1: Hearing loss. *American Journal of Nursing, 106,* 40–49.

Wang, R. (2001). Syndromic ear anomalies and renal ultrasounds. *Pediatrics, 108,* 1–8.

Wittmann-Price, R., & Pope, K. (2002). Universal newborn hearing screening. *American Journal of Nursing, 102,* 71–77.

Yueh, B., Shapiro, N., MacLean, C. H., & Shekelle, P. G. (2003). Screening and management of adult hearing loss in primary care. *Journal of the American Medical Association, 289,* 1976–1985.

Nose, Mouth, and Throat

Written by **Carolyn Jarvis**, PhD, APN, CNP
Adapted by **Barbara Wilson-Keates**, RN, MS

Electronic Resources

On Evolve *evolve*

http://evolve.elsevier.com/Canada/Jarvis/examination/

- Interactive Case Studies
- Physical Examination Audio and Printable Summaries
- Bedside Assessment Summary Checklists
- Complete Physical Examination Form
- Nursing Diagnoses Boxes
- Health Promotion Guides
- Quick Assessments for 20 Common Conditions
- Multiple Choice Review Questions
- Chapter Objectives
- Appendices
- Weblinks

On the Companion CD

- Interactive Case Studies with Heart and Lung Sounds
- Health Promotion Guides
- Quick Assessments for 20 Common Conditions
- Head-to-Toe Physical Examination Video Clips

STRUCTURE AND FUNCTION

NOSE

The **nose** is the first segment of the respiratory system. It warms, moistens, and filters the inhaled air, and it is the sensory organ for smell. The external nose is shaped like a triangle with one side attached to the face (Fig. 16-1). On its leading edge, the superior part is the *bridge* and the free corner is the *tip.* The oval openings at the base of the triangle are the *nares;* just inside, each naris widens into the *vestibule.* The *columella* divides the two nares and is continuous inside with the nasal septum. The *ala* is the lateral outside wing of the nose on either side. The upper third of the external nose is made up of bone; the rest is cartilage.

Inside, the **nasal cavity** is much larger than the external nose would indicate (Fig. 16-2). It extends back over the roof of the mouth. The anterior edge of the cavity is lined with numerous coarse nasal hairs, or vibrissae. The rest of the cavity is lined with a blanket of ciliated mucous membrane. The nasal hairs filter the coarsest matter from inhaled air, whereas the mucous blanket filters out dust and bacteria. Nasal mucosa appears redder than oral mucosa because of the rich blood supply present to warm the inhaled air.

The nasal cavity is divided medially by the **septum** into two slitlike air passages. The anterior part of the septum holds a rich vascular network, *Kiesselbach's plexus,* the most common site of nosebleeds. In many people, the nasal septum is not absolutely straight and may deviate toward one passage.

The lateral walls of each nasal cavity contain three parallel bony projections—the superior, middle, and inferior **turbinates.** They increase the surface area so that more blood vessels and mucous membranes are available to warm, humidify, and filter the inhaled air. Underlying each turbinate

is a cleft, the **meatus,** which is named for the turbinate above. The sinuses drain into the middle meatus, and tears from the nasolacrimal duct drain into the inferior meatus.

The olfactory receptors (hair cells) lie at the roof of the nasal cavity and in the upper one third of the septum. These receptors for smell merge into the olfactory nerve, cranial nerve I, which transmits to the temporal lobe of the brain. Although it is not necessary for human survival, the sense of smell adds to nutrition by enhancing the pleasure and taste of food.

The **paranasal sinuses** are air-filled pockets within the cranium (Fig. 16-3). They communicate with the nasal cavity and are lined with the same type of ciliated mucous membrane. They lighten the weight of the skull bones, serve as resonators for sound production, and provide mucus, which drains into the nasal cavity. The sinus openings are narrow and easily occluded, which may cause inflammation or sinusitis.

Two pairs of sinuses are accessible to examination: the **frontal** sinuses in the frontal bone above and medial to the orbits and the **maxillary** sinuses in the maxilla (cheekbone) along the side walls of the nasal cavity. The other two sets are smaller and deeper: the **ethmoid** sinuses between the orbits and the **sphenoid** sinuses deep within the skull in the sphenoid bone.

Only the maxillary and ethmoid sinuses are present at birth. The maxillary sinuses reach full size after all permanent teeth have erupted. The ethmoid sinuses grow rapidly between 6 and 8 years of age and after puberty. The frontal sinuses are absent at birth, are fairly well developed between 7 and 8 years of age, and reach full size after puberty. The sphenoid sinuses are minute at birth and develop after puberty.

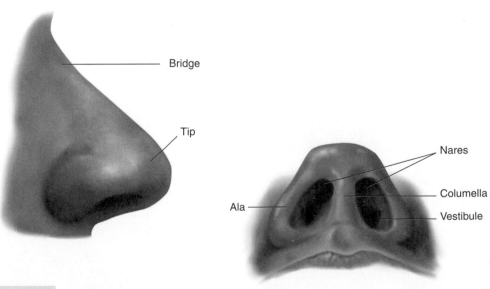

Bridge

Tip

Nares

Columella

Ala

Vestibule

Fig. 16-1 Nasal structures.

© Pat Thomas, 2006.

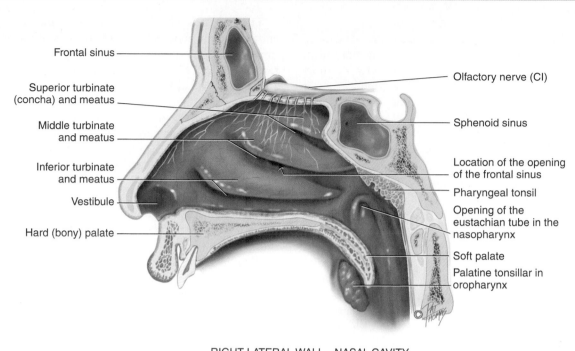

RIGHT LATERAL WALL—NASAL CAVITY

Fig. 16-2

© Pat Thomas, 2006.

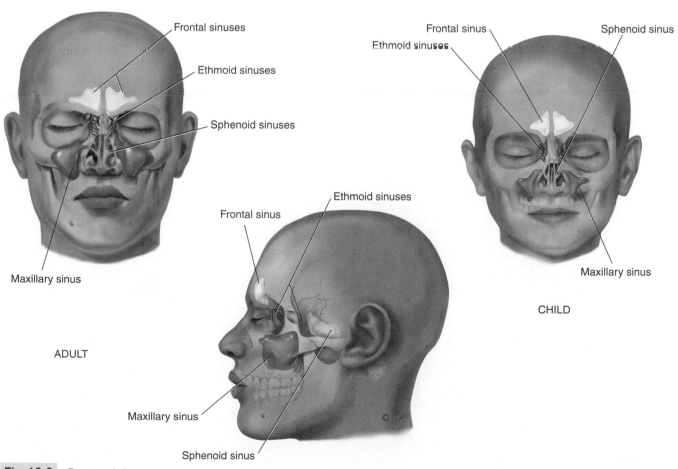

Fig. 16-3   Paranasal sinuses.

© Pat Thomas, 2006.

MOUTH

The mouth is the first segment of the digestive system and an airway for the respiratory system. The **oral cavity** is a short passage bordered by the lips, palate, cheeks, and tongue. It contains the teeth and gums, tongue, and salivary glands (Fig. 16-4).

The lips are the anterior border of the oral cavity—the transition zone from the outer skin to the inner mucous membrane lining the oral cavity. The arching roof of the mouth is the palate; it is divided into two parts. The anterior **hard palate** is made up of bone and is a whitish colour. Posterior to this is the **soft palate,** an arch of muscle that is pinker and mobile. The **uvula** is the free projection hanging down from the middle of the soft palate. The cheeks are the side walls of the oral cavity.

The floor of the mouth consists of the horseshoe-shaped mandible bone, the tongue, and underlying muscles. The **tongue** is a mass of striated muscle arranged in a crosswise pattern so that it can change shape and position. The papillae are the rough, bumpy elevations on its dorsal surface. Note the larger vallate papillae in an inverted V shape across the posterior base of the tongue, and do not confuse them with abnormal growths. Underneath, the ventral surface of the tongue is smooth and shiny and has prominent veins. The **frenulum** is a midline fold of tissue that connects the tongue to the floor of the mouth.

The tongue's ability to change shape and position enhances its functions in mastication, swallowing, cleansing the teeth, and speech. The tongue also functions in taste sensation. Microscopic taste buds are in the papillae at the back and along the sides of the tongue and on the soft palate.

The mouth contains three pairs of salivary glands (Fig. 16-5). The largest, the **parotid** gland, lies within the cheeks in front of the ear extending from the zygomatic arch down to the angle of the jaw. Its duct, Stensen's duct, runs forward to open on the buccal mucosa opposite the second molar. The **submandibular** gland is the size of a walnut. It lies beneath the mandible at the angle of the jaw. Wharton's duct runs up and forward to the floor of the mouth and opens at either side of the frenulum. The smallest, the almond-shaped **sublingual** gland, lies within the floor of the mouth under the tongue. It has many small openings along the sublingual fold under the tongue.

The glands secrete saliva, the clear fluid that moistens and lubricates the food bolus, starts digestion, and cleans and protects the mucosa.

Adults have 32 **permanent** teeth—16 in each arch. Each tooth has three parts: the crown, the neck, and the root. The gums (gingivae) collar the teeth. They are thick fibrous tissues covered with mucous membrane. The gums are different from the rest of the oral mucosa because of their pale pink colour and stippled surface.

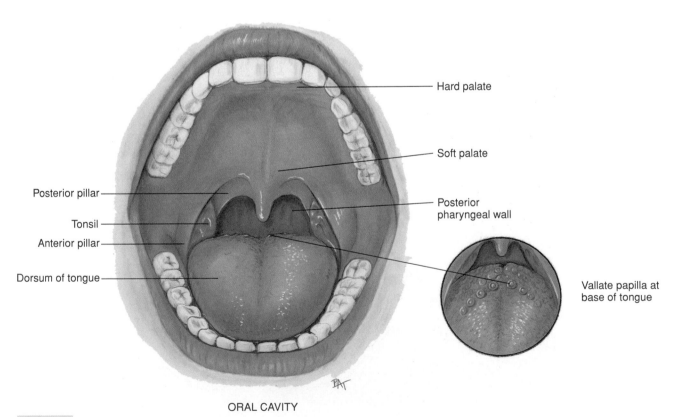

Hard palate

Soft palate

Posterior pillar

Tonsil

Anterior pillar

Dorsum of tongue

Posterior pharyngeal wall

Vallate papilla at base of tongue

ORAL CAVITY

Fig. 16-4

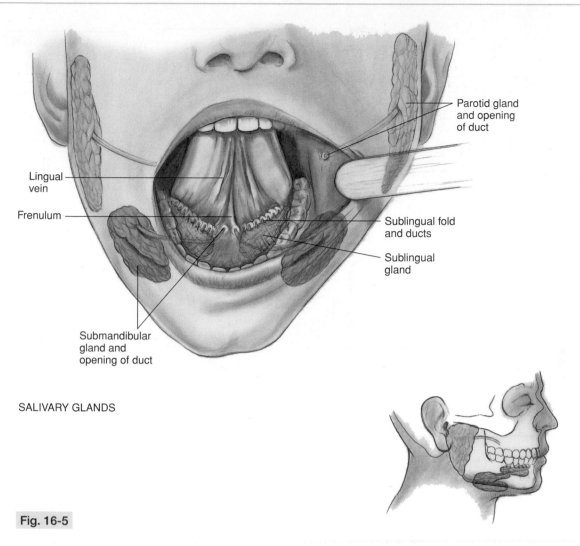

Parotid gland
and opening
of duct

Lingual
vein

Frenulum

Sublingual fold
and ducts

Sublingual
gland

Submandibular
gland and
opening of duct

SALIVARY GLANDS

Fig. 16-5

THROAT

The throat, or pharynx, is the area behind the mouth and nose. The **oropharynx** is separated from the mouth by a fold of tissue on each side, the anterior tonsillar pillar. Behind the folds are the **tonsils,** each a mass of lymphoid tissue. The tonsils are the same colour as the surrounding mucous membrane, although they look more granular, and their surface shows deep crypts. Tonsillar tissue enlarges during childhood until puberty and then involutes. The posterior pharyngeal wall is seen behind these structures. Some small blood vessels may show on it.

The **nasopharynx** is continuous with the oropharynx, although it is above the oropharynx and behind the nasal cavity. The pharyngeal tonsils (adenoids) and the eustachian tube openings are located here (see Fig. 16-2).

The oral cavity and throat have a rich lymphatic network. Review the lymph nodes and their drainage patterns in Chapter 13 and keep this in mind when evaluating the mouth.

DEVELOPMENTAL CARE

Infants and Children

In the infant, salivation starts at 3 months. The baby will drool periodically for a few months before learning to swallow the saliva. This drooling does not herald the eruption of the first tooth, although many parents think it does.

The teeth, both sets, begin development in utero. Children have 20 **deciduous,** or temporary, teeth. These erupt between 6 months and 24 months of age. All 20 teeth should appear by 2½ years of age. The deciduous teeth are lost beginning at age 6 years through age 12 years. They are replaced by the permanent teeth, starting with the central incisors (Fig. 16-6). The permanent teeth appear earlier in girls than in boys, and they erupt earlier in children of African descent than in children of European descent.

The nose develops during adolescence, along with the secondary sex characteristics. This growth starts at age 12 or 13 years, reaching full growth at age 16 years in females and age 18 years in males.

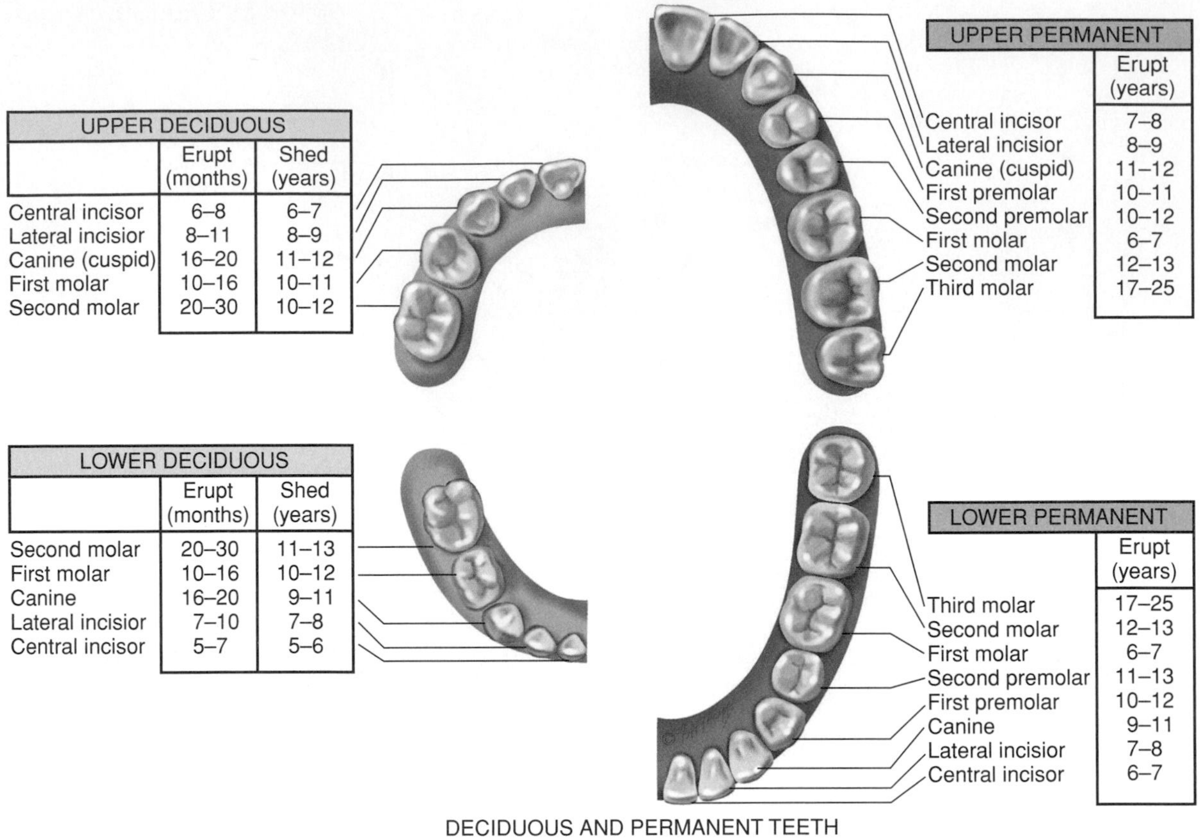

UPPER DECIDUOUS		
	Erupt (months)	Shed (years)
Central incisor	6–8	6–7
Lateral incisior	8–11	8–9
Canine (cuspid)	16–20	11–12
First molar	10–16	10–11
Second molar	20–30	10–12

UPPER PERMANENT	
	Erupt (years)
Central incisor	7–8
Lateral incisior	8–9
Canine (cuspid)	11–12
First premolar	10–11
Second premolar	10–12
First molar	6–7
Second molar	12–13
Third molar	17–25

LOWER DECIDUOUS		
	Erupt (months)	Shed (years)
Second molar	20–30	11–13
First molar	10–16	10–12
Canine	16–20	9–11
Lateral incisior	7–10	7–8
Central incisor	5–7	5–6

LOWER PERMANENT	
	Erupt (years)
Third molar	17–25
Second molar	12–13
First molar	6–7
Second premolar	11–13
First premolar	10–12
Canine	9–11
Lateral incisior	7–8
Central incisor	6–7

DECIDUOUS AND PERMANENT TEETH

Fig. 16-6

© Pat Thomas, 2006.

The Pregnant Female

Nasal stuffiness and epistaxis may occur during pregnancy as a result of increased vascularity in the upper respiratory tract. Also, the gums may be hyperemic and softened and may bleed with normal toothbrushing. Contrary to superstitious folklore, no evidence exists that pregnancy causes tooth decay or loss.

The Aging Adult

A gradual loss of subcutaneous fat starts during later middle adult years, making the nose appear more prominent in some people. The nasal hairs grow coarser and stiffer and may not filter the air as well. The hairs protrude and may cause itching and sneezing. Many older people clip these hairs, thinking them unsightly, but this practice can cause infection. The sense of smell may diminish because of a decrease in the number of olfactory nerve fibres. The decrease in the sensation of smell begins after age 60 years, and it continues progressively with age (Edelstein, 1996).

In the oral cavity, the soft tissues atrophy and the epithelium thins, especially in the cheek and tongue. This results in loss of taste buds, with about an 80% reduction in taste functioning. Further impairments to taste include a decrease in salivary secretion that is needed to dissolve flavouring agents, and the presence of upper dentures that cover secondary taste sites (Kane et al., 2003).

Atrophic tissues ulcerate easily, which places the older person at risk for infections such as oral moniliasis. An increased risk of malignant oral lesions is also present.

Many dental changes occur with aging. The tooth surface is abraded. The gums begin to recede and the teeth begin to erode at the gum line. A smooth V-shaped cavity forms around the neck of the tooth, exposing the nerve and making the tooth hypersensitive. Some tooth loss may occur from bone resorption (osteoporosis), which decreases the inner tooth structure and its outer support. Natural tooth loss is exacerbated by years of inadequate dental care, decay, poor oral hygiene, and tobacco use.

If tooth loss occurs, the remaining teeth drift, causing **malocclusion.** The stress of chewing with maloccluding teeth causes further problems: (1) excessive bone resorption with further tooth loss occurs, (2) muscle imbalance results from a mandible and maxilla now out of alignment, which produces muscle spasms, tenderness of muscles of mastication, and chronic headaches, and (3) the temporomandibular joint is stressed, leading to osteoarthritis, pain, and inability to fully open the mouth.

Diminished senses of taste and smell decrease the older person's interest in food and may contribute to malnutrition. Saliva production decreases; saliva acts as a solvent for food flavours and helps move food around the mouth. Decreased saliva also reduces the mouth's self-cleaning property. The major cause of decreased saliva flow is not the aging process itself but the use of medications that have anticholinergic effects. More than 250 medications have a side effect of dry mouth.

The absence of some teeth and trouble with mastication encourage the older person to eat soft foods (usually high in carbohydrates) and to decrease meat and fresh vegetable intake. This produces a risk of nutritional deficit for protein, vitamins, and minerals.

CULTURAL AND SOCIAL CONSIDERATIONS

Bifid, or **cleft uvula**, a condition in which the uvula is either completely or partially split, is more commonly found in Aboriginal people and people of Asian descent (Overfield, 1995). The occurrence in people of European or African descent is rare. **Cleft lip** and **cleft palate** are most common in Aboriginal people and people of Asian descent and least common in people of African descent (Overfield, 1995). Torus palatinus, a bony ridge running down the middle of the hard palate, is also more common in Aboriginal people and people of Asian descent (Overfield, 1995).

Leukoedema, a greyish-white benign lesion occurring on the buccal mucosa, may be present in people of African descent. Oral hyperpigmentation also varies according to ethnocultural groups. Usually absent at birth, hyperpigmentation increases with age. By 50 years of age, 10% of people of European descent and 50 to 90% of people of African descent show oral hyperpigmentation, a condition that is believed to be caused by a lifetime of accumulation of postinflammatory oral changes (Overfield, 1995).

Although it is rare for a baby of European descent to be born with teeth (one in 3000), the incidence rises to one or two in 100 among Canadian Inuit infants (Overfield, 1995). The size of teeth varies widely, with the teeth of people of European descent being the smallest, followed by people of African descent, then people of Asian descent and Aboriginal people. Large teeth cause some ethnocultural groups to have prognathic, or protruding, jaws, a condition that is seen more frequently in people of African or Asian descent. The condition is normal and does not reflect an orthodontic problem.

Across Canada, Aboriginal people generally have higher rates of periodontal disease and dental decay than does the general Canadian population. Poorer oral health is influenced by changes from traditional diets to ones higher in processed and sugary foods, lack of access to fluoridated water, and lack of access to comprehensive dental health services. The last two factors are particularly evident in remote areas (Health Canada, 2005). Consequently, restorative dental care, such as fillings, is more prevalent than dental health promotion activities among Aboriginal people (40% versus 8%; Health Canada, 2001).

The First Nations and Inuit Regional Health Survey (RHS) (1997) indicated that almost 50% of surveyed adults reported needing dental treatment, and nearly 25% had dental pain or another dental problem during the preceding month. Over 40% of First Nation and Inuit adults had not received dental care in the past year. The 2002–2003 RHS survey showed that almost 20% of children had never received dental care and among First Nation and Inuit children under 3 years of age, 12% had prevalence of baby bottle tooth decay. As a result, First Nation and Inuit children have a greater prevalence of dental caries, malocclusion, and baby bottle tooth decay than other Canadian children.

Various socioeconomic variables are correlated with poor dental health. Individuals from lower-income households have a greater prevalence of edentulism, periodontal disease, dental pain, and chewing difficulties than do people from higher-income households. Consequently, lower-income individuals report poorer oral health–related quality of life than do Canadians from higher-income groups (Locker, 2007).

Access to comprehensive dental health care continues to be a major barrier to oral health promotion and maintenance for many Canadians. Aboriginal people, recent immigrants, individuals from lower socioeconomic groups, and Canadians living in rural and/or remote areas are less likely to have access to regular, comprehensive dental care. In addition, many Canadians lack adequate dental coverage and may not be able to pay dental care expenses. Inability to access regular and affordable dental care in their own communities is thought to result in poorer oral and overall health status for these Canadians.

Recent immigration may also potentially impact dental health (Lai et al., 2007). Language and cultural differences, lack of familiarity with the healthcare and dental care systems, and limited financial resources may prevent immigrants from accessing dental care services. At time of immigration, immigrant adolescents had a higher prevalence of dental decay than did nonimmigrant adolescents (15% versus 4%). Dental health status improved as time in Canada increased, possibly due to provincially funded dental promotion programs. However, adolescent immigrants did not attain the same oral health status as did Canadian-born adolescents (Locker et al., 1998).

SUBJECTIVE DATA

Nose

1. Discharge
2. Frequent colds (upper respiratory infections)
3. Sinus pain
4. Trauma
5. Epistaxis (nosebleeds)
6. Allergies
7. Altered smell

Mouth and Throat

1. Sores or lesions
2. Sore throat
3. Bleeding gums
4. Toothache
5. Hoarseness
6. Dysphagia
7. Altered taste
8. Smoking, alcohol consumption
9. Self-care behaviours
   Dental care pattern
   Dentures or appliances

Examiner Asks	Rationale

Subjective Data

Nose

1. Discharge. Any **nasal discharge** or runny nose? Continuous?
- Is the discharge watery, purulent, mucoid, bloody?

Rhinorrhea occurs with colds, allergies, sinus infection, trauma.

2. Frequent colds (upper respiratory infections). Any unusually frequent or severe colds? How often do these occur?

Most people have occasional colds; thus, asking this more precise question yields more meaningful data.

3. Sinus pain. Any **sinus pain** or sinusitis? How is this treated?
- Do you have chronic postnasal drip?

4. Trauma. Ever had any **trauma** or a blow to the nose?
- Can you breathe through your nose? Is either side obstructed?

Trauma may cause deviated septum, which may cause nares to be obstructed.

5. Epistaxis (nosebleeds). Any nosebleeds? How often?
- How much bleeding—about 5 mL or does it pour out?
- Colour of the blood—red or brown? Clots?
- From one nostril or both?
- Aggravated by nose-picking or scratching?
- How do you treat the nosebleeds? Are they difficult to stop?

Epistaxis occurs with trauma, vigorous nose blowing, foreign body.

Person should sit up with head tilted forward, pinch nose between thumb and forefinger for 5 to 15 minutes.

6. Allergies. Any **allergies** or hay fever? To what are you allergic (e.g., pollen, dust, pets)?
- How was this determined?
- What type of environment makes it worse? Can you avoid exposure?
- Use inhalers, nasal spray, nose drops? How often? Which type?
- How long have you used this?

"Seasonal" rhinitis if due to pollen; "perennial" if allergen is dust.

Misuse of over-the-counter nasal medications irritates the mucosa, causing rebound swelling, a common problem.

7. Altered smell. Experienced any change in sense of smell?

Sense of smell diminished with cigarette smoking or chronic allergies.

Mouth and Throat

1. Sores or lesions. Noticed any **sores** or **lesions** in the mouth, or on the tongue or gums?
- How long have you had it? Ever had this lesion before?
- Is it single or multiple?
- Does it seem to be associated with stress, season change, food?
- How have you treated the sore? Applied any local medication?

History helps determine whether oral lesions have infectious, traumatic, immunological, or malignant etiology. Periodontal disease is thought to be associated with cardiovascular diseases, diabetes, pulmonary infections, and osteoporosis (Meurman et al., 2004; Renvert, 2003).

2. Sore throat. How about **sore throats?** How frequently do you get them? Have a sore throat now? When did it start?
- Is it associated with cough, fever, fatigue, decreased appetite, headache, postnasal drip, or hoarseness?
- Is it worse when arising? What is the humidity level in the room where you sleep? Any dust or smoke inhaled at work?
- Usually get a throat culture for the sore throats? Were any documented as streptococcal?
- How have you treated this sore throat: medication, gargling? How effective are these? Have your tonsils or adenoids been taken out?

Untreated strep throat may lead to the complication of rheumatic fever.

3. Bleeding gums. Any **bleeding gums?** How long have you had this?

A little bleeding is normal if just starting to floss. More frequent bleeding from brushing or flossing may indicate periodontal disease or a clotting disorder.

Examiner Asks	Rationale
4. Toothache. Any **toothache?** Do your teeth seem sensitive to hot, cold? Have you lost any teeth?	
5. Hoarseness. Any **hoarseness,** voice change? For how long? • Feel as though you have to clear your throat? Or have a "lump in your throat?" • Use your voice a lot at work, recreation? • Does the hoarseness seem associated with a cold, sore throat?	A disorder of the larynx with many causes, such as overuse of the voice, upper respiratory infection, chronic inflammation, lesions, or a neoplasm.
6. Dysphagia. Any difficulty swallowing? How long have you had it? • Feel like food gets stopped at a certain point? • Any pain with this?	**Dysphagia** occurs with pharyngitis, gastroesophageal reflux disease, pharyngitis, stroke and other neurological diseases, esophageal cancer.
7. Altered taste. Any change in sense of taste?	
8. Smoking, alcohol consumption. Do you smoke? Pipe or cigarettes? Smokeless tobacco? How many packs per day? For how many years? • When was your last alcoholic drink? How much alcohol did you drink that time? How much alcohol do you usually drink?	Chronic tobacco use is associated with tooth loss, coronal and root caries, and periodontal disease in older adults. Chronic tobacco use in any form and heavy alcohol consumption greatly increase risk of oral and pharyngeal cancers.
9. Self-care behaviours. Tell me about your daily dental care. How often do you use a toothbrush and floss? • Last dental examination? Do dental problems affect which foods you eat? • Do you have a dental appliance: braces, bridge, headgear? • Wear dentures? All the time? How long have you had this set? How do they fit? • Any sores or irritation on the palate or gums? • Any problems with talking—Do the dentures whistle or drop? Can you chew all foods with them? How do you clean them? • Do you have dental coverage?	Assess self-care behaviours for oral hygiene. Regular dental screening, usually every 6 months, is necessary for the promotion and maintenance of oral health. Dentists may recommend more frequent checkups, depending on oral and overall health. However, dental benefit plans may only provide coverage for dental screening and cleaning every 9 months. Lesions may arise from ill-fitting dentures, or the presence of dentures may mask the eruption of a new lesion. Many Canadians do not have coverage and this may impact self-care behaviours.

Additional History for Infants and Children

Examiner Asks	Rationale
1. Does the child have any mouth infections or sores, such as thrush or canker sores? How frequently do these occur?	
2. Does the child have frequent sore throat, or tonsillitis? How often? How are these treated? Have they ever been documented as streptococcal infections?	
3. Did the child's teeth erupt about on time? • Do the teeth seem straight to you? • Is the child using a bottle? How often during the day? Does the child go to sleep with a bottle at night? • Have you noticed any thumb-sucking after the child's secondary teeth came in? • Have you noticed the child grinding his or her teeth? Does this happen at night?	Eruption is delayed with Down syndrome, cretinism, and rickets, and may impair nutrition. Malocclusion. Prolonged use of a bottle increases risk for tooth decay and middle ear infections. Prolonged thumb-sucking (after age 6 to 7 years) may affect occlusion. Bruxism usually occurs in sleep, from dental problems, nervous tension.

Subjective Data

Examiner Asks	Rationale
4. Self-care behaviours. How are the child's dental habits? Use a toothbrush regularly? How often does the child see a dentist? • Do you use fluoridated water or fluoride supplement?	Evaluate child's self-care. When baby teeth have erupted (age 2 to 3 years), begin regular 6-month dental checkups to evaluate self-care and identify potential problems. To prevent fluorosis, adults should brush teeth of children under 3 years of age, using a smear of toothpaste. Children under 6 years of age should use a pea-sized portion of toothpaste.
Additional History for the Aging Adult	
1. Any dryness in the mouth? Are you taking any medications? (Note prescribed and over-the-counter medications.)	**Xerostomia** (dry mouth) is a side effect of many drugs: antidepressants, anticholinergics, antispasmodics, antihypertensives, antipsychotics, bronchodilators.
2. Have you had any loss of teeth? Can you chew all types of food?	Note a decrease in eating meat, fresh vegetables, and cleansing foods such as apples.
3. Are you able to care for your own teeth or dentures?	Self-care may be decreased by physical disability (arthritis), vision loss, confusion, or depression.
4. Noticed a change in your sense of taste or smell?	Some people add extra salt and sugar to enhance food when taste begins to wane. Also, diminished smell may decrease the person's ability to detect food spoilage, natural gas leaks, or smoke from a fire.

OBJECTIVE DATA

PREPARATION

Position the person sitting up straight with his or her head at your eye level. If the person wears dentures, offer a paper towel and ask the person to remove them.

EQUIPMENT NEEDED

Otoscope with short, wide-tipped nasal speculum attachment
Penlight
Two tongue blades
Cotton gauze pad (10 × 10 cm)
Gloves
Occasionally: long-stem light attachment for otoscope

Normal Range of Findings

INSPECT AND PALPATE THE NOSE

External Nose

Normally, the nose is symmetrical, in the midline, and in proportion to other facial features (Fig. 16-7). Inspect for any deformity, asymmetry, inflammation, or skin lesions. If an injury is reported or suspected, palpate gently for any pain or break in contour.

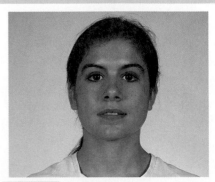

Fig. 16-7

Normal Range of Findings

Test the patency of the nostrils by pushing each nasal wing shut with your finger while asking the person to sniff inward through the other naris. This reveals any obstruction, which later is explored using the nasal speculum. The sense of smell, mediated by cranial nerve I, is usually not tested in a routine examination. The procedure for assessing smell is presented with cranial nerve testing in Chapter 23.

Nasal Cavity

Attach the short wide-tipped speculum to the otoscope head and insert this combined apparatus into the nasal vestibule, avoiding pressure on the nasal septum. Gently lift up the tip of the nose with your finger before inserting.

View each nasal cavity with the person's head erect and then with the head tilted back. Inspect the nasal mucosa, noting its normal red colour and smooth moist surface (Fig. 16-8). Note any swelling, discharge, bleeding, or foreign body.

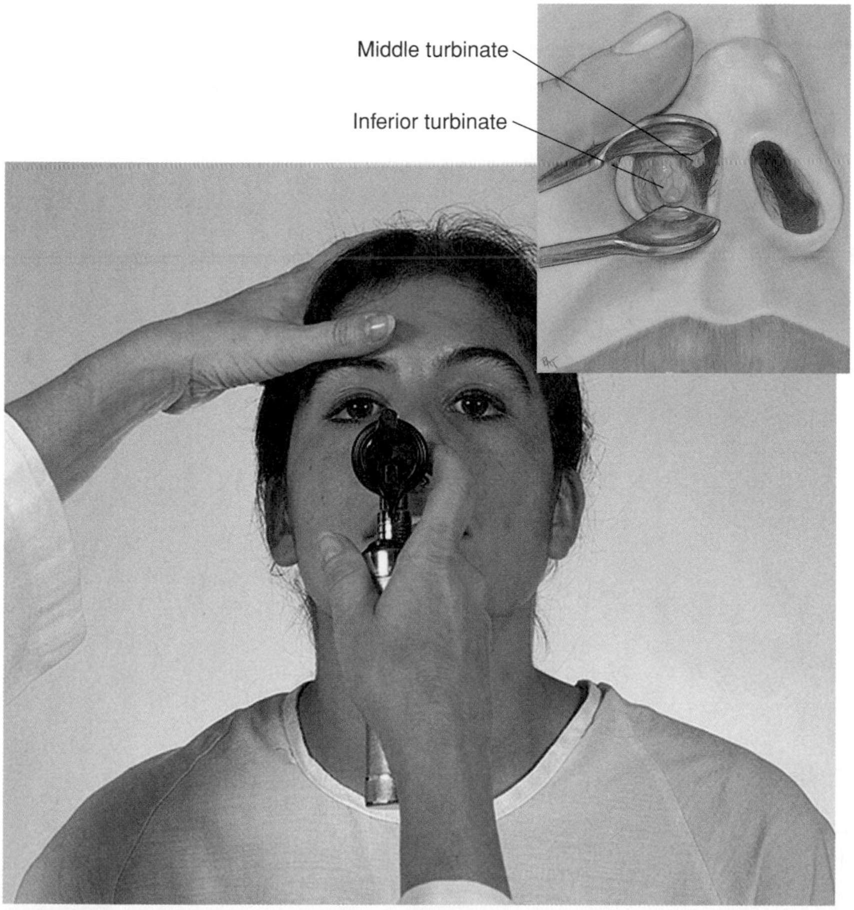

Abnormal Findings

Absence of sniff indicates obstruction (e.g., common cold, nasal polyps, rhinitis).

Rhinitis—nasal mucosa is swollen and bright red with an upper respiratory infection.

Discharge is common with rhinitis and sinusitis, varying from watery and copious to thick, purulent, and green-yellow.

With chronic allergy, mucosa looks swollen, boggy, pale, and grey.

Middle turbinate
Inferior turbinate

Fig. 16-8

Objective Data

Objective Data

Normal Range of Findings	Abnormal Findings

Observe the nasal septum for deviation (Fig. 16-9). A deviated septum is common and is not significant unless air flow is obstructed. (If present in a hospitalized patient, document the deviated septum in the event that the person needs nasal suctioning or a nasogastric tube.) Also note any perforation or bleeding in the septum.

A deviated septum looks like a hump or shelf in one nasal cavity.

Perforation is seen as a spot of light from penlight shining in other naris and occurs with cocaine use.

Epistaxis commonly comes from anterior septum (Table 16-1 on p. 395).

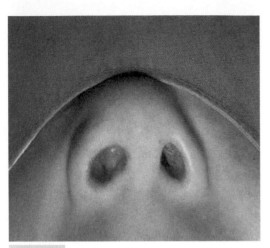

Fig. 16-9

Inspect the turbinates, the bony ridges curving down from the lateral walls. The superior turbinate will not be in your view, but the middle and inferior turbinates appear the same light red colour as the nasal mucosa. Note any swelling but do not try to push the speculum past it. Turbinates are quite vascular and tender if touched.

Note any polyps, benign growths that accompany chronic allergy, and distinguish them from the normal turbinates.

Polyps are smooth, pale grey, avascular, mobile, nontender (see Table 16-1, p. 395).

PALPATE THE SINUS AREAS

Using your thumbs, press over the frontal sinuses below the eyebrows (Fig. 16-10, A) and over the maxillary sinuses below the cheekbones (Fig. 16-10, B). Take care not to press directly on the eyeballs. The person should feel firm pressure but no pain.

Sinus areas are tender to palpation in persons with chronic allergies and acute infection (sinusitis).

A   B

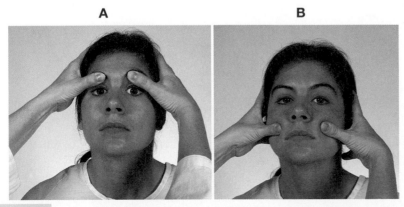

Fig. 16-10

Normal Range of Findings	Abnormal Findings

Transillumination

You may use this technique when you suspect sinus inflammation, although it is of limited usefulness. Darken the examining room. Affix a strong narrow light to the end of the otoscope and hold it deep under the superior orbital ridge against the location of the frontal sinus area (Fig. 16-11). Cover with your hand. A diffuse red glow is a normal response. It comes from the light shining through the air in the healthy sinus.

An inflamed sinus filled with fluid does not transilluminate.

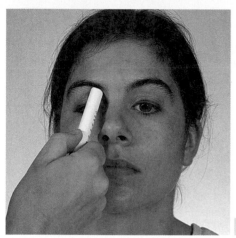

Fig. 16-11

You may use the same technique with the maxillary sinuses, providing the person has no upper denture that would impede the light. Ask the person to tilt the head back and open the mouth. Shine the light on each cheek just under the inner corner of the eye. Note a dull glow inside the mouth on the hard palate as the light transmits through the sinuses. Healthy sinuses contain air and may light up symmetrically. But be aware that asymmetry is not a reliable sign of sinus inflammation because many healthy sinuses normally will not transilluminate.

A significant finding is one sinus illuminated and the other clouded. If one has fluid, it looks darker than the healthy one.

INSPECT THE MOUTH

Begin with anterior structures and move posteriorly. Use a tongue blade to retract structures and a bright light for optimal visualization.

Lips

Inspect the lips for colour, moisture, cracking, or lesions. Retract the lips and note their inner surface as well (Fig. 16-12). Individuals with darker complexions may normally have bluish lips and a dark line on the gingival margin.

In light-skinned people: circumoral pallor occurs with shock and anemia; cyanosis with hypoxemia and chilling; cherry red lips with carbon monoxide poisoning, acidosis from aspirin poisoning, or ketoacidosis.

Cheilitis (perlèche)—cracking at the corners.

Herpes simplex, other lesions (see Table 16-2, p. 397).

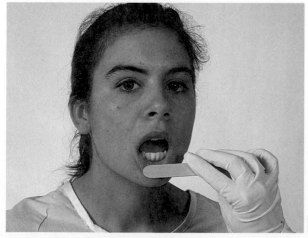

Fig. 16-12

Normal Range of Findings	Abnormal Findings

Objective Data

Teeth and Gums

The condition of the teeth is an index of the person's general health. Your examination should not replace the regular dental examination, but you should note any diseased, absent, loose, or abnormally positioned teeth. The teeth normally look white, straight, and evenly spaced, and clean and free of debris or decay.

Compare the number of teeth with the number expected for the person's age. Ask the person to bite as if chewing something and note alignment of upper and lower jaw. Normal occlusion in the back is the upper teeth resting directly on the lowers; in the front, the upper incisors slightly override the lower incisors.

Normally, the gums look pink or coral with a stippled (dotted) surface. The gum margins at the teeth are tight and well defined. Check for swelling; retraction of gingival margins; and spongy, bleeding, or discolored gums. Individuals with darker complexions may normally have a dark melanotic line along the gingival margin.

Discolored teeth appear brown with excessive fluoride use, yellow with tobacco use.

Grinding down of tooth surface.

Plaque—soft debris.

Caries—decay.

Malocclusion (poor biting relationship), protrusion of upper or lower incisors (Table 16-3, p. 398).

Gingival hyperplasia (see Table 16-3, p. 398), crevices between teeth and gums, pockets of debris.

Gums bleed with slight pressure, indicating gingivitis.

Dark line on gingival margins occurs with lead and bismuth poisoning.

Tongue

Check the tongue for colour, surface characteristics, and moisture. The colour is pink and even. The dorsal surface is normally roughened from the papillae. A thin white coating may be present. Ask the person to touch the tongue to the roof of the mouth. Its ventral surface looks smooth, glistening, and shows veins. Saliva is present.

Beefy red swollen tongue. Smooth glossy areas (Table 16-5, p. 401).

Enlarged tongue occurs with intellectual disability, hypothyroidism, acromegaly; a small tongue accompanies malnutrition.

Dry mouth occurs with dehydration, fever; tongue has deep vertical fissures.

Saliva is decreased while the person is taking anticholinergic and other medications.

Excess saliva and drooling occur with gingivostomatitis and neurological dysfunction.

With a glove,* hold the tongue with a cotton gauze pad for traction and swing the tongue out and to each side (Fig. 16-13). Inspect for any white patches or lesions—normally none are present. If any occur, palpate these lesions for induration.

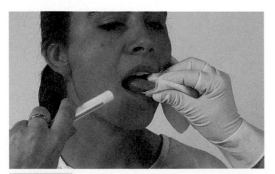

Fig. 16-13

*Always wear gloves to examine mucous membranes. This follows Routine Practices to prevent the spread of possible communicable disease.

Normal Range of Findings	Abnormal Findings

Normal Range of Findings

Inspect carefully the entire U-shaped area under the tongue behind the teeth. Oral malignancies are most likely to develop here. Note any white patches, nodules, or ulcerations. If lesions are present, or with any person over 50 years old or with a positive history of smoking or alcohol use, use your gloved hand to palpate the area. Place your other hand under the jaw to stabilize the tissue and to "capture" any abnormality (Fig. 16-14). Note any induration.

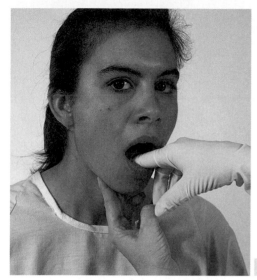

Fig. 16-14

Buccal Mucosa

Hold the cheek open with a wooden tongue blade, and check the buccal mucosa for colour, nodules, or lesions. It looks pink, smooth, and moist, although patchy hyperpigmentation is common and normal in dark-skinned people.

An expected finding is **Stensen's duct,** the opening of the parotid salivary gland. It looks like a small dimple opposite the upper second molar. You also may see a raised occlusion line on the buccal mucosa parallel with the level the teeth meet. This is caused by the teeth closing against the cheek.

A larger patch also may be present along the buccal mucosa. This is **leuko-edema,** a benign greyish opaque area, more common in people of African or South Asian descent. When it is mild, the patch disappears as you stretch the cheeks. The severity of the condition increases with age, looking greyish white and thickened. The cause of the condition is unknown. Do not mistake leuko-edema for oral infections such as candidiasis (thrush).

Fordyce's granules are small, isolated white or yellow papules on the mucosa of cheek, tongue, and lips (Fig. 16-15). These little sebaceous cysts are painless and not significant.

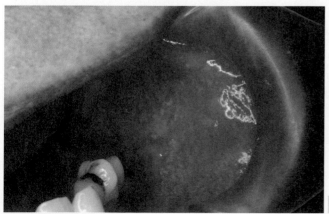

Fig. 16-15

Abnormal Findings

Any lesion or ulcer persisting for more than 2 weeks must be investigated.

An indurated area may be a mass or lymphadenopathy, and it must be investigated.

Dappled brown patches are present with Addison's disease (chronic adrenal insufficiency).

Orifice of Stensen's duct looks red with mumps.

Koplik's spots—early prodromal (early warning) sign of measles.

The chalky white raised patch of **leukoplakia** is abnormal (Table 16-4, p. 400).

Objective Data

Normal Range of Findings	Abnormal Findings

Palate

Shine your light up to the roof of the mouth. The more anterior hard palate is white with irregular transverse rugae. The posterior soft palate is pinker, smooth, and upwardly movable. A normal variation is a nodular bony ridge down the middle of the hard palate, a **torus palatinus** (Fig. 16-16). This benign growth arises after puberty and is a more common finding in Aboriginal people and people of African or Asian descent. In Figure 16-16 a mirror is used to reflect the image of the torus palatinus, which lies in the roof of the mouth.

The hard palate appears yellow with jaundice. In dark-skinned people with jaundice, it may look yellow, muddy yellow, or green-brown.

Oral Kaposi's sarcoma is the most common early lesion in people with acquired immune deficiency syndrome (AIDS) (Table 16-6, p. 403).

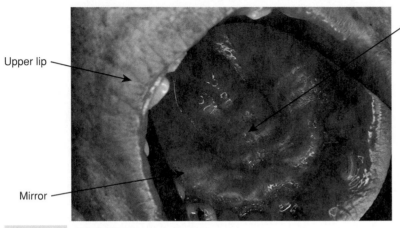

Upper lip

Torus in upper hard palate

Mirror

Fig. 16-16   Torus palatinus (viewed with a mirror).

Observe the uvula; it normally looks like a fleshy pendant hanging in the midline (Fig. 16-17). Ask the person to say "ahhh" and note the soft palate and uvula rise in the midline. This tests one function of cranial nerve X, the vagus nerve.

A *bifid* uvula looks like it is split in two; more common in Aboriginal people (see Table 16-6, p. 403).

Any deviation to the side or absent movement indicates nerve damage, which also occurs with poliomyelitis and diphtheria.

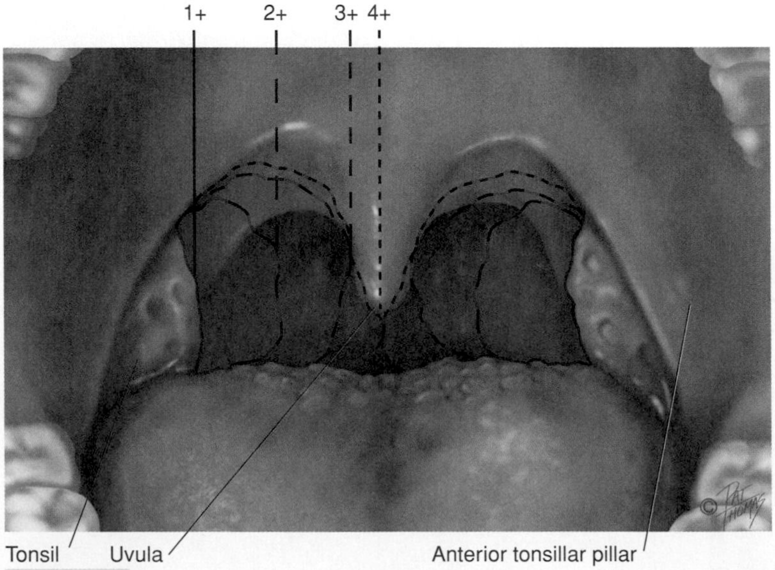

1+   2+   3+ 4+

Tonsil   Uvula   Anterior tonsillar pillar

Fig. 16-17   © Pat Thomas, 2006.

Normal Range of Findings	Abnormal Findings

INSPECT THE THROAT

With your light, observe the oval, rough-surfaced **tonsils** behind the anterior tonsillar pillar (see Fig. 16-17). Their colour is the same pink as the oral mucosa, and their surface is peppered with indentations, or crypts. In some people the crypts collect small plugs of whitish cellular debris. This does not indicate infection. However, there should be no exudate on the tonsils. Tonsils are graded in size as follows:

1+ Visible
2+ Halfway between tonsillar pillars and uvula
3+ Touching the uvula
4+ Touching each other

You may normally see 1+ or 2+ tonsils in healthy people, especially in children, because lymphoid tissue is proportionately enlarged until puberty.

Enlarge your view of the posterior pharyngeal wall by depressing the tongue with a tongue blade (Fig. 16-18). Push down halfway back on the tongue; if you push on its tip, the tongue will hump up in back. Press slightly off-centre to avoid eliciting the gag reflex. You can help the person whose gag reflex is easily triggered by offering a tongue blade to depress his or her own tongue. (Some people can lower their own tongue so the tongue blade is not needed.) Scan the posterior wall for colour, exudate, or lesions. When finished, discard the tongue blade.

With an acute infection, tonsils are bright red, swollen, and may have exudate or large white spots.

A white membrane covering the tonsils may accompany infectious mononucleosis, leukemia, and diphtheria.

Tonsils are enlarged to 2+, 3+, or 4+ with an acute infection.

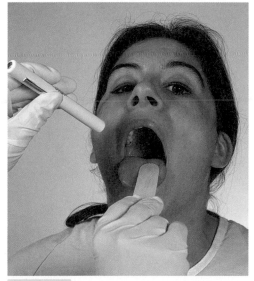

Fig. 16-18

Although usually it is not done in the screening examination, touching the posterior wall with the tongue blade elicits the gag reflex. This tests cranial nerves IX and X, the glossopharyngeal and vagus.

Objective Data

Normal Range of Findings

Test cranial nerve XII, the hypoglossal nerve, by asking the person to stick out the tongue. It should protrude in the midline. Children enjoy this request! Note any tremor, loss of movement, or deviation to the side.

During the examination, notice any breath odour, *halitosis.* This is common and usually is due to a local cause, such as poor oral hygiene, consumption of odoriferous foods, alcohol consumption, heavy smoking, or dental infection. Occasionally it may indicate a systemic disease.

 ## DEVELOPMENTAL CARE

Infants and Children

Because the oral examination is intrusive for the infant or young child, the timing is best toward the end of the complete examination, along with the ear examination. But if any crying episodes occur earlier, seize the opportunity to examine the open mouth and oropharynx.

As with the ear examination, let the parent help position the child. Place the infant supine on the examining table, with the arms restrained (Fig. 16-19). The older infant and toddler may be held on the parent's lap with one of the parent's

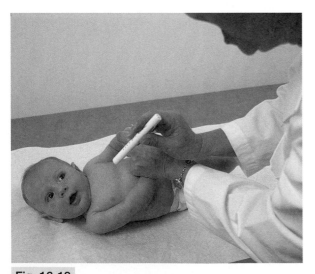

Fig. 16-19

Abnormal Findings

With cranial nerve XII damage, the tongue deviates *toward* the paralyzed side.

A fine tremor of the tongue occurs with hyperthyroidism, a coarse tremor with cerebral palsy and alcoholism.

Diabetic ketoacidosis produces a sweet, fruity breath odour; this acetone smell also occurs in children with malnutrition or dehydration. Others are an ammonia breath odour with uremia; a musty odour with liver disease; a foul, fetid odour with dental or respiratory infections; alcohol odour with alcohol ingestion or chemicals; a mouse-like smell of the breath with diphtheria.

Normal Range of Findings	Abnormal Findings

hands holding the arms down and the other hand securing the child's head against the parent's chest. Although not often needed, the parent's leg can reach over and capture the child's legs between the parent's own (Fig. 16-20).

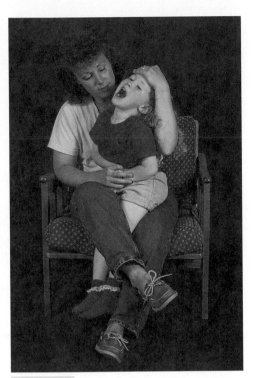

Fig. 16-20

Use a game to help prepare the young child. Encourage the preschool child to use a tongue blade to look into a puppet's mouth. Or place a mirror so that the child can look into the mouth while you do. The school-age child is usually co-operative and loves to show off missing or new teeth (Fig. 16-21).

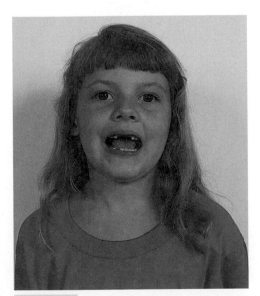

Fig. 16-21

Objective Data

Normal Range of Findings	**Abnormal Findings**

Be discriminating in your use of the tongue blade. It may be necessary for a full view of oral structures, but it produces a strong gag reflex in the infant. You may avoid the tongue blade completely with a co-operative preschooler and school-age child. Try asking the young child to open the mouth "as big as a lion" and to move the tongue in different directions. To enlarge your view of the oropharynx, ask the child to stick out the tongue and "pant like a dog."

At some point, you will encounter an unco-operative young child who clenches the teeth and refuses to open the mouth. If all your other efforts have failed, slide the tongue blade along the buccal mucosa and turn it between the back teeth. Push down to depress the tongue. This stimulates the gag reflex, and the child opens the mouth wide for a few seconds. You will have a *brief* look at the throat. Make the most of it.

Nose. The newborn may have milia across the nose. The nasal bridge may be flat in Aboriginal children and children of Asian or African descent. There should be no nasal flaring or narrowing with breathing.

> Nasal flaring in the infant indicates respiratory distress.
>
> A transverse ridge across the nose occurs in a child with chronic allergy from wiping the nose upward with palm (see Table 13-3 on p. 293). Nasal narrowing on inhalation is seen with chronic nasal obstruction and mouth breathing.
>
> Inability to pass catheter through nasal cavity indicates choanal atresia, which needs immediate intervention (see Table 16-1 on p. 395).

It is essential to determine the patency of the nares in the immediate newborn period because most newborns are obligate nose breathers. Nares blocked with amniotic fluid are suctioned gently with a bulb syringe. If obstruction is suspected, a small-lumen (5 to 10 Fr) catheter is passed down each naris to confirm patency.

Avoid the nasal speculum when examining the infant and young child. Instead, gently push up the tip of the nose with your thumb while using your other hand to shine the light into the naris. With a toddler, be alert for the possibility of a foreign body lodged in the nasal cavity (see Table 16-1).

Only in children older than 8 years do you need to palpate the child's sinus areas. In younger children, sinus areas are too small for palpation.

Mouth and Throat. A normal finding in infants is the **sucking tubercle**, a small pad in the middle of the upper lip from friction of breast- or bottle-feeding. Note the number of teeth and whether it is appropriate for the child's age. Also note pattern of eruption, position, condition, and hygiene. Use this guide for children under 2 years old; the child's age in months minus the number 6 should equal the expected number of deciduous teeth. Normally, all 20 deciduous teeth are in by 2½ years. Saliva is present after 3 months of age and shows in excess with teething children.

> No teeth by age 1 year.
>
> Discolored teeth appear yellow or yellow-brown with infants taking tetracycline or whose mothers took the drug during the last trimester; appear green or black with excessive iron ingestion, although this reverses when the iron is stopped. White specks may indicate a child getting too much fluoride (fluorosis). A cosmetic condition, it is not health threatening.
>
> Malocclusion: upper or lower dental arch is out of alignment.
>
> Ankyloglossia, a short lingual frenulum, can limit tongue protrusion and impair speech development (see Table 16-5, p. 401).
>
> Trauma may indicate child abuse from forced feeding of bottle or spoon.
>
> A high-arched palate is usually normal in the newborn, but a very narrow or high arch also occurs with Turner's syndrome, Ehlers-Danlos syndrome, Marfan syndrome, and Treacher Collins syndrome, or develops in the mouth-breather in chronic allergies.

Mobility should allow the tongue to extend at least as far as the alveolar ridge.

Note any bruising or laceration on the buccal mucosa or gums of the infant or young child.

On the palate, **Epstein pearls** are a normal finding in newborns and infants (Fig. 16-22). They are small, whitish, glistening, pearly papules along the median raphe of the hard palate and on the gums, where they look like teeth. They are small retention cysts and disappear in the first few weeks.

Normal Range of Findings	Abnormal Findings

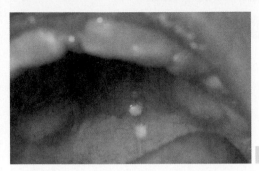

Fig. 16-22   Epstein pearls.

Bednar aphthae are traumatic areas or ulcers on the posterior hard palate on either side of the midline. They result from abrasions while sucking.

The tonsils are not visible in the newborn. They gradually enlarge during childhood, remaining proportionately larger until puberty. Tonsils appear still larger if the infant is crying or gagging. Normally the newborn can produce a strong, lusty cry.

Insert your gloved finger into the baby's mouth and palpate the hard and soft palates as the baby sucks. The sucking reflex can be elicited in infants up to 12 months old.

The Pregnant Female

Gum hypertrophy (surface looks smooth and stippling disappears) may occur normally at puberty or during pregnancy (pregnancy gingivitis).

The Aging Adult

The nose may appear more prominent on the face from a loss of subcutaneous fat. In the edentulous person the mouth and lips fold in, giving a "purse-string" appearance. The teeth may look slightly yellowed, although the colour is uniform. Yellowing results from the dentin visible through worn enamel. The surface of the incisors may show vertical cracks from a lifetime of exposure to extreme temperatures. The teeth may look longer as the gum margins recede.

The surfaces look worn down or abraded. Old dental work deteriorates, especially at the gum margins. The teeth loosen with bone resorption and may move with palpation.

The tongue looks smoother as a result of papillary atrophy. The older adult's buccal mucosa is thinned and may look shinier, as though it were "varnished."

Objective Data

Summary Checklist: Nose, Mouth, and Throat Examination

   For a PDA-downloadable version, go to http://evolve.elsevier.com/Canada/Jarvis/examination/.

Nose
1. **Inspect nose for**
   Symmetry, deformity, or lesions
2. **Palpation**
   Test patency of each nostril
3. **Inspect with nasal speculum**
   Nasal mucosa—note colour and integrity
   Septum—deviation, perforation, or bleeding

Turbinates—colour, exudates, swelling, or polyps
4. **Palpate the sinus areas**
   Note any tenderness

Mouth and Throat
1. **Inspect with penlight**
   Lips, teeth, and gums—note colour, whether structures are intact, any lesions

Palate and uvula—note integrity and mobility as person phonates
Grade tonsils
Pharyngeal wall—note colour, any exudates, or lesions
2. **Palpation**
   When indicated in adults, bimanual palpation of mouth
   With the neonate, palpate for integrity of the palate and to assess sucking reflex

Objective Data

Promoting Health: Smokeless Tobacco and Cancer Risk

Smokeless (Tobacco) Does Not Mean Harmless!

Smokeless tobacco (SLT) carries significant health risks and should not be viewed as a safe substitute for smoking. SLT, like cigarettes, contains nicotine and can lead to nicotine addiction and dependence.

Two types of SLT are commonly used in Canada. The first type, chewing tobacco, comes in loose leaf, plug, and twist forms, and as the name implies, it is chewed. The leaves are air cured, shredded into flakes, and treated with sweet flavouring solutions. Snuff, the second type, is finely ground tobacco that is either dry or moist. Dry snuff is inhaled through the nose. Moist snuff, sold in small, proportioned, tea bag pouches, is taken orally. It is popular because the tobacco stays in one place and generates less saliva. Most users of chewing tobacco and moist snuff place the product between their gingival and buccal mucosa, suck on the tobacco, and spit out the juices. In addition, a Scandinavian-style SLT called snus is now available in Canada. Similar to chewing tobacco and moist snuff, it is less noticeable because it does not need to be spat out.

Over 3000 chemicals, including 28 carcinogens, have been identified in SLT. Holding one pinch of SLT in your mouth for 30 minutes typically delivers as much nicotine as three cigarettes. Consequently, the health consequences of nicotine from smoking are also found in SLT users. Nicotine may play a role in the pathogenesis of diseases, including coronary artery and peripheral vascular diseases, hypertension, peptic ulcer disease, and fetal mortality and morbidity.

The use of SLT has also been associated with an even greater risk of oral cancer than smoking. Early signs of oral cancer include:

- An ulcer or sore that does not heal
- White or red patches
- A prolonged sore throat or feeling that something is in the throat

- Difficulty chewing
- Unexplained bleeding
- Numbness or tingling
- Restricted movement of the tongue or jaw
- A small lump or thickening in the lip, tongue, floor or roof, cheeks, gums, tonsil

Pain is rarely an early symptom of oral cancer, which is why a thorough examination of the mouth is important. There may also be an increased risk of cancers of the pharynx, larynx, esophagus, stomach, and pancreas. Besides oral cancer, SLT use is associated with other oral effects. Because tobacco has an unpleasant taste, many brands are heavily sweetened with sugars. This concentrated sugar is then held in the mouth next to the teeth, promoting tooth decay. Other oral health effects of SLT use include leukoplakia, periodontal disease, dental caries, and delayed wound healing. In addition, tobacco leaves contain gritty materials that wear down the surfaces of teeth, exacerbating the problem. Further, the gritty materials scratch the soft tissues in the mouth, allowing the nicotine and other chemicals to enter directly into the bloodstream. The flavouring salts found in SLT also contribute to abnormal blood pressure and kidney disease.

SLT use is higher among Aboriginal people, athletes (primarily baseball players), men, and individuals living in rural areas. In 2005, 9% of Canadian youth aged 15 to 24 reported having used SLT, compared with 25% of adults aged 25 or over. Adolescents who use SLT are more likely to become cigarette smokers. Across Canada 13% of males, compared with 2% of females, have reported using SLT. SLT is used more often in the Prairie provinces.

SLT is not a healthy alternative to smoking, nor should it be encouraged for smokers who find themselves in smoke-free zones. As with smoking, it is never too late to quit and best never to start.

❧— DOCUMENTATION AND CRITICAL THINKING —❧

Sample Charting

SUBJECTIVE

Nose: No history of discharge, sinus problems, obstruction, epistaxis, or allergy. Colds one to two per year, mild. Fractured nose during high-school sports, treated by MD.

Mouth and Throat: No pain, lesions, bleeding gums, toothache, dysphagia, or hoarseness. Occasional sore throat with colds. Tonsillectomy, age 8. Smokes cigarettes 1 PPD X 9 years. Alcohol—one to two drinks socially, about 2 X/month. Visits dentist annually, dental hygienist 2 X/year, flosses daily. No dental appliance.

OBJECTIVE

Nose: Symmetrical, no deformity or skin lesions. Nares patent. Mucosa pink, no discharge, lesions, or polyps; no septal deviation or perforation. Sinuses—no tenderness to palpation.

Mouth: Can clench teeth. Mucosa and gingivae pink, no masses or lesions. Teeth are all present, straight, and in good repair. Tongue smooth, pink, no lesions, protrudes in midline, no tremor.

Throat: Mucosa pink, no lesions or exudate. Uvula rises in midline on phonation. Tonsils out. Gag reflex present.

ASSESSMENT

Structures intact and appear healthy

Focused Assessment: Clinical Case Study 1

Brad D., a 34-year-old electrician, seeks care for "sore throat for 2 days."

SUBJECTIVE

- 2 days PTA experienced sudden onset of sore throat, swollen glands, fever 38.3°C, occasional shaking chills, extreme fatigue.
- Today—symptoms remain. Cough productive of yellow sputum. Treated self with aspirin for minimal relief. Unable to eat last 2 days because "throat on fire." Taking adequate fluids, on bed rest. Not aware of exposure to other sick persons. Does not smoke.

OBJECTIVE

Ears: Tympanic membranes pearl grey with landmarks intact.

Nose: No discharge. Mucosa pink, no swelling.

Mouth: Mucosa and gingivae pink, no lesions.

Throat: Tonsils 3+. Pharyngeal wall bright red with yellow-white exudate, exudate also on tonsils.

Neck: Enlarged anterior cervical nodes bilaterally, painful to palpation. No other lymph adenopathy.

Chest: Resonant to percussion throughout. Breath sounds clear anterior and posterior. No adventitious sounds.

ASSESSMENT

Pharyngitis
Pain R/T inflammation
Imbalanced nutrition: less than body requirements R/T dysphagia

Continued

Focused Assessment: Clinical Case Study 2

Calvin W., a 53-year-old male, is in the hospital awaiting coronary bypass surgery for coronary artery disease. He is allergic to dust and animal hair. As part of a preoperative teaching plan for coughing and deep breathing, a respiratory assessment is performed.

SUBJECTIVE

* States understanding of reason for admission to hospital and extent of coronary artery disease. Unaware of details of surgical procedure and postoperative care. Interested: "I do better when I know what I'm dealing with." History of exertional angina after walking one short block or climbing one flight of stairs, treats self with nitroglycerine. Does not smoke. Chronic watery nasal discharge, "comes and goes, but present most of the time."

OBJECTIVE

Nose: Only R naris patent. Mucosa grey and boggy bilaterally. L naris has mobile, grey, nontender mass, obstructing view of turbinates and rest of nasal cavity.

Mouth and Throat: Mucosa pink, no lesions. Uvula midline, rises on phonation. Tonsils absent. No lumps or lesions on palpation.

Chest: Thorax symmetrical, AP < transverse diameter, respirations 18/min, effortless. Resonant to percussion. Breath sounds are clear. No adventitious sounds.

ASSESSMENT

L nasal mass, possibly polyp

Deficient knowledge for surgery and expected postoperative course R/T lack of exposure

Focused Assessment: Clinical Case Study 3

Esther V. is a 61-year-old professor who has been admitted to the hospital for chemotherapy for carcinoma of the breast. This is her fifth day in the hospital. An oral assessment is performed when she complains of "soreness and a white coating" in the mouth.

SUBJECTIVE

* Felt soreness on tongue and cheeks during night. Now pain persists, and E.V. can see a "white coating" on tongue and cheeks. "I'm worried. Is this more cancer?"

OBJECTIVE

E.V. generally appears restless and overly aware.

Oral mucosa pink. Large white, cheesy patches covering most of dorsal surface of tongue and buccal mucosa. Will scrape off with tongue blade, revealing red eroded area beneath.

Bleeds with slight contact. Posterior pharyngeal wall pink, no lesions. Patches are soft to palpation. No palpable lymph nodes.

ASSESSMENT

Oral lesion, appears as candidiasis

Impaired oral mucous membrane R/T effects of chemotherapy

Pain R/T infectious process

Anxiety R/T threat to health status

Nursing Diagnoses Commonly Associated With Nose, Mouth, and Throat Disorders

All nursing diagnoses can be found on the Evolve Web site at **http://evolve.elsevier.com/Canada/Jarvis/examination**.

Documentation and Critical Thinking

ABNORMAL FINDINGS

| TABLE 16-1 | **Abnormalities of the Nose** |

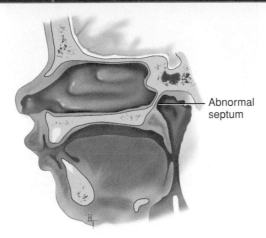

Abnormal septum

Choanal Atresia

A bony or membranous septum between the nasal cavity and the pharynx of the newborn. When the condition is bilateral, it requires the immediate insertion of an oral airway to prevent asphyxia because most newborns are obligate nose breathers. When the condition is unilateral, the infant may be asymptomatic until the onset of the first respiratory infection.

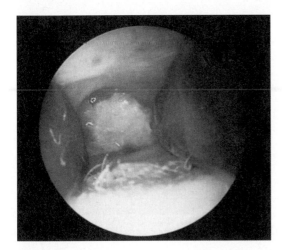

Foreign Body

Children particularly are apt to put an object up the nose (here, yellow plastic foam), producing unilateral mucopurulent drainage and foul odour. Because some risk for aspiration exists, removal should be prompt.

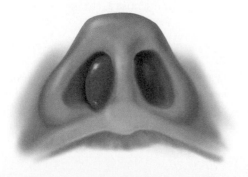

Epistaxis

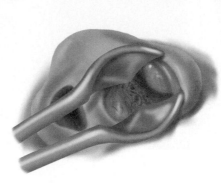

The most common site of a nosebleed is Kiesselbach's plexus in the anterior septum. It may be spontaneous from a local cause, or a sign of underlying illness. Causes include nose picking, forceful coughing or sneezing, fracture, foreign body, rhinitis, heavy exertion, or a coagulation disorder. Bleeding from the anterior septum is easily controlled and rarely severe. A posterior hemorrhage is less common (<10%) but is more profuse, harder to manage, and more serious.

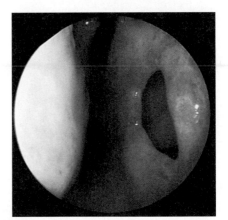

Perforated Septum

A hole in the septum, usually in the cartilaginous part, may be caused by snorting cocaine, chronic infection, trauma from continual picking of crusts, or nasal surgery. It is seen directly, or as a spot of light when the penlight is directed into the other naris.

◀ **Furuncle**

A small boil located in the skin or mucous membrane; appears red and swollen, and is quite painful. Avoid any manipulation or trauma that may spread the infection.

Continued

TABLE 16-1   Abnormalities of the Nose—cont'd

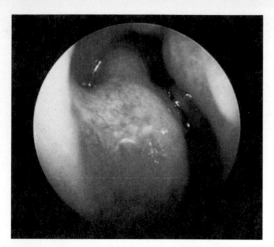

Acute Rhinitis

The first sign is a clear, watery discharge, rhinorrhea, which later becomes purulent. This is accompanied by sneezing and swollen mucosa, which causes nasal obstruction. Turbinates are dark red and swollen.

Reprinted from Fireman, P. (1995). Atlas of allergies, (2nd ed.), Mosby, by permission of the publisher.

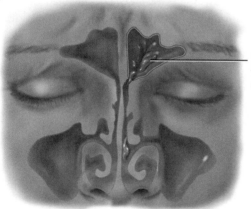

Infected frontal sinus

Sinusitis

Facial pain, after upper respiratory infection; signs include red swollen nasal mucosa, swollen turbinates, and purulent discharge. Person also has fever, chills, malaise. With maxillary sinusitis, dull throbbing pain occurs in cheeks and teeth on the same side, and pain with palpation is present. With frontal sinusitis, pain is above the supraorbital ridge.

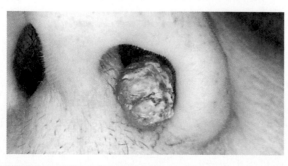

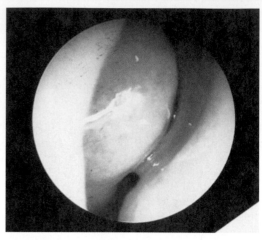

Allergic Rhinitis

Rhinorrhea, itching of nose and eyes, lacrimation, nasal congestion, and sneezing are present. Note serous edema and swelling of turbinates to fill the air space. Turbinates are usually pale (although may appear violet), and their surface looks smooth and glistening. May be seasonal or perennial, depending on allergen. Individual often has a strong family history of seasonal allergies.

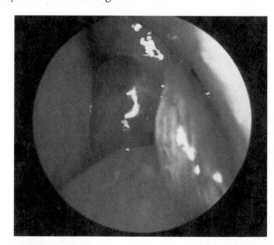

Nasal Polyps

Smooth, pale grey nodules, which are overgrowths of mucosa, most commonly caused by chronic allergic rhinitis. May be stalked. A common site is protrusion from the middle meatus. Often multiple, they are mobile and nontender in contrast to turbinates. They may obstruct air passageways as they get larger. Symptoms include the absence of a sense of smell and a "valve that moves" in the nose as the person breathes.

◀ **Carcinoma**

This appears grey-white and nontender. It may produce slow bloody unilateral discharge, in contrast to the profuse bleeding that accompanies epistaxis. It is not a common lesion.

TABLE 16-2 | **Abnormalities of the Lips**

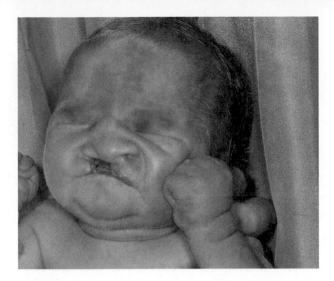

Cleft Lip

Maxillofacial clefts are the most common congenital deformities of the head and neck. The incidence varies widely among ethnocultural groups, with a higher frequency among Aboriginal people than among people of European descent. Although reliable birth registry is not present in all countries, birth records do show a relatively high incidence in Scandinavia and middle European countries (e.g., 1 in 550 in Denmark and Finland, 1 in 575 in Poland and the former Czechoslovakia [Bluestone, Stool, and Kenna, 1996]). Early treatment preserves the functions of speech and language formation and deglutition (swallowing).

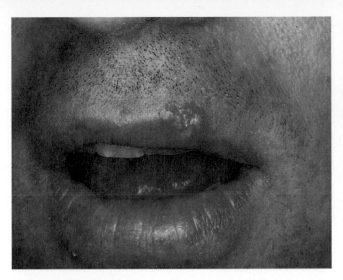

Herpes Simplex 1

"Cold sores" are groups of clear vesicles with a surrounding indurated erythematous base. These evolve into pustules, which rupture, weep, crust, and heal in 4 to 10 days. The most likely site is the lip–skin junction; infection often recurs in same site. Caused by the herpes simplex virus (HSV-1), the lesion is highly contagious and is spread by direct contact. Recurrent herpes infections may be precipitated by sunlight, fever, colds, allergy. It is a very common lesion, affecting 50% of adults.

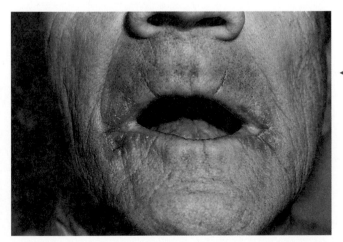

◄ Angular Cheilitis (Stomatitis, Perlèche)

Erythema, scaling, and shallow, and painful fissures at the corners of the mouth occur with excess salivation and *Candida* infection. Cheilitis is often seen in edentulous persons and in those with poorly fitting dentures causing folding in of corners of the mouth, creating a warm, moist environment favouring the growth of yeast.

Continued

TABLE 16-2	**Abnormalities of the Lips—cont'd**

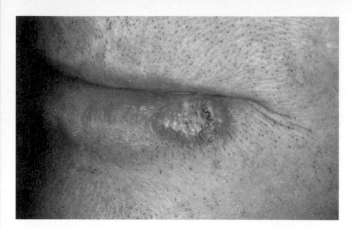

Carcinoma

The initial lesion is round and indurated, and then it becomes crusted and ulcerated with an elevated border. The majority occur between the outer and middle thirds of the lip. Any lesion that is still unhealed after 2 weeks should be referred.

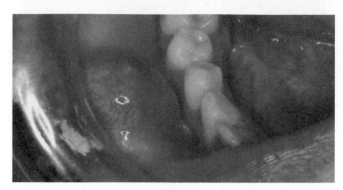

Retention "Cyst" (Mucocele)

A round, well-defined translucent nodule that may be very small or up to 1 or 2 cm. It is a pocket of mucus that forms when a duct of a minor salivary gland ruptures. The benign lesion also may occur on the buccal mucosa, on the floor of the mouth, or under the tip of the tongue.

ABNORMAL FINDINGS
FOR ADVANCED PRACTICE

TABLE 16-3	**Abnormalities of the Teeth and Gums**

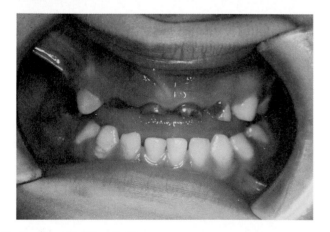

Baby Bottle Tooth Decay

Destruction of numerous deciduous teeth may occur in older infants and toddlers who take a bottle of milk, juice, or sweetened drink to bed and prolong bottle-feeding past the age of 1 year. Liquid pools around the upper front teeth. Mouth bacteria act on carbohydrates in the liquid, especially sucrose, forming metabolic acids. Acids break down tooth enamel and destroy its protein.

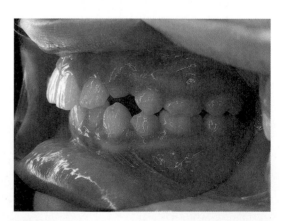

Malocclusion

Upper or lower dental arches are not in alignment and incisors protrude from developmental problem of mandible or maxilla, or incompatibility between jaw size and tooth size. The condition increases risk of facial deformity, negative body image, chewing problems, or speech dysfluency.

| TABLE 16-3 | Abnormalities of the Teeth and Gums—cont'd |

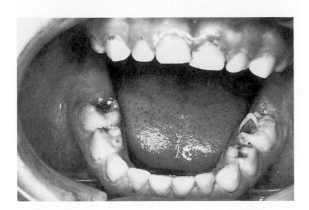

Dental Caries

Progressive destruction of tooth. Decay initially looks chalky white. Later, it turns brown or black and forms a cavity. Early decay is apparent only on X-ray. Susceptible sites are tooth surfaces where food debris, bacterial plaque, and saliva collect.

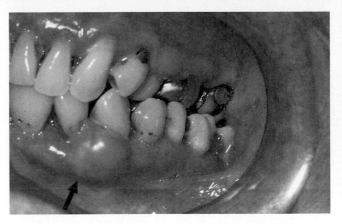

Epulis

A nontender, fibrous nodule of the gum, seen emerging between the teeth; an inflammatory response to injury or hemorrhage.

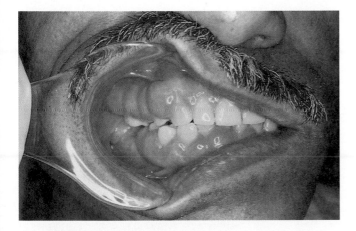

Gingival Hyperplasia

Painless enlargement of the gums, sometimes overreaching the teeth. This occurs with puberty, pregnancy, leukemia, and with long therapeutic use of phenytoin (Dilantin).

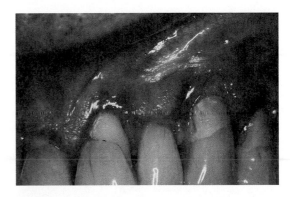

Gingivitis

Gum margins are red, swollen, and bleed easily. This case is severe; gingival tissue has desquamated, exposing roots of teeth. Inflammation is usually due to poor dental hygiene or vitamin C deficiency. The condition may occur in pregnancy and puberty because of changing hormonal balance.

◀ ### Meth Mouth

Illicit methamphetamine abuse (crystal meth, meth ice) leads to extensive dental caries, gingivitis, tooth cracking, and edentulism. Methamphetamine causes vasoconstriction and decreased saliva, and its use increases the urge to consume sugars and starches and to give up oral hygiene. Absence of the buffering saliva leads to increased acidity in the mouth, and the increased plaque encourages bacterial growth. These conditions and the presence of carbohydrates set up an oral environment prone to caries, cracking of enamel, and the damage seen here.

From Neville, B.W., et al. (2009). Oral and maxillofacial pathology, (3rd ed.). St. Louis, MO: Saunders. In press.

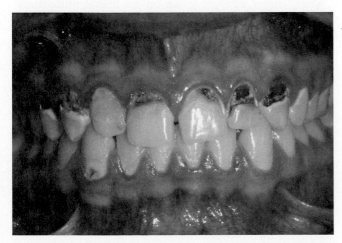

Abnormal Findings

TABLE 16-4   Abnormalities of the Buccal Mucosa

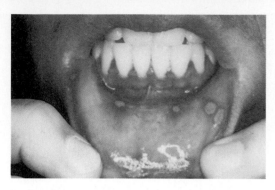

Aphthous Ulcers

A "canker sore" is a vesicle at first, then a small, round, "punched-out" ulcer with white base surrounded by a red halo. It is quite painful and lasts for 1 to 2 weeks. The cause is unknown, although it is associated with stress, fatigue, and food allergy. It is common, affecting 20 to 60% of the population.

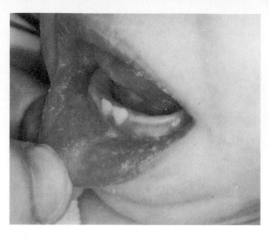

Koplik's Spots

Small blue-white spots with irregular red halo scattered over mucosa opposite the molars. An early sign, and pathognomonic, of measles.

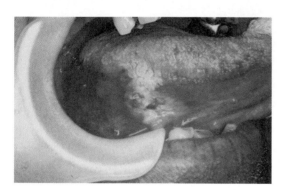

Leukoplakia

Chalky white, thick, raised patch with well-defined borders. The lesion is firmly attached and does not scrape off. It may occur on the lateral edges of tongue. It is due to chronic irritation, and occurs more frequently with heavy smoking and heavy alcohol use. Lesions are precancerous, and the person should be referred. (Here, the lesion is associated with squamous carcinoma.)

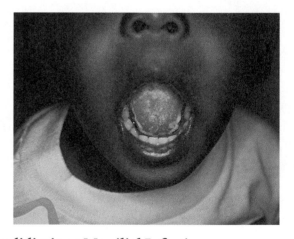

Candidiasis or Monilial Infection

A white, cheesy, curdlike patch on the buccal mucosa and tongue. It scrapes off, leaving raw, red surface that bleeds easily. Termed "thrush" in the newborn. It is an opportunistic infection that occurs after the use of antibiotics or corticosteroids, and in immunosuppressed persons.

TABLE 16-5	Abnormalities of the Tongue

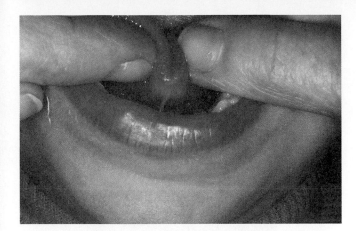

Ankyloglossia

Also known as tongue-tie. A short lingual frenulum, here fixing the tongue tip to the floor of the mouth and gums. This limits mobility and will affect speech (pronunciation of a, d, n) if the tongue tip cannot be elevated to the alveolar ridge. A congenital defect.

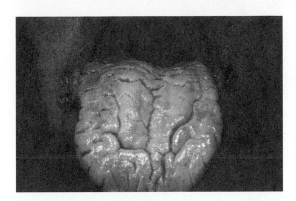

Fissured or Scrotal Tongue

Deep furrows divide the papillae into small irregular rows. The condition occurs in 5% of the general population and in Down syndrome. The incidence increases with age. (Vertical, or longitudinal, fissures also occur with dehydration because of reduced volume of the tongue.)

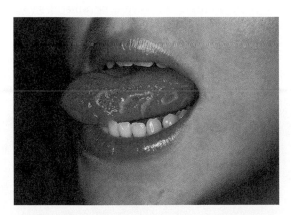

Geographic Tongue (Migratory Glossitis)

Pattern of normal coating interspersed with bright red, shiny, circular bald areas with raised pearly borders. Pattern resembles a map, and changes in a few days. Not significant, and its cause is not known.

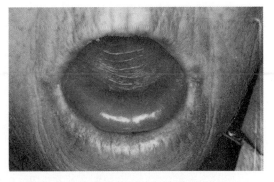

Smooth, Glossy Tongue (Atrophic Glossitis)

The surface is slick and shiny; the mucosa thins and looks red from decreased papillae. Accompanied by dryness of tongue and burning. Occurs with vitamin B_{12} deficiency (pernicious anemia), folic acid deficiency, and iron deficiency anemia. Here, also note angular cheilitis.

Continued

TABLE 16-5 | **Abnormalities of the Tongue—cont'd**

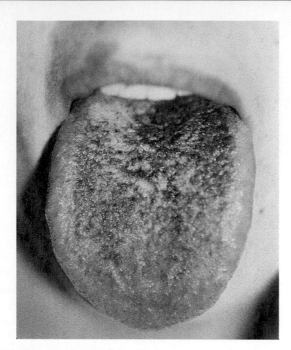

Black Hairy Tongue

This is not really hair but the elongation of filiform papillae and painless overgrowth of mycelial threads of fungus infection on the tongue. Colour varies from black-brown to yellow. It occurs after use of antibiotics, which inhibit normal bacteria and allow proliferation of fungus.

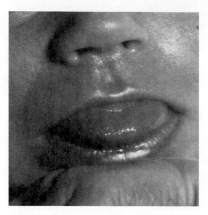

Enlarged Tongue (Macroglossia)

The tongue is enlarged and may protrude from the mouth. The condition is not painful but may impair speech development. Here, it occurs with Down syndrome; it also occurs with cretinism, myxedema, acromegaly. Also a transient swelling can occur with local infections.

Carcinoma   ▶

An ulcer with rolled edges; indurated. Occurs particularly at sides, base, and under the tongue. When it is in the floor of the mouth, it may cause painful movement or limited movement of the tongue. Risk of early metastasis is present because of rich lymphatic drainage. Heavy smoking and heavy alcohol use place persons at greater risk.

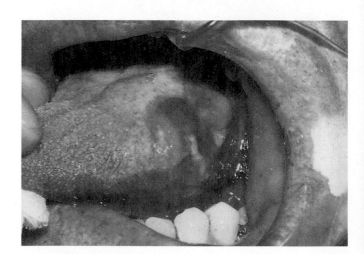

TABLE 16-6   Abnormalities of the Oropharynx

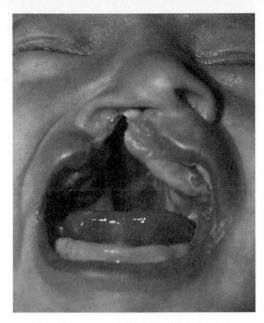

Cleft Palate

A congenital defect, the failure of fusion of the maxillary processes. Wide variation occurs in the extent of cleft formation, from upper lip only, palate only, uvula only, to cleft of the nostril and the hard and soft palates.

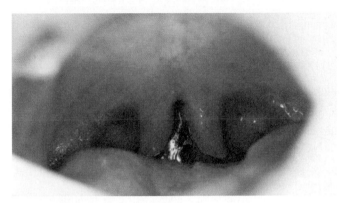

Bifid Uvula

The uvula looks partly severed. May indicate a submucous cleft palate, which feels like a notch at the junction of the hard and soft palates. The submucous cleft palate may affect speech development because it prevents necessary air trapping. The incidence of bifid uvula is higher among Aboriginal people.

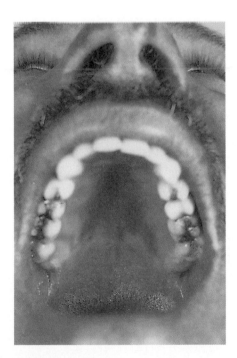

Oral Kaposi's Sarcoma

Bruiselike, dark red or violet, confluent macule, usually on the hard palate, may be on soft palate or gingival margin. Oral lesions may be among the earliest lesions to develop with AIDS.

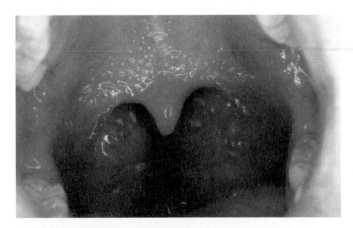

Acute Tonsillitis and Pharyngitis

Bright red throat; swollen tonsils; white or yellow exudate on tonsils and pharynx; swollen uvula; and enlarged, tender anterior cervical and tonsillar nodes. Accompanied by severe sore throat, painful swallowing, fever >38.3°C of sudden onset.

Caution: One cannot discriminate bacterial from viral infection on clinical data alone; all sore throats need a throat culture. Bacterial pharyngitis caused by group A β-hemolytic *Streptococcus,* if untreated, may lead to the complication of rheumatic fever. This is a serious complex illness characterized by fever, malaise, swollen joints, rash, and scarring on the heart valves.

BIBLIOGRAPHY

Adams, C. (2006). Poststroke complications and risk factors: Implications for primary care nurse practitioners. *Journal for Nurse Practitioners, 2*, 533–539, 546.

Alper, C., Myers, E. N., & Eibline, D. E. (2001). *Decision-making in ear, nose, and throat disorders*. Philadelphia, PA: W.B. Saunders.

Andreae, M. (2004). How to recognize and manage herpes simplex virus type 1 infections. *Contemporary Pediatrics, 21*, 41–60.

Armengol, C., Hendley, O., & Schlager, T. (2006). An office-based guide to diagnosing streptococcal pharyngitis. *Contemporary Pediatrics, 23*, 64–70.

Bernstein, J. (2006). Making the distinction between allergic rhinitis and nonallergic rhinitis. *Journal of Respiratory Diseases, 27*, 281.

Bluestone, C. D., Stool, S. E., Alper, C. M., Arjmand, E. M., Casselbrant, M. L., Dohar, J. E., et al. (2002). *Pediatric otolaryngology* (4th ed.). Philadelphia, PA: W.B. Saunders.

Brothwell, D. R., Carbonell, V. M., & Goose, D. H. (1963). Congenital absence of teeth in human populations. In D. R. Brothwell (Ed.), *Dental anthropology*. New York, NY: Pergamon Press.

Burgess, J. (2006). Painful oral lesions: What to look for, how to treat, part 1. *Consultant, 46*, 1497–1504.

Canadian Dental Association. (2005). Retrieved from http://www.cda-adc.ca

Curtis, E. K. (2006). Meth mouth: A review of methamphetamine use and its oral manifestations. *General Dentistry, 54*, 125–129.

Dahlin, C. (2004). Oral complications at the end of life. *American Journal of Nursing, 104*, 40–48.

Eccles, R. (2005). Understanding the symptoms of the common cold and influenza. *Lancet Infectious Disease, 5*, 718–725.

Edelstein, D. R. (1996). Aging of the normal nose in adults. *Laryngoscope, 106*(Suppl. 81), 1–25.

First Nations and Inuit Regional Longitudinal Health Survey. *RHS 1997: The pilot survey*. Retrieved June 5, 2008, from http://rhs-ers.ca/english/pilot-survey.asp

First Nations and Inuit Regional Longitudinal Health Survey. *RHS 2002/03: Phase 1*. Retrieved June 5, 2008, from http://rhs-ers.ca/english/phase1.asp

Gleason, M., et al. (2006). Childhood allergic rhinitis: Using clinical clues and optimizing management. *American Journal for Nurse Practitioners, 10*, 45–53.

Gupta, A., Hawrych, A., & Wilson, W. R. (2001). Cocaine-induced sinonasal destruction. *Otolaryngology—Head and Neck Surgery, 124*, 480.

Habel, A., Elhadi, N., Sommerlad, B., & Powell, J. (2006). Delayed detection of cleft palate: An audit of newborn examination. *Archives of Disease in Childhood, 91*, 238–240.

Harrison, R. L., & Davis, D. W. (1996). Dental malocclusion in native children of British Columbia, Canada. *Community Dentistry and Oral Epidemiology, 24*, 217–221.

Hayden, M. (2004). Rhinitis. *Nurse Practitioner, 29*, 27–39.

Health Canada. (2001). *Non-insured health benefits program: 1999–2000 annual report*. Ottawa, ON: Public Works and Government Services Canada.

Health Canada. (2005). *A statistical profile on the health of First Nations in Canada for the year 2000*. Ottawa, ON: Author.

Huang, S. (2006). Nasal allergy and sinus infection: The link and therapeutic implications. *Consultant, 46*, 1357–1365.

Kadish, H. (2005). Ear and nose foreign bodies. *Clinical Pediatrics, 44*, 665–670.

Kane, R. L., Ouslander, J. G., & Abrass, I. E. (2003). *Essentials of clinical geriatrics* (5th ed.). New York, NY: McGraw-Hill.

Lai, D. W., & Hui, N. T. A. (2007). Use of dental care by elderly Chinese immigrants in Canada. *American Association of Public Health Dentistry, 67*(1), 55–59.

Lash, A. A. (2001). Sjögren's syndrome: Pathogenesis, diagnosis, and treatment. *Nurse Practitioner, 26*, 50–58.

Laskin, D., Giglio, J. A., & Rippert, E. T. (2003). Differential diagnosis of tongue lesions. *Quintessence International, 34*, 331–342.

Locker, D. (2007). Disparities in oral health–related quality of life in a population of Canadian children. *Community Dentistry and Oral Epidemiology, 35*, 348–356.

Locker, D., Clarke, M., & Murray, H. (1998). Oral health status of Canadian-born and immigrant adolescents in North York, Ontario. *Community Dentistry and Oral Epidemiology, 26*, 177–181.

Merritt, L. (2005). Part 1: Understanding the embryology and genetics of cleft lip and palate. *Advances in Neonatal Care, 5*, 64–71.

Meurman, J., Sanz, M., & Janket, S. (2004). Oral health, atherosclerosis, and cardiovascular disease. *Critical Reviews in Oral Biology and Medicine, 15*, 403–413.

Morris, H. (2006). Managing dysphagia in older people. *Primary Health Care, 16*, 34–36.

Myers, N. E., Compliment, J. M., Post, J. C., & Buchinsky, F. D. (2006). Tonsilloliths: A common finding in pediatric patients. *Nurse Practitioner, 31*, 53–54.

Overfield, T. (1995). *Biologic variation in health and illness: Race, age, and sex differences* (2nd ed.). New York, NY: CRC Press.

Renvert, S. (2003). Destructive periodontal disease in relation to diabetes mellitus, cardiovascular disease, osteoporosis and respiratory disease. *Oral Health Preventive Dentistry, 1*(Suppl. 1): 341–357.

Statistics Canada. (2001). *The health of Inuit children: Fact sheet*. Retrieved June 5, 2008, from http://www.statcan.ca/english/freepub/89-627-XIE/89-627-XIE2007002.pdf

Westergren, A. (2006). Detection of eating difficulties after stroke: A systematic review. *International Nursing Review, 53*, 143–149.

Wright, W. (2005). Viral or acute bacterial rhinosinusitis? *Nurse Practitioner, 30*, 31–43.

Breasts and Regional Lymphatics

Written by **Carolyn Jarvis**, PhD, APN, CNP
Adapted by **Denise S. Tarlier**, PhD, MSN, NP(F)

Electronic Resources

On Evolve *evolve*

http://evolve.elsevier.com/Canada/Jarvis/examination/
- Interactive Case Studies
- Physical Examination Audio and Printable Summaries
- Bedside Assessment Summary Checklists
- Complete Physical Examination Form
- Nursing Diagnoses Boxes
- Health Promotion Guides
- Quick Assessments for 20 Common Conditions
- Multiple Choice Review Questions
- Chapter Objectives
- Appendices
- Weblinks

On the Companion CD

- Interactive Case Studies with Heart and Lung Sounds
- Health Promotion Guides
- Quick Assessments for 20 Common Conditions
- Head-to-Toe Physical Examination Video Clips

Structure and Function

STRUCTURE AND FUNCTION

The breasts, or mammary glands, are present in both females and males, although in the male they are rudimentary throughout life. The female breasts are accessory reproductive organs whose function is to produce milk for nourishing the newborn.

SURFACE ANATOMY

The **breasts** lie anterior to the pectoralis major and serratus anterior muscles (Fig. 17-1). The breasts are located between the second and sixth ribs, extending from the side of the sternum to the midaxillary line. The superior lateral corner of breast tissue, called the axillary **tail of Spence,** projects up and laterally into the axilla.

The **nipple** is just below the centre of the breast. It is rough, round, and usually protuberant; its surface looks wrinkled and indented with tiny milk duct openings. The **areola** surrounds the nipple for a 1- to 2-cm radius. In the areola are small elevated sebaceous glands, called Montgomery's glands. These secrete a protective lipid material during lactation. The areola also has smooth muscle fibres that cause nipple erection when stimulated. Both the nipple and areola are more darkly pigmented than the rest of the breast surface; the colour varies from pink to brown depending on the person's skin colour and parity.

INTERNAL ANATOMY

The breast is composed of (1) glandular tissue, (2) fibrous tissue including the suspensory ligaments, and (3) adipose tissue (Fig. 17-2). The **glandular tissue** contains 15 to 20 lobes radiating from the nipple, and these are composed of lobules. Within each lobule are clusters of alveoli that produce milk. Each lobe empties into a lactiferous duct. The 15 to

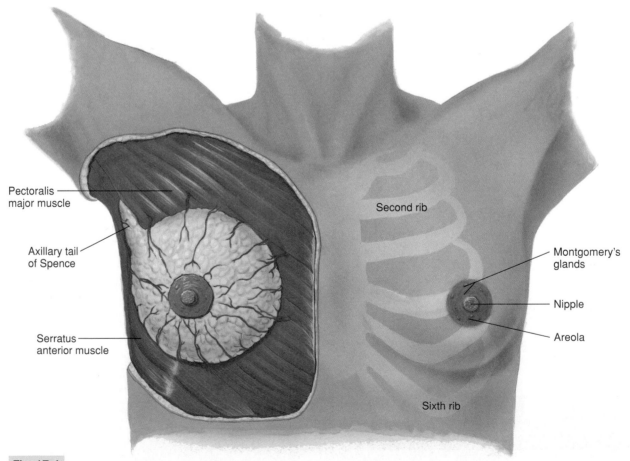

Pectoralis
major muscle

Axillary tail
of Spence

Serratus
anterior muscle

Second rib

Montgomery's
glands

Nipple

Areola

Sixth rib

Fig. 17-1

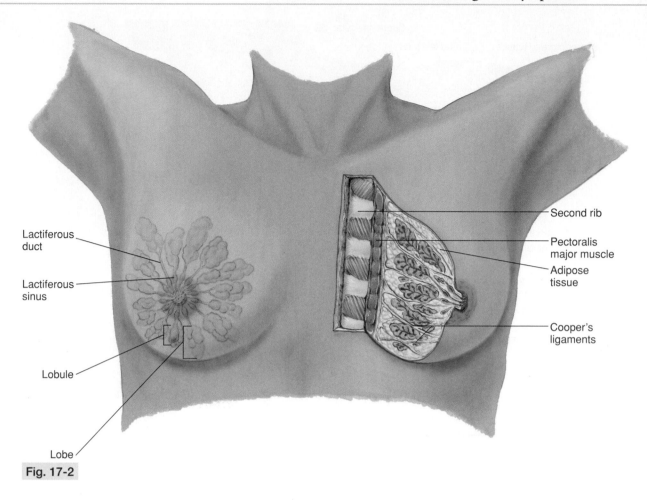

Lactiferous
duct

Lactiferous
sinus

Lobule

Lobe

Second rib

Pectoralis
major muscle

Adipose
tissue

Cooper's
ligaments

Fig. 17-2

20 lactiferous ducts form a collecting duct system converging toward the nipple. There, the ducts form ampullae, or lactiferous sinuses, behind the nipple, which are reservoirs for storing milk.

The suspensory ligaments, or **Cooper's ligaments,** are fibrous bands extending vertically from the surface to attach on chest wall muscles. These support the breast tissue. They become contracted in cancer of the breast, producing pits or dimples in the overlying skin.

The lobes are embedded in **adipose tissue.** These layers of subcutaneous and retromammary fat actually provide most of the bulk of the breast. The relative proportion of glandular, fibrous, and fatty tissue varies depending on age, cycle, pregnancy, lactation, and general nutritional state.

The breast may be divided into four quadrants by imaginary horizontal and vertical lines intersecting at the nipple (Fig. 17-3). This makes a convenient map to describe clinical findings. In the upper outer quadrant, note the axillary **tail of Spence,** the cone-shaped breast tissue that projects up into the axilla, close to the pectoral group of axillary lymph nodes. The upper outer quadrant is the site of most breast tumours.

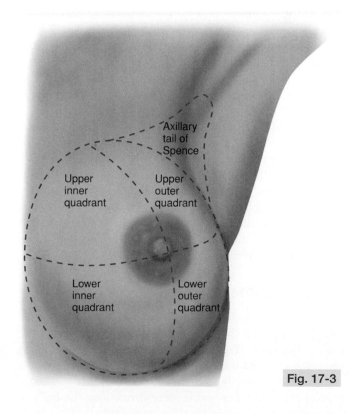

Axillary
tail of
Spence

Upper
inner
quadrant

Upper
outer
quadrant

Lower
inner
quadrant

Lower
outer
quadrant

Fig. 17-3

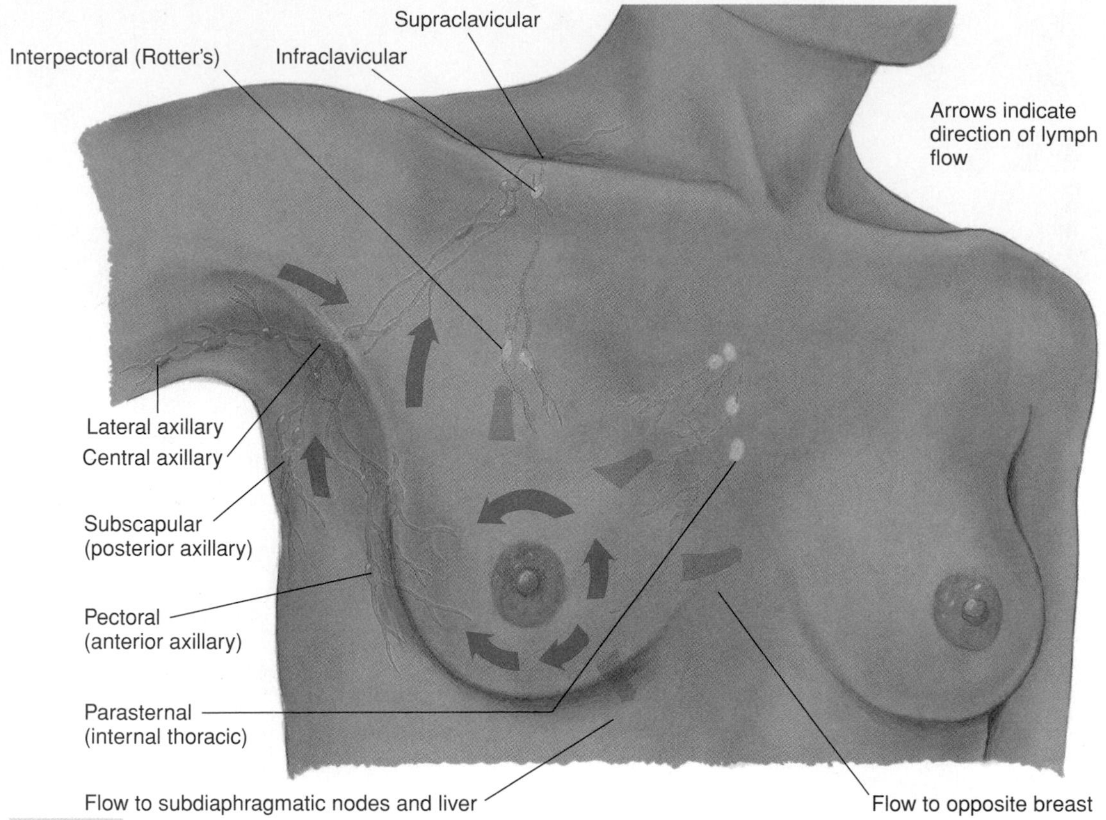

Interpectoral (Rotter's)   Infraclavicular   Supraclavicular

Arrows indicate direction of lymph flow

Lateral axillary
Central axillary
Subscapular (posterior axillary)
Pectoral (anterior axillary)
Parasternal (internal thoracic)

Flow to subdiaphragmatic nodes and liver

Flow to opposite breast

Fig. 17-4

LYMPHATICS

The breast has extensive lymphatic drainage. Most of the lymph, more than 75%, drains into the ipsilateral (same side) axillary nodes. Four groups of axillary nodes are present (Fig. 17-4):

1. **Central axillary nodes**—high up in the middle of the axilla, over the ribs and serratus anterior muscle. These receive lymph from the other three groups of nodes.
2. **Pectoral** (anterior)—along the lateral edge of the pectoralis major muscle, just inside the anterior axillary fold.
3. **Subscapular** (posterior)—along the lateral edge of the scapula, deep in the posterior axillary fold.
4. **Lateral**—along the humerus, inside the upper arm.

From the central axillary nodes, drainage flows up to the infraclavicular and supraclavicular nodes.

A smaller amount of lymphatic drainage does not take these channels but flows directly up to the infraclavicular group, deep into the chest, or into the abdomen, or directly across to the opposite breast.

💮 DEVELOPMENTAL CARE

During embryonic life, ventral epidermal ridges, or "milk lines," are present; these curve down from the axilla to the groin bilaterally (Fig. 17-5). The breast develops along the ridge over the thorax, and the rest of the ridge usually atrophies. Occasionally a **supernumerary nipple** (i.e., an extra nipple) persists and is visible somewhere along the track of the mammary ridge (see Fig. 17-8 on p. 415).

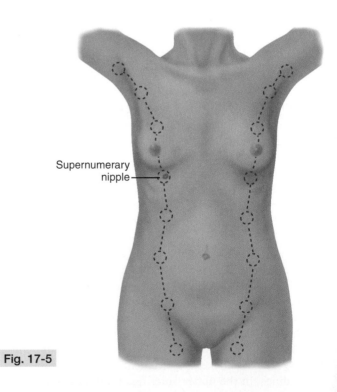

Supernumerary nipple

Fig. 17-5

At birth, the only breast structures present are the lactiferous ducts within the nipple. No alveoli have developed. Little change occurs until puberty.

The Adolescent

At puberty the estrogen hormones stimulate breast changes. The breasts enlarge, mostly as a result of extensive fat deposition. The duct system also grows and branches, and masses of small, solid cells develop at the duct endings. These are potential alveoli.

Occasionally, one breast may grow faster than the other, producing a temporary asymmetry. This may cause some distress; reassurance is necessary. Tenderness is common also. Although the age of onset varies widely, the five stages of breast development follow this classic description of sexual maturity rating, or **Tanner staging** (Table 17-1).

Full development from stage 2 to stage 5 takes an average of 3 years, although the range is 1.5 to 6 years. During this time, pubic hair develops, and axillary hair appears 2 years after the onset of pubic hair. The beginning of breast development precedes **menarche** (beginning of menstruation) by about 2 years. Menarche occurs in breast development stage 3 or 4, usually just after the peak of the adolescent growth spurt around age 12 years. Note the relationship of these events (Fig. 17-6). This aids in assessing the development of adolescent girls and increases their knowledge about their own development.

Breasts of the nonpregnant woman change with the ebb and flow of hormones during the monthly menstrual cycle.

TABLE 17-1	Sexual Maturity Rating in Girls
Stage	
1 Preadolescent: Only a small elevated nipple	
2 Breast bud stage: A small mound of breast and nipple develops; the areola widens	
3 The breast and areola enlarge; the nipple is flush with the breast surface	
4 The areola and nipple form a secondary mound over the breast	
5 Mature breast: Only the nipple protrudes; the areola is flush with the breast contour (the areola may continue as a secondary mound in some normal women)	

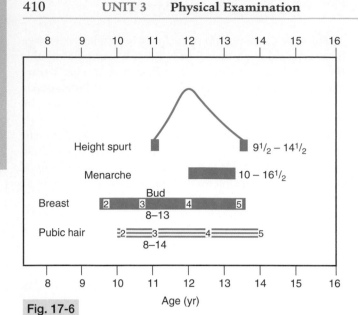

Fig. 17-6

Nodularity increases from midcycle up to menstruation. During the 3 to 4 days before menstruation, the breasts feel full, tight, heavy, and occasionally sore. The breast volume is smallest on days 4 to 7 of the menstrual cycle.

The Pregnant Female

During pregnancy, breast changes start during the second month and are an early sign of pregnancy for most women. Pregnancy stimulates the expansion of the ductal system and supporting fatty tissue as well as development of the true secretory alveoli. Thus the breasts enlarge and feel more nodular. The nipples are larger, darker, and more erectile. The areolae become larger and grow a darker brown as pregnancy progresses, and the tubercles become more prominent. (The brown colour fades after lactation, but the areolae never return to the original colour.) A venous pattern is prominent over the skin surface (see Fig. 29-4 on p. 835).

After the fourth month, **colostrum** may be expressed. This thick yellow fluid is the precursor for milk, containing the same amount of protein and lactose but practically no fat. The breasts produce colostrum for the first few days after delivery. It is rich with antibodies that protect the newborn against infection, so breastfeeding is important. Milk production (lactation) begins 1 to 3 days post partum. The whitish colour is from emulsified fat and calcium caseinate.

The Aging Female

After menopause, ovarian secretion of estrogen and progesterone decreases, which causes the breast glandular tissue to atrophy. This is replaced with fibrous connective tissue. The fat envelope atrophies also, beginning in the middle years and becoming marked in the eighth and ninth decades. These changes decrease breast size and elasticity so the breasts droop and sag, looking flattened and flabby. Drooping is accentuated by the kyphosis in some older women.

The decreased breast size makes inner structures more prominent. A breast lump may have been present for years but is suddenly palpable. Around the nipple the lactiferous ducts are more palpable and feel firm and stringy because of fibrosis and calcification. The axillary hair decreases.

THE MALE BREAST

The male breast is a rudimentary structure consisting of a thin disk of undeveloped tissue underlying the nipple. The areola is well developed, although the nipple is relatively very small. During adolescence, it is common for the breast tissue to temporarily enlarge, producing **gynecomastia.** This condition is usually unilateral and temporary. Reassurance is necessary for the adolescent male, whose attention is riveted on his body image. Gynecomastia may reappear in the aging male and may be due to testosterone deficiency.

CULTURAL AND SOCIAL CONSIDERATIONS

Few health initiatives across Canada have been taken up by the public in the way that women's breast screening has. Long-term, proactive public awareness initiatives and access to screening measures such as mammography are paying off in declining mortality rates due to breast cancer (National Cancer Institute of Canada [NCIC], 2007). Women with breast cancer are being diagnosed at earlier stages of cancer development, receiving treatment sooner, and surviving longer. Despite these successes, breast cancer remains the most common cancer among women in Canada, and is the second most common cause of cancer-related death (NCIC, 2007).

The lifetime risk of being diagnosed with breast cancer in Canada is approximately one in nine women (Wilkinson, 2007). Women who have a first-degree relative with breast cancer have a one in seven annual risk or one in six (lifetime) risk (Wilkinson, 2007). Incidence and mortality rates for breast cancer, and related risk factors, are heavily influenced by socioeconomic level, ethnocultural background, rural locations, and inequities in access to health services. Genetic factors are also implicated as risk factors but to a lesser extent: only 5 to 10% of cancers have an identifiable breast cancer gene (*BRCA1* or *BRCA2*).

There is a growing focus among researchers and healthcare professionals on how these influences, along with an identified lack of culturally safe health service options, present barriers to women's access to and use of healthcare resources. For example, researchers Ahmad et al. (2005) found that offering "socioculturally tailored and language-specific health education materials" (p. 575) to South Asian immigrant women residing in Toronto not only increased women's knowledge of breast cancer but also improved self-efficacy and uptake of clinical breast examination (CBE). Similarly, research shows that Aboriginal women are more likely to access and understand breast cancer education when it is culturally relevant and respectful and offered in easily understood language (Friedman et al., 2007).

Some studies have found that a diet rich in certain fats has a strong promoting effect on breast cancer and that breast cancer is less common in countries where the diet is low in total fat, low in polyunsaturated fat, and low in saturated fat (Buzdar, 2006). Although the relationship of breast cancer to dietary fat is not clear at this time, it is known that reducing the intake of dietary fat in postmenopausal women has a subsequent reduced risk of invasive breast cancer (Prentice et al., 2006). The relationship between high-fat diets and breast cancer has implications for Canadians who consume a "typical" high-fat North American–style diet and, in particular, for those who lack the socioeconomic resources to eat a more nutritious diet. For example, Aboriginal people living in Canada's far northern and remote communities may not be able to make more nutritious food choices due to both the high cost and the lack of availability of such foods in their communities.

SUBJECTIVE DATA

Breast

1. Pain
2. Lump
3. Discharge
4. Rash
5. Swelling
6. Trauma
7. History of breast disease
8. Surgery
9. Self-care behaviours
   Perform breast self-examination
   Last mammogram

Axilla

1. Tenderness, lump, or swelling
2. Rash

In Western culture the female breasts signify more than their primary purpose of lactation. Women are surrounded by messages that feminine norms of beauty and desirability are enhanced by and dependent on the size of the breasts and their appearance. More recently, women leaders have tried to refocus this attitude, stressing women's self-worth as individual human beings, not as stereotyped sexual objects. The intense cultural emphasis is gradually changing, yet the breasts still are crucial to a woman's self-concept and her perception of her femininity. Matters pertaining to the breast affect a woman's body image and generate deep emotional responses.

This emotionality may take strong forms that you observe as you discuss the woman's history. One woman may be acutely embarrassed talking about her breasts, as evidenced by lack of eye contact, minimal response, nervous gestures, or inappropriate humour. Another woman may talk wryly and disparagingly about the size or development of her breasts. A young adolescent is acutely aware of her own development in relation to her peers. Or, a woman who has found a breast lump may come to you with fear, high anxiety, and even panic. Although many breast lumps are benign, women initially assume the worst possible outcome—cancer, disfigurement, and death. While you are collecting the subjective data, tune in to cues for these behaviours that call for a straightforward and reasoned attitude.

Examiner Asks	Rationale
Breast	

1. Pain. Any **pain** or tenderness in the breasts? When did you first notice it?
 • Where is the pain? Localized or all over?
   Is the painful spot sore to touch? Do you feel a burning or pulling sensation?
 • Is the pain cyclical? Any relation to your menstrual period?
 	
 • Is the pain brought on by strenuous activity, especially involving one arm; a change in activity; manipulation during sex; part of underwire bra; exercise?
	Mastalgia occurs with trauma, inflammation, infection, and benign breast disease.
	   Cyclical pain is common with normal breasts, oral contraceptives, and benign breast (fibrocystic) disease.
	   Is pain related to specific cause?

2. Lump. Ever noticed a **lump** or **thickening** in the breast? Where? • When did you first notice it? Changed at all since then? • Does the lump have any relation to your menstrual period? • Noticed any change in the overlying skin: redness, warmth, dimpling, swelling?	Carefully explore the presence of any lump. A lump present for many years and exhibiting no change may not be serious but still should be explored. Approach any recent change or new lump with suspicion.

Subjective Data

Examiner Asks	Rationale
3. Discharge. Any **discharge** from the nipple? • When did you first notice this? • What colour is the discharge? • Consistency—thick or runny? • Odour?	**Galactorrhea.** Note medications that may cause clear nipple discharge: oral contraceptives, phenothiazines, diuretics, digitalis, steroids, methyldopa, calcium channel blockers. Bloody or blood-tinged discharge always is significant. Any discharge with a lump is significant.
4. Rash. Any **rash** on the breast? • When did you first notice this? • Where did it start? On the nipple, areola, or surrounding skin?	Paget's disease starts with a small crust on the nipple apex, then spreads to areola. Eczema or other dermatitis rarely starts at nipple unless it is due to breastfeeding. It usually starts on the areola or surrounding skin and then spreads to the nipple.
5. Swelling. Any **swelling** in the breasts? In one spot or all over? • Related to your menstrual period, pregnancy, or breastfeeding? • Any change in bra size?	
6. Trauma. Any **trauma** or injury to the breasts? • Did it result in any swelling, lump, or break in skin?	A lump from an injury is due to local hematoma or edema and should resolve shortly. Or, trauma may cause a woman to feel the breast and find a lump that really was there before.
7. History of breast disease. Any history of breast disease yourself? • What type? How was this diagnosed? • When did this occur? • How is it being treated? • Any breast cancer in your family? Who? Sister, mother, maternal grandmother, maternal aunts, daughter? • At what age did this relative have breast cancer?	Past breast cancer increases the risk of recurrent cancer (Table 17-2, p. 414). The presence of benign breast disease makes the breasts more difficult to examine; the general lumpiness conceals a new lump. Breast cancer occurring before menopause in certain family members increases risk for this woman (see Table 17-2, p. 414).
8. Surgery. Have you ever had **surgery** on your breasts? Was this a biopsy? What were the biopsy results? • Mastectomy? Mammoplasty—augmentation or reduction?	
9. Routine breast health behaviours. • Do you have your breasts examined regularly (at least every 2 years) by a trained healthcare professional? • Have you ever had mammography, a screening X-ray examination of the breasts? • (If age 40 to 49) Have you ever discussed your risk of breast cancer and the risks and benefits of mammography with a healthcare professional? • (If age 50 to 69) Do you have a mammogram regularly (at least every 2 years)? When was your last mammogram? • (If over age 70) Have you discussed routine breast cancer screening with a healthcare professional? • Have you ever discussed breast self-examination, or BSE, with a healthcare professional? (If not) Would you be interested in learning about the benefits and risks of BSE? • Have you ever been taught BSE? Do you currently perform BSE? • (If so) I would like you to show me your technique after I complete your examination.	Recommended routine breast health behaviours for Canadian women include the complementary screening approaches of CBE, mammography, and possibly BSE (Canadian Cancer Society [CCS], 2008). There is some variation among the provinces and territories regarding the recommended frequency of screening and the age at which healthcare coverage for routine preventive screening measures commences. The CCS breast cancer screening guidelines suggest that: • Women aged 40 to 69 have CBE by a trained healthcare professional at least once every 2 years • Women aged 40 to 49 discuss their risk of breast cancer and the risks and benefits

Examiner Asks	Rationale
• (If not) If you decide you would like to practise BSE following a discussion of the benefits and risks, I will teach you the technique.	of routine mammography screening with their healthcare professional • Women aged 50 to 69 have a screening mammogram every 2 years • Women aged 70 and older discuss routine breast cancer screening with their healthcare professional The Canadian Task Force on Preventive Health Care recommends screening mammography starting at either age 40 or 50 (Ringash, 2001), based on individual risk assessment and personal choice, after being informed of the potential benefits and risks (e.g., unnecessary biopsies).

Axilla

1. Tenderness, lump, or swelling. Any **tenderness** or **lump** in the underarm area?
- Where? When did you first notice this?

Breast tissue extends up into the axilla. Also, the axilla contains many lymph nodes.

2. Rash. Any axillary **rash?** Please describe it.
- Seem to be a reaction to deodorant?

Additional History for the Preadolescent

1. Have you noticed your breasts changing?
- How long has this been happening?

2. Many girls notice other changes in their bodies, too, that come with growing up. What have you noticed?
- What do you think about all this?

Developing breasts are the most obvious sign of puberty and the focus of attention for most girls, especially in comparison to peers. Assess each girl's perception of her own development, provide teaching and reassurance as indicated.

Additional History for the Pregnant Female

1. Have you noticed any enlargement or fullness in the breasts?
- Is there any tenderness or tingling?

- Do you have a history of inverted nipples?

Breast changes are expected and normal during pregnancy. Assess the woman's knowledge and provide reassurance.

Inverted nipples may need special care in preparation for breastfeeding.

2. Are you planning to breastfeed your baby?

Breastfeeding provides the perfect food and antibodies for the baby, decreases risk of ear infections, promotes bonding, and provides relaxation.

Additional History for the Menopausal Woman

1. Have you noticed any change in the breast contour, size, or firmness? (Note: Change may not be as apparent to obese woman or to the woman whose earlier pregnancies already have produced breast changes.)

Decreased estrogen level causes decreased firmness. Rapid decrease in estrogen level causes actual shrinkage.

Risk Factor Profile for Breast Cancer

Breast cancer is the second major cause of death from cancer in women. However, early detection and improved treatment have increased survival rates. The 5-year survival rate for stage I and II breast cancers is 96% and 86%, respectively (based on Ontario data; national staging data are not yet available). Survival rates are lower for cancers diagnosed at stages III or IV (NCIC, 2007). Note the risk factors listed in Table 17-2.

Examiner Asks

Risk Factors That Cannot Be Changed	Modifiable Risk Factors
Female sex, age >50 years	Nulliparity or first child after age
Personal history of breast cancer	30 years
Mutation of *BRCA1* and *BRCA2* genes	Recent oral contraceptive use
First-degree relative with breast or ovarian	Postmenopausal hormone therapy
cancer (mother, sister, daughter)	(especially combined estrogen and
Previous breast biopsy with *atypical* hyper-	progesterone therapy)
plasia, or *breast disease without* atypia or	Not breastfeeding
usual hyperplasia	Alcohol intake of ≥1 drink daily
Previous breast irradiation	Obesity (especially after menopause)
Menstruation before age 12 years or meno-	and high-fat diet
pause after age 50 years	Physical inactivity

TABLE 17-2   Breast Cancer Risk Factors

Data adapted from Canadian Cancer Society. Retrieved February, 2008 from http://www.cancer.ca.

Rationale

The best way to detect a person's risk for breast cancer is by asking the right history questions. Table 17-2 highlights risk factors for breast cancer, and from these you can fashion your questions. Be aware that most breast cancers occur in women with no identifiable risk factors except sex and age. Just because a woman does not report the cited risk factors does not mean that you or she should fail to consider breast cancer seriously.

OBJECTIVE DATA

PREPARATION

The woman is sitting up facing the examiner. An alternative draping method is to use a short gown, open at the back, and lift it up to the woman's shoulders during inspection. During palpation, when the woman is supine, cover one breast with the gown while examining the other. Be aware that many women are embarrassed to have their breasts examined; use a sensitive but matter-of-fact approach.

After your examination, be prepared to teach the woman breast self-examination.

EQUIPMENT NEEDED

Small pillow
Ruler marked in centimetres
Pamphlet or teaching aid for BSE

Normal Range of Findings

INSPECT THE BREASTS

General Appearance

Note symmetry of size and shape (Fig. 17-7). It is common to have a slight asymmetry in size; often the left breast is slightly larger than the right.

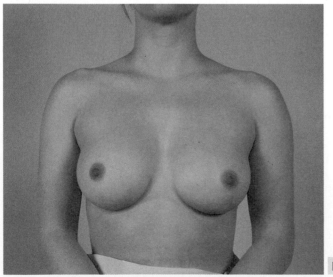

Fig. 17-7

Abnormal Findings

A sudden increase in the size of one breast signifies inflammation or new growth.

Normal Range of Findings	Abnormal Findings

Skin

The skin normally is smooth and of even colour. Note any localized areas of redness, bulging, or dimpling. Also, note any skin lesions or focal vascular pattern. A fine blue vascular network is visible normally during pregnancy. Pale linear striae, or stretch marks, often follow pregnancy.

Normally no edema is present. Edema exaggerates the hair follicles, giving a "pig-skin" or "orange-peel" look (also called *peau d'orange*).

Hyperpigmentation.
Redness and heat with inflammation.
Unilateral dilated superficial veins in a nonpregnant woman.
Edema (see Table 17-3, p. 428).

Lymphatic Drainage Areas

Observe the axillary and supraclavicular regions. Note any bulging, discoloration, or edema.

Nipple

The nipples should be symmetrically placed on the same plane on the two breasts. Nipples usually protrude, although some are flat and some are inverted. They tend to stay in their original condition. Distinguish a recently retracted nipple from one that has been inverted for many years or since puberty. Normal nipple inversion may be unilateral or bilateral and usually can be pulled out (i.e., it is not fixed).

Note any dry scaling, any fissure or ulceration, and bleeding or other discharge.

A **supernumerary nipple** is a normal and common variation (Fig. 17-8). An extra nipple along the embryonic "milk line" on the thorax or abdomen is a congenital finding. Usually, it is 5 to 6 cm below the breast near the midline and has no associated glandular tissue. It looks like a mole, although a close look reveals a tiny nipple and areola. It is not significant; merely distinguish it from a mole.

Deviation in pointing (see Table 17-3, p. 428).

Recent nipple retraction signifies acquired disease (see Table 17-3, p. 428).

Explore any discharge, especially in the presence of a breast mass.

Rarely, additional glandular tissue, called a supernumerary breast, is present.

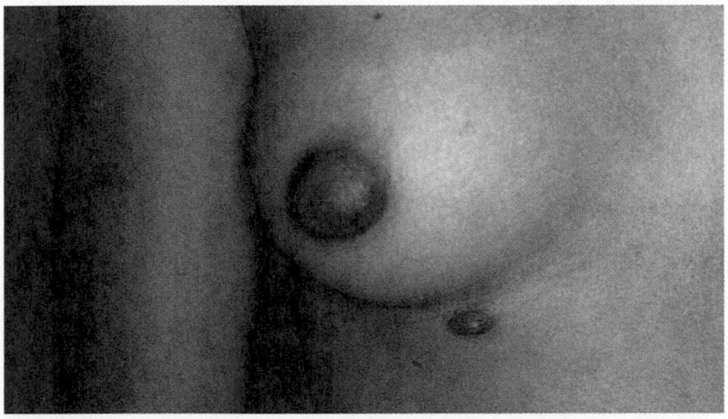

Fig. 17-8   Supernumerary nipple and areolar complex.

Manoeuvres to Screen for Retraction

Direct the woman to change position while you check the breasts for skin retraction signs. First ask her to lift the arms slowly over the head. Both breasts should move up symmetrically (Fig. 17-9).

Retraction signs are due to fibrosis in the breast tissue, usually caused by growing neoplasms. The fibrosis shortens with time, causing contrasting signs with the normally loose breast tissue.
Note a lag in movement of one breast.

Normal Range of Findings	**Abnormal Findings**

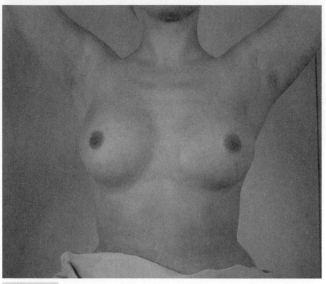

Fig. 17-9   Retraction manoeuvre.

Next ask her to push her hands onto her hips (Fig. 17-10) and then to push her two palms together (Fig. 17-11). These manoeuvres contract the pectoralis major muscle. A slight lifting of both breasts will occur.

Note a dimpling or a pucker, which indicates skin retraction (see Table 17-3, p. 428).

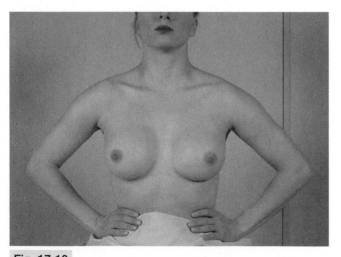

Fig. 17-10

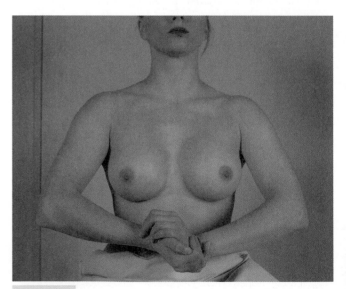

Fig. 17-11

Ask the woman with large pendulous breasts to lean forward while you support her forearms. Note the symmetrical free-forward movement of both breasts (Fig. 17-12).

Normal Range of Findings	Abnormal Findings
	Note fixation to chest wall or skin retraction (see Table 17-3, p. 428).

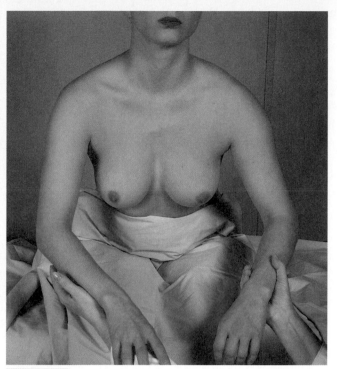

Fig. 17-12

INSPECT AND PALPATE THE AXILLAE

Examine the axillae while the woman is sitting. Inspect the skin, noting any rash or infection. Lift the woman's arm and support it yourself, so that her muscles are loose and relaxed. Use your right hand to palpate the left axilla (Fig. 17-13). Reach your fingers high into the axilla. Move them firmly down in four directions: (1) down the chest wall in a line from the middle of the axilla, (2) along the anterior border of the axilla, (3) along the posterior border, and (4) along the inner aspect of the upper arm. Move the woman's arm through the range of motion to increase the surface area you can reach.

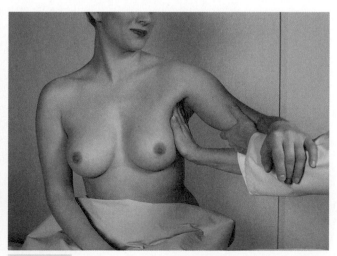

Fig. 17-13

Objective Data

Normal Range of Findings

Usually nodes are not palpable, although you may feel a small, soft, non-tender node in the central group. Expect some tenderness when palpating high in the axilla. Note any enlarged and tender lymph nodes.

PALPATE THE BREASTS

Help the woman to a supine position. Tuck a small pad under the side to be palpated and raise her arm over her head. These manoeuvres will flatten the breast tissue and displace it medially. Any significant lumps will then feel more distinct (Fig. 17-14).

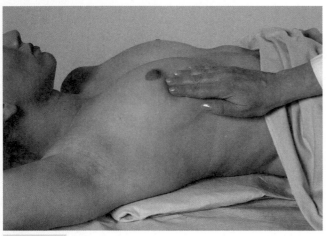

Fig. 17-14

Use the pads of your first three fingers and make a gentle rotary motion on the breast. Vary your pressure so you are palpating light, medium, and deep tissues in each location. The vertical strip pattern (Fig. 17-15, *A*) currently is recommended as the best to detect a breast mass, but two other patterns are in common use: from the nipple palpating out to the periphery as if following spokes on a wheel and palpating in concentric circles out to the periphery (Fig. 17-15, *B* and *C*).

Abnormal Findings

Nodes enlarge with any local infection of the breast, arm, or hand, and with breast cancer metastases.

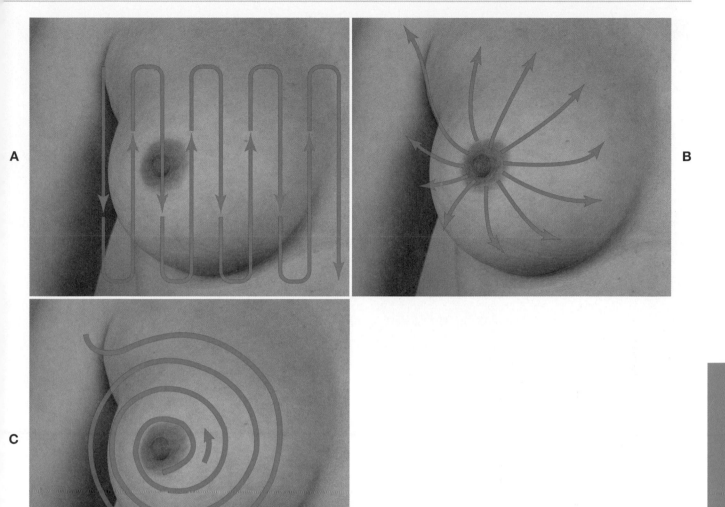

Fig. 17-15   A, Vertical strip pattern of palpation. B, Spokes-on-a-wheel pattern of palpation. C, Concentric circles pattern of palpation.

Normal Range of Findings	Abnormal Findings
For the vertical strip pattern, start high in the axilla and palpate down just lateral to the breast. Proceed in overlapping vertical lines ending at the sternal edge. In every pattern, take care to palpate every square centimetre of the breast and to examine the tail of Spence high into the axilla. Be consistent and thorough in your approach to each woman.	
In nulliparous women, normal breast tissue feels firm, smooth, and elastic. After pregnancy, the tissue feels softer and looser. Premenstrual engorgement is normal from increasing progesterone. This consists of a slight enlargement, a tenderness to palpation, and a generalized nodularity; the lobes feel prominent and their margins more distinct.	Heat, redness, and swelling in nonlactating and nonpostpartum breasts indicate inflammation.
Also, normally you may feel a firm transverse ridge of compressed tissue in the lower quadrants. This is the **inframammary ridge,** and it is especially noticeable in large breasts. Do not confuse it with an abnormal lump.	

Objective Data

Normal Range of Findings

After palpating over the four breast quadrants, palpate the nipple (Fig. 17-16). Note any induration or subareolar mass. With your thumb and forefinger, gently depress the nipple tissue into the well behind the areola. The tissue should move inward easily. If the woman reports spontaneous nipple discharge, press the areola inward with your index finger—repeat from a few different directions. If any discharge appears, note its colour and consistency.

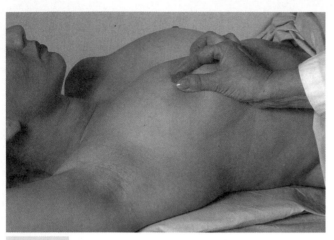

Fig. 17-16

For the woman with large pendulous breasts, you may palpate by using a bimanual technique (Fig. 17-17). The woman is in a sitting position, leaning forward. Support the inferior part of the breast with one hand. Use your other hand to palpate the breast tissue against your supporting hand.

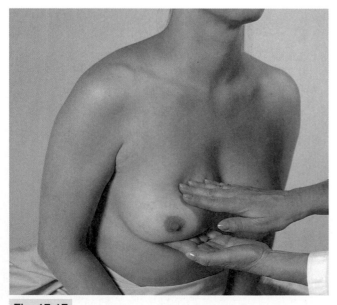

Fig. 17-17

Abnormal Findings

Except in pregnancy and lactation, discharge is abnormal (see Table 17-6, p. 431). Note the number of discharge droplets and the quadrant(s) producing them. Blot the discharge on a white gauze pad to ascertain its colour. Test any abnormal discharge for the presence of blood.

Normal Range of Findings	Abnormal Findings

If the woman mentions a breast lump that she has discovered herself, examine the unaffected breast first to learn a baseline of normal consistency for this woman. If you do feel a lump or mass, note these characteristics (Fig. 17-18):

1. **Location**—Using the breast as a clock face, describe the distance in centimetres from the nipple (e.g., "7:00, 2 cm from the nipple"). Or diagram the breast in the woman's record and mark in the location of the lump.
2. **Size**—Judge in centimetres in three dimensions: width × length × thickness.
3. **Shape**—State whether the lump is oval, round, lobulated, or indistinct.
4. **Consistency**—State whether the lump is soft, firm, or hard.
5. **Movable**—Is the lump freely movable, or is it fixed when you try to slide it over the chest wall?
6. **Distinctness**—Is the lump solitary or multiple?
7. **Nipple**—Is it displaced or retracted?
8. **Note the skin over the lump**—Is it erythematous, dimpled, or retracted?
9. **Tenderness**—Is the lump tender to palpation?
10. **Lymphadenopathy**—Are any regional lymph nodes palpable?

See Tables 17-4 and 17-5 (pp. 429 and 430) for description of common breast lumps with these characteristics.

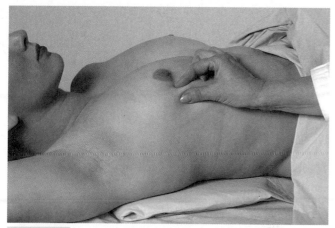

Fig. 17-18

TEACH THE BREAST SELF-EXAMINATION

BSE is no longer routinely recommended to Canadian women (Society of Obstetricians and Gynaecologists of Canada [SOGC], 2006). This recommendation was initially presented in 2001 but has been slow to gain broad acceptance due largely to women's perception that BSE offers control over their own health. However, the available evidence supports that BSE does not decrease mortality associated with breast cancer and carries the risk of potentially increasing benign biopsy rates (SOGC, 2006). Therefore, BSE is currently not recommended as a screening technique.

If, after a full discussion with a healthcare professional of the risks and benefits of BSE, a woman makes an informed decision to perform BSE, she should be taught to perform BSE proficiently, and her proficiency should be evaluated and ensured by the healthcare professional. Teach BSE after completing your own assessment. You need to focus your skill and concentration on the examination, and you may be diverted by teaching at the same time. The same is true for the woman. She waits to hear that your examination of her affirms that she is healthy. Once reassured, she can relax about the findings and concentrate on your teaching. Ask her to return-demonstrate her technique so that you may evaluate her proficiency.

Objective Data

Normal Range of Findings	Abnormal Findings

Help each woman establish a regular schedule of self-care. The best time to conduct BSE is right after the menstrual period, or the fourth through seventh day of the menstrual cycle, when the breasts are the smallest and least congested. Advise the pregnant or menopausal woman who is not having menstrual periods to select a familiar date to examine her breasts each month, for example, her birth date or the day the rent is due.

Stress that self-examination will familiarize the woman with her own breasts and their normal variation. Emphasize the absence of lumps (not the presence of them). However, do encourage her to report any unusual finding promptly.

While teaching, focus on the positive aspects of BSE. Avoid citing frightening mortality statistics about breast cancer. This may generate excessive fear and denial that actually obstructs a woman's self-care action. Rather, be selective in your choice of factual material:

- The majority of women will never get breast cancer.
- The great majority of breast lumps are benign.
- Early detection of breast cancer is important; if the cancer is not invasive, the survival rate is close to 100%.

Emphasize self-care through knowledge of risk factors and early referral for any suspicious findings.

Keep your teaching simple! The simpler the plan, the more likely the person will comply. Describe the correct technique and rationale and the expected findings to note as the woman inspects her own breasts (Fig. 17-19). Teach the woman to do this in front of a mirror while she is disrobed to the waist. At home, she can start palpation in the shower, where soap and water assist palpation. Then palpation should be performed while lying supine. Encourage the woman to palpate her own breasts while you are there to monitor her technique. Use the return demonstration to assess her technique and understanding of the procedure.

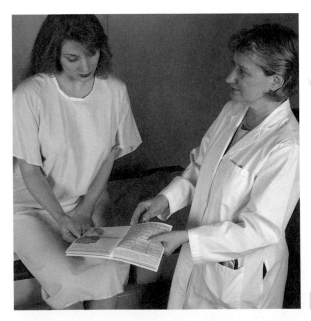
Fig. 17-19

Many examiners use a simulated breast model so that the woman can palpate a "lump." Pamphlets are helpful reinforcers; give the woman two pamphlets to take home and encourage her to give one to a relative or friend. This may promote discussion, which is reinforcing.

Normal Range of Findings	Abnormal Findings

THE MALE BREAST

Your examination of the male breast can be much more abbreviated, but do not omit it. Combine the breast examination with that of the anterior thorax. Inspect the chest wall, noting the skin surface and any lumps or swelling. Palpate the nipple area for any lump or tissue enlargement (Fig. 17-20). It should feel even, with no nodules. Palpate the axillary lymph nodes.

The incidence of breast cancer in men is 1%, or approximately 170 cases per year (CCS, 2008).

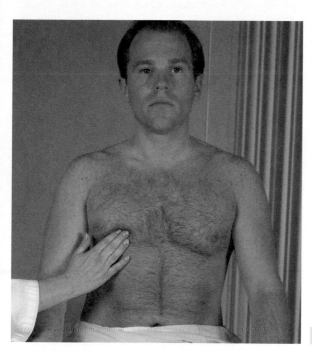

Fig. 17-20

The normal male breast has a flat disc of undeveloped breast tissue beneath the nipple. **Gynecomastia** is an enlargement of this breast tissue, making it clinically distinguishable from the other tissues in the chest wall (Fig. 17-21). It feels like a smooth, firm, movable disc. This occurs normally during puberty. It usually affects only one breast and is temporary. The adolescent is acutely aware of his body image. Reassure him that this change is normal, common, and temporary. In contrast, an obese male has an increase of fatty, not glandular, tissue.

Gynecomastia also occurs with use of anabolic steroids, some medications, and some disease states. See Table 17-8, p. 433.

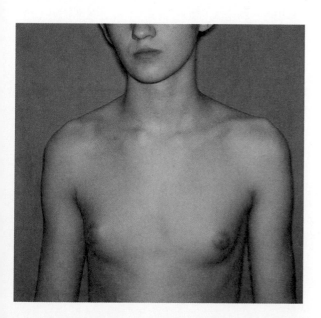

Fig. 17-21
Adolescent
gynecomastia.

Objective Data

Normal Range of Findings	Abnormal Findings

 DEVELOPMENTAL CARE

Infants and Children

In the neonate, the breasts may be enlarged and visible due to maternal estrogen crossing the placenta. They may secrete a clear or white fluid, called "witch's milk." These signs are not significant and are resolved within a few days to a few weeks.

Note the position of the nipples on the prepubertal child. They should be symmetrical, just lateral to the midclavicular line, between the fourth and fifth ribs. The nipple is flat, and the areola is darker pigmented.

Premature thelarche is early breast development with no other hormone-dependent signs (pubic hair, menses).

The Adolescent

Adolescent breast development usually begins on an average between 8 and 10 years of age. Expect some asymmetry during growth. (Distinguish breast development from extra adipose tissue present in obese children.) Record the stage of development using Tanner's staging described on p. 411. Use the chart to teach the adolescent normal developmental stages and to assure her of her own normal progress.

Note precocious development, occurring before age 8 years. It is usually normal but also occurs with thyroid dysfunction, stilbestrol ingestion, or ovarian or adrenal tumour.

Note delayed development, occurring with hormonal failure or anorexia nervosa beginning before puberty, or with severe malnutrition.

With maturing adolescents, palpate the breasts as you would with the adult. The breasts normally feel firm and uniform. Note any mass.

At this age a mass is almost always a benign fibroadenoma or a cyst (see Table 17-4, p. 429).

The Pregnant Female

A delicate blue vascular pattern is visible over the breasts. The breasts increase in size, as do the nipples. Jagged linear stretch marks, or striae, may develop if the breasts have a large increase. The nipples also become darker and more erectile. The areolae widen; grow darker; and contain the small, scattered, elevated Montgomery's glands. On palpation, the breasts feel more nodular, and thick yellow colostrum can be expressed after the first trimester.

The Lactating Female

Colostrum changes to milk production around the third postpartum day. At this time, the breasts may become engorged, appearing enlarged, reddened, and shiny and feeling warm and hard. Frequent nursing helps drain the ducts and sinuses and stimulate milk production. Nipple soreness is normal, appearing around the twentieth nursing, lasting 24 to 48 hours, then disappearing rapidly. The nipples may look red and irritated. They may even crack but will heal rapidly if kept dry and exposed to air. Again, frequent nursings are the best treatment for nipple soreness.

One section of the breast surface appearing red and tender indicates a plugged duct (see Table 17-7, p. 432).

The Aging Female

On inspection, the breasts look pendulous, flattened, and sagging. Nipples may be retracted but can be pulled outward. On palpation, the breasts feel more granular, and the terminal ducts around the nipple feel more prominent and stringy. Thickening of the inframammary ridge at the lower breast is normal, and it feels more prominent with age.

Because atrophy causes shrinkage of normal glandular tissue, cancer detection is somewhat easier. Any palpable lump that cannot be positively identified as a normal structure should be referred.

Normal Range of Findings	Abnormal Findings

Reinforce the value of routine breast health behaviours. Women over 50 years old have an increased risk of breast cancer. Older women may have problems with arthritis, limited range of motion, or decreased vision that may inhibit self-care. Suggest aids to the self-examination; for example, talcum powder helps fingers glide over skin.

Summary Checklist: Breasts and Regional Lymphatics Examination

For a PDA-downloadable version, go to http://evolve.elsevier.com/Canada/Jarvis/examination/.

1. **Inspect breasts** as the woman sits, raises arms overhead, pushes hands on hips, leans forward
2. **Inspect** the supraclavicular and infraclavicular areas
3. **Palpate the axillae** and regional lymph nodes
4. With woman supine, **palpate the breast tissue,** including tail of Spence, the nipples, and areolae
5. **Discuss routine breast health behaviours.**

Promoting Health: Assessing Breast Cancer Risk

New Breast Cancer Screening Tool

During a breast examination, the opportunity often arises to review the individual's breast self-examination technique and dates for scheduled mammograms. It is also an opportunity to assess the individual's breast cancer risk, including family history.

The use of breast cancer risk assessment tools in the clinical setting has the potential to improve health substantially by reducing breast cancer incidence through cancer prevention and by more effective early detection programs for high-risk individuals. The *Gail Model* is widely used for calculating individual risk estimates for breast cancer. This model takes into account identified risk factors, including current age, age at menarche, age at first live birth, and family history of breast cancer in first-degree relatives. It also calculates 5-year and lifetime cumulative absolute risk estimates for the individual. It is easy to complete and many computer-based data programs are available to clinicians. However, the ability of the *Gail Model* to identify the subgroup of women with family cancer histories suggestive of hereditary breast cancer syndromes, such as BRCA1 and BRCA2, has come under question.

The *Pedigree Assessment Tool (PAT)* was developed to identify this subgroup of women and can be used along with the Gail Model to screen for breast cancer risk. The PAT score is calculated by adding the points assigned to every family member, including second- and third-degree relatives, with a breast or ovarian cancer diagnosis. Further, points are calculated for bilateral disease, the occurrence of both breast and ovarian cancers, and for the age at diagnosis. A separate score is calculated for the individual's maternal and paternal family histories. The higher of the two scores is used. The specific inclusion of both sides of a women's family is important because many women often disregard or overlook paternal lineage altogether when thinking about or reporting family history of breast cancer.

A computer software program that collects all the relevant risk factor data and calculations of *Gail Model* estimates and the *PAT* score is available. The program is easily used, requires little or no knowledge of breast cancer risk assessment, and is available at no cost from http://www.osfhealth.com.

Hoskins, K.F., Zwaagstra, A., & Ranz, M. (2006). Validation of a tool for identifying women at high risk for hereditary breast cancer in population-based screening. *Cancer, 107,* 1769–1776.

Objective Data

❖➤ DOCUMENTATION AND CRITICAL THINKING ◄❖

Sample Charting

FEMALE

SUBJECTIVE

States no breast pain, lump, discharge, rash, swelling, or trauma. No history of breast disease herself; does have mother with fibrocystic disease. No history of breast surgery. Never been pregnant. Last CBE 1 yr ago. Mammogram yearly, due next month.

OBJECTIVE

Inspection: Breasts symmetrical. Skin smooth with even colour and no rash or lesions. Arm movement shows no dimpling or retractions. No nipple discharge, no lesions.
Palpation: Breast contour and consistency firm and homogeneous. No masses or tenderness. No lymphadenopathy.

ASSESSMENT

Healthy breast structure
Knowledgeable regarding breast screening recommendations

MALE

SUBJECTIVE

No pain, lump, rash, or swelling.

OBJECTIVE

No masses or tenderness. No lymphadenopathy.

Focused Assessment: Clinical Case Study 1

J.G. is a 32-year-old female high-school teacher, married, with no children. She reports good health until finding "lump in my right breast 2 weeks ago."

SUBJECTIVE

- 2 weeks PTA—noticed lump in R breast on self-examination. Lump firm, nonmovable area "the size of a quarter," in upper outer quadrant of breast, tender on touch only. No skin changes, no nipple discharge, on no medications. Last breast exam by MD 3 months before was reported normal. Did not notice lump on previous self-examination 1 month before. No history of breast disease in self or family.
- 2 days PTA—saw MD, who confirmed presence of lump and recommended biopsy as outpatient. Last menstrual period 1/25/(2½ weeks PTA). States the last 2 days has been so nervous has been unable to sleep well or to concentrate at work: "I just know it's cancer."

OBJECTIVE

Voice trembling and breathless during history. Sitting posture stiff and rigid. B/P 148/78. Temp 37°C, pulse 92, resp 16.
Inspection: Breasts symmetrical, nipples everted. No skin lesions, no dimpling, no retraction, no fixation.
Palpation: Left breast firm, no mass, no tenderness, no discharge. Right breast firm, with 2 cm × 2 cm × 1 cm mass at 10:00 position, 5 cm from the nipple. Lump is firm, oval, with smooth discrete borders, nonmovable, tender to palpation. No other mass. No discharge. No lymphadenopathy.

ASSESSMENT

Lump in R breast
Anxiety

Documentation and Critical Thinking

Focused Assessment: Clinical Case Study 2

D.B. is a 62-year-old female bank comptroller, married, with no children. History of hypertension, managed by diuretic medication and diet. No other health problems until yearly company physical examination 3 days PTA, when NP "found a lump in my right breast."

SUBJECTIVE

- 3 days PTA—NP noted lump in R breast during yearly physical examination. NP did not describe lump but told D.B. it was "serious" and needed immediate biopsy. D.B. has not felt it herself. States has noted no skin changes, no nipple discharge. No previous history of breast disease. Mother died age 54 years of breast cancer; no other relative with breast disease. D.B. has had no term pregnancies; two spontaneous abortions, ages 28, 31 years. Menopause completed at age 52 years.
- Married 43 years. States husband supportive, but "I just can't talk to him about this. I can't even go near him now."

OBJECTIVE

Inspection: Breasts symmetrical when sitting, arms down. Nipples flat. No lesions, no discharge. As lifts arms, left breast elevates, right breast stays fixed. Dimple in right breast, 9:00 position, apparent at rest and with muscle contraction. Leaning forward reveals left breast falls free, right breast flattens.

Palpation: Left breast feels soft and granular throughout, no mass. Right breast soft and granular, with large, stony hard mass in outer quadrant. Lump is 5 cm × 4 cm × 2 cm, at 9:00 position, 3 cm from nipple. Borders irregular, mass fixed to tissues, no pain with palpation.

One firm, palpable lymph node in centre of right axilla. No palpable nodes on the left.

ASSESSMENT

Lump in R breast

Situational stress R/T breast lump

Nursing Diagnoses Commonly Associated With Breast Disorders

All nursing diagnoses can be found on the Evolve Web site at **http://evolve.elsevier.com/Canada/Jarvis/examination/.**

Documentation
and Critical Thinking

━━ ❧ ━━ ABNORMAL FINDINGS ━━ ❧ ━━

| TABLE 17-3 | Signs of Retraction and Inflammation in the Breast |

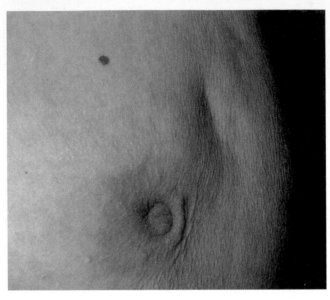

Dimpling

The shallow dimple (also called a skin tether) shown here is a sign of skin retraction. Cancer causes fibrosis, which contracts the suspensory ligaments. The dimple may be apparent at rest, with compression, or with lifting of the arms. Also note the distortion of the areola here as the fibrosis pulls the nipple toward it.

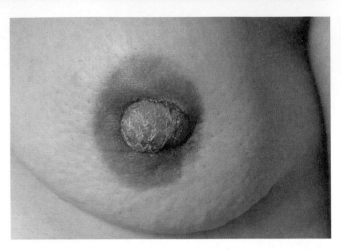

Edema (Peau d'Orange)

Lymphatic obstruction produces edema. This thickens the skin and exaggerates the hair follicles, giving a pig-skin or orange-peel look. This condition suggests cancer. Edema usually begins in the skin around and beneath the areola, the most dependent area of the breast. Also note nipple infiltration here.

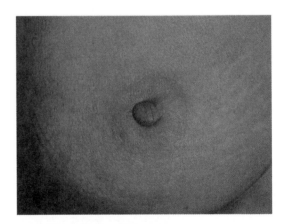

Deviation in Nipple Pointing

An underlying cancer causes fibrosis in the mammary ducts, which pulls the nipple angle toward it. Here, note the swelling behind the right nipple and that the nipple tilts laterally.

Nipple Retraction

The retracted nipple looks flatter and broader, like an underlying crater. A recent retraction suggests cancer, which causes fibrosis of the whole duct system and pulls in the nipple. It also may occur with benign lesions such as ectasia of the ducts. Do not confuse retraction with the normal long-standing type of nipple inversion, which has no broadening and is not fixed.

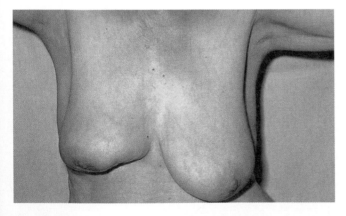

Fixation

Asymmetry, distortion, or decreased mobility with the elevated arm manoeuvre. As cancer becomes invasive, the fibrosis fixes the breast to the underlying pectoral muscles. Here, note the right breast is held against the chest wall.

TABLE 17-4 | Breast Lump

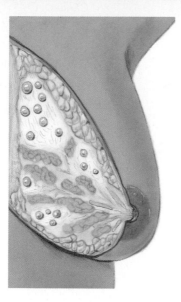

◀ **Benign Breast Disease (Formerly Fibrocystic Breast Disease)**

Multiple tender masses. "Fibrocystic disease" is a meaningless term because it covers too many entities. Actually, six diagnostic categories exist, based on symptoms and physical findings (Love & Lindsey, 2005):

- Swelling and tenderness (cyclical discomfort)
- Mastalgia (severe pain, both cyclical and noncyclical)
- Nodularity (significant lumpiness, both cyclical and noncyclical)
- Dominant lumps (including cysts and fibroadenomas)
- Nipple discharge (including intraductal papilloma and duct ectasia)
- Infections and inflammations (including subareolar abscess, lactational mastitis, breast abscess, and Mondor's disease)

About 50% of all women have some form of benign breast disease. Nodularity occurs bilaterally; regular, firm nodules that are mobile, well demarcated, and feel rubbery, like small water balloons. Pain may be dull, heavy, and cyclical or just before menses as nodules enlarge. Some women have nodularity but no pain, and vice versa. Cysts are discrete, fluid-filled sacs. Dominant lumps and nipple discharge must be investigated carefully and may need biopsy to rule out cancer. Nodularity itself is not premalignant but may produce difficulty in detecting other cancerous lumps.

Cancer

Solitary unilateral nontender mass. Single focus in one area, although it may be interspersed with other nodules. Solid, hard, dense, and fixed to underlying tissues or skin as cancer becomes invasive. Borders are irregular and poorly delineated. Grows constantly. Often painless, although the person may have pain. Most common in upper outer quadrant. Usually found in women 30 to 80 years of age; increased risk in ages 40 to 44 years and in women older than 50 years. As cancer advances, signs include firm or hard irregular axillary nodes; skin dimpling; nipple retraction, elevation, and discharge.

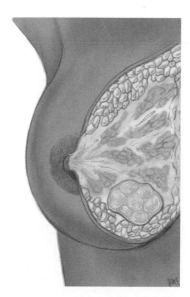

Fibroadenoma

Solitary nontender mass. A category of benign breast disease that deserves mention because of its frequency and characteristic appearance. Solid, firm, rubbery, and elastic. Round, oval, or lobulated; 1 to 5 cm. Freely movable, slippery; fingers slide it easily through tissue. Most common between 15 and 30 years of age but can occur up to age 55 years. Grows quickly and constantly. Benign, although it must be diagnosed by biopsy.

TABLE 17-5	Differentiating Breast Lumps		
	Fibroadenoma	Benign Breast Disease	Cancer
Likely age	15–30 years, can occur up to 55 years	30–55 years, decreases after menopause	30–80 years, risk increases after 50 years
Shape	Round, lobular	Round, lobular	Irregular, star shaped
Consistency	Usually firm, rubbery	Firm to soft, rubbery	Firm to stony hard
Demarcation	Well demarcated, clear margins	Well demarcated	Poorly defined
Number	Usually single	Usually multiple, may be single	Single
Mobility	Very mobile, slippery	Mobile	Fixed
Tenderness	Usually none	Tender, usually increases before menses, may be noncyclical	Usually none, can be tender
Skin retraction	None	None	Usually
Pattern of growth	Grows quickly and constantly	Size may increase or decrease rapidly	Grows constantly
Risk to health	None; they are benign—must diagnose by biopsy	Benign, although general lumpiness may mask other cancerous lump	Serious, needs early treatment

ABNORMAL FINDINGS
FOR ADVANCED PRACTICE

TABLE 17-6 | **Abnormal Nipple Discharge**

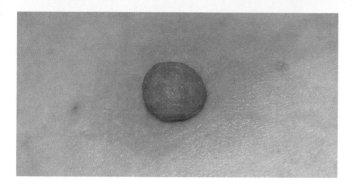

Mammary Duct Ectasia

Pastelike matter in subareolar ducts produces sticky, purulent discharge that may be white, grey, brown, green, or bloody. A light green, single duct discharge is shown here. Caused by stagnation of cellular debris and secretions in the ducts, leading to obstruction, inflammation, and infection. Occurs in women who have lactated; usually occurs in perimenopause.

Itching, burning, or drawing pain occurs around nipple. May have subareolar redness and swelling. Ducts are palpable as rubbery, twisted tubules under areola. May have palpable mass, soft or firm, poorly delineated. Not malignant, but needs biopsy.

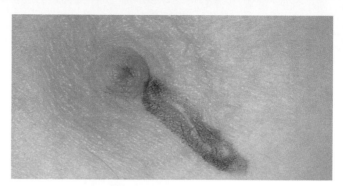

Intraductal Papilloma

Serous or serosanguineous discharge, which is spontaneous, unilateral, or from a single duct. Lesion consists of tiny tumours, 2 to 3 mm. Often there is a palpable nodule in the underlying duct (highlighted here). Papillomas affect women 40 to 60 years of age; most are benign. Refer any bloody discharge for careful evaluation, including biopsy, to rule out cancer.

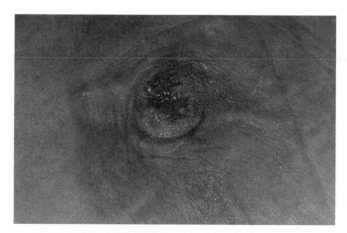

Paget's Disease (Intraductal Carcinoma)

Early lesion has unilateral, clear, yellow discharge and dry, scaling crusts, friable at nipple apex. Spreads outward to areola with erythematous halo on areola and crusted, eczematous, retracted nipple. Later lesion shows nipple reddened, excoriated, ulcerated, with bloody discharge when surface is eroded, and an erythematous plaque surrounding the nipple. Symptoms include tingling, burning, itching.

Except for the redness and occasional cracking from initial breastfeeding, any dermatitis of the nipple area must be carefully explored and referred immediately.

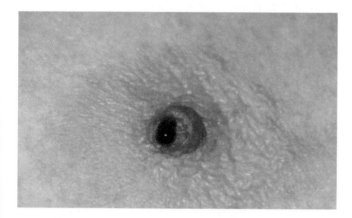

Carcinoma

Bloody nipple discharge that is unilateral and from a single duct requires further investigation. Although there was no palpable lump associated with the discharge shown here, mammography revealed a 1-cm, centrally located, ill-defined mass.

TABLE 17-7	Disorders Occurring During Lactation

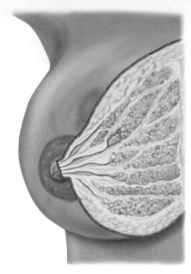

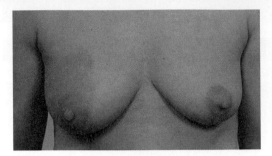

Mastitis

This is uncommon; an inflammatory mass before abscess formation. Usually occurs in single quadrant. Area is red, swollen, tender, very hot, and hard, here forming outward from areola upper edge, in right breast. Also the woman has a headache, malaise, fever, chills and sweating, increased pulse, flulike symptoms. May occur during first 4 months of lactation from infection or from stasis from plugged duct. Treat with rest, local heat to area, antibiotics, and frequent nursing to keep breast as empty as possible. Must not wean now or the breast will become engorged and the pain will increase. Mother's antibiotic not harmful to infant. Usually resolves in 2 to 3 days.

Plugged Duct

A fairly common and not serious condition. One milk duct is clogged. One section of the breast is tender; may be reddened. No infection. It is important to keep breast as empty as possible and milk flowing. The woman should nurse her baby frequently, on affected side first to ensure complete emptying, and manually express any remaining milk. A plugged duct usually resolves in less than 1 day.

Breast Abscess ▶

A rare complication of generalized infection (e.g., mastitis) if untreated. A pocket of pus accumulates in one local area. Here extensive nipple edema, and abscess is "pointing" at 3:00 on areolar margin. Must temporarily discontinue nursing on affected breast; manually express milk and discard. Continue to nurse on unaffected side. Treat with antibiotics, surgical incision, and drainage.

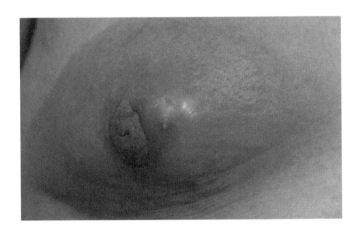

TABLE 17-8	Abnormalities in the Male Breast

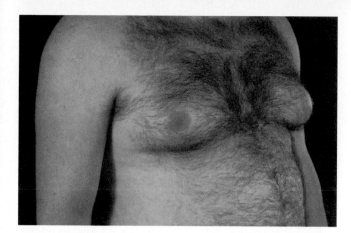

Gynecomastia

Noninflammatory enlargement of male breast tissue. This is physiological at puberty, unilateral, usually mild and transient. Gynecomastia occurs commonly in aging males because of changing hormone levels. It is bilateral and may be tender.

It also occurs bilaterally from hormone stimulation (e.g., on estrogen for cancer of prostate); Cushing's syndrome; cirrhosis of liver as unable to metabolize estrogen completely; leukemia occasionally; and sometimes with medication—digitalis, isoniazid, spironolactone, phenothiazines, and marijuana; testicular tumour, lung cancer; adrenal disease; and thyrotoxicosis.

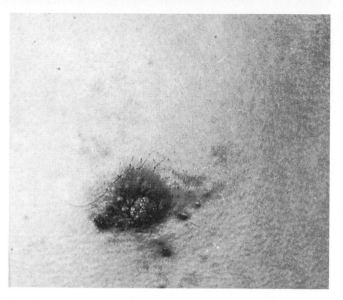

Carcinoma

Fewer than 1% of all breast cancer occurs in men. The lesion is a hard, irregular, nontender mass, most often directly under the areola, fixed to the area, and may have nipple retraction. Mass is noticeable early because of minimal breast tissue. There is also early spread to axillary lymph nodes due to minimal breast tissue. The ulcerating mass shown here had been present for $3\frac{1}{2}$ years and is advanced carcinoma.

BIBLIOGRAPHY

Ahmad, F., Cameron, J. I., & Stewart, D. E. (2005). A tailored intervention to promote breast cancer screening among South Asian immigrant women. *Social Science & Medicine, 60*, 575–586.

Boehmke, M., & Dickerson, S. (2006). The diagnosis of breast cancer: Transition from health to illness. *Oncology Nursing Forum, 33*, 1121–1127.

Buzdar, A. (2006). Dietary modification and risk of breast cancer. *Journal of the American Medical Association, 295*, 691–692.

Canadian Cancer Society. (2007). *Causes of breast cancer.* Retrieved February 14, 2008, from http://www.cancer.ca/ccs/internet/standardpf/0,3182,3172_10175_272579_langId-en,00.html

Canadian Cancer Society. (2008). *Early detection and screening for breast cancer.* Retrieved February 14, 2008, from http://www.cancer.ca/ccs/internet/standard/0,3182,3172_10175_74544430_langId-en,00.html

Colditz, G. A., & Rosner, B. (2000). Cumulative risk of breast cancer to age 70 years according to risk factor status: Data from the Nurses' Health Study. *American Journal of Epidemiology, 152*, 950–964.

Fowler, B. (2006). Social processes used by African American women in making decisions about mammography screening. *Journal of Nursing Scholarship, 38*, 247–254.

Friedman, D. B., & Hoffman-Goetz, L. (2007). Assessing cultural sensitivity of breast cancer information for older Aboriginal women. *Journal of Cancer Education: The Official Journal of the American Association for Cancer Education, 22*(2), 112–118.

Hall, I. J., Newman, B., Millikan, R. C., & Moorman, P. G. (2000). Body size and breast cancer risk in black women and white women. *American Journal of Epidemiology, 151*, 754–764.

Jacobs, E. A., Karavolos, K., Rathouz, P. J., Ferris, T. G., & Powell, L. H. (2005). Limited English proficiency and breast and cervical cancer screening in a multiethnic population. *American Journal of Public Health, 95*, 1410–1416.

Johnson, P. (2002). Breast lumps in the adolescent female. *Journal of Pediatric Health Care, 16*, 43–48.

Johnson, P. (2003). Inflammatory breast cancer in primary care. *Nurse Practitioner, 28*, 57–59.

Klein, S. (2005). Evaluation of palpable breast masses. *American Family Physician, 71*, 1731–1738.

Kramer, M. S., Chalmers, B., Hodnett, E. D., Sevkovskaya, Z., Dzikovick, I., Shapiro, S., et al. (2001). Promotion of Breastfeeding Intervention Trial (PROBIT): a randomized trial in the Republic of Belarus. *Journal of the American Medical Association, 285*, 413–420.

Love, S., & Lindsey, K. (2005). *Dr. Susan Love's breast book* (4th ed.). Cambridge, MA: Da Capo Lifelong Books.

Mitchell, J., Mathews, H., & Mayne, L. (2005). Differences in breast self-examination techniques between Caucasian and African American elderly women. *Journal of Women's Health, 14*, 476–484.

Morrell, R. M., Halyard, M. Y., Schild, S. E., Ali, M. S., Gunderson, L. L., & Pockaj, B. A. (2005). Breast cancer–related lymphedema. *Mayo Clinic Proceedings, 80*, 1480–1484.

National Cancer Institute of Canada. (2007). *Breast cancer statistics, 2007.* Retrieved February 13, 2008, from http://www.ncic.cancer.ca/ncic/internet/standard/0,3621,84658243_85787780_1834604849_langId-en,00.html

Pagano-Therrien, J., & Katz, D. L. (2003). The low-down on low-carbohydrate diets. *Nurse Practitioner, 28*, 5, 14.

Pasacreta, J., Jacobs, L., & Cataldo, J. (2002). Genetic testing for breast and ovarian cancer risk: The psychosocial issues. *American Journal of Nursing, 102*, 40–47.

Prentice, R. L., Caan, B., Chlebowski, R. T., Patterson, R., Kuller, L. H., Ockene, J. K., et al. (2006). Low-fat dietary pattern and risk of invasive breast cancer: the Women's Health Initiative Randomized Controlled Dietary Modification Trial. *Journal of the American Medical Association, 295*, 629–642.

Psyrri, A., & Burtness, B. (2005). Pregnancy associated breast cancer. *Cancer Journal, 11*, 83–95.

Public Health Agency of Canada. (1999). *Breast cancer in Canada.* Retrieved April 18, 2008, from http://www.phac-aspc.gc.ca/publicat/updates/breast-99_e.html

Ringash, J. (2001). Preventive health care, 2001 update: Screening mammography among women aged 40–49 years at average risk of breast cancer. *Canadian Medical Association, 164*, 469–476.

Sandstrom-Wakeling, S. K., Nied, L., Gambino, K., Zak, M., & Duffy, E. (2003). The importance of mammography screening in elderly women. *Nurse Practitioner, 28*, 50–54.

Saslow, D., Hannan, J., Osuch, J., Alciati, M. H., Baines, C., Barton, M., et al. (2004). Clinical breast examination: Practical recommendations for optimizing performance and reporting, *CA: A Cancer Journal for Clinicians, 54*, 327–334.

Simonian, K., Brown, S. E., Sanders, D. B., Kidd, C. Y., Murillo, V. E., Garcia, R., et al. (2004). Promoting breast cancer screening to women of color. *Nurse Practitioner, 29*, 45–46.

Smith, E. D., Phillips, J. M., & Price, M. M. (2001). Screening and early detection among racial and ethnic minority women. *Seminars in Oncology Nursing, 17*, 159–170.

Tanner, J. M. (1962). *Growth at adolescence* (2nd ed.). Oxford, UK: Blackwell Scientific.

Wilkinson, S. (2007). Breast cancer: Lived experience and feminist action. In O. Hankivsky, M. Morrow, & C. Varcoe (Eds.), *Women's health in Canada: Critical theory and policy* (408–434). Toronto, ON: University of Toronto Press.

Wirfält, E., Mattison, I., Gullberg, B., Olsson, H., & Berglund, G. (2005). Fat from different foods show diverging relations with breast cancer risk in postmenopausal women. *Nutrition and Cancer 53*, 135–143.

Wood, R., Giuliano, K. K., & Liu, L. M. (2004). Challenges in mammography screening for older women. *Nurse Practitioner, 29*, 12–13.

Wu, T., Bancroft, J., & Guthrie, B. (2005). An integrative review on breast cancer screening practice and correlates among Chinese, Korean, Filipino, and Asian American Women. *Health Care for Women International, 26*, 225–246.

Yamamoto, D. S., & Viale, P. H. (2006). Does every breast lump need to be worked up despite previous diagnoses? *Clinical Journal of Oncology Nursing, 10*, 821–823.

Zimmerman, V. (2002). BRCA gene mutations and cancer. *American Journal of Nursing, 102*, 28–36.

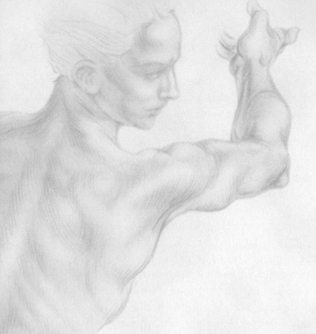

Chapter Eighteen

Thorax and Lungs

Written by **Carolyn Jarvis**, PhD, APN, CNP
Adapted by **June MacDonald-Jenkins**, RN, BScN, MSc

Electronic Resources

On Evolve *evolve*

http://evolve.elsevier.com/Canada/Jarvis/examination/

- Interactive Case Studies
- Physical Examination Audio and Printable Summaries
- Bedside Assessment Summary Checklists
- Complete Physical Examination Form
- Nursing Diagnoses Boxes
- Health Promotion Guides
- Quick Assessments for 20 Common Conditions
- Multiple Choice Review Questions
- Chapter Objectives
- Appendices
- Weblinks

On the Companion CD

- Interactive Case Studies with Heart and Lung Sounds
- Health Promotion Guides
- Quick Assessments for 20 Common Conditions
- Head-to-Toe Physical Examination Video Clips

STRUCTURE AND FUNCTION

POSITION AND SURFACE LANDMARKS

The **thoracic cage** is a bony structure with a conical shape, which is narrower at the top (Fig. 18-1). It is defined by the **sternum,** 12 pairs of **ribs,** and 12 thoracic **vertebrae.** Its "floor" is the **diaphragm,** a musculotendinous septum that separates the thoracic cavity from the abdomen. The first seven ribs attach directly to the sternum via their costal cartilages; ribs 8, 9, and 10 attach to the costal cartilage above, and ribs 11 and 12 are "floating," with free palpable tips. The **costochondral junctions** are the points at which the ribs join their cartilages. They are not palpable.

Anterior Thoracic Landmarks

Surface landmarks on the thorax are signposts for underlying respiratory structures. Knowledge of landmarks will help you localize a finding and will facilitate communication of your findings to others.

Suprasternal Notch. Feel this hollow U-shaped depression just above the sternum, in between the clavicles.

Sternum. The "breastbone" has three parts—the manubrium, the body, and the xiphoid process. Walk your fingers down the manubrium a few centimetres until you feel a distinct bony ridge, the manubriosternal angle.

Manubriosternal Angle. Often called the sternal angle or the "angle of Louis," this is the articulation of the manubrium and body of the sternum, and it is continuous with the second rib. The angle of Louis is a useful place to start counting ribs, which helps localize a respiratory finding horizontally. Identify the angle of Louis, palpate lightly to the second rib, and slide down to the second intercostal space. Each intercostal space is numbered by the rib above it. Continue counting down the ribs in the middle of the hemithorax, not close to the sternum where the costal cartilages lie too close together to count. You can palpate easily down to the tenth rib.

The angle of Louis also marks the site of tracheal bifurcation into the right and left main bronchi; it corresponds with the upper border of the atria of the heart, and it lies above the fourth thoracic vertebra on the back.

Costal Angle. The right and left costal margins form an angle where they meet at the xiphoid process. Usually 90 degrees or less, this angle increases when the rib cage is chronically overinflated, as in emphysema.

Posterior Thoracic Landmarks

Counting ribs and intercostal spaces on the back is a bit harder due to the muscles and soft tissue surrounding the ribs and spinal column (Fig. 18-2).

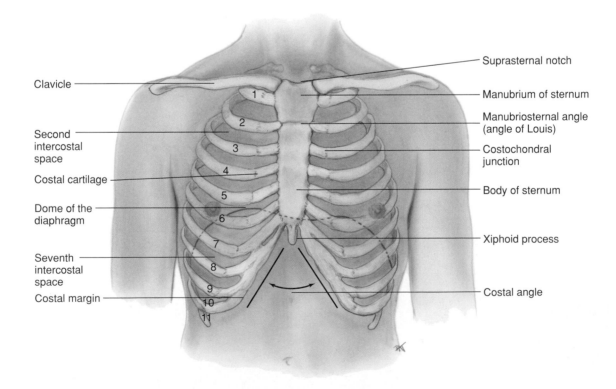

Clavicle

Second intercostal space

Costal cartilage

Dome of the diaphragm

Seventh intercostal space

Costal margin

Suprasternal notch

Manubrium of sternum

Manubriosternal angle (angle of Louis)

Costochondral junction

Body of sternum

Xiphoid process

Costal angle

ANTERIOR THORACIC CAGE

Fig. 18-1

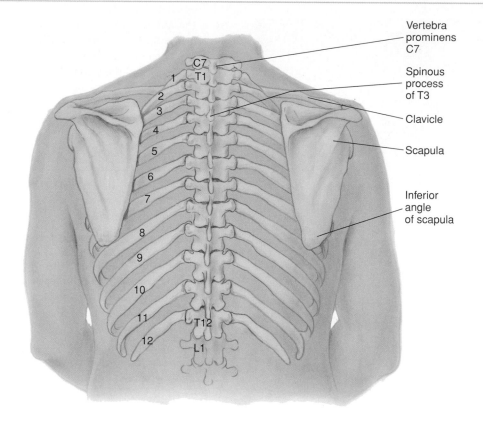

Vertebra prominens C7

Spinous process of T3

Clavicle

Scapula

Inferior angle of scapula

POSTERIOR THORACIC CAGE

Fig. 18-2

Vertebra Prominens. Start here. Flex your head and feel for the most prominent bony spur protruding at the base of the neck. This is the spinous process of C7. If two bumps seem equally prominent, the upper one is C7 and the lower one is T1.

Spinous Processes. Count down these knobs on the vertebrae, which stack together to form the spinal column. Note that the spinous processes align with their same numbered ribs only down to T4. After T4, the spinous processes angle downward from their vertebral body and overlie the vertebral body and rib below.

Inferior Border of the Scapula. The scapulae are located symmetrically in each hemithorax. The lower tip is usually at the seventh or eighth rib.

Twelfth Rib. Palpate midway between the spine and the person's side to identify its free tip.

Reference Lines

Use the reference lines to pinpoint a finding vertically on the chest. On the anterior chest, note the **midsternal** line and the **midclavicular** line. The midclavicular line bisects the centre of each clavicle at a point halfway between the palpated sternoclavicular and acromioclavicular joints (Fig. 18-3).

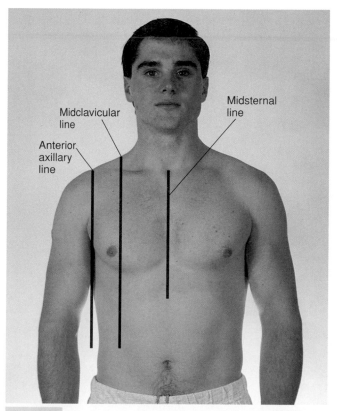

Midclavicular line

Anterior axillary line

Midsternal line

Fig. 18-3

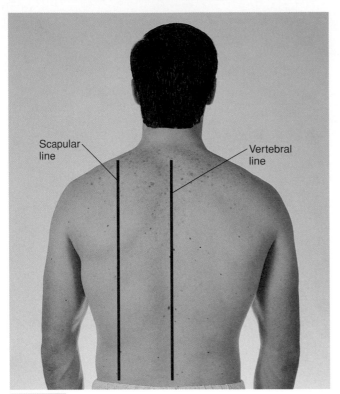

Scapular line

Vertebral line

Fig. 18-4

The posterior chest wall has the **vertebral** (or midspinal) line and the **scapular** line, which extends through the inferior angle of the scapula when the arms are at the sides of the body (Fig. 18-4).

Lift up the person's arm 90 degrees, and divide the lateral chest by three lines: The **anterior axillary** line extends down

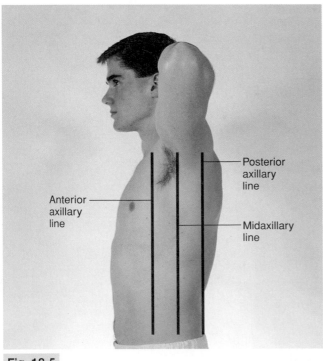

Anterior axillary line

Posterior axillary line

Midaxillary line

Fig. 18-5

from the anterior axillary fold where the pectoralis major muscle inserts; the **posterior axillary** line continues down from the posterior axillary fold where the latissimus dorsi muscle inserts; and the **midaxillary** line runs down from the apex of the axilla and lies between and parallel to the other two (Fig. 18-5).

THE THORACIC CAVITY

The **mediastinum** is the middle section of the thoracic cavity containing the esophagus, trachea, heart, and great vessels. The right and left **pleural cavities,** on either side of the mediastinum, contain the lungs.

Lung Borders. In the anterior chest, the **apex,** or highest point, of lung tissue is 3 or 4 cm above the inner third of the clavicles. The **base,** or lower border, rests on the diaphragm at about the sixth rib in the midclavicular line. Laterally, lung tissue extends from the apex of the axilla down to the seventh or eighth rib. Posteriorly, the location of C7 marks the apex of lung tissue, and T10 usually corresponds to the base. Deep inspiration expands the lungs, and their lower border drops to the level of T12.

Lobes of the Lungs

The lungs are paired but not precisely symmetrical structures (Fig. 18-6). The right lung is shorter than the left lung because of the underlying liver. The left lung is narrower than the right lung because the heart bulges to the left. The right lung has three lobes, and the left lung has two lobes. These lobes are not arranged in horizontal bands like dessert layers in a parfait glass. Rather, they stack in diagonal sloping segments and are separated by **fissures** that run obliquely through the chest.

Anterior. On the anterior chest, the **oblique** (the major or diagonal) fissure crosses the fifth rib in the midaxillary line and terminates at the sixth rib in the midclavicular line. The right lung also contains the **horizontal** (minor) fissure, which divides the right upper and middle lobes. This fissure extends from the fifth rib in the right midaxillary line to the third intercostal space or fourth rib at the right sternal border.

Posterior. The most remarkable point about the posterior chest is that it is almost all lower lobe (Fig. 18-7). The upper lobes occupy a smaller band of tissue from their apices at T1 down to T3 or T4. At this level, the lower lobes begin, and their inferior border reaches down to the level of T10 on expiration and to T12 on inspiration. Note that the right middle lobe does not project onto the posterior chest at all. If the person abducts the arms and places the hands on the back of the head, the division between upper and lower lobes corresponds to the medial border of the scapulae.

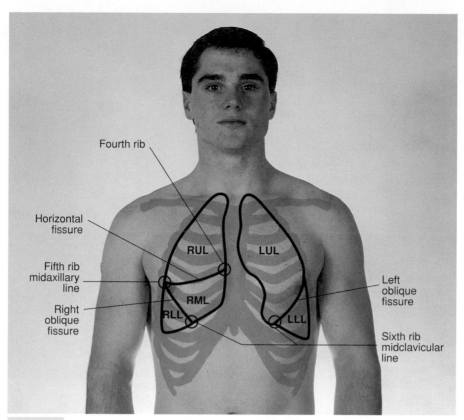

Fourth rib

Horizontal fissure

Fifth rib midaxillary line

Right oblique fissure

RUL

LUL

RML

RLL

LLL

Left oblique fissure

Sixth rib midclavicular line

Fig. 18-6

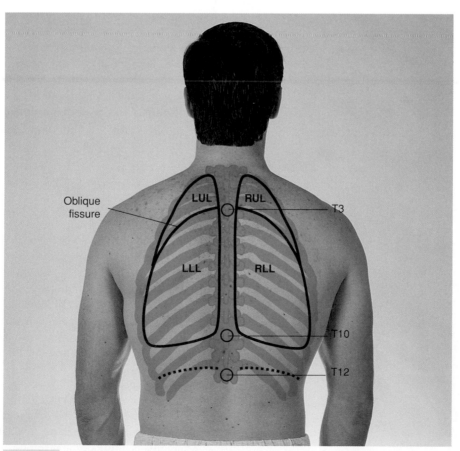

Oblique fissure

LUL

RUL

T3

LLL

RLL

T10

T12

Fig. 18-7

Lateral. Laterally, lung tissue extends from the apex of the axilla down to the seventh or eighth rib. The right upper lobe extends from the apex of the axilla down to the horizontal fissure at the fifth rib (Fig. 18-8). The right middle lobe extends from the horizontal fissure down and forward to the sixth rib at the midclavicular line. The right lower lobe continues from the fifth rib to the eighth rib in the midaxillary line.

The left lung contains only two lobes, upper and lower (Fig. 18-9). These are seen laterally as two triangular areas separated by the oblique fissure. The left upper lobe extends from the apex of the axilla down to the fifth rib at the midaxillary line. The left lower lobe continues down to the eighth rib in the midaxillary line.

Using these landmarks, take a marker and try tracing the outline of each lobe on a willing partner. Take special note of the three points that commonly confuse beginning examiners:
1. The left lung has no middle lobe.
2. The anterior chest contains mostly upper and middle lobe with very little lower lobe.
3. The posterior chest contains almost all lower lobe.

Pleurae

The thin, slippery **pleurae** form an envelope between the lungs and the chest wall (Fig. 18-10). The **visceral** pleura lines the outside of the lungs, dipping down into the fissures. It is continuous with the **parietal** pleura lining the inside of the chest wall and diaphragm.

The inside of the envelope, the pleural cavity, is a potential space filled only with a few millilitres of lubricating fluid. It

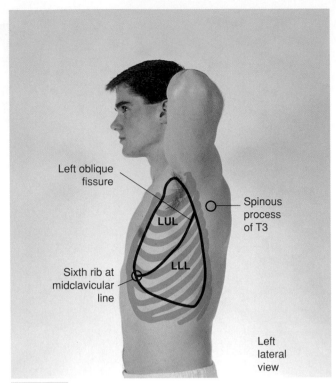

Fig. 18-9

normally has a vacuum, or negative pressure, which holds the lungs tightly against the chest wall. The lungs slide smoothly and noiselessly up and down during respiration, lubricated by a few millilitres of fluid. Think of this as similar to two glass slides with a drop of water between them; although it is difficult to separate the slides, they slide smoothly back and forth. The pleurae extend about 3 cm below the level of the lungs, forming the **costodiaphragmatic recess.** This is a potential space; when it abnormally fills with air or fluid, it compromises lung expansion.

Trachea and Bronchial Tree

The **trachea** lies anterior to the esophagus and is 10 to 11 cm long in the adult. It begins at the level of the cricoid cartilage in the neck and bifurcates just below the sternal angle into the right and left main bronchi. Posteriorly, tracheal bifurcation is at the level of T4 or T5. The right main bronchus is shorter, wider, and more vertical than the left main bronchus.

The **trachea** and **bronchi** transport gases between the environment and the lung parenchyma. They constitute the *dead space,* or space that is filled with air but is not available for gaseous exchange. This is about 150 mL in the adult. The bronchial tree also protects alveoli from small particulate matter in the inhaled air. The bronchi are lined with goblet cells, which secrete mucus that entraps the particles. The bronchi are lined with cilia, which sweep the particles upward where they can be swallowed or expelled.

An **acinus** is a functional respiratory unit that consists of the bronchioles, alveolar ducts, alveolar sacs, and the alveoli.

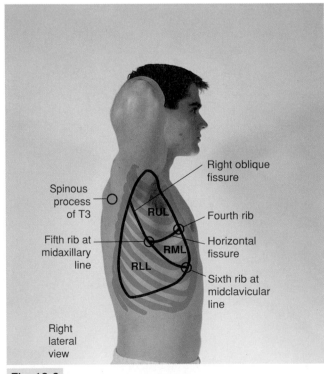

Fig. 18-8

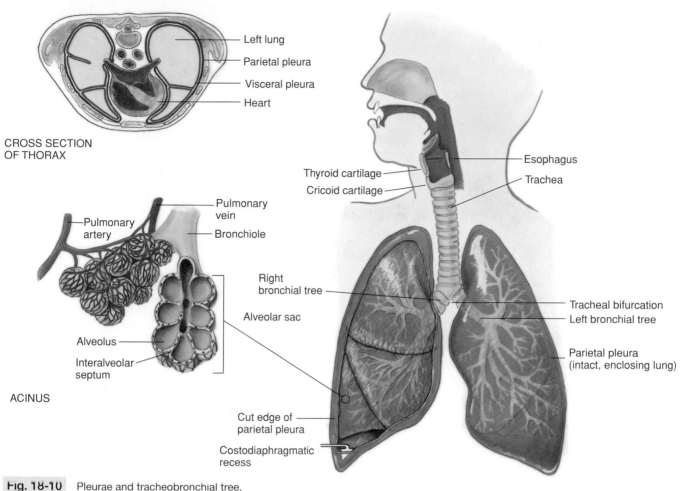

CROSS SECTION
OF THORAX

ACINUS

Fig. 18-10   Pleurae and tracheobronchial tree.

Gaseous exchange occurs across the respiratory membrane in the alveolar duct and in the millions of alveoli. Note how the alveoli are clustered like grapes around each alveolar duct. This creates millions of interalveolar septa (walls) that tremendously increase the working space available for gas exchange. This bunched arrangement creates a surface area for gas exchange that is as large as a tennis court.

MECHANICS OF RESPIRATION

There are four major functions of the respiratory system: (1) supplying oxygen to the body for energy production, (2) removing carbon dioxide as a waste product of energy reactions, (3) maintaining homeostasis (acid–base balance) of arterial blood, and (4) maintaining heat exchange (less important in humans).

By supplying oxygen to the blood and eliminating excess carbon dioxide, respiration maintains the pH or the acid–base balance of the blood. The body tissues are bathed by blood that normally has a narrow acceptable range of pH. Although a number of compensatory mechanisms regulate the pH, the lungs help maintain the balance by adjusting the level of carbon dioxide through respiration. That is, hypoventilation (slow, shallow breathing) causes carbon dioxide to build up in the blood, and hyperventilation (rapid, deep breathing) causes carbon dioxide to be blown off.

Control of Respirations

Normally, our breathing pattern changes without our awareness in response to cellular demands. This involuntary control of respirations is mediated by the respiratory centre in the brainstem (pons and medulla). The major feedback loop is humoral regulation, or the change in carbon dioxide and oxygen levels in the blood, and, less importantly, the hydrogen ion level. The *normal stimulus to breathe* for most of us is an increase of carbon dioxide in the blood, or **hypercapnia.** A decrease of oxygen in the blood (**hypoxemia**) also increases respirations but is less effective than hypercapnia.

Changing Chest Size

Respiration is the physical act of breathing; air rushes into the lungs as the chest size increases (inspiration) and is expelled from the lungs as the chest recoils (expiration). The mechanical expansion and contraction of the chest cavity alters the size of the thoracic container in two dimensions: (1) the vertical diameter lengthens or shortens, which is

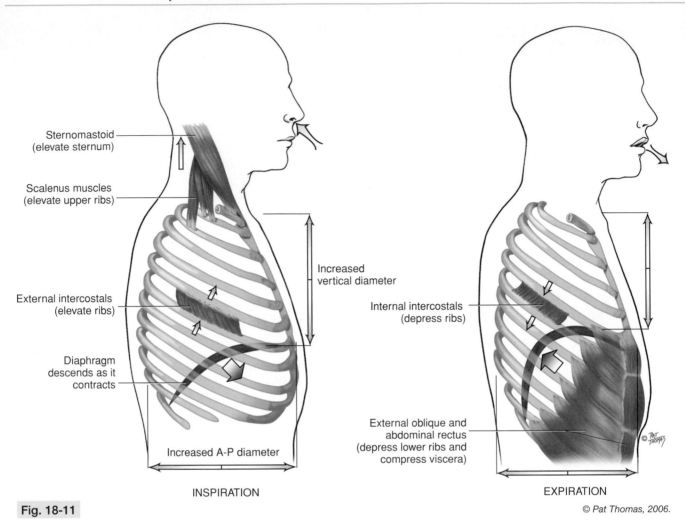

Sternomastoid
(elevate sternum)

Scalenus muscles
(elevate upper ribs)

External intercostals
(elevate ribs)

Diaphragm
descends as it
contracts

Increased
vertical diameter

Increased A-P diameter

INSPIRATION

Fig. 18-11

Internal intercostals
(depress ribs)

External oblique and
abdominal rectus
(depress lower ribs and
compress viscera)

EXPIRATION

© Pat Thomas, 2006.

accomplished by downward or upward movement of the diaphragm, and (2) the anteroposterior diameter increases or decreases, which is accomplished by elevation or depression of the ribs (Fig. 18-11).

In inspiration, increasing the size of the thoracic container creates a slightly negative pressure in relation to the atmosphere, so air rushes in to fill the partial vacuum. The major muscle responsible for this increase is the diaphragm. During inspiration, contraction of the bell-shaped diaphragm causes it to descend and flatten. This lengthens the vertical diameter. Intercostal muscles lift the sternum and elevate the ribs, making them more horizontal. This increases the anteroposterior diameter.

Expiration is primarily passive. As the diaphragm relaxes, elastic forces within the lung, chest cage, and abdomen cause it to dome up. All this squeezing creates a relatively positive pressure within the alveoli, and the air flows out.

Forced inspiration, such as that after heavy exercise or occurring pathologically with respiratory distress, commands the use of the accessory neck muscles to heave up the sternum and rib cage. These neck muscles are the sternomastoids, the scaleni, and the trapezii. In forced expiration, the abdominal muscles contract powerfully to push the abdominal viscera forcefully in and up against the diaphragm, making it dome upward and squeeze against the lungs.

DEVELOPMENTAL CARE

Infants and Children

During the first 5 weeks of fetal life, the primitive lung bud emerges; by 16 weeks, the conducting airways reach the same number as in the adult; at 32 weeks, **surfactant,** the complex lipid substance needed for sustained inflation of the air sacs, is present in adequate amounts; and by birth, the lungs have 70 million primitive alveoli ready to start the job of respiration.

Breath is life. When the newborn inhales the first breath, the lusty cry that follows reassures anxious parents that their baby is all right (Fig. 18-12). The baby's body systems all develop in utero, but the respiratory system alone does not function until birth. Birth demands its instant performance.

When the cord is cut, blood is cut off from the placenta, and it gushes into the pulmonary circulation. Relatively less resistance exists in the pulmonary arteries than in the aorta, so the foramen ovale in the heart closes just after birth. (See the discussion of fetal circulation in Chapter 19.) The ductus arteriosus (linking the pulmonary artery and the aorta) contracts and closes some hours later, and pulmonary and systemic circulation are functional.

Respiratory development continues throughout childhood, with increases in the diameter and length of airways and in the size and number of alveoli, reaching the adult range of 300 million by adolescence.

The relatively smaller size and immaturity of children's pulmonary systems and the presence of older caregivers who smoke result in enormous vulnerability and increased risks to child health. Prenatal exposure results in chronic hypoxia and low birth weight. Postnatal exposure to environmental tobacco smoke (ETS) is linked to increased rates of otitis media, respiratory tract infections, and childhood asthma (DiFranza et al., 2004). Other conditions associated with ETS exposure include sudden infant death syndrome, negative behavioural and cognitive functioning, and increased rates of adolescent smoking.

The Pregnant Female

The enlarging uterus elevates the diaphragm 4 cm during pregnancy. This decreases the vertical diameter of the thoracic cage, but this decrease is compensated for by an increase in the horizontal diameter. The increase in estrogen level relaxes the chest cage ligaments. This allows an increase in the transverse diameter of the chest cage by 2 cm, and the costal angle widens. The total circumference of the chest cage increases by 6 cm. Although the diaphragm is elevated, it is not fixed. It moves with breathing even more during

pregnancy, which results in an increase in tidal volume (Cunningham et al., 2005).

The growing fetus increases the oxygen demand on the mother's body. This is met easily by the increasing tidal volume (deeper breathing). Little change occurs in the respiratory rate. An increased awareness of the need to breathe develops, even early in pregnancy, and some pregnant women may interpret this as dyspnea, although structurally nothing is wrong.

The Aging Adult

In the aging adult, the costal cartilages become calcified, which produces a less mobile thorax. Respiratory muscle strength declines after age 50 years and continues to decrease into the 70s. A more significant change is the decrease in elastic properties within the lungs, making them less distensible and lessening their tendency to contract and recoil. In all, the aging lung is a more rigid structure that is harder to inflate.

These changes result in an increase in small airway closure, and that yields a *decreased vital capacity* (the maximum amount of air that a person can expel from the lungs after first filling the lungs to maximum) and an *increased residual volume* (the amount of air remaining in the lungs even after the most forceful expiration).

With aging, histological changes (i.e., a gradual loss of intra-alveolar septa and a decreased number of alveoli) also occur, so less surface area is available for gas exchange. Also, the lung bases become less ventilated as a result of the closing off of a number of airways. This increases the older person's risk of dyspnea with exertion beyond his or her usual workload.

The histological changes also increase the older person's risk of postoperative pulmonary complications. That is, the older person has a greater risk of postoperative atelectasis and infection from a decreased ability to cough, a loss of protective airway reflexes, and increased secretions.

CULTURAL AND SOCIAL CONSIDERATIONS

A disproportionately large number of **tuberculosis** (TB) cases were reported in 2007 among immigrants, accounting for 67% of all reported cases in Canada. Canadian-born non-Aboriginal and Canadian-born Aboriginal cases made up 12% and 20%, respectively. In 2006, 1621 cases (5 per 100,000 populations) of new active and relapsed TB were reported to the Canadian Tuberculosis Reporting System. Rates have been consistently highest in Nunavut, with lowest rates in the Maritime provinces. The three most populous provinces (British Columbia, Ontario, and Quebec) account for 76% of total reported cases (Public Health Agency of Canada [PHAC], 2006).

In 2005, 2.7 million Canadians were identified as active **asthma** cases. The two most important preventable risk factors for respiratory disease are tobacco smoke (both personal and second-hand) and air quality (indoor and outdoor). Asthma was a contributing factor in approximately 10% of

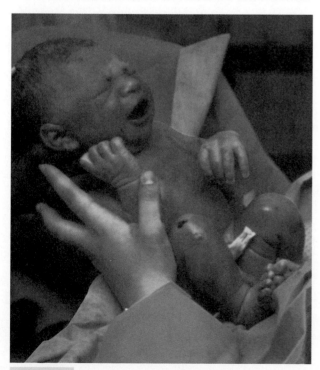

Fig. 18-12

the admissions for children under the age of 5 and 8% for those aged 5 to 14 years (PHAC, 2007).

Respiratory diseases, including lung cancer, are a major cause of death in Canada. Among major health problems, respiratory diseases (excluding lung cancer) ranked fourth (10.3%) in the total proportion of direct healthcare costs.

Maternal smoking during pregnancy contributes to preterm birth, the major factor associated with the development of respiratory distress syndrome in infants. All Canadians are affected by the quality of the air that they breathe, but the effects are more severe on those who live with a respiratory disease (PHAC, 2007).

SUBJECTIVE DATA

1. Cough
2. Shortness of breath
3. Chest pain with breathing

4. History of respiratory infections
5. Smoking history

6. Environmental exposure
7. Self-care behaviours

Examiner Asks	Rationale
1. Cough. Do you have a **cough?** When did it start? Gradual or sudden? • How long have you had it? • How often do you cough? At any special time of day or just on arising? Cough wake you up at night?	Some conditions have a characteristic timing of a cough: • Continuous throughout day—acute illness (e.g., respiratory infection) • Afternoon/evening—may reflect exposure to irritants at work • Night—postnasal drip, sinusitis • Early morning—chronic bronchial inflammation of smokers
• Do you cough up any phlegm or sputum? How much? What colour is it?	• Chronic bronchitis is characterized by a history of productive cough for 3 months of the year for 2 years in a row. **Hemoptysis.**
• Cough up any blood? Does this look like streaks or frank blood? Does the sputum have a foul odour?	Some conditions have characteristic sputum production: white or clear mucoid—colds, bronchitis, viral infections; yellow or green—bacterial infections; rust coloured—tuberculosis, pneumococcal pneumonia; pink, frothy—pulmonary edema, some sympathomimetic medications have a side effect of pink-tinged mucus.
• How would you describe your cough: hacking, dry, barking, hoarse, congested, bubbling?	Some conditions have a characteristic cough: *Mycoplasma* pneumonia—hacking; early heart failure—dry; croup—barking; colds, bronchitis, pneumonia—congested.
• Cough seem to come with anything: activity, position (lying), fever, congestion, talking, anxiety? • Activity make it better or worse? • What treatment have you tried? Prescription or over-the-counter medications, vaporizer, rest, position change?	Assess effectiveness of coping strategies.
• Does the cough bring on anything: chest pain, ear pain? Is it tiring? Are you concerned about it?	Note severity.
2. Shortness of breath. Ever had any **shortness of breath (SOB)** or hard-breathing spells? What brings it on? How severe is it? How long does it last?	Determine how much activity precipitates the SOB—state specific number of blocks walked, number of stairs.

Examiner Asks	Rationale
• Is it affected by position, such as lying down?	**Orthopnea** is difficulty breathing when supine. State number of pillows needed to achieve comfort (e.g., "two-pillow orthopnea").
• Occur at any specific time of day or night?	**Paroxysmal nocturnal dyspnea** is awakening from sleep with SOB and needing to be upright to achieve comfort. Diaphoresis. Cyanosis.
• Shortness of breath episodes associated with night sweats? • Or cough, chest pain, or bluish colour around lips or nails? Wheezing sound? • Episodes seem to be related to food, pollen, dust, animals, season, or emotion? • What do you do in a hard-breathing attack? Take a special position, or use pursed-lip breathing? Use any oxygen, inhalers, or medications? • How does the SOB affect your work or home activities? Getting better or worse or staying about the same?	Asthma attacks may be associated with a specific allergen or extreme cold, anxiety. Assess effect of coping strategies and the need for more teaching. Assess effect on activities of daily living.
3. **Chest pain with breathing.** Any **chest pain with breathing?** Please point to the exact location. • When did it start? Constant, or does it come and go? • Describe the pain: burning, stabbing? • Brought on by respiratory infection, coughing, or trauma? Is it associated with fever, deep breathing, unequal chest inflation? • What have you done to treat it? Medication or heat application?	
4. **History of respiratory infections.** Any **past history** of breathing trouble or lung diseases such as bronchitis, emphysema, asthma, pneumonia? • Any unusually frequent or unusually severe colds? • Any family history of allergies, tuberculosis, or asthma?	Consider sequelae after these conditions. Because most people have had some colds, it is more meaningful to ask about excess number or severity. Assess possible risk factors.
5. **Smoking history.** Do you **smoke** cigarettes or cigars? At what age did you start? How many packs per day do you smoke now? For how long? • Have you ever tried to quit? What helped? Why do you think it did not work? What activities do you associate with smoking? • Live with someone who smokes?	State number of packs per day and the number of years smoked. Most people already know they should quit smoking. Instead of admonishing, assess smoking behaviour and ways to modify daily smoking activities.
6. **Environmental exposure.** Are there any **environmental conditions** that may affect your breathing? Where do you work? At a factory, chemical plant, coal mine, farm, outdoors in a heavy traffic area? • Do anything to protect your lungs, such as wear a mask or have the ventilatory system checked at work? Do anything to monitor your exposure? Have periodic examinations, pulmonary function tests, radiographic examination?	Pollution exposure. Farmers may be at risk for grain inhalation and pesticide inhalation. "Farmer's lung" (**extrinsic allergic alveolitis**) occurs in about 2 to 10% of farm workers, depending on the region. The disease is most common in Canada in regions with wet weather at harvest time. Coal miners have a risk of pneumoconiosis. Stone cutters, miners, potters—silicosis. Other irritants: asbestos, radon. Assess **self-care** measures.

Subjective Data

Examiner Asks	Rationale
• Do you know what specific symptoms to note that may signal breathing problems?	General symptoms: cough, SOB. Some gases produce specific symptoms: carbon monoxide—dizziness, headache, fatigue; sulphur dioxide—cough, congestion.
7. Self-care behaviours. Last tuberculosis skin test, chest radiographic study, pneumonia or influenza immunization?	Self-care measures.

Additional History for Infants and Children

1. Has the child had any frequent or very severe colds?

Limit of four to six uncomplicated upper respiratory infections per year is expected in early childhood.

2. Is there any history of allergy in the family?
  • (For child under 2 years of age): At what age were new foods introduced? Was the child breastfed or bottle-fed?

Consider new foods or formula as possible allergens.

3. Does the child have a cough? Seem congested? Have noisy breathing or wheezing? (Further questions similar to those listed in the section on adults.)

Screen for onset, and follow course of childhood chronic respiratory problems: asthma, bronchitis.

4. What measures have you taken to child-proof your home? Yard? Is there any risk of the child inhaling or swallowing toxic substances?
  • Has anyone taught you emergency care measures in case of accidental choking or a hard-breathing spell?

Young child is at risk for accidental aspiration, poisoning, and injury.

Assess knowledge level of parents and caregivers.

5. Any smokers in the home or in the car with child?

ETS increases the risk of ear and respiratory infections in children (DiFranza et al., 2004).

Additional History for the Aging Adult

1. Have you noticed any SOB or fatigue with your daily activities?

Older adults have a less efficient respiratory system (decreased vital capacity, less surface area for gas exchange), so they have less tolerance for activity.

2. Tell me about your usual amount of physical activity.

May have reduced capacity to perform exercise because of pulmonary function deficits of aging.

Sedentary or bedridden people are at risk for respiratory dysfunction.

3. (For those with a history of chronic obstructive pulmonary disease [COPD], lung cancer, or tuberculosis): How are you getting along each day? Any weight change in the last 3 months? How much?
  • How about energy level? Do you tire more easily? How does your illness affect you at home? At work?

Assess coping strategies.

Activities may decrease because of increasing SOB or pain.

4. Do you have any chest pain with breathing?

Some older adults feel pleuritic pain less intensely than younger adults.

  • Any chest pain after a bout of coughing? After a fall?

Precisely localized sharp pain (points to it with one finger)—consider fractured rib or muscle injury.

OBJECTIVE DATA

PREPARATION

Ask the person to sit upright and the male to disrobe to the waist. For the female, leave the gown on and open at the back. When examining the anterior chest, lift up the gown and drape it on her shoulders rather than removing it completely. This promotes comfort by giving her the feeling of being somewhat clothed. These provisions will ensure further comfort: a warm room, a warm diaphragm end piece, and a private examination time with no interruptions.

For smooth choreography in a complete examination, begin the respiratory examination just after palpating the thyroid gland when you are standing behind the person. Perform the inspection, palpation, percussion, and auscultation on the posterior and lateral thorax. Then move to face the person, and repeat the four manoeuvres on the anterior chest. This avoids repetitiously moving front to back around the person.

Finally, clean your stethoscope end piece with an alcohol wipe. Because your stethoscope touches many people, it could be a possible vector for both aerobic and anaerobic bacteria. Cleaning with an alcohol wipe is very effective.

EQUIPMENT NEEDED

Stethoscope
Small ruler, marked in centimetres
Marking pen
Alcohol wipe

Normal Range of Findings	Abnormal Findings

INSPECT THE POSTERIOR CHEST

Thoracic Cage

Note the **shape and configuration** of the chest wall. The spinous processes should appear in a straight line. The thorax is symmetrical, in an elliptical shape, with downward sloping ribs, about 45 degrees relative to the spine. The scapulae are placed symmetrically in each hemithorax.

The anteroposterior diameter should be less than the transverse diameter. The ratio of anteroposterior to transverse diameter is from 1:2 to 5:7.

The neck muscles and trapezius muscles should have developed normally for age and occupation.

Note the **position** the person takes to breathe. This includes a relaxed posture and the ability to support one's own weight with arms comfortably at the sides or in the lap.

Assess the **skin colour and condition.** Colour should be consistent with the person's genetic background, with allowance for sun-exposed areas on the chest and the back. No cyanosis or pallor should be present. Note any lesions. Inquire as to any change in a nevus on the back, for example, where the person may have difficulty monitoring (see Chapter 12).

Abnormal Findings

Skeletal deformities may limit thoracic cage excursion: scoliosis, kyphosis (see Table 18-3, p. 465).

Anteroposterior = transverse diameter, or "barrel chest." Ribs are horizontal, chest appears as if held in continuous inspiration. This occurs in chronic emphysema from hyperinflation of the lungs (see Table 18-3, p. 465).

Neck muscles are hypertrophied in chronic obstructive pulmonary disease (COPD) from aiding in forced respirations.

People with COPD often sit in a tripod position, leaning forward with arms braced against their knees, chair, or bed. This gives them leverage so that their rectus abdominis, intercostal, and accessory neck muscles all can aid in expiration.

PALPATE THE POSTERIOR CHEST

Symmetrical Expansion

Confirm **symmetrical chest expansion** by placing your warmed hands on the posterolateral chest wall with thumbs at the level of T9 or T10. Slide your hands medially to pinch up a small fold of skin between your thumbs (Fig. 18-13).

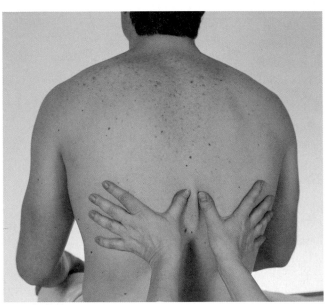

Fig. 18-13

Ask the person to take a deep breath. Your hands serve as mechanical amplifiers; as the person inhales deeply, your thumbs should move apart symmetrically. Note any lag in expansion.

Unequal chest expansion occurs with marked atelectasis or pneumonia; with thoracic trauma such as fractured ribs; or with pneumothorax.

Pain accompanies deep breathing when the pleurae are inflamed.

Tactile Fremitus

Assess **tactile** (or **vocal**) **fremitus.** Fremitus is a palpable vibration. Sounds generated from the larynx are transmitted through patent bronchi and through the lung parenchyma to the chest wall, where you feel them as vibrations.

Use either the palmar base (the ball) of the fingers or the ulnar edge of one hand, and touch the person's chest while he or she repeats the words "ninety-nine" or "blue moon." These are resonant phrases that generate strong vibrations. Start over the lung apices, and palpate from one side to another (Fig. 18-14).

Objective Data

Normal Range of Findings

Abnormal Findings

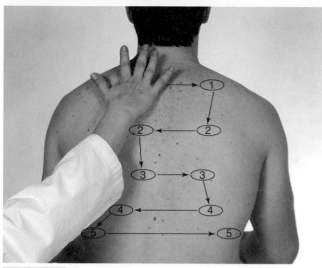

Fig. 18-14

Fremitus varies among persons, but symmetry is most important; the vibrations should feel the same in the corresponding area on each side. However, just between the scapulae, fremitus may feel stronger on the right side than on the left side because the right side is closer to the bronchial bifurcation. Avoid palpating over the scapulae because bone damps sound transmission.

The following factors affect the normal intensity of tactile fremitus:

- Relative location of bronchi to the chest wall.

    Normally, fremitus is most prominent between the scapulae and around the sternum, sites where the major bronchi are closest to the chest wall. Fremitus normally decreases as you progress down because more and more tissue impedes sound transmission.

- Thickness of the chest wall.

    Fremitus feels greater over a thin chest wall than over an obese or heavily muscular one where thick tissue damps the vibration.

- Pitch and intensity.

    A loud, low-pitched voice generates more fremitus than does a soft, high-pitched one.

Note any areas of abnormal fremitus. Sound is conducted better through a uniformly dense structure than through a porous one, which changes in shape and solidity (as does the lung tissue during normal respiration). Thus conditions that increase the density of lung tissue make a better conducting medium for sound vibrations and increase tactile fremitus.

Using the fingers, gently **palpate the entire chest wall.** This enables you to note any areas of tenderness, to note skin temperature and moisture, to detect any superficial lumps or masses, and to explore any skin lesions noted on inspection.

Decreased fremitus occurs when anything obstructs transmission of vibrations (e.g., obstructed bronchus, pleural effusion or thickening, pneumothorax, or emphysema). Any barrier that comes between the sound and your palpating hand will decrease fremitus.

Increased fremitus occurs with compression or consolidation of lung tissue (e.g., lobar pneumonia). This is present only when the bronchus is patent and when the consolidation extends to the lung surface. Note that only gross changes increase fremitus. Small areas of early pneumonia do not significantly affect fremitus.

Rhonchal fremitus is palpable with thick bronchial secretions.

Pleural friction fremitus is palpable with inflammation of the pleura (see Table 18-5, p. 465).

Crepitus is a coarse crackling sensation palpable over the skin surface. It occurs in subcutaneous emphysema when air escapes from the lung and enters the subcutaneous tissue, as after open thoracic injury or surgery.

Normal Range of Findings	Abnormal Findings

PERCUSS THE POSTERIOR CHEST

Lung Fields

Determine the **predominant note over the lung fields.** Start at the apices and percuss the band of normally resonant tissue across the tops of both shoulders (Fig. 18-15). Then, percussing in the interspaces, make a side-to-side comparison all the way down the lung region. Percuss at 5-cm intervals. Avoid the damping effect of the scapulae and ribs.

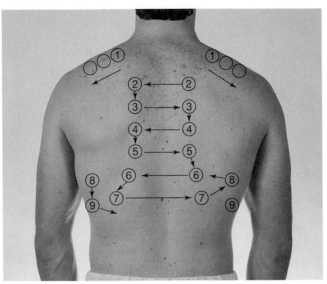

Fig. 18-15

Resonance is the low-pitched, clear, hollow sound that predominates in healthy lung tissue in the adult (Fig. 18-16). However, resonance is a relative term and has no constant standard. The resonant note may be modified somewhat in the athlete with a heavily muscular chest wall and in the heavily obese adult in whom subcutaneous fat produces scattered dullness.

Hyperresonance is a lower-pitched, booming sound found when too much air is present, as in emphysema or pneumothorax.

A **dull** note (soft, muffled thud) signals abnormal density in the lungs, as with pneumonia, pleural effusion, atelectasis, or tumour.

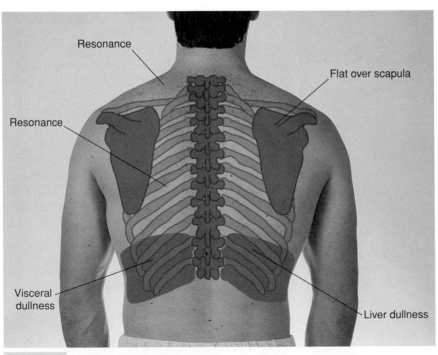

Resonance

Flat over scapula

Resonance

Visceral dullness

Liver dullness

Fig. 18-16   Expected percussion notes.

Objective Data

Normal Range of Findings

The depth of penetration of percussion has limits. Percussion sets into motion only the outer 5 to 7 cm of tissue. It will not penetrate to reveal any change in density deeper than that. Also, an abnormal finding must be 2 to 3 cm wide to yield an abnormal percussion note. Lesions smaller than that are not detectable by percussion.

Diaphragmatic Excursion

Determine **diaphragmatic excursion** (Fig. 18-17, *A*). Percuss to map out the lower lung border, both in expiration and in inspiration. First, ask the person to "exhale and hold it" briefly while you percuss down the scapular line until the sound changes from resonant to dull on each side. This estimates the level of the diaphragm separating the lungs from the abdominal viscera. It may be somewhat higher on the right side (about 1 to 2 cm) because of the presence of the liver. Mark the spot.

Now ask the person to "take a deep breath and hold it." Continue percussing down from your first mark, and mark the level where the sound changes to dull on this deep inspiration. Measure the difference. This diaphragmatic excursion should be equal bilaterally and measure about 3 to 5 cm in adults, although it may be up to 7 to 8 cm in well-conditioned people (Fig. 18-17, *B*).

Abnormal Findings

Note any abnormally high level of dullness and absence of excursion. These occur with pleural effusion (fluid in the space between the visceral and parietal pleura) or atelectasis of the lower lobes.

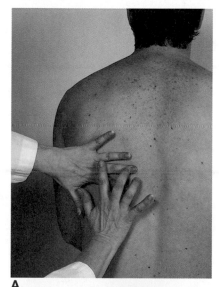

A

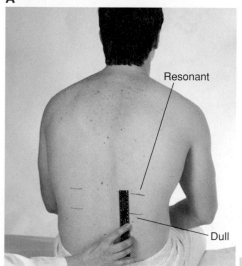

Resonant

Dull

Fig. 18-17

B

Objective Data

Often, the beginning examiner becomes so involved in the subtle differences of percussion notes that he or she extends the patient's limits of breathholding. Always hold your own breath when you ask your patient to. When you run out of air, the other person surely has, too, especially if that person has a respiratory problem.

AUSCULTATE THE POSTERIOR CHEST

The passage of air through the tracheobronchial tree creates a characteristic set of noises that are audible through the chest wall. These noises also may be modified by obstruction within the respiratory passageways or by changes in the lung parenchyma, the pleura, or the chest wall.

Breath Sounds

Evaluate the presence and quality of **normal breath sounds.** The person is sitting, leaning forward slightly, with arms resting comfortably across the lap. Instruct the person to breathe through the mouth, a little bit deeper than usual, but to stop if he or she begins to feel dizzy. Be careful to monitor the breathing throughout the examination and allow times for the person to rest and breathe normally. The person is usually willing to comply with your instructions in an effort to please you and to be a "good patient." Watch that he or she does not hyperventilate to the point of fainting.

Hold the flat diaphragm end piece of the stethoscope firmly on the person's chest wall. Listen to at least one full respiration in each location. Side-to-side comparison is most important.

Do not confuse background noise with lung sounds. Become familiar with these extraneous noises that may be confused with lung pathology if not recognized:

1. Examiner's breathing on stethoscope tubing
2. Stethoscope tubing bumping together
3. Patient shivering
4. Patient's hairy chest; movement of hairs under stethoscope sounds like crackles (rales) (see p. 469)—minimize this by pressing harder or by wetting the hair with a damp cloth
5. Rustling of paper gown or paper drapes

While standing behind the person, listen to the following lung areas—posterior from the apices at C7 to the bases (around T10) and laterally from the axilla down to the seventh or eighth rib. Use the sequence illustrated in Fig. 18-18.

Normal Range of Findings	Abnormal Findings

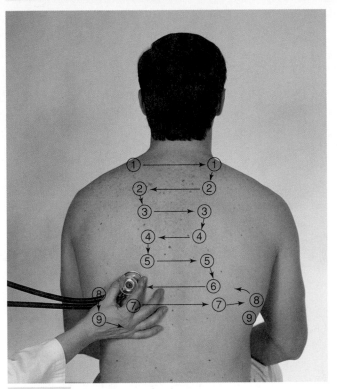

Fig. 18-18   Sequence for auscultation.

Continue to visualize approximate locations of the lobes of each lung so that you correlate your findings to anatomical areas. As you listen, think (1) what AM I hearing over this spot? and (2) what should I expect to be hearing? You should expect to hear three types of normal breath sounds in the adult and older child: **bronchial** (sometimes called tracheal or tubular), **bronchovesicular,** and **vesicular.** Study the characteristics of these normal breath sounds presented in Table 18-1.

TABLE 18-1	Characteristics of Normal Breath Sounds				
	Pitch	Amplitude	Duration	Quality	Normal Location
BRONCHIAL (TRACHEAL)	High	Loud	Inspiration < expiration	Harsh, hollow tubular	Trachea and larynx
BRONCHOVESICULAR	Moderate	Moderate	Inspiration = expiration	Mixed	Over major bronchi, where fewer alveoli are located: posterior, between scapulae especially on right; anterior, around upper sternum in first and second intercostal spaces
VESICULAR	Low	Soft	Inspiration > expiration	Rustling, like the sound of the wind in the trees	Over peripheral lung fields, where air flows through smaller bronchioles and alveoli

Objective Data

Normal Range of Findings

Note the normal location of the three types of breath sounds on the chest wall of the adult or older child (Figs. 18-19 and 18-20).

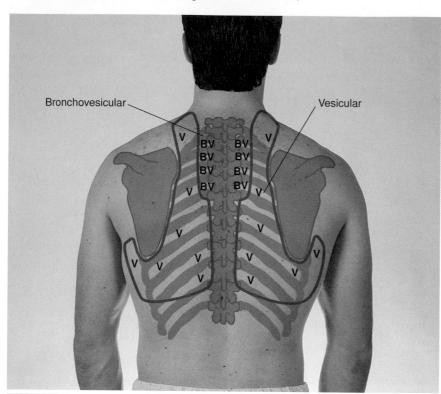

Fig. 18-19

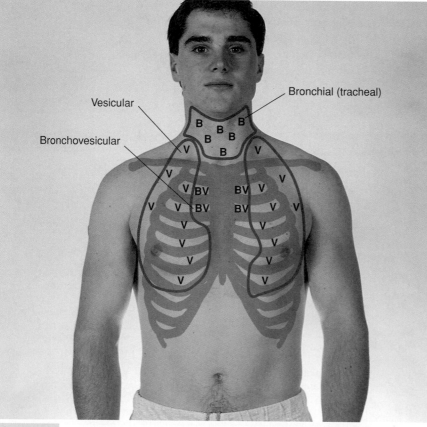

Fig. 18-20

Abnormal Findings

Decreased or **absent breath sounds** occur:

1. When the bronchial tree is obstructed at some point by secretions, mucus plug, or a foreign body
2. In emphysema as a result of loss of elasticity in the lung fibres and decreased force of inspired air; also the lungs are already hyperinflated so the inhaled air does not make as much noise
3. When anything obstructs transmission of sound between the lung and your stethoscope, such as pleurisy or pleural thickening, or air (pneumothorax) or fluid (pleural effusion) in the pleural space

A silent chest means no air is moving in or out, which is an ominous sign.

Increased breath sounds mean that sounds are louder than they should be (e.g., bronchial sounds are abnormal when they are heard over an abnormal location, the peripheral lung fields). They have a high-pitched tubular quality, with a prolonged expiratory phase and a distinct pause between inspiration and expiration. They sound very close to your stethoscope, as if they were right *in* the tubing close to your ear. They occur when consolidation (e.g., pneumonia) or compression (e.g., fluid in the intrapleural space) yields a dense lung area that enhances the transmission of sound from the bronchi. When the inspired air reaches the alveoli, it hits solid lung tissue that conducts sound more efficiently to the surface.

Normal Range of Findings	Abnormal Findings

Adventitious Sounds

Note the presence of any **adventitious sounds.** These are added sounds that are *not* normally heard in the lungs. If present, they are heard as being superimposed on the breath sounds. They are caused by moving air colliding with secretions in the tracheobronchial passageways or by the popping open of previously deflated airways. Sources differ as to the classification and nomenclature of these sounds (see Table 18-6, p. 469), but **crackles** (or rales) and **wheeze** (or rhonchi) are terms commonly used by most examiners.

One type of adventitious sound, **atelectatic crackles,** is not pathological. These are short, popping, crackling sounds that sound like fine crackles but do not last beyond a few breaths. When sections of alveoli are not fully aerated (as in people who are asleep, or in older adults), they deflate slightly and accumulate secretions. Crackles are heard when these sections are expanded by a few deep breaths. Atelectatic crackles are heard only in the periphery, usually in dependent portions of the lungs, and disappear after the first few breaths or after a cough.

In the past, persons were asked to "take a deep breath and blow it out hard" to screen for the presence of wheezing. However, this manoeuvre is futile because slight wheezing may occur on maximal forced exhalation in healthy people.

Study Table 18-6, p. 469, for a complete description of these abnormal adventitious breath sounds.

During normal tidal flow, high-pitched wheeze occurs with asthma.

Voice Sounds

Determine the quality of **voice sounds** or **vocal resonance.** The spoken voice can be auscultated over the chest wall just as it can be felt in tactile fremitus described earlier. Ask the person to repeat a phrase such as "ninety-nine" while you listen over the chest wall. Normal voice transmission is soft, muffled, and indistinct; you can hear sounds through the stethoscope but cannot distinguish exactly what is being said. Pathology that increases lung density enhances transmission of voice sounds.

Eliciting voice sounds is usually not done in routine examination. Rather, these are supplemental manoeuvres that are performed if you suspect lung pathology on the basis of earlier data. When they are performed, you are testing for possible presence of **bronchophony, egophony,** and **whispered pectoriloquy** (Table 18-7, p. 471).

Consolidation or compression of lung tissue will enhance the voice sounds, making the words more distinct.

INSPECT THE ANTERIOR CHEST

Note the **shape and configuration** of the chest wall. The ribs are sloping downward with symmetrical interspaces. The costal angle is within 90 degrees. Development of abdominal muscles is as expected for the person's age, weight, and athletic condition.

Note the person's **facial expression.** The facial expression should be relaxed and benign, indicating unconscious effort of breathing.

Barrel chest has horizontal ribs and costal angle >90 degrees.

Hypertrophy of abdominal muscles occurs in chronic emphysema.

Tense, strained, tired facies present in COPD.

The person with COPD may purse the lips in a whistling position. By exhaling slowly and against a narrow opening, the pressure in the bronchial tree remains positive, and fewer airways collapse.

Assess the **level of consciousness.** The person should be alert and co-operative.

Cerebral hypoxia may be reflected by excessive drowsiness or by anxiety, restlessness, and irritability.

Note skin **colour and condition.** The lips and nail beds are free of cyanosis or unusual pallor. The nails are of normal configuration. Explore any skin lesions.

Clubbing of distal phalanx occurs with chronic respiratory disease.

Objective Data

Normal Range of Findings	**Abnormal Findings**

Assess the quality of **respirations.** Normal relaxed breathing is automatic and effortless, regular and even, and produces no noise. The chest expands symmetrically with each inspiration. Note any localized lag on inspiration.

No retraction or bulging of the interspaces should occur on inspiration.

Normally, accessory muscles are not used to augment respiratory effort. However, with very heavy exercise, the accessory neck muscles (scalene, sternomastoid, trapezius) are used momentarily to enhance inspiration.

The respiratory rate is within normal limits for the person's age (see Table 9-3, p. 161) and the pattern of breathing is regular. Occasional sighs normally punctuate breathing.

PALPATE THE ANTERIOR CHEST

Palpate **symmetrical chest expansion.** Place your hands on the anterolateral wall with the thumbs along the costal margins and pointing toward the xiphoid process (Fig. 18-21).

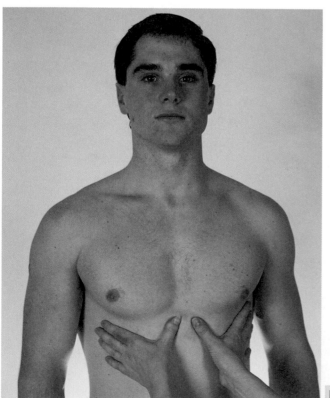

Fig. 18-21

Abnormal Findings

Cutaneous angiomas (spider nevi) associated with liver disease or portal hypertension may be evident on the chest.

Noisy breathing occurs with severe asthma or chronic bronchitis.

Unequal chest expansion occurs when part of the lung is obstructed or collapsed, as with pneumonia, or when guarding to avoid postoperative incisional pain or pleurisy pain.

Retraction suggests obstruction of respiratory tract or that increased inspiratory effort is needed, as in atelectasis. Bulging indicates trapped air as in forced expiration associated with emphysema or asthma.

Accessory muscles are used in acute airway obstruction and massive atelectasis.

Rectus abdominis and internal intercostal muscles are used to force expiration in COPD.

Tachypnea and hyperventilation, bradypnea and hypoventilation, periodic breathing (see Table 18-4, p. 466).

Abnormally wide costal angle with little inspiratory variation occurs with emphysema.

Normal Range of Findings	Abnormal Findings
Ask the person to take a deep breath. Watch your thumbs move apart symmetrically, and note smooth chest expansion with your fingers. Any limitation in thoracic expansion is easier to detect on the anterior chest because greater range of motion exists here with breathing.	A lag in expansion occurs with atelectasis, pneumonia, and postoperative guarding. A palpable grating sensation with breathing indicates pleural friction fremitus (see Table 18-5, p. 468).

Assess **tactile (vocal) fremitus.** Begin palpating over the lung apices in the supraclavicular areas (Fig. 18-22). Compare vibrations from one side to the other as the person says "ninety-nine." Avoid palpating over female breast tissue because breast tissue normally damps sounds.

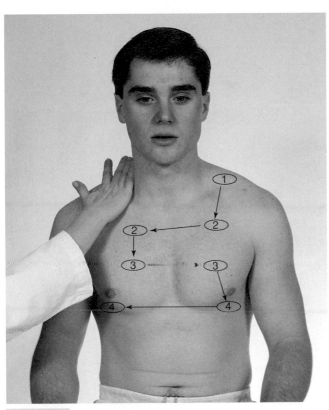

Fig. 18-22 Assess tactile fremitus.

Palpate the anterior chest wall to note any tenderness (normally none is present) and to detect any superficial lumps or masses (again, normally none is present). Note skin mobility and turgor, and note skin temperature and moisture.

PERCUSS THE ANTERIOR CHEST

Begin percussing the apices in the supraclavicular areas. Then, percussing the interspaces and comparing one side to the other, move down the anterior chest.

Interspaces are easier to palpate on the anterior chest than on the back. Do not percuss directly over female breast tissue because this would produce a dull note. Shift the breast tissue over slightly using the edge of your stationary hand. In females with large breasts, percussion may yield little useful data. With all people, use the sequence illustrated in Figure 18-23.

Normal Range of Findings	Abnormal Findings

Objective Data

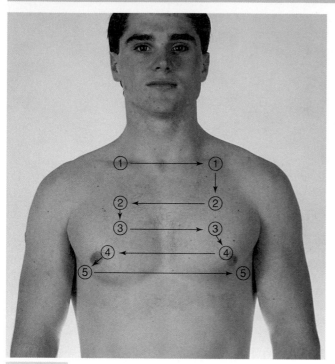

Fig. 18-23   Sequence for percussion and auscultation.

Note the borders of cardiac dullness normally found on the anterior chest, and do not confuse these with suspected lung pathology (Fig. 18-24). In the right hemithorax the upper border of liver dullness is located in the fifth intercostal space in the right midclavicular line. On the left, tympany is evident over the gastric space.

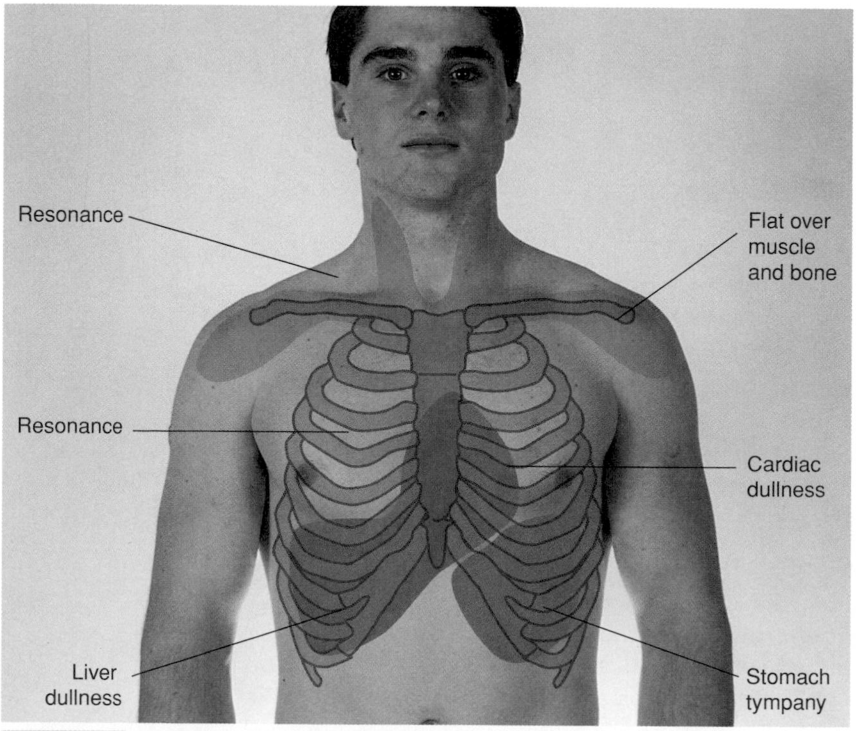

Lungs are hyperinflated with chronic emphysema, resulting in hyperresonance where you would expect cardiac dullness.

Resonance

Resonance

Flat over muscle and bone

Cardiac dullness

Liver dullness

Stomach tympany

Fig. 18-24   Expected percussion notes.

Normal Range of Findings	Abnormal Findings

AUSCULTATE THE ANTERIOR CHEST

Breath Sounds

Auscultate the lung fields over the anterior chest from the apices in the supra-clavicular areas down to the sixth rib. Progress from side to side as you move downward, and listen to one full respiration in each location. Use the sequence indicated for percussion. Do not place your stethoscope directly over the female breast. Displace the breast and listen directly over the chest wall.

Evaluate normal breath sounds, noting any abnormal breath sounds and any adventitious sounds. If the situation warrants, assess the voice sounds on the anterior chest.

> Study Table 18-8, p. 472, for a complete description of abnormal respiratory conditions.

Measurement of Pulmonary Function Status

The **forced expiratory time** is the number of seconds it takes for the person to exhale from total lung capacity to residual volume. It is a screening measure of air flow obstruction. Although the test usually is not performed in the respiratory assessment, it is useful when you wish to screen for pulmonary function.

Ask the person to inhale the deepest breath possible and then to blow it all out hard, as quickly as possible, with the mouth open. Listen with your stethoscope over the sternum. The normal time for full expiration is 4 seconds or less.

> A forced expiration of 6 seconds or more occurs with obstructive lung disease. Refer this person for more precise pulmonary function studies.

The **pulse oximeter** is a noninvasive method to assess arterial oxygen saturation (SpO_2) and is described in Chapter 9. A healthy person with no lung disease and no anemia normally has an SpO_2 of 97 to 98%. However, every SpO_2 result must be evaluated in the context of the person's hemoglobin level, acid–base balance, and ventilatory status

The **6-minute distance (6MD) walk** is a safer, simple, inexpensive, clinical measure of functional status in aging adults (Enright, 2003). The 6MD is used as an outcome measure for people in pulmonary rehabilitation because it mirrors conditions that are used in everyday life. Locate a flat-surfaced corridor that has little foot traffic, is wide enough to permit comfortable turns, and has a controlled environment. Ensure that the person is wearing comfortable shoes, and equip him or her with a pulse oximeter to monitor oxygen saturation. Ask the person to set his or her own pace to cover as much ground as possible in 6 minutes, and assure the person it is all right to slow down or to stop to rest at any time. Use a stopwatch to time the walk. A person who walks >300 m in 6 minutes is more likely to engage in activities of daily living.

> Ask the person to stop the walk if you measure an SpO_2 below 85 to 88% or if extreme breathlessness occurs.

✤ DEVELOPMENTAL CARE

Infants and Children

To prepare, let the parent hold an infant supported against the chest or shoulder. Do not let the usual sequence of the physical examination restrain you; seize the opportunity with a sleeping infant to inspect and then to listen to lung sounds next. This way you can concentrate on the breath sounds before the baby wakes up and possibly cries. The crying does not have to be a problem for you, though, because it actually enhances palpation of tactile fremitus and auscultation of breath sounds.

A child may sit upright on the parent's lap. Offer the stethoscope and let the child handle it. This reduces any fear of the equipment. Promote the child's participation; school-age children usually are delighted to hear their own breath sounds when you place the stethoscope properly. While listening to breath sounds, ask the young child to take a deep breath and "blow out" your penlight

Normal Range of Findings	Abnormal Findings

while you hold the stethoscope with your other hand. Time your letting go of the penlight button so the light goes off after the child blows. Or ask the child to "pant like a dog" while you auscultate.

Inspection. The infant has a rounded thorax with an equal anteroposterior-to-transverse chest diameter (Fig. 18-25). By age 6 years, the thorax reaches the adult ratio of 1:2 (anteroposterior-to-transverse diameter). The newborn's chest circumference is 30 to 36 cm and is 2 cm smaller than the head circumference until 2 years of age. The chest wall is thin with little musculature. The ribs and the xiphoid are prominent; you can see as well as feel the sharp tip of the xiphoid process. The thoracic cage is soft and flexible.

Note a barrel shape persisting after age 6 years, which may develop with chronic asthma or cystic fibrosis.

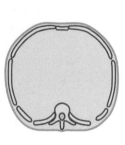
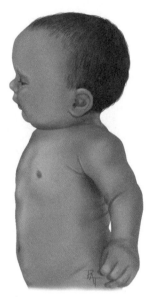

Fig. 18-25   Round thorax in an infant.

In male and female newborns, the breasts may look enlarged by the second or third day from maternal estrogen. Occasionally a white fluid, sometimes referred to by the slang expression "witch's milk," can be expressed. This resolves within a week.

In some children, "Harrison groove" occurs normally. This is a horizontal groove in the rib cage at the level of the insertion of the diaphragm, extending from the sternum to the midaxillary line.

The newborn's first respiratory assessment is part of the **Apgar scoring system** to measure the successful transition to extrauterine life (Table 18-2). The five standard parameters are scored at 1 minute and at 5 minutes after birth. A 1-minute Apgar with a total score of 7 to 10 indicates a newborn in good condition, needing only suctioning of the nose and mouth and otherwise routine care.

Harrison groove also occurs with rickets from the pull of the diaphragm on weakened ribs.

In the immediate newborn period, depressed respirations are due to maternal drugs, interruption of the uterine blood supply, or obstruction of the tracheobronchial tree by mucus or fluid.

A 1-minute Apgar score with a total score of 3 to 6 indicates a moderately depressed newborn needing more resuscitation and subsequent close observation. A score of 0 to 2 indicates a severely depressed newborn needing full resuscitation, ventilatory assistance, and subsequent intensive care.

Objective Data

TABLE 18-2	Apgar Scoring System			
	2	1	0	
Heart rate	Over 100	Slow (below 100)	Absent	_____
Respiratory effort	Good, sustained cry; regular respirations	Slow, irregular, shallow	Absent	_____
Muscle tone	Active motion, spontaneous flexion	Some flexion of extremities; some resistance to extension	Limp, flaccid	_____
Reflex irritability (response to catheter nares)	Sneeze, cough, cry	Grimace, frown	No response	_____
Colour	Completely pink	Body pink, extremities pale	Cyanotic, pale	_____
			Total score	_____

Normal Range of Findings

The infant breathes through the nose rather than the mouth and is an obligate nose breather until 3 months. Slight flaring of the lower costal margins may occur with respirations, but normally no flaring of the nostrils and no sternal retractions or intercostal retractions occur. The diaphragm is the newborn's major respiratory muscle. Intercostal muscles are not well developed. Thus you observe the abdomen bulge with each inspiration but see little thoracic expansion.

Count the respiratory rate for 1 full minute. Normal rates for the newborn are 30 to 40 breaths per minute but may spike up to 60 per minute. Obtain the most accurate respiratory rate by counting when the infant is asleep because infants reach rapid rates with very little excitation when awake. The respiratory pattern may be irregular when extremes in room temperature occur or with feeding or sleeping. Brief periods of apnea less than 10 or 15 seconds are common. This periodic breathing is more common in premature infants.

Palpation. Palpate symmetrical chest expansion by encircling the infant's thorax with both hands. Further palpation should yield no lumps, masses, or crepitus, although you may feel the costochondral junctions in some normal infants.

Percussion. Percussion is of limited usefulness in the newborn and especially in the premature newborn because the adult's fingers are too large in relation to the tiny chest. The percussion note of hyperresonance occurs normally in the infant and young child because of the relatively thin chest wall. Anything less than hyperresonance would have the same clinical significance as dullness in the adult. If measured, diaphragmatic excursion measures about one to two rib interspaces in children.

Auscultation. Auscultation normally yields bronchovesicular breath sounds in the peripheral lung fields of the infant and young child up to age 5 to 6 years. Their relatively thin chest walls with underdeveloped musculature do not damp the sound as do the thicker walls of adults, so breath sounds are louder and harsher.

Abnormal Findings

Marked retractions of sternum and intercostal muscles indicate increased inspiratory effort, as in atelectasis, pneumonia, asthma, and acute airway obstruction.

Rapid respiratory rates accompany pneumonia, fever, pain, heart disease, and anemia.

In an infant, tachypnea of 50 to 100 per minute during sleep may be an early sign of heart failure.

Asymmetrical expansion occurs with diaphragmatic hernia or pneumothorax.

Crepitus is palpable around a fractured clavicle, which may occur with difficult forceps delivery.

Rachitic rosary—prominent round knobs at costochondral junctions—is seen in infants with rickets or scurvy.

Diminished breath sounds occur with pneumonia, atelectasis, pleural effusion, or pneumothorax.

Objective Data

Normal Range of Findings	Abnormal Findings

Fine crackles are the adventitious sounds commonly heard in the immediate newborn period from opening of the airways and clearing of fluid. Because the newborn's chest wall is so thin, transmission of sounds is enhanced, and sound is heard easily all over the chest, making localization of breath sounds a problem. Even bowel sounds are easily heard in the chest. Try using the smaller pediatric diaphragm end piece, or place the bell over the infant's interspaces and not over the ribs. Use the pediatric diaphragm on an older infant or toddler (Fig. 18-26).

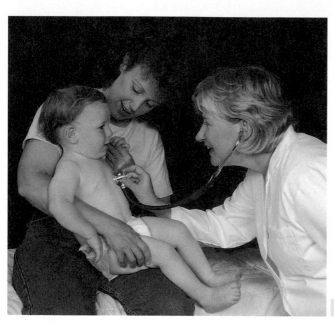

Fig. 18-26

The Pregnant Female

The thoracic cage may appear wider, and the costal angle may feel wider than in the nonpregnant state. Respirations may be deeper, although this can be quantified only with pulmonary function tests.

The Aging Adult

The chest cage commonly shows an increased anteroposterior diameter, giving a round barrel shape, and **kyphosis** or an outward curvature of the thoracic spine (see Table 18-3, p. 465). The person compensates by holding the head extended and tilted back. You may palpate marked bony prominences because of decreased subcutaneous fat. Chest expansion may be somewhat decreased with the older person, although it still should be symmetrical. The costal cartilages become calcified with aging, resulting in a less mobile thorax.

The older person may fatigue easily, especially during auscultation when deep mouth breathing is required. Take care that this person does not hyperventilate and become dizzy. Allow brief rest periods or quiet breathing. If the person does feel faint, holding the breath for a few seconds will restore equilibrium.

The Acutely Ill Person

Ask a second examiner to hold the person's arms and to support him or her in the upright position. If no one else is available, you need to roll the person from side to side, examining the uppermost half of the thorax. This obviously prevents you from comparing findings from one side to another. Also, side flexion of the trunk alters percussion findings because the ribs of the upward side may flex closer together.

Abnormal Findings

Persistent fine crackles that are scattered over the chest occur with pneumonia, bronchiolitis, or atelectasis.

Crackles only in upper lung fields occur with cystic fibrosis; crackles only in lower lung fields occur with heart failure.

Expiratory wheezing occurs with lower airway obstruction (e.g., asthma or bronchiolitis). When unilateral, it may be due to foreign body aspiration.

Persistent peristaltic sounds with diminished breath sounds on the same side may indicate diaphragmatic hernia.

Stridor is a high-pitched inspiratory crowing sound heard without the stethoscope, occurring with upper airway obstruction (e.g., croup, foreign body aspiration, or acute epiglottitis).

Objective Data

Summary Checklist: Thorax and Lung Examination

 For a PDA-downloadable version, go to http://evolve.elsevier.com/Canada/Jarvis/examination/.

1. Inspection
Thoracic cage
Respirations
Skin colour and condition
Person's position
Facial expression
Level of consciousness

2. Palpation
Confirm symmetrical expansion
Assess tactile fremitus
Detect any lumps, masses, tenderness

3. Percussion
Percuss over lung fields
Estimate diaphragmatic excursion

4. Auscultation
Assess normal breath sounds
Note any abnormal breath sounds
If so, perform bronchophony, whispered pectoriloquy, egophony
Note any adventitious sounds

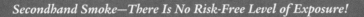

Promoting Health: Environmental Tobacco Smoke (ETS)

Secondhand Smoke—There Is No Risk-Free Level of Exposure!

Secondhand smoke, also referred to as environmental tobacco smoke (ETS), is a mixture of *sidestream smoke,* the smoke from the burning end of a cigarette, pipe, or cigar, and *mainstream smoke,* the smoke exhaled from the lungs of the smoker. Health Canada has determined that there is no safe level of exposure to the carcinogens found in cigarette smoke. Exposure to secondhand smoke, which is primarily involuntary, increases risk for adverse health effects. Further, the general public's exposure to secondhand smoke, for both smokers and others, is much higher than most people realize.

Secondhand smoke is especially harmful to young children, increasing respiratory infection rates, inner ear infections, and aggravation of asthma. In 2006, 15% of Canadian households reported at least one person who smoked inside the home every day or almost every day. Of those households without someone regularly smoking inside the home, 86% did not allow smoking inside their home.

Since 2001, provincial legislation in Canada has been implemented to restrict smoking in the workplace. In addition to the increase in the prevalence of smoke-free and smoke-restricted workplaces, many provincial and territorial governments have enacted legislation requiring public places to be smoke free: Northwest Territories, Prince Edward Island, Nunavut, New Brunswick, and Manitoba in 2004; Saskatchewan, Newfoundland, and Labrador in 2005; Ontario, Quebec, and Nova Scotia in 2006; and Alberta and British Columbia in 2007. Not all provinces have enacted 100% smoke-free legislation, but many provinces such as Alberta and British Columbia have implemented some of the most aggressive nonsmoking laws in the country.

Secondhand smoke contains hundreds of chemicals known to be toxic or carcinogenic, including formaldehyde, benzene, vinyl chloride, arsenic, and cyanide. It can linger in the air for hours long after the cigarette, cigar, or pipe has been extinguished and is involuntarily inhaled by nonsmokers.

Exposure to secondhand smoke places nonsmokers at risk for the same diseases as active smoking does. Nonsmokers exposed to secondhand smoke are 25% more likely to have heart disease and 20% more likely to have lung cancer than those nonsmokers not exposed to smoke. Separating smokers from nonsmokers, cleaning the air indoors, and ventilating buildings do not eliminate the exposure risk to nonsmokers. However, eliminating smoking in indoor spaces does fully protect the nonsmoker.

Levels of ETS in restaurants and bars that allow smoking can be two to five times higher than levels of ETS in residences with active smokers. When workplaces across Canada initiated smoke-free policies, workplace productivity increased and absenteeism decreased. The Ontario Tobacco Research Unit has recently released the results of a report that examined the sales tax data from the city of Ottawa before and after the implementation of its 100% smoke-free bylaw on August 1, 2001. Results showed that the bylaw had no negative impact on bar and restaurant sales. Health Canada has recently developed *Smoke-Free Public Places: You Can Get There*, a guide to planning, implementing, and evaluating nonsmoking by-laws (visit http://www.hc-sc.gc.ca/hl-vs/pubs/tobac-tabac/sfpp-fslp/index_e.html).

Where do you start? First, do not smoke or allow smoking in your home. Tell smokers that you do mind if they smoke indoors. Ask them to go outside while they smoke. It is important to protect children from the harmful effects of second-hand smoke, as research has demonstrated that children have an especially high risk of health problems from exposure. Children breathe in more air relative to their body weight—which means they absorb more tobacco smoke—their immune systems are less developed, and they have less power and ability to complain about being around secondhand smoke. The Canadian Lung Association has just launched a national strategy to ban smoking in vehicles with children. Starting in January 2008, Canadians will take part in the campaign by visiting www.cleanairforkids.ca to send a message directly to their provincial representatives, health ministers, and premiers.

❖— DOCUMENTATION AND CRITICAL THINKING —❖

Sample Charting

SUBJECTIVE

No cough, shortness of breath, or chest pain with breathing. No history of respiratory diseases. Has "one or no" colds per year. Has never smoked. Works in well-ventilated office—smoking co-workers are restricted to smoke in lounge. Last TB skin test 4 years PTA, negative. Never had chest radiography.

OBJECTIVE

Inspection: AP < transverse diameter. Respirations 16/min, relaxed and even.
Palpation: Chest expansion symmetrical. Tactile fremitus equal bilaterally. No tenderness to palpation. No lumps or lesions.
Percussion: Resonant to percussion over lung fields. Diaphragmatic excursion 5 cm bilaterally.
Auscultation: Vesicular breath sounds clear over lung fields. No adventitious sounds.

ASSESSMENT

Intact thoracic structures
Lung sounds clear

Focused Assessment: Clinical Case Study

Thomas G. is a 58-year-old, thin, male traffic patrolman who appears older than stated age. Face is anxious and tense, although in no acute distress at this time. Seeks care for "increasing SOB and fatigue in last couple months."

SUBJECTIVE

- 1 year PTA—noticed more "winded" than usual when walking >3–4 blocks. Early morning cough present daily × 10 years, but now increased sputum production to 2 T per morning, frothy white.
- 6 mo. PTA—had a "cold" with severe harsh coughing, productive of "½ cup" thick white sputum per day. Noted midsternal chest pain (mild) with cough. Lasted 2 weeks. Treated self with humidifier and OTC cough syrup—minimal relief.
- 3 mo. PTA—noticed increasing SOB with less activity. Fatigue and SOB when working outside during traffic rush hours. Unable to take evening walks (usually 2–3 blocks) due to SOB and fatigue. Has two-pillow orthopnea. Wakes 3–4 times during night.
- Now—feels he is "worse and needs some help." Continues with two-pillow orthopnea. Unable to walk >2 blocks or climb >1 flight stairs without resting. Unable to blow out birthday candles on cake last week. Morning cough productive of "¼ cup" thin white sputum, cough continues sporadically during day.
- No chest pain, hemoptysis, night sweats, or paroxysmal nocturnal dyspnea. No history of allergies, hospitalizations, or injuries to chest. No family history of TB, allergies, asthma, or cancer. Smokes cigarettes 2 packs per day × 30 years. Alcohol < 1 six-pack beer/week summer months only.

OBJECTIVE

Inspection: Sitting on side of bed with arms propped on bedside table. Resp. resting 24/min, regular, shallow with prolonged expiration; resp. 34/min ambulating. Increased use of accessory muscles, AP = transverse diameter with widening of costal angle, slightly flushed face, tense expression.
Palpation: Minimal but symmetrical chest expansion. Tactile fremitus = bilaterally. No lumps, masses, or tenderness to palpation.
Percussion: Diaphragmatic excursion is 1 cm and = bilaterally. Hyperresonance over lung fields.
Auscultation: Breath sounds diminished. Expiratory wheeze throughout posterior chest, R > L. No crackles.

ASSESSMENT

Chronic and increasing SOB
Ineffective airway clearance R/T bronchial secretions and obstruction
Activity intolerance R/T imbalance between oxygen supply and demand
Insomnia R/T dyspnea and decreased mobility
Anxiety R/T change in health status

Nursing Diagnoses Commonly Associated With the Thorax and Lungs/Respiratory Disorders

All nursing diagnoses can be found on the Evolve Web site at **http://evolve.elsevier.com/Canada/Jarvis/examination/**.

——— ABNORMAL FINDINGS ———

TABLE 18-3	Configurations of the Thorax

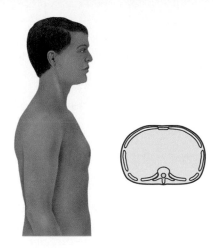

Normal Adult (for comparison)

The thorax has an elliptical shape with an anteroposterior-to-transverse diameter of 1:2 to 5:7.

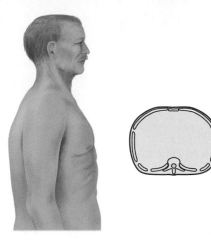

Barrel Chest

Note equal anteroposterior-to-transverse diameter and that ribs are horizontal instead of the normal downward slope. This is associated with normal aging and also with chronic emphysema and asthma as a result of hyperinflation of lungs.

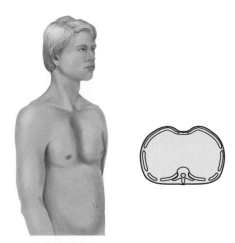

Pectus Excavatum

A markedly sunken sternum and adjacent cartilages (also called funnel breast). Depression begins at second intercostal space, becoming depressed most at junction of xiphoid with body of sternum. More noticeable on inspiration. Congenital, usually not symptomatic. When severe, sternal depression may cause embarrassment and a negative self-concept. Surgery may be indicated.

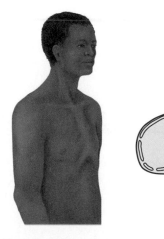

Pectus Carinatum

A forward protrusion of the sternum, with ribs sloping back at either side and vertical depressions along costochondral junctions (pigeon breast). Less common than pectus excavatum, this minor deformity requires no treatment. If severe, surgery may be indicated.

Continued

TABLE 18-3	Configurations of the Thorax—cont'd

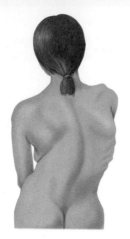 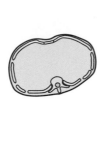   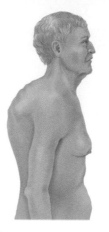 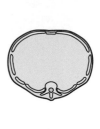

Scoliosis

A lateral S-shaped curvature of the thoracic and lumbar spine, usually with involved vertebrae rotation. Note unequal shoulder and scapular height and unequal hip levels, rib interspaces flared on convex side. More prevalent in adolescent age groups, especially girls. Mild deformities are asymptomatic. If severe (>45 degrees) deviation is present, scoliosis may reduce lung volume; then person is at risk for impaired cardiopulmonary function. Primary impairment is cosmetic deformity, negatively affecting self-image. Refer early for treatment, often surgery.

Kyphosis

An exaggerated posterior curvature of the thoracic spine (humpback) that causes significant back pain and limited mobility. Severe deformities impair cardiopulmonary function. If the neck muscles are strong, compensation occurs by hyperextension of head to maintain level of vision.

Kyphosis has been associated with aging, especially the familiar "dowager's hump" of postmenopausal osteoporotic women. However, it is common well before menopause. It is related to physical fitness; women with adequate exercise habits are less likely to have kyphosis.

TABLE 18-4	Respiration Patterns[1]

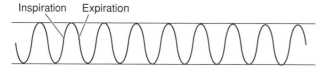   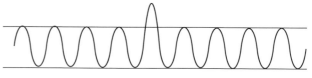

Normal Adult (for Comparison)

Rate—10 to 20 breaths per minute.
Depth—500 mL to 800 mL.
Pattern—even.
The ratio of pulse to respirations is fairly constant, about 4:1. Both values increase as a normal response to exercise, fear, or fever.
Depth—air moving in and out with each respiration.

Sigh

Occasional sighs punctuate the normal breathing pattern and are purposeful to expand alveoli. Frequent sighs may indicate emotional dysfunction. Frequent sighs also may lead to hyperventilation and dizziness.

[1]Assess the (1) rate, (2) depth (tidal volume), and (3) pattern.

TABLE 18-4	Respiration Patterns—cont'd

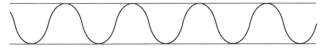

Tachypnea

Rapid shallow breathing. Increased rate >24 per minute. This is a normal response to fever, fear, or exercise. Rate also increases with respiratory insufficiency, pneumonia, alkalosis, pleurisy, and lesions in the pons.

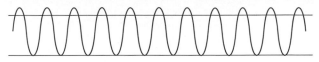

Hyperventilation

Increase in both rate and depth. Normally occurs with extreme exertion, fear, or anxiety. Also occurs with diabetic ketoacidosis (Kussmaul's respirations), hepatic coma, salicylate overdose (producing a respiratory alkalosis to compensate for the metabolic acidosis), lesions of the midbrain, and alteration in blood gas concentration (either an increase in carbon dioxide or decrease in oxygen). Hyperventilation blows off carbon dioxide, causing a decreased level in the blood (alkalosis).

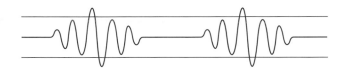

Bradypnea

Slow breathing. A decreased but regular rate (less than 10 per minute), as in drug-induced depression of the respiratory centre in the medulla, increased intracranial pressure, and diabetic coma.

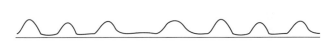

Hypoventilation

An irregular shallow pattern caused by an overdose of narcotics or anaesthetics. May also occur with prolonged bed rest or conscious splinting of the chest to avoid respiratory pain.

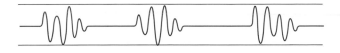

Cheyne-Stokes Respiration

A cycle in which respirations gradually wax and wane in a regular pattern, increasing in rate and depth and then decreasing. The breathing periods last 30 to 45 seconds, with periods of apnea (20 seconds) alternating the cycle. The most common cause is severe heart failure; other causes are renal failure, meningitis, drug overdose, and increased intracranial pressure. Occurs normally in infants and aging persons during sleep.

Biot's Respiration

Similar to Cheyne-Stokes respiration, except that the pattern is irregular. A series of normal respirations (three to four) is followed by a period of apnea. The cycle length is variable, lasting anywhere from 10 seconds to 1 minute. Seen with head trauma, brain abscess, heat stroke, spinal meningitis, and encephalitis.

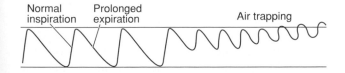

◀ Chronic Obstructive Breathing

Normal inspiration and prolonged expiration to overcome increased airway resistance. In a person with chronic obstructive lung disease, any situation calling for increased heart rate (exercise) may lead to dyspneic episode (air trapping) because then the person does not have enough time for full expiration.

TABLE 18-5	Abnormal Tactile Fremitus

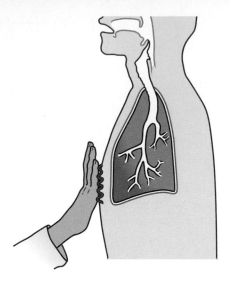

Increased Tactile Fremitus

Occurs with conditions that increase the density of lung tissue, thereby making a better conducting medium for vibrations (e.g., compression or consolidation [pneumonia]). There must be a patent bronchus, and consolidation must extend to lung surface for increased fremitus to be apparent.

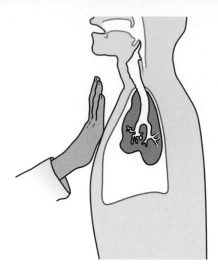

Decreased Tactile Fremitus

Occurs when anything obstructs transmission of vibrations (e.g., an obstructed bronchus, pleural effusion or thickening, pneumothorax, and emphysema). Any barrier that gets in the way of the sound and your palpating hand decreases fremitus.

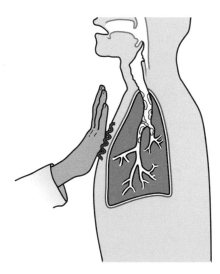

Rhonchal Fremitus

Vibration felt when inhaled air passes through thick secretions in the larger bronchi. This may decrease somewhat by coughing.

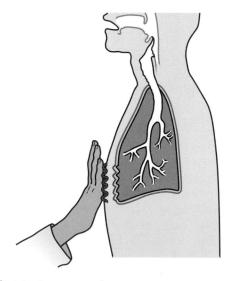

Pleural Friction Fremitus

Produced when inflammation of the parietal or visceral pleura causes a decrease in the normal lubricating fluid. Then the opposing surfaces make a coarse grating sound when rubbed together during breathing. Although this sound is best detected by auscultation, it may sometimes be palpable and feels like two pieces of leather grating together. It is synchronous with respiratory excursion. Also called a palpable friction rub.

TABLE 18-6	Adventitious Lung Sounds		
Sound	Description	Mechanism	Clinical Example

Discontinuous Sounds

These are discrete, crackling sounds.

Crackles—fine (formerly called rales)	Discontinuous, high-pitched, short crackling, popping sounds heard during inspiration that are not cleared by coughing; you can simulate this sound by rolling a strand of hair between your fingers near your ear, or by moistening your thumb and index finger and separating them near your ear	Inhaled air collides with previously deflated airways; airways suddenly pop open, creating crackling sound as gas pressures between the two compartments equalize (Forgacs, 1978b)	*Late inspiratory crackles* occur with restrictive disease: pneumonia, heart failure, and interstitial fibrosis *Early inspiratory crackles* occur with obstructive disease: chronic bronchitis, asthma, and emphysema *Posturally induced crackles* (PICs) are fine crackles that appear with a change from sitting to the supine position, or with a change from supine to supine with legs elevated. PICs that appear after acute myocardial infarction have been associated with increased mortality (Deguchi et al., 1993)
Crackles—coarse (coarse rales)	Loud, low-pitched, bubbling and gurgling sounds that start in early inspiration and may be present in expiration; may decrease somewhat by suctioning or coughing but will reappear shortly—sounds like opening a Velcro fastener	Inhaled air collides with secretions in the trachea and large bronchi	Pulmonary edema, pneumonia, pulmonary fibrosis, and a depressed cough reflex in the terminally ill
Atelectatic crackles (atelectatic rales)	Sounds like fine crackles but do not last and are not pathological; disappear after the first few breaths; heard in axillae and bases (usually dependent) of lungs	When sections of alveoli are not fully aerated, they deflate and accumulate secretions. Crackles are heard when these sections re-expand with a few deep breaths	In aging adults, bedridden persons, or in persons just aroused from sleep
Pleural friction rub	A very superficial sound that is coarse and low pitched; it has a grating quality as if two pieces of leather are being rubbed together; sounds just like crackles, but *close* to the ear; sounds louder if you push the stethoscope harder onto the chest wall; sound is inspiratory and expiratory	Caused when pleurae become inflamed and lose their normal lubricating fluid; their opposing roughened pleural surfaces rub together during respiration; heard best in anterolateral wall where greatest lung mobility exists	Pleuritis, accompanied by pain with breathing (rub disappears after a few days if pleural fluid accumulates and separates pleurae)

Continued

TABLE 18-6	Adventitious Lung Sounds—cont'd		
Sound	Description	Mechanism	Clinical Example
Continuous Sounds These are connected, musical sounds.			
Wheeze—high-pitched (sibilant)	High-pitched, musical squeaking sounds that sound polyphonic (multiple notes as in a musical chord); predominate in expiration but may occur in both expiration and inspiration	Air squeezed or compressed through passageways narrowed almost to closure by collapsing, swelling, secretions, or tumours; the passageway walls oscillate in apposition between the closed and barely open positions; the resulting sound is similar to that from a vibrating reed (Forgacs, 1978b)	Diffuse airway obstruction from acute asthma or chronic emphysema
Wheeze—low-pitched (sonorous rhonchi)	Low-pitched; monophonic single note, musical snoring, moaning sounds; they are heard throughout the cycle, although they are more prominent on expiration; may clear somewhat by coughing	Air flow obstruction as described by the vibrating reed mechanism above; the pitch of the wheeze cannot be correlated to the size of the passageway that generates it	Bronchitis, single bronchus obstruction from airway tumour
Stridor	High-pitched, monophonic, inspiratory, crowing sound, louder in neck than over chest wall	Originating in larynx or trachea, upper airway obstruction from swollen, inflamed tissues or lodged foreign body	Croup and acute epiglottitis in children, foreign body inhalation, and obstructed airway may be life threatening

ABNORMAL FINDINGS
FOR ADVANCED PRACTICE

TABLE 18-7	Voice Sounds	
Technique	Normal Finding	Abnormal Finding
Bronchophony Ask the person to repeat "ninety-nine" while you listen with the stethoscope over the chest wall; listen especially if you suspect pathology	Normal voice transmission is soft, muffled, and indistinct; you can hear sound through the stethoscope but cannot distinguish exactly what is being said	Pathology that increases lung density will enhance transmission of voice sounds; you auscultate a clear "ninety-nine" The words are more distinct than normal and sound close to your ear

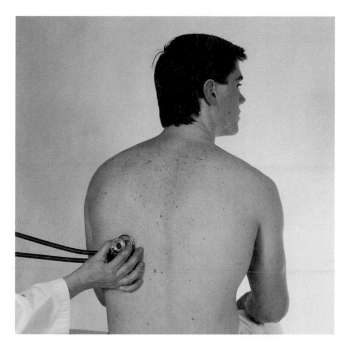

Egophony (Greek: the voice of a goat) Auscultate the chest while the person phonates a long "ee-ee-ee-ee" sound	Normally, you should hear "ee-eeeeee" through your stethoscope	Over area of consolidation or compression, the spoken "eeee" sound changes to a bleating long "aaaaa" sound
Whispered Pectoriloquy Ask the person to whisper a phrase like "one-two-three" as you auscultate	The normal response is faint, muffled, and almost inaudible	With only small amounts of consolidation, the whispered voice is transmitted very clearly and distinctly, although still somewhat faint; it sounds as if the person is whispering right into your stethoscope, "one-two-three"

TABLE 18-8 | **Assessment of Common Respiratory Conditions**

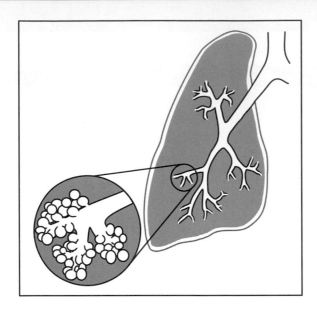

◀ **Normal Lung (for comparison)**

Inspection Anteroposterior < transverse diameter, relaxed posture, normal musculature; rate 10 to 18 breaths per minute, regular, no cyanosis or pallor.

Palpation Symmetrical chest expansion. Tactile fremitus present and equal bilaterally, diminishing toward periphery. No lumps, masses, or tenderness.

Percussion Resonant. Diaphragmatic excursion 3 to 5 cm and equal bilaterally.

Auscultation Vesicular over peripheral fields. Broncho-vesicular parasternally (anterior) and between scapulae (posterior). Infant and young child—bronchovesicular throughout.

Adventitious Sounds None.

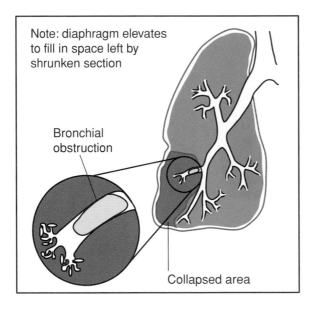

Note: diaphragm elevates to fill in space left by shrunken section

Bronchial obstruction

Collapsed area

◀ **Atelectasis (Collapse)**

Condition Collapsed shrunken section of alveoli, or an entire lung, as a result of (1) airway obstruction (e.g., the bronchus is completely blocked by thick exudate, aspirated foreign body, or tumour), the alveolar air beyond it is gradually absorbed by the pulmonary capillaries, and the alveolar walls cave in; (2) compression on the lung; and (3) lack of surfactant (hyaline membrane disease).

Inspection Cough. Lag on expansion on affected side. Increased respiratory rate and pulse. Possible cyanosis.

Palpation Chest expansion decreased on affected side. Tactile fremitus decreased or absent over area. With large collapse, tracheal shift toward affected side.

Percussion Dull over area (remainder of thorax sometimes may have hyperresonant note).

Auscultation Breath sounds decreased vesicular or absent over area. Voice sounds variable, usually decreased or absent over affected area.

Adventitious Sounds None if bronchus is obstructed. Occasional fine crackles if bronchus is patent.

TABLE 18-8   Assessment of Common Respiratory Conditions—cont'd

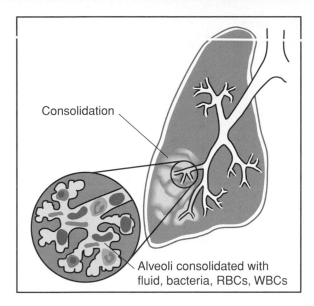

Consolidation

Alveoli consolidated with fluid, bacteria, RBCs, WBCs

◀ **Lobar Pneumonia**

Condition Infection in lung parenchyma leaves alveolar membrane edematous and porous, so red blood cells and white blood cells pass from blood to alveoli. Alveoli progressively fill up (become consolidated) with bacteria, solid cellular debris, fluid, and blood cells, all of which replace alveolar air. This results in decreased surface area of the respiratory membrane, which causes hypoxemia.

Inspection Increased respiratory rate. Guarding and lag on expansion on affected side. Children—sternal retraction, nasal flaring.

Palpation Chest expansion decreased on affected side. Tactile fremitus increased if bronchus patent, decreased if bronchus obstructed.

Percussion Dull over lobar pneumonia.

Auscultation Breath sounds louder with patent bronchus, as if coming directly from larynx. Voice sounds have increased clarity, bronchophony, egophony, whispered pectoriloquy present. Children—diminished breath sounds may occur early in pneumonia.

Adventitious Sounds Crackles, fine to medium.

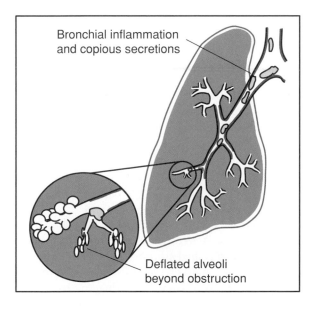

Bronchial inflammation and copious secretions

Deflated alveoli beyond obstruction

◀ **Bronchitis**

Condition Proliferation of mucous glands in the passageways, resulting in excessive mucus secretion. Inflammation of bronchi with partial obstruction of bronchi by secretions or constrictions. Sections of lung distal to obstruction may be deflated. Bronchitis may be acute or chronic with recurrent productive cough. Chronic bronchitis is usually caused by cigarette smoking.

Inspection Hacking, rasping cough productive of thick mucoid sputum. Chronic—dyspnea, fatigue, cyanosis, possible clubbing of fingers.

Palpation Tactile fremitus normal.

Percussion Resonant.

Auscultation Normal vesicular. Voice sounds normal. Chronic—prolonged expiration.

Adventitious Sounds Crackles over deflated areas. May have wheeze.

Continued

TABLE 18-8   Assessment of Common Respiratory Conditions—cont'd

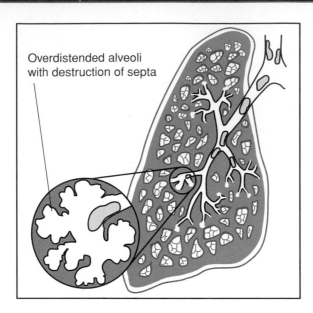

Overdistended alveoli with destruction of septa

◀ **Emphysema**

Condition Caused by destruction of pulmonary connective tissue (elastin, collagen); characterized by permanent enlargement of air sacs distal to terminal bronchioles and rupture of interalveolar walls. This increases airway resistance, especially on expiration—producing a hyperinflated lung and an increase in lung volume. Cigarette smoking accounts for 80 to 90% of cases of emphysema.

Inspection Increased anteroposterior diameter. Barrel chest. Use of accessory muscles to aid respiration. Tripod position. Shortness of breath, especially on exertion. Respiratory distress. Tachypnea.

Palpation Decreased tactile fremitus and chest expansion.

Percussion Hyperresonant. Decreased diaphragmatic excursion.

Auscultation Decreased breath sounds. May have prolonged expiration. Muffled heart sounds resulting from overdistension of lungs.

Adventitious Sounds Usually none; occasionally, wheeze.

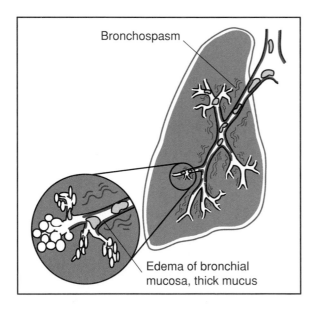

Bronchospasm

Edema of bronchial mucosa, thick mucus

◀ **Asthma (Reactive Airway Disease)**

Condition An allergic hypersensitivity to certain inhaled allergens (pollen), irritants (tobacco, ozone), microorganisms, stress, or exercise that produces a complex response characterized by bronchospasm, and inflammation, edema in walls of bronchioles, and secretion of highly viscous mucus into airways. These factors greatly increase airway resistance, especially during expiration, and produce the symptoms of wheezing, dyspnea, and chest tightness.

Inspection During severe attack: increased respiratory rate, shortness of breath with audible wheeze, use of accessory neck muscles, cyanosis, apprehension, retraction of intercostal spaces. Expiration laboured, prolonged. When chronic may have barrel chest.

Palpation Tactile fremitus decreased, tachycardia.

Percussion Resonant. May be hyperresonant if chronic.

Auscultation Diminished air movement. Breath sounds decreased, with prolonged expiration. Voice sounds decreased.

Adventitious Sounds Bilateral wheezing on expiration, sometimes inspiratory and expiratory wheezing.

TABLE 18-8 | Assessment of Common Respiratory Conditions—cont'd

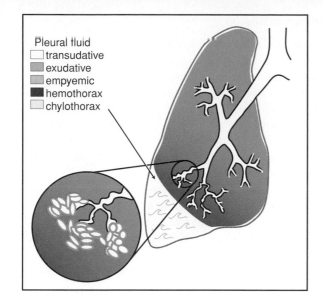

◀ Pleural Effusion (Fluid) or Thickening

Condition Collection of excess fluid in the intrapleural space, with compression of overlying lung tissue. Effusion may contain watery capillary fluid (transudative), protein (exudative), purulent matter (empyemic), blood (hemothorax), or milky lymphatic fluid (chylothorax). Gravity settles fluid in dependent areas of thorax. Presence of fluid subdues all lung sounds.

Inspection Increased respirations, dyspnea; may have dry cough, tachycardia, cyanosis, abdominal distension.

Palpation Tactile fremitus decreased or absent. Tracheal shift away from affected side. Chest expansion decreased on affected side.

Percussion Dull to flat. No diaphragmatic excursion on affected side.

Auscultation Breath sounds decreased or absent. Voice sounds decreased or absent. When remainder of lung is compressed near the effusion, may have bronchial breath sounds over the compression along with bronchophony, egophony, whispered pectoriloquy.

Adventitious Sounds None.

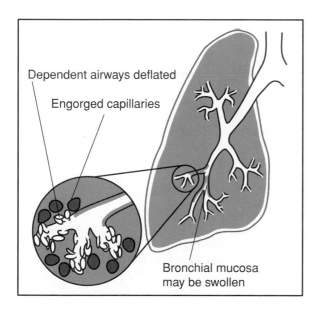

◀ Heart Failure

Condition Pump failure with increasing pressure of cardiac overload causes pulmonary congestion or an increased amount of blood present in pulmonary capillaries. Dependent air sacs are deflated. Pulmonary capillaries engorged. Bronchial mucosa may be swollen.

Inspection Increased respiratory rate, shortness of breath on exertion, orthopnea, paroxysmal nocturnal dyspnea, nocturia, ankle edema, pallor in light-skinned people.

Palpation Skin moist, clammy. Tactile fremitus normal.

Percussion Resonant.

Auscultation Normal vesicular. Heart sounds include S_3 gallop.

Adventitious Sounds Crackles at lung bases.

Continued

| TABLE 18-8 | **Assessment of Common Respiratory Conditions—cont'd** |

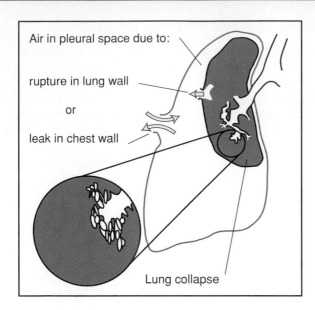

Air in pleural space due to:

rupture in lung wall

or

leak in chest wall

Lung collapse

◀ **Pneumothorax**

Condition Free air in pleural space causes partial or complete lung collapse. Air in pleural space neutralizes the usual negative pressure present; thus lung collapses. Usually unilateral. Pneumothorax can be (1) **spontaneous** (air enters pleural space through rupture in lung wall), (2) **traumatic** (air enters through opening or injury in chest wall), or (3) **tension** (trapped air in pleural space increases, compressing lung and shifting mediastinum to the unaffected side).

Inspection Unequal chest expansion. If large, tachypnea, cyanosis, apprehension, bulging in interspaces.

Palpation Tactile fremitus decreased or absent. Tracheal shift to opposite side (unaffected side). Chest expansion decreased on affected side. Tachycardia, decreased blood pressure (BP).

Percussion Hyperresonant. Decreased diaphragmatic excursion.

Auscultation Breath sounds decreased or absent. Voice sounds decreased or absent.

Adventitious Sounds None.

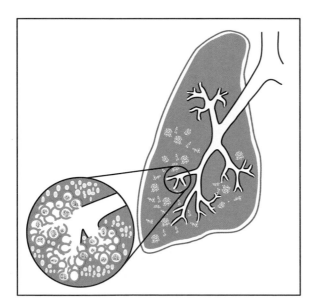

◀ *Pneumocystis jiroveci (P. carinii)* **Pneumonia**

Condition This virulent form of pneumonia is a protozoal infection associated with AIDS. The parasite *P. jiroveci* (*P. carinii*) is common in Canada and harmless to most people, except to the immunocompromised, in whom a diffuse interstitial pneumonitis ensues. Greater than 75% of children are seropositive by the age of 4, which suggests a high background exposure to the organism. Cysts containing the organism and macrophages form in alveolar spaces, alveolar walls thicken, and the disease spreads to bilateral interstitial infiltrates of foamy, protein-rich fluid.

Inspection Anxiety, shortness of breath, dyspnea on exertion, malaise are common; also tachypnea; fever; a dry, nonproductive cough; intercostal retractions in children; cyanosis.

Palpation Decreased chest expansion.

Percussion Dull over areas of diffuse infiltrate.

Auscultation Breath sounds may be diminished.

Adventitious Sounds Crackles may be present but often are absent.

TABLE 18-8 | **Assessment of Common Respiratory Conditions—cont'd**

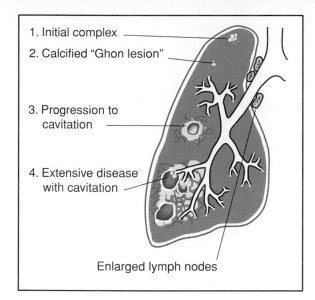

1. Initial complex
2. Calcified "Ghon lesion"
3. Progression to cavitation
4. Extensive disease with cavitation

Enlarged lymph nodes

◀ Tuberculosis

Condition Inhalation of tubercle bacilli into the alveolar wall starts: (1) Initial complex is acute inflammatory response—macrophages engulf bacilli but do not kill them. Tubercle forms around bacilli; (2) scar tissue forms, lesion calcifies and shows on radiograph; (3) reactivation of previously healed lesion. Dormant bacilli now multiply, producing necrosis, cavitation, and caseous lung tissue (cheeselike); (4) extensive destruction as lesion erodes into bronchus, forming air-filled cavity. Apex usually has the most damage.

Subjective Initially asymptomatic, showing as positive skin test or on radiograph. Progressive tuberculosis involves weight loss, anorexia, easy fatigability, low-grade afternoon fevers, night sweats. May have pleural effusion, recurrent lower respiratory infections.

Inspection Cough initially nonproductive, later productive of purulent, yellow-green sputum, may be blood tinged. Dyspnea, orthopnea, fatigue, weakness.

Palpation Skin moist at night from night sweats.

Percussion Resonant initially. Dull over any effusion.

Auscultation Normal or decreased vesicular breath sounds.

Adventitious Sounds Crackles over upper lobes common, persist following full expiration and cough.

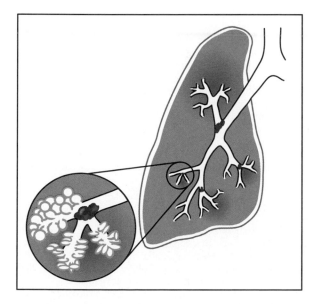

◀ Pulmonary Embolism

Condition Undissolved materials (e.g., thrombus, or air bubbles, fat globules) originating in legs or pelvis, detach and travel through venous system returning blood to right heart and lodge to occlude pulmonary vessels. Over 95% arise from deep vein thrombi in lower legs as a result of stasis of blood, vessel injury, or hypercoaguability. Pulmonary occlusion results in ischemia of downstream lung tissue, increased pulmonary artery pressure, decreased cardiac output, and hypoxia. Rarely, a saddle embolus in bifurcation of pulmonary arteries leads to sudden death from hypoxia. More often, small to medium pulmonary branches occlude, leading to dyspnea. These may resolve by fibrolytic activity.

Subjective Chest pain, worse on deep inspiration, dyspnea.

Inspection Apprehensive, restless, anxiety, mental status changes, cyanosis, tachypnea, cough, hemoptysis, PaO_2 <80 on pulse oximetry. Arterial blood gases show respiratory alkalosis.

Palpation Diaphoresis, hypotension.

Auscultation Tachycardia, accentuated pulmonic component of S_2 heart sound.

Adventitious Sounds Crackles, wheezes.

Continued

Abnormal Findings

| TABLE 18-8 | Assessment of Common Respiratory Conditions—cont'd |

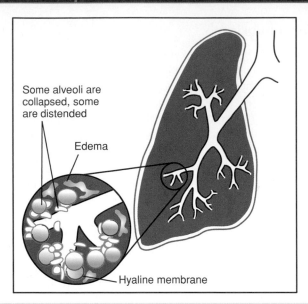

Some alveoli are collapsed, some are distended

Edema

Hyaline membrane

◀ Acute Respiratory Distress Syndrome (ARDS)

Condition An acute pulmonary insult (trauma, gastric acid aspiration, shock, sepsis) damages alveolar capillary membrane, leading to increased permeability of pulmonary capillaries and alveolar epithelium, and to pulmonary edema. Gross examination (autopsy) would show dark red, firm, airless tissue, with some alveoli collapsed, and hyaline membranes lining the distended alveoli.

Subjective Acute onset of dyspnea, apprehension.

Inspection Restlessness, disorientation, rapid shallow breathing, productive cough, thin frothy sputum, retractions of intercostal spaces and sternum. Decreased PaO_2, blood gases show respiratory alkalosis, radiographs show diffuse pulmonary infiltrates, a late sign is cyanosis.

Palpation Hypotension.

Auscultation Tachycardia.

Adventitious Sounds Crackles, rhonchi.

BIBLIOGRAPHY

Akinbami, L. J., Rhodes, J. C., & Lara, M. (2005). Racial and ethnic differences in asthma diagnosis among children who wheeze. *Pediatrics, 115,* 1254–1260.

Canadian Centre for Occupational Health and Safety. (2006). *Diseases, disorders and injuries: Farmer's lung.* Hamilton, ON: Author.

Canadian Lung Association. (2008). *Lung Association to launch Clean Air for Kids Campaign on January 23.*

Centers for Disease Control and Prevention. (2004). *Trends in tuberculosis, 1998–2003.* Retrieved from http://www.cdc.gov/mmwr/preview/mmwrhtml/mm5310a2

Centers for Disease Control and Prevention. (2006). Trends in tuberculosis—United States, 2005. *Morbidity and Mortality Weekly Reports (MMWR), 55z,* 305–308. Retrieved from http://www.cdc.gov/mmwr/preview/mmwrhtml/mm5511a3.htm#top

Charlebois, D. (2005). Early recognition of pulmonary embolism. *Cardiovascular Nursing, 20,* 254–259.

Chen, E., Herman, C., & Rodgers, D. (2006). Symptom perception in childhood asthma: The role of anxiety and asthma severity. *Health Psychology, 25,* 389–391.

Conboy-Ellis, K. (2006). Asthma pathogenesis and management. *Nurse Practitioner, 31,* 24–39.

Cunningham, F. G., Leveno, K. J., Bloom, S. L., Hauth, J. C., Gilstrap, L. C., & Wenstrom, K. D. (2005). *Williams' obstetrics* (22nd ed.). New York: McGraw-Hill Professional.

de Boer, M., Bruijnesteijn van Coppenraet, L., Gaasbeek, A., et al. (2007). An outbreak of *Pneumocystis jiroveci* pneumonia with 1 predominant genotype among renal transplant recipients: Interhuman transmission or a common environmental source? *Clinical Infectious Diseases, 44,* 1143–1149.

Deguchi, F., Hirakawa, S., Gotoh, K., Yagi, Y., & Ohshima, S. (1993). Prognostic significance of posturally induced crackles: Long term follow-up of patients after recovery from acute myocardial infarction. *Chest, 103,* 1457–1462.

DiFranza, J. R., Aligne, A., & Weitzman, M. (2004). Prenatal and postnatal environmental tobacco smoke exposure and children's health. *Pediatrics, 113,* 1007–1015.

Enright, P. L. (2003). The six-minute walk test. *Respiratory Care, 48,* 783–785.

Forgacs, P. (1978a). *Lung sounds.* London: Ballière Tindall.

Forgacs, P. (1978b). The functional basis of pulmonary sounds. *Chest, 73,* 399–405.

Goldberg, H., & Peters, J. (2006). Life-threatening asthma, part 1: Identifying the risk factors, *Consultant, 46,* 609–612.

Goldrick, B. A. (2004). Respiratory syncytial virus. *American Journal of Nursing, 104,* 55–56.

Goldrick, B. A. (2005). Update: Tuberculosis in the United States. *American Journal of Nursing, 105,* 85–86.

Health Canada. (2006). *Second hand smoke.* Retrieved February 5, 2008, from http://www.hc-sc.gc.ca/hl-vs/tobac-tabac/second/index_e.html

Holm, K., & Foreman, M. (2006). Analysis of measures of functional and cognitive ability for aging adults with cardiac and vascular disease. *Cardiovascular Nursing, 21,* 40–47.

Holman, M. (2005). Obstructive sleep apnea syndrome: Implications for primary care. *Nurse Practitioner, 30,* 39–43.

Koschel, M. J. (2004). Pulmonary embolism. *American Journal of Nursing, 104,* 46–50.

Kum-Nji, P., Meloy, L., & Herrod, H. G. (2006). Environmental tobacco smoke exposure: prevalence and mechanisms of causation of infection in children. *Pediatrics, 117,* 1745–1754.

Loudon, R. G. (1987). The lung exam. *Clinics in Chest Medicine, 8,* 265–272.

Miskovich-Riddle, L., & Keresztes, P. A. (2006). CAP management guidelines. *Nurse Practitioner, 31,* 43–55.

Mody, L., Rongjun, S., & Bradley, S. F. (2006). Assessment of pneumonia in older adults: Effect of functional status. *Journal of the American Geriatric Society, 54,* 1062–1067.

Moore, B. A., Augustson, E. M., & Moser, R. P. (2004). Respiratory effects of marijuana and tobacco use in a U.S. sample. *General Internal Medicine, 20,* 33–37.

Murphy, K. R., Cecil, B., & Server, N. L. (2004). Helping patients breathe easier. *Nurse Practitioner, 29,* 39–57.

Pauwels, R. A., & Rabe, K. F. (2004). Burden and clinical features of chronic obstructive pulmonary disease. *Lancet, 364,* 613–620.

Public Health Agency of Canada. (2006). *Tuberculosis in Canada, 2006.* Ottawa, ON: Health Canada.

Public Health Agency of Canada. (2007). *Life and breathe: Respiratory disease in Canada.* Ottawa: Health Canada.

Rosenthal, L. D. (2006). Carbon monoxide poisoning. *American Journal of Nursing, 106,* 40–47.

Ryan, B. (2005). Pneumothorax. *Cardiovascular Nursing, 20,* 251–253.

Schneiderman, H., & Kagan, J. M. (2006). Resumption of cigarette smoking manifested by "tar" and nicotine staining of hair: The Kagan sign. *Consultant, 46,* 1489–1496.

Simon, B. M. (2007). Lung cancer diagnosis in primary care. *Nurse Practitioner, 32,* 43–49.

Steinbis, S. (2004). What you should know about pulmonary hypertension. *Nurse Practitioner, 29,* 8–19.

Taylor, M. M. (2005). ARDS diagnosis and management. *Dimensions in Critical Care Nursing, 24,* 197–207.

Wright, W. L. (2005). Viral or acute bacterial rhinosinusitis? Determining the difference. *Nurse Practitioner, 30,* 31–43.

Heart and Neck Vessels

Written by **Carolyn Jarvis**, PhD, APN, CNP
Adapted by **June MacDonald-Jenkins**, RN, BScN, MSc

Electronic Resources ————————➤

On Evolve *evolve*

http://evolve.elsevier.com/Canada/Jarvis/examination/

- Interactive Case Studies
- Physical Examination Audio and Printable Summaries
- Bedside Assessment Summary Checklists
- Complete Physical Examination Form
- Nursing Diagnoses Boxes
- Health Promotion Guides
- Quick Assessments for 20 Common Conditions
- Multiple Choice Review Questions
- Chapter Objectives
- Appendices
- Weblinks

On the Companion CD

- Interactive Case Studies with Heart and Lung Sounds
- Health Promotion Guides
- Quick Assessments for 20 Common Conditions
- Head-to-Toe Physical Examination Video Clips

Structure and Function

STRUCTURE AND FUNCTION

The cardiovascular system consists of the **heart,** a muscular pump, and the **blood vessels.** The blood vessels are arranged in two continuous loops, the *pulmonary circulation* and the *systemic circulation* (Fig. 19-1). When the heart contracts, it pumps blood simultaneously into both loops.

POSITION AND SURFACE LANDMARKS

The **precordium** is the area on the anterior chest overlying the heart and great vessels (Fig. 19-2). The great vessels are the major arteries and veins connected to the heart. The heart and the great vessels are located between the lungs in the middle third of the thoracic cage, called the **mediastinum.** The heart extends from the second to the fifth intercostal space and from the right border of the sternum to the left midclavicular line.

Think of the heart as an upside-down triangle in the chest. The "top" of the heart is the broader *base,* and the "bottom" is the *apex,* which points down and to the left (Fig. 19-3). During contraction, the apex beats against the chest wall, producing an apical impulse. This is palpable in most people, normally at the fifth intercostal space, 7 to 9 cm from the midsternal line.

Inside the body, the heart is rotated so that its right side is anterior and its left side is mostly posterior. Of the heart's four chambers, the right ventricle forms the greatest area of anterior cardiac surface. The left ventricle lies behind the right ventricle and forms the apex and slender area of the left border. The right atrium lies to the right and above the right ventricle and forms the right border. The left atrium is located posteriorly, with only a small portion, the left atrial appendage, showing anteriorly.

The **great vessels** lie bunched above the base of the heart. The **superior** and **inferior venae cavae** return unoxygenated venous blood to the right side of the heart. The **pulmonary artery** leaves the right ventricle, bifurcates, and carries the venous blood to the lungs. The **pulmonary veins** return the freshly oxygenated blood to the left side of the heart, and the **aorta** carries it out to the body. The aorta ascends from the left ventricle, arches back at the level of the sternal angle, and descends behind the heart.

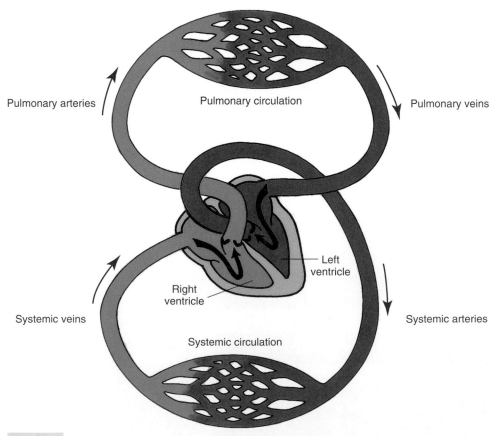

Pulmonary arteries

Pulmonary circulation

Pulmonary veins

Left ventricle

Right ventricle

Systemic veins

Systemic arteries

Systemic circulation

Fig. 19-1

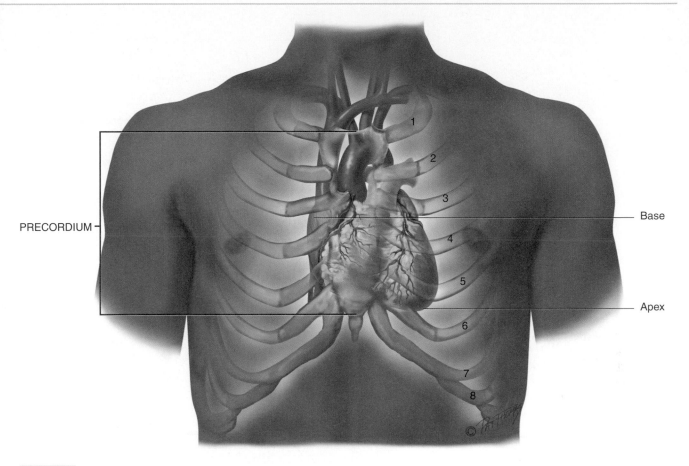

Fig. 19-2

© Pat Thomas, 2006.

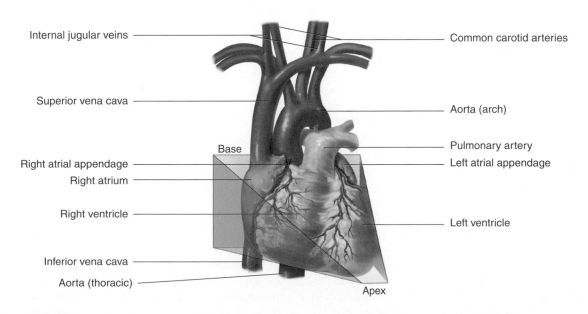

Fig. 19-3

© Pat Thomas, 2006.

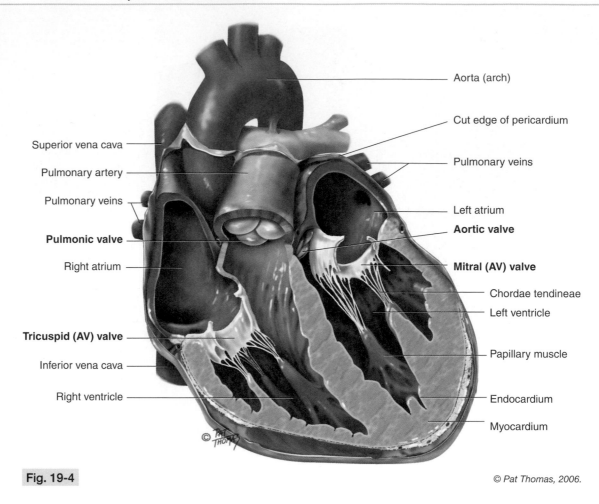

| Aorta (arch) |
| Cut edge of pericardium |
| Pulmonary veins |
| Left atrium |
| **Aortic valve** |
| **Mitral (AV) valve** |
| Chordae tendineae |
| Left ventricle |
| Papillary muscle |
| Endocardium |
| Myocardium |

Superior vena cava
Pulmonary artery
Pulmonary veins
Pulmonic valve
Right atrium
Tricuspid (AV) valve
Inferior vena cava
Right ventricle

Fig. 19-4

© Pat Thomas, 2006.

HEART WALL, CHAMBERS, AND VALVES

The **heart wall** has numerous layers. The **pericardium** is a tough, fibrous, double-walled sac that surrounds and protects the heart (see its cut edge in Fig. 19-4). It has two layers that contain a few millilitres of serous *pericardial fluid*. This ensures smooth, friction-free movement of the heart muscle. The pericardium is adherent to the great vessels, esophagus, sternum, and pleurae and is anchored to the diaphragm. The **myocardium** is the muscular wall of the heart; it does the pumping. The **endocardium** is the thin layer of endothelial tissue that lines the inner surface of the heart chambers and valves.

The common metaphor is to think of the heart as a pump. But consider that the heart is actually *two* pumps; the right side of the heart pumps blood into the lungs, and the left side of the heart simultaneously pumps blood into the body. The two pumps are separated by an impermeable wall, the septum. Each side has an **atrium** and a **ventricle.** The atrium (Latin for "anteroom") is a thin-walled reservoir for holding blood, and the thick-walled ventricle is the muscular pumping chamber. (It is common to use the following abbreviations to refer to the chambers: *RA*, right atrium; *RV*, right ventricle; *LA*, left atrium; and *LV*, left ventricle.)

The four **chambers** are separated by swinging doorlike structures, called *valves*, whose main purpose is to prevent backflow of blood. The valves are unidirectional; they can only open one way. The valves open and close *passively* in response to pressure gradients in the moving blood.

There are four **valves** in the heart (see Fig. 19-4). The two **atrioventricular** (AV) valves separate the atria and the ventricles. The right AV valve is the **tricuspid,** and the left AV valve is the bicuspid or **mitral** valve (so named because it resembles a bishop's mitred cap). The valves' thin leaflets are anchored by collagenous fibres (**chordae tendineae**) to papillary muscles embedded in the ventricle floor. The AV valves open during the heart's filling phase, or **diastole,** to allow the ventricles to fill with blood. During the pumping phase, or **systole,** AV valves close to prevent regurgitation of blood back up into the atria. The papillary muscles contract at this time, so that the valve leaflets meet and unite to form a perfect seal without turning themselves inside out.

The **semilunar** (SL) valves are set between the ventricles and the arteries. Each valve has three cusps that look like half moons. The SL valves are the **pulmonic** valve in the right side of the heart and the **aortic** valve in the left side of the heart. They open during pumping, or **systole,** to allow blood to be ejected from the heart.

Note that no valves are present between the vena cava and the right atrium, or between the pulmonary veins and the left atrium. For this reason, abnormally high pressure in the left side of the heart gives a person symptoms of pulmonary congestion, and abnormally high pressure in the right side of the heart shows in the neck veins and abdomen.

DIRECTION OF BLOOD FLOW

Think of an unoxygenated red blood cell being drained downstream into the vena cava. It is swept along with the flow of venous blood and follows the route illustrated in Fig. 19-5.

1. From liver to right atrium (RA) through inferior vena cava
   Superior vena cava drains venous blood from the head and upper extremities
   From RA, venous blood travels through tricuspid valve to right ventricle (RV)
2. From RV, venous blood flows through pulmonic valve to pulmonary artery
   Pulmonary artery delivers unoxygenated blood to lungs

3. Lungs oxygenate blood
   Pulmonary veins return fresh blood to LA
4. From LA, arterial blood travels through mitral valve to LV
   LV ejects blood through aortic valve into aorta
5. Aorta delivers oxygenated blood to body

Remember that the circulation is a continuous loop. The blood is kept moving along by continually shifting pressure gradients. The blood flows from an area of higher pressure to one of lower pressure.

CARDIAC CYCLE

The rhythmic movement of blood through the heart is the **cardiac cycle.** It has two phases, **diastole** and **systole.** In **diastole,** the ventricles relax and fill with blood. This takes up two thirds of the cardiac cycle. The heart's contraction is **systole.** During systole, blood is pumped from the ventricles and fills the pulmonary and systemic arteries. This is one third of the cardiac cycle.

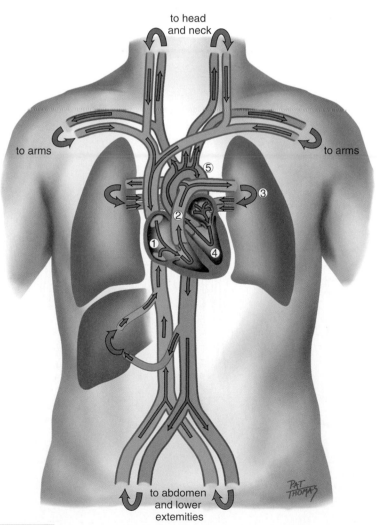

to head and neck

to arms

to arms

to abdomen and lower extremities

Fig. 19-5

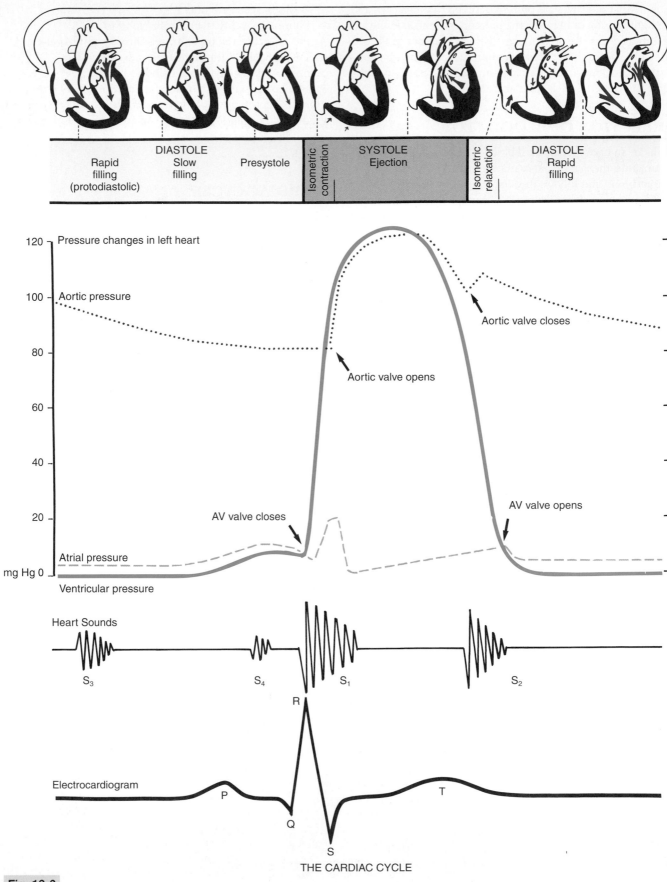

DIASTOLE			Isometric contraction	SYSTOLE	Isometric relaxation	DIASTOLE
Rapid filling (protodiastolic)	Slow filling	Presystole		Ejection		Rapid filling

Pressure changes in left heart

Aortic pressure

Aortic valve closes

Aortic valve opens

AV valve closes

AV valve opens

Atrial pressure

mg Hg 0

Ventricular pressure

120
100
80
60
40
20

Heart Sounds

S₃   S₄   S₁   S₂

R

Electrocardiogram

P

Q

S

T

THE CARDIAC CYCLE

Fig. 19-6

Diastole. In diastole, the ventricles are relaxed, and the AV valves, (i.e., the tricuspid and mitral) are open (Fig. 19-6). (Opening of the normal valve is acoustically silent.) The pressure in the atria is higher than that in the ventricles, so blood pours rapidly into the ventricles. This first passive filling phase is called **early** or **protodiastolic filling.**

Toward the end of diastole, the atria contract and push the last amount of blood (about 25% of stroke volume) into the ventricles. This active filling phase is called **presystole,** or **atrial systole,** or sometimes the "atrial kick." It causes a small rise in left ventricular pressure. (Note that atrial systole occurs during ventricular diastole, a confusing but important point.)

Systole. Now so much blood has been pumped into the ventricles that ventricular pressure is finally higher than that in the atria, so the mitral and tricuspid valves swing shut. The closure of the AV valves contributes to the first heart sound (S_1) and signals the beginning of systole. The AV valves close to prevent any regurgitation of blood back up into the atria during contraction.

For a very brief moment, all four valves are closed. The ventricular walls contract. This contraction against a closed system works to build pressure inside the ventricles to a high level (**isometric contraction**). Consider first the left side of the heart. When the pressure in the ventricle finally exceeds pressure in the aorta, the aortic valve opens and blood is ejected rapidly.

After the ventricle's contents are ejected, its pressure falls. When pressure falls below pressure in the aorta, some blood flows backward toward the ventricle, causing the aortic valve to swing shut. This closure of the semilunar valves causes the second heart sound (S_2) and signals the end of systole.

Diastole Again. Now all four valves are closed and the ventricles relax (called **isometric** or **isovolumic relaxation**).

Meanwhile, the atria have been filling with blood delivered from the lungs. Atrial pressure is now higher than the relaxed ventricular pressure. The mitral valve drifts open and diastolic filling begins again.

Events in the Right and Left Sides. The same events are happening in the right side of the heart, but pressures in the right side of the heart are much lower than those of the left side because less energy is needed to pump blood to its destination, the pulmonary circulation. Also, events occur just slightly later in the right side of the heart because of the route of myocardial depolarization. As a result, two distinct components to each of the heart sounds exist, and sometimes you can hear them separately. In the first heart sound, the mitral component (M_1) closes just before the tricuspid component (T_1). And with S_2, aortic closure (A_2) occurs slightly before pulmonic closure (P_2).

HEART SOUNDS

Events in the cardiac cycle generate sounds that can be heard through a stethoscope over the chest wall. These include normal heart sounds and, occasionally, extra heart sounds and murmurs (Fig. 19-7).

Normal Heart Sounds

The **first heart sound** (S_1) occurs with closure of the AV valves and thus signals the beginning of systole. The mitral component of the first sound (M_1) slightly precedes the tricuspid component (T_1), but you usually hear these two components fused as one sound. You can hear S_1 over all the precordium, but usually it is loudest at the apex.

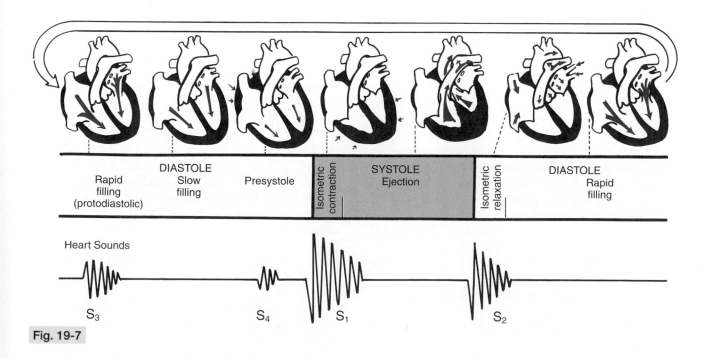

| Rapid filling (protodiastolic) | DIASTOLE Slow filling | Presystole | Isometric contraction | SYSTOLE Ejection | Isometric relaxation | DIASTOLE Rapid filling |

Heart Sounds

S_3 S_4 S_1 S_2

Fig. 19-7

The **second heart sound** (S_2) occurs with closure of the semilunar valves and signals the end of systole. The aortic component of the second sound (A_2) slightly precedes the pulmonic component (P_2). Although it is heard over all the precordium, S_2 is loudest at the base.

Effect of Respiration. The volume of right and left ventricular systole is just about equal, but this can be affected by respiration. To learn this, consider the phrase:

MoRe to the Right heart,
Less to the Left

That means that during inspiration, intrathoracic pressure is decreased. This pushes more blood into the vena cava, increasing venous return to the right side of the heart, which increases right ventricular stroke volume. The increased volume prolongs right ventricular systole and delays pulmonic valve closure.

Meanwhile on the left side, a greater amount of blood is sequestered in the lungs during inspiration. This momentarily decreases the amount returned to the left side of the heart, decreasing left ventricular stroke volume. The decreased volume shortens left ventricular systole and allows the aortic valve to close a bit earlier. When the aortic valve closes significantly earlier than the pulmonic valve, you can hear the two components separately. This is a *split* S_2.

Extra Heart Sounds

Third Heart Sound (S_3). Normally diastole is a silent event. However, in some conditions, ventricular filling creates vibrations that can be heard over the chest. These vibrations are S_3. The S_3 occurs when the ventricles are resistant to filling during the early rapid filling phase (protodiastole). This occurs immediately after S_2, when the AV valves open and atrial blood first pours into the ventricles. (See a complete discussion of S_3 in Table 19-7 on p. 516.)

Fourth Heart Sound (S_4). The S_4 occurs at the end of diastole, at presystole, when the ventricle is resistant to filling. The atria contract and push blood into a noncompliant ventricle. This creates vibrations that are heard as S_4. The S_4 occurs just before S_1.

Murmurs

Blood circulating through normal cardiac chambers and valves usually makes no noise. However, some conditions create turbulent blood flow and collision currents. These result in a murmur, much like a pile of stones or a sharp turn in a stream creates a noisy water flow. A murmur is a gentle, blowing, swooshing sound that can be heard on the chest wall. Conditions resulting in a murmur are as follows:

1. Velocity of blood increases (flow murmur) (e.g., in exercise, thyrotoxicosis)
2. Viscosity of blood decreases (e.g., in anemia)
3. Structural defects in the valves (narrowed valve, incompetent valve) or unusual openings occur in the chambers (dilated chamber, wall defect)

Characteristics of Sound

All heart sounds are described by:
1. Frequency (pitch)—heart sounds are described as high pitched or low pitched, although these terms are relative because all are low-frequency sounds, and you need a high-quality stethoscope to hear them
2. Intensity (loudness)—loud or soft
3. Duration—very short for heart sounds; silent periods are longer
4. Timing—systole or diastole

CONDUCTION

Of all organs, the heart has a unique ability—automaticity. The heart can contract by itself, independent of any signals or stimulation from the body. The heart contracts in response to an electrical current conveyed by a conduction system (Fig. 19-8). Specialized cells in the sinoatrial (SA) node near the superior vena cava initiate an electrical impulse. (Because the SA node has an intrinsic rhythm, it is the "pacemaker.") The current flows in an orderly sequence, first across the atria to the AV node low in the atrial septum. There, it is delayed slightly so that the atria have time to contract before the ventricles are stimulated. Then, the impulse travels to the bundle of His, the right and left bundle branches, and then through the ventricles.

The electrical impulse stimulates the heart to do its work, which is to contract. A small amount of electricity spreads to the body surface, where it can be measured and recorded on the electrocardiogram (ECG). The ECG waves are arbitrarily labeled PQRST, which stand for the following elements:

P wave—depolarization of the atria
P–R interval—from the beginning of the P wave to the beginning of the QRS complex (the time necessary for atrial depolarization plus time for the impulse to travel through the AV node to the ventricles)
QRS complex—depolarization of the ventricles
T wave—repolarization of the ventricles

Electrical events slightly *precede* the mechanical events in the heart. The ECG juxtaposed on the cardiac cycle is illustrated in Figure 19-8.

PUMPING ABILITY

In the resting adult, the heart normally pumps between 4 and 6 L of blood per minute throughout the body. This **cardiac output (CO)** equals the volume of blood in each systole (called the stroke volume [SV]) times the number of beats per minute (rate [R]). This is described as follows:

$$CO = SV \times R$$

The heart can alter its cardiac output to adapt to the metabolic needs of the body. Preload and afterload affect the heart's ability to increase cardiac output.

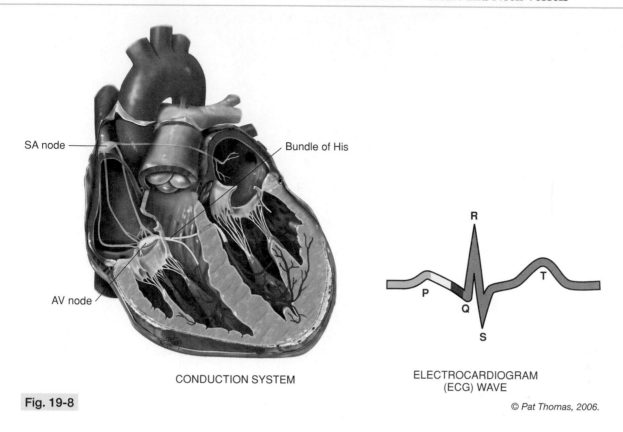

SA node

Bundle of His

AV node

R

P

Q

S

T

CONDUCTION SYSTEM

ELECTROCARDIOGRAM
(ECG) WAVE

Fig. 19-8

© Pat Thomas, 2006.

Preload is the venous return that builds during diastole. It is the length to which the ventricular muscle is stretched at the end of diastole just before contraction (Fig. 19-9).

When the volume of blood returned to the ventricles is increased (as when exercise stimulates skeletal muscles to contract and force more blood back to the heart), the muscle bundles are stretched beyond their normal resting state to accommodate it. The force of this switch is the preload. According to the Frank-Starling law, the greater the stretch, the stronger is the heart's contraction. This increased con-

tractility results in an increased volume of blood ejected (increased stroke volume).

Afterload is the opposing pressure the ventricle must generate to open the aortic valve against the higher aortic pressure. It is the resistance against which the ventricle must pump its blood. Once the ventricle is filled with blood, the ventricular end diastolic pressure is 5 to 10 mm Hg, whereas that in the aorta is 70 to 80 mm Hg. To overcome this difference, the ventricular muscle *tenses* (isovolumic contraction). After the aortic valve opens, rapid ejection occurs.

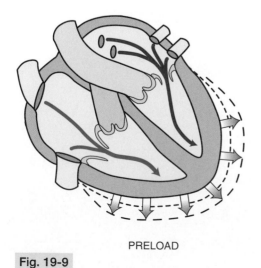

PRELOAD

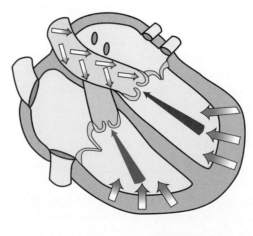

AFTERLOAD

Fig. 19-9

© Pat Thomas, 2006.

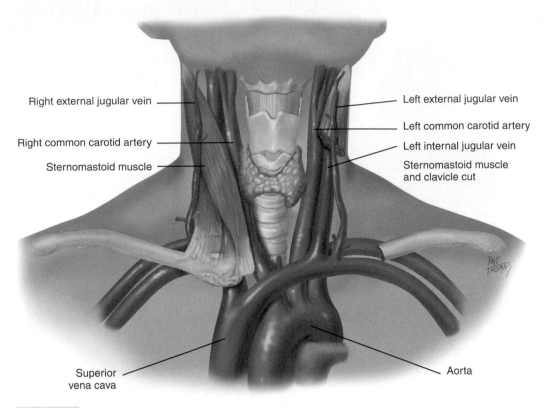

Fig. 19-10

NECK VESSELS

THE NECK VESSELS

Cardiovascular assessment includes the survey of vascular structures in the neck—the carotid artery and the jugular veins (Fig. 19-10). These vessels reflect the efficiency of cardiac function.

The Carotid Artery Pulse

Chapter 9 describes the pulse as a pressure wave generated by each systole pumping blood into the aorta. The carotid artery is a central artery—that is, it is close to the heart. Its timing closely coincides with ventricular systole. (Assessment of the peripheral pulses is found in Chapter 20, and blood pressure assessment is found in Chapter 9.)

The **carotid artery** is located in the groove between the trachea and the sternomastoid muscle, medial to and alongside that muscle. Note the characteristics of its waveform (Fig. 19-11): a smooth rapid upstroke, a summit that is rounded and smooth, and a downstroke that is more gradual and that has a dicrotic notch caused by closure of the aortic valve (marked D in the figure).

Jugular Venous Pulse and Pressure

The **jugular veins** empty unoxygenated blood directly into the superior vena cava. Because no cardiac valve exists to separate the superior vena cava from the right atrium, the jugular veins give information about activity on the right side of the heart. Specifically, they reflect filling pressure and volume changes. Because volume and pressure increase when the right side of the heart fails to pump efficiently, the jugular veins expose this.

Two jugular veins are present in each side of the neck (see Fig. 19-10). The larger **internal jugular** lies deep and medial to the sternomastoid muscle. It is usually not visible, although its diffuse pulsations may be seen in the sternal notch when the person is supine. The **external jugular** vein is more superficial; it lies lateral to the sternomastoid muscle, above the clavicle.

Although an arterial pulse is caused by a forward propulsion of blood, the jugular pulse is different. The jugular pulse results from a backwash, a waveform moving backward caused by events upstream. The jugular pulse has five components, as shown in Fig 19-12.

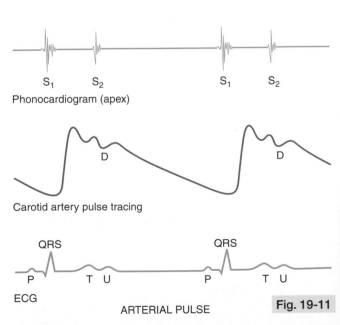

Phonocardiogram (apex)

Carotid artery pulse tracing

ECG

ARTERIAL PULSE

Fig. 19-11

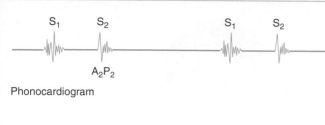

Phonocardiogram

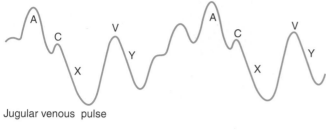

Jugular venous pulse

QRS

P   T   P   T

ECG

VENOUS PULSE

Fig. 19-12

The five components of the jugular venous pulse occur because of events in the right side of the heart. The A wave reflects atrial contraction because some blood flows backward to the vena cava during right atrial contraction. The C wave, or ventricular contraction, is backflow from the bulging upward of the tricuspid valve when it closes at the beginning of ventricular systole (not from the neighbouring carotid artery pulsation). Next, the X descent shows atrial relaxation when the right ventricle contracts during systole and pulls the bottom of the atria downward. The V wave occurs with passive atrial filling because of the increasing volume in the right atria and increased pressure. Finally, the Y descent reflects passive ventricular filling when the tricuspid valve opens and blood flows from the RA to the RV.

✿ DEVELOPMENTAL CARE

Infants and Children

The fetal heart functions early; it begins to beat at the end of 3 weeks' gestation. The lungs are nonfunctional, but the fetal circulation compensates for this (Fig. 19-13). Oxygenation

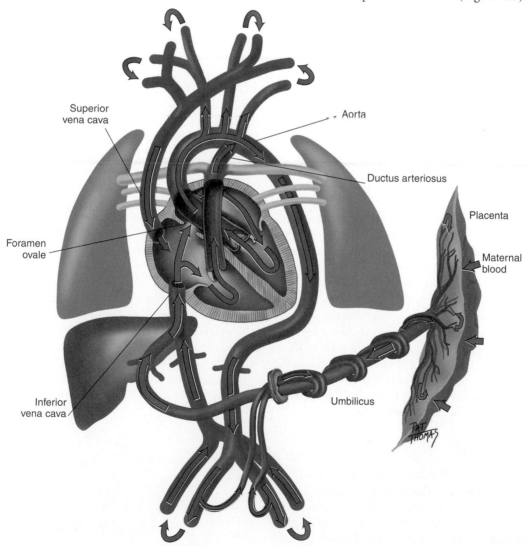

FETAL CIRCULATION

Fig. 19-13

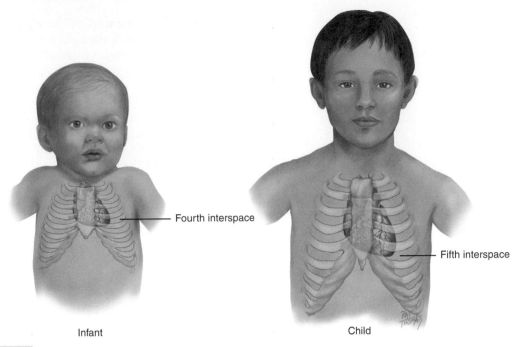

Fourth interspace

Fifth interspace

Infant

Child

Fig. 19-14   HEART'S POSITION IN THE CHEST

takes place at the placenta, and the arterial blood is returned to the right side of the heart. There is no point in pumping all this freshly oxygenated blood through the lungs, so it is rerouted in two ways. First, about two thirds of it is shunted through an opening in the atrial septum, the **foramen ovale,** into the left side of the heart, where it is pumped out through the aorta. Second, the rest of the oxygenated blood is pumped by the right side of the heart out through the pulmonary artery, but it is detoured through the **ductus arteriosus** to the aorta. Because they are both pumping into the systemic circulation, the right and left ventricles are equal in weight and muscle wall thickness.

Inflation and aeration of the lungs at birth produces circulatory changes. Now the blood is oxygenated through the lungs rather than through the placenta. The foramen ovale closes within the first hour because of the new lower pressure in the right side of the heart than in the left side. The ductus arteriosus closes later, usually within 10 to 15 hours of birth. Now, the LV has the greater workload of pumping into the systemic circulation, so that when the baby has reached 1 year of age, the LV's mass increases to reach the adult ratio of 2:1, LV to RV.

The heart's position in the chest is more horizontal in the infant than in the adult; thus the apex is higher, located at the fourth left intercostal space (Fig. 19-14). It reaches the adult position when the child reaches 7 years of age.

The Pregnant Female

Blood volume increases by 30 to 40% during pregnancy, with the most rapid expansion occurring during the second trimester. This creates an increase in stroke volume and cardiac output and an increased pulse rate of 10 to 15 beats per minute. Despite the increased cardiac output, arterial blood pressure decreases in pregnancy as a result of peripheral vasodilation. The blood pressure drops to its lowest point during the second

trimester, then rises after that. The blood pressure varies with the person's position, as described on p. 511.

The Aging Adult

It is difficult to isolate the "aging process" of the cardiovascular system per se because it is so closely interrelated with lifestyle, habits, and diseases. We now know that lifestyle is a modifying factor in the development of cardiovascular disease; smoking, diet, alcohol use, exercise patterns, and stress have an influence on coronary artery disease. Lifestyle also affects the aging process; cardiac changes once thought to be due to aging are partially due to the sedentary lifestyle accompanying aging (Fig. 19-15). What is left to be attributed to the aging process alone?

Hemodynamic Changes with Aging

- From age 20 to 60 years, systolic blood pressure increases by about 20 mm Hg, and by another 20 mm Hg between ages 60 and 80 years (Wei, 1992). This is due to stiffening of the large arteries, which, in turn is due to calcification of vessel walls (arteriosclerosis). This stiffening creates an increase in pulse wave velocity because the less compliant arteries cannot store the volume ejected.

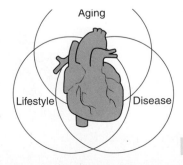

Aging

Lifestyle   Disease

Fig. 19-15

- The overall size of the heart does not increase with age, but left ventricular wall thickness increases. This is an adaptive mechanism to accommodate the vascular stiffening mentioned earlier that creates an increased workload on the heart.
- No significant change in diastolic pressure occurs with age. A rising systolic pressure with a relatively constant diastolic pressure increases the pulse pressure (the difference between the two).
- No change in resting heart rate occurs with aging.
- Cardiac output at rest is not changed with aging.
- There is a decreased ability of the heart to augment cardiac output with exercise. This is shown by a decreased maximum heart rate with exercise and diminished sympathetic response. Noncardiac factors also cause a decrease in maximum work performance with aging: decrease in skeletal muscle performance, increase in muscle fatigue, increased sense of dyspnea. Chronic exercise conditioning will modify many of the aging changes in cardiovascular function (Zipes et al., 2005).

Arrhythmias. The presence of supraventricular and ventricular arrhythmias increases with age. Ectopic beats are common in aging people; although these are usually asymptomatic in healthy older people, they may compromise cardiac output and blood pressure when disease is present.

Tachyarrhythmias may not be tolerated as well in older people. The myocardium is thicker and less compliant, and early diastolic filling is impaired at rest (Wei, 1992). Thus, it may not tolerate a tachycardia as well because of shortened diastole. Also, tachyarrhythmias may further compromise a vital organ whose function has already been affected by aging or disease. For example, a ventricular tachycardia produces a 40 to 70% decrease in cerebral blood flow. Although a younger person may tolerate this, an older person with cerebrovascular disease may experience syncope (Cheitlin and Zipes, 2001).

ECG. Age-related changes in the ECG occur as a result of histological changes in the conduction system. These changes include:

- Prolonged P–R interval (first-degree AV block) and prolonged Q–T interval, but the QRS interval is unchanged
- Left axis deviation from age-related mild LV hypertrophy and fibrosis in left bundle branch
- Increased incidence of bundle branch block

Although the hemodynamic changes associated with aging alone do not seem severe or portentous, the fact remains that the incidence of cardiovascular disease increases with age. The incidence of coronary artery disease increases sharply with advancing age and accounts for about half of the deaths of older people. Hypertension (systolic >140 mm Hg and diastolic >90 mm Hg) and heart failure also increase with age. Certainly, lifestyle habits (smoking, chronic alcohol use, lack of exercise, poor diet) play a significant role in the acquisition of heart disease. Also, increasing the physical activity of older adults—even at a moderate level—is associated with a reduced risk of death from cardiovascular diseases and respiratory illnesses. Both points underscore the need for health education as an important treatment parameter.

CULTURAL AND SOCIAL CONSIDERATIONS

In Canada the prevalence of **death** due to cardiovascular disease (CVD) is sharply decreasing on an annual basis, yet the incidence of CVD continues to grow. Better medications, early intervention, and public health awareness are some of the contributing factors to the reduction in deaths. According to Statistics Canada (2004c), men and women in Canada have almost equal death rates from CVD, a trend noted over the past 10 years. Interestingly, as cardiovascular death rates have diminished (31.9%), cancer rates have increased (29.5%), quite possibly to surpass CVD as the primary killer of Canadians.

The prevalence of heart disease and stroke is higher in adults of African descent than in any other ethnic group: 44.6% for men and 49% for women as opposed to 37.2% for men and 35% for women of European descent. These differences in prevalence show the crucial need to improve early detection, screening, and treatment (Heart and Stroke Foundation, 2003). Socioeconomic factors also influence the incidence of CVD in Canadians. Income and employment, ability to afford a nutritious diet, access to resources, and extended healthcare plans all affect the ability of the patient with CVD to implement a comprehensive treatment plan. Statistics Canada (2004a) reported that income differences alone accounted for 6400 premature deaths from CVD.

The major risk factors for heart disease and stroke are high blood pressure, smoking, high cholesterol levels, obesity, physical inactivity, and diabetes. In addition, for some women, the use of oral contraceptives and the presence of postmenopausal hormones are risk factors.

High Blood Pressure (HBP). Over one fifth of Canadians have hypertension. A dramatic increase in the number of Canadians diagnosed and treated for high blood pressure has been noted in the past 10 years; this has been primarily attributed to national education programs such as the Canadian Hypertension Education Program, initiated in 1999 (Onysko et al., 2006).

Smoking. The Canadian Tobacco Use Monitoring Survey found a slight decline in the overall prevalence of smoking in Canada in 2004 (Statistics Canada, 2004b). An estimated 5.1 million Canadians or 20% of the population aged 15 and older, reported smoking daily or occasionally in 2004. As before, among Canadians aged 15 and older, more men (22%) smoked than women (17%).

Serum Cholesterol. During childhood (ages 4 to 19), children and adolescents of African descent have higher total cholesterol, higher low-density lipoprotein (LDL) cholesterol, and higher high-density lipoprotein (HDL) cholesterol (the "good" cholesterol) than do children and adolescents of Euro-Canadian descent. These differences reverse during adulthood when individuals of African descent have lower serum cholesterol levels than do Euro-Canadians.

Obesity. Overweight is defined by a body mass index (BMI) of 25 kg/m^2 or higher and obesity by a BMI of 30 kg/m^2 or higher. These problems have reached epidemic proportions in Canada. Canadian women are more overweight than men at a rate of 64% versus 53% nationally. Childhood challenges with being overweight and obese are of national concern, with 25% of females and 29% of males between the ages of 2 and 17 years weighing in above the national average body mass index.

Diabetes. Over 2 million Canadians have diabetes, and it is estimated that the prevalence will increase significantly in the next 10 years, in part because 77% of new Canadians, including Hispanics, Asians, South Asians, and those of African descent, come from populations that are at higher risk for type 2 diabetes.

Across Canada the prevalence of diabetes in males is higher than in that of females. Approximately 80% of people with diabetes die as a result of heart disease or stroke. A growing incidence of type 2 diabetes occurs in children from high-risk populations. Recent data suggest that a child born in the year 2000 stands a one in three chance of being diagnosed with diabetes in his or her lifetime. Childhood obesity rates and lifestyle choices are considered significant contributing factors (Canadian Diabetes Association, 2007).

SUBJECTIVE DATA

1. Chest pain
2. Dyspnea
3. Orthopnea
4. Cough

5. Fatigue
6. Cyanosis or pallor
7. Edema
8. Nocturia

9. Past cardiac history
10. Family cardiac history
11. Personal habits (cardiac risk factors)

Examiner Asks	Rationale
1. Chest pain. Any **chest pain** or tightness? • Onset: When did it start? How long have you had it *this* time? Had this type of pain before? How often? • Location: Where did the pain start? Does the pain radiate to any other spot? • Character: How would you describe it? Crushing, stabbing, burning, viselike? (Allow the person to offer adjectives before you suggest them.) (Note if uses clenched fist to describe pain.)	Angina, an important cardiac symptom, occurs when heart's vascular supply cannot keep up with metabolic demand. Chest pain also may have pulmonary, musculoskeletal, or gastrointestinal origin; it is important to differentiate. A squeezing "clenched fist" sign is characteristic of angina, but the symptoms below may be anginal equivalents in the absence of chest pain (Reigle, 2005).
• Pain brought on by: activity—what type; rest; emotional upset; after eating; during sexual intercourse; with cold weather? • Any associated symptoms: sweating, ashen grey or pale skin, heart skips beat, shortness of breath, nausea or vomiting, racing of heart?	Diaphoresis, cold sweats, pallor, greyness. Palpitations, dyspnea, nausea, tachycardia, fatigue.
• Pain made worse by moving the arms or neck, breathing, lying flat? • Pain relieved by rest or nitroglycerine? How many tablets?	Try to differentiate pain of cardiac versus noncardiac origin.
2. Dyspnea. Any shortness of breath? • What type of activity, and how much, brings on shortness of breath? How much activity brought it on 6 months ago? • Onset: Does the shortness of breath come on unexpectedly? • Duration: constant or does it come and go? • Seem to be affected by position: lying down? • Awaken you from sleep at night?	**Dyspnea** on exertion (DOE)—quantify exactly (e.g., DOE after walking two level blocks). Paroxysmal. Constant or intermittent. Recumbent. Paroxysmal nocturnal dyspnea (PND) occurs with heart failure. Lying down increases volume of intrathoracic blood, and the weakened heart cannot accommodate the increased load. Classically, the person awakens after 2 hours of sleep with the perception of needing fresh air.
• Does the shortness of breath interfere with activities of daily living?	
3. Orthopnea. How many pillows do you use when sleeping or lying down?	Orthopnea is the need to assume a more upright position to breathe. Note the exact number of pillows used.

Examiner Asks	Rationale

4. **Cough.** Do you have a **cough?**
   - Duration: How long have you had it?
   - Frequency: Is it related to time of day?
   - Type: dry, hacking, barky, hoarse, or congested?
   - Do you cough up mucus? Colour? Any odour? Blood tinged?

Sputum production, mucoid or purulent. Hemoptysis is often a pulmonary disorder but also occurs with mitral stenosis.

   - Associated with: activity, position (lying down), anxiety, talking?
   - Does activity make it better or worse (sit, walk, exercise)?
   - Relieved by rest or medication?

5. **Fatigue.** Do you seem to tire easily? Able to keep up with your family and co-workers?
   - Onset: When did fatigue start? Sudden or gradual? Has any *recent* change occurred in energy level?
   - Fatigue related to time of day: all day, morning, evening?

Fatigue from decreased cardiac output is worse in the evening, whereas fatigue from anxiety or depression occurs all day or is worse in the morning.

6. **Cyanosis or pallor.** Ever noted your facial skin turn blue or ashen?

Cyanosis or **pallor** occurs with myocardial infarction or low cardiac output states as a result of decreased tissue perfusion.

7. **Edema.** Any swelling of your feet and legs?
   - Onset: When did you first notice this?
   - Any recent change?
   - What time of day does the swelling occur? Do your shoes feel tight at the end of day?

Edema is dependent when caused by heart failure.

Cardiac edema is worse at evening and better in morning after elevating legs all night.

   - How much swelling would you say there is? Are both legs equally swollen?
   - Does the swelling go away with: rest, elevation, after a night's sleep?
   - Any associated symptoms, such as shortness of breath? If so, does the shortness of breath occur before leg swelling or after?

8. **Nocturia.** Do you awaken at night with an urgent need to urinate? How long has this been occurring? Any recent change?

Nocturia—Recumbency at night promotes fluid reabsorption and excretion; this occurs with heart failure in the person who is ambulatory during the day.

9. **Cardiac history.** Any **past history** of: hypertension, elevated cholesterol or triglycerides, heart murmur, congenital heart disease, rheumatic fever or unexplained joint pains as child or youth, recurrent tonsillitis, anemia?
   - Ever had heart disease? When was this? Treated by medication or heart surgery?
   - Last ECG, stress ECG, serum cholesterol measurement, other heart tests?

10. **Family cardiac history.** Any **family history** of: hypertension, obesity, diabetes, coronary artery disease (CAD), sudden death at younger age?

11. **Personal habits (cardiac risk factors).**
   - Nutrition: Please describe your usual daily diet. (Note if this diet is representative of the basic food groups, the amount of calories, cholesterol, and any additives such as salt.) What is your usual weight? Has there been any recent change?
   - Smoking: Do you smoke cigarettes or other tobacco? At what age did you start? How many packs per day? For how many years have you smoked this amount? Have you ever tried to quit? If so, how did this go?

Risk factors for CAD—Collect data regarding elevated cholesterol, elevated blood pressure, random plasma glucose level value >11.1 mmol/L or known diabetes mellitus, obesity, cigarette smoking, low activity level, and length of any hormone replacement therapy for postmenopausal women.

Subjective Data

- Alcohol: How much alcohol do you usually drink each week, or each day? When was your last drink? What was the number of drinks that episode? Have you ever been told you had a drinking problem?
- Exercise: What is your usual amount of exercise each day or week? What type of exercise (state type or sport)? If a sport, what is your usual amount (light, moderate, heavy)?
- Drugs: Do you take any antihypertensives, β-blockers, calcium channel blockers, digoxin, diuretics, aspirin and anticoagulants, over-the-counter drugs, or street drugs?

Additional History for Infants

1. How was the mother's health during pregnancy: any unexplained fever, rubella first trimester, other infection, hypertension, drugs taken?

2. Have you noted any cyanosis while nursing, crying? Is the baby able to eat, nurse, or finish bottle without tiring?

> To screen for heart disease in an infant, note fatigue during feeding. Infants with heart failure take fewer ounces each feeding; become dyspneic with sucking; may be diaphoretic, then fall into exhausted sleep; awaken after a short time hungry again.

3. **Growth:** Has this baby grown as expected by growth charts and about the same as siblings or peers?

> Poor weight gain.

4. **Activity:** Were this baby's motor milestones achieved as expected? Is the baby able to play without tiring? How many naps does the baby take each day? How long does a nap last?

Additional History for Children

1. **Growth:** Has this child grown as expected by growth charts?

> Poor weight gain.

2. **Activity:** Is this child able to keep up with siblings or age mates? Is the child willing or reluctant to go out to play? Is the child able to climb stairs, ride a bike, walk a few blocks? Does the child squat to rest during play or to watch television, or assume a knee-chest position while sleeping? Have you noted "blue spells" during exercise?

> Fatigue. Record specific limitations.
>
> Cyanosis.

3. Has the child had any unexplained joint pains or unexplained fever?

4. Does the child have frequent headaches, nosebleeds?

5. Does the child have frequent respiratory infections? How many per year? How are they treated? Have any of these proved to be streptococcal infections?

6. **Family history:** Does the child have a sibling with heart defect? Is anyone in the child's family known to have chromosomal abnormalities, such as Down syndrome?

Additional History for the Pregnant Female

1. Have you had any high blood pressure during this or earlier pregnancies?
   - What was your usual blood pressure level before pregnancy? How has your blood pressure been monitored during the pregnancy?
   - If high blood pressure, what treatment has been started?

Examiner Asks	Rationale
• Any associated symptoms: weight gain, protein in urine, swelling in feet, legs, or face?	
2. Have you had any faintness or dizziness with this pregnancy?	

Additional History for the Aging Adult

1. Do you have any known heart or lung disease: hypertension, CAD, chronic emphysema, or bronchitis?
  • What efforts to treat this have been started?
  • Usual symptoms changed recently? Does your illness interfere with activities of daily living?

2. Do you take any medications for your heart, such as water, blood pressure, or heart pills? Are you aware of side effects? Have you recently stopped taking your medication? Why?

> Noncompliance may be related to side effects or lack of finances.

3. Environment: Does your home have any stairs? How often do you need to climb them? Does this have any effect on activities of daily living?

 — **OBJECTIVE DATA** —

PREPARATION

To evaluate the carotid arteries, the person can be sitting up. To assess the jugular veins and the precordium, the person should be supine with the head and chest slightly elevated.

Stand on the person's right side; this will facilitate your hand placement and auscultation of the precordium.

The room must be warm—chilling makes the person uncomfortable, and shivering interferes with heart sounds. Take scrupulous care to ensure *quiet*; heart sounds are very soft, and any ambient room noise masks them.

Ensure the female's privacy by keeping her breasts draped. The female's left breast overrides part of the area you will need to examine. Gently displace the breast upward, or ask the woman to hold it out of the way.

When performing a regional cardiovascular assessment, use this order:
1. Pulse and blood pressure (see Chapter 9)
2. Extremities (see Chapter 20)
3. Neck vessels
4. Precordium

The logic of this order is that you will begin observations peripherally and move in toward the heart. For choreography of these steps in the complete physical examination, see Chapter 27.

EQUIPMENT NEEDED

Marking pen
Small centimetre ruler
Stethoscope with diaphragm and bell end
    pieces
Alcohol wipe (to clean end piece)

Normal Range of Findings	Abnormal Findings
THE NECK VESSELS	
Palpate the Carotid Artery	
Located central to the heart, the carotid artery yields important information about cardiac function.	

Normal Range of Findings

Abnormal Findings

Palpate each carotid artery medial to the sternomastoid muscle in the neck (Fig. 19-16). Avoid excessive pressure on the carotid sinus area higher in the neck; excessive vagal stimulation here could slow down the heart rate, especially in older adults. Take care to palpate gently. Palpate only one carotid artery at a time to avoid compromising arterial blood to the brain.

Carotid sinus hypersensitivity is the condition in which pressure over the carotid sinus leads to a decreased heart rate, decreased BP, and cerebral ischemia with syncope. This may occur in older adults with hypertension or occlusion of the carotid artery.

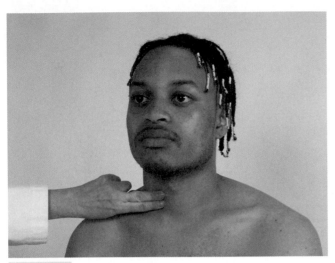

Fig. 19-16

Feel the contour and amplitude of the pulse. Normally the contour is smooth with a rapid upstroke and slower downstroke, and the normal strength is 2+ or moderate (see Chapter 20). Your findings should be the same bilaterally.

Diminished pulse feels small and weak (decreased stroke volume).

Increased pulse feels full and strong (hyperkinetic states) (see Table 20-1, p. 547).

Auscultate the Carotid Artery

For persons middle-aged or older, or who show symptoms or signs of cardiovascular disease, auscultate each carotid artery for the presence of a **bruit** (pronounced bru'-ee) (Fig. 19-17). This is a blowing, swishing sound indicating blood flow turbulence; normally none is present.

A bruit indicates turbulence due to a local vascular cause, such as atherosclerotic narrowing.

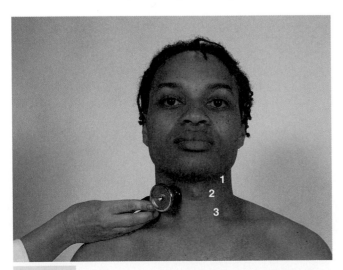

Fig. 19-17

Normal Range of Findings

Keep the neck in a neutral position. Lightly apply the bell of the stethoscope over the carotid artery at three levels: (1) the angle of the jaw, (2) the midcervical area, and (3) the base of the neck (see Fig. 19-17). Avoid compressing the artery because this could create an artificial bruit, and it could compromise circulation if the carotid artery is already narrowed by atherosclerosis. Ask the person to take a breath, exhale, and hold it briefly while you listen so that tracheal breath sounds do not mask or mimic a carotid artery bruit. (Holding the breath on inhalation will also tense the levator scapulae muscles, which makes it hard to hear the carotids.) Sometimes you can hear normal heart sounds transmitted to the neck; do not confuse these with a bruit.

Inspect the Jugular Venous Pulse

From the jugular veins you can assess the **central venous pressure** (CVP) and thus judge the heart's efficiency as a pump. Although the external jugular vein is easier to see, the internal (especially the right) jugular vein is attached more directly to the superior vena cava and thus is more reliable for assessment. You cannot see the internal jugular vein itself, but you can see its pulsation.

Position the person supine anywhere from a 30- to a 45-degree angle, wherever you can best see the pulsations. In general, the higher the venous pressure is, the higher the position you need. Remove the pillow to avoid flexing the neck; the head should be in the same plane as the trunk. Turn the person's head slightly away from the examined side, and direct a strong light tangentially onto the neck to highlight pulsations and shadows.

Note the external jugular veins overlying the sternomastoid muscle. In some persons, the veins are not visible at all, whereas in others they are full in the supine position. As the person is raised to a sitting position, these external jugulars flatten and disappear, usually at 45 degrees.

Now look for pulsations of the internal jugular veins in the area of the suprasternal notch or around the origin of the sternomastoid muscle around the clavicle. You must be able to distinguish internal jugular vein pulsation from that of the carotid artery. It is easy to confuse them because they lie close together. Use the guidelines shown in Table 19-1.

Abnormal Findings

A carotid bruit is audible when the lumen is occluded by ½ to ⅔. Bruit loudness increases as the atherosclerosis worsens until the lumen is occluded by ⅔. After that, bruit loudness decreases. When the lumen is completely occluded, the bruit disappears. Thus absence of a bruit does not ensure absence of a carotid lesion.

A murmur sounds much the same but is caused by a cardiac disorder. Some aortic valve murmurs (aortic stenosis) radiate to the neck and must be distinguished from a local bruit.

Unilateral distension of external jugular veins is due to local cause (kinking or aneurysm).

Full distended external jugular veins above 45 degrees signify increased CVP as with heart failure.

TABLE 19-1	Characteristics of Jugular Versus Carotid Pulsations	
	Internal Jugular Pulse	Carotid Pulse
1. Location	Lower, more lateral, under or behind the sternomastoid muscle	Higher and medial to this muscle
2. Quality	Undulant and diffuse, two visible waves per cycle	Brisk and localized, one wave per cycle
3. Respiration	Varies with respiration; its level descends during inspiration when intrathoracic pressure is decreased	Does not vary
4. Palpable	No	Yes
5. Pressure	Light pressure at the base of the neck easily obliterates	No change
6. Position of person	Level of pulse drops and disappears as the person is brought to a sitting position	Unaffected

Normal Range of Findings	Abnormal Findings

Estimate the Jugular Venous Pressure

Think of the jugular veins as a CVP manometer attached directly to the right atrium. You can "read" the CVP at the highest level of pulsations (Fig. 19-18). Use the angle of Louis (sternal angle) as an arbitrary reference point, and compare it with the highest level of venous pulsation. Hold a vertical ruler on the sternal angle. Align a straight edge on the ruler like a T-square, and adjust the level of the horizontal straight edge to the level of pulsation. Read the level of intersection on the vertical ruler; normal jugular venous pulsation is 2 cm or less above the sternal angle. Also state the person's position, for example, "internal jugular vein pulsations 3 cm above sternal angle when elevated 30 degrees."

Elevated pressure is a level of pulsation that is more than 3 cm above the sternal angle while at 45 degrees. This occurs with heart failure.

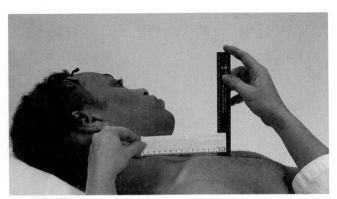

Fig. 19-18

If you cannot find the internal jugular veins, use the external jugular veins and note the point where they look collapsed. Be aware that the technique of estimating venous pressure is difficult and is not always a reliable predictor of CVP. Consistency in grading among examiners is difficult to achieve.

If venous pressure is elevated, or if you suspect heart failure, perform **hepatojugular reflux** (Fig. 19-19). Position the person comfortably supine and instruct him or her to breathe quietly through an open mouth. Hold your right hand on the right upper quadrant of the person's abdomen just below the rib cage. Watch the level of jugular pulsation as you push in with your hand. Exert firm sustained pressure for 30 seconds. This empties venous blood out of the liver sinusoids and adds its volume to the venous system. If the heart is able to pump this additional volume (i.e., if no elevated CVP is present), the jugular veins will rise for a few seconds, then recede back to previous level.

If heart failure is present, the jugular veins will elevate and stay elevated as long as you push.

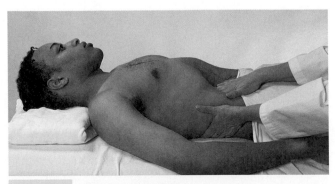

Fig. 19-19   Hepatojugular reflux.

Normal Range of Findings	Abnormal Findings

THE PRECORDIUM

Inspect the Anterior Chest

Arrange tangential lighting to accentuate any flicker of movement.

Pulsations. You may or may not see the **apical impulse,** the pulsation created as the left ventricle rotates against the chest wall during systole. When visible, it occupies the fourth or fifth intercostal space, at or inside the midclavicular line. It is easier to see in children and in those with thinner chest walls.

> A **heave** or **lift** is a sustained forceful thrusting of the ventricle during systole. It occurs with ventricular hypertrophy as a result of increased workload. A right ventricular heave is seen at the sternal border; a left ventricular heave is seen at the apex (see Table 19-8, p. 518).

Palpate the Apical Impulse

(This used to be called the *point of maximal impulse,* or PMI. Because some abnormal conditions may cause a maximal impulse to be felt elsewhere on the chest, use the term **apical impulse** specifically for the apex beat.)

Localize the apical impulse precisely by using one finger pad (Fig. 19-20, *A*). Asking the person to "exhale and then hold it" aids the examiner in locating the pulsation. You may need to roll the person midway to the left to find it; note that this also displaces the apical impulse farther to the left (Fig. 19-20, *B*).

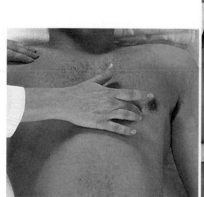
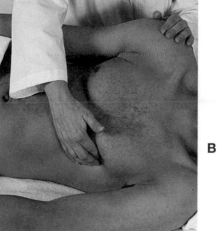

A   **B**

Fig. 19-20   The apical impulse.

Note:
- *Location*—The apical impulse should occupy only one interspace, the fourth or fifth, and be at or medial to the midclavicular line
- *Size*—Normally 1 × 2 cm
- *Amplitude*—Normally a short, gentle tap
- *Duration*—Short, normally occupies only first half of systole

Cardiac enlargement:
- Left ventricular dilatation (volume overload) displaces impulse down and to left, and increases size more than one space.
- Increased force and duration but no change in location occurs with left ventricular hypertrophy and no dilatation (pressure overload) (see Table 19-8, p. 518).

The apical impulse is palpable in about half of adults. It is not palpable in obese persons or in persons with thick chest walls. With high cardiac output states (anxiety, fever, hyperthyroidism, anemia), the apical impulse increases in amplitude and duration.

Not palpable with pulmonary emphysema due to overriding lungs.

Normal Range of Findings	Abnormal Findings

Palpate Across the Precordium

Using the palmar aspects of your four fingers, gently palpate the apex, the left sternal border, and the base, searching for any other pulsations (Fig. 19-21). Normally none occur. If any are present, note the timing. Use the carotid artery pulsation as a guide, or auscultate as you palpate.

A **thrill** is a palpable vibration. It feels like the throat of a purring cat. The thrill signifies turbulent blood flow and accompanies loud murmurs. Absence of a thrill, however, does not necessarily rule out the presence of a murmur.

Accentuated first and second heart sounds and extra heart sounds also may cause abnormal pulsations.

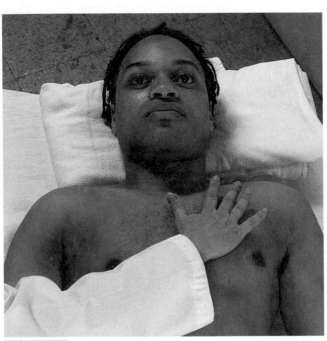

Fig. 19-21

Percussion

Percussion is used to outline the heart's borders, but it is often displaced by chest X-rays or echocardiography, which are much more accurate methods of detecting heart enlargement. When the right ventricle enlarges, it does so in the anteroposterior diameter, which is better seen on X-ray film. Also, percussion is of limited usefulness with the female breast tissue or in an obese person or a person with a muscular chest wall.

However, there are times when your percussing hands are the only tools you have with you, such as in an outpatient setting, extended care facility, or the person's home. When you need to search for cardiac enlargement, place your stationary finger in the person's fifth intercostal space over on the left side of the chest near the anterior axillary line. Slide your stationary hand toward yourself, percussing as you go, and note the change of sound from resonance over the lung to dull (over the heart). Normally, the left border of cardiac dullness is at the midclavicular line in the fifth interspace and slopes in toward the sternum as you progress upward, so that by the second interspace the border of dullness coincides with the left sternal border. The right border of dullness normally matches the sternal border.

Cardiac enlargement is due to increased ventricular volume or wall thickness; it occurs with hypertension, CAD, heart failure, and cardiomyopathy.

Normal Range of Findings	Abnormal Findings

Auscultation

Identify the auscultatory areas where you will listen. These include the four traditional valve "areas" (Fig. 19-22). The valve areas are not over the actual anatomical locations of the valves but are the sites on the chest wall where sounds produced by the valves are best heard. The sound radiates with the direction of blood flow. The valve areas are:

- Second right interspace—aortic valve area
- Second left interspace—pulmonic valve area
- Left lower sternal border—tricuspid valve area
- Fifth interspace at around left midclavicular line—mitral valve area

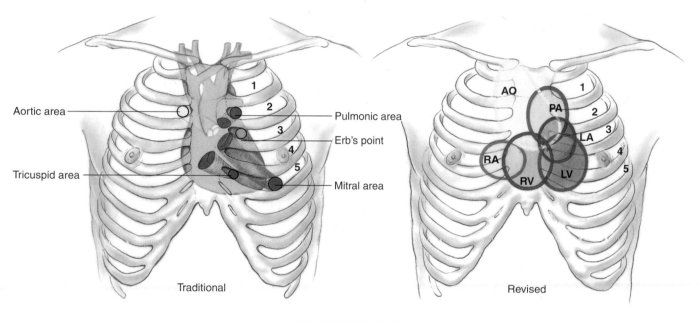

AUSCULTATORY AREAS

Fig. 19-22

Do not limit your auscultation to only four locations. Sounds produced by the valves may be heard all over the precordium. (For this reason, many experts even discourage the naming of the valve areas.) Thus, learn to inch your stethoscope in a rough Z pattern, from the base of the heart across and down, then over to the apex. Or start at the apex and work your way up. Include the sites shown in Figure 19-22.

Recall the characteristics of a high-quality stethoscope (see Chapter 8). Clean the end pieces with an alcohol wipe; you will use both end pieces. Although all heart sounds are low frequency, the diaphragm is for relatively higher-pitched sounds, and the bell is for relatively lower-pitched ones.

Before you begin, alert the person: "I always listen to the heart in a number of places on the chest. Just because I am listening a long time, it does not necessarily mean that something is wrong."

After you place the stethoscope, try closing your eyes briefly to tune out any distractions. Concentrate, and listen selectively to *one sound at a time*. Consider that at least two, and perhaps three or four, sounds may be happening in less than 1 second. You cannot process everything at once. Begin with the diaphragm end piece and use the following routine: (1) note the rate and rhythm, (2) identify S_1 and S_2, (3) assess S_1 and S_2 separately, (4) listen for extra heart sounds, and (5) listen for murmurs.

Objective Data

Normal Range of Findings

Note the Rate and Rhythm. The rate ranges normally from 60 to 100 beats per minute. (Review the full discussion of the pulse in Chapter 9 and the normal rates across age groups.) The rhythm should be regular, although **sinus arrhythmia** occurs normally in young adults and children. With sinus arrhythmia, the rhythm varies with the person's breathing, increasing at the peak of inspiration and slowing with expiration. Note any other irregular rhythm. If one occurs, check if it has any pattern, or if it is totally irregular.

When you notice any irregularity, check for a **pulse deficit** by auscultating the apical beat while simultaneously palpating the radial pulse. Count a serial measurement (one after the other) of apical beat and radial pulse. Normally, every beat you hear at the apex should perfuse to the periphery and be palpable. The two counts should be identical. When different, subtract the radial rate from the apical and record the remainder as the pulse deficit.

Identify S_1 and S_2. This is important because S_1 is the start of systole and thus serves as the reference point for the timing of all other cardiac sounds. Usually, you can identify S_1 instantly because you hear a pair of sounds close together (lub-dup), and S_1 is the first of the pair. This guideline works, except in the cases of the tachyarrhythmias (rates >100 per minute). Then the diastolic filling time is shortened, and the beats are too close together to distinguish. Other guidelines to distinguish S_1 from S_2 are:

- S_1 is louder than S_2 at the apex; S_2 is louder than S_1 at the base.
- S_1 coincides with the carotid artery pulse. Feel the carotid gently as you auscultate at the apex; the sound you hear as you feel each pulse is S_1 (Fig. 19-23).
- S_1 coincides with the R wave (the upstroke of the QRS complex) if the person is on an ECG monitor.

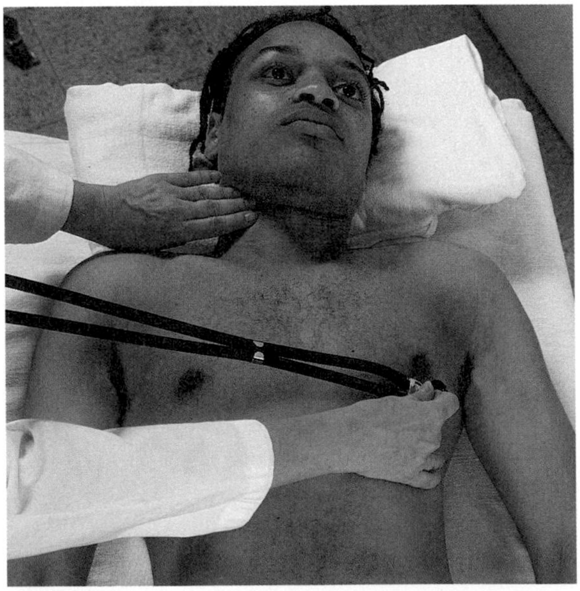

Fig. 19-23

Listen to S_1 and S_2 Separately. Note whether each heart sound is normal, accentuated, diminished, or split. Inch your diaphragm across the chest as you do this.

Abnormal Findings

Premature beat—an isolated beat is early, or a pattern occurs in which every third or fourth beat sounds early.

Irregularly irregular—no pattern to the sounds; beats come rapidly and at random intervals.

A **pulse deficit** signals a weak contraction of the ventricles; it occurs with atrial fibrillation, premature beats, and heart failure.

Normal Range of Findings	Abnormal Findings

Normal Range of Findings

First Heart Sound (S₁). Caused by closure of the AV valves, S₁ signals the beginning of systole. You can hear it over the entire precordium, although it is loudest at the apex (Fig. 19-24). (Sometimes the two sounds are equally loud at the apex, because S₁ is lower pitched than S₂.)

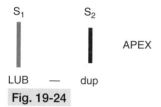

Fig. 19-24

You can hear S₁ with the diaphragm with the person in any position and equally well during inspiration and expiration. A split S₁ is normal, but it occurs rarely. A split S₁ means you are hearing the mitral and tricuspid components separately. It is audible in the tricuspid valve area, the left lower sternal border. The split is very rapid, with the two components only 0.03 second apart.

Second Heart Sound (S₂). The S₂ is associated with closure of the semilunar valves. You can hear it with the diaphragm, over the entire precordium, although S₂ is loudest at the base (Fig. 19-25).

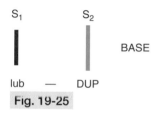

Fig. 19-25

Splitting of S₂. A split S₂ is a normal phenomenon that occurs toward the end of inspiration in some people. Recall that closure of the aortic and pulmonic valves is nearly synchronous. Because of the effects of respiration on the heart described earlier, inspiration separates the timing of the two valves' closure, and the aortic valve closes 0.06 seconds before the pulmonic valve. Instead of one DUP, you hear a split sound—T-DUP (Fig. 19-26). During expiration, synchrony returns, and the aortic and pulmonic components fuse together. A split S₂ is heard only in the pulmonic valve area, the second left interspace.

SPLITTING OF THE SECOND HEART SOUND

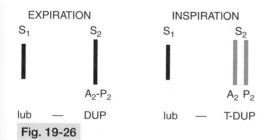

Fig. 19-26

When you first hear the split S₂, do *not* be tempted to ask the person to hold his or her breath so that you can concentrate on the sounds. Breath holding will only equalize ejection times in the right and left sides of the heart and cause the split to go away. Instead, concentrate on the split as you watch the person's chest rise up and down with breathing. The split S₂ occurs about every fourth heartbeat, fading in with inhalation and fading out with exhalation.

Abnormal Findings

Causes of accentuated or diminished S₁ (see Table 19-3, p. 513).

Both heart sounds are diminished with conditions that place an increased amount of tissue between the heart and your stethoscope: emphysema (hyperinflated lungs), obesity, pericardial fluid.

Accentuated or diminished S₂ (see Table 19-4, p. 514).

A **fixed split** is unaffected by respiration; the split is always there.

A **paradoxical split** is the opposite of what you would expect; the sounds fuse on inspiration and split on expiration (see Table 19-5, p. 514).

Objective Data

Normal Range of Findings	Abnormal Findings

Focus on Systole, Then on Diastole, and Listen for any Extra Heart Sounds. Listen with the diaphragm, then switch to the bell, covering all auscultatory areas (Fig. 19-27). Usually, these are silent periods. When you do detect an extra heart sound, listen carefully to note its timing and characteristics. During systole, the **midsystolic click** (which is associated with mitral valve prolapse) is the most common extra sound (see Table 19-6, p. 515). The third and fourth heart sounds occur in diastole; either may be normal or abnormal (see Table 19-7, p. 516).

A pathological S_3 (ventricular gallop) occurs with heart failure and volume overload; a pathological S_4 (atrial gallop) occurs with CAD (see Table 19-7, p. 516, for a full description).

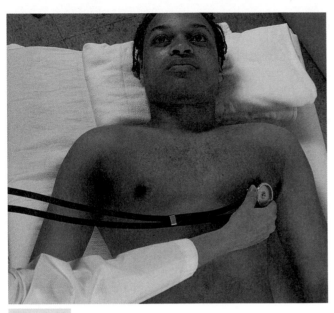

Fig. 19-27

Listen for Murmurs. A murmur is a blowing, swooshing sound that occurs with turbulent blood flow in the heart or great vessels. Except for the innocent murmurs described, murmurs are abnormal. If you hear a murmur, describe it by indicating these following characteristics:

Timing. It is crucial to define the murmur by its occurrence in systole or diastole. You must be able to identify S_1 and S_2 accurately to do this. Try to further describe the murmur as being in early, mid-, or late systole or diastole; throughout the cardiac event (termed pansystolic or holosystolic/pandiastolic or holodiastolic); and whether it obscures or muffles the heart sounds.

Loudness. Describe the intensity in terms of six "grades." For example, record a grade ii murmur as "II/VI."

Grade I—barely audible, heard only in a quiet room and then with difficulty
Grade II—clearly audible, but faint
Grade III—moderately loud, easy to hear
Grade IV—loud, associated with a thrill palpable on the chest wall
Grade V—very loud, heard with one corner of the stethoscope lifted off the chest wall
Grade VI—loudest, still heard with entire stethoscope lifted just off the chest wall

Pitch. Describe the pitch as high, medium, or low. The pitch depends on the pressure and the rate of blood flow producing the murmur.

Murmurs may be due to congenital defects and acquired valvular defects. Study Tables 19-9 and 19-10, pp. 519 and 521, for a complete description.

A systolic murmur may occur with a normal heart or with heart disease; a diastolic murmur always indicates heart disease.

Normal Range of Findings	Abnormal Findings
Pattern. The intensity may follow a pattern during the cardiac phase, growing louder (crescendo), tapering off (decrescendo), or increasing to a peak and then decreasing (crescendo–decrescendo, or diamond shaped). Because the whole murmur is just milliseconds long, it takes practice to diagnose any pattern.	
Quality. Describe the quality as musical, blowing, harsh, or rumbling.	The murmur of mitral stenosis is rumbling, whereas that of aortic stenosis is harsh (see Table 19-10, p. 521).
Location. Describe the area of maximum intensity of the murmur (where it is best heard) by noting the valve area or intercostal spaces.	
Radiation. The murmur may be transmitted downstream in the direction of blood flow and may be heard in another place on the precordium, the neck, the back, or the axilla.	

Posture. Some murmurs disappear or are enhanced by a change in position.
  Some murmurs are common in healthy children or adolescents and are termed *innocent* or *functional.* **Innocent** indicates having no valvular or other pathological cause; **functional** is due to increased blood flow in the heart (e.g., in anemia, fever, pregnancy, hyperthyroidism). The contractile force of the heart is greater in children. This increases blood flow velocity. The increased velocity plus a smaller chest measurement makes an audible murmur.
  The innocent murmur is generally soft (grade II), midsystolic, short, crescendo–decrescendo, and with a vibratory or musical quality ("vooot" sound like fiddle strings). Also, the innocent murmur is heard at the second or third left intercostal space and disappears with sitting, and the young person has no associated signs of cardiac dysfunction.
  Although it is important to distinguish innocent murmurs from pathological ones, it is best to suspect all murmurs as pathological until they are proved otherwise. Diagnostic tests such as electrocardiography, phonocardiography, and echocardiography are needed to establish an accurate diagnosis.	

Change Position. After auscultating in the supine position, roll the person toward his or her left side. Listen with the bell at the apex for the presence of any diastolic filling sounds (i.e., the S_3 or S_4) (Fig. 19-28).	S_3 and S_4, and the murmur of mitral stenosis sometimes may be heard only when on the left side.

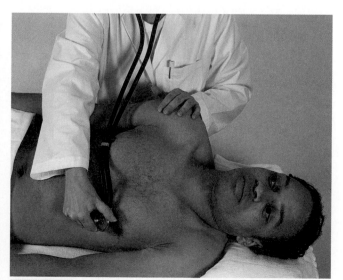

Fig. 19-28

Objective Data

Normal Range of Findings	Abnormal Findings

Ask the person to sit up, lean forward slightly, and exhale. Listen with the diaphragm firmly pressed at the base, right, and left sides. Check for the soft, high-pitched, early diastolic murmur of aortic or pulmonic regurgitation (Fig. 19-29).

Murmur of aortic regurgitation sometimes may be heard only when the person is leaning forward in the sitting position.

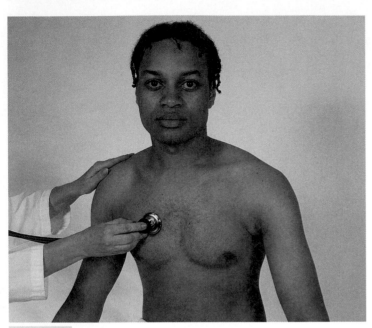

Fig. 19-29

🌱 DEVELOPMENTAL CARE

Infants

The transition from fetal to pulmonic circulation occurs in the immediate newborn period. Fetal shunts normally close within 10 to 15 hours but may take up to 48 hours. Thus, you should assess the cardiovascular system during the first 24 hours and again in 2 to 3 days.

Note any extracardiac signs that may reflect heart status (particularly in the skin), liver size, and respiratory status. The skin colour should be pink to pinkish brown, depending on the infant's genetic heritage. If cyanosis occurs, determine its first appearance—at or shortly after birth versus after the neonatal period. Normally, the liver is not enlarged, and the respirations are not laboured. Also, note the expected parameters of weight gain throughout infancy.

Failure of shunts to close (e.g., patent ductus arteriosus [PDA], atrial septal defect [ASD]); see Table 19-9, p. 519.

Cyanosis at or just after birth signals oxygen desaturation of congenital heart disease (Table 19-9, p. 519).

The most important signs of heart failure in an infant are persistent tachycardia, tachypnea, and liver enlargement. Engorged veins, gallop rhythm, and pulsus alternans also are signs. Respiratory crackles (rales) is an important sign in adults but not in infants.

Failure to thrive occurs with cardiac disease.

Palpate the apical impulse to determine the size and position of the heart. Because the infant's heart has a more horizontal placement, expect to palpate the apical impulse at the fourth intercostal space just lateral to the midclavicular line. It may or may not be visible.

The apex is displaced with:
- Cardiac enlargement, shifts to the left
- Pneumothorax, shifts away from affected side
- Diaphragmatic hernia, shifts usually to right because this hernia occurs more often on the left
- Dextrocardia, a rare anomaly in which the heart is located on right side of chest

Normal Range of Findings

The heart rate is best auscultated because radial pulses are hard to count accurately. Use the small (pediatric size) diaphragm and bell (Fig. 19-30). The heart rate may range from 100 to 180 per minute immediately after birth, then stabilize to an average of 120 to 140 per minute. Infants normally have wide fluctuations with activity, from 170 per minute or more with crying or being active to 70 to 90 per minute with sleeping. Variations are greatest at birth and are even more so with premature babies (see Table 9-2, p. 157).

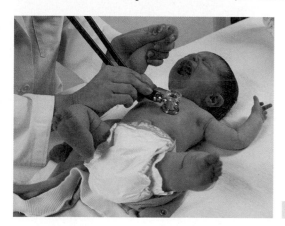

Fig. 19-30

Expect the heart rhythm to have sinus arrhythmia, the phasic speeding up or slowing down with the respiratory cycle.

Rapid rates make it more challenging to evaluate heart sounds. Expect heart sounds to be louder in infants than in adults because of the infant's thinner chest wall. Also, S_2 has a higher pitch and is sharper than S_1. Splitting of S_2 just after the height of inspiration is common, not at birth, but beginning a few hours after birth.

Murmurs in the immediate newborn period do not necessarily indicate congenital heart disease. Murmurs are relatively common in the first 2 to 3 days because of fetal shunt closure. These murmurs are usually grade I or II, are systolic, accompany no other signs of cardiac disease, and disappear in 2 to 3 days. The murmur of PDA is a continuous machinery murmur, which disappears by 2 to 3 days. On the other hand, absence of a murmur in the immediate newborn period does not ensure a perfect heart; congenital defects can be present that are not signalled by an early murmur. It is best to listen frequently and to note and describe any murmur according to the characteristics listed on p. 504.

To help facilitate the assessment of an infant, it is suggested that you listen to the heart sounds while the infant is quiet. This may mean that you need to alter the traditional sequence of assessment.

Children

Note any extracardiac or cardiac signs that may indicate heart disease: poor weight gain, developmental delay, persistent tachycardia, tachypnea, dyspnea on exertion, cyanosis, and clubbing. Note that clubbing of fingers and toes usually does not appear until late in the first year, even with severe cyanotic defects.

The apical impulse is sometimes visible in children with thin chest walls. Note any obvious bulge or any heave—these are not normal.

Abnormal Findings

Persistent tachycardia is >200 per minute in newborns, or >150 per minute in infants.

Bradycardia is <90 per minute in newborns or <60 in older infants or children. This causes a serious drop in cardiac output because the small muscle mass of their hearts cannot increase stroke volume significantly.

Investigate any irregularity except sinus arrhythmia.

Fixed split S_2 indicates atrial septal defect (see Table 19-9, p. 519).

Persistent murmur after 2 to 3 days, holosystolic murmurs or those that last into diastole, and those that are loud—all warrant further evaluation.

A precordial bulge to the left of the sternum with a hyperdynamic precordium signals cardiac enlargement. The bulge occurs because the cartilaginous rib cage is more compliant.

A substernal heave occurs with right ventricular enlargement, and an apical heave occurs with left ventricular hypertrophy.

Objective Data

Normal Range of Findings	Abnormal Findings

Normal Range of Findings

Palpate the apical impulse: in the fourth intercostal space to the left of the midclavicular line until age 4 years; at the fourth interspace at the midclavicular line from age 4 to 6 years; and in the fifth interspace to the right of the midclavicular line at age 7 years (Fig. 19-31).

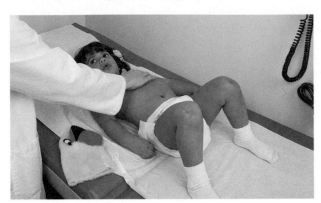

Fig. 19-31

The average heart rate slows as the child grows older, although it is still variable with rest or activity (see Table 9-2, 157).

The heart rhythm remains characterized by sinus arrhythmia. Physiological S_3 is common in children (see Table 19-7, p. 516). It occurs in early diastole, just after S_2, and is a dull soft sound that is best heard at the apex.

A **venous hum**—due to turbulence of blood flow in the jugular venous system—is common in healthy children and has no pathological significance. It is a continuous, low-pitched, soft hum that is heard throughout the cycle, although it is loudest in diastole. Listen with the bell over the supraclavicular fossa at the medial third of the clavicle, especially on the right, or over the upper anterior chest.

The venous hum is usually not affected by respiration, may sound louder when the child stands, and is easily obliterated by occluding the jugular veins in the neck with your fingers.

Heart murmurs that are innocent (or functional) in origin are very common through childhood. Some studies indicate that they have a 30% occurrence, and others state that nearly all children may demonstrate a murmur at some time. Most innocent murmurs have these characteristics: soft, relatively short systolic ejection murmur; medium pitch; vibratory; best heard at the left lower sternal or midsternal border, with no radiation to the apex, base, or back.

For the child whose murmur has been shown to be innocent, it is very important that the parents understand this completely. They need to believe that this murmur is just a "noise" and has no pathological significance. Otherwise, the parents may become overprotective and limit activity for the child, which may result in the child developing a negative self-concept.

The Pregnant Female

The vital signs usually yield an increase in resting pulse rate of 10 to 15 beats per minute and a drop in blood pressure from the normal prepregnancy level. The BP decreases to its lowest point during the second trimester and then slowly rises during the third trimester. The BP varies with position. It is usually lowest in left lateral recumbent position, a bit higher when supine, and highest when sitting (Cunningham et al., 2005).

Inspection of the skin often shows a mild hyperemia in light-skinned women because the increased cutaneous blood flow tries to eliminate the excess heat generated by the increased metabolism. Palpation of the apical impulse is higher and lateral compared with the normal position, as the enlarging uterus elevates the diaphragm and displaces the heart up and to the left and rotates it on its long axis.

Abnormal Findings

The apical impulse moves laterally with cardiac enlargement.

Thrill (palpable vibration).

This latter manoeuvre helps differentiate the venous hum from other cardiac murmurs (e.g., PDA).

Distinguish innocent murmurs from pathological ones. This may involve referral to another examiner or the performance of diagnostic tests such as electrocardiography or ultrasonography.

Suspect pregnancy-induced hypertension with a sustained rise of 30 mm Hg systolic or 15 mm Hg diastolic under basal conditions.

Normal Range of Findings	Abnormal Findings

Auscultation of the heart sounds shows changes caused by the increased blood volume and workload:

- Heart sounds

    Exaggerated splitting of S_1 and increased loudness of S_1

    A loud, easily heard S_3

- Heart murmurs

    A systolic murmur in 90%, which disappears soon after delivery

    A soft, diastolic murmur heard transiently in 19%

    A continuous murmur from breast vasculature in 10% (Cunningham et al., 2005)

The last-mentioned murmur is termed a **mammary souffle** (pronounced soof′ f′l), which occurs near term or when the mother is lactating; it is due to increased blood flow through the internal mammary artery. The murmur is heard in the second, third, or fourth intercostal space; it is continuous, although it is accented in systole. You can obliterate it by pressure with the stethoscope or one finger lateral to the murmur.

Murmurs of aortic valve disease cannot be obliterated.

The ECG has no changes except for a slight left axis deviation due to the change in the heart's position.

The Aging Adult

A gradual rise in systolic blood pressure is common in older persons; the diastolic blood pressure stays fairly constant with a resulting widening of pulse pressure. Some older adults experience **orthostatic hypotension,** a sudden drop in blood pressure when rising to sit or stand.

Use caution in palpating and auscultating the carotid artery. Avoid pressure in the carotid sinus area, which could cause a reflex slowing of the heart rate. Also, pressure on the carotid artery could compromise circulation if the artery is already narrowed by atherosclerosis.

When measuring jugular venous pressure, view the right internal jugular vein. The aorta stiffens, dilates, and elongates with aging, which may compress the left neck veins and obscure pulsations on the left side (Fleg, 1990).

The chest often increases in anteroposterior diameter in older persons. This makes it more difficult to palpate the apical impulse and to hear the splitting of S_2. The S_4 often occurs in older people with no known cardiac disease. Systolic murmurs are common, occurring in over 50% of older people (Fleg, 1990).

The S_3 is associated with heart failure and is always abnormal over 40 years of age (see Table 19-7, p. 516).

Occasional premature ectopic beats are common and do not necessarily indicate underlying heart disease. When in doubt, obtain an ECG. However, consider that the ECG only records for 1 isolated minute in time and may need to be supplemented by a test of 24-hour ambulatory heart monitoring.

Objective Data

Summary Checklist: Heart and Neck Vessels Examination

 For a PDA-downloadable version, go to http://evolve.elsevier.com/Canada/Jarvis/examination/.

Neck

1. Carotid pulse—observe and palpate
2. Observe jugular venous pulse
3. Estimate jugular venous pressure

Precordium

1. Inspection and palpation

    Describe location of apical impulse

    Note any heave (lift) or thrill

2. Auscultation

    Identify anatomical areas where you listen

    Note rate and rhythm of heartbeat

    Identify S_1 and S_2 and note any variation

    Listen in systole and diastole for any extra heart sounds

Listen in systole and diastole for any murmurs

Repeat sequence with bell

Listen at the apex with person in left lateral position

Listen at the base with person in sitting position

Objective Data

Promoting Health: Women and Heart Attack

The Heart Truth: Women and Heart Attacks

When someone complains of chest pain or pain radiating down the left arm, almost everyone thinks "heart attack." After all, these are the symptoms that typically occur. Aren't they? Well, yes and no. In the past it was believed that women experienced different warning signs than men. The Heart and Stroke Foundation notes that this may not actually be the case. Both women and men may experience typical or atypical symptoms, such as nausea; sweating; pain in the arm, throat, or jaw; or pain that is unusual. *However*, women may describe their pain differently than men. Nevertheless, the most common symptom in women is still chest pain.

Many of the symptoms women experienced are easily attributable to something else, other than the heart, and are therefore often ignored. Scientific evidence now shows that women tend to minimize the significance of the symptoms of cardiac disease. However, part of this may be due to a lack of awareness.

Heart disease is the leading cause of death in women older than 55 years. Women tend to be safeguarded from heart disease prior to menopause because of the protective effect of naturally occuring estrogen, but not always. For example, premenopausal women with diabetes have a similar risk to that of men of the same age because diabetes cancels out the protective effect that estrogen provides to premenopausal women.

Some factors directly influence a woman's risk of cardiovascular disease. During a woman's reproductive life cycle, from about age 12 to 50, the naturally occurring estrogen provides a protective effect on women's cardiovascular health. However, estrogen's protective effect can change, depending on a variety of factors and conditions.

Oral contraceptives are much safer now than the forms used in the past. In women under the age of 35 who do not smoke, contraceptive use does not increase the risk of stroke. However, in a small proportion of women, oral contraceptives increase the risk of high blood pressure and blood clots. The risk increases if the person smokes or already has high blood pressure or other risk factors for heart disease or stroke.

During the menopausal transition, which occurs around age 51, a woman's risk of heart disease and stroke increases. During this period the ovaries slowly decrease the production of the hormone estrogen, which as previously mentioned has a protective effect on the heart. A menopausal woman may experience an increase in LDL or "bad" cholesterol and triglyceride levels and a decrease in HDL or "good" cholesterol. She may also show a tendency toward higher blood pressure. Reduced estrogen levels may also increase body fat above the waist, have harmful effects on the way blood clots, and affect the way the body metabolizes sugar, a precursor condition to diabetes.

Until recently it was thought that hormone replacement therapy (HRT) could help reduce the risk of cardiac disease in menopausal women. However, recent studies have shown that taking certain types of hormones (estrogen with progestin) can actually increase the risk of heart attack, stroke, blood clots, and breast cancer for some women. As a result of these studies, hormone therapy is no longer recommended to prevent heart disease, although it may be helpful for some women in treating other symptoms of menopause, such as hot flashes. Women should always consult their physician for recommendations regarding HRT.

Naturally occurring estrogen also helps to keep cholesterol levels in a healthy range. But, overall, 45% of Canadian women between the ages of 18 and 74 have cholesterol levels that are too high. After menopause, as estrogen levels drop, the incidence of developing high cholesterol increases. Among women between the ages of 65 and 74, an alarming 80% have cholesterol levels that are unhealthy. A healthcare professional should be consulted about how often cholesterol levels should be checked.

Exercise and weight control are paramount to mitigating the risk of heart disease. Inactive women have twice the risk of developing heart disease than active women. Thirty minutes of physical activity, four to six times a week, helps to keep the heart strong and prevent heart disease. Even losing a small amount of extra weight can also help reduce the risk.

The Heart Truth is a national awareness and prevention campaign launched recently in the United States about heart disease in women. The Canadian Heart and Stroke foundation adopted this US-based initiative in February, 2008 due to its overwhelming success. The Heart Truth campaign introduced the *Red Dress* as the national symbol for women and heart disease awareness. Since its introduction, many women have taken ownership of the symbol.

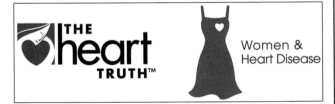

For more information about women and heart disease, consult the following Web sites:

Canadian Health Network: http://canadian-health-network.ca
Heart and Stroke Foundation of Canada: www.heartandstroke.ca
American Heart Association: www.americanheart.org

⇨— DOCUMENTATION AND CRITICAL THINKING —⇦

Sample Charting

SUBJECTIVE

No chest pain, dyspnea, orthopnea, cough, fatigue, or edema. No personal history of hypertension, abnormal blood tests, heart murmur, or rheumatic fever. Last ECG 2 yr PTA, result normal. No stress ECG or other heart tests.

Family history: father with obesity, smoking, and hypertension, treated c̄ diuretic medication. No other family history significant for cardiovascular disease.

Personal habits: diet balanced in 4 food groups, 2 to 3 regular coffee/day; no smoking; alcohol, 1 to 2 beers occasionally on weekend; exercise, runs 5 km, 3 to 4 ×/week; no prescription or OTC medications or street drugs.

OBJECTIVE

Neck: Carotids 2+ and = bilaterally. Internal jugular vein pulsations present when supine, and disappear when elevated to a 45-degree position.
Precordium: Inspection. No visible pulsations, no heave or lift.
Palpation: Apical impulse in fifth ICS at left midclavicular line, no thrill.
Auscultation: Rate 68 beats per minute, rhythm regular, S_1–S_2 are normal, not diminished or accentuated, no S_3, no S_4 or other extra sounds, no murmurs.

ASSESSMENT

Neck vessels healthy by inspection and auscultation
Heart sounds normal

Focused Assessment: Clinical Case Study

Mr. N.V. is a 53-year-old Euro-Canadian male woodcutter admitted to the CCU at Toronto General Hospital (TGH) with chest pain.

SUBJECTIVE

- 1 year PTA—N.V. admitted to TGH with crushing substernal chest pain, radiating to L shoulder, accompanied by nausea, vomiting, diaphoresis.
- Diagnosed as MI, hospitalized 7 days, discharged with nitroglycerine prn for anginal pain.
- Did not return to work. Activity included walking 2 km/d, hunting. Had occasional episodes of chest pain with exercise, relieved by rest.
- 1 day PTA—had increasing frequency of chest pain, about every 2 hours, lasting few minutes, saw pain as warning to go to MD.
- Day of admission—severe substernal chest pain ("like someone sitting on my chest") unrelieved by rest. Saw personal MD; while in office had episode of chest pain as last year's, accompanied by diaphoresis, no N & V or SOB, relieved by 1 nitroglycerine. Transferred to TGH by paramedics. No further pain since admission 2 hours ago.
- Family hx—mother died of MI at age 57.
- Personal habits—smokes 1½ pack cigarettes daily × 34 years, no alcohol, diet—trying to limit fat and fried food, still high in added salt.

OBJECTIVE

Extremities: Skin pink, no cyanosis. Upper extrem.—capillary refill sluggish, no clubbing. Lower extrem.—no edema, no hair growth 10 cm below knee bilaterally.
Pulses—

carotid	brachial	radial	femoral	popliteal	P.T.	D.P.	
2+	2+	2+	2+	0	0	1+	all = bilaterally

B/P R arm 104/66
Neck: External jugulars flat. Internal jugular pulsations present when supine and absent when elevated to 45 degrees.
Precordium: Inspection. Apical impulse visible fifth ICS, 7 cm left of midsternal line, no heave.
Palpation: Apical impulse palpable in fifth and sixth ICS. No thrill.

Continued

Auscultation: Apical rate 92 regular, S_1–S_2 are normal, not diminished or accentuated, no S_3 or S_4, grade III/VI systolic murmur present at left lower sternal border.

ASSESSMENT

Substernal chest pain
Systolic murmur
Ineffective tissue perfusion R/T interruption in flow
Decreased cardiac output R/T reduction in stroke volume

Nursing Diagnoses Commonly Associated With Cardiovascular Disorders

All nursing diagnoses can be found on the Evolve Web site at **http://evolve.elsevier.com/Canada/Jarvis/examination/.**

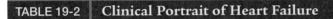

─ ABNORMAL FINDINGS ─

| TABLE 19-2 | Clinical Portrait of Heart Failure |

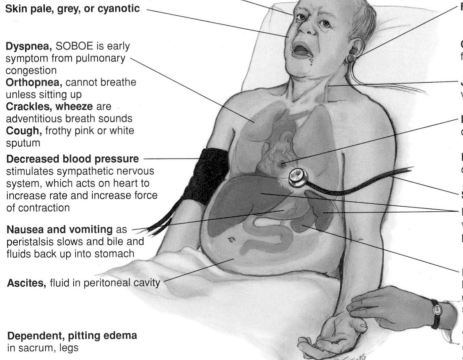

Dilated pupils, a sympathetic nervous system response

Skin pale, grey, or cyanotic

Dyspnea, SOBOE is early symptom from pulmonary congestion
Orthopnea, cannot breathe unless sitting up
Crackles, wheeze are adventitious breath sounds
Cough, frothy pink or white sputum

Decreased blood pressure stimulates sympathetic nervous system, which acts on heart to increase rate and increase force of contraction

Nausea and vomiting as peristalsis slows and bile and fluids back up into stomach

Ascites, fluid in peritoneal cavity

Dependent, pitting edema in sacrum, legs

Anxiety, gasping from pulmonary congestion

Falling O_2 saturation

Confusion, unconsciousness from decreased O_2 to brain

Jugular vein distension from venous congestion

Infarct, may be cause of decreased cardiac output

Fatigue, weakness from decreased cardiac output

S_3 gallop, tachycardia
Enlarged spleen and liver from venous congestion, which causes pressure on breathing

Decreased urine output as kidneys compensate for decreased CO by retaining sodium and H_2O

Weak pulse
Cool, moist skin as peripheral vasoconstriction shunts blood to vital organs

Decreased cardiac output occurs when the heart fails as a pump, and the circulation becomes backed up and congested.

Signs and symptoms of heart failure come from two basic mechanisms: (1) the heart's inability to pump enough blood to meet the metabolic demands of the body, and (2) the kidney's compensatory mechanisms of abnormal retention of sodium and water to compensate for the decreased cardiac output. This increases blood volume and venous return, which causes further congestion.

Onset of heart failure may be: (1) *acute,* as following a myocardial infarction when direct damage to the heart's contracting ability has occurred; or (2) *chronic,* as with hypertension, when the ventricles must pump against chronically increased pressure.

ABNORMAL FINDINGS
FOR ADVANCED PRACTICE

TABLE 19-3	Variations in S_1

The intensity of S_1 depends on three factors: (1) position of AV valve at the start of systole, (2) structure of the valve leaflets, and (3) how quickly pressure rises in the ventricle.

	Factor	Examples
Loud (Accentuated) S_1 S_1 S_2	1. Position of AV valve at start of systole—wide open and no time to drift together	Hyperkinetic states where blood velocity is increased: exercise, fever, anemia, hyperthyroidism
	2. Change in valve structure—calcification of valve, needs increasing ventricular pressure to close the valve against increased atrial pressure	Mitral stenosis with leaflets still mobile
Faint (Diminished) S_1 S_1 S_2	1. Position of AV valve—delayed conduction from atria to ventricles. Mitral valve drifts shut before ventricular contraction closes it	First-degree heart block (prolonged PR interval)
	2. Change in valve structure—extreme calcification, which limits mobility	Mitral insufficiency
	3. More forceful atrial contraction into noncompliant ventricle; delays or diminishes ventricular contraction	Severe hypertension—systemic or pulmonary
Varying Intensity of S_1 S_1 S_2 S_1 S_2	1. Position of AV valve varies before closing from beat to beat	Atrial fibrillation—irregularly irregular rhythm
	2. Atria and ventricles beat independently	Complete heart block with changing PR interval
Split S_1 S_1 S_2 T M	Mitral and tricuspid components are heard separately	Normal but uncommon

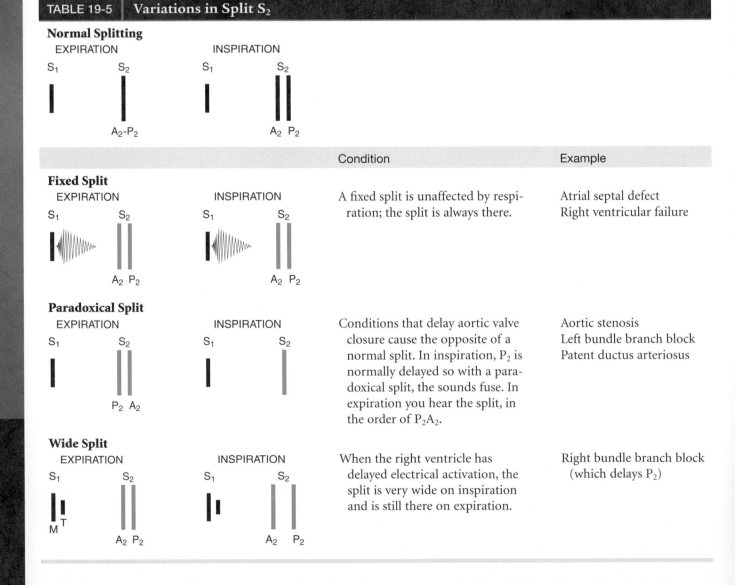

TABLE 19-4	Variations in S$_2$	
	Condition	Example
Accentuated S$_2$	1. Higher closing pressure	Systemic hypertension, ringing or booming S$_2$
	2. Exercise and excitement increase pressure in aorta	
	3. Pulmonary hypertension	Mitral stenosis, heart failure
	4. Semilunar valves calcified but still mobile	Aortic or pulmonic stenosis
Diminished S$_2$	1. A fall in systemic blood pressure causes a decrease in valve strength	Shock
	2. Semilunar valves thickened and calcified, with decreased mobility	Aortic or pulmonic stenosis

TABLE 19-5	Variations in Split S$_2$	
Normal Splitting		
	Condition	Example
Fixed Split	A fixed split is unaffected by respiration; the split is always there.	Atrial septal defect Right ventricular failure
Paradoxical Split	Conditions that delay aortic valve closure cause the opposite of a normal split. In inspiration, P$_2$ is normally delayed so with a paradoxical split, the sounds fuse. In expiration you hear the split, in the order of P$_2$A$_2$.	Aortic stenosis Left bundle branch block Patent ductus arteriosus
Wide Split	When the right ventricle has delayed electrical activation, the split is very wide on inspiration and is still there on expiration.	Right bundle branch block (which delays P$_2$)

TABLE 19-6	Systolic Extra Sounds

Early systolic   Mid-/late systolic
   Ejection click   Midsystolic (mitral) click
   Aortic prosthetic valve sounds

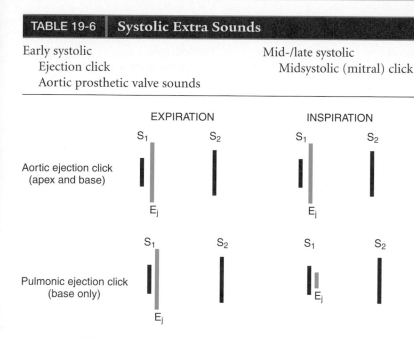

Ejection Click

The ejection click occurs early in systole at the start of ejection because it results from opening of the semilunar valves. Normally, the SL valves open silently, but in the presence of stenosis (e.g., aortic stenosis, pulmonic stenosis) their opening makes a sound. It is short and high pitched, with a click quality, and is heard better with the diaphragm.

   The aortic ejection click is heard at the second right interspace and apex and may be loudest at the apex. Its intensity does not change with respiration. The pulmonic ejection click is best heard in the second left interspace and often grows softer with inspiration.

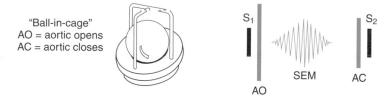

Aortic Prosthetic Valve Sounds

As a sequela of modern technological intervention for heart problems, some people now have *iatrogenically* induced heart sounds. The opening of an aortic ball-in-cage prosthesis (e.g., Starr-Edwards prosthesis) produces an early systolic sound. This sound is less intense with a tilting disc prosthesis (e.g., Bjork-Shiley prosthesis) and is absent with a tissue prosthesis (e.g., porcine).

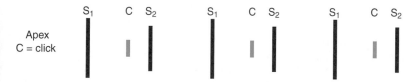

Midsystolic Click

Although it is systolic, this is not an ejection click. It is associated with **mitral valve prolapse,** in which the mitral valve leaflets not only close with contraction but balloon back up into the left atrium. During ballooning, the sudden tensing of the valve leaflets and the chordae tendineae creates the click.

   The sound occurs in mid- to late systole and is short and high pitched, with a click quality. It is best heard with the diaphragm, at the apex, but also may be heard at the left lower sternal border. The click usually is followed by a systolic murmur. The click and murmur move with postural change; when the person assumes a squatting position, the click may move closer to S_2, and the murmur may sound louder and delayed. The Valsalva manoeuvre also moves the click closer to S_2.

TABLE 19-7	Diastolic Extra Sounds

Early diastole	Mid-diastole	Late diastole
Opening snap	Third heart sound	Fourth heart sound
Mitral prosthetic valve sound	Summation sound ($S_3 + S_4$)	Pacemaker-induced sound

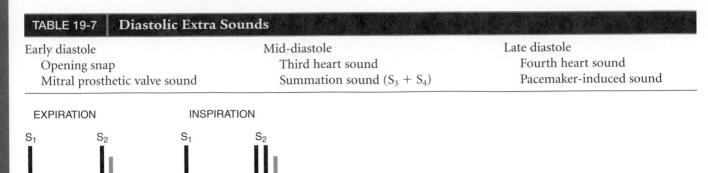

Opening Snap

Normally the opening of the AV valves is silent. In the presence of stenosis, increasingly higher atrial pressure is required to open the valve. The deformed valve opens with a noise: the opening snap. It is sharp and high pitched, with a snapping quality. It sounds after S_2 and is best heard with the diaphragm at the third or fourth left interspace at the sternal border, less well at the apex.

The opening snap usually is not an isolated sound. As a sign of mitral stenosis, the opening snap usually ushers in the low-pitched diastolic rumbling murmur of that condition.

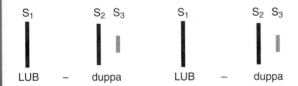

Mitral Prosthetic Valve Sound

An iatrogenic sound, the opening of a ball-in-cage mitral prosthesis gives an early diastolic sound: an opening click just after S_2. It is loud, is heard over the whole precordium, and is loudest at the apex and left lower sternal border.

Third Heart Sound

The S_3 is a ventricular filling sound. It occurs in early diastole during the rapid filling phase. Your hearing quickly accommodates to the S_3, so it is best heard when you listen initially. It sounds after S_2 but later than an opening snap would be. It is a dull, soft sound, and it is low pitched, like "distant thunder." It is heard best in a quiet room, at the apex, with the bell held lightly (just enough to form a seal), and with the person in the left lateral position.

The S_3 can be confused with a split S_2. Use these guidelines to distinguish the S_3:
- *Location*—The S_3 is heard at the apex or left lower sternal border; the split S_2 is heard at the base.
- *Respiratory variation*—The S_3 does not vary in timing with respirations; the split S_2 does.
- *Pitch*—The S_3 is lower pitched; the pitch of the split S_2 stays the same.

The S_3 may be normal (physiological) or abnormal (pathological). The **physiological S_3** is heard frequently in children and young adults; it occasionally may persist after age 40 years, especially in women. The normal S_3 usually disappears when the person sits up.

In adults, the S_3 is usually abnormal. The **pathological S_3** is also called a **ventricular gallop** or an S_3 gallop, and it persists when sitting up. The S_3 indicates decreased compliance of the ventricles, as in heart failure. The S_3 may be the earliest sign of heart failure. The S_3 may originate from either the left or the right ventricle; a left-sided S_3 is heard at the apex in the left lateral position, and a right-sided S_3 is heard at the left lower sternal border with the person supine and is louder on inspiration.

The S_3 occurs also with conditions of volume overload, such as mitral regurgitation and aortic or tricuspid regurgitation. The S_3 is also found in high cardiac output states in the absence of heart disease, such as hyperthyroidism, anemia, and pregnancy. When the primary condition is corrected, the gallop disappears.

Abnormal Findings

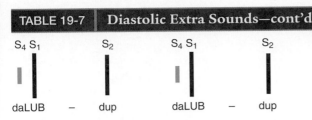

TABLE 19-7	Diastolic Extra Sounds—cont'd

Fourth Heart Sound

The S$_4$ is a ventricular filling sound. It occurs when the atria contract late in diastole. It is heard immediately before S$_1$. This is a very soft sound, of very low pitch. You need a good bell, and you must listen for it. It is heard best at the apex, with the person in left lateral position.

A **physiological S$_4$** may occur in adults older than 40 or 50 years with no evidence of cardiovascular disease, especially after exercise.

A **pathological S$_4$** is termed an **atrial gallop** or an S$_4$ gallop. It occurs with decreased compliance of the ventricle (e.g., coronary artery disease, cardiomyopathy) and with systolic overload (afterload), including outflow obstruction to the ventricle (aortic stenosis) and systemic hypertension. A left-sided S$_4$ occurs with these conditions. It is heard best at the apex, in the left lateral position.

A right-sided S$_4$ is less common. It is heard at the left lower sternal border and may increase with inspiration. It occurs with pulmonary stenosis or pulmonary hypertension.

Summation Sound

When both the pathological S$_3$ and S$_4$ are present, a quadruple rhythm is heard. Often, in cases of cardiac stress, one response is tachycardia. During rapid rates, the diastolic filling time shortens and the S$_3$ and S$_4$ move closer together. They sound superimposed in mid-diastole, and you hear one loud, prolonged, summated sound, often louder than either S$_1$ or S$_2$.

EXTRACARDIAC SOUNDS

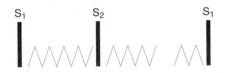

Pericardial Friction Rub

Inflammation of the precordium gives rise to a friction rub. The sound is high pitched and scratchy, like sandpaper being rubbed. It is best heard with the diaphragm, with the person sitting up and leaning forward, and with the breath held in expiration.

A friction rub can be heard any place on the precordium but usually is best heard at the apex and left lower sternal border, places where the pericardium comes in close contact with the chest wall. Timing may be systolic and diastolic. The friction rub of pericarditis is common during the first week after a myocardial infarction and may last only a few hours.

TABLE 19-8 | **Abnormal Pulsations on the Precordium**

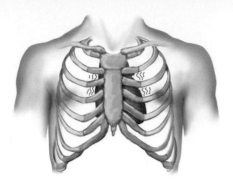

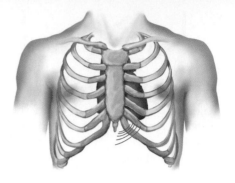

Base

A **thrill** in the second and third right interspaces occurs with severe aortic stenosis and systemic hypertension.

A **thrill** in the second and third left interspaces occurs with pulmonic stenosis and pulmonic hypertension.

Left Sternal Border

A **lift (heave)** occurs with right ventricular hypertrophy, as found in pulmonic valve disease, pulmonic hypertension, and chronic lung disease. You feel a diffuse lifting impulse during systole at the left lower sternal border. It may be associated with retraction at the apex because the left ventricle is rotated posteriorly by the enlarged right ventricle.

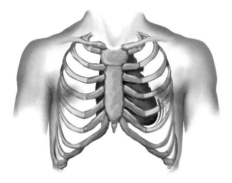

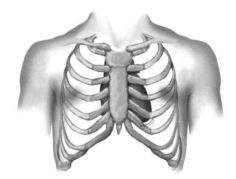

Apex

Cardiac enlargement displaces the apical impulse laterally and over a wider area when left ventricular hypertrophy and dilatation are present. This is **volume overload,** as in mitral regurgitation, aortic regurgitation, and left-to-right shunts.

Apex

The apical impulse is increased in force and duration but is not necessarily displaced to the left when left ventricular hypertrophy occurs alone without dilatation. This is **pressure overload,** as found in aortic stenosis or systemic hypertension.

Images © Pat Thomas, 2006.

TABLE 19-9	**Congenital Heart Defects**

	Description	Clinical Data

Patent Ductus Arteriosus (PDA)

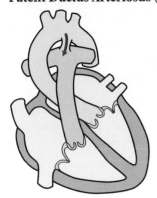

Persistence of the channel joining left pulmonary artery to aorta. This is normal in the fetus and usually closes spontaneously within hours of birth.

S: Usually no symptoms in early childhood; growth and development are normal.

O: Blood pressure has wide pulse pressure and bounding peripheral pulses from rapid runoff of blood into low-resistance pulmonary bed during diastole. Thrill often palpable at left upper sternal border. The continuous murmur heard in systole and diastole is called a machinery murmur.

Atrial Septal Defect (ASD)

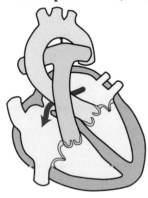

Abnormal opening in the atrial septum, resulting usually in left-to-right shunt and causing large increase in pulmonary blood flow.

S: Defect is remarkably well tolerated. Symptoms in infant are rare; growth and development normal. Children and young adults have mild fatigue and DOE.

O: Sternal lift often present. S_2 has fixed split, with P_2 often louder than A_2. Murmur is systolic, ejection, medium pitch, best heard at base in second left interspace. Murmur caused not by shunt itself but by increased blood flow through pulmonic valve.

Ventricular Septal Defect (VSD)

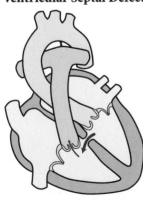

Abnormal opening in septum between the ventricles, usually subaortic area. The size and exact position vary considerably.

S: Small defects are asymptomatic. Infants with large defects have poor growth, slow weight gain; later look pale, thin, delicate. May have feeding problems; DOE; frequent respiratory infections; and when the condition is severe, heart failure.

O: Loud, harsh holosystolic murmur, best heard at left lower sternal border, may be accompanied by thrill. Large defects also have soft diastolic murmur at apex (mitral flow murmur) due to increased blood flow through mitral valve.

S, Subjective data; *O*, objective data.

Images © Pat Thomas, 2006.
Continued

TABLE 19-9	Congenital Heart Defects—cont'd

	Description	Clinical Data

Tetralogy of Fallot

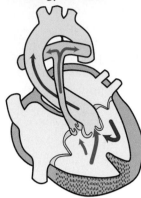

Four components: (1) right ventricular outflow stenosis, (2) VSD, (3) right ventricular hypertrophy, and (4) overriding aorta. *Result:* Shunts a lot of venous blood directly into aorta away from pulmonary system, so blood never gets oxygenated.

S: Severe cyanosis, not in first months of life but develops as infant grows and RV outflow (i.e., pulmonic) stenosis gets worse. Cyanosis with crying and exertion at first, then at rest. Uses squatting posture after starts walking. DOE common. Development is slowed.

O: Thrill palpable at left lower sternal border. S_1 normal; S_2 has A_2 loud and P_2 diminished or absent. Murmur is systolic, loud, crescendo–decrescendo.

Coarctation of the Aorta

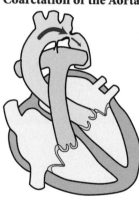

Severe narrowing of descending aorta, usually at the junction of the ductus arteriosus and the aortic arch, just distal to the origin of the left subclavian artery. Results in increased work load on left ventricle.

Associated with defects of aortic valve in most cases, as well as associated patent ductus arteriosus; and associated ventricular septal defect.

S: In infants with associated lesions or symptoms, diagnosis occurs in first few months as symptoms of heart failure develop. For asymptomatic children and adolescents, growth and development are normal. Diagnosis usually accidental due to blood pressure findings. Adolescents may complain of vague lower extremity cramping that is worse with exercise.

O: Upper extremity hypertension over 20 mm Hg higher than lower extremity measures is a hallmark of coarctation. Another important sign is absent or greatly diminished femoral pulses. A systolic murmur is heard best at the left sternal border, radiating to the back.

S, Subjective data; O, objective data.

Images © Pat Thomas, 2006.

TABLE 19-10 | Murmurs Due to Valvular Defects

Midsystolic Ejection Murmurs
Due to forward flow through semilunar valves

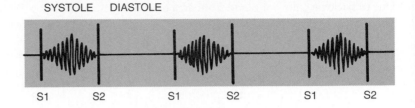

SYSTOLE   DIASTOLE

S1   S2   S1   S2   S1   S2

	Description	Clinical Data
Aortic Stenosis 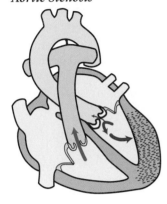	Calcification of aortic valve cusps restricts forward flow of blood during systole; LV hypertrophy develops.	S: Fatigue, DOE, palpitation, dizziness, fainting, anginal pain. O: Pallor, slow diminished radial pulse, low blood pressure, and auscultatory gap are common. Apical impulse sustained and displaced to left. Thrill in systole over second and third right z interspaces and right side of neck. S_1 normal, often ejection click present, often paradoxical split S_2, S_4 present with LV hypertrophy. Murmur: Loud, harsh, midsystolic, crescendo–decrescendo, loudest at second right interspace, radiates widely to side of neck, down left sternal border, or apex.
Pulmonic Stenosis 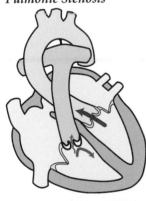	Calcification of pulmonic valve restricts forward flow of blood.	O: Thrill in systole at second and third left interspace, ejection click often present after S_1, diminished S_2 and usually with wide split, S_4 common with RV hypertrophy. Murmur: Systolic, medium pitch, coarse, crescendo–decrescendo (diamond shape), best heard at second left interspace, radiates to left and neck.

S, Subjective data; *O*, objective data.

Stenosis images © Pat Thomas, 2006.

Continued

TABLE 19-10	Murmurs Due to Valvular Defects—cont'd

Pansystolic Regurgitant Murmurs

Due to backward flow of blood from area of higher pressure to one of lower pressure.

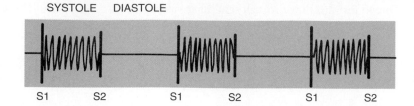

SYSTOLE   DIASTOLE

S1   S2   S1   S2   S1   S2

	Description	Clinical Data
Mitral Regurgitation 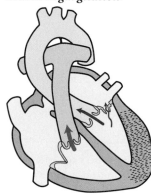	Stream of blood regurgitates back into LA during systole through incompetent mitral valve. In diastole, blood passes back into LV again along with new flow; results in LV dilatation and hypertrophy.	S: Fatigue, palpitation, orthopnea, PND. O: Thrill in systole at apex. Lift at apex. Apical impulse displaced down and to left. S_1 diminished, S_2 accentuated, S_3 at apex often present. Murmur: Pansystolic, often loud, blowing, best heard at apex, radiates well to left axilla.
Tricuspid Regurgitation 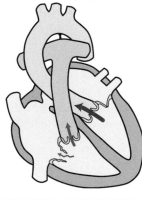	Backflow of blood through incompetent tricuspid valve into RA.	O: Engorged pulsating neck veins, liver enlarged. Lift at sternum if RV hypertrophy present, often thrill at left lower sternal border. Murmur: Soft, blowing, pansystolic, best heard at left lower sternal border, increases with inspiration.

S, Subjective data; *O*, objective data.

Regurgitation images © Pat Thomas, 2006.

TABLE 19-10   Murmurs Due to Valvular Defects—cont'd

Diastolic Rumbles of AV Valves

Filling murmurs at low pressures, best heard with bell lightly touching skin

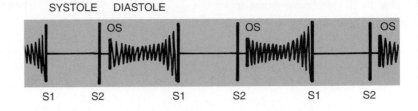

	Description	Clinical Data
Mitral Stenosis 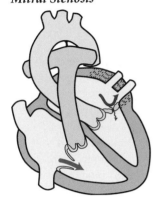	Calcified mitral valve will not open properly, impedes forward flow of blood into LV during diastole. Results in LA enlarged and LA pressure increased.	S: Fatigue, palpitations, DOE, orthopnea, occasional PND or pulmonary edema. O: Diminished, often irregular arterial pulse. Lift at apex, diastolic thrill common at apex. S_1 accentuated; opening snap after S_2 heard over wide area of precordium, followed by murmur. Murmur: Low-pitched diastolic rumble, best heard at apex, with person in left lateral position; does not radiate.
Tricuspid Stenosis 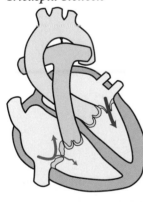	Calcification of tricuspid valve impedes forward flow into RV during diastole.	O: Diminished arterial pulse, jugular venous pulse prominent. Murmur: Diastolic rumble; best heard at left lower sternal border; louder in inspiration.

S, Subjective data; *O,* objective data.

Stenosis images © Pat Thomas, 2006.

Continued

TABLE 19-10	Murmurs Due to Valvular Defects—cont'd

Early Diastolic Murmurs

Due to SL valve incompetence

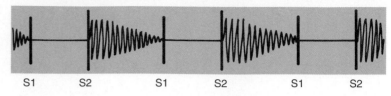

SYSTOLE   DIASTOLE

S1   S2   S1   S2   S1   S2

	Description	Clinical Data
Aortic Regurgitation 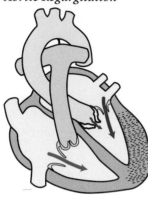	Stream of blood regurgitates back through incompetent aortic valve into LV during diastole. LV dilatation and hypertrophy due to increased LV stroke volume. Rapid ejection of large stroke volume into poorly filled aorta, then rapid runoff in diastole as part of blood pushed back into LV.	S: Only minor symptoms for many years, then rapid deterioration: DOE, PND, angina, dizziness. O: Bounding "water–hammer" pulse in carotid, brachial, and femoral arteries. Blood pressure has wide pulse pressure. Pulsations in cervical and suprasternal areas, apical impulse displaced to left and down, apical impulse feels brief. Murmur starts almost simultaneously with S_2: soft high-pitched, blowing diastolic, decrescendo, best heard at third left interspace at base, as person sits up and leans forward, radiates down.
Pulmonic Regurgitation 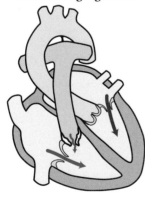	Backflow of blood through incompetent pulmonic valve, from pulmonary artery to RV.	Murmur has same timing and characteristics as that of aortic regurgitation, and is hard to distinguish on physical examination.

S, Subjective data; *O,* objective data.

Regurgitation images © Pat Thomas, 2006.

BIBLIOGRAPHY

American Heart Association. (2006). *Populations and cardiovascular disease.* Retrieved from http://www.americanheart.org/presenter

American Heart Association. (2007). *2007 heart disease and stroke statistics.* Retrieved February, 2007, from http://www.american-heart.org/downloadable/heart

Anderson, J., & Kessenich, C. R. (2001). Women and coronary heart disease. *Nurse Practitioner, 26,* 12–33.

Artinian, N. (2003). The psychosocial aspects of heart failure. *American Journal of Nursing, 103,* 32–43.

Boie, E. (2005). Initial evaluation of chest pain. *Emergency Medicine Clinics of North America, 23,* 937–957.

Caboral, M., & Mitchell, J. (2003). New guidelines for heart failure: Focus on prevention. *Nurse Practitioner, 28,* 13–25.

Canadian Diabetes Association. (2007). *About diabetes: the prevalence and cost of diabetes.* Retrieved April 18, 2008, from http://www.diabetes.ca/Section_About/prevalence.asp

Carroll, M. D, Lacher, D. A., Sorlie, P. D., Cleeman, J. I., Gordon, D. J., Wolz, M., et al. (2005). Trends in serum lipids and lipoproteins of adults, 1960–2002. *Journal of the American Medical Association, 294,* 1773–1781.

Carter, T., & Brooks, C. (2005). Pericarditis: Inflammation or infarction? *Journal of Cardiovascular Nursing, 20,* 239–244.

Cunningham, F. G., Leveno, K. J., Bloom, S. L., Hauth, J. C., Gilstrap, L. C., & Wenstrom, K. D. (2005). *Williams' obstetrics* (22nd ed.). New York, NY: McGraw-Hill Professional.

Cushman, M., Kuller, L., Prentice, R., Rodabough, R., Psaty, B., Stafford, R., et al. (2004). Estrogen plus progestin and risk of venous thrombosis. *Journal of the American Medical Association, 292,* 1573–1580.

DeVon, H. A., & Ryan, C. J. (2005). Chest pain and associated symptoms of acute coronary syndromes. *Journal of Cardiovascular Nursing, 20,* 232–238.

Dobbenga-Rhodes, Y. A., & Prive, A. M. (2006). Assessment and evaluation of the woman with cardiac disease during pregnancy. *Journal of Perinatal and Neonatal Nursing, 20,* 295–302.

Efre, A. (2004). Gender bias in acute myocardial infarction. *Nurse Practitioner, 29,* 42–57.

Fink, A. (2006). Endocarditis after valve replacement surgery. *American Journal of Nursing, 106,* 40–52.

Fleg, J. L. (1990). Diagnostic evaluations. In W. B. Abrams & R. Berkow (Eds.), *The Merck manual of geriatrics.* Rahway, NJ: Merck, Sharp, and Dohme.

Grenier, M. C., Gagnon, K., Genest, J., Jr., Durand, J., & Durand, L.G. (1998). Clinical comparison of acoustic and electronic stethoscopes and design of a new electronic stethoscope. *American Journal of Cardiology, 81,* 653–656.

Haro, L. H, Decker, W. W., Boie, E. T., & Wright, R. S. (2006). Initial approach to the patient who has chest pain. *Cardiology Clinics, 24,* 1–17.

Hayek, E., Gring, C., & Griffin, B. (2005). Mitral valve prolapse. *Lancet, 365,* 507–518.

Heart and Stroke Foundation. (2003). *The growing burden of heart disease and stroke in Canada, 2003.* Ottawa, ON: Author.

Heart and Stroke Foundation of Canada. (2008). *Women's unique risk factors.* Toronto, ON: Author.

Holcomb, S. (2005). Recognizing and managing anemia. *Nurse Practitioner, 30,* 16–33.

Holman, J. (2005a). Preoperative evaluation: Priorities and pointers, part 1: Cardiac assessment. *Consultant, 45,* 1296–1301.

Holman, J. (2005b). Preoperative evaluation: Priorities and pointers, part 2. *Consultant, 45,* 1307–1314.

Hsia, J., Criqui, M., Rodabough, R., Langer, R., Resnick, H., Phillips, L., et al. (2004). Estrogen plus progestin and the risk of peripheral arterial disease. *Circulation, 109,* 620–626.

Klein, D. G. (2005). Thoracic aortic aneurysms. *Journal of Cardiovascular Nursing, 20,* 245–250.

Kliegman, R. M., Behrman, R. E., Jenson, H. B., & Stanton, B. F. (2007). *Nelson textbook of pediatrics* (18th ed.). Philadelphia, PA: Saunders.

Klieman, L., Hyde, S., & Berra, K. (2006). Cardiovascular disease risk reduction in older adults. *Journal of Cardiovascular Nursing, 21,* 527–539.

Mangione, S., & Nieman, L. Z. (1997). Cardiac auscultatory skills of internal medicine and family practice trainees. *Journal of the American Medical Association, 278,* 717–722.

National Center for Health Statistics. (2006). *Health, United States, 2005 with chartbook on trends in the health of Americans* (DHHS Publication No. 2005-1232). Hyattsville, MD: Author.

Office of Minority Health, Public Health Service, Department of Health and Human Services. (1990). *Heart disease, stroke, and minorities: Closing the gap.* Washington, DC: Government Printing Office.

Onysko, J., Maxwell, C., Eliasziw, M., Zhang, J. X., Johansen, H., & Campbell, N. R. C. (2006). Large increases in hypertension diagnosis and treatment in Canada after a healthcare professional education program. *Hypertension, 48,* 853–860.

Patel, D., & Wasserman, A. (2005). Chest pain: Is it life-threatening or benign? *Consultant, 45,* 21–28.

Perloff, J. K. (2000). *Physical examination of the heart and circulation* (3rd ed.). Philadelphia, PA: W.B. Saunders.

Public Health Agency of Canada. (2006). *Are women at risk for heart disease?* Ottawa, ON: Health Canada.

Raphael, D. (2004). *Introduction to the social determinants of health; Canadian perspectives.* Toronto, ON: Canadian Scholars' Press, Inc.

Rasmusson, K. (2006). Heart failure epidemic boiling on the surface. *Nurse Practitioner, 31,* 12–23.

Reigle, J. (2005). Evaluating the patient with chest pain: The value of a comprehensive history. *Journal of Cardiovascular Nursing, 20,* 226–231.

Scheetz, L. (2006). Aortic dissection. *American Journal of Nursing, 106,* 55–59.

Statistics Canada. (2004a). *Canadian community survey, 2004.* Ottawa, ON: Author.

Statistics Canada. (2004b). *Canadian tobacco use monitoring survey.* Ottawa, ON: Author.

Statistics Canada. (2004c). *Mortality: Summary list of causes 2004.* Ottawa, ON: Author.

Statistics Canada. (2006). Adult obesity. *Health Report, 17*(3), 9–25.

Taylor, M. (2005). Coarctation of the aorta: A critical catch for newborn well-being. *Nurse Practitioner, 30,* 34–45.

Tilkian, A. G., & Conover, M. B. (2001). *Understanding heart sounds and murmurs with an introduction to lung sounds* (4th ed.). Philadelphia, PA: W.B. Saunders.

Wei, J. Y. (1992). Age and the cardiovascular system. *New England Journal of Medicine, 327,* 1735–1739.

Yancy, C. (2005). Heart failure in African Americans. *American Journal of Cardiology, 96,* 3i–12i.

Yusuf, S., Hawken, S., Ounpuu, S., Dans, T., Avezum, A., Lanas, F., et al. (2004). Effect of potentially modifiable risk factors associated with myocardial infarction in 52 countries (the INTERHEART study): Case-control study. *Lancet, 364,* 937–952.

Zipes, D., et al. (2005). *Braunwald's heart disease: A textbook of cardiovascular medicine* (7th ed.). Philadelphia, PA: W.B. Saunders.

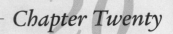

Chapter Twenty

Peripheral Vascular System and Lymphatic System

Written by **Carolyn Jarvis**, PhD, APN, CNP
Adapted by **June MacDonald-Jenkins**, RN, BScN, MSc

Structure and Function, p. 528

Arteries
Veins
Venous Flow
Lymphatics

Subjective Data, p. 533

Health History Questions

Objective Data, p. 534

Preparation
Inspect and Palpate the Arms
Inspect and Palpate the Legs
Summary Checklist: Peripheral Vascular Examination

Documentation and Critical Thinking, p. 545

Abnormal Findings, p. 547

Abnormal Findings for Advanced Practice, p. 548

Electronic Resources

On Evolve *evolve*

http://evolve.elsevier.com/Canada/Jarvis/examination/
- Interactive Case Studies
- Physical Examination Audio and Printable Summaries
- Bedside Assessment Summary Checklists
- Complete Physical Examination Form
- Nursing Diagnoses Boxes
- Health Promotion Guides
- Quick Assessments for 20 Common Conditions
- Multiple Choice Review Questions
- Chapter Objectives
- Appendices
- Weblinks

On the Companion CD

- Interactive Case Studies with Heart and Lung Sounds
- Health Promotion Guides
- Quick Assessments for 20 Common Conditions
- Head-to-Toe Physical Examination Video Clips

STRUCTURE AND FUNCTION

The vascular system consists of the vessels of the body. Vessels are tubes for transporting fluid, such as the blood or lymph. Any disease in the vascular system creates problems with delivery of oxygen and nutrients to the tissues or elimination of waste products from cellular metabolism.

ARTERIES

The heart pumps freshly oxygenated blood through the arteries to all body tissues. The pumping heart makes this a high-pressure system. The artery walls are strong, tough, and tense to withstand pressure demands. Arteries contain elastic fibres, which allow their walls to stretch with systole and recoil with diastole. Arteries also contain muscle fibres (vascular smooth muscle, or VSM), which control the amount of blood delivered to the tissues. The VSM contracts or dilates, which changes the diameter of the arteries to control the rate of blood flow.

Each heartbeat creates a pressure wave, which makes the arteries expand and then recoil. It is the recoil that propels blood through like a wave. All arteries have this pressure wave, or **pulse,** throughout their length, but you can feel it only at body sites where the artery lies close to the skin and over a bone. The arteries described in the following sections are accessible to examination.

Temporal Artery. The temporal artery is palpated in front of the ear, as discussed in Chapter 13 in the head and neck section.

Carotid Artery. The carotid artery is palpated in the groove between the sternomastoid muscle and the trachea and is covered in Chapter 19 in the section on great vessels.

Arteries in the Arm. The major artery supplying the arm is the **brachial** artery, which runs in the biceps–triceps furrow of the upper arm and surfaces at the antecubital fossa in the elbow medial to the biceps tendon (Fig. 20-1). Immediately below the elbow, the brachial artery bifurcates into the **ulnar** and **radial** arteries. These run distally and form two arches supplying the hand; these are called the *superficial* and *deep palmar arches.* The radial pulse lies just medial to the radius at the wrist; the ulnar artery is in the same relation to the ulna, but it is deeper and often difficult to feel.

Arteries in the Leg. The major artery to the leg is the **femoral** artery, which passes under the inguinal ligament (Fig. 20-2). The femoral artery travels down the thigh. At the lower thigh, it courses posteriorly; then it is termed the **popliteal** artery. Below the knee, the popliteal artery divides. The anterior tibial artery travels down the front of the leg on to the dorsum of the foot, where it becomes the **dorsalis pedis.** In back of the leg, the **posterior tibial** artery travels down behind the medial malleolus and in the foot forms the plantar arteries.

The function of the arteries is to supply oxygen and essential nutrients to the tissues. **Ischemia** is a deficient supply of oxygenated arterial blood to a tissue caused by obstruction of a blood vessel. A complete blockage leads to death of the distal tissue. A partial blockage creates an insufficient supply, and the ischemia may be apparent only at exercise when oxygen needs increase.

VEINS

The course of veins parallels that of arteries, but the body has more veins, and they lie closer to the skin surface. The following veins are accessible to examination.

Jugular Veins. Assessment of the jugular veins is presented in Chapter 19.

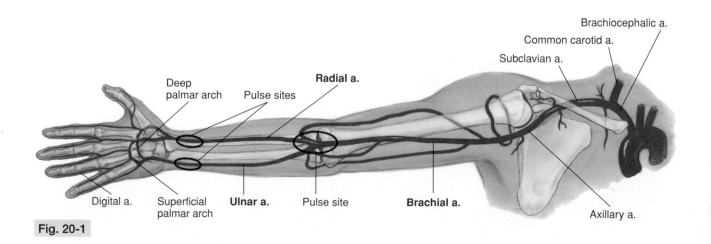

Deep palmar arch Pulse sites **Radial a.**

Brachiocephalic a.
Common carotid a.
Subclavian a.

Digital a. Superficial palmar arch **Ulnar a.** Pulse site **Brachial a.**

Axillary a.

Fig. 20-1

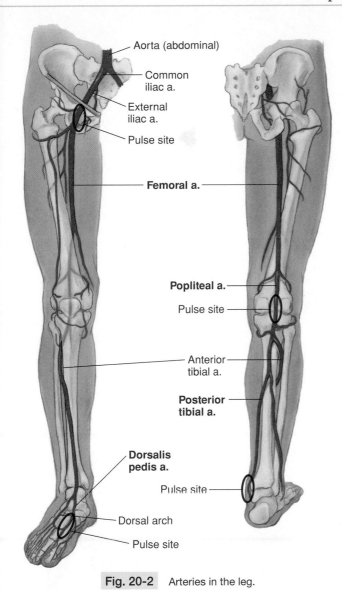

Fig. 20-2 Arteries in the leg.

the thigh. The small saphenous vein, outside the leg, starts on the lateral side of the dorsum of the foot and ascends behind the lateral malleolus, up the back of the leg, where it joins the popliteal vein.

3. **Perforators** (not illustrated) are connecting veins that join the two sets. They also have one-way valves that route blood from the superficial into the deep veins.

VENOUS FLOW

Veins drain the deoxygenated blood and its waste products from the tissues and return it to the heart. Unlike the arteries, veins are a low-pressure system. Because veins do not have a pump to generate their blood flow, the veins need a

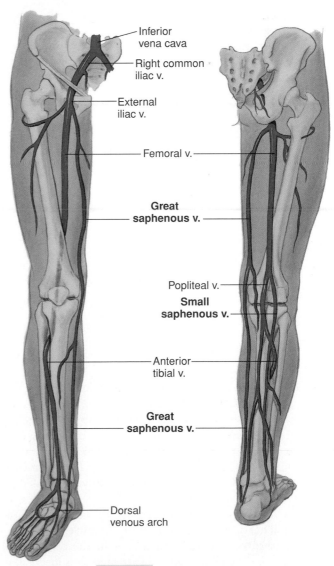

Fig. 20-3 Veins in the leg.

Veins in the Arm. Each arm has two sets of veins: superficial and deep. The superficial veins are in the subcutaneous tissue and are responsible for most of the venous return.

Veins in the Leg. The legs have three types of veins (Fig. 20-3).

1. The **deep veins** run alongside the deep arteries and conduct most of the venous return from the legs. These are the **femoral** and **popliteal** veins. As long as these veins remain intact, the superficial veins can be excised without harming the circulation.

2. The **superficial veins** are the **great** and **small saphenous** veins. The great saphenous vein, inside the leg, starts at the medial side of the dorsum of the foot. You can see it ascend in front of the medial malleolus; then it crosses the tibia obliquely and ascends along the medial side of

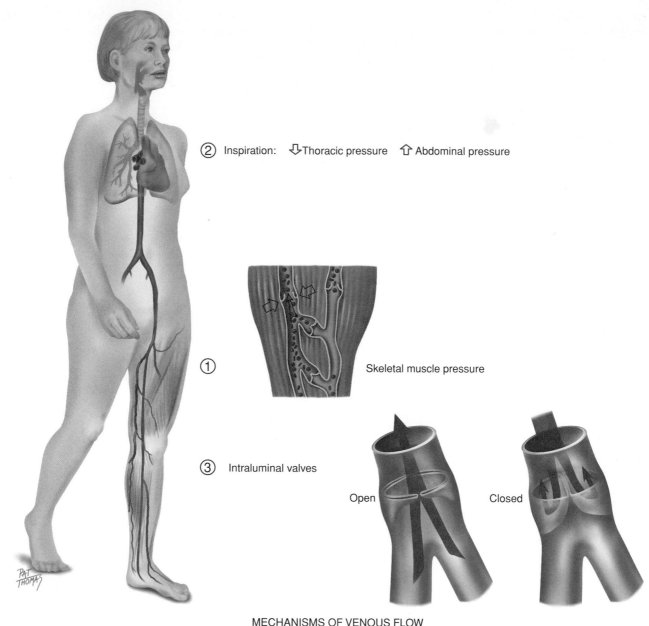

(2) Inspiration: ⬇Thoracic pressure   ⬆ Abdominal pressure

Skeletal muscle pressure

(1)

(3) Intraluminal valves

Open   Closed

MECHANISMS OF VENOUS FLOW

Fig. 20-4

mechanism to keep blood moving (Fig. 20-4). This is accomplished by (1) the contracting skeletal muscles that milk the blood proximally, back toward the heart; (2) the pressure gradient caused by breathing, in which inspiration makes the thoracic pressure decrease and the abdominal pressure increase; and (3) the intraluminal valves, which ensure unidirectional flow. Each valve is a paired semilunar pocket that opens toward the heart and closes tightly when filled to prevent back flow of blood.

In the legs, this mechanism is called the "calf pump," or "peripheral heart." While walking, the calf muscles alternately contract (systole) and relax (diastole). In the contraction phase, the gastrocnemius and soleus muscles squeeze the veins and direct the blood flow proximally. Because of the valves, venous blood flows just one way—toward the heart.

Besides the presence of intraluminal valves, venous structure differs from arterial structure. Because venous pressure is lower, walls of the veins are thinner than those of the arteries. Veins have a larger diameter and are more distensible; they can expand and hold more blood when blood volume increases. This is a compensatory mechanism to reduce stress on the heart. Because of this ability to stretch, veins are called **capacitance vessels.**

Efficient venous return is dependent on contracting skeletal muscles, competent valves in the veins, and a patent lumen. Problems with any of these three elements lead to venous stasis. At risk for venous disease are people who undergo prolonged standing, sitting, or bed rest because they do not benefit from the milking action that walking accomplishes. Hypercoagulable states and vein wall trauma are other factors that increase risk for venous disease. Also, dilated and tortuous (varicose) veins create **incompetent valves,** wherein the lumen is so wide the valve cusps cannot approximate. This condition increases venous pressure, which further dilates the vein. Some people have a genetic predisposition to varicose veins, but obesity and pregnancy are risk factors.

LYMPHATICS

The lymphatics form a completely separate vessel system, which retrieves excess fluid from the tissue spaces and returns it to the bloodstream (Fig. 20-5). During circulation of the blood, somewhat more fluid leaves the capillaries than the veins can absorb. Without lymphatic drainage, fluid would build up in the interstitial spaces and produce edema.

The vessels drain into two main trunks, which empty into the venous system at the subclavian veins (see Fig. 20-5):

1. The **right lymphatic duct** empties into the right subclavian vein. It drains the right side of the head and neck, right arm, right side of thorax, right lung and pleura, right side of the heart, and right upper section of the liver.
2. The **thoracic duct** drains the rest of the body. It empties into the left subclavian vein.

The functions of the lymphatic system are (1) to conserve fluid and plasma proteins that leak out of the capillaries, (2) to form a major part of the immune system that defends the body against disease, and (3) to absorb lipids from the intestinal tract.

The processes of the immune system are complicated and not fully understood. The immune system detects and

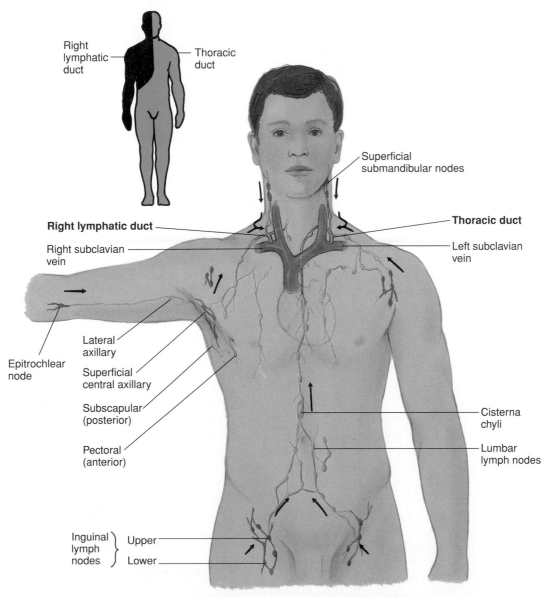

Right lymphatic duct

Thoracic duct

Superficial submandibular nodes

Right lymphatic duct

Thoracic duct

Right subclavian vein

Left subclavian vein

Epitrochlear node

Lateral axillary

Superficial central axillary

Subscapular (posterior)

Pectoral (anterior)

Cisterna chyli

Lumbar lymph nodes

Inguinal lymph nodes { Upper Lower

LYMPHATIC DUCTS AND DRAINAGE PATTERNS

Fig. 20-5

eliminates foreign pathogens, both those that come in from the environment and those arising from inside (abnormal or mutant cells). It accomplishes this by phagocytosis (digestion) of the substances by neutrophils and monocytes or macrophages and by production of specific antibodies or specific immune responses by the lymphocytes.

The lymphatic vessels have a unique structure. Lymphatic capillaries start as microscopic open-ended tubes, which siphon interstitial fluid. The capillaries converge to form vessels. The vessels, like veins, drain into larger ones. The vessels have valves, so flow is one way from the tissue spaces into the bloodstream. The many valves make the vessels look beaded. The flow of lymph is slow compared with that of the blood. Lymph flow is propelled by contracting skeletal muscles, by pressure changes secondary to breathing, and by contraction of the vessel walls themselves.

Lymph nodes are small oval clumps of lymphatic tissue located at intervals along the vessels. Most nodes are arranged in groups, both deep and superficial, in the body. Nodes filter the fluid before it is returned to the bloodstream and filter out micro-organisms that could be harmful to the body. The pathogens are exposed to lymphocytes in the lymph nodes. The lymphocytes mount an antigen-specific response to eliminate the pathogens. With local inflammation, the nodes in that area become swollen and tender.

The superficial groups of nodes are accessible to inspection and palpation and give clues to the status of the lymphatic system:

- **Cervical nodes** drain the head and neck and are described in Chapter 13.
- **Axillary nodes** drain the breast and upper arm. They are described in Chapter 17.
- The **epitrochlear node** is in the antecubital fossa and drains the hand and lower arm.
- The **inguinal nodes** in the groin drain most of the lymph of the lower extremity, the external genitalia, and the anterior abdominal wall.

Related Organs

The spleen, tonsils, and thymus aid the lymphatic system (Fig. 20-6). The **spleen** is located in the left upper quadrant of the abdomen. It has four functions: (1) to destroy old red blood cells, (2) to produce antibodies, (3) to store red blood cells, and (4) to filter micro-organisms from the blood.

The **tonsils** (palatine, adenoid, and lingual) are located at the entrance to the respiratory and gastrointestinal tracts and respond to local inflammation.

The **thymus** is the flat, pink-grey gland located in the superior mediastinum behind the sternum and in front of the aorta. It is relatively large in the fetus and young child and atrophies after puberty. It is important in developing the T lymphocytes of the immune system in children, but it serves no function in adults. The T and B lymphocytes originate in the bone marrow and mature in the lymphoid tissue.

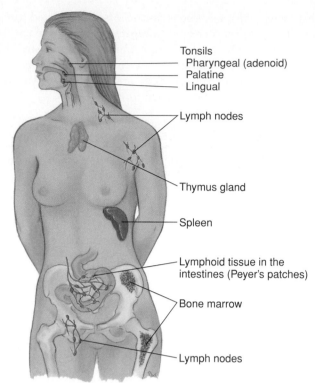

Tonsils
Pharyngeal (adenoid)
Palatine
Lingual

Lymph nodes

Thymus gland

Spleen

Lymphoid tissue in the intestines (Peyer's patches)

Bone marrow

Lymph nodes

RELATED ORGANS IN IMMUNE SYSTEM
Fig. 20-6

DEVELOPMENTAL CARE

Infants and Children

The lymphatic system has the same function in children as in adults. Lymphoid tissue has a unique growth pattern compared with other body systems (Fig. 20-7). It is well developed at birth and grows rapidly until age 10 or 11 years. By age 6 years, the lymphoid tissue reaches adult size; it surpasses adult size by puberty, and then it slowly atrophies. It is possible that the excessive antigen stimulation in children causes the early rapid growth.

Lymph nodes are relatively large in children, and the superficial ones often are palpable even when the child is healthy. With infection, excessive swelling and hyperplasia occur. Enlarged tonsils are familiar signs in respiratory infections. The excessive lymphoid response also may account for the common childhood symptom of abdominal pain with seemingly unrelated problems such as upper respiratory infections (Johnson et al., 1978). Possibly the inflammation of mesenteric lymph nodes produces the abdominal pain.

The Pregnant Female

Hormonal changes cause vasodilatation and the resulting drop in blood pressure described in Chapter 19. The growing uterus obstructs drainage of the iliac veins and the inferior vena cava. This condition causes low blood flow and increases venous pressure. This, in turn, causes dependent edema, varicosities in the legs and vulva, and hemorrhoids.

The Aging Adult

Peripheral blood vessels grow more rigid with age, resulting in a condition called **arteriosclerosis.** This condition produces the rise in systolic blood pressure discussed in Chapter 9. Do not confuse this process with another one, **atherosclerosis,** or the deposition of fatty plaques on the intima of the arteries.

Aging produces a progressive enlargement of the intramuscular calf veins. Prolonged bed rest, prolonged sitting, and heart failure increase the risk of deep venous thrombosis and subsequent pulmonary embolism. These conditions are common in aging and also occur after myocardial infarction (MI). However, care for MI now includes early mobilization and low-dose anticoagulant medication, which reduce the risk of pulmonary embolism.

Loss of lymphatic tissue leads to fewer numbers of lymph nodes in older people and to a decrease in the size of remaining nodes.

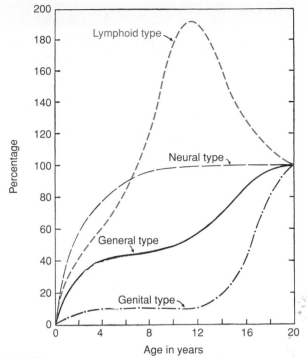

Fig. 20-7   Comparison of growth rates of three types of tissues in the body.

SUBJECTIVE DATA

1. Leg pain or cramps
2. Skin changes on arms or legs
3. Swelling in the arms or legs
4. Lymph node enlargement
5. Medications

Examiner Asks	Rationale
1. Leg pain or cramps. Any leg pain (cramps)? Where? • Describe the type of pain; is it burning, aching, cramping, stabbing? Did this come on gradually or suddenly? • Is it aggravated by activity, walking? • How many blocks (stairs) does it take to produce this pain?	Peripheral vascular disease (PVD)—see Table 20-3, p. 549. **Claudication distance** is the number of blocks walked or stairs climbed to produce pain.
• Has this amount changed recently? • Is the pain worse with elevation? Worse with cool temperatures? • Does the pain wake you up at night?	Note sudden decrease in claudication distance or pain not relieved by rest. Night leg pain is common in aging adults. It may indicate the ischemic rest pain of PVD, severe night muscle cramping (usually the calf), or restless leg syndrome.
• Any recent change in exercise, a new exercise, increasing exercise?	Pain of musculoskeletal origin rather than vascular.
• What relieves this pain: dangling, walking, rubbing? Is the leg pain associated with any skin changes? • Is it associated with any change in sexual function (males)?	Aortoiliac occlusion is associated with impotence (Leriche syndrome).
• Any history of vascular problems, heart problems, diabetes, obesity, pregnancy, smoking, trauma, prolonged standing, or bed rest?	

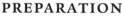

Examiner Asks	Rationale
2. Skin changes on arms or legs. Any **skin changes** in arms or legs? What colour: redness, pallor, blueness, brown discolorations? • Any change in temperature—excess warmth or coolness? • Do your leg veins look bulging and crooked? How have you treated these? Do you use support hose? • Any leg sores or ulcers? Where on the leg? Any pain with the leg ulcer?	Coolness is associated with arterial disease. Varicose veins. Leg ulcers occur with chronic arterial and chronic venous disease (see Table 20-4, p. 550).
3. Swelling in the arms or legs. Swelling in one or both legs? When did this swelling start? • What time of day is the swelling at its worst: morning, or after up most of day? • Does the swelling come and go, or is it constant? • What seems to bring it on: trauma, standing all day, sitting? • What relieves swelling: elevation, support hose? • Is swelling associated with pain, heat, redness, ulceration, hardened skin?	**Edema** is bilateral when caused by a systemic problem such as heart failure or unilateral when the result of a local obstruction or inflammation.
4. Lymph node enlargement. Any "swollen glands" (lumps, kernels)? Where in body? How long have you had them? • Any recent change? • How do they feel to you: hard, soft? • Are the swollen glands associated with pain, or local infection?	Enlarged lymph nodes occur with infection, malignancies, and immunological diseases.
5. Medications. What medications are you taking (e.g., oral contraceptives, hormone replacement)?	

OBJECTIVE DATA

PREPARATION

During a complete physical examination, examine the arms at the very beginning when you are checking the vital signs—the person is sitting. Examine the legs directly after the abdominal examination while the person is still supine. Then stand the person up to evaluate the leg veins.

Examination of the arms and legs includes peripheral vascular characteristics (following here), the skin (see Chapter 12), musculoskeletal findings (see Chapter 22), and neurological findings (see Chapter 23). A method of integrating these steps is discussed in Chapter 27.

Room temperature should be about 22°C (72°F) and draftless to prevent vasodilatation or vasoconstriction.

Use inspection and palpation. Compare your findings with the opposite extremity.

EQUIPMENT NEEDED

Occasionally need:
Paper tape measure
Tourniquet or blood pressure cuff
Stethoscope
Doppler ultrasonic stethoscope

Normal Range of Findings	Abnormal Findings
INSPECT AND PALPATE THE ARMS Lift both the person's hands in your hands. Inspect, then turn the person's hands over, noting colour of skin and nailbeds; temperature, texture, and turgor of skin; and the presence of any lesions, edema, or clubbing. Use the **profile sign** (viewing the finger from the side) to detect early clubbing. The normal nail bed angle is 160 degrees. (See Chapter 12 for a full discussion of skin colour, lesions, and clubbing.)	Flattening of angle and clubbing (diffuse enlargement of terminal phalanges) occur with congenital cyanotic heart disease and cor pulmonale.

Normal Range of Findings	Abnormal Findings

With the person's hands near the level of his or her heart, check **capillary refill.** This is an index of peripheral perfusion and cardiac output. Depress and blanch the nail beds; release and note the time for colour return. Usually, the vessels refill within a fraction of a second. Consider it normal if the colour returns in less than 1 or 2 seconds. Note conditions that can skew your findings: a cool room, decreased body temperature, cigarette smoking, peripheral edema, and anemia.

The two arms should be symmetrical in size.

Refill lasting more than 1 or 2 seconds signifies vasoconstriction or decreased cardiac output (hypovolemia, heart failure, shock). The hands are cold, clammy, and pale.

Edema of upper extremities occurs when lymphatic drainage is obstructed, which may occur after breast surgery (see Table 20-2, p. 548).

Note the presence of any scars on hands and arms. Many occur normally with usual childhood abrasions or with occupations involving hand tools.

Needle tracks in antecubital fossae occur with IV drug use; linear scars in wrists may signify past self-inflicted injury.

Palpate both radial pulses, noting rate, rhythm, elasticity of vessel wall, and equal force (Fig. 20-8). Grade the force (amplitude) on a three-point scale:

3+, increased, full, bounding
2+, **normal**
1+, weak
0, absent

Full, bounding pulse (3+) occurs with hyperkinetic states (exercise, anxiety, fever), anemia, and hyperthyroidism.

Weak, "thready" pulse occurs with shock and peripheral arterial disease. See Table 20-1 on p. 547 for illustrations of these and irregular pulse rhythms.

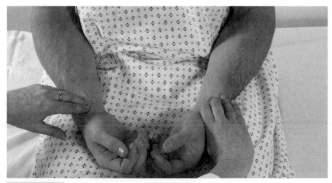

Fig. 20-8

It usually is not necessary to palpate the ulnar pulses. If indicated, palpate along the medial side of the inner forearm (Fig. 20-9), although the ulnar pulses often are not palpable in the normal person.

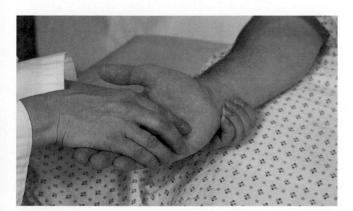

Fig. 20-9

Objective Data

Normal Range of Findings	Abnormal Findings

Palpate the brachial pulses—their force should be equal bilaterally (Fig. 20-10).

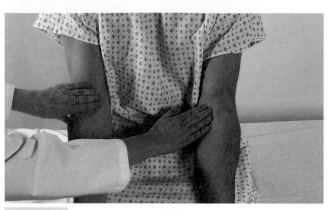

Fig. 20-10

Check the epitrochlear lymph node in the depression above and behind the medial condyle of the humerus. Do this by "shaking hands" with the person and reaching your other hand under the person's elbow to the groove between the biceps and triceps muscles, above the medial epicondyle (Fig. 20-11). This node is not palpable normally.

An enlarged epitrochlear node occurs with infection of the hand or forearm.

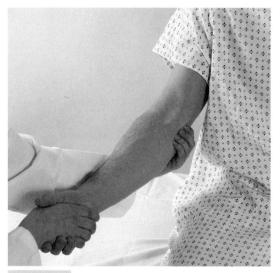

Fig. 20-11

The **modified Allen test** is used to evaluate the adequacy of collateral circulation prior to cannulating the radial artery (Fig. 20-12). (A) Firmly occlude both the ulnar and radial arteries of one hand while the person makes a fist several times. This causes the hand to blanch. (B) Ask the person to open the hand without hyperextending it; then release pressure on the ulnar artery while maintaining pressure on the radial artery. Adequate circulation is suggested by a return to the hand's normal colour in approximately 2 to 5 seconds. Although this test is simple and useful, it is relatively crude and subject to error—that is, you must occlude both arteries uniformly with 5 kg (11 lb) of pressure for the test to be accurate (Fuhrman et al., 1992; Gelberman et al., 1981).

(C) Pallor persists or a sluggish return to colour suggests occlusion of the collateral arterial flow. Avoid radial artery cannulation until adequate circulation is shown.

Normal Range of Findings	Abnormal Findings

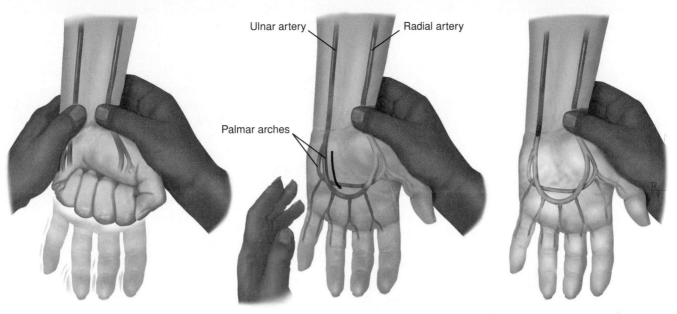

Ulnar artery   Radial artery

Palmar arches

Ⓐ Depress radial and ulnar arteries—
   person opens and closes fist

Ⓑ Normal—
   blood returns via ulnar artery

Ⓒ Occluded ulnar artery—
   no blood return

Fig. 20-12

INSPECT AND PALPATE THE LEGS

Uncover the legs while keeping the genitalia draped. Inspect both legs together, noting skin colour, hair distribution, venous pattern, size (swelling or atrophy), and any skin lesions or ulcers.

Normally hair covers the legs. Even if leg hair is shaved, you will still note hair on the dorsa of the toes.

The venous pattern normally is flat and barely visible. Note obvious varicosities, although these are best assessed while standing.

Both legs should be symmetrical in size without any swelling or atrophy. If the lower legs look asymmetrical or if deep venous thrombosis is suspected, measure the calf circumference with a nonstretchable tape measure (Fig. 20-13). Measure at the widest point, taking care to measure the other leg in exactly the same place—the same number of centimetres down from the patella or other landmark. If lymphedema is suspected, measure also at the ankle, distal calf, knee, and thigh. Record your findings in centimetres.

Pallor with vasoconstriction; erythema with vasodilatation; cyanosis.

Malnutrition: thin, shiny atrophic skin, thick-ridged nails, loss of hair, ulcers, gangrene. Malnutrition, pallor, and coolness occur with arterial insufficiency.

Diffuse bilateral edema occurs with systemic illnesses.

Acute, unilateral, painful swelling and asymmetry of calves of 1 cm or more is abnormal; refer the person to determine whether deep venous thrombosis is present.

Asymmetry of 1 to 3 cm occurs with mild lymphedema; 3 to 5 cm with moderate lymphedema; and more than 5 cm with severe lymphedema (see Table 20-2, p. 548).

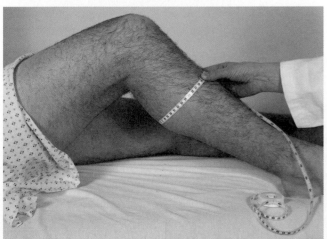

Fig. 20-13

Objective Data

Objective Data

Normal Range of Findings

In the presence of skin discoloration, skin ulcers, or gangrene, note the size and the exact location.

Palpate for temperature along the legs down to the feet, comparing symmetrical spots (Fig. 20-14). The skin should be warm and equal bilaterally. Bilateral cool feet may be due to environmental factors such as cool room temperature, apprehension, and cigarette smoking. If any increase in temperature is present higher up the leg, note if it is gradual or abrupt.

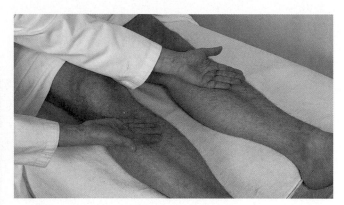

Fig. 20-14

Flex the person's knee, then gently compress the gastrocnemius (calf) muscle anteriorly against the tibia; no tenderness should be present. Or you may sharply dorsiflex the foot toward the tibia. Flexing the knee first exerts pressure on the posterior tibial vein. Normally this does not cause pain.

Palpate the inguinal lymph nodes. It is not unusual to find palpable nodes that are small (1 cm or less), movable, and nontender.

Palpate these peripheral arteries in both legs: femoral, popliteal, dorsalis pedis, and posterior tibial. Grade the force on the four-point scale. Locate the **femoral arteries** just below the inguinal ligament halfway between the pubis and anterior superior iliac spines (Fig. 20-15). To help expose the femoral area, particularly in obese people, ask the person to bend his or her knees to the side in a frog-like position. Press firmly and then slowly release, noting the pulse tap under your fingertips. Should this pulse be weak or diminished, auscultate the site for a bruit.

Abnormal Findings

Brown discoloration occurs with chronic venous stasis due to hemosiderin deposits from red blood cell degradation.

Venous ulcers occur usually at medial malleolus because of bacterial invasion of poorly drained tissues (see Table 20-4 on p. 550).

With arterial deficit, ulcers occur on tips of toes, metatarsal heads, and lateral malleoli.

A unilateral cool foot or leg or a sudden temperature drop as you move down the leg occurs with arterial deficit.

Calf pain with these manoeuvres is a positive **Homans' sign,** which occurs in about 20% of cases of deep vein thrombosis. This test was once considered a significant finding but has lost its impact due to **low sensitivity** in predicting the actual presence of a clot. A positive Homans' is also present in a variety of other conditions such as muscle injury, Achilles tendonitis, and plantar muscle injury. Venous ultrasonography is considered the **highly sensitive** diagnostic test to determine the presence or absence of a clot. Keep in mind that about half of all patients experiencing DVT have no clinically detectable signs or symptoms.

Enlarged nodes, tender, or fixed in area.

A bruit occurs with turbulent blood flow, indicating partial occlusion (see Table 20-5, p. 552).

Normal Range of Findings	Abnormal Findings

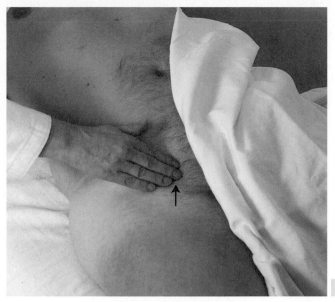

Fig. 20-15

The **popliteal pulse** is a more diffuse pulse and can be difficult to localize. With the leg extended but relaxed, anchor your thumbs on the knee, and curl your fingers around into the popliteal fossa (Fig. 20-16). Press your fingers forward hard to compress the artery against the bone (the lower edge of the femur or the upper edge of the tibia). Often it is just lateral to the medial tendon.

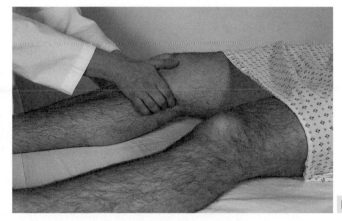

Fig. 20-16

If you have difficulty, turn the person prone and lift up the lower leg (Fig. 20-17). Let the leg relax against your arm and press in deeply with your two thumbs. Often a normal popliteal pulse is impossible to palpate.

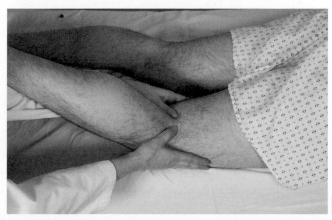

Fig. 20-17

Objective Data

Normal Range of Findings	Abnormal Findings

For the **posterior tibial** pulse, curve your fingers around the medial malleolus (Fig. 20-18). You will feel the tapping right behind it in the groove between the malleolus and the Achilles tendon. If you cannot, try passive dorsiflexion of the foot to make the pulse more accessible.

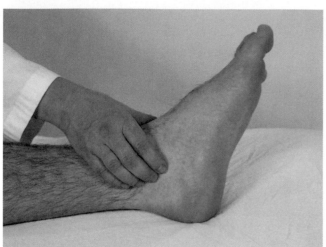

Fig. 20-18
Posterior tibial pulse.

The **dorsalis pedis** pulse requires a very light touch. Normally it is just lateral to and parallel with the extensor tendon of the big toe (Fig. 20-19). Do not mistake the pulse in your own fingertips for that of the person.

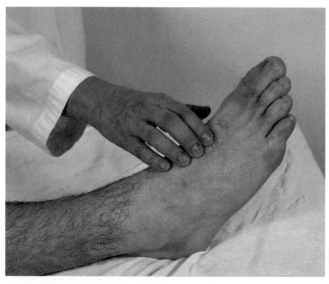

Fig. 20-19
Dorsalis pedis pulse.

In adults over 45 years, occasionally either the dorsalis pedis or the posterior tibial pulse may be hard to find, but not both on the same foot.

Check for pretibial edema. Firmly depress the skin over the tibia or the medial malleolus for 5 seconds and release (Fig. 20-20, *A*). Normally, your finger should leave no indentation, although a pit commonly is seen if the person has been standing all day or during pregnancy.

If pitting edema is present, grade it on the following scale:
1+ Mild pitting, slight indentation, no perceptible swelling of the leg
2+ Moderate pitting, indentation subsides rapidly
3+ Deep pitting, indentation remains for a short time, leg looks swollen
4+ Very deep pitting, indentation lasts a long time, leg is very swollen

Bilateral, dependent, pitting edema occurs with heart failure, diabetic neuropathy, and hepatic cirrhosis (Fig. 20-20, *B*).

Unilateral edema occurs with occlusion of a deep vein. Unilateral or bilateral edema occurs with lymphatic obstruction. With these factors, it is "brawny" or nonpitting and feels hard to the touch.

Normal Range of Findings

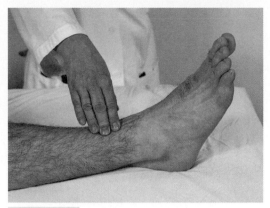

Fig. 20-20A   Check pretibial edema.

This scale is subjective and qualitative. The amount of pressure used is arbitrary, as is the judgement of the depth and rate of pitting. Clinicians need a standard quantified scale to ensure consistent clinical measurements and management. Many classify the edema by measuring the depth of the pitting in centimetres (1+ = 1 cm, 2+ = 2 cm, etc.) (Welsh et al., 1996).

Some measure with a millimetre scale, others by an increase in weight; still others try to quantify the rate of time the pitting remains after release of pressure. Check with your institution to determine a consistently used scale.

Ask the person to stand so that you can assess the venous system. Note any visible, dilated, and tortuous veins.

Manual Compression Test

While the person is still standing, test the length of the varicose vein to determine whether its valves are competent (Fig. 20-21). Place one hand on the lower part of the varicose vein, and compress the vein with your other hand about 15 to 20 cm higher. Competent valves will prevent a wave transmission and your distal (lower) fingers will feel no change.

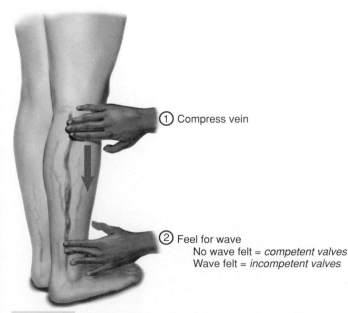

① Compress vein

② Feel for wave
   No wave felt = *competent valves*
   Wave felt = *incompetent valves*

Fig. 20-21   Manual compression test.   © *Pat Thomas, 2006.*

Abnormal Findings

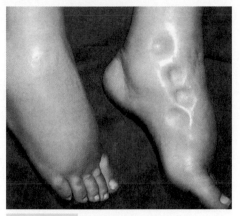

Fig. 20-20B   Pitting edema.

Varicosities occur in the saphenous veins (see Table 20-4, p. 550).

A palpable wave transmission occurs when the valves are incompetent.

Objective Data

Normal Range of Findings	Abnormal Findings

Colour Changes

If you suspect an arterial deficit, raise the legs about 30 cm off the table and ask the person to wag the feet for about 30 seconds to drain off venous blood (Fig. 20-22). The skin colour now reflects only the contribution of arterial blood. A light-skinned person's feet normally will look a little pale but still should be pink. A dark-skinned person's feet are more difficult to evaluate, but the soles should reveal extreme colour change.

Elevational pallor (marked) indicates arterial insufficiency.

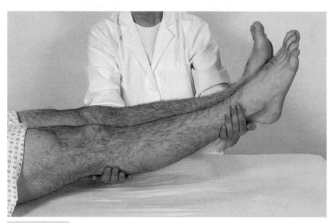

Fig. 20-22

Now have the person sit up with the legs over the side of the table (Fig. 20-23). Compare the colour of both feet. Note the time it takes for colour to return to the feet. Normally, this is 10 seconds or less. Note also the time it takes for the superficial veins around the feet to fill—the normal time is about 15 seconds. This test is unreliable if the person has concomitant venous disease with incompetent valves.

Dependent rubour (deep blue-red colour) occurs with severe arterial insufficiency. Chronic hypoxia produces a loss of vaso-motor tone and a pooling of blood in the veins.

Delayed venous filling occurs with arterial insufficiency.

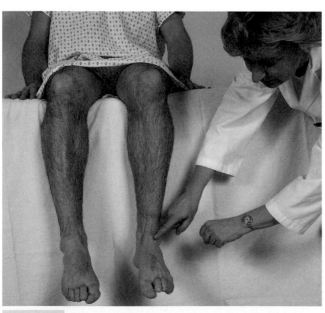

Fig. 20-23

Normal Range of Findings	Abnormal Findings

Test the lower legs for strength (see Chapter 22). Test the lower legs for sensation (see Chapter 23).

Motor loss occurs with severe arterial deficit.

Sensory loss occurs with arterial deficit, especially diabetes.

The Doppler Ultrasonic Stethoscope

Use the Doppler ultrasonic stethoscope device to detect a weak peripheral pulse, to monitor blood pressure in infants or children, or to measure a low blood pressure or blood pressure in a lower extremity (Fig. 20-24). This device magnifies pulsatile sounds from the heart and blood vessels. Position the person supine, with the legs externally rotated so you can reach the medial ankles easily. Place a drop of coupling gel on the end of the hand-held transducer. Place the transducer over a pulse site, swiveled at a 45-degree angle. Apply very light pressure; locate the pulse site by the swishing, whooshing sound.

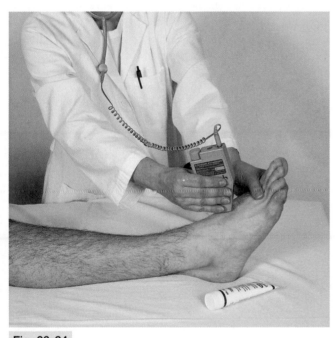

Fig. 20-24

The Ankle-Brachial Index (ABI)

Use of the Doppler stethoscope is a highly specific, noninvasive, and readily available way to determine the extent of peripheral vascular disease. Apply a regular arm blood pressure cuff above the ankle and determine the systolic pressure in either the posterior tibial or dorsalis pedis artery. Then divide that figure by the systolic pressure of the brachial artery.   *(Continued on next page)*

Objective Data

Normal Range of Findings	Abnormal Findings
(Take brachial systolic pressures in both arms and use the higher measurement.) The normal ankle pressure is slightly greater than or equal to the brachial pressure; thus, a normal ABI is usually 1.0 to 1.2. For example,	An ABI of 90% or less indicates the presence of peripheral arterial disease:

$$\frac{132 \text{ ankle systolic pressure}}{124 \text{ arm systolic pressure}} = 1.06 \text{ or } 106\%, \text{ indicating no flow reduction}$$

- 0.90 to 0.70—mild claudication
- 0.70 to 0.40—moderate to severe claudication
- 0.40 to 0.30—severe claudication, usually with rest pain except in the presence of diabetic neuropathy
- <0.30—ischemia, with impending loss of tissue

In people with diabetes mellitus, the ABI may be less reliable because of calcification (which makes their arteries noncompressible) and may give a falsely high measurement (Khan et al., 2006).

DEVELOPMENTAL CARE

Infants and Children

Transient acrocyanosis and skin mottling at birth are discussed in Chapter 12. Pulse force should be normal and symmetrical. Pulse force also should be the same in the upper and lower extremities.

Weak pulses occur with vasoconstriction of diminished cardiac output.

Full, bounding pulses occur with patent ductus arteriosus as a result of the large left-to-right shunt.

Diminished or absent femoral pulses while upper extremity pulses are normal suggest coarctation of aorta.

Palpable lymph nodes occur often in healthy infants and children. They are small, firm (shotty), mobile, and nontender. They may be the sequelae of past infection, such as inguinal nodes from a diaper rash or cervical nodes from a respiratory infection. Vaccinations also can produce local lymphadenopathy. Note characteristics of any palpable nodes and whether they are local or generalized.

Enlarged, warm, tender nodes indicate current infection. Look for source of infection.

The Pregnant Female

Expect diffuse bilateral pitting edema in the lower extremities, especially at the end of the day and into the third trimester. Varicose veins in the legs also are common in the third trimester.

The Aging Adult

The dorsalis pedis and posterior tibial pulse may become more difficult to find. Trophic changes associated with arterial insufficiency (thin, shiny skin, thick-ridged nails, loss of hair on lower legs) also occur normally with aging.

Summary Checklist: Peripheral Vascular Examination

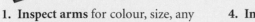 For a PDA-downloadable version, to http://evolve.elsevier.com/Canada/Jarvis/examination/.

1. **Inspect arms** for colour, size, any lesions
2. **Palpate pulses:** radial, brachial
3. **Check** epitrochlear node
4. **Inspect legs** for colour, size, any lesions, trophic skin changes
5. **Palpate the skin for temperature** of feet and legs
6. **Palpate inguinal nodes**
7. **Palpate pulses:** femoral, popliteal, posterior tibial, dorsalis pedis

---

Promoting Health: Foot Care

Take Care of Your Feet!

Foot problems often herald more serious health conditions such as arthritis, diabetes, and nerve or circulatory disorders. Healthcare professionals should not only remember to examine the feet for common foot problems but also be prepared to explain what "good" foot care really means. Too often healthcare professionals will advise good foot care but do not take the time to explain what "good" foot care entails.

Good foot care entails the following:
- Checking your feet every day.
  - If individuals are unable to see the bottoms of their feet, they need to be instructed to use a mirror or to ask someone to help them.
  - Each foot should be examined for red spots or sensitive areas, discoloration of skin or nails, ingrown nails, pain, cuts, swelling, or blisters. A good time to examine feet is after a shower or bath. Feet should be dried carefully, especially between the toes.
  - Toenails should be kept trimmed, straight across, and filed at the edges with an emery board or nail file.
  - Although freshly applied nail polish does not increase the number of bacteria, chipped nail polish may support the growth of larger numbers of organisms on nails. This is especially important for individuals who already are at risk for infection.
- Keeping the blood flowing to your feet.
  - It is important to keep blood circulating to one's feet. This is accomplished by increasing activity. Walking is one of the best exercises for overall circulation.
  - When an individual is not able to walk, putting the feet up when sitting or lying down, stretching, wiggling toes, having a gentle foot massage, and a warm foot bath are great alternatives.

- Do not cross legs for long periods of time.
- Do not smoke.
- Wearing shoes that fit and are comfortable.
  - Wear comfortable shoes that fit well. The size of our feet changes as we age, so it is important to be measured each time we buy new shoes. The best time to measure feet is toward the end of the day, when feet tend to be the largest.
  - Another thing to remember is that most individuals have one foot that is larger than the other. It is recommended that shoes are fit to the larger foot. Further, just as we have different body shapes, our feet have different shapes too.
  - It is important to select shoes that are shaped like one's feet. The ball of the foot should fit comfortably into the widest part of the shoe and toes should not be crowded.
  - For women, low-heeled shoes are safer and less damaging than high-heeled shoes.
- Keeping skin soft and smooth.
  - A thin coat of skin lotion over the tops and bottoms of one's feet helps to keep skin soft and smooth. However, this extra moisture should not go between toes.
  - Use mild soap.
  - Be careful about adding oils to bath water. They can make your feet and the bathtub both very slippery.

For more information on foot care, consult the following:

Canadian Diabetes Association. *Foot care a step toward good health.* Retrieved from http://www.diabetes.ca/files/footcare now.pdf

Canadian Podiatric Medical Society. http://www.podiatrycanada.org/

College of Family Physicians of Canada. *Diabetes and your body: How to take care of your eyes and feet.* Retrieved from http://www.cfpc.ca

---

DOCUMENTATION AND CRITICAL THINKING

Sample Charting

SUBJECTIVE

No leg pain, no skin changes, no swelling or lymph node enlargement. No history of heart or vascular problems, diabetes, or obesity. Does not smoke. On no medications.

OBJECTIVE

Inspection: Extremities have pink-tan colour without redness, cyanosis, or any skin lesions. Extremity size is symmetrical without swelling or atrophy.
Palpation: Temperature is warm and = bilaterally. All pulses present, 2+ and = bilaterally. No lymphadenopathy.

ASSESSMENT

Healthy tissue integrity
Effective tissue perfusion

Continued

Focused Assessment: Clinical Case Study

James K. is a 43-year-old, married male city sanitation worker, admitted to Queen Elizabeth II Medical Centre today for "bypass surgery tomorrow to fix my aorta and these black toes."

SUBJECTIVE

- 6 yr PTA: motorcycle accident with handle bars jammed into groin. Treated and released at local hospital. No apparent injury, although M.D. now thinks accident may have precipitated present stenosis of aorta.
- 1 yr PTA: radiating pain in right calf on walking 1½ km (1 mile). Pain relieved by stopping walking.
- 3 months PTA: problems with sex, unable to maintain erection during intercourse.
- 1 month PTA: leg pain present after walking two blocks. Numbness and tingling in right foot and calf. Tips of three toes on right foot look black. Saw M.D. Diagnostic studies showed stenosis of aorta "below vessels that go to my kidneys."
- Present: leg pain at rest, constant and severe, worse at night, partially relieved by dangling leg over side of bed.
- History: no history of heart or vessel disease, hypertension, diabetes, obesity.
- Personal habits: smokes cigarettes three packs/day × 23 years. Now cut down to 1 ppd.
- Walking is part of occupation, although has been driving city truck last 3 months due to leg pain. On no medications.

OBJECTIVE

Inspection: Lower extremity size = bilaterally with no swelling or atrophy. No varicosities. Colour L leg pink, R leg pink when supine, but marked pallor to R foot on elevation. Black gangrene at tips of R second, third, fourth toes. Leg hair present but absent on involved toes.

Palpation: R foot cool and temperature gradually warms as proceed palpating up R leg.

Pulses: Femorals, both 1+; popliteals, both O; posterior tibial, both O but present with Doppler; dorsalis pedis O, but left dorsalis pedis is present with Doppler, and right is not present with Doppler.

ASSESSMENT

Ischemic rest pain R leg
Ineffective tissue perfusion R/T interruption of flow
Impaired tissue integrity R/T altered circulation
Activity intolerance R/T leg pain
Sexual dysfunction R/T effects of disease

Nursing Diagnoses Commonly Associated With Peripheral Vascular System and Lymphatic Disorders

All nursing diagnoses can be found on the Evolve Web site at **http://evolve.elsevier.com/Canada/Jarvis/examination/.**

ABNORMAL FINDINGS

TABLE 20-1	Variations in Arterial Pulse
Description	**Associated With**

Weak, "Thready" Pulse—1+
Hard to palpate, need to search for it, may fade in and out, easily obliterated by pressure.

Decreased cardiac output; peripheral arterial disease; aortic valve stenosis

Full, Bounding Pulse—3+
Easily palpable, pounds under your fingertips.

Hyperkinetic states (exercise, anxiety, fever), anemia, hyperthyroidism

Water–Hammer (Corrigan's) Pulse—3+
Greater than normal force, then collapses suddenly.

Aortic valve regurgitation; patent ductus arteriosus

Pulsus Bigeminus
Rhythm is coupled, every other beat comes early, or normal beat followed by premature beat. Force of premature beat is decreased because of shortened cardiac filling time.

Conduction disturbance (e.g., premature ventricular contraction, premature atrial contraction)

Pulsus Alternans
Rhythm is regular, but force varies with alternating beats of large and small amplitude.

Heart failure

Pulsus Paradoxus
Beats have weaker amplitude with inspiration, stronger with expiration. Best determined during blood pressure measurement; reading decreases (>10 mm Hg) during inspiration and increases with expiration.

Any condition that blocks venous return to the right side of the heart, or blocks left ventricular filling (e.g., cardiac tamponade; constrictive pericarditis, pulmonary embolism)

Pulsus Bisferiens
Each pulse has two strong systolic peaks, with a dip in between. Best assessed at the carotid artery.

Aortic valve stenosis plus regurgitation

ABNORMAL FINDINGS
FOR ADVANCED PRACTICE

TABLE 20-2	Peripheral Vascular Disease in the Arms

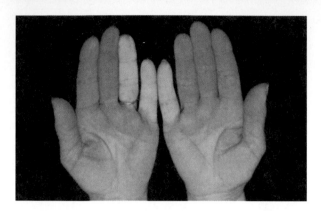

◄ **Raynaud's Phenomenon**

Episodes of abrupt progressive tricolour change of the fingers in response to cold, vibration, or stress: first white (pallor) from arteriospasm and resulting deficit in supply; then blue (cyanosis) from slight relaxation of the spasm that allows a slow trickle of blood through the capillaries and increased oxygen extraction of hemoglobin; finally red (rubour) due to return of blood into the dilated capillary bed or reactive hyperemia.

May have cold, numbness, or pain along with pallor or cyanosis stage; then burning, throbbing pain, swelling along with rubour. Lasts minutes to hours; occurs bilaterally.

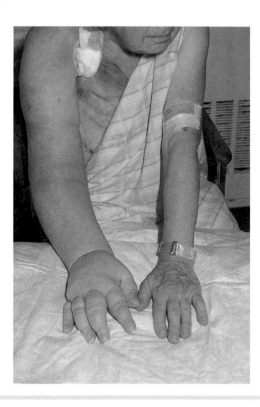

◄ **Lymphedema**

Removal of lymph nodes with breast surgery, or damage to lymph nodes and channels with radiation therapy for breast cancer; can impede drainage of lymph. Protein-rich lymph builds up in the interstitial spaces, which further raises local colloid oncotic pressure and promotes more fluid leakage. Stagnant lymphatic fluid can lead to infection, delayed wound healing, chronic inflammation, and fibrosis of surrounding tissue. Chronic lymphedema is unilateral swelling, nonpitting brawny edema, with overlying skin indurated, and is psychologically demoralizing as a threat to body image and is a constant reminder of the cancer.

TABLE 20-3	History Profiles of Pain of Peripheral Vascular Disease	
Symptom Analysis	Chronic Arterial Symptoms	Acute Arterial Symptoms
Location	Deep muscle pain, usually in calf, but may be lower leg or dorsum of foot	Varies, distal to occlusion, may involve entire leg
Character	Intermittent claudication, feels like "cramp," "numbness and tingling," "feeling of cold"	Throbbing
Onset and duration	Chronic pain, onset gradual after exertion	Sudden onset (within 1 hr)
Aggravating factors	Activity (walking, stairs) "Claudication distance" is specific number of blocks, stairs it takes to produce pain Elevation (rest pain indicates severe involvement)	
Relieving factors	Rest (usually within 2 min [e.g., standing]) Dangling (severe involvement)	
Associated symptoms	Cool pale skin	Six Ps: pain, pallor, pulselessness, paresthesia, poikilothermia (coldness), paralysis (indicates severe)
Those at risk	Older adults, more males than females, inherited predisposition, history of hypertension, smoking, diabetes, hypercholesterolemia, obesity, vascular disease	History of vascular surgery; arterial invasive procedure; abdominal aneurysm (emboli); trauma, including injured arteries, chronic atrial fibrillation
	Chronic Venous Symptoms	Acute Venous Symptoms
Location	Calf, lower leg	Calf
Character	Aching, tiredness, feeling of fullness	Intense, sharp; deep muscle tender to touch
Onset and duration	Chronic pain, increases at end of day	Sudden onset (within 1 hr)
Aggravating factors	Prolonged standing, sitting	Pain may increase with sharp dorsiflexion of foot
Relieving factors	Elevation, lying, walking	
Associated symptoms	Edema, varicosities, weeping ulcers at ankles	Red, warm, swollen leg
Those at risk	Those with a job with prolonged standing or sitting; obesity; pregnancy; prolonged bed rest; history of heart failure, varicosities, or thrombophlebitis; veins crushed by trauma or surgery	

Abnormal Findings

TABLE 20-4	**Peripheral Vascular Disease in the Legs**

Chronic Arterial Insufficiency	Chronic Venous Insufficiency

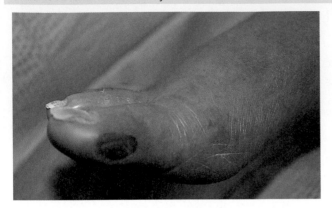

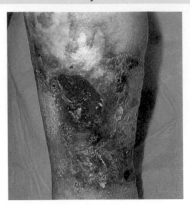

Arteriosclerosis—Ischemic Ulcer

Buildup of fatty plaques on intima (atherosclerosis) plus hardening and calcification of arterial wall (arteriosclerosis).

S: Deep muscle pain in calf or foot, claudication (pain with walking), pain at rest indicates worsening of condition.

O: Coolness, pallor, elevational pallor, and dependent rubour; diminished pulses; systolic bruits; trophic skin; signs of malnutrition (thin, shiny skin, thick-ridged nails, absence of hair, atrophy of muscles); xanthoma formation; distal gangrene.

Ulcers occur at toes, metatarsal heads, heels, lateral ankle, and are characterized by pale ischemic base, well-defined edges, and no bleeding.

Diabetes hastens changes described above, with generalized dysfunction in all arterial areas: peripheral, coronary, cerebral, retina, kidney. Peripheral involvement is associated with diabetic neuropathy and local infection.

Venous (Stasis) Ulcer

After acute deep vein thrombosis or chronic incompetent valves in deep veins.

S: Aching pain in calf or lower leg, worse at end of the day, worse with prolonged standing or sitting.

O: Firm brawny edema; coarse, thickened skin; pulses normal; brown pigment discoloration; petechiae; dermatitis. Venous stasis causes increased venous pressure, which then causes red blood cells (RBCs) to leak out of veins and into the skin. As these RBCs break down, they leave hemosiderin (iron deposits) behind, which are the brown pigment deposits.

Ulcers occur at medial malleolus and are characterized by bleeding, uneven edges.

S, Subjective data; *O,* objective data.

TABLE 20-4	Peripheral Vascular Disease in the Legs—cont'd
Chronic Venous Disease	Acute Venous Disease

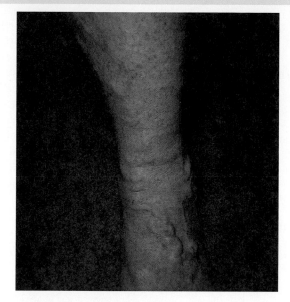

Superficial Varicose Veins

Incompetent valves permit reflux of blood, producing dilated, tortuous veins. Unremitting hydrostatic pressure causes distal valves to be incompetent and causes worsening of the varicosity.

Over age 45 years, occurrence is three times more common in women than in men.

S: Aching, heaviness in calf, easy fatigability, night leg or foot cramps.
O: Dilated, tortuous veins.

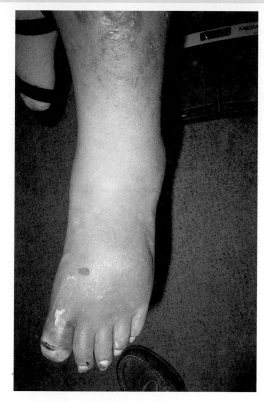

Deep Vein Thrombophlebitis

A deep vein is occluded by a thrombus, causing inflammation, blocked venous return, cyanosis, and edema. Cause may be prolonged bed rest; history of varicose veins; trauma; infection; cancer; and, in younger women, the use of oral estrogenic contraceptives (Dockery, 1997).

S: Sudden onset of intense, sharp, deep muscle pain, may increase with sharp dorsiflexion of foot.
O: Increased warmth; swelling (to compare swelling, observe the usual shoe size as in above photo); redness; dependent cyanosis is mild or may be absent; tender to palpation; Homans' sign is present only in few cases.

Requires emergency referral because of risk of pulmonary embolism.

TABLE 20-5	Peripheral Artery Disease

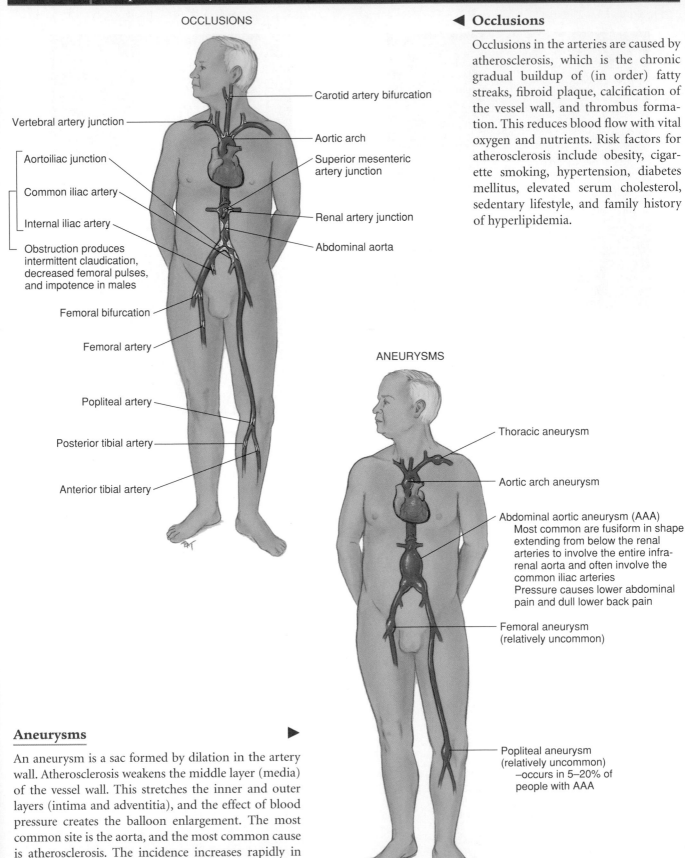

OCCLUSIONS

Vertebral artery junction

Aortoiliac junction

Common iliac artery

Internal iliac artery

Obstruction produces intermittent claudication, decreased femoral pulses, and impotence in males

Femoral bifurcation

Femoral artery

Popliteal artery

Posterior tibial artery

Anterior tibial artery

Carotid artery bifurcation

Aortic arch

Superior mesenteric artery junction

Renal artery junction

Abdominal aorta

ANEURYSMS

Thoracic aneurysm

Aortic arch aneurysm

Abdominal aortic aneurysm (AAA)
Most common are fusiform in shape extending from below the renal arteries to involve the entire infrarenal aorta and often involve the common iliac arteries
Pressure causes lower abdominal pain and dull lower back pain

Femoral aneurysm (relatively uncommon)

Popliteal aneurysm (relatively uncommon) –occurs in 5–20% of people with AAA

◀ Occlusions

Occlusions in the arteries are caused by atherosclerosis, which is the chronic gradual buildup of (in order) fatty streaks, fibroid plaque, calcification of the vessel wall, and thrombus formation. This reduces blood flow with vital oxygen and nutrients. Risk factors for atherosclerosis include obesity, cigarette smoking, hypertension, diabetes mellitus, elevated serum cholesterol, sedentary lifestyle, and family history of hyperlipidemia.

Aneurysms   ▶

An aneurysm is a sac formed by dilation in the artery wall. Atherosclerosis weakens the middle layer (media) of the vessel wall. This stretches the inner and outer layers (intima and adventitia), and the effect of blood pressure creates the balloon enlargement. The most common site is the aorta, and the most common cause is atherosclerosis. The incidence increases rapidly in men over 55 years and women over 70 years; the overall occurrence is four to five times more frequent in men.

BIBLIOGRAPHY

Bowling, J. C. R., & Dowd, P. M. (2003). Raynaud's disease. *Lancet, 361,* 2078–2080.

Brown, J. (2003). A clinically useful method for evaluating lymphedema. *Clinical Journal of Oncology Nursing, 8,* 35–38.

Chant, T. (2004). Peripheral vascular disease. *Primary Health Care, 14,* 29–34.

Dockery, G. L. (1997). *Cutaneous disorders of the lower extremity.* Philadelphia, PA: W.B. Saunders.

Fahey, V. A. (2004). *Vascular nursing* (4th ed.). Philadelphia, PA: W.B. Saunders.

Federman, D. G., Kravetz, J. D., Bravata, D. M., & Kirsner, R. S. (2006). Peripheral arterial disease. *Postgraduate Medicine, 119,* 21–27.

Fox, J. C., Otarodifard, K., & Deavers, M. (2006). Diagnostic and therapeutic keys to deep vein thrombosis. *Emergency Medicine, 38,* 14–20.

Fuhrman, T. M., Pippin, W. D., Talmage, L. A., & Reilley, T. E. (1992). Evaluation of collateral circulation of the hand. *Journal of Clinical Monitoring, 8,* 28–32.

Gelberman, R. H., & Blasingame, J. P. (1981). The timed Allen test. *Journal of Trauma, 21,* 477–479.

Gupta, A. (2006). Intermittent claudication. *Geriatric Medicine, 36,* 22–25.

Gould, S. D., & Spandorfer, J. M. (2005). Unilateral leg swelling: Clues to cause and ways to treat. *Patient Care, 39,* 49–55.

Joshua, A. M., Celermajer, D. S., & Stockler, M. R. (2005). Beauty is in the eye of the examiner: Reaching agreement about physical signs and their value. *Internal Medicine Journal 35,* 178–187.

Khan, N. A., Rahim, S. A., Anand, S. S., Simel, D. L., & Panju, A. (2006). Does the clinical examination predict lower extremity peripheral arterial disease? *Journal of the American Medical Association, 295,* 536–545.

McDermott, M. M. (1999). Ankle brachial index as a predictor of outcomes in peripheral arterial disease. *Journal of Laboratory and Clinical Medicine, 133,* 33–40.

Morrell, R. M., Halyard, M. Y., Schild, S. E., Ali, M. S., Gunderson, L. L., Pockaj, B. A. (2005). Breast cancer–related lymphedema. *Mayo Clinic Proceedings, 80,* 1480–1484.

Oka, R. K. (2006). Peripheral arterial disease in older adults. *Journal of Cardiovascular Nursing, 21,* 515–520.

Olson, K. W. P., & Treat-Jacobson, D. (2004). Symptoms of peripheral arterial disease. *Journal of Vascular Nursing, 22,* 72–77.

Perrodin, J. P. (2001). Noninvasive assessment of the peripheral vascular system: Hand-held Doppler, oscillometry, and air plethysmography. *Acute Care Perspectives, 10,* 13–15.

Reilly, A., & Snyder, B. (2005). Raynaud phenomenon. *American Journal of Nursing, 105,* 56–66.

Rice, K. L. (2005). How to measure ankle/brachial index. *Nursing, 35*(1), 56–57.

Scarvelis, D., & Wells, P. S. (2006). Diagnosis and treatment of deep vein thrombosis. *Canadian Medical Association Journal, 175,* 1087–1092.

Sieggreen, M. (2005). Lower extremity arterial and venous ulcers. *Nursing Clinics of North America, 40,* 391–410.

Sieggreen, M. (2006). A contemporary approach to peripheral arterial disease. *Nurse Practitioner, 31,* 14–26.

Sieggreen, M. Y., & Line, R. A. (2004). Arterial insufficiency and ulceration. *Nurse Practitioner, 29,* 46–52.

Slack, C. B., & Landis, C. A. (2006). Improving outcomes for restless legs syndrome. *Nurse Practitioner, 31,* 27–37.

Stevens, L. M. (2006). Peripheral arterial disease. *Journal of the American Medical Association, 295*(5), 584.

Urbano, F. L. (2001). Homans' sign in the diagnosis of deep venous thrombosis. *Hospital Physician, 37,* 22–24.

U.S. Preventive Services Task Force. (2006). Screening for peripheral arterial disease: Recommendation statement. *American Family Physician, 73,* 497–500.

Welsh, J. R., Arzouman, J. M., & Holm, K. (1996). Nurses' assessment and documentation of peripheral edema. *Clinical Nurse Specialist, 10,* 7–10.

Wigley, F. M. (2002). Raynaud's phenomenon. *New England Journal of Medicine, 347,* 1001–1007.

Williams, A. F. (2006). How to recognize lymphoedema. *Practical Nursing, 17,* 228–232.

Zipes, D., Libby, P., Bonow, R., & Braunwald, E. (2005). *Braunwald's heart disease: A textbook of cardiovascular medicine* (7th ed.). Philadelphia, PA: Saunders.

The Abdomen

Written by **Carolyn Jarvis**, PhD, APN, CNP
Adapted by **Marian Luctkar-Flude**, RN, MScN

Electronic Resources

On Evolve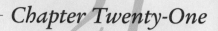

http://evolve.elsevier.com/Canada/Jarvis/examination/

- Interactive Case Studies
- Physical Examination Audio and Printable Summaries
- Bedside Assessment Summary Checklists
- Complete Physical Examination Form
- Nursing Diagnoses Boxes
- Health Promotion Guides
- Quick Assessments for 20 Common Conditions
- Multiple Choice Review Questions
- Chapter Objectives
- Appendices
- Weblinks

On the Companion CD

- Interactive Case Studies with Heart and Lung Sounds
- Health Promotion Guides
- Quick Assessments for 20 Common Conditions
- Head-to-Toe Physical Examination Video Clips

STRUCTURE AND FUNCTION

SURFACE LANDMARKS

The **abdomen** is a large oval cavity extending from the diaphragm down to the brim of the pelvis. It is bordered in back by the vertebral column and paravertebral muscles and at the sides and front by the lower rib cage and abdominal muscles (Fig. 21-1). Four layers of large, flat muscles form the ventral abdominal wall. These are joined at the midline by a tendinous seam, the **linea alba.** One set, the **rectus abdominis,** forms a strip extending the length of the midline, and its edge is often palpable.

INTERNAL ANATOMY

Inside the abdominal cavity, all the internal organs are called the **viscera.** It is important that you know the location of these organs so well that you could draw a map of them on the skin (Fig. 21-2). You must be able to visualize each organ that you listen to or palpate through the abdominal wall.

The **solid viscera** are those that maintain a characteristic shape (liver, pancreas, spleen, adrenal glands, kidneys, ovaries, and uterus). The liver fills most of the right upper quadrant (RUQ) and extends over to the left midclavicular line. The lower edge of the liver and the right kidney may normally be palpable. The ovaries normally are palpable only on bimanual examination during the pelvic examination.

The shape of the **hollow viscera** (stomach, gallbladder, small intestine, colon, and bladder) depends on the contents. They usually are not palpable, although you may feel a colon distended with feces or a bladder distended with urine. The stomach is just below the diaphragm, between the liver and spleen. The gallbladder rests under the posterior surface of the liver, just lateral to the right midclavicular line. Note that the small intestine is located in all four quadrants. It extends from the stomach's pyloric valve to the ileocecal valve in the right lower quadrant (RLQ), where it joins the colon.

The **spleen** is a soft mass of lymphatic tissue on the posterolateral wall of the abdominal cavity, immediately under the diaphragm (Fig. 21-3). It lies obliquely with its long axis behind and parallel to the tenth rib, lateral to the midaxillary line. Its width extends from the ninth to the eleventh ribs, about 7 cm. It is not palpable normally. If it becomes enlarged, its lower pole moves downward and toward the midline.

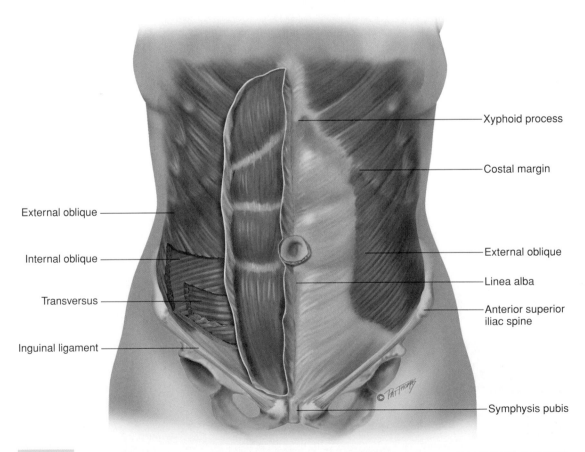

External oblique

Internal oblique

Transversus

Inguinal ligament

Xyphoid process

Costal margin

External oblique

Linea alba

Anterior superior iliac spine

Symphysis pubis

Fig. 21-1

© Pat Thomas, 2006.

Structure and Function

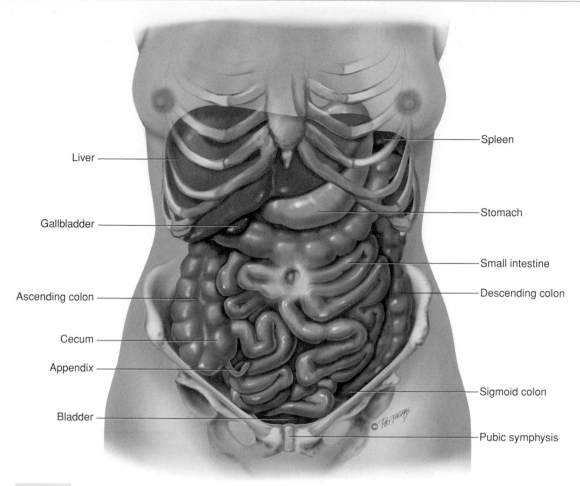

Liver

Gallbladder

Ascending colon

Cecum

Appendix

Bladder

Spleen

Stomach

Small intestine

Descending colon

Sigmoid colon

Pubic symphysis

Fig. 21-2

© Pat Thomas, 2006.

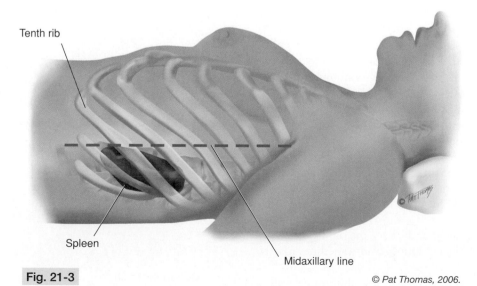

Tenth rib

Spleen

Midaxillary line

Fig. 21-3

© Pat Thomas, 2006.

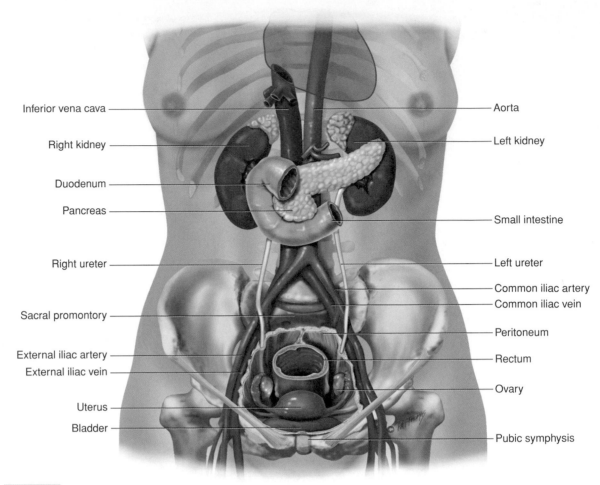

Inferior vena cava
Right kidney
Duodenum
Pancreas
Right ureter
Sacral promontory
External iliac artery
External iliac vein
Uterus
Bladder

Aorta
Left kidney
Small intestine
Left ureter
Common iliac artery
Common iliac vein
Peritoneum
Rectum
Ovary
Pubic symphysis

Fig. 21-4

© Pat Thomas, 2006.

The **aorta** is just to the left of midline in the upper part of the abdomen (Fig. 21-4). It descends behind the peritoneum and at 2 cm below the umbilicus, it bifurcates into the right and left common iliac arteries opposite the fourth lumbar vertebra. You can palpate the aortic pulsations easily in the upper anterior abdominal wall. The right and left iliac arteries become the femoral arteries in the groin area. Their pulsations are easily palpated as well, at a point halfway between the anterior superior iliac spine and the symphysis pubis.

The **pancreas** is a soft, lobulated gland located behind the stomach. It stretches obliquely across the posterior abdominal wall to the left upper quadrant (LUQ).

The bean-shaped **kidneys** are retroperitoneal, or posterior to the abdominal contents (Fig. 21-5). They are well protected by the posterior ribs and musculature. The twelfth rib forms an angle with the vertebral column, the **costovertebral angle.** The left kidney lies here at the eleventh and twelfth ribs.

Because of the placement of the liver, the right kidney rests 1 to 2 cm lower than the left kidney and sometimes may be palpable.

For convenience in description, the abdominal wall is divided into **four quadrants** by a vertical and a horizontal

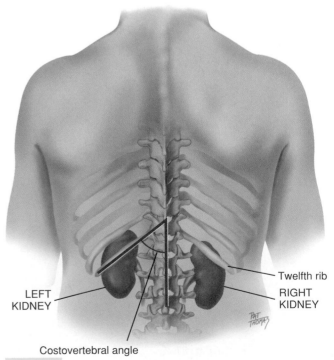

LEFT
KIDNEY

Twelfth rib

RIGHT
KIDNEY

Costovertebral angle

Fig. 21-5

line bisecting the umbilicus (Fig. 21-6). (An older, more complicated scheme divided the abdomen into nine regions. Although the old system generally is not used, some regional names persist, such as **epigastric** for the area between the costal margins, **umbilical** for the area around the umbilicus, and **hypogastric** or **suprapubic** for the area above the pubic bone.)

The anatomical location of the organ by quadrants is

RIGHT UPPER QUADRANT (RUQ)
Liver
Gallbladder
Duodenum
Head of pancreas
Right kidney and adrenal
Hepatic flexure of colon
Part of ascending and transverse colon

LEFT UPPER QUADRANT (LUQ)
Stomach
Spleen
Left lobe of liver
Body of pancreas
Left kidney and adrenal
Splenic flexure of colon
Part of transverse and descending colon

RIGHT LOWER QUADRANT (RLQ)
Cecum
Appendix
Right ovary and tube
Right ureter
Right spermatic cord

LEFT LOWER QUADRANT (LLQ)
Part of descending colon
Sigmoid colon
Left ovary and tube
Left ureter
Left spermatic cord

MIDLINE
Aorta
Uterus (If enlarged)
Bladder (if distended)

 DEVELOPMENTAL CARE

Infants and Children

In the newborn, the umbilical cord shows prominently on the abdomen. It contains two arteries and one vein. The liver takes up proportionately more space in the abdomen at birth than in later life. In healthy term neonates, the lower edge may be palpated 0.5 to 2.5 cm below the right costal margin. Age-related values of expected liver span are listed in the Objective Data section. The urinary bladder is located higher in the abdomen than in the adult. It lies between the symphysis and the umbilicus. Also, during early childhood the abdominal wall is less muscular, so the organs may be easier to palpate.

The Pregnant Female

Nausea and vomiting, or "morning sickness," is an early sign of pregnancy for most pregnant women, starting between the first and second missed periods. The cause is unknown but may be due to hormone changes such as the production of human chorionic gonadotropin (hCG). Another symptom is "acid indigestion" or heartburn (pyrosis) caused by esophageal reflux. Gastrointestinal motility decreases, which prolongs gastric emptying time. The decreased motility causes more water to be reabsorbed from the colon, which leads to constipation. The constipation, as well as increased venous pressure in the lower pelvis, may lead to hemorrhoids.

The enlarging uterus displaces the intestines upward and posteriorly. Bowel sounds are diminished. The appendix is

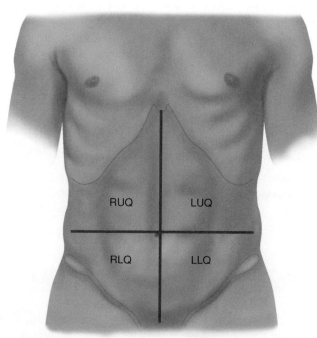

Four quadrants

Fig. 21-6

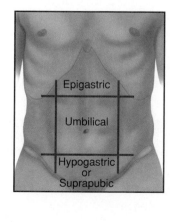

Epigastric
Umbilical
Hypogastric or Suprapubic

displaced upward and to the right. Skin changes on the abdomen, such as striae and linea nigra, are discussed later in this chapter and in Chapter 12.

The Aging Adult

Aging alters the appearance of the abdominal wall. During and after middle age, some fat accumulates in the suprapubic area in females as a result of decreased estrogen levels. Males also show some fat deposits in the abdominal area, resulting in the "spare tire" or "bay window." This accentuates in adults with a more sedentary lifestyle.

With further aging, adipose tissue is redistributed away from the face and extremities and to the abdomen and hips. The abdominal musculature relaxes.

Changes of aging occur in the gastrointestinal system but do not significantly affect function as long as no disease is present.

- Salivation decreases, causing a dry mouth and a decreased sense of taste. Further changes are discussed in Chapter 16.
- Esophageal emptying is delayed. If an aging person is fed in the supine position, this increases risk of aspiration.
- Gastric acid secretion decreases with aging. This may cause pernicious anemia (because it interferes with vitamin B_{12} absorption), iron deficiency anemia, and malabsorption of calcium.
- The incidence of gallstones increases with age, occurring in up to 20% of Canadian women and 10% of men by age 60.
- Liver size decreases with age, particularly after 80 years, although most liver function remains normal. Drug metabolism by the liver is impaired, in part because by age 60 to 80 years blood flow through the liver is decreased by 55 to 60% (Katzung, 2006). Therefore, the liver metabolism that is responsible for the enzymatic oxidation, reduction, and hydrolysis of drugs is substantially decreased with age. Prolonged liver metabolism causes increased side effects (e.g., older people taking benzodiazepines scored lower on functional status measures and had increased risk of hip fracture) (Reid et al., 1998).
- Older people frequently report constipation. However, a greater number use laxatives regularly (up to 30% of healthy older people) than actually are constipated (<10% of healthy, ambulatory, older adults). This is due to a concern about how often a healthy person should defecate (true constipation is less often than every third day) and confusing the passage of hard or small stools, the feeling of incomplete evacuation, or the need to strain at stool for constipation.

Of those older adults who actually are constipated, two thirds have slowed passage in the distal colon and delayed rectal emptying. Common causes of constipation include decreased physical activity, inadequate intake of water, a low-fibre diet, side effects of medications, irritable bowel syndrome, bowel obstruction, hypothyroidism, inadequate toilet facilities (i.e., difficulty ambulating to the toilet may cause the person to deliberately retain the stool until it becomes hard and difficult to pass).

CULTURAL AND SOCIAL CONSIDERATIONS

Lactase is the digestive enzyme necessary for absorption of the carbohydrate lactose (milk sugar). In some individuals, lactase activity is high at birth but declines to low levels by adulthood. These people are **lactose intolerant** and have abdominal pain, bloating, and flatulence when milk products are consumed. Lactose intolerance affects as much as 70% of the world's population. The prevalence of lactose intolerance is higher in Canadian Aboriginals and Canadians of African, Asian, Middle Eastern, or South American descent, and rarer in Canadians of European descent.

Infectious diseases such as hepatitis A and gastrointestinal illnesses are often related to socioeconomic factors such as inadequate housing, sewage, and water-treatment facilities. These conditions are often present in Aboriginal communities (National Aboriginal Health Organization, 2003). Government cutbacks have contributed to improper monitoring and operating practices, such as those that resulted in the contamination of the drinking water in Walkerton, Ontario, in 2000. Seven people died and 2300 people became ill as a result of bacterial infection, primarily with *Escherichia coli* O157:H7 (Ministry of the Attorney General, 2002).

SUBJECTIVE DATA

1. Appetite
2. Dysphagia
3. Food intolerance

4. Abdominal pain
5. Nausea/vomiting
6. Bowel habits

7. Abdominal history
8. Medications
9. Nutritional assessment

Examiner Asks	Rationale
1. Appetite. • Any change in **appetite?** Is this a loss of appetite? • Any change in weight? How much weight gained or lost? Over what time period? Is the weight loss due to diet?	**Anorexia** is a loss of appetite that occurs with gastrointestinal disease, a side effect to some medications, with pregnancy, or with psychological disorders.

Examiner Asks	Rationale
2. Dysphagia. • Any difficulty swallowing? When did you first notice this?	**Dysphagia** occurs with disorders of the throat or esophagus.
3. Food intolerance. • Are there any foods you cannot eat? What happens if you do eat them: allergic reaction, heartburn, belching, bloating, indigestion? • Do you use antacids? How often?	**Food intolerance** (e.g., lactase deficiency resulting in bloating or excessive gas after taking milk products). **Pyrosis** (heartburn), a burning sensation in esophagus and stomach, from reflux of gastric acid. Eructation (belching).
4. Abdominal pain. • Any **abdominal pain?** Please point to it. • Is the pain in one spot or does it move around? • How did it start? How long have you had it? • Constant or does it come and go? Occur before or after meals? Does it peak? When? • How would you describe the character: cramping (colic type), burning in pit of stomach, dull, stabbing, aching? • Is the pain relieved by food, or worse after eating? • Is the pain associated with: menstrual period or irregularities, stress, dietary indiscretion, fatigue, nausea and vomiting, gas, fever, rectal bleeding, frequent urination, vaginal or penile discharge? • What makes the pain worse: food, position, stress, medication, activity? • What have you tried to relieve pain: rest, heating pad, change in position, medication?	Abdominal pain may be *visceral* from an internal organ (dull, general, poorly localized), *parietal* from inflammation of overlying peritoneum (sharp, precisely localized, aggravated by movement), or *referred* from a disorder in another site (see Table 21-2 on p. 586). Aggravating factors. Alleviating factors.
5. Nausea or vomiting. • Any **nausea** or **vomiting?** How often? How much comes up? What is the colour? Is there an odour? • Is it bloody? • Is the nausea and vomiting associated with colicky pain, diarrhea, fever, chills? • What foods did you eat in the last 24 hours? Where? At home, school, restaurant? Is there anyone else in the family with same symptoms in last 24 hours?	Nausea/vomiting is a common side effect of many medications, with gastrointestinal disease, early pregnancy. Hematemesis occurs with stomach or duodenal ulcers and esophageal varices. Consider food poisoning.
6. Bowel habits. • How often do you have a **bowel movement?** • What is the colour? Consistency? • Any diarrhea or constipation? How long? • Any recent change in bowel habits? • Use laxatives? Which ones? How often do you use them?	Assess usual **bowel habits.** Black stools may be tarry due to occult blood (melena) from gastrointestinal bleeding or nontarry from iron medications. Grey stools occur with hepatitis. Red blood in stools occurs with gastrointestinal bleeding or localized bleeding around the anus.
7. Abdominal history. • Any **history** of gastrointestinal problems: ulcer, gallbladder disease, hepatitis/jaundice, appendicitis, colitis, hernia? • Ever had any operations in the abdomen? Please describe. • Any problems after surgery? • Any abdominal X-ray studies? How were the results?	

Subjective Data

Examiner Asks	Rationale

8. Medications.
- What **medications** are you currently taking?
- How about alcohol—How much would you say you drink each day? Each week? When was your last alcoholic drink?
- How about cigarettes—Do you smoke? How many packs per day? How long have your smoked?

Peptic ulcer disease occurs with frequent use of nonsteroidal anti-inflammatory drugs (NSAIDs), alcohol, smoking, and *Helicobacter pylori* infection.

9. Nutritional assessment.
- Now I would like to ask you about your diet. Please tell me all the food you ate yesterday, starting with breakfast.

Nutritional assessment, via 24-hour recall (see Chapter 11 for a complete discussion).

Additional History for Infants and Children

1. Are you breast- or bottle-feeding the baby? If bottle-feeding, how does baby tolerate the formula?

2. What table foods have you introduced? How does the infant tolerate the food?

Consider a new food as a possible allergen. Adding only one new food at a time to the infant's diet helps identify allergies.

3. How often does your toddler/child eat? Does he or she eat regular meals? How do you feel about your child's eating problems?
- Please describe all that your child had to eat yesterday, starting with breakfast. What foods does the child eat for snacks?

- Does toddler or child ever eat nonfoods: grass, dirt, paint chips?

Irregular eating patterns are common, and a source of parental anxiety. As long as child shows normal growth and development and only nutritious foods are offered, parents may be reassured.

Pica: Although a toddler may attempt nonfoods at some time, he or she should recognize edibles by age 2 years.

4. Does your child have constipation: How long?
- What are the number of stools per day? Stools per week?
- How much water, juice is in the diet?
- Does the constipation seem to be associated with toilet training?
- What have you tried to treat the constipation?

5. Does the child have abdominal pain? Please describe what you have noticed and when it started.

This symptom is hard to assess with young children. Many conditions of unrelated organ systems are associated with vague abdominal pain (e.g., otitis media). They cannot articulate specific symptoms and often focus on "the tummy." Abdominal pain accompanies inflammation of the bowel, constipation, urinary tract infection, and anxiety.

6. For the overweight child: How long has weight been a problem?
- At what age did the child first seem overweight? Did any change in diet pattern occur then?
- Describe the diet pattern now.
- Do any others in family have similar problem?
- How does child feel about his or her own weight?

Reduced physical activity and poor food marketing practices contribute to current obesity epidemic (Keith, 2006).

Family history of obesity.

Assess body image.

Examiner Asks	Rationale

Additional History for Adolescents

1. What do you eat at regular meals? Do you eat breakfast? What do you eat for snacks?

Adolescent takes control of eating and may reject family values (e.g., skipping breakfast, consuming junk foods, pop). The only control parents have is to control what food is in the house.

- How many calories do you figure you consume?

You probably cannot change adolescent eating pattern, but you can supply nutritional facts.

2. What is your exercise pattern?

Boys need an average 4000 cal/day to maintain weight; more calories if exercise is pursued. Girls need 20% fewer calories and the same nutrients as boys. Fast food is high in fat, calories, and salt and has no fibre.

3. If weight is less than body requirements: How much have you lost? By diet, exercise, or how?

Screen any extremely thin teenage girl for **anorexia nervosa,** a serious psychosocial disorder that includes loss of appetite, voluntary starvation, and grave weight loss. This person may augment weight loss by purging (self-induced vomiting) and use of laxatives.

- How do you feel? Tired, hungry? How do you think your body looks?

Denial of these feelings is common. Though thin, this person insists she looks fat, "disgusting." Distorted body image.

- What is your activity pattern?

The anorectic may have healthy activity and exercise but often is hyperactive.

- Is the weight loss associated with any other body change, such as menstrual irregularity?

Amenorrhea is common with anorexia nervosa.

- What do your parents say about your eating? Your friends?

This is a family problem involving control issues. Anyone at risk warrants immediate referral to an M.D. or psychologist.

Additional History for the Aging Adult

1. How do you acquire your groceries and prepare your meals?

Assess risk for nutritional deficit: limited access to grocery store, income, or cooking facilities; physical disability (impaired vision, decreased mobility, decreased strength, neurological deficit).

2. Do you eat alone or share meals with others?

Assess risk for nutritional deficit if living alone; may not bother to prepare all meals; social isolation; depression.

3. Please tell me all that you had to eat yesterday, starting with breakfast.

Note: Twenty-four-hour recall may not be sufficient because daily pattern may vary. Attempt week-long diary of intake. Food pattern may be different in the month if monthly income (e.g., Old Age Security pension cheque) runs out.

- Do you have any trouble swallowing these foods?
- What do you do right after eating: walk, take a nap?

Examiner Asks	Rationale
4. How often do your bowels move? • If the person reports constipation: What do you mean by constipation? How much liquid is in your diet? How much bulk or fibre? • Do you take anything for constipation, such as laxatives? Which ones? How often? • What medications do you take?	Consider gastrointestinal side effects (e.g., nausea, upset stomach, anorexia, dry mouth).

 ━━━ OBJECTIVE DATA ━━━

PREPARATION

The lighting should include a strong overhead light and a secondary stand light. Expose the abdomen so that it is fully visible. Drape the genitalia and female breasts.

The following measures will enhance abdominal wall relaxation:

- The person should have emptied the bladder, saving a urine specimen if needed.
- Keep the room warm to avoid chilling and tensing of muscles.
- Position the person supine, with the head on a pillow, the knees bent or on pillow, and the arms at the sides or across the chest. (Note: Discourage the person from placing his or her arms over the head because this tenses abdominal musculature.)
- To avoid abdominal tensing, the stethoscope end piece must be warm, your hands must be warm, and your fingernails must be very short.
- Inquire about any painful areas. Examine such an area last to avoid any muscle guarding.
- Finally, learn to use distraction: enhance muscle relaxation through breathing exercises; emotive imagery; your low, soothing voice; and the person relating his or her abdominal history while you palpate.

EQUIPMENT NEEDED

Stethoscope
Small centimeter ruler
Skin-marking pen
Alcohol wipe (to clean end piece)

Normal Range of Findings	Abnormal Findings
### INSPECT THE ABDOMEN #### Contour Stand on the person's right side and look down on the abdomen. Then stoop or sit to gaze across the abdomen. Your head should be slightly higher than the abdomen. Determine the profile from the rib margin to the pubic bone. The contour describes the nutritional state and normally ranges from flat to rounded (Fig. 21-7).	Scaphoid abdomen, protuberant abdomen, abdominal distension (see also Table 21-1, p. 586).

Normal Range of Findings	Abnormal Findings

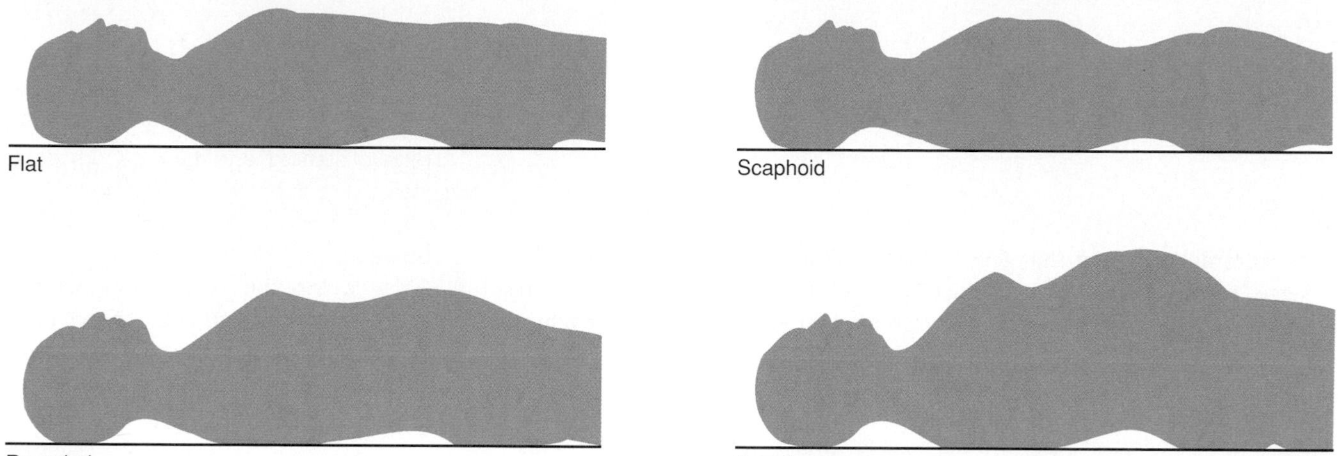

Flat

Scaphoid

Rounded

Protuberant

Fig. 21-7

Symmetry

Shine a light across the abdomen toward you, or shine it lengthwise across the person. The abdomen should be symmetrical bilaterally (Fig. 21-8). Note any localized bulging, visible mass, or asymmetrical shape. Even small bulges are highlighted by shadow. Step to the foot of the examination table to recheck symmetry.

Bulges, masses.
Hernia—protrusion of abdominal viscera through abnormal opening in muscle wall (see Table 21-3, p. 589).

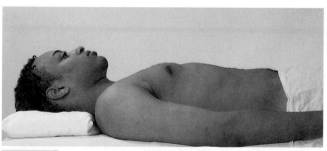

Fig. 21-8

Ask the person to take a deep breath to further highlight any change. The abdomen should stay smooth and symmetrical. Or ask the person to perform a sit-up without pushing up with his or her hands.

Note any localized bulging.
Hernia, enlarged liver or spleen may show.

Umbilicus

Normally it is midline and inverted, with no sign of discoloration, inflammation, or hernia. It becomes everted and pushed upward with pregnancy.

The umbilicus is a common site for piercings in young women. The site should not be red or crusted.

Everted with acites, or underlying mass (see Table 21-1, p. 586).
Deeply sunken with obesity.
Enlarged and everted with umbilical hernia.
Bluish periumbilical color occurs with intra-abdominal bleeding (Cullen's sign).

Normal Range of Findings	Abnormal Findings

Skin

The surface is smooth and even, with homogeneous colour. This is a good area to judge pigment because it is often protected from sun.

Redness with localized inflammation.

Jaundice (shows best in natural daylight).

Skin glistening and taut occurs with ascites.

One common pigment change is **striae** (lineae albicantes), silvery white, linear, jagged marks about 1 to 6 cm long (Fig. 21-9). They occur when elastic fibres in the reticular layer of the skin are broken after rapid or prolonged stretching, as in pregnancy or excessive weight gain. Recent striae are pink or blue; then they turn silvery white.

Striae also occur with ascites.

Striae look purple-blue with Cushing's syndrome (excess adrenocortical hormone causes the skin to be fragile and easily broken from normal stretching).

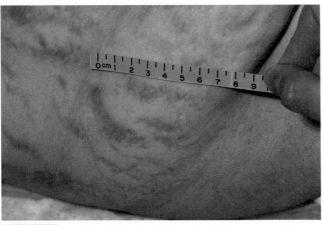

Fig. 21-9   Striae.

Pigmented nevi (moles), circumscribed brown macular or papular areas, are common on the abdomen.

Unusual colour or change in shape of mole (see Chapter 12).

Petechiae.

Normally, no lesions are present, although you may note well-healed surgical scars. If a scar is present, draw its location in the person's record, indicating the length in centimetres (Fig. 21-10). (Note: Infrequently, a person forgets a past operation while providing the history. If you note a scar, ask about it.) A surgical scar alerts you to the possible presence of underlying adhesions and excess fibrous tissue.

Cutaneous angiomas (spider nevi) occur with portal hypertension or liver disease.

Lesions, rashes (see Chapter 12).

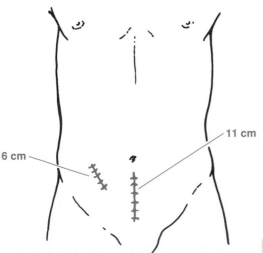

6 cm

11 cm

Fig. 21-10

Normal Range of Findings	Abnormal Findings

Veins usually are not seen, but a fine venous network may be visible in thin persons.

Good skin turgor reflects healthy nutrition. Gently pinch up a fold of skin; then release to note the skin's immediate return to original position.

Prominent, dilated veins occur with portal hypertension, cirrhosis, ascites, or vena caval obstruction. Veins are more visible with malnutrition as a result of thinned adipose tissue.

Poor turgor occurs with dehydration, which often accompanies gastrointestinal disease.

Pulsation or Movement

Normally, you may see the pulsations from the aorta beneath the skin in the epigastric area, particularly in thin persons with good muscle wall relaxation. Respiratory movement also shows in the abdomen, particularly in males. Finally, waves of peristalsis sometimes are visible in very thin persons. They ripple slowly and obliquely across the abdomen.

Marked pulsation of aorta occurs with widened pulse pressure (e.g., hypertension, aortic insufficiency, thyrotoxicosis) and with aortic aneurysm.

Marked visible peristalsis, together with a distended abdomen, indicates intestinal obstruction.

Hair Distribution

The pattern of pubic hair growth normally has a diamond shape in adult males and an inverted triangle shape in adult females (see Chapters 24 and 26).

Patterns alter with endocrine or hormone abnormalities, chronic liver disease.

Demeanour

A comfortable person is relaxed quietly on the examining table and has a benign facial expression and slow, even respirations.

Restlessness and constant turning to find comfort occur with the colicky pain of gastroenteritis or bowel obstruction.

Absolute stillness, resisting any movement, occurs with the pain of peritonitis.

Knees flexed up; facial grimacing; and rapid, uneven respirations also indicate pain.

AUSCULTATE BOWEL SOUNDS AND VASCULAR SOUNDS

Depart from the usual examination sequence and auscultate the abdomen next. This is done because percussion and palpation can increase peristalsis, which would give a false interpretation of bowel sounds. Use the diaphragm end piece because bowel sounds are relatively high pitched. Hold the stethoscope lightly against the skin; pushing too hard may stimulate more bowel sounds (Fig. 21-11). Begin in the RLQ at the ileocecal valve area because bowel sounds are normally always present here.

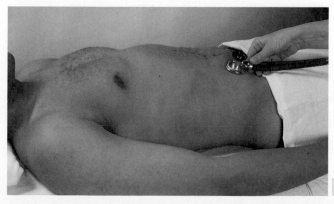

Fig. 21-11

Objective Data

Normal Range of Findings	Abnormal Findings

Bowel Sounds

Note the character and frequency of bowel sounds. Bowel sounds originate from the movement of air and fluid through the small intestine. Depending on the time elapsed since eating, a wide range of normal sounds can occur. Bowel sounds are high-pitched, gurgling, cascading sounds, occurring irregularly anywhere from 5 to 30 times per minute. Do not bother to count them. Judge if they are normal, hypoactive, or hyperactive.

One type of hyperactive bowel sounds is fairly common. This is the hyperperistalsis when you feel your "stomach growling," termed **borborygmus.** A perfectly "silent abdomen" is uncommon; you must listen for 5 minutes by your watch before deciding bowel sounds are completely absent.

Two distinct patterns of abnormal bowel sounds may occur:
1. **Hyperactive sounds** are loud, high-pitched, rushing, tinkling sounds that signal increased motility.
2. **Hypoactive or absent sounds** follow abdominal surgery or with inflammation of the peritoneum (see Table 21-4, p. 590).

Vascular Sounds

As you listen to the abdomen, note the presence of any vascular sounds or **bruits.** Using firmer pressure, check over the aorta and the renal arteries, iliac, and femoral arteries, especially in people with hypertension (Fig. 21-12). Usually, no such sound is present. Note: If a bruit is heard over the aorta, you should NOT palpate the area for fear of rupturing a possible aortic aneurysm.

Note location, pitch, and timing of a vascular sound.

A systolic bruit is a pulsatile blowing sound and occurs with stenosis or occlusion of an artery.

Venous hum and peritoneal friction rub are rare (see Table 21-5, p. 591).

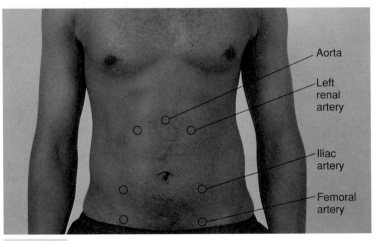

Aorta

Left renal artery

Iliac artery

Femoral artery

Fig. 21-12

PERCUSS GENERAL TYMPANY, LIVER SPAN, AND SPLENIC DULLNESS

Percuss to assess the relative density of abdominal contents, to locate organs, and to screen for abnormal fluid or masses.

General Tympany

First, percuss lightly in all four quadrants to determine the prevailing amount of tympany and dullness (Fig. 21-13). Move clockwise. Tympany should predominate because air in the intestines rises to the surface when the person is supine.

Dullness occurs over a distended bladder, adipose tissue, fluid, or a mass.

Hyperresonance is present with gaseous distension.

Abnormal Findings

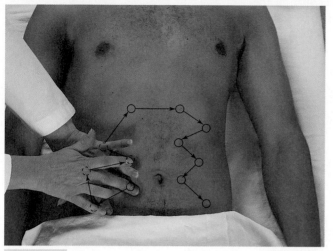

Fig. 21-13

Liver Span

Next, percuss to map out the boundaries of certain organs. Measure the height of the liver in the right midclavicular line. (For a consistent placement of the midclavicular line landmark, remember to palpate the acromioclavicular and the sternoclavicular joints and judge the line at a point midway between the two.)

Begin in the area of lung resonance, and percuss down the interspaces until the sound changes to a dull quality (Fig. 21-14). Mark the spot, usually in the fifth intercostal space. Then find abdominal tympany and percuss up in the midclavicular line. Mark where the sound changes from tympany to a dull sound, normally at the right costal margin.

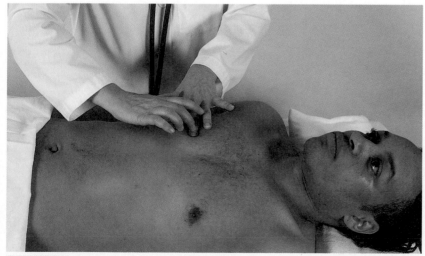

Fig. 21-14

Normal Range of Findings

Measure the distance between the two marks; the normal liver span in the adult ranges from 6 to 12 cm (Fig. 21-15). The height of the liver span correlates with the height of the person; taller people have longer livers. Also males have a larger liver span than females of the same height. Overall, the mean liver span is 10.5 cm for males and 7 cm for females.

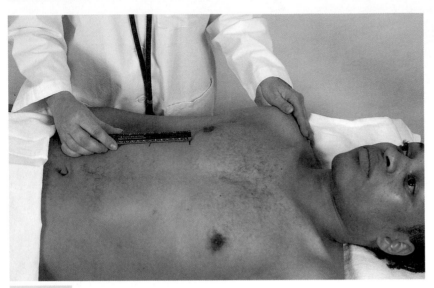

Fig. 21-15

One variation occurs in people with chronic emphysema, in which the liver is displaced downward by the hyperinflated lungs. Although you hear a dull percussion note well below the right costal margin, the overall span is still within normal limits.

Clinical estimation of liver span is important to screen for hepatomegaly and to monitor changes in liver size. However, this measurement is a gross estimate; the liver span may be underestimated because of inaccurate detection of the upper border.

Scratch Test. One final technique is the *scratch test*, which may help define the liver border when the abdomen is distended or the abdominal muscles are tense. Place your stethoscope over the liver. With one fingernail, scratch short strokes over the abdomen, starting in the RLQ and moving progressively up toward the liver (Fig. 21-16). When the scratching sound in your stethoscope becomes magnified, you will have crossed the border from over a hollow organ to a solid one.

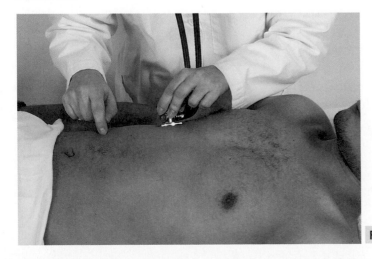

Fig. 21-16

Abnormal Findings

An enlarged liver span indicates liver enlargement or **hepatomegaly.**

Accurate detection of liver borders is confused by dullness above the fifth intercostal space, which occurs with lung disease (e.g., pleural effusion or consolidation). Accurate detection at the lower border is confused when dullness is pushed up with ascites or pregnancy or with gas distension in colon, which obscures lower border.

Normal Range of Findings	Abnormal Findings

Splenic Dullness

Often the spleen is obscured by stomach contents, but you may locate it by percussing for a dull note from the ninth to eleventh intercostal space just behind the left midaxillary line (Fig. 21-17). The area of splenic dullness normally is not wider than 7 cm in the adult and should not encroach on the normal tympany over the gastric air bubble.

Now percuss in the lowest interspace in the left *anterior* axillary line. Tympany should result. Ask the person to take a deep breath. Normally, tympany remains through full inspiration.

A dull note forward of the midaxillary line indicates enlargement of the spleen, as occurs with mononucleosis, trauma, and infection.

In this site, the *anterior* axillary line, a change in percussion from tympany to a dull sound with full inspiration is a **positive spleen percussion sign,** indicating splenomegaly. This method will detect mild to moderate splenomegaly before the spleen becomes palpable, as in mononucleosis, malaria, or hepatic cirrhosis.

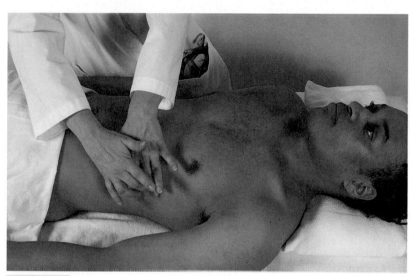

Fig. 21-17

Costovertebral Angle Tenderness

Indirect fist percussion causes the tissues to vibrate instead of producing a sound. To assess the kidney, place one hand over the twelfth rib at the costovertebral angle on the back (Fig. 21-18). Thump that hand with the ulnar edge of your other fist. The person normally feels a thud but no pain. (Although this step is explained here with percussion techniques, its usual sequence in a complete examination is with thoracic assessment, when the person is sitting up and you are standing behind.)

Sharp pain occurs with inflammation of the kidney or paranephric area.

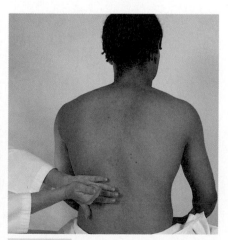

Fig. 21-18

Normal Range of Findings	Abnormal Findings

Special Procedures

At times, you may suspect that a person has ascites (free fluid in the peritoneal cavity) because of a distended abdomen, bulging flanks, and an umbilicus that is protruding and displaced downward. You can differentiate ascites from gaseous distension by performing two percussion tests.

Fluid Wave. First, test for a **fluid wave** by standing on the person's right side. Place the ulnar edge of another examiner's hand or the patient's own hand firmly on the abdomen in the midline (Fig. 21-19). (This will stop transmission across the skin of the upcoming tap.) Place your left hand on the person's right flank. With your right hand, reach across the abdomen and give the left flank a firm strike.

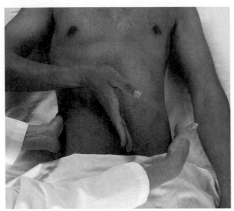

Fig. 21-19
Fluid wave.

If ascites is present, the blow will generate a fluid wave through the abdomen and you will feel a distinct tap on your left hand. If the abdomen is distended from gas or adipose tissue, you will feel no change.

Shifting Dullness. The second test for ascites is percussing for **shifting dullness.** In a supine person, ascitic fluid settles by gravity into the flanks, displacing the air-filled bowel upward. You will hear a tympanitic note as you percuss over the top of the abdomen because gas-filled intestines float over the fluid (Fig. 21-20). Then percuss down the side of the abdomen. If fluid is present, the note will change from tympany to dull as you reach its level. Mark this spot.

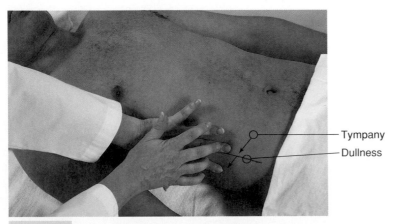

— Tympany
— Dullness

Fig. 21-20

Ascites occurs with heart failure, portal hypertension, cirrhosis, hepatitis, pancreatitis, and cancer.

A positive fluid wave test occurs with large amounts of ascitic fluid.

Normal Range of Findings	Abnormal Findings

Now turn the person onto the right side (roll the person toward you) (Fig. 21-21). The fluid will gravitate to the dependent (in this case, right) side, displacing the lighter bowel upward. Begin percussing the upper side of the abdomen and move downward. The sound changes from tympany to a dull sound as you reach the fluid level, but this time the level of dullness is higher, upward toward the umbilicus. This **shifting level of dullness** indicates the presence of fluid.

Both tests, fluid wave and shifting dullness, are not completely reliable. Ultra-sonography study is the definitive tool.

Shifting dullness is positive with a large volume of ascitic fluid: it will not detect less than 500 mL of fluid.

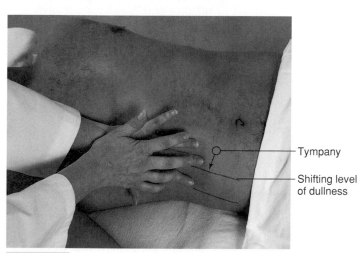

Tympany

Shifting level of dullness

Fig. 21-21

PALPATE SURFACE AND DEEP AREAS

Perform palpation to judge the size, location, and consistency of certain organs and to screen for an abnormal mass or tenderness. Review comfort measures on p. 564. Because most people are naturally inclined to protect the abdomen, you need to use additional measures to enhance complete muscle relaxation:

1. Bend the person's knees.
2. Keep your palpating hand low and parallel to the abdomen. Holding the hand high and pointing down would make anyone tense up.
3. Teach the person to breathe slowly (in through the nose, and out through the mouth).
4. Keep your own voice low and soothing. Conversation may relax the person.
5. Try "emotive imagery." For example, you might say, "Now I want you to imagine you are dozing on the beach, with the sun warming your muscles and the sound of the waves lulling you to sleep. Let yourself relax."
6. With a very ticklish person, keep the person's hand under your own with your fingers curled over his or her fingers. Move both hands around as you palpate; people are not ticklish to themselves.
7. Alternatively, perform palpation just after auscultation. Keep the stethoscope in place and curl your fingers around it, palpating as you pretend to auscultate. People do not perceive a stethoscope as a ticklish object. You can slide the stethoscope out when the person is used to being touched.

Objective Data

| **Normal Range of Findings** | **Abnormal Findings** |

Light and Deep Palpation

Begin with **light palpation.** With the first four fingers close together, depress the skin about 1 cm (Fig. 21-22). Make a gentle rotary motion, sliding the fingers and skin together. Then lift the fingers (do not drag them) and move clockwise to the next location around the abdomen. The objective here is not to search for organs but to form an overall impression of the skin surface and superficial musculature. Save the examination of any identified tender areas until last. This method avoids pain and the resulting muscle rigidity that would obscure deep palpation later in the examination.

Muscle guarding.
Rigidity.
Large masses.
Tenderness.

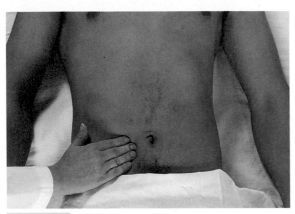

Fig. 21-22

As you circle the abdomen, discriminate between voluntary muscle guarding and involuntary rigidity. **Voluntary guarding** occurs when the person is cold, tense, or ticklish. It is bilateral, and you will feel the muscles relax slightly during exhalation. Use the relaxation measures to try to eliminate this type of guarding, or it will interfere with deep palpation. If the rigidity persists, it is probably involuntary.

Involuntary rigidity is a constant board-like hardness of the muscles. It is a protective mechanism accompanying acute inflammation of the peritoneum. It may be unilateral, and the same area usually becomes painful when the person increases intra-abdominal pressure by attempting a sit-up.

Now perform **deep palpation** using the same technique described earlier, but push down about 5 to 8 cm (Fig. 21-23). Moving clockwise, explore the entire abdomen.

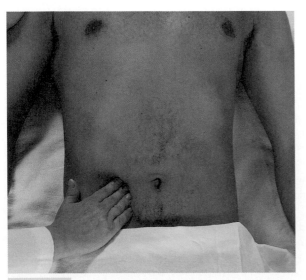

Fig. 21-23

Objective Data

Normal Range of Findings	Abnormal Findings

Normal Range of Findings

To overcome the resistance of a very large or obese abdomen, use a bimanual technique. Place your two hands on top of each other (Fig. 21-24). The top hand does the pushing; the bottom hand is relaxed and can concentrate on the sense of palpation. With either technique, note the location, size, consistency, and mobility of any palpable organs and the presence of any abnormal enlargement, tenderness, or masses.

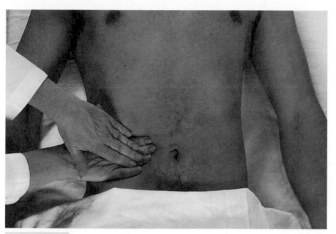

Fig. 21-24

Making sense of what you are feeling is more difficult than it looks. Inexperienced examiners complain that the abdomen "all feels the same," as if they are pushing their hand into a soft sofa cushion. It helps to memorize the anatomy and visualize what is under each quadrant as you palpate. Also remember that some structures are normally palpable, as illustrated in Figure 21-25.

Abnormal Findings

Tenderness occurs with local inflammation, with inflammation of the peritoneum or underlying organ, and with an enlarged organ whose capsule is stretched.

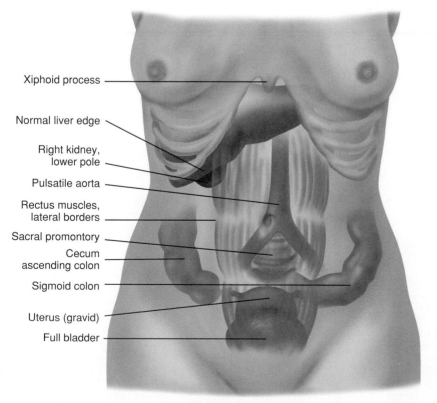

Xiphoid process

Normal liver edge

Right kidney, lower pole

Pulsatile aorta

Rectus muscles, lateral borders

Sacral promontory

Cecum ascending colon

Sigmoid colon

Uterus (gravid)

Full bladder

NORMALLY PALPABLE STRUCTURES

Fig. 21-25

Objective Data

Normal Range of Findings	Abnormal Findings

Mild tenderness normally is present when palpating the sigmoid colon. Any other tenderness should be investigated.

If you identify a mass, first distinguish it from a normally palpable structure or an enlarged organ. Then note the following:

1. Location
2. Size
3. Shape
4. Consistency (soft, firm, hard)
5. Surface (smooth, nodular)
6. Mobility (including movement with respirations)
7. Pulsatility
8. Tenderness

Liver

Next, palpate for specific organs, beginning with the liver in the RUQ (Fig. 21-26). Place your left hand under the person's back parallel to the eleventh and twelfth ribs and lift up to support the abdominal contents. Place your right hand on the RUQ, with fingers parallel to the midline. Push deeply down and under the right costal margin. Ask the person to take a deep breath. It is normal to feel the edge of the liver bump your fingertips as the diaphragm pushes it down during inhalation. It feels like a firm regular ridge. Often, the liver is not palpable and you feel nothing firm.

Except with a depressed diaphragm, a liver palpated more than 1 to 2 cm below the right costal margin is enlarged. Record the number of centimetres it descends and note its consistency (hard, nodular) and tenderness (see Table 21-6, p. 591).

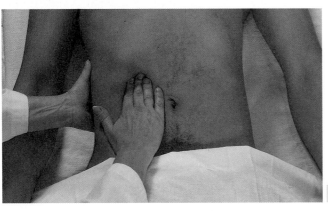

Fig. 21-26

Hooking Technique. An alternative method of palpating the liver is to stand up at the person's shoulder and swivel your body to the right so that you face the person's feet (Fig. 21-27). Hook your fingers over the costal margin from above. Ask the person to take a deep breath. Try to feel the liver edge bump your fingertips.

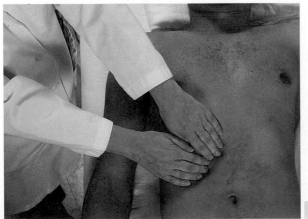

Fig. 21-27

Normal Range of Findings	Abnormal Findings

Spleen

Normally, the spleen is not palpable and must be enlarged three times its normal size to be felt. To search for it, reach your left hand over the abdomen and behind the left side at the eleventh and twelfth ribs (Fig. 21-28, *A*). Lift up for support. Place your right hand obliquely on the LUQ with the fingers pointing toward the left axilla and just inferior to the rib margin. Push your hand deeply down and under the left costal margin and ask the person to take a deep breath. You should feel nothing firm.

The spleen enlarges with mononucleosis and trauma (see Table 21-6, p. 591). If you feel an enlarged spleen, refer the person but do not continue to palpate it. An enlarged spleen is friable and can rupture easily with overpalpation.

Describe the number of centimetres it extends below the left costal margin.

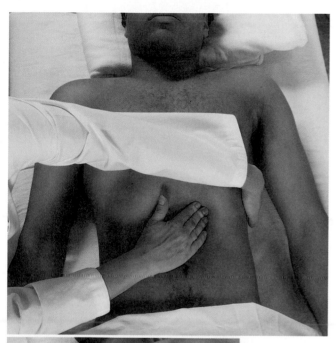

A

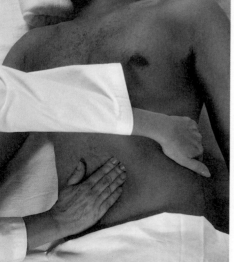

B

Fig. 21-28

When enlarged, the spleen slides out and bumps your fingertips. It can grow so large that it extends into the lower quadrants. When this condition is suspected, start low so you will not miss it. An alternative position is to roll the person onto his or her right side to displace the spleen more forward and downward (Fig. 21-28, *B*). Then palpate as described earlier.

Objective Data

Normal Range of Findings	Abnormal Findings

Kidneys

Search for the right kidney by placing your hands together in a "duck-bill" position at the person's right flank (Fig. 21-29, *A*). Press your two hands together firmly (you need deeper palpation than that used with the liver or spleen) and ask the person to take a deep breath. In most people, you will feel no change. Occasionally, you may feel the lower pole of the right kidney as a round, smooth mass slide between your fingers. Either condition is normal.

Enlarged kidney.
Kidney mass.

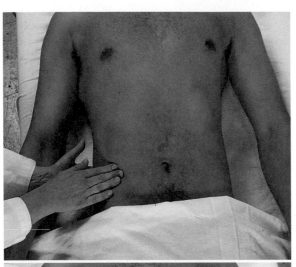

A

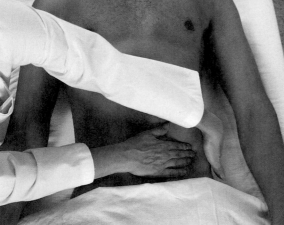

B

Fig. 21-29

The left kidney sits 1 cm higher than the right kidney and is not palpable normally. Search for it by reaching your left hand across the abdomen and behind the left flank for support (Fig. 21-29, *B*). Push your right hand deep into the abdomen and ask the person to breathe deeply. You should feel no change with the inhalation.

Aorta

Using your opposing thumb and fingers, palpate the aortic pulsation in the upper abdomen slightly to the left of midline (Fig. 21-30). Normally, it is 2.5 to 4 cm wide in the adult and pulsates in an anterior direction.

Widened with aneurysm (see Tables 21-5 and 21-6, p. 591).
Prominent lateral pulsation with aortic aneurysm.

Note: If a bruit was heard on auscultation, you should NOT palpate the area for fear of rupturing an aortic aneurysm.

Normal Range of Findings	Abnormal Findings

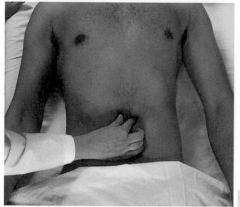

Fig. 21-30

Special Procedures for Advanced Practice

Rebound Tenderness (Blumberg's Sign). Assess rebound tenderness when the person reports abdominal pain or when you elicit tenderness during palpation. Choose a site away from the painful area. Hold your hand 90 degrees, or perpendicular, to the abdomen. Push down slowly and deeply (Fig. 21-31, *A*); then lift up *quickly* (Fig. 21-31, *B*). This makes structures that are indented by palpation rebound suddenly. A normal, or negative, response is no pain on release of pressure. Perform this test at the end of the examination, because it can cause severe pain and muscle rigidity.

Pain on release of pressure confirms rebound tenderness, which is a reliable sign of peritoneal inflammation. Peritoneal inflammation accompanies appendicitis.

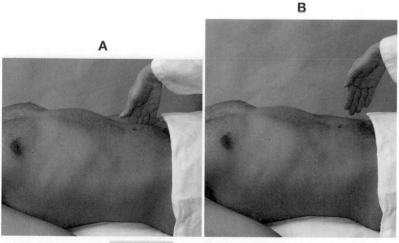

B

A

Fig. 21-31   Rebound tenderness.

Inspiratory Arrest (Murphy's Sign). Normally, palpating the liver causes no pain. In a person with inflammation of the gallbladder, or cholecystitis, pain occurs. Hold your fingers under the liver border. Ask the person to take a deep breath. A normal response is to complete the deep breath without pain.

When the test is positive, as the descending liver pushes the inflamed gallbladder onto the examining hand, the person feels sharp pain and abruptly stops inspiration midway.

Iliopsoas Muscle Test. Perform the iliopsoas muscle test when the acute abdominal pain of appendicitis is suspected. With the person supine, lift the right leg straight up, flexing at the hip (Fig. 21-32); then push down over the lower part of the right thigh as the person tries to hold the leg up. When the test is negative, the person feels no change.

When the iliopsoas muscle is inflamed (which occurs with an inflamed or perforated appendix), pain is felt in the RLQ.

Objective Data

Normal Range of Findings	Abnormal Findings

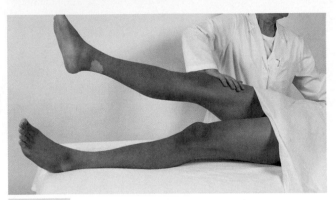

Fig. 21-32   Iliopsoas muscle test.

Obturator Test. The obturator test also is performed when appendicitis is suspected. With the person supine, lift the right leg, flexing at the hip and 90 degrees at the knee (Fig. 21-33). Hold the ankle and rotate the leg internally and externally. A negative or normal response is no pain.

A perforated appendix irritates the obturator muscle, producing pain.

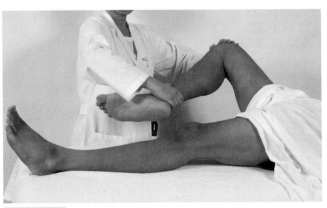

Fig. 21-33   Obturator test.

 DEVELOPMENTAL CARE

The Infant

Inspection. The contour of the abdomen is protuberant because of the immature abdominal musculature. The skin contains a fine, superficial venous pattern. This may be visible in lightly pigmented children up to the age of puberty.

Inspect the umbilical cord throughout the neonatal period. At birth, it is white and contains two umbilical arteries and one vein surrounded by mucoid connective tissue, called Wharton's jelly. The umbilical stump dries within a week, hardens, and falls off by 10 to 14 days. Skin covers the area by 3 to 4 weeks.

The abdomen should be symmetrical, although two bulges are common. You may note an **umbilical hernia.** It appears at 2 to 3 weeks and is especially prominent when the infant cries. The hernia reaches maximum size at 1 month (up to 2.5 cm) and usually disappears by 1 year. Another common variation is **diastasis recti,** a separation of the rectus muscles with a visible bulge along the midline. The condition is more common with infants of African descent, and it usually disappears by early childhood.

Scaphoid shape occurs with dehydration.
Dilated veins.

The presence of only one artery signals the risk of congenital defects.
Inflammation.
Drainage after cord falls off.

Refer any umbilical hernia larger than 2.5 cm (see Table 21-3, p. 589); continuing to grow after 1 month; or lasting for more than 2 years in a child of European descent or for more than 7 years in a child of African descent.
Refer diastasis recti lasting more than 6 years.

Normal Range of Findings	Abnormal Findings

The abdomen shows respiratory movement. The only other abdominal movement you should note is occasional peristalsis, which may be visible because of the thin musculature.

Marked peristalsis with pyloric stenosis (see Table 21-4, p. 590).

Auscultation. Auscultation yields only bowel sounds, the metallic tinkling of peristalsis. No vascular sounds should be heard.

Bruit.
Venous hum.

Percussion. Percussion finds tympany over the stomach (the infant swallows some air with feeding) and dullness over the liver. Percussing the spleen is not done. The abdomen sounds tympanitic, although it is normal to percuss dullness over the bladder. This dullness may extend up to the umbilicus.

Palpation. Aid palpation by flexing the baby's knees with one hand while palpating with the other (Fig. 21-34). Alternatively, you may hold the upper back and flex the neck slightly with one hand. Offer a pacifier to a crying baby.

The liver fills the RUQ. It is normal to feel the liver edge at the right costal margin or 1 to 2 cm below. Normally, you may palpate the spleen tip and both kidneys and the bladder. Also easily palpated are the cecum in the RLQ, and the sigmoid colon, which feels like a sausage in the left inguinal area.

Make note of the newborn's first stool, a sticky, greenish black meconium stool within 24 hours of birth. By the fourth day, stools of breastfed babies are golden yellow, pasty, and smell like sour milk, whereas those of formula-fed babies are brown-yellow, firmer, and more fecal smelling.

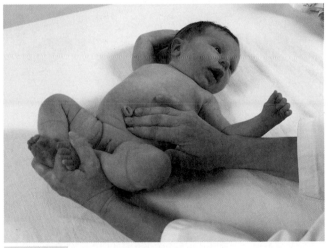

Fig. 21-34

The Child

Under age 4 years, the abdomen looks protuberant when the child is both supine and standing. After age 4 years, the potbelly remains when standing because of lumbar lordosis, but the abdomen looks flat when supine. Normal movement on the abdomen includes respirations, which remain abdominal until 7 years of age.

A scaphoid abdomen is associated with dehydration or malnutrition.

Under 7 years of age, the absence of abdominal respirations occurs with inflammation of the peritoneum.

To palpate the abdomen, position the young child on the parent's lap as you sit knee to knee with the parent (Fig. 21-35). Flex the knees up, and elevate the head slightly. The child can "pant like a dog" to further relax abdominal muscles. Hold your entire palm flat on the abdominal surface for a moment before starting palpation. This accustoms the child to being touched. If the child is very ticklish, hold his or her hand under your own as you palpate; or apply the stethoscope and palpate around it.

Objective Data

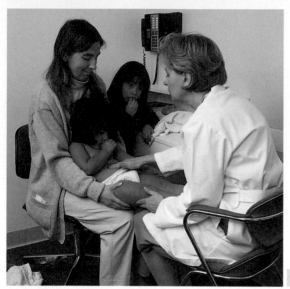

Fig. 21-35

The liver remains easily palpable 1 to 2 cm below the right costal margin. The edge is soft and sharp and moves easily. On the left, the spleen also is easily palpable with a soft, sharp, movable edge. Usually you can feel 1 to 2 cm of the right kidney and the tip of the left kidney. Percussion of the liver span measures about 3.5 cm at age 2 years, 5 cm at age 6 years, and 6 to 7 cm during adolescence.

In assessing abdominal tenderness, remember that the young child often answers this question affirmatively no matter how the abdomen actually feels. Use objective signs to aid assessment, such as a cry changing in pitch as you palpate, facial grimacing, moving away from you, and guarding.

The school-age child has a slim abdominal shape as he or she loses the pot-belly. This slimming trend continues into adolescence. The adolescent is easily embarrassed with exposure of the abdomen, and adequate draping is necessary. The physical findings are the same as those listed for the adult.

The Aging Adult

On inspection, you may note increased deposits of subcutaneous fat on the abdomen and hips because it is redistributed away from the extremities. The abdominal musculature is thinner and has less tone than that of the younger adult, so in the absence of obesity you may note peristalsis.

Because of the thinner, softer abdominal wall, the organs may be easier to palpate (in the absence of obesity). The liver is easier to palpate. Normally, you will feel the liver edge at or just below the costal margin. With distended lungs and a depressed diaphragm, the liver is palpated lower, descending 1 to 2 cm below the costal margin with inhalation. The kidneys are easier to palpate.

Abdominal rigidity with acute abdominal conditions is less common in aging.

With an acute abdomen, the aging person often complains of less pain than a younger person would.

Summary Checklist: Abdomen Examination

 For a PDA-downloadable version, go to http://evolve.elsevier.com/Canada/Jarvis/examination/.

1. **Inspection**
   Contour
   Symmetry
   Umbilicus
   Skin
   Pulsation or movement
   Hair distribution
   Demeanour

2. **Auscultation**
   Bowel sounds
   Note any vascular sounds

3. **Percussion**
   Percuss all four quadrants
   Percuss borders of liver, spleen

4. **Palpation**
   Light palpation in all four quadrants
   Deeper palpation in all four quadrants
   Palpate for liver, spleen, kidneys

Promoting Health: Hepatitis Risk

How's Your Liver Doing?

The liver is the largest organ in the body. It has an immense capacity to heal and regenerate, but that capacity is not infinite. Unfortunately, signs of severe liver damage or disease usually do not become apparent until the liver has been significantly harmed. The best protection for the liver is to prevent damage *before* it occurs!

There are many measures an individual can follow to protect the liver:

- **Practice safe sex.** Do not have unprotected sex with a male or female.
- **Don't share items that may have bodily fluids on them.** This means needles, razors, nail clippers, cuticle scissors, and toothbrushes. If getting a tattoo, make sure that a new bottle of ink is opened and used for only one individual.
- **Be aware of your environment.** Be careful with aerosol cleaners. Make sure rooms are well ventilated. Wear a mask, hat, or protective clothing when using insecticides, fungicides, paint, or other toxic chemicals. The liver can be damaged by what you breathe or absorb through your skin.
- **Watch your diet and weight.** Obesity can cause a condition called nonalcoholic fatty liver disease, which may include cirrhosis.
- **Travel wisely.** Visit a travel medicine clinic before travelling. If travelling to an area with an increased rate of hepatitis A, such as Mexico, Central America, and the Caribbean, get vaccinated, avoid eating uncooked food, including raw vegetables, avoid drinking unboiled or unbottled water (including ice cubes), and brush your teeth with boiled or bottled water.
- **Use medications wisely.** Only use prescription and over-the-counter medications when needed. Be sure to take only the recommended doses.
- **Do not mix medications without consulting a healthcare professional.** Mixing certain medications can form toxic compounds that can cause liver damage. Be certain that all medications, including over-the-counter and herbal preparations, are discussed with a healthcare professional.
- **Drink alcohol in moderation.** More than one drink a day for women or two drinks a day for men over many years may be enough to lead to cirrhosis. A cirrhotic liver shrinks to a fraction of its former size and ability.
- **Do not mix medications and alcohol.** Acetaminophen can be toxic to the liver even if one drinks alcohol in moderation.
- **Do not use illegal drugs.** Cocaine is one of many illegal drugs known to cause liver damage.
- **Get vaccinated.** A vaccine is available for both hepatitis A and hepatitis B. Universal immunization of children and adolescents against hepatitis B is now part of the publicly funded vaccine programs offered in all Canadian provinces and territories.

- **Be aware of your risk for hepatitis.** Six hepatitis viruses have been identified, but three—hepatitis A (HAV), hepatitis B (HBV), and hepatitis C (HCV)—cause about 90% of acute hepatitis cases in Canada. The incidence of HAV has been estimated at 2.9 cases for every 100,000 persons in Canada; the incidence of HBV is higher at approximately 4.9 cases for every 100,000 persons; and the incidence of HCV is highest at between 10 and 20 cases per 100,000 persons per year.

  - HAV is primarily spread through food or water contaminated by feces from an infected person. **Risk factors for HAV include:**
    - Eating food that has been prepared by someone who is infected with HAV and who has poor hygiene
    - Eating raw or undercooked shellfish (such as oysters or clams)
    - Eating uncooked food, including unpeeled fruits and vegetables
    - Travelling to HAV-endemic areas
    - Having homosexual relations
    - Sharing a household with an HAV-infected person

  - HBV is primarily spread through contact with infected blood or bodily fluids. **Risk factors for HBV include:**
    - Having unprotected sex, especially with someone who is infected with HBV or whose sexual history is unknown
    - Sharing needles or other drug use equipment, including spoons, water, and cotton, to inject illegal drugs
    - Handling blood or bodily fluids as a routine part of your job. This includes nurses and other healthcare professionals. It also includes morticians and embalmers
    - Getting body piercings or tattoos from a site using poor infection control practices
    - Travelling to HBV-endemic areas
    - Sharing a household with an HBV-infected person
    - Being on dialysis

  - HCV is primarily spread through contact with infected blood. **Risk factors for HCV include:**
    - Receiving a transfusion before 1992 or experiencing clotting factors before 1987
    - Using illegal IV drugs or intranasal cocaine
    - Handling blood or bodily fluids as a routine part of your job
    - Being on dialysis
    - Getting body piercings or tattoos from a site using poor infection control practices
    - Sharing a household with an HCV infected person

DOCUMENTATION AND CRITICAL THINKING

Sample Charting

SUBJECTIVE

States appetite is good with no recent change, no dysphagia, no food intolerance, no pain, no nausea/vomiting. Has one formed BM/day. Takes vitamins, no other prescribed or over-the-counter medication. No history of abdominal disease, injury, or surgery. Diet recall of last 24 hours listed at end of history.

OBJECTIVE

Inspection: Abdomen flat, symmetrical with no apparent masses. Skin smooth with no striae, scars, or lesions.
Auscultation: Bowel sounds present, no bruits.
Percussion: Tympany predominates in all four quadrants, liver span is 8 cm in right midclavicular line. Splenic dullness located at tenth intercostal space in left midaxillary line.
Palpation: Abdomen soft, no organomegaly, no masses, no tenderness.

ASSESSMENT

Healthy abdomen, bowel sounds present

Focused Assessment: Clinical Case Study 1

George E. is a 58-year-old unemployed, divorced male with chronic alcoholism who enters the chemical dependency treatment centre.

SUBJECTIVE

* For 6 months PTA has been drinking 500 mL whisky/d.
* Last alcohol use 1 week PTA, with "5 or 6" drinks that episode.
* Estranged from family, lives alone. Makes a few meals on hot plate. States never has appetite. Has fatigue and weakness.

OBJECTIVE

Inspection: Appears older than stated age. Oriented, although verbal response time slowed. Weight loss of 5.5 kg in last 3 months. Abdomen protuberant, symmetrical, no visible masses. Poor skin turgor. Dilated venous pattern over abdominal wall. Hair sparse in axillary, pubic area.
Auscultation: Bowel sounds present. No vascular sounds.
Percussion: Tympany predominates over abdomen. Liver span is 16 cm in right midclavicular line. No fluid wave. No shifting dullness.
Palpation: Soft. Liver palpable 10 cm below right costal margin, smooth and nontender. No other organomegaly or masses.

ASSESSMENT

Alcohol dependence, severe, with physiological dependence
Imbalanced nutrition: less than body requirements R/T impaired absorption
Ineffective coping R/T effects of chronic alcoholism
Social isolation

Focused Assessment: Clinical Case Study 2

Edith J. is a 63-year-old, retired homemaker with a history of lung cancer with metastasis to the liver.

SUBJECTIVE

- Feeling "puffy and bloated" for the past week. States unable to get comfortable. Also short of breath "all the time now." Difficulty sleeping. "I feel like crying all the time now."

OBJECTIVE

Inspection: Weight increase of 3.7 kg in 1 week. Abdomen is distended with everted umbilicus and bulging flanks. Girth at umbilicus is 85 cm. Prominent dilated venous pattern present over abdomen.
Auscultation: Bowel sounds present, no vascular sounds.
Percussion: When supine, tympany present at dome of abdomen, dullness over flanks. Shifting dullness present. Positive fluid wave present. Liver span is 12 cm in right midclavicular line.
Palpation: Abdominal wall firm, able to feel liver with deep palpation at 6 cm below right costal margin. Liver feels firm, nodular, nontender. 4+ pitting edema in both ankles.

ASSESSMENT

Ascites
Grieving
Ineffective breathing pattern R/T increased intra-abdominal pressure
Pain R/T distended abdomen
Risk for impaired skin integrity: R/T ascites, edema, and faulty metabolism
Insomnia

Focused Assessment: Clinical Case Study 3

Dan G. is a 17-year-old male high-school student who enters the emergency department having had abdominal pain for 2 days.

SUBJECTIVE

- Two days PTA Dan noted general abdominal pain in umbilical region. Now pain is sharp and severe, and Dan points to location in right lower quadrant.
- No BM for 2 days. Nausea and vomiting off and on 1 day.

OBJECTIVE

Inspection: BP 112/70, temp 38°C, pulse 116, resp 18.
Lying on side with knees drawn up under chin. Resists any movement. Face tight and occasionally grimacing. Cries out with any sudden movement.
Auscultation: No bowel sounds present. No vascular sounds.
Percussion: Tympany. Percussion over RLQ leads to tenderness.
Palpation: Abdominal wall is rigid and boardlike. Extreme tenderness to palpation in RLQ.
Rebound tenderness is present in RLQ. Positive iliopsoas muscle test.

ASSESSMENT

Acute abdominal pain in RLQ
Nausea

Nursing Diagnoses Commonly Associated With Abdominal Disorders

All nursing diagnoses can be found on the Evolve Web site at **http://evolve.elsevier.com/Canada/Jarvis/examination/**.

ABNORMAL FINDINGS

TABLE 21-1 | Abdominal Distension[1]

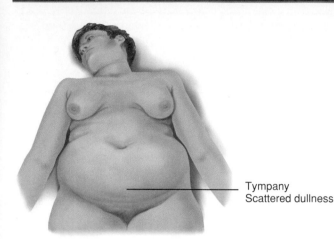

Obesity

Inspection. Uniformly rounded. Umbilicus sunken (it adheres to peritoneum, and layers of fat are superficial to it).
Auscultation. Normal bowel sounds.
Percussion. Tympany. Scattered dullness over adipose tissue.
Palpation. Normal. May be hard to feel through thick abdominal wall.

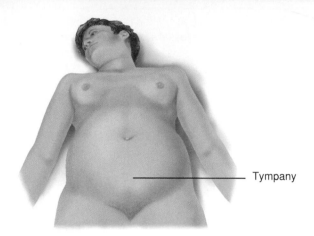

Air or Gas

Inspection. Single round curve.
Auscultation. Depends on cause of gas (e.g., decreased or absent bowel sounds with ileus); hyperactive with early intestinal obstruction.
Percussion. Tympany over large area.
Palpation. May have muscle spasm of abdominal wall.

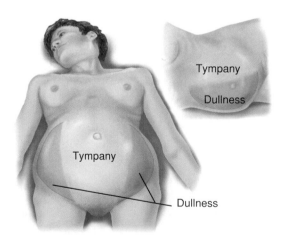

Ascites

Inspection. Single curve. Everted umbilicus. Bulging flanks when supine. Taut, glistening skin, recent weight gain, increase in abdominal girth.
Auscultation. Normal bowel sounds over intestines. Diminished over ascitic fluid.
Percussion. Tympany at top where intestines float. Dull over fluid. Produces fluid wave and shifting dullness.
Palpation. Taut skin and increased intra-abdominal pressure limit palpation.

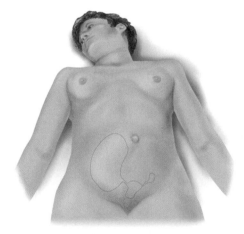

Ovarian Cyst (Large)

Inspection. Curve in lower half of abdomen, midline. Everted umbilicus.
Auscultation. Normal bowel sounds over upper abdomen where intestines pushed superiorly.
Percussion. Top dull over fluid. Intestines pushed superiorly. Large cyst produces fluid wave and shifting dullness.
Palpation. Transmits aortic pulsation while ascites does not.

[1]A mnemonic device to recall the common causes of abdominal distension is the seven Fs: fat, flatus, fluid, fetus, feces, fetal growth, and fibroid.

TABLE 21-1	Abdominal Distension—cont'd

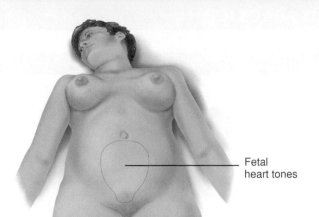

Fetal heart tones

Pregnancy[2]

Inspection. Single curve. Umbilicus protruding. Breasts engorged.
Auscultation. Fetal heart tones. Bowel sounds diminished.
Percussion. Tympany over intestines. Dull over enlarging uterus.
Palpation. Fetal parts. Fetal movements.

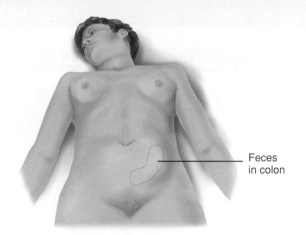

Feces in colon

Feces

Inspection. Localized distension.
Auscultation. Normal bowel sounds.
Percussion. Tympany predominates. Scattered dullness over fecal mass.
Palpation. Plastic- or rope-like mass with feces in intestines.

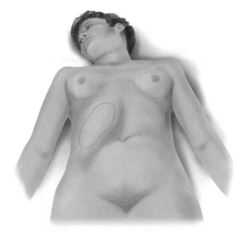

Tumour

Inspection. Localized distension.
Auscultation. Normal bowel sounds.
Percussion. Dull over mass if reaches up to skin surface.
Palpation. Define borders. Distinguish from enlarged organ or normally palpable structure.

[2]Obviously a normal finding, pregnancy is included for comparison of conditions causing abdominal distension.

ABNORMAL FINDINGS
FOR ADVANCED PRACTICE

TABLE 21-2 | **Common Sites of Referred Abdominal Pain**

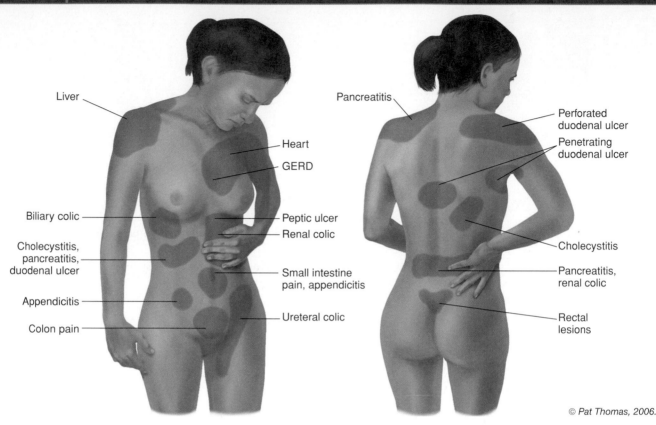

© Pat Thomas, 2006.

When a person gives a history of abdominal pain, the pain's location may not necessarily be directly over the involved organ. That is because the human brain has no felt image for internal organs. Rather, pain is referred to a site where the organ was located in fetal development. Although the organ migrates during fetal development, its nerves persist in referring sensations from the former location. The following are examples, not a complete list.

Liver. Hepatitis may have mild to moderate, dull pain in right upper quadrant or epigastrium, along with anorexia, nausea, malaise, low-grade fever.

Esophagus. Gastroesophageal reflux disease (GERD) is a complex of symptoms of esophagitis, including burning pain in midepigastrium or behind lower sternum that radiates upward, or "heartburn." Occurs 30 to 60 minutes after eating; aggravated by lying down or bending over.

Gallbladder. Cholecystitis is biliary colic, sudden pain in right upper quadrant that may radiate to right or left scapula, and that builds over time, lasting 2 to 4 hours, after ingestion of fatty foods, alcohol, or caffeine. Associated with nausea and vomiting, and positive Murphy's sign or sudden stop in inspiration with RUQ palpation.

Pancreas. Pancreatitis has acute, boring midepigastric pain radiating to the back and sometimes to the left scapula or flank, severe nausea, and vomiting.

Duodenum. Duodenal ulcer typically has dull, aching, gnawing pain, does not radiate, may be relieved by food, and may awaken the person from sleep.

Stomach. Gastric ulcer pain is dull, aching, gnawing epigastric pain, usually brought on by food, radiates to back or substernal area. Pain of perforated ulcer is burning epigastric pain of sudden onset that refers to one or both shoulders.

Appendix. Appendicitis typically starts as dull, diffuse pain in periumbilical region that later shifts to severe, sharp, persistent pain and tenderness localized in RLQ (McBurney's point). Pain is aggravated by movement, coughing, deep breathing; associated with anorexia, then nausea and vomiting, fever.

Kidney. Kidney stones prompt a sudden onset of severe, colicky flank or lower abdominal pain.

Small intestine. Gastroenteritis has diffuse, generalized abdominal pain, with nausea, diarrhea.

Colon. Large bowel obstruction has moderate, colicky pain of gradual onset in lower abdomen, bloating. Irritable bowel syndrome (IBS) has sharp or burning, cramping pain over a wide area; does not radiate. Brought on by meals, relieved by bowel movement.

Abnormal Findings

TABLE 21-3	Abnormalities on Inspection

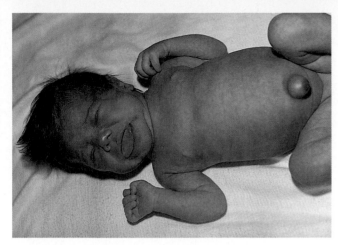

◀ Umbilical Hernia

Umbilical hernia is a soft, skin-covered mass, which is the protrusion of the omentum or intestine through a weakness or incomplete closure in the umbilical ring. It is accentuated by increased intra-abdominal pressure as with crying, coughing, vomiting, or straining, but the bowel rarely incarcerates or strangulates. It is more common in infants of African or Asian descent, and premature infants. Most umbilical hernias resolve spontaneously by 1 year; parents should avoid affixing a belt or coin at the hernia because this will not help closure and may cause contact dermatitis.

In an adult, it occurs with pregnancy, chronic ascites, or from chronic intrathoracic pressure (e.g., asthma, chronic bronchitis).

Epigastric Hernia (not illustrated)

A small, fatty nodule at epigastrium in midline, through the linea alba. Usually one can feel it rather than observe it. May be palpable only when standing.

Incisional Hernia (not illustrated)

A bulge near an old operative scar that may not show when person is supine but is apparent when the person increases intra-abdominal pressure by a sit-up, stand, or Valsalva manoeuvre.

Diastasis Recti (not illustrated)

Diastasis recti, or a midline longitudinal ridge, is a separation of the abdominal rectus muscles. Ridge is revealed when intra-abdominal pressure is increased by raising head while supine. Occurs congenitally and as a result of pregnancy or marked obesity in which prolonged distension or a decrease in muscle tone has occurred. It is not clinically significant.

TABLE 21-4 | Abnormal Bowel Sounds

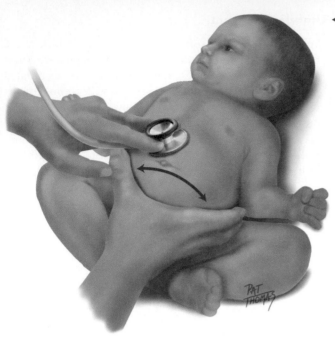

◄ Succussion Splash

Unrelated to peristalsis, this is a very loud splash auscultated over the upper abdomen when the infant is rocked side to side. It indicates increased air and fluid in the stomach, as seen with pyloric obstruction or large hiatus hernia.

Marked peristalsis, together with projectile vomiting in the newborn, suggests pyloric stenosis, an obstruction of the stomach's pyloric valve. Pyloric stenosis is a congenital defect and appears in the second or third week. After feeding, pronounced peristaltic waves cross from left to right, leading to projectile vomiting. Then one can palpate an olive-sized mass in the RUQ midway between the right costal margin and umbilicus. Refer promptly because of the risk of weight loss.

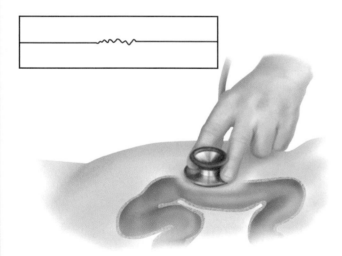

Hypoactive Bowel Sounds

Diminished or absent bowel sounds signal decreased motility as a result of inflammation as seen with peritonitis, from paralytic ileus as following abdominal surgery, or from late bowel obstruction. Occurs also with pneumonia.

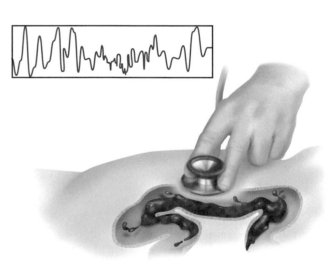

Hyperactive Bowel Sounds

Loud, gurgling sounds, "borborygmi," signal increased motility. They occur with early mechanical bowel obstruction (high-pitched), gastroenteritis, brisk diarrhea, laxative use, and subsiding paralytic ileus.

TABLE 21-5	Abdominal Friction Rubs and Vascular Sounds

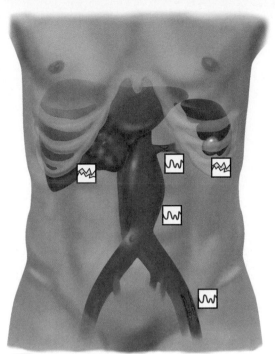

◢ **Peritoneal Friction Rub**

A rough, grating sound, like two pieces of leather rubbed together, indicates peritoneal inflammation. Occurs rarely. Usually occurs over organs with a large surface area in contact with the peritoneum.

Liver—friction rub over lower right rib cage, from abscess or metastatic tumour.

Spleen—friction rub over lower left rib cage in left anterior axillary line, from abscess, infection, or tumour.

Vascular Sounds

Arterial—a **bruit** indicates turbulent blood flow, as found in constricted, abnormally dilated, or tortuous vessels. Listen with the bell. Occurs with the following three conditions:

Aortic aneurysm—murmur is harsh, systolic, or continuous and accentuated with systole. Note in person with hypertension.

Renal artery stenosis—murmur is midline or toward flank, soft, low-to-medium pitch.

Partial occlusion of femoral arteries

Venous hum—occurs rarely. Heard in periumbilical region. Originates from inferior vena cava. Medium pitch, continuous sound, pressure on bell may obliterate it. May have palpable thrill. Occurs with portal hypertension and cirrhotic liver.

◈ Peritoneal friction rub

◈ Vascular sounds

TABLE 21-6	Abnormalities on Palpation of Enlarged Organs

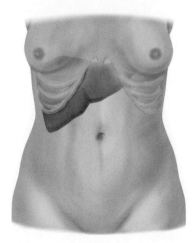

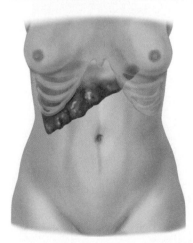

Enlarged Liver

An enlarged, smooth, and nontender liver occurs with fatty infiltration, portal obstruction or cirrhosis, high obstruction of inferior vena cava, and lymphocytic leukemia.

The liver feels enlarged and smooth but is tender to palpation with early heart failure, acute hepatitis, or hepatic abscess.

Enlarged Nodular Liver

An enlarged and nodular liver occurs with late portal cirrhosis, metastatic cancer, or tertiary syphilis.

Continued

Abnormal Findings

TABLE 21-6 | **Abnormalities on Palpation of Enlarged Organs—cont'd**

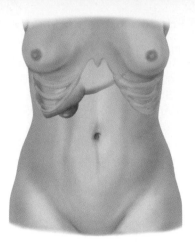

Enlarged Gallbladder

An enlarged, tender gallbladder suggests acute cholecystitis. Feel it behind the liver border as a smooth and firm mass like a sausage, although it may be difficult to palpate because of involuntary rigidity of abdominal muscles. The area is exquisitely painful to fist percussion, and inspiratory arrest (Murphy's sign) is present.

An enlarged, nontender gallbladder also feels like a smooth, sausagelike mass. It occurs when the gallbladder is filled with stones, as with common bile duct obstruction.

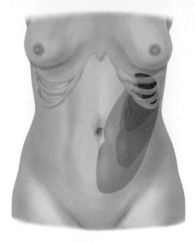

Enlarged Spleen

Because any enlargement superiorly is stopped by the diaphragm, the spleen enlarges down and to the midline. When extreme, it can extend down to the left pelvis. It retains the splenic notch on the medial edge. When splenomegaly occurs with acute infections (mononucleosis), it is moderately enlarged and soft, with rounded edges. When the result of a chronic cause, the enlargement is firm or hard, with sharp edges. An enlarged spleen is usually not tender to palpation; it is tender only if the peritoneum is also inflamed.

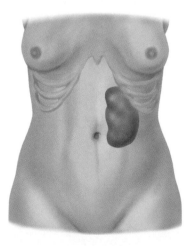

Enlarged Kidney

Enlarged with hydronephrosis, cyst, or neoplasm. May be difficult to distinguish an enlarged kidney from an enlarged spleen because they have a similar shape. Both extend forward and down. However, the spleen may have a sharp edge, whereas the kidney never does. The spleen retains the splenic notch, whereas the kidney has no palpable notch. Percussion over the spleen is dull, whereas over the kidney it is tympanitic because of the overriding bowel.

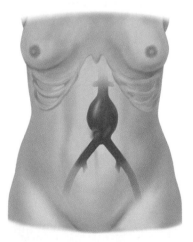

Aortic Aneurysm

Most aortic aneurysms (more than 95%) are located below the renal arteries and extend to the umbilicus. About 80% of these are detectable during routine physical examination. You will hear a bruit. Femoral pulses are present but decreased. An aortic aneurysm is at great risk of rupture. If you hear a bruit, you should **not** palpate the area, for fear of rupturing the aneurysm.

Additional information on abdominal aneurysm is illustrated in Table 20-5, p. 552.

BIBLIOGRAPHY

Alexander, D., Schaffer, S., & Zeilman, C. (2003). Noninfectious liver disorders: Assessment and diagnosis. *Nurse Practitioner, 28*, 12–27.

Banning, M. (2006). *Helicobacter pylori*: Pathophysiology, assessment and treatment. *Gastrointestinal Nursing, 4*, 28–33.

Baron, M. (2002). Crohn disease in children. *American Journal of Nursing, 102*, 26–35.

Bohrn, M., & Siewert, B. (2004). Acute abdominal pain: What not to miss. *Patient Care, 38*, 31–39.

British Nutrition Foundation. *Food allergy and intolerance*. In *Canadian health network: Aboriginal peoples*. Retrieved February 2, 2008, from http://hcsweb11.canadian-healthnetwork.ca/servlet/ContentServer?cid=1047415457298&pagename=CHN-RCS/Page/SearchPageTemplate&c=Page&subjectID=402&lang=En

Canadian Liver Foundation. *Gallstones*. Retrieved January 13, 2008, from http://www.liver.ca/Liver_Disease/Adult_Liver_Diseases/Gallstones.aspx

Canadian Liver Foundation. (2000). Hepatitis C: Medical information update. *Canadian Journal of Public Health, 91*, S4–S9.

Croghan, A., & Heitkemper, M. M. (2005). Recognizing and managing patients with irritable bowel syndrome. *Journal of the American Academy of Nurse Practitioners, 17*, 51–59.

Cronin, C., & Terra, R. P. (2005). *What is lactose intolerance?* Retrieved February 2, 2008, from http://www.bchealthguide.org/kbase/topic/mini/hw177971/overview.htm

Despins, L., Kivlahan, C., & Cox, K. (2005). Acute pancreatitis: Diagnosis and treatment of a potentially fatal condition. *American Journal of Nursing, 105*, 54–57.

Durston, S. (2005). What you need to know about viral hepatitis. *Nursing, 35*, 36–42.

Fox, M., & Forgacs, I. (2006). Gastro-esophageal reflux disease. *British Medical Journal, 332*, 88–93.

Ganong, W. F. (2005). *Review of medical physiology* (22nd ed.). New York, NY: McGraw-Hill, Inc.

Gendall, K., Joyce, P., & Carter, F. (2005). Childhood gastrointestinal complaints in women with bulimia nervosa. *International Journal of Eating Disorders, 37*, 256–260.

Health Canada. (2000). The Hepatitis C Prevention, Support and Research Program: Health Canada initiatives on hepatitis C. *Canadian Journal of Public Health, 91*, S27–S29.

Health Canada. (2003). Hepatitis A fact sheet. In *Bloodborne Pathogens Section, Blood Safety Surveillance and Health Care Acquired Infections Division*. Retrieved January 17, 2008, from http://www.phac-aspc.gc.ca/hcai-iamss/bbp-pts/hepatitis/hep_a_e.html

Health Canada. (2003). Hepatitis B fact sheet. In *Bloodborne Pathogens Section, Blood Safety Surveillance and Health Care Acquired Infections Division*. Retrieved January 17, 2008, from http://www.phac-aspc.gc.ca/hcai-iamss/bbp-pts/hepatitis/hep_b_e.html

Health Canada. (2003). Hepatitis C fact sheet. In *Bloodborne Pathogens Section, Blood Safety Surveillance and Health Care Acquired Infections Division*. Retrieved January 17, 2008, from http://www.phac-aspc.gc.ca/hcai-iamss/bbp-pts/hepatitis/hep_c_e.html

Health Canada. (2005). Common immunologic problems: Lactose intolerance. In *First Nations and Inuit Health: Pediatric clinical practice guidelines for nurses in primary care*. Retrieved February 2, 2008, from http://www.hc-sc.gc.ca/fnih-spni/pubs/nursing-infirm/2001_ped_guide/chap_17b_e.html

Hendrickson, A. (2002). *Lactose intolerance or milk allergy?* Retrieved February 2, 2008, from http://www.homefamily.net/index.php?/categories/foodnutrition/lactose_intolerance_or_milk_allergy/

Iosue, K. (2002). Chronic hepatitis: Latest treatment options. *Nurse Practitioner, 27*, 32–49.

Jacobson, B. C., Somers, S. C., Fuchs, C. S., Kelly, C. P., & Camargo, C. A., Jr. (2006). Body-mass index and symptoms of gastroesophageal reflux in women. *New England Journal of Medicine, 354*, 2340–2348, 2405–2408.

Katzung, B. G. (2006). *Basic and clinical pharmacology* (10th ed.). New York, NY: McGraw-Hill Medical.

Keith, S. W., Redden, D. T., & Katzmarzyk, P. T. (2006). Putative contributors to the secular increase in obesity. *International Journal of Obesity, 30*, 1585–1594.

Krahn, M. (1994). Hepatitis B immunization in childhood. In Canadian Task Force on the Periodic Health Examination (Eds.), *Canadian guide to clinical preventive health care* (pp. 397–404). Ottawa, ON: Health Canada.

Landzberg, B. (2006). Celiac disease: Could you be missing this diagnosis? *Consultant, 46*, 1458–1465.

Lawson, E. E., Grand, R. J., Neff, R. K., & Cohen, L. F. (1978). Clinical estimation of liver span in infants and children. *Archives of Pediatric and Adolescent Medicine, 132*, 474–476.

Longstreth, G. (2006). Functional dyspepsia—Managing the conundrum. *New England Journal of Medicine, 354*, 791–793.

Madsen, D., Sebolt, T., Cullen, L., Folkedahl, B., Mueller, T., Richardson, C., et al. (2005). Listening to bowel sounds: An evidence-based practice project. *American Journal of Nursing, 105*, 40–50.

Malagelada, J. (2006). A symptom-based approach to making a positive diagnosis of irritable bowel syndrome with constipation. *International Journal of Clinical Practice, 60*, 57–63.

Miller, S., & Alpert, P. (2006). Assessment and differential diagnosis of abdominal pain. *Nurse Practitioner, 31*, 39–47.

Minister of Public Works and Government Services Canada. (2006). *Canadian immunization guide* (7th ed). Ottawa, ON: Health Canada.

Ministry of the Attorney General. (2002). *Report of the Walkerton Commission of Inquiry*. Retrieved April 5, 2008, from http://www.attorneygeneral.jus.gov.on.ca/english/about/pubs/walkerton/

Molle, E. (2005). Caring for older adults: Getting down to the lower GI tract. *Nursing, 35*, 20–21.

National Aboriginal Health Organization. (2003). *Canada's environment agenda and implications for Aboriginal peoples*. Retrieved April 5, 2008, from http://www.naho.ca/english/publications/BN059_environment.pdf

Park, J., Akhtar, R., & Dietrich, D. (2006). Chronic hepatitis C: Latest diagnosis and treatment guidelines. *Consultant, 46*, 463–468.

Patrick, D. M., Buxton, J. A., Bigham, M., & Mathias, R. G. (2000). Public health and hepatitis C. *Canadian Journal of Public Health, 91*, S18–S21.

Ray, S. W., Secrest, J., Ch'ien, A. P. Y., & Corey, R. S. (2002). Managing gastroesophageal reflux disease. *Nurse Practitioner, 27*, 36–55.

Reid, L. D., Johnson, R. E., & Gettman, D. A. (1998). Benzodiazepine exposure and functional status in older people. *Journal of the American Geriatric Society, 46*, 71–76.

Riben, P., Bailey, G., Hudson, S., McCulloch, K., Dignan, T., & Martin, D. (2000). Hepatitis C in Canada's First Nations and Inuit populations: An unknown burden. *Canadian Journal of Public Health, 91*, S16–S17.

Sambaziotis, H., & Dinsmoor, M. J. (2005). Diagnostic puzzler: A simple UTI that wasn't so simple. *Contemporary OB/GYN, 50*, 89–92.

Stone, J. K., Wyman, J. F., & Salisbury, S. A. (1999). *Clinical gerontological nursing—A guide to advanced practice* (2nd ed.). Philadelphia, PA: Saunders.

Torpy, J. M. (2006). Irritable bowel syndrome. *Journal of the American Medical Association, 295*, 960.

Walker, B. (2004). Assessing gastrointestinal infections. *Nursing, 34*, 48–52.

Wilson, T. (2005). The ABCs of hepatitis. *Nurse Practitioner, 30*, 12–23.

Wollner, T. (2004). Eradicate *H. pylori* with effective treatment regimens. *Nurse Practitioner, 29*, 40–44.

Wu, J., Zou, S., & Giulivi, A. (2001). Hepatitis A and its control. *Canada Communicable Diseases Report, 27S3*.

Zhang, J., Zou, S., & Giulivi, A. (2001). Hepatitis B in Canada. *Canada Communicable Diseases Report, 27S3*.

Zou, S., Tepper, M., & Giulivi, A. (2000). Current status of Hepatitis C in Canada. *Canadian Journal of Public Health, 91*, S10–S15.

Chapter Twenty-Two

Musculoskeletal System

Written by **Carolyn Jarvis**, PhD, APN, CNP
Adapted by **Marian Luctkar-Flude**, RN, MScN

Electronic Resources

On Evolve *evolve*

http://evolve.elsevier.com/Canada/Jarvis/examination/

- Interactive Case Studies
- Physical Examination Audio and Printable Summaries
- Bedside Assessment Summary Checklists
- Complete Physical Examination Form
- Nursing Diagnoses Boxes
- Health Promotion Guides
- Quick Assessments for 20 Common Conditions
- Multiple Choice Review Questions
- Chapter Objectives
- Appendices
- Weblinks

On the Companion CD

- Interactive Case Studies with Heart and Lung Sounds
- Health Promotion Guides
- Quick Assessments for 20 Common Conditions
- Head-to-Toe Physical Examination Video Clips

STRUCTURE AND FUNCTION

The musculoskeletal system consists of the body's **bones, joints,** and **muscles.** Humans need this system (1) for *support* to stand erect, and (2) for *movement.* The musculoskeletal system also functions (3) to encase and *protect* the inner vital organs (e.g., brain, spinal cord, heart), (4) to *produce* the red blood cells in the bone marrow (hematopoiesis), and (5) as a *reservoir* for *storage* of essential minerals such as calcium and phosphorus in the bones.

COMPONENTS OF THE MUSCULOSKELETAL SYSTEM

The skeleton is the bony framework of the body. It has 206 bones, which support the body like the posts and beams of a building. **Bone** and cartilage are specialized forms of connective tissue. Bone is hard, rigid, and very dense. Its cells are continually turning over and remodelling. The **joint** (or articulation) is the place of union of two or more bones. Joints are the functional units of the musculoskeletal system because they permit the mobility needed for activities of daily living.

Nonsynovial or Synovial Joints

In **nonsynovial** joints, the bones are united by fibrous tissue or cartilage and are immovable (e.g., the sutures in the skull) or only slightly movable (e.g., the vertebrae). **Synovial** joints are freely movable because they have bones that are separated from each other and are enclosed in a joint cavity (Fig. 22-1). This cavity is filled with a lubricant, or synovial fluid. Just like grease on gears, synovial fluid allows sliding of opposing surfaces, and this sliding permits movement.

In synovial joints, a layer of resilient **cartilage** covers the surface of opposing bones. Cartilage is avascular; it receives nourishment from synovial fluid that circulates during joint movement. It is a very stable connective tissue with a slow cell turnover. It has a tough, firm consistency, yet is flexible. This cartilage cushions the bones and gives a smooth surface to facilitate movement.

The joint is surrounded by a fibrous capsule and is supported by ligaments. **Ligaments** are fibrous bands running directly from one bone to another that strengthen the joint and help prevent movement in undesirable directions. A **bursa** is an enclosed sac filled with viscous synovial fluid, much like a joint. Bursae are located in areas of potential friction (e.g., subacromial bursa of the shoulder, prepatellar bursa of the knee) and help muscles and tendons glide smoothly over bone.

Muscles

Muscles account for 40 to 50% of the body's weight. When they contract, they produce movement. Muscles are of three types: skeletal, smooth, and cardiac. This chapter is concerned with **skeletal,** or voluntary, muscles, which are under conscious control.

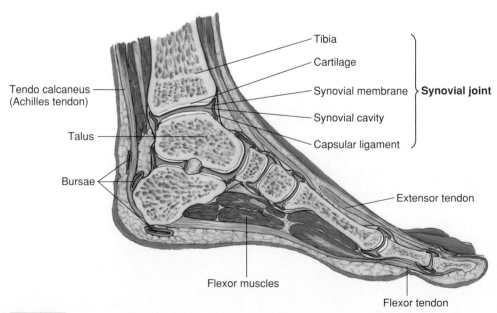

Tibia
Cartilage
Synovial membrane   } **Synovial joint**
Synovial cavity
Capsular ligament

Tendo calcaneus (Achilles tendon)

Talus

Bursae

Extensor tendon

Flexor muscles

Flexor tendon

Fig. 22-1

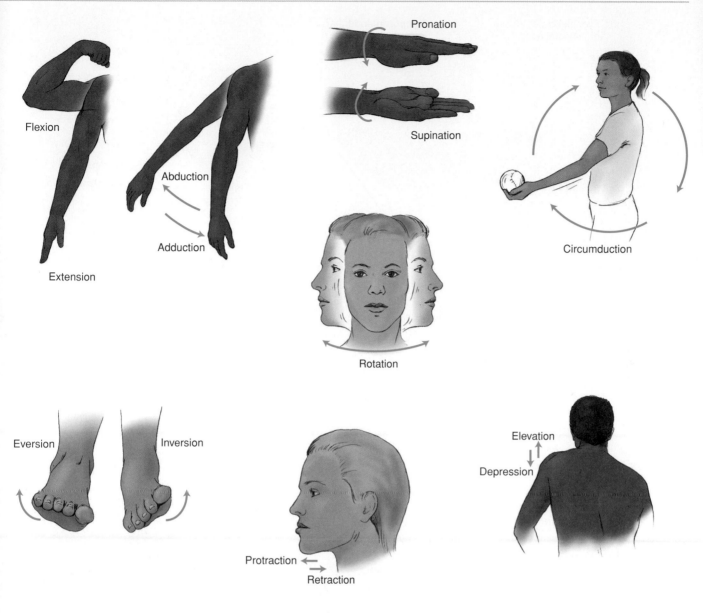

SKELETAL MUSCLE MOVEMENTS

Fig. 22-2

© Pat Thomas, 2006.

Each **skeletal muscle** is composed of bundles of muscle fibres, or **fasciculi.** The skeletal muscle is attached to bone by a **tendon**—a strong fibrous cord. Skeletal muscles produce the following movements (Fig. 22-2):

1. Flexion—bending a limb at a joint
2. Extension—straightening a limb at a joint
3. Abduction—moving a limb away from the midline of the body
4. Adduction—moving a limb toward the midline of the body
5. Pronation—turning the forearm so that the palm is down
6. Supination—turning the forearm so that the palm is up
7. Circumduction—moving the arm in a circle around the shoulder
8. Inversion—moving the sole of the foot inward at the ankle
9. Eversion—moving the sole of the foot outward at the ankle
10. Rotation—moving the head around a central axis
11. Protraction—moving a body part forward and parallel to the ground
12. Retraction—moving a body part backward and parallel to the ground
13. Elevation—raising a body part
14. Depression—lowering a body part

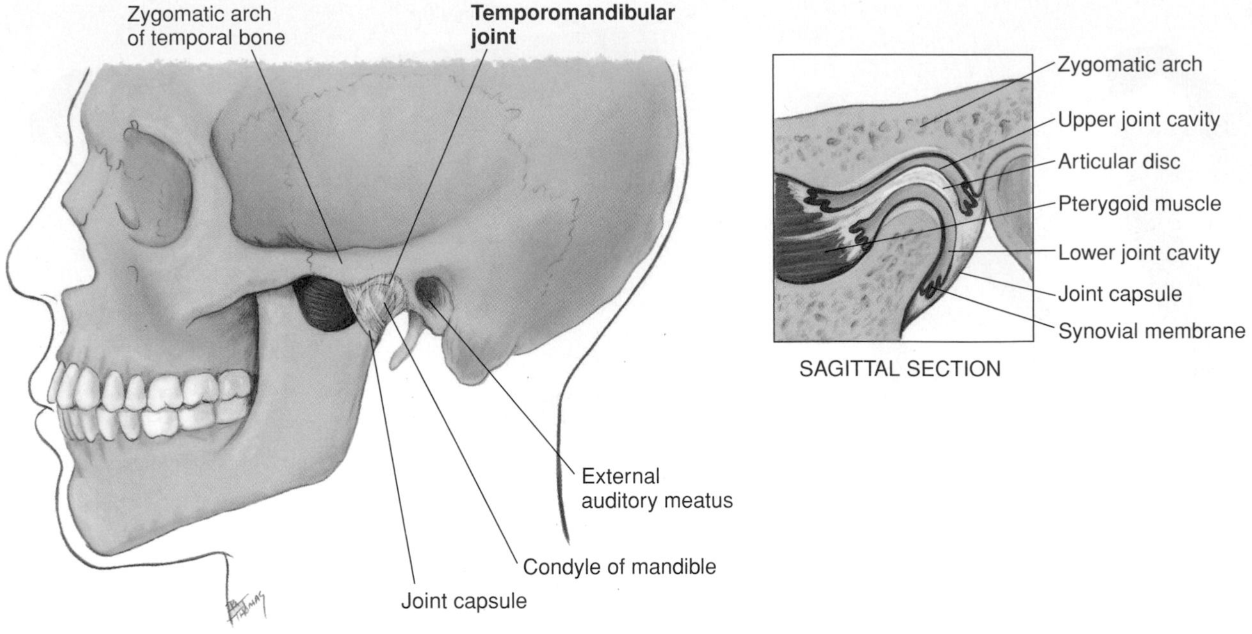

Zygomatic arch
of temporal bone

**Temporomandibular
joint**

Zygomatic arch

Upper joint cavity

Articular disc

Pterygoid muscle

Lower joint cavity

Joint capsule

Synovial membrane

SAGITTAL SECTION

External
auditory meatus

Condyle of mandible

Joint capsule

Fig. 22-3

Temporomandibular Joint

The temporomandibular joint (TMJ) is the articulation of
the mandible and the temporal bone (Fig. 22-3). You can feel
it in the depression anterior to the tragus of the ear. The TMJ
permits jaw function for speaking and chewing. The joint
allows three motions: (1) hinge action to open and close the
jaws, (2) gliding action for protrusion and retraction, and
(3) gliding action for side-to-side movement of the lower jaw.

Spine

The **vertebrae** are 33 connecting bones stacked in a vertical
column (Fig. 22-4). You can feel their spinous processes in a
furrow down the midline of the back. The furrow has paravertebral muscles mounded on either side down to the
sacrum, where it flattens. Humans have 7 cervical, 12 thoracic, 5 lumbar, 5 sacral, and 3 to 4 coccygeal vertebrae. The
following surface landmarks will orient you to their levels:

* The spinous processes of C7 and T1 are prominent at the
  base of the neck.
* The inferior angle of the scapula normally is at the level of
  the interspace between T7 and T8.
* An imaginary line connecting the highest point on each
  iliac crest crosses L4.
* An imaginary line joining the two symmetrical dimples
  that overlie the posterior superior iliac spines crosses the
  sacrum.

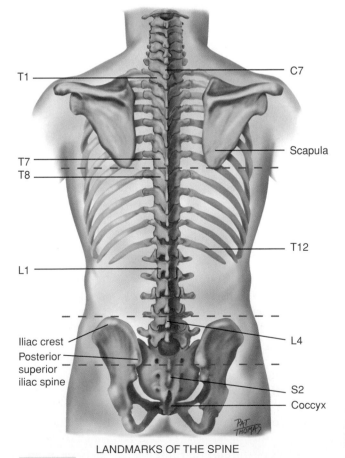

T1

C7

Scapula

T7
T8

T12

L1

Iliac crest

Posterior
superior
iliac spine

L4

S2

Coccyx

LANDMARKS OF THE SPINE

Fig. 22-4

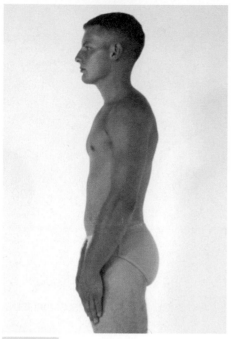

Fig. 22-5

A lateral view shows that the vertebral column has four curves (a double-S shape) (Fig. 22-5). The cervical and lumbar curves are concave (inward or anterior), and the thoracic and sacrococcygeal curves are convex. The balanced or compensatory nature of these curves, together with the resilient intervertebral discs, allows the spine to absorb a great deal of shock.

The **intervertebral discs** are elastic fibrocartilaginous plates that constitute one fourth of the length of the column (Fig. 22-6). Each disc centre has a **nucleus pulposus,** made of soft, semifluid, mucoid material that has the consistency of toothpaste in the young adult. The discs cushion the spine like a shock absorber and help it move. As the spine moves, the elasticity of the discs allows compression on one side, with compensatory expansion on the other. Sometimes compression can be too great. The disc then can rupture, and the nucleus pulposus can herniate out of the vertebral column, compressing on the spinal nerves and causing pain.

The unique structure of the spine enables both upright posture and flexibility for motion. The motions of the vertebral column are flexion (bending forward), extension (bending back), abduction (to either side), and rotation.

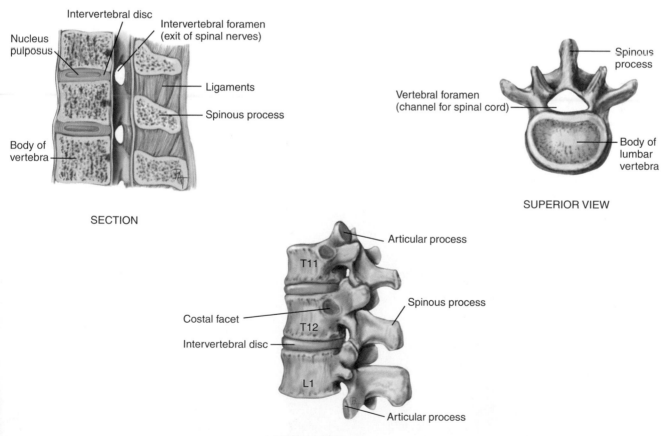

Nucleus pulposus

Intervertebral disc

Intervertebral foramen (exit of spinal nerves)

Ligaments

Spinous process

Body of vertebra

SECTION

Spinous process

Vertebral foramen (channel for spinal cord)

Body of lumbar vertebra

SUPERIOR VIEW

Articular process

T11

Costal facet

T12

Spinous process

Intervertebral disc

L1

Articular process

LATERAL VIEW

Fig. 22-6

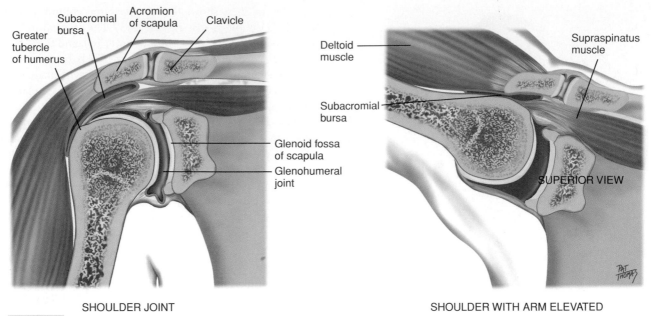

SHOULDER JOINT   SHOULDER WITH ARM ELEVATED

Fig. 22-7

Shoulder

The **glenohumeral joint** is the articulation of the humerus with the glenoid fossa of the scapula (Fig. 22-7). Its ball-and-socket action allows great mobility of the arm on many axes. The joint is enclosed by a group of four powerful muscles and tendons that support and stabilize it. Together these are called the **rotator cuff** of the shoulder. The large **subacromial bursa** helps during abduction of the arm so that the greater tubercle of the humerus moves easily under the acromion process of the scapula.

The bones of the shoulder have palpable landmarks to guide your examination (Fig. 22-8). The scapula and the clavicle connect to form the shoulder girdle. You can feel the

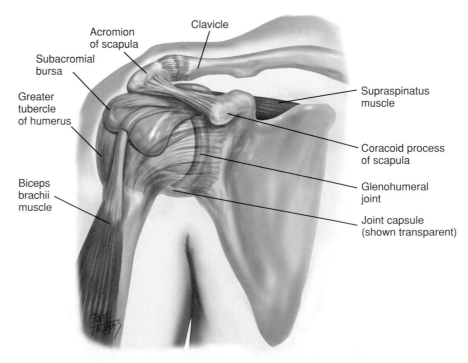

BONY LANDMARKS OF THE SHOULDER—ANTERIOR VIEW

Fig. 22-8

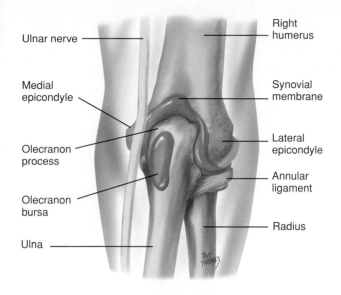

RIGHT ELBOW—POSTERIOR VIEW

Fig. 22-9

Elbow

The elbow joint contains the three bony articulations of the humerus, radius, and ulna of the forearm (Fig. 22-9). Its hinge action moves the forearm (radius and ulna) on one plane, allowing flexion and extension. The olecranon bursa lies between the olecranon process and the skin.

Palpable landmarks are the **medial** and **lateral epicondyles** of the humerus and the large **olecranon process** of the ulna in between them. The sensitive ulnar nerve runs between the olecranon process and the medial epicondyle.

The radius and ulna articulate with each other at two radioulnar joints, one at the elbow and one at the wrist. These move together to permit pronation and supination of the hand and forearm.

Wrist and Carpals

Of the body's 206 bones, over half are in the hands and feet. The wrist or **radiocarpal joint** is the articulation of the radius (on the thumb side) and a row of carpal bones (Fig. 22-10). Its condyloid action permits movement in two planes at right angles: flexion and extension, and side-to-side deviation. You can feel the groove of this joint on the dorsum of the wrist.

The **midcarpal** joint is the articulation between the two parallel rows of carpal bones. It allows flexion, extension, and some rotation. The **metacarpophalangeal** and the **interphalangeal** joints permit finger flexion and extension. The flexor tendons of the wrist and hand are enclosed in synovial sheaths.

bump of the scapula's **acromion process** at the very top of the shoulder. Move your fingers in a small circle outward, down, and around. The next bump is the **greater tubercle** of the humerus a few centimetres down and laterally, and from that the **coracoid process** of the scapula is a few centimetres medially. These surround the deeply situated joint.

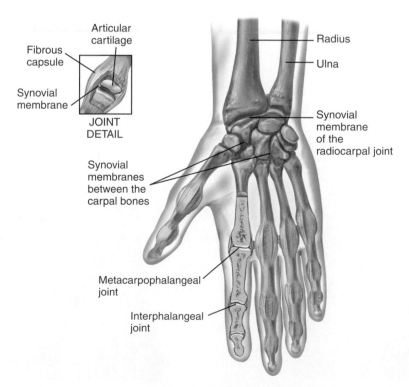

BONES OF THE HAND—PALMAR VIEW

Fig. 22-10

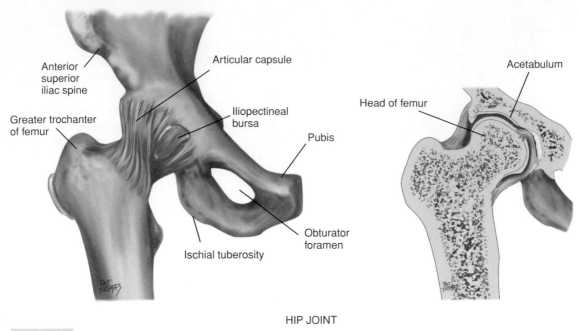

HIP JOINT

Fig. 22-11

Hip

The hip joint is the articulation between the acetabulum and the head of the femur (Fig. 22-11). As in the shoulder, ball-and-socket action permits a wide range of motion (ROM) on many axes. The hip has somewhat less ROM than the shoulder, but it has more stability befitting its weight-bearing function. Hip stability is due to powerful muscles that spread over the joint, a strong fibrous articular capsule, and the very deep insertion of the head of the femur. Three bursae facilitate movement.

Palpation of these bony landmarks will guide your examination. You can feel the entire iliac crest, from the **anterior superior iliac spine** to the posterior. The **ischial tuberosity** lies under the gluteus maximus muscle and is palpable when the hip is flexed. The **greater trochanter** of the femur is nor-

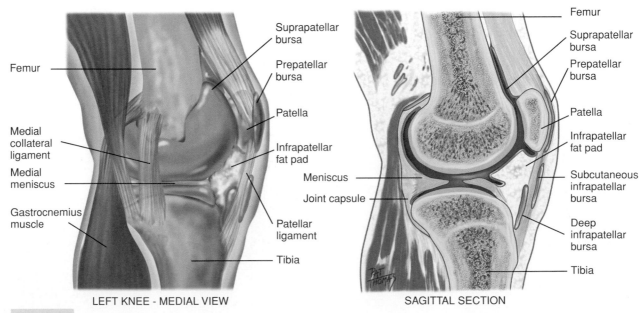

LEFT KNEE - MEDIAL VIEW   SAGITTAL SECTION

Fig. 22-12

mally the width of the person's palm below the iliac crest and halfway between the anterior superior iliac spine and the ischial tuberosity. Feel it, when the person is standing, in a flat depression on the upper lateral side of the thigh.

Knee

The knee joint is the articulation of three bones—the femur, the tibia, and the patella (kneecap)—in one common articular cavity (Fig. 22-12). It is the largest joint in the body and is complex. It is a hinge joint, permitting flexion and extension of the lower leg on a single plane.

The knee's synovial membrane is the largest in the body. It forms a sac at the superior border of the patella, called the **suprapatellar pouch,** which extends up as much as 6 cm behind the quadriceps muscle. Two wedge-shaped cartilages, called the **medial** and **lateral menisci,** cushion the tibia and femur. The joint is stabilized by two sets of ligaments. The **cruciate ligaments** (not shown) criss-cross within the knee; they give anterior and posterior stability and help control rotation. The **collateral ligaments** connect the joint at both sides; they give medial and lateral stability and prevent dislocation. Numerous bursae prevent friction. One, the **prepatellar bursa,** lies between the patella and the skin. The **infrapatellar fat pad** is a small, triangular fat pad below the patella behind the patellar ligament.

Landmarks of the knee joint start with the large **quadriceps** muscle, which you can feel on your anterior and lateral thigh (Fig. 22-13). The muscle's four heads merge into a common tendon that continues down to enclose the round bony patella. Then the tendon inserts down on the **tibial tuberosity,** which you can feel as a bony prominence in the midline. Move to the sides and a bit superiorly, and note the lateral and medial condyles of the tibia. Superior to these on either side of the patella are the medial and lateral epicondyles of the femur.

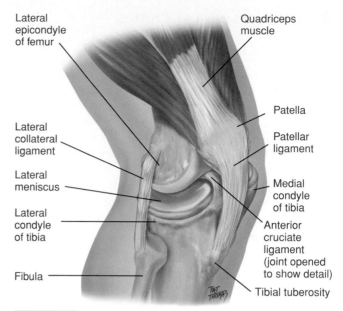

Fig. 22-13   LANDMARKS OF THE RIGHT KNEE JOINT

Ankle and Foot

The ankle or **tibiotalar joint** is the articulation of the tibia, fibula, and talus (Fig. 22-14). It is a hinge joint, limited to flexion (dorsiflexion) and extension (plantar flexion) on one plane. Landmarks are two bony prominences on either side—the **medial malleolus** and the **lateral malleolus.** Strong, tight medial and lateral ligaments extend from each malleolus onto the foot. These help the lateral stability of the ankle joint, although they may be torn in eversion or inversion sprains of the ankle.

Joints distal to the ankle give additional mobility to the foot. The subtalar joint permits inversion and eversion of the foot. The foot has a longitudinal arch, with weight-bearing distributed between the parts that touch the ground—the heads of the metatarsals and the calcaneus (heel).

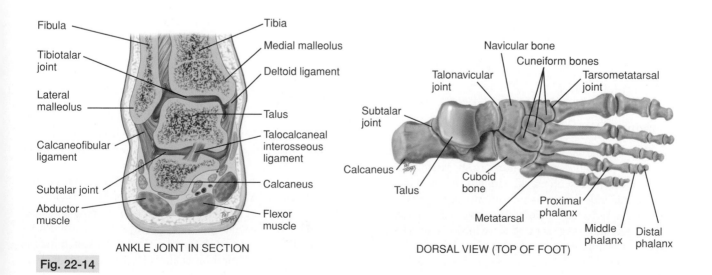

ANKLE JOINT IN SECTION

DORSAL VIEW (TOP OF FOOT)

Fig. 22-14

❧ DEVELOPMENTAL CARE

Infants and Children

By 3 months' gestation, the fetus has formed a "scale model" of the skeleton that is made up of cartilage. During succeeding months in utero, the cartilage ossifies into true bone and starts to grow. Bone growth continues after birth—rapidly during infancy and then steadily during childhood—until adolescence, when both boys and girls undergo a rapid growth spurt.

Long bones grow in two dimensions. They increase in width or diameter by deposition of new bony tissue around the shafts. Lengthening occurs at the **epiphyses,** or growth plates. These specialized growth centres are transverse discs located at the ends of long bone. Any trauma or infection at this location puts the growing child at risk for bone deformity. This longitudinal growth continues until closure of the epiphyses; the last closure occurs at about age 20 years.

Skeletal contour changes are apparent at the vertebral column. At birth the spine has a single C-shaped curve. At 3 to 4 months, the baby raising its head from the prone position develops the anterior curve in the cervical neck region. From 1 year to 18 months, standing erect develops the anterior curve in the lumbar region.

Although the skeleton contributes to linear growth, muscles and fat are significant for weight increase. Individual muscle fibres grow through childhood, but growth is marked during the adolescent growth spurt. At this time, muscles respond to increased secretion of growth hormone, to adrenal androgens, and in boys, to further stimulation by testosterone. Muscles vary in size and strength in different people. This is due to genetic programming, nutrition, and exercise. All through life, muscles increase with use and atrophy with disuse.

Developmental dysplasia of the hip (DDH) refers to a number of congenital abnormalities of the hip joint including dislocated hip and subluxed hip. The Canadian Task Force on Preventive Health Care (Patel et al., 2001) recommends clinical examination of the hips in the periodic health examination of all infants during the first week of life, in the first month, and then at 2, 4, 6, 9, and 12 months of age, by a trained clinician. Potential risk factors for DDH include having a first-degree relative with DDH, breech delivery, or clinical evidence of joint instability. Females are more predisposed than males to DDH, and Canadian Aboriginal people have a high risk for DDH.

The Pregnant Female

Increased levels of circulating hormones (estrogen, relaxin from the corpus luteum, and corticosteroids) cause increased mobility in the joints. Increased mobility in the sacroiliac, sacrococcygeal, and symphysis pubis joints in the pelvis contributes to the noticeable changes in maternal posture. The most characteristic change is progressive **lordosis,** which compensates for the enlarging fetus; otherwise, the centre of balance would shift forward. Lordosis compensates by shifting the weight farther back on the lower extremities. This shift in balance, in turn, creates strain on the low back muscles, which in some women is felt as low back pain during late pregnancy.

Anterior flexion of the neck and slumping of the shoulder girdle are other postural changes that compensate for the lordosis. These upper back changes may put pressure on the ulnar and median nerves during the third trimester. Nerve pressure creates aching, numbness, and weakness in the upper extremities in some women.

The Aging Adult

With aging, loss of bone matrix (resorption) occurs more rapidly than does new bone growth (deposition). The net effect is a loss of bone density, or **osteoporosis.** Although some degree of osteoporosis is nearly universal, females have it more than males, and people of European descent more than people of African descent. A list of the major and minor risk factors for osteoporosis is given in Table 22-1.

Postural changes are evident with aging, and decreased height is the most noticeable. Long bones do not shorten with age. Decreased height is due to shortening of the vertebral column. This is caused by loss of water content and thinning of the intervertebral discs, which occurs more in the middle years. Also, decreased height is caused by a decrease in height of individual vertebrae, which occurs in later years due to osteoporosis.

Both men and women can expect a progressive decrease in height beginning at age 40 years in males and age 43 years in females, although this is not significant until age 60 years (Cline et al., 1989). A greater decrease occurs in the 70s and 80s as a result of osteoporotic collapse of the vertebrae. The result is a shortening of the trunk and comparatively long extremities. Other postural changes are kyphosis, and a backward head tilt to compensate for the kyphosis, and a slight flexion of hips and knees.

The distribution of subcutaneous fat changes through life. Usually, men and women gain weight in their 40s and 50s. The contour is different, even if the weight is the same as when younger. They begin to lose fat in the face and deposit it in the abdomen and hips. In the 80s and 90s, fat further decreases in the periphery, noticeably in the forearms and over the abdomen and hips.

Loss of subcutaneous fat leaves bony prominences more marked (e.g., tips of vertebrae, ribs, iliac crests), and body hollows deeper (e.g., cheeks, axillae). An absolute loss in muscle mass occurs; some muscles decrease in size, and some atrophy, producing weakness. The contour of muscles becomes more prominent, and muscle bundles and tendons feel more distinct.

It has become more apparent that lifestyle affects musculoskeletal changes. A sedentary lifestyle hastens the musculoskeletal changes of aging. However, physical exercise increases skeletal mass. This helps prevent or delay osteoporosis. Physical activity delays or prevents bone loss in postmenopausal and older women (Ebrahim et al., 1997; Gregg et al., 1998).

TABLE 22-1	Factors That Identify People Who Should Be Assessed for Osteoporosis	
Major Risk Factors	**Minor Risk Factors**
Age	Rheumatoid arthritis
Vertebral compression fracture	Past history of clinical hyperthyroidism
Fragility fracture after age 40	Chronic anticonvulsant therapy
Family history of osteoporotic fracture (especially maternal hip fracture)	Low dietary calcium intake
	Smoking
Systemic glucocorticoid therapy of >3 months' duration	Excessive alcohol intake
Malabsorption syndrome	Excessive caffeine intake
Primary hyperparathyroidism	Weight <57 kg
Propensity to fall	Weight loss >10% of weight at age 25
Osteopenia apparent on X-ray film	Chronic heparin therapy
Hypogonadism	
Early menopause (before age 45)	

CULTURAL AND SOCIAL CONSIDERATIONS

Arthritis is one of the most prevalent chronic health conditions and a leading cause of pain, physical disability, and healthcare utilization in Canada (Health Canada, 2003). According to the 2000 Canadian Community Health Survey, arthritis and other rheumatic conditions affected approximately one in six Canadians aged 15 years and over, and two thirds of those affected were women. The prevalence of arthritis increases with increasing age; however, nearly three in five people with arthritis were younger than 65 years of age. Arthritis was the most prevalent chronic condition reported by Canadian Aboriginal people, affecting approximately 19% of the population. After adjusting for differing age distributions, the prevalence was even higher, at 27% as compared with 16% in the non-Aboriginal Canadian population. Aboriginal people

with arthritis reported higher rates of disability than did non-Aboriginals with arthritis. This may be due to a higher prevalence of specific types of arthritis such as rheumatoid arthritis (RA) among Aboriginal people. Aboriginal Canadians are also reported to have an earlier age of onset of RA than have non-Aboriginal Canadians (Peschken et al., 1999).

Hip fractures are a serious consequence of falls in older adults. Over 28,000 hospitalizations for hip fracture occurred in Canada in 2005–2006, with 88% of these involving patients aged 65 years and older (Canadian Institute for Health Information, 2006). Women are twice as likely as men to fracture a hip. Hip fractures can result in loss of mobility and independence, financial difficulties, increased healthcare service utilization, and mortality. Similarly, older adults accounted for the majority of hip and knee joint replacements in Canada in 2004–2005. Across the country, efforts have been initiated to reduce wait times for hip and joint replacement surgeries.

SUBJECTIVE DATA

1. Joints
   Pain
   Stiffness
   Swelling, heat, redness
   Limitation of movement

2. Muscles
   Pain (cramps)
   Weakness

3. Bones
   Pain
   Deformity

   Trauma (fractures, sprains, dislocations)

4. Functional assessment (activities of daily living [ADLs])

5. Self-care behaviours

Examiner Asks	Rationale
1. Joints.	
• Any problems with your joints? Any **pain?**	**Joint pain** and loss of function are the most common musculoskeletal concerns that prompt a person to seek care.
• Location: Which joints? On one side or both sides?	Rheumatoid arthritis (RA) involves symmetrical joints; other musculoskeletal illnesses involve isolated or unilateral joints.

Subjective Data

Examiner Asks	Rationale

Subjective Data

- Quality: What does the pain feel like: aching, stiff, sharp or dull, shooting?
- Severity: How strong is the pain?
- Onset: When did this pain start?
- Timing: What time of day does the pain occur? How long does it last? How often does it occur?

- Is the pain aggravated by movement, rest, position, weather? Is the pain relieved by rest, medications, application of heat or ice?

- Is the pain associated with chills, fever, recent sore throat, trauma, repetitive activity?

- Any **stiffness** in your joints?

- Any **swelling, heat, redness** in the joints?
- Any **limitation of movement** in any joint? Which joint?
- Which activities give you problems? (See Functional Assessment, p. 638.)

Rationale:

Exquisitely tender with acute inflammation.

RA pain is worse in morning when arising; osteoarthritis is worse later in the day; tendinitis is worse in morning, improves during the day.

Movement increases most joint pain except in RA, in which movement decreases pain.

Joint pain 10 to 14 days after an untreated strep throat suggests rheumatic fever. Joint injury occurs from trauma, repetitive motion.

RA stiffness occurs in morning and after rest periods.

Suggests acute inflammation.

Decreased ROM may be due to joint injury to cartilage or capsule, or to muscle contracture.

2. Muscles.

- Any problems in the muscles, such as any **pain** or **cramping?** Which muscles?
- If in calf muscles: Does the pain occur with walking? Does it go away with rest?
- Are your muscle aches associated with fever, chills, the "flu"?
- Any **weakness** in muscles?
- Location: Where is the weakness? How long have you noticed weakness?

- Do the muscles look smaller there?

Rationale:

Myalgia is usually felt as cramping or aching.

Suggests intermittent claudication (see Chapter 20).

Viral illness often includes myalgia.

Weakness may involve musculoskeletal or neurological systems (see Chapters 22 and 23).

Atrophy.

3. Bones.

- Any **bone pain?** Is the pain affected by movement?
- Any **deformity** of any bone or joint? Is the deformity due to injury or trauma? Does the deformity affect ROM?
- Any **accidents** or **trauma** ever affected the bones or joints: fractures, joint strain, sprain, dislocation? Which ones?
- When did this occur? What treatment was given? Any problems or limitations now as a result?
- Any back pain? In which part of your back? Is pain felt anywhere else, like shooting down leg?
- Any numbness and tingling? Any limping?

Rationale:

Fracture causes sharp pain that increases with movement. Other bone pain usually feels "dull" and "deep" and is unrelated to movement.

4. Functional assessment.
Do your joint (muscle, bone) problems create any limits on your usual activities of daily living (ADLs)? Which ones? (Note: Ask about each category; if the person answers "yes," ask specifically about each activity in category.)

- Bathing—getting in and out of the tub, turning faucets?
- Toileting—urinating, defacating, able to get self on and off toilet, wipe self?
- Dressing—doing buttons, zipper, fasten opening behind neck, pulling dress or sweater over head, pulling up pants, tying shoes, getting shoes that fit?
- Grooming—shaving, brushing teeth, brushing or fixing hair, applying makeup?

Rationale:

Functional assessment screens the safety of independent living, the need for home healthcare services, and quality of life (see Chapter 30).

Assess any self-care deficit.

Examiner Asks	Rationale
• Eating—preparing meals, pouring liquids, cutting up foods, bringing food to mouth, drinking?	
• Mobility—walking, walking up or down stairs, getting in and out of bed, getting out of house?	Impaired physical mobility.
• Communicating—talking, using phone, writing?	Impaired verbal communication.

5. Self-care behaviours. Any occupational hazards that could affect the muscles and joints? Does your work involve heavy lifting? Or any repetitive motion or chronic stress to joints? Any efforts to alleviate these?

Assess risk for back pain or carpal tunnel syndrome.

Self-care behaviours.

- Tell me about your exercise program. Describe the type of exercise, frequency, the warm-up program.
- Any pain during exercise? How do you treat it?
- Have you had any recent weight gain? Please describe your usual daily diet. (Note the person's usual caloric intake, all four food groups, daily amount of protein, calcium.)
- Are you taking any medications for musculoskeletal system: aspirin, anti-inflammatory, muscle relaxant, pain reliever?
- If person has chronic disability or crippling illness: How has your illness affected:
  Your interaction with family?
  Your interaction with friends?
  The way you view yourself?

Assess for:
- Self-esteem disturbance
- Loss of independence
- Body image disturbance
- Role performance disturbance
- Social isolation

Additional History for Infants and Children

1. Were you told about any trauma to infant during labour and delivery? Did the baby come head first? Was there a need for forceps?

Traumatic delivery increases risk for fractures (e.g., humerus, clavicle).

2. Did the baby need resuscitation?

Period of anoxia may result in hypotonia of muscles.

3. Were the baby's motor milestones achieved at about the same time as siblings or age-mates?

4. Has your child ever broken any bones? Any dislocations? How were these treated?

5. Have you ever noticed any bone deformity? Spinal curvature? Unusual shape of toes or feet? At what age? Have you ever sought treatment for any of these?

Additional History for Adolescents

1. Involved in any sports at school or after school? How frequently (times per week)?

Assess safety of sport for child. Note if child's height and weight are adequate for the particular sport (e.g., football).

2. Do you use any special equipment? Does any training program exist for your sport?

Use of safety equipment and presence of adult supervision decrease risk of sports injuries.

3. What is the nature of your daily warm-up?

Lack of adequate warm-up increases risk of sports injury.

Subjective Data

Examiner Asks	Rationale
4. What do you do if you get hurt?	Students may not report injury or pain for fear of participation in sport being restricted.
5. How does your sport fit in with other school demands and other activities?	

Additional History for the Aging Adult

Use the functional assessment history questions in Chapter 5 (pp. 78 to 80) to elicit any loss of function, self-care deficit, or safety risk that may occur as a process of aging or musculoskeletal illness. (Review the complete functional assessment in Chapter 30.)

1. Any change in weakness over the past months or years?

2. Any increase in falls or stumbling over the past months or years?

3. Do you use any mobility aids to help you get around: cane, walker?

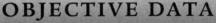 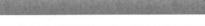

OBJECTIVE DATA

PREPARATION

The purpose of the musculoskeletal examination is to assess function for ADLs and to screen for any abnormalities. You already will have considerable data regarding ADLs through the history. Note additional ADL data as the person goes through the motions necessary for an examination: gait, posture, how the person sits in a chair, raises from chair, takes off jacket, manipulates small object such as a pen, raises from supine position.

A **screening** musculoskeletal examination suffices for most people:
- Inspection and palpation of joints integrated with each body region
- Observation of ROM as person proceeds through motions described earlier
- Age-specific screening measures, such as Ortolani's sign for infants or scoliosis screening for adolescents

A **complete** musculoskeletal examination, as described in this chapter, is appropriate for persons with articular disease, a history of musculoskeletal symptoms, or any problems with ADLs.

Make the person comfortable before and throughout the examination. Drape for full visualization of the body part you are examining without needlessly exposing the person.

Take an orderly approach—head to toe, proximal to distal.

Support each joint at rest. Muscles must be soft and relaxed to assess the joints under them accurately. Take care when examining any inflamed area where rough manipulation could cause pain and muscle spasm. To avoid this, use firm support, gentle movement, and gentle return to a relaxed state.

Compare corresponding paired joints. Expect symmetry of structure and function and normal parameters for that joint.

EQUIPMENT NEEDED
Tape measure
Goniometer, to measure joint angles
Skin marking pen

Normal Range of Findings	Abnormal Findings

ORDER OF THE EXAMINATION

Inspection

Note the **size** and **contour** of the joint. Inspect the skin and tissues over the joints for **colour, swelling,** and any **masses** or **deformity.** Presence of swelling is significant and signals joint irritation.

Swelling may be due to excess joint fluid (effusion), thickening of the synovial lining, inflammation of surrounding soft tissue (bursae, tendons), or bony enlargement.

Deformities include dislocation (one or more bones in a joint being out of position), **subluxation** (partial dislocation of a joint), **contracture** (shortening of a muscle leading to limited ROM of joint), or **ankylosis** (stiffness or fixation of a joint).

Palpation

Palpate each joint, including its skin for temperature, its muscles, bony articulations, and area of joint capsule. Note any heat, tenderness, swelling, or masses. Joints normally are not tender to palpation. If any tenderness does occur, try to localize it to specific anatomical structures (e.g., skin, muscles, bursae, ligaments, tendons, fat pads, or joint capsule).

The synovial membrane normally is not palpable. When thickened, it feels "doughy" or "boggy." A small amount of fluid is present in the normal joint, but it is not palpable.

Palpable fluid is abnormal. Because fluid is contained in an enclosed sac, if you push on one side of the sac, the fluid will shift and cause a visible bulging on another side.

Range of Motion

Ask for **active ROM** while stabilizing the body area proximal to that being moved. With each joint familiarize yourself with the type and its normal ROM so that you can recognize limitations. If you see a limitation, gently attempt **passive motion.** Anchor the joint with one hand while your other hand slowly moves it to its limit. The normal ranges of active and passive motions should be the same.

If any limitation or any increase in ROM occurs, use a goniometer to measure the angles precisely (Fig. 22-15). First, extend the joint to neutral or 0 degrees. Centre the 0 point of the goniometer on the joint. Keep the fixed arm of the goniometer on the 0 line, and use the movable arm to measure; then flex the joint and measure through the goniometer to determine the angle of greatest flexion.

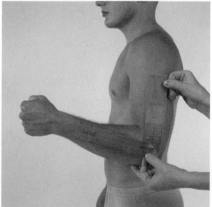

Fig. 22-15

Normal Range of Findings	Abnormal Findings

Joint motion normally causes no tenderness, pain, or crepitation. Do not confuse crepitation with the normal discrete "crack" heard as a tendon or ligament slips over bone during motion, such as when you do a knee bend.

Crepitation is an audible and palpable crunching or grating that accompanies movement. It occurs when the articular surfaces in the joints are roughened, as with rheumatoid arthritis (see Table 22-2, p. 641).

Muscle Testing

Test the strength of the prime mover muscle groups for each joint. Repeat the motions you elicited for active ROM. Now ask the person to flex and hold as you apply opposing force. Muscle strength should be equal bilaterally and should fully resist your opposing force. (Note: Muscle status and joint status are interdependent and should be interpreted together. Chapter 23 discusses the examination of muscles for size and development, tone, and presence of tenderness.)

A wide variability of strength exists among people. You may wish to use a grading system from no voluntary movement to full strength, as shown.

Grade	Description	% Normal	Assessment
5	Full ROM against gravity, full resistance	100	Normal
4	Full ROM against gravity, some resistance	75	Good
3	Full ROM with gravity	50	Fair
2	Full ROM with gravity eliminated (passive motion)	25	Poor
1	Slight contraction	10	Trace
0	No contraction	0	Zero

TEMPOROMANDIBULAR JOINT

With the person seated, **inspect** the area just anterior to the ear. Place the tips of your first two fingers in front of each ear and ask the person to open and close the mouth. Drop your fingers into the depressed area over the joint, and note smooth motion of the mandible. An audible and palpable snap or click occurs in many healthy people as the mouth opens (Fig. 22-16).

Swelling looks like a round bulge over the joint, although it must be moderate or marked to be visible.

Crepitus and pain occur with temporomandibular joint dysfunction.

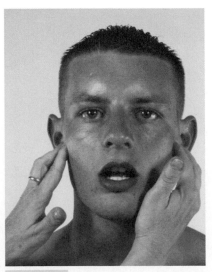

Fig. 22-16

Normal Range of Findings	Abnormal Findings

Ask the person to:

INSTRUCTIONS TO PERSON	MOTION AND EXPECTED RANGE
• Open mouth maximally.	Vertical motion. You can measure the space between the upper and lower incisors. Normal is 3 to 6 cm, or three fingers inserted sideways.
• Partially open mouth, thrust lower jaw, and move it side to side.	Lateral motion. Normal extent is 1 to 2 cm (Fig. 22-17).
• Stick out lower jaw.	Protrusion without deviation.

Lateral motion may be lost earlier and more significantly than vertical motion.

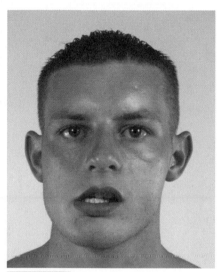

Fig. 22-17

Palpate the contracted temporalis and masseter muscles as the person clenches the teeth. Compare right and left sides for size, firmness, and strength. Ask the person to move the jaw forward and laterally against your resistance, and to open mouth against your resistance. This also tests the integrity of cranial nerve V (trigeminal).

CERVICAL SPINE

Inspect the alignment of head and neck. The spine should be straight and the head erect. **Palpate** the spinous processes and the sternomastoid, trapezius, and paravertebral muscles. They should feel firm, with no muscle spasm or tenderness.

Head tilted to one side.
Asymmetry of muscles.
Tenderness and hard muscles with muscle spasm.

Normal Range of Findings	Abnormal Findings

Ask the person to perform these motions (Fig. 22-18):*

INSTRUCTIONS TO PERSON
- Touch chin to chest.
- Lift the chin toward the ceiling.
- Move each ear toward the corresponding shoulder. Do not lift up the shoulder.
- Turn the chin toward each shoulder.

MOTION AND EXPECTED RANGE
Flexion of 45 degrees (Fig. 22-18, A).
Hyperextension of 55 degrees.
Lateral bending of 40 degrees (Fig. 22-18, B).

Rotation of 70 degrees (Fig. 22-18, C).

Limited ROM.

Pain with movement.

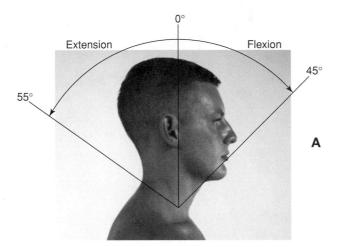

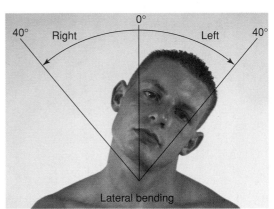

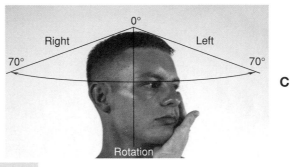

Fig. 22-18

Ask the person to repeat the motions while applying opposing force. The person normally can maintain flexion against your full resistance. This also tests the integrity of cranial nerve XI (spinal).

The person cannot hold flexion.

UPPER EXTREMITY

Shoulders

Inspect and compare both shoulders posteriorly and anteriorly. Check the size and contour of the joint, and compare shoulders for equality of bony landmarks. Normally, no redness, muscular atrophy, deformity, or swelling is present. Check the anterior aspect of the joint capsule and the subacromial bursa for abnormal swelling.

Redness.
Inequality of bony landmarks.
Atrophy, shows as lack of fullness.
Dislocated shoulder loses the normal rounded shape and looks flattened laterally.

*Do not attempt if you suspect neck trauma.

Normal Range of Findings	Abnormal Findings

Abnormal Findings

Swelling from excess fluid is best seen anteriorly. Considerable fluid must be present to cause a visible distension because the capsule normally is loose (see Table 22-3, p. 642).

Swelling of subacromial bursa is localized under deltoid muscle and may be accentuated when the person tries to abduct the arm.

If the person reports any shoulder pain, ask that he or she point to the spot with the hand of the unaffected side. Be aware that shoulder pain may be due to local causes, or it may be referred pain from a hiatal hernia or a cardiac or pleural condition, which could be potentially serious. Pain from a local cause is reproducible during the examination by palpation or motion.

While standing in front of the person, **palpate** both shoulders, noting any muscular spasm or atrophy, swelling, heat, or tenderness. Start at the clavicle and methodically explore the acromioclavicular joint, scapula, greater tubercle of the humerus, area of the subacromial bursa, the biceps groove, and the anterior aspect of the glenohumeral joint. Palpate the pyramid-shaped axilla; no adenopathy or masses should be present.

Swelling.
Hard muscles with muscle spasm.
Tenderness or pain.

Test ROM by asking the person to perform four motions (Fig. 22-19). Cup one hand over the shoulder during ROM to note any crepitation; normally none is present.

INSTRUCTIONS TO PERSON

- With arms at sides and elbows extended, move both arms forward and up in wide vertical arcs, then move them back.
- Rotate arms internally behind back, place back of hands as high as possible toward the scapulae.

MOTION AND EXPECTED RANGE

Forward flexion of 180 degrees.
    Hyperextension up to 50 degrees (Fig. 22-19, A).

Internal rotation of 90 degrees (Fig. 22-19, B).

Limited ROM.
Asymmetry.
Pain with motion.

Crepitus with motion.
Rotator cuff lesions may cause limited ROM, pain, and muscle spasm during abduction, whereas forward flexion stays fairly normal.

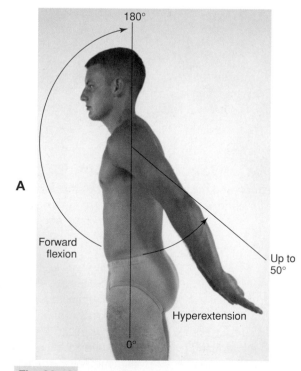

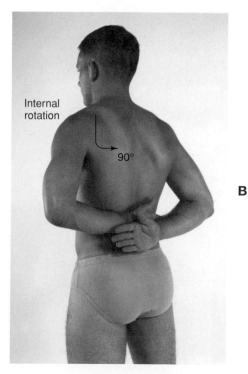

Fig. 22-19

Continued

Normal Range of Findings	Abnormal Findings

- With arms at sides and elbows extended, raise both arms in wide arcs in the coronal plane. Touch palms together above head.
- Touch both hands behind the head with elbows flexed and rotated posteriorly.

Abduction of 180 degrees.
Adduction of 50 degrees
    (Fig. 22-19, *C*).

External rotation of 90 degrees
    (Fig. 22-19, *D*).

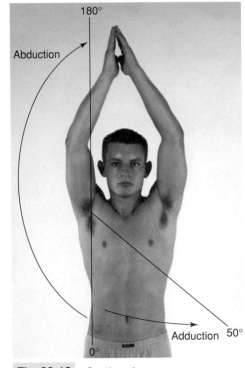

C

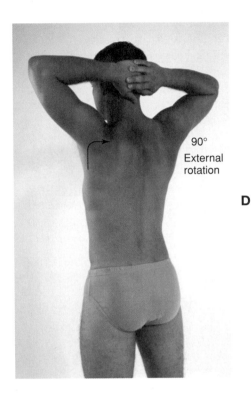

D

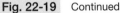

Fig. 22-19   Continued

Test the strength of the shoulder muscles by asking the person to shrug the shoulders, flex them forward and up, and abduct them against your resistance. The shoulder shrug also tests the integrity of cranial nerve XI, the spinal accessory.

Elbow

Inspect the size and contour of the elbow in both flexed and extended positions. Look for any deformity, redness, or swelling. Check the olecranon bursa and the normally present hollows on either side of the olecranon process for abnormal swelling.

Palpate with the person's elbow flexed about 70 degrees and as relaxed as possible (Fig. 22-20). Use your left hand to support the person's left forearm and palpate the extensor surface of the elbow—the olecranon process and the medial and lateral epicondyles of humerus—with your right thumb and fingers.

Subluxation of the elbow shows the forearm dislocated posteriorly.

Swelling and redness of olecranon bursa are localized and easy to observe because of the close proximity of the bursa to skin.

Effusion or synovial thickening shows first as a bulge or fullness in groove on either side of the olecranon process, and it occurs with gouty arthritis.

Epicondyles, head of radius, and tendons are common sites of inflammation and local tenderness, or "tennis elbow."

Normal Range of Findings	Abnormal Findings

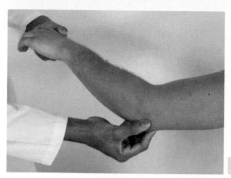

Fig. 22-20

With your thumb in the lateral groove and your index and middle fingers in the medial groove, palpate either side of the olecranon process using varying pressure. Normally, present tissues and fat pads feel fairly solid. Check for any synovial thickening, swelling, nodules, or tenderness.

Palpate the area of the olecranon bursa for heat, swelling, tenderness, consistency, or nodules.

Soft, boggy, or fluctuant swelling in both grooves occurs with synovial thickening or effusion.

Local heat or redness (signs of inflammation) can extend beyond synovial membrane.

Subcutaneous nodules are raised, firm, and nontender, and overlying skin moves freely. Common sites are in the olecranon bursa and along extensor surface of the ulna. These nodules occur with RA (see Table 22-4, p. 643).

Test ROM by asking the person to:

INSTRUCTIONS TO PERSON	MOTION AND EXPECTED RANGE
• Bend and then straighten the elbow (Fig. 22-21).	Flexion of 150 to 160 degrees; extension at 0. Some healthy people lack 5 to 10 degrees of full extension, and others have 5 to 10 degrees of hyperextension.
• Hold the hand midway; then touch touch front and back sides of hand to table.	Movement of 90 degrees in pronation and supination (Fig. 22-22).

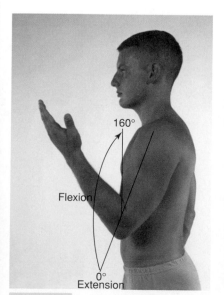

Fig. 22-21

160°

Flexion

0°
Extension

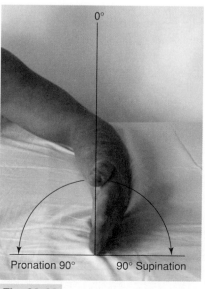

Fig. 22-22

0°

Pronation 90°   90° Supination

Normal Range of Findings	Abnormal Findings

While testing **muscle strength,** stabilize the person's arm with one hand (Fig. 22-23). Have the person flex the elbow against your resistance applied just proximal to the wrist. Then ask the person to extend the elbow against your resistance.

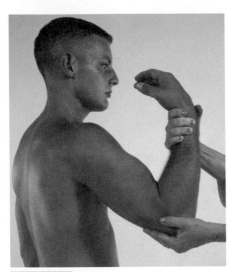

Fig. 22-23

Wrist and Hand

Inspect the hands and wrists on the dorsal and palmar sides, noting position, contour, and shape. The normal functional position of the hand shows the wrist in slight extension. This way the fingers can flex efficiently, and the thumb can oppose them for grip and manipulation. The fingers lie straight in the same axis as the forearm. Normally, no swelling or redness, deformity, or nodules are present.

The skin looks smooth with knuckle wrinkles present and no swelling or lesions. Muscles are full, with the palm showing a rounded mound proximal to the thumb (the **thenar eminence**) and a smaller rounded mound proximal to the little finger.

Palpate each joint in the wrist and hands. Facing the person, support the hand with your fingers under it, and palpate the wrist firmly with both your thumbs on its dorsum (Fig. 22-24). Make sure the person's wrist is relaxed and in straight alignment. Move your palpating thumbs side to side to identify the normal depressed areas that overlie the joint space. Use gentle but firm pressure. Normally the joint surfaces feel smooth, with no swelling, bogginess, nodules, or tenderness.

Subluxation of wrist.
Ulnar deviation; fingers list to ulnar side.
Ankylosis; wrist in extreme flexion.
Dupuytren's contracture; flexion contracture of finger(s).

Swan-neck or boutonnière deformity in fingers.
Atrophy of the thenar eminence (see Table 22-5, p. 644).
Ganglion in wrist.
Synovial swelling on dorsum.
Generalized swelling.
Tenderness.

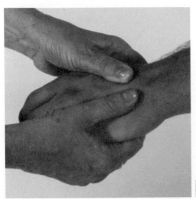

Fig. 22-24

| **Normal Range of Findings** | **Abnormal Findings** |

Palpate the metacarpophalangeal joints with your thumbs, just distal to and on either side of the knuckle (Fig. 22-25).

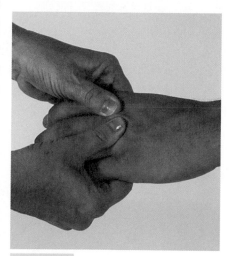

Fig. 22-25

Use your thumb and index finger in a pinching motion to palpate the sides of the interphalangeal joints (Fig. 22-26). Normally, no synovial thickening, tenderness, warmth, or nodules are present.

Heberden's and Bouchard's nodes are hard and nontender and occur with osteoarthritis (see Table 22-5, p. 644).

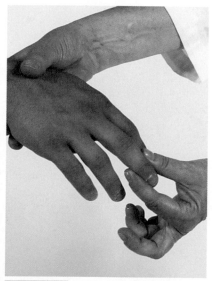

Fig. 22-26

Normal Range of Findings	Abnormal Findings

Test ROM (Fig. 22-27) by asking the person to:

INSTRUCTIONS TO PERSON	MOTION AND EXPECTED RANGE
• Bend the hand up at the wrist.	Hyperextension of 70 degrees (Fig. 22-27, *A*).
• Bend hand down at the wrist.	Palmar flexion of 90 degrees.
• Bend the fingers up and down at metacarpophalangeal joints.	Flexion of 90 degrees. Hyperextension of 30 degrees (Fig. 22-27, *B*).
• With palms flat on table, turn them outward and in.	Ulnar deviation of 50 to 60 degrees, and radial deviation of 20 degrees (Fig. 22-27, *C*).
• Spread fingers apart; make a fist.	Abduction of 20 degrees; fist tight. The responses should be equal bilaterally (Fig. 22-27, *D, E*).
• Touch the thumb to each finger and to the base of little finger.	The person is able to perform, and the responses are equal bilaterally (Fig. 22-27, *F*).

Loss of ROM here is the most common and most significant functional loss of the wrist.
  Limited motion.
  Pain on movement.

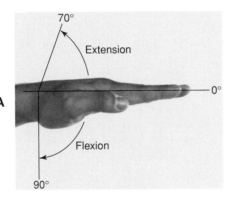

A

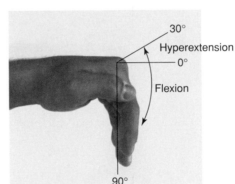

B

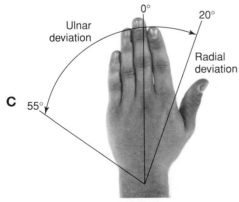

C

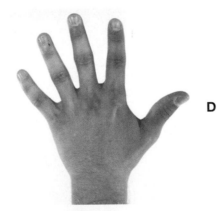

D

E

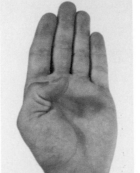

F

Fig. 22-27

Normal Range of Findings	Abnormal Findings

Normal Range of Findings

For **muscle testing,** position the person's forearm supinated (palm up) and resting on a table (Fig. 22-28). Stabilize by holding your hand at the person's midforearm. Ask the person to flex the wrist against your resistance at the palm.

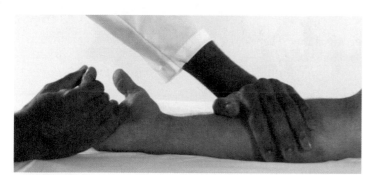

Fig. 22-28

Phalen's Test. Ask the person to hold both hands back to back while flexing the wrists 90 degrees. Acute flexion of the wrist for 60 seconds produces no symptoms in the normal hand (Fig. 22-29).

Tinel's Sign. Direct percussion of the location of the median nerve at the wrist produces no symptoms in the normal hand (Fig. 22-30).

Abnormal Findings

Phalen's test reproduces numbness and burning in a person with carpal tunnel syndrome (see Table 22-5, p. 644).

In carpal tunnel syndrome, percussion of the median nerve produces burning and tingling along its distribution, which is a positive Tinel's sign.

Objective Data

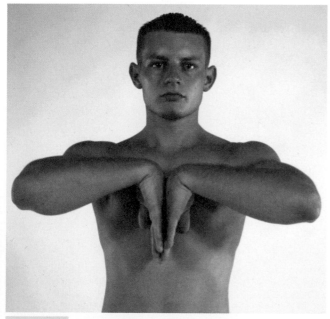

Fig. 22-29   Phalen's test.

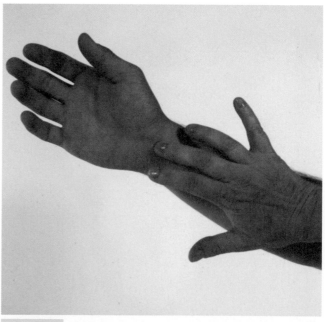

Fig. 22-30   Tinel's sign.

LOWER EXTREMITY

Hip

Inspect the hip joint together with the spine a bit later in the examination as the person stands. At that time, note symmetrical levels of iliac crests, gluteal folds, and equal-sized buttocks. A smooth, even gait reflects equal leg lengths and functional hip motion.

Help the person into the supine position, and **palpate** the hip joints. The joints should feel stable and symmetrical, with no tenderness or crepitance.

Pain with palpation.
Crepitation.

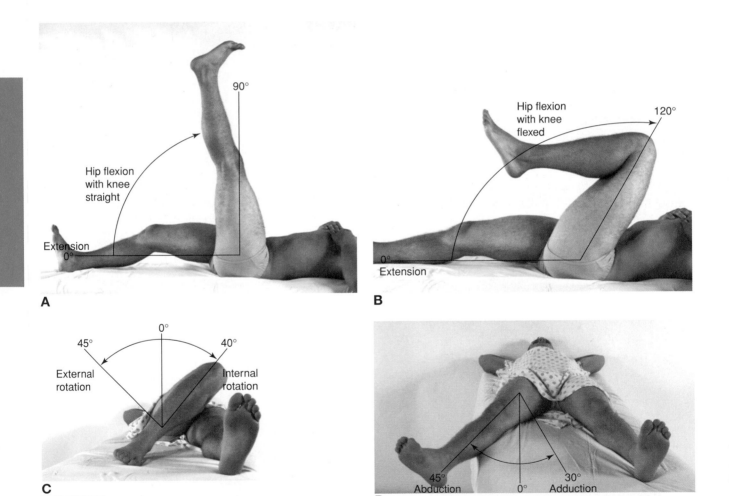

Fig. 22-31

Normal Range of Findings	Abnormal Findings

Assess **ROM** (Fig. 22-31) by asking the person to:

INSTRUCTIONS TO PERSON	MOTION AND EXPECTED RANGE
• Raise each leg with knee extended.	Hip flexion of 90 degrees (Fig. 22-31, *A*).
• Bend each knee up to the chest while keeping the other leg straight.	Hip flexion of 120 degrees. The opposite thigh should remain on the table (Fig. 22-31, *B*).
• Flex knee and hip to 90 degrees. Stabilize by holding the thigh with one hand and the ankle with the other hand. Swing the foot outward. Swing the foot inward. (Foot and thigh move in opposite directions.)	Internal rotation of 40 degrees. External rotation of 45 degrees (Fig. 22-31, *C*).
• Swing leg laterally, then medially, with knee straight. Stabilize pelvis by pushing down on the opposite anterior superior iliac spine.	Abduction of 40 to 45 degrees. Adduction of 20 to 30 degrees (Fig. 22-31, *D*).
• When standing (later in examination), swing straight leg back behind body. Stabilize pelvis to eliminate exaggerated lumbar lordosis. The most efficient way is to ask person to bend over the table and support the trunk on the table, or lie prone on the table.	Hyperextension of 15 degrees when stabilized.

Limited motion.
Pain with motion.
Flexion flattens the lumbar spine; if this reveals a flexion deformity in the opposite hip, it represents a positive *Thomas test.*

Limited internal rotation of hip is an early and reliable sign of hip disease.

Limitation of abduction of the hip while supine is the most common motion dysfunction found in hip disease.

Knee

The person should remain supine with legs extended, although some examiners prefer the knees to be flexed and dangling for **inspection.** The skin normally looks smooth, with even colouring and no lesions.

Shiny and atrophic skin.
Swelling or inflammation (see Table 22-6, p. 647).
Lesions (e.g., psoriasis).

Inspect lower leg alignment. The lower leg should extend in the same axis as the thigh.

Angulation deformity:
• Genu varum (bow legs) (see p. 634)
• Genu valgum (knock knees)
• Flexion contracture

Inspect the knee's shape and contour. Normally, distinct concavities, or hollows, are present on either side of the patella. Check them for any sign of fullness or swelling. Note other locations, such as the prepatellar bursa and the suprapatellar pouch, for any abnormal swelling.

Hollows disappear; then they may bulge with synovial thickening or effusion.

Check the quadriceps muscle in the anterior thigh for any atrophy. Because it is the prime mover of knee extension, this muscle is important for joint stability during weight-bearing.

Atrophy occurs with disuse or chronic disorders. First, it appears in the medial part of the muscle, although it is difficult to note because the vastus medialis is relatively small.

Objective Data

Normal Range of Findings	Abnormal Findings

Improve **palpation** with the person's knee in the supine position with complete relaxation of the quadriceps muscle. Start high on the anterior thigh, about 10 cm above the patella. Palpate with your left thumb and fingers in a grasping fashion (Fig. 22-32). Proceed down toward the knee, exploring the region of the suprapatellar pouch. Note the consistency of the tissues. The muscles and soft tissues should feel solid, and the joint should feel smooth, with no warmth, tenderness, thickening, or nodularity.

Feels fluctuant or boggy with synovitis of suprapatellar pouch.

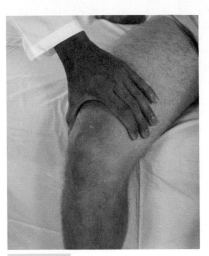

Fig. 22-32

When swelling occurs, you need to distinguish whether it is due to soft tissue swelling or increased fluid in the joint. The tests for the bulge sign and ballottement of the patella aid this assessment.

Bulge Sign. For swelling in the suprapatellar pouch, the bulge sign confirms the presence of small amounts of fluid as you try to move the fluid from one side of the joint to the other. Firmly stroke up on the medial aspect of the knee two or three times to displace any fluid (Fig. 22-33, *A*). Tap the lateral aspect (Fig. 22-33, *B*). Watch the medial side in the hollow for a distinct bulge from a fluid wave. Normally none is present.

The bulge sign occurs with very small amounts of effusion, 4 to 8 mL, from fluid flowing across the joint (Fig. 22-33, *C*).

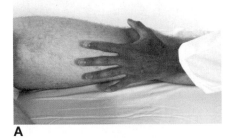

A

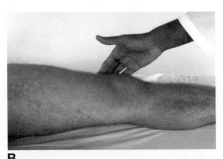

B

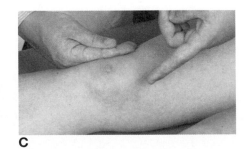

C

Fig. 22-33   Bulge sign.

Normal Range of Findings	Abnormal Findings

Ballottement of the Patella. This test is reliable when larger amounts of fluid are present. Use your left hand to compress the suprapatellar pouch to move any fluid into the knee joint. With your right hand, push the patella sharply against the femur. If no fluid is present, the patella is already snug against the femur (Fig. 22-34, *A*).

If fluid has collected, your tap on the patella moves it through the fluid, and you will hear a tap as the patella bumps up on the femoral condyles (Fig. 22-34, *B*).

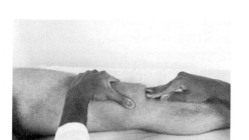

A

Fig. 22-34   Ballottement.

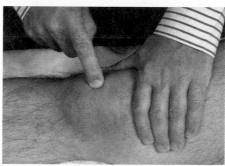

B

Continue palpation, and explore the tibiofemoral joint (Fig. 22-35). Note smooth joint margins and absence of pain. Palpate the infrapatellar fat pad and the patella. Check for crepitus by holding your hand on the patella as the knee is flexed and extended. Some crepitus in an otherwise-asymptomatic knee is not uncommon.

Irregular bony margins occur with osteoarthritis.

Pain at joint line.

Pronounced crepitus is significant and occurs with degenerative diseases of the knee.

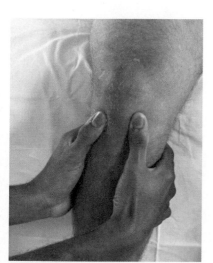

Fig. 22-35

Objective Data

Objective Data

Normal Range of Findings	Abnormal Findings

Normal Range of Findings

Check ROM (Fig. 22-36) by asking the person to:

INSTRUCTIONS TO PERSON	MOTION AND EXPECTED RANGE
• Bend each knee.	Flexion of 130 to 150 degrees.
• Extend each knee.	A straight line of 0 degrees in some persons; a hyperextension of 15 degrees in others.
• Ambulate. (Check knee ROM during ambulation.)	

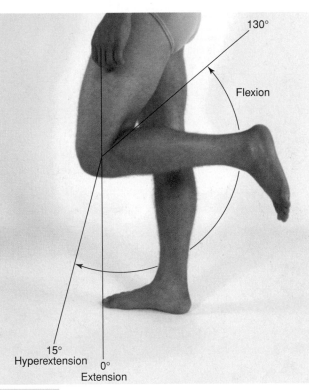

Fig. 22-36

Check **muscle strength** by asking the person to maintain knee flexion while you oppose by trying to pull the leg forward. Muscle extension is demonstrated by the person successfully rising from a seated position in a low chair or rising from a squat without using the hands for support.

Special Test for Meniscal Tears

McMurray's Test. Perform this test when the person has reported a history of trauma followed by locking, giving way, or local pain in the knee. Position the person supine as you stand on the affected side. Hold the heel and flex the knee and hip. Place your other hand on the knee with fingers on the medial side. Rotate the leg in and out to loosen the joint. Externally rotate the leg and push a valgus (inward) stress on the knee. Then slowly extend the knee. Normally the leg extends smoothly with no pain (Fig. 22-37).

Abnormal Findings

Limited ROM.
Contracture.
Pain with motion.
Limp.
Sudden locking—the person is unable to extend the knee fully. This usually occurs with a painful and audible "pop" or "click." Sudden buckling, or "giving way," occurs with ligament injury, which causes weakness and instability.

If you hear or feel a "click," McMurray's test is positive for a torn meniscus.

Normal Range of Findings	Abnormal Findings

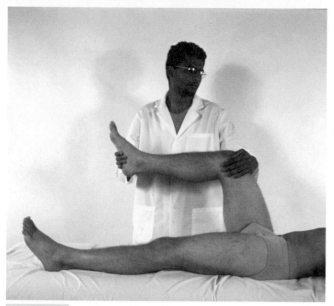

Fig. 22-37   McMurray's test.

Ankle and Foot

Inspect while the person is in a sitting, non–weight-bearing position, as well as when standing and walking. Compare both feet, noting position of feet and toes, contour of joints, and skin characteristics. The foot should align with the long axis of the lower leg; an imaginary line would fall from midpatella to between the first and second toes.

Weight-bearing should fall on the middle of the foot, from the heel, along the midfoot, to between the second and third toes. Most feet have a longitudinal arch, although that can vary normally from "flat feet" to a high instep.

The toes point straight forward and lie flat. The ankles (malleoli) are smooth bony prominences. Normally the skin is smooth, with even colouring and no lesions. Note the locations of any calluses or bursal reactions because they reveal areas of abnormal friction. Examining well-worn shoes helps assess areas of wear and accommodation.

Support the ankle by grasping the heel with your fingers while palpating with your thumbs (Fig. 22-38). Explore the joint spaces. They should feel smooth and depressed, with no fullness, swelling, or tenderness.

Hallux valgus (see Table 22-7, p. 648).
Hammertoes. Claw toes.
Swelling or inflammation.
Calluses. Ulcers.

Swelling or inflammation.
Tenderness.

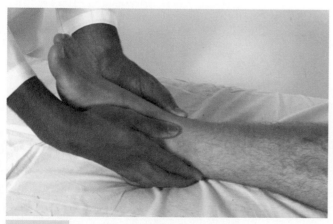

Fig. 22-38

Objective Data

Objective Data

Normal Range of Findings	Abnormal Findings

Palpate the metatarsophalangeal joints between your thumb on the dorsum and your fingers on the plantar surface (Fig. 22-39).

Swelling or inflammation; tenderness.

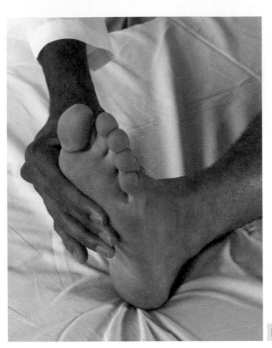

Fig. 22-39

Using a pinching motion of your thumb and forefinger, palpate the interphalangeal joints on the medial and lateral sides of the toes.

Test ROM (Fig. 22-40) by asking the person to:

INSTRUCTIONS TO PERSON	MOTION AND EXPECTED RANGE
• Point toes toward the floor.	Plantar flexion of 45 degrees.
• Point toes toward your nose.	Dorsiflexion of 20 degrees (Fig. 22-40, *A*).
• Turn soles of feet out, then in. (Stabilize the ankle with one hand, hold heel with the other to test the subtalar joint.)	Eversion of 20 degrees. Inversion of 30 degrees (Fig. 22-40, *B*).
• Flex and straighten toes.	

Limited ROM.
Pain with motion.

Assess **muscle strength** by asking the person to maintain dorsiflexion and plantar flexion against your resistance.

Unable to hold flexion.

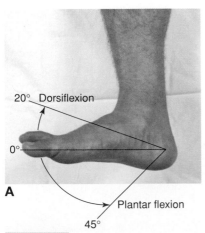

A

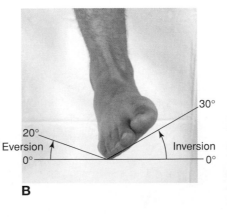

B

Fig. 22-40

Normal Range of Findings

SPINE

The person should be standing, draped in a gown open at the back. Place yourself far enough back so that you can see the entire back. **Inspect** and note whether the spine is straight by following an imaginary vertical line from the head through the spinous processes and down through the gluteal cleft, and by noting equal horizontal positions for the shoulders, scapulae, iliac crests, and gluteal folds, and equal spaces between arm and lateral thorax on the two sides (Fig. 22-41, *A*). The person's knees and feet should be aligned with the trunk and should be pointing forward.

A difference in shoulder elevation and in level of scapulae and iliac crests occur with scoliosis (see Table 22-8, p. 650).

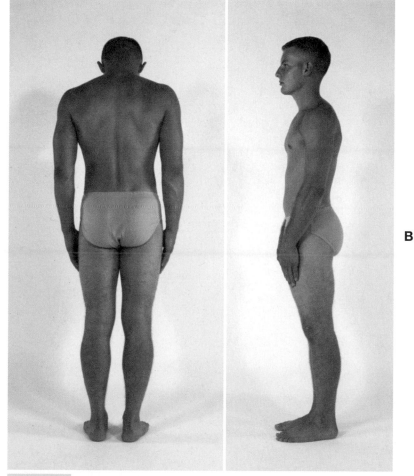

A   **B**

Fig. 22-41

From the side, note the normal convex thoracic curve and concave lumbar curve (Fig. 22-41, *B*). An enhanced thoracic curve, or kyphosis, is common in aging people. A pronounced lumbar curve, or lordosis, is common in obese people.

Lateral tilting and forward bending occur with a herniated nucleus pulposus (see Table 22-8, p. 650).

Normal Range of Findings	Abnormal Findings

Normal Range of Findings

Palpate the spinous processes. Normally they are straight and not tender. Palpate the paravertebral muscles; they should feel firm with no tenderness or spasm.

Check **ROM** of the spine by asking the person to bend forward and touch the toes (Fig. 22-42). Look for flexion of 75 to 90 degrees and smoothness and symmetry of movement. Note that the concave lumbar curve should disappear with this motion, and the back should have a single convex C-shaped curve.

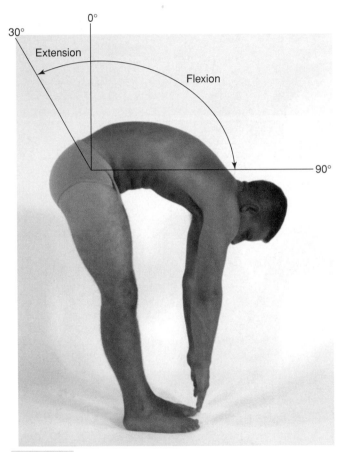

Fig. 22-42

If you suspect a spinal curvature during inspection, this may be more clearly seen when the person touches the toes. While the person is bending over, mark a dot on each spinous process. When the person resumes standing, the dots should form a straight vertical line.

Abnormal Findings

Spinal curvature.
Tenderness. Spasm of paravertebral muscles.

If the dots form a slight S-shape when the person stands, a spinal curve is present.

Normal Range of Findings

Abnormal Findings

Stabilize the pelvis with your hands. Check ROM (Fig. 22-43) by asking the person to:

INSTRUCTIONS TO PERSON
- Bend sideways.

- Bend backward.
- Twist shoulders to one side, then the other.

MOTION AND EXPECTED RANGE
Lateral bending of 35 degrees (Fig. 22-43, *A*).
Hyperextension of 30 degrees.
Rotation of 30 degrees, bilaterally. (Fig. 22-43, *B*).

Limited ROM.

Pain with motion.

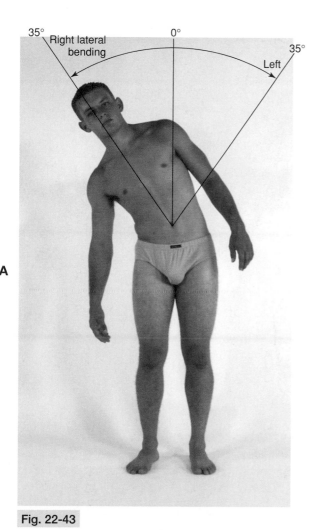

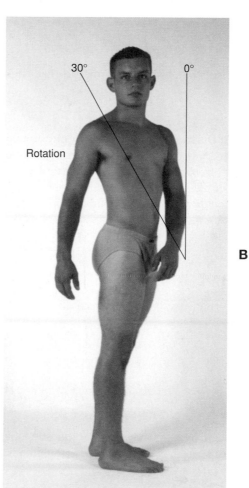

A

B

Fig. 22-43

These manoeuvres reveal only gross restriction. Movement is still possible even if some spinal fusion has occurred.

Finally, ask the person to walk on his or her toes for a few steps; then return walking on the heels.

Straight Leg Raising or LaSegue's Test. These manoeuvres reproduce back and leg pain and help confirm the presence of a herniated nucleus pulposus. Straight leg raising while keeping the knee extended normally produces no pain. Raise the affected leg just short of the point where it produces pain. Then dorsiflex the foot (Fig. 22-44).

Normal Range of Findings	**Abnormal Findings**

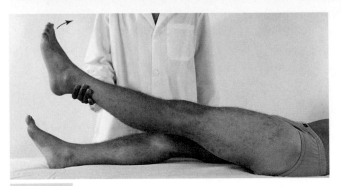

Fig. 22-44

LaSegue's test is positive if it reproduces sciatic pain. If lifting the affected leg reproduces sciatic pain, it confirms the presence of a herniated nucleus pulposus.

Raise the unaffected leg while leaving the other leg flat. Inquire about the involved side.

If lifting the unaffected leg reproduces sciatic pain, it strongly suggests a herniated nucleus pulposus.

Measure Leg Length Discrepancy. Perform this measurement if you need to determine whether one leg is shorter than the other. For *true leg length,* measure between *fixed* points, from the anterior iliac spine to the medial malleolus, crossing the medial side of the knee (Fig. 22-45). Normally these measurements are equal or within 1 cm, indicating no true bone discrepancy.

Unequal leg lengths.

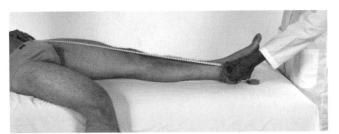

Fig. 22-45

Sometimes the true leg length is equal, but the legs still look unequal. For *apparent leg length,* measure from a nonfixed point (the umbilicus) to a fixed point (medial malleolus) on each leg.

True leg lengths are equal, but apparent leg lengths unequal—this condition occurs with pelvic obliquity or adduction or flexion deformity in the hip.

DEVELOPMENTAL CARE

Review the developmental milestones discussed in Chapter 2. Keep handy a concise chart of the usual sequence of motor development so that you can refer to expected findings for the age of each child you are examining. Use the Denver II test to identify the fine and gross motor skills for the child's age.

Because some overlap exists between the musculoskeletal and neurological examinations, assessment of muscle tone, resting posture, and motor activity are discussed in the next chapter.

Infants

Examine the infant with the infant fully undressed and lying on the back. Take care to place the newborn on a warming table to maintain body temperature.

Normal Range of Findings	Abnormal Findings

Feet and Legs. Start with the feet and work your way up the extremities. Note any *positional deformities,* a residual of fetal positioning. Often the newborn's feet are not held straight but in a varus (apart) or valgus (together) position. It is important to distinguish whether this position is flexible (and thus usually self-correctable) or fixed. Scratch the outside of the bottom of the foot. If the deformity is self-correctable, the foot assumes a normal right angle to the lower leg. Or immobilize the heel with one hand and gently push the forefoot to the neutral position with the other hand. If you can move it to neutral position, it is flexible.

A true deformity is fixed and assumes a right angle only with forced manipulation or not at all.

Note the relationship of the forefoot to the hindfoot. Commonly, the hindfoot is in alignment with the lower leg and just the forefoot angles inward. This forefoot adduction is *metatarsus adductus.* It is usually present at birth and usually resolves spontaneously by age 3 years.

Metatarsus varus—adduction and inversion of forefoot.

Talipes equinovarus (see Table 22-9, p. 651).

Check for *tibial torsion,* a twisting of the tibia. Place the child's feet flat on the table, and push to flex up the knees. With the patella and the tibial tubercle in a straight line, place your fingers on the malleoli. In an infant, note whether a line connecting the four malleoli is parallel to the table.

More than 20 degrees of deviation; or if lateral malleolus is anterior to medial malleolus, it indicates tibial torsion.

Tibial torsion may originate from intrauterine positioning and then may be exacerbated at a later age by continuous sitting in a reverse tailor position, the "TV squat." This is sitting with the buttocks on the floor and the lower legs splayed back and out on either side.

Hips. Check the hips for *congenital dislocation.* The most reliable method is the **Ortolani manoeuvre,** which should be done at every professional visit until the infant is 1 year old. With the infant supine, flex the knees holding your thumbs on the inner mid-thighs, and your fingers outside on the hips touching the greater trochanters. Adduct the legs until your thumbs touch (Fig. 22-46, A). Then gently lift and *abduct* the legs, moving the knees apart and down so their lateral aspects touch the table (Fig. 22-46, B). This normally feels smooth and produces no sound.

With a dislocated hip, the head of the femur is not cupped in the acetabulum but rests posterior to it.

Hip instability feels like a clunk as the head of the femur pops back into place. This is a *positive Ortolani sign* and warrants referral.

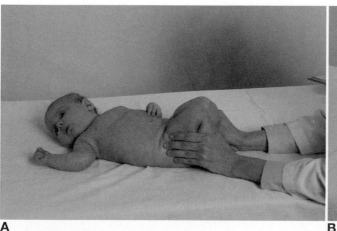
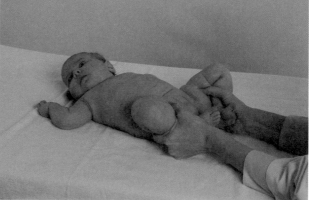

A   **B**

Fig. 22-46   The Ortolani manoeuvre.

Normal Range of Findings	Abnormal Findings

The **Allis test** also is used to check for hip dislocation by comparing leg lengths (Fig. 22-47). Place the baby's feet flat on the table and flex the knees up. Scan the tops of the knees; normally they are at the same elevation.

Finding one knee significantly lower than the other is a positive indication of Allis' sign and suggests hip dislocation.

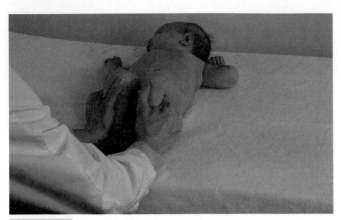

Fig. 22-47   Allis test.

Note the gluteal folds. Normally they are equal on both sides. However, some asymmetry may occur in healthy children.

Unequal gluteal folds may accompany hip dislocation after 2 to 3 months of age.

Hands and Arms. Inspect the hands, noting shape, number, and position of fingers and palmar creases.

Polydactyly is the presence of extra fingers or toes. Syndactyly is webbing between adjacent fingers or toes (see Table 22-5, p. 644).

A simian crease is a single palmar crease that occurs with Down syndrome, accompanied by short broad fingers, incurving of little fingers, and low-set thumbs.

Palpate the length of the clavicles because the clavicle is the bone most frequently fractured during birth. The clavicles should feel smooth, regular, and without crepitus. Also note equal ROM of arms during Moro's reflex.

Fractured clavicle: Note irregularity at the fracture site, crepitus, and angulation. The site has rapid callus formation with a palpable lump within a few weeks. Observe limited arm ROM and unilateral response to Moro's reflex.

Back. Lift up the infant and examine the back. Note the normal single C curve of the newborn's spine (Fig. 22-48). By 2 months of age, the infant can lift the head while prone. This builds the concave cervical spinal curve and indicates normal forearm strength. Inspect the length of the spine for any tuft of hair, dimple in midline, cyst, or mass. Normally none are present.

A tuft of hair over a dimple in the midline may indicate spina bifida.

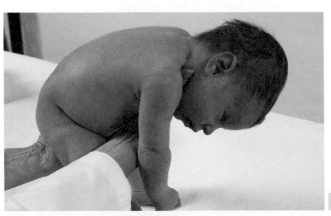

Fig. 22-48

Normal Range of Findings

Observe ROM through spontaneous movement of extremities.

Test muscle strength by lifting up the infant with your hands under the axillae (Fig. 22-49). A baby with normal muscle strength wedges securely between your hands.

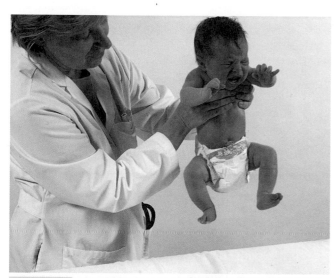

Fig. 22-49

Preschool- and School-Age Children

Once the infant learns to crawl and then to walk, the waking hours show perpetual motion. This is convenient for your musculoskeletal assessment; you can observe the muscles and joints during spontaneous play before a table-top examination. Most young children enjoy showing off their physical accomplishments. For specific motions, coax the toddler: "Show me how you can walk to Mom," "Climb the step stool." Ask the preschooler to hop on one foot or to jump.

Back. While the child is standing, note the posture. From behind, you should note a "plumb line" from the back of the head, along the spine, to the middle of the sacrum. Shoulders are level within 1 cm, and scapulae are symmetrical. From the side, lordosis is common throughout childhood, appearing more pronounced in children with a protuberant abdomen.

Abnormal Findings

A small dimple in the midline—anywhere from the head to the coccyx—suggests dermoid sinus.

Mass, for example, meningocele.

A baby who starts to "slip" between your hands shows weakness of the shoulder muscles.

Lordosis is marked in muscular dystrophy and rickets.

Objective Data

Normal Range of Findings	Abnormal Findings

Legs and Feet. Anteriorly, note the leg position. A "bowlegged" stance *(genu varum)* is a lateral bowing of the legs (Fig. 22-50, *A*). It is present when you measure a persistent space of more than 2.5 cm between the knees when the medial malleoli are together. Genu varum is normal for 1 year after the child begins to walk. The child may walk with a waddling gait. This resolves with growth; no treatment is indicated.

Genu varum also occurs in rickets.

"Knock knees" *(genu valgum)* are present when there is a span of more than 2.5 cm between the medial malleoli when the knees are together (Fig. 22-50, *B*). It occurs normally between 2 and 3½ years of age. Also, treatment is not indicated. (Note: To remember the two conditions, remember to link the r's and g's: genu va**r**um—knees apa**r**t; genu val**g**um—knees to**g**ether.)

Genu valgum also occurs in rickets, poliomyelitis, and syphilis.

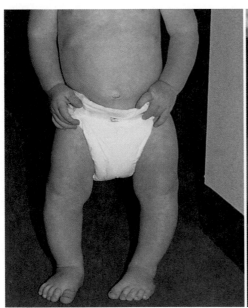 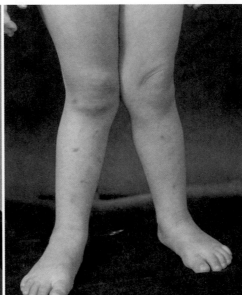

Fig. 22-50   A, Genu varum.   B, Genu valgum.

Often, parents tell you they are concerned about the child's foot development. The most common questions are about "flatfeet" and "pigeon toes." Flatfoot *(pes planus)* is pronation, or turning in, of the medial side of the foot. The young child may look flatfooted because the normal longitudinal arch is concealed by a fat pad until age 3 years. When standing begins, the child takes a broad-based stance, which causes pronation. Thus pronation is common between 12 and 30 months. You can see it best from behind the child, where the medial side of the foot drops down and in.

Pronation beyond 30 months.

Pigeon toes, or toeing in, are demonstrated when the child tends to walk on the lateral side of the foot, and the longitudinal arch looks higher than normal. It often starts as a forefoot adduction, which usually corrects spontaneously by age 3 years, as long as the foot is flexible.

Toeing in from forefoot adduction that is fixed, or lasts beyond age 3 years.
Toeing in from tibial torsion.

Normal Range of Findings

Check the child's gait while walking away from and toward you. Let the child wear socks because a cold tile floor will distort the usual gait. From 1 to 2 years of age, expect a broad-based gait, with arms out for balance. Weight-bearing falls on the inside of the foot. From 3 years of age, the base narrows and the arms are kept closer to the sides. Inspect the shoes for spots of greatest wear to aid your judgement of the gait. Normally the shoes wear more on the outside of the heel and the inside of the toe.

Check **Trendelenburg's sign** to screen progressive subluxation of the hip (Fig. 22-51). Watching from behind, ask the child to stand on one leg, then the other. Note the iliac crests; they should stay level when weight is shifted.

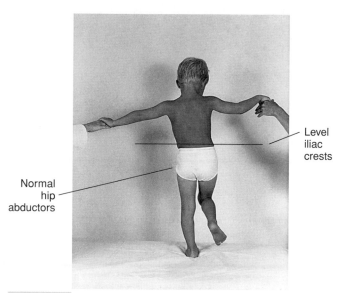

Normal hip abductors

Level iliac crests

Fig. 22-51

The child may sit for the remainder of the examination. Start with the feet and hands of the child from 2 to 6 years of age because the child is happy to show these off, and proceed through the examination as described earlier.

Particularly, check the arm for full ROM and presence of pain. Look for subluxation of the elbow (head of the radius). This occurs most often between 2 and 4 years of age as a result of forceful removal of clothing or dangling while adults suspend the child by the hands.

Palpate the bones, joints, and muscles of the extremities as described in the adult examination.

Abnormal Findings

Limp, usually caused by trauma, fatigue, or hip disease.

Abnormal gait patterns (see Chapter 23).

The sign occurs with severe subluxation of one hip. When the child stands on the good leg, the pelvis looks level. When the child stands on the affected leg, the pelvis drops toward the "good" side.

Inability to supinate the hand while the arm is flexed, together with pain in elbow, indicates subluxation of the head of the radius.

Pain or tenderness in extremities is usually caused by trauma or infection.

Fractures are usually due to trauma and are exhibited as an inability to use the area, a deformity, or an excess motion in the involved bone with pain and crepitation.

Enlargement of the tibial tubercles with tenderness suggests Osgood-Schlatter disease (see Table 22-6, p. 647).

Objective Data

Normal Range of Findings	Abnormal Findings

Adolescents

Proceed with musculoskeletal examination as with for the adult, with special attention to spinal posture. Kyphosis is common during adolescence because of chronic poor posture. Be aware of the risk of sports-related injuries with the adolescent because sports participation and competition often peak in this age group.

The Canadian Task Force on Preventive Health Care (Goldbloom, 1994) concluded that there was insufficient evidence to recommend the routine screening of asymptomatic adolescents for idiopathic scoliosis; however, periodic visual inspection of the backs of adolescents seen for other reasons is reasonable.

Inspect for scoliosis with the *forward bend test* (Fig. 22-52). Seat yourself behind the standing child, and ask the child to stand with the feet shoulder-width apart, and bend forward slowly to touch the toes. Expect a straight vertical spine while standing and also while bending forward. Posterior ribs should be symmetrical, with equal elevation of shoulders, scapulae, and iliac crests. You may wish to mark each spinous process with a felt marker. The lineup of ink dots highlights even a subtle curve.

Scoliosis is most apparent during the preadolescent growth spurt. Asymmetry suggests scoliosis—ribs hump up on one side as child bends forward, and with unequal landmark elevation (see Table 22-8, p. 650).

Objective Data

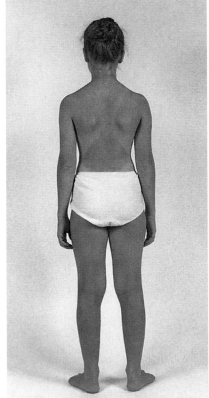
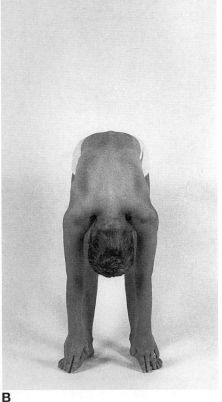

A   **B**

Fig. 22-52

Normal Range of Findings	Abnormal Findings

The Pregnant Female

Proceed through the examination described in the adult section. Expected postural changes in pregnancy include progressive lordosis and, toward the third trimester, anterior cervical flexion, kyphosis, and slumped shoulders (Fig. 22-53, *A*). At full term, the protuberant abdomen and the relaxed mobility in the joints create the characteristic "waddling" gait (Fig. 22-53, *B*).

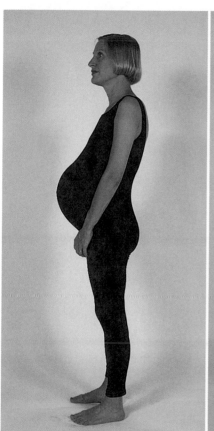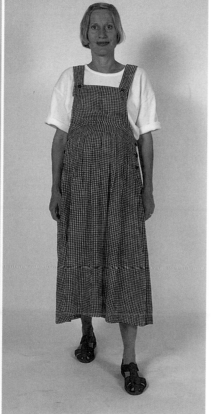

A   **B**

Fig. 22-53

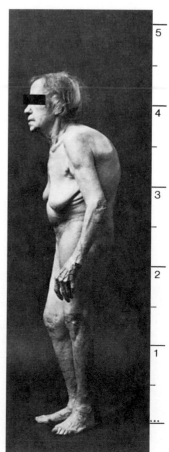

Fig. 22-54

The Aging Adult

Postural changes include a decrease in height, more apparent in the eighth and ninth decades (Fig. 22-54). "Lengthening of the arm–trunk axis" describes this shortening of the trunk with comparatively long extremities. Kyphosis is common, with a backward head tilt to compensate. This creates the outline of a figure "3" when you view this older adult from the left side. Slight flexion of hips and knees is also common.

Objective Data

Normal Range of Findings	Abnormal Findings

Contour changes include a decrease of fat in the body periphery and fat deposition over the abdomen and hips. The bony prominences become more marked.

With most older adults, ROM testing is done as described earlier. ROM and muscle strength are much the same as with the younger adult, provided no musculoskeletal illnesses or arthritic changes are present.

Functional Assessment. In the case of those with advanced aging changes, arthritic changes, or musculoskeletal disability, perform a **functional assessment for ADLs.** This applies the ROM and muscle strength assessments to the accomplishment of specific activities. You need to determine adequate and safe performance of functions essential for independent home life. See Chapter 30 for further assessments.

INSTRUCTIONS TO PERSON	COMMON ADAPTATION FOR AGING CHANGES
1. Walk (with shoes on).	Shuffling pattern; swaying; arms out to help balance; broader base of support; person may watch feet.
2. Climb up stairs.	Person holds onto hand rail; may haul body up with it; may lead with favoured (stronger) leg.
3. Walk down stairs.	Holds hand rail, sometimes with both hands. If the person is weak, he or she may descend sideways, lowering the weaker leg first. If the person is unsteady, he or she may watch feet.
4. Pick up object from floor.	Person often bends at waist instead of bending knees; holds onto furniture for support while bending or straightening.
5. Rise up from sitting in chair.	Person uses arms to push off chair arms, upper trunk leans forward before body straightens, feet planted wide in broad base of support.
6. Rise up from lying in bed.	May roll to one side, push with arms to lift up torso, grab bedside table to increase leverage.

Summary Checklist: Musculoskeletal Examination

 For a PDA-downloadable version, go to http://evolve.elsevier.com/Canada/Jarvis/examination/.

For each joint to be examined:
1. **Inspection**
   Size and contour of joint
   Skin colour and characteristics
2. **Palpation of joint area**
   Skin
   Muscles

Bony articulations
Joint capsule
3. **ROM**
   Active
   Passive (if limitation in active ROM is present)

Measure with goniometer (if abnormality in ROM is present)
4. **Muscle testing**

Promoting Health: Preventing Osteoporosis

Don't Overlook Osteoporosis

Bone is a living tissue that continually grows and changes. Every day old bone dissolves and is replaced with new, stronger bone. Up until a person is 30 years old, new bone appears at a faster rate than the bone disappears. But as we age, the opposite begins to occur. When this happens, bones can become "spongy," weak, and more likely to break with even the slightest of twists or bumps. This condition is called osteoporosis. The bones of the wrist, hip, and spine are most often affected.

Osteoporosis is more common in women than in men and more common in individuals of European descent. It has been estimated that one in four women and one in eight men in Canada have osteoporosis. Postmenopausal women are especially vulnerable because of hormonal changes. Further, osteoporosis occurs more often in slender people. It tends to run in families, but lifestyle choices can increase the risk of osteoporosis even in individuals without a family history. A person whose calcium intake is low, lacks exercise, smokes, or consumes alcohol is at higher risk for developing osteoporosis.

Osteoporosis Canada (Brown et al., 2002) recommends that all women older than 50 be assessed for the presence of risk factors for osteoporosis. Bone mineral density (BMD) testing is used to diagnose osteoporosis and predict fracture risk. BMD is recommended for all women age 65 and older; for those who have had a fragility fracture after age 40 (including wrist, vertebral, and hip fractures); for those with a family history of osteoporotic fracture (especially maternal hip fracture); and for those who have been on systemic glucocorticoid therapy >3 months.

Prevention of osteoporosis is important because there is no cure, only treatment for osteoporosis. The gold standard for treatment of osteoporosis has traditionally been hormone replacement therapy (HRT), which has been shown to prevent bone loss and to improve bone mineralization. However, new research indicates that HRT may carry an increased risk for breast cancer and myocardial infarction in women. Alternative therapies that include exercise and diet provide similar, if not equal, benefits for women who are at risk for osteoporosis.

Recommendations for Bone Health

1. **DIET.** The bottom line is that you need the daily recommended amounts of calcium and vitamin D.
    a. **Drink milk.** Low-fat and skim milk, nonfat yogurt, and reduced-fat cheese are healthy sources of calcium. Fortified milk products also contain vitamin D, which is needed to absorb calcium.
    b. **Go fish.** Salmon and sardines, which are canned with their bones, are also rich in calcium. Also, oily fish such as mackerel are rich in vitamin D.
    c. **Eat greens with gusto.** Leafy green vegetables have a lot of calcium. Fill up on broccoli, kale, Swiss chard, turnip greens, and bok choy. In addition to the calcium, you will also get the benefits of potassium and vitamin K, which help block calcium loss from bones.
    d. **Try soy.** Soy contains calcium and plant estrogens. Try substituting soy flour for regular flour in recipes, nibbling on soybean "nuts," or drinking soy milk.
    e. **Limit caffeine.** Caffeine causes the body to excrete calcium more readily. Caffeine is present in coffee, tea, hot chocolate, and many types of pop (e.g., cola).
    f. **Eat onions.** Although onions are not known to have any nutritive value, they appear to reduce the bone breakdown process that can lead to osteoporosis.

2. **EXERCISE.** The key here is to participate in weight-bearing activities. Your bones and muscles must work against gravity to have a bone-building effect. A regular program of weight-bearing exercise for at least 30 minutes three times a week is recommended as the minimum. Try walking, low-impact aerobics, dancing, or stationary cycling. The bonus: by improving your posture, balance, and flexibility, exercise also reduces your risk of falls. Do not forget sunshine either. Sunshine helps the body produce vitamin D. About 15 minutes of exposure to sunshine a day is all that is needed to maintain a good vitamin D supply.

3. **LIFESTYLE.** Avoid smoking and excessive alcohol, and seek help for depression. Smokers have twice the risk of spinal and hip fractures. Further, fractures heal more slowly in smokers and are more apt to heal improperly. Too much alcohol prevents your body from absorbing calcium. And do not let depression linger. Seek help. Research has shown that women with clinical depression have lower bone densities.

4. **MEDICAL OPTIONS.** Talk to your healthcare professional about bone health. Although many people consider osteoporosis prevention to be important, less than half discuss the topic with healthcare professionals or undergo bone density screening. Ask that your height be measured on an annual basis. A loss of 2 to 5 cm is an early sign of undiagnosed vertebral fractures and osteoporosis. Seek treatment for those conditions that can jeopardize bone density, including thyroid disease, certain intestinal and kidney diseases, and some cancers. Also, remember that some medications may contribute to bone loss, for example, corticosteroids, anticoagulants, thyroid supplements, and certain anticonvulsants.

5. **SUPPLEMENTS.** When appropriate, take supplemental calcium. Adults need 1000 mg of elemental calcium a day during their middle-age years. The need rises to 1500 to 2000 mg daily after menopause in women and after age 65 years in men. Most people do not get enough calcium in their diets, and supplements may help make up the difference. Make sure the supplement contains vitamin D, which helps your body absorb the calcium. The recommended daily dose of vitamin D is 800 IU for individuals aged 50 and older.

Objective Data

◈—— DOCUMENTATION AND CRITICAL THINKING ——◈

Sample Charting

SUBJECTIVE

Reports no joint pain, stiffness, swelling, or limitation. No muscle pain or weakness. No history of bone trauma or deformity. Able to manage all usual daily activities with no physical limitations. Occupation involves no musculoskeletal risk factors. Exercise pattern is brisk walk 1½ km (1 mile) 5×/week.

OBJECTIVE

Joints and muscles symmetrical; no swelling, masses, deformity; normal spinal curvature. No tenderness to palpation of joints; no heat, swelling, or masses. Full ROM; movement smooth, no crepitance, no tenderness. Muscle strength—able to maintain flexion against resistance and without tenderness.

ASSESSMENT

Muscles and joints—healthy and functional

Focused Assessment: Clinical Case Study

M.T. is a 45-year-old female salesperson with a diagnosis of rheumatoid arthritis 3 years PTA, who seeks care now for "swelling and burning pain in my hands" for 1 day.

SUBJECTIVE

- M.T. was diagnosed as having rheumatoid arthritis at age 41 years by staff at this agency. Since that time, her "flare-ups" seem to come every 6 to 8 months. Acute episodes involve hand joints and are treated with aspirin, which gives relief. Typically experiences morning stiffness, lasting ½ to 1 hour. Joints feel warm, swollen, tender. Has had weight loss of 7 kg (15 lb) over last 4 years and feels fatigued much of the time. States should rest more, but "I can't take the time." Daily exercises have been prescribed but does not do them regularly. Takes aspirin for acute flare-ups, feels better in a few days, decreases dose herself.

OBJECTIVE

Body joints within normal limits with exception of joints of wrist and hands. Radiocarpal, metacarpophalangeal, and proximal interphalangeal joints are red, swollen, tender to palpation. Spindle-shaped swelling of proximal interphalangeal joints of third digit right hand and second digit left hand; ulnar deviation of metacarpophalangeal joints.

ASSESSMENT

Acute pain R/T inflammation
Impaired physical mobility R/T inflammation
Deficient knowledge about aspirin treatment R/T lack of exposure
Noncompliance with exercise program R/T lack of perceived benefits of treatment
Noncompliance with advised rest periods R/T lack of perceived benefits of treatment

Nursing Diagnoses Commonly Associated With Musculoskeletal Disorders

All nursing diagnoses can be found on the Evolve Web site at **http://evolve.elsevier.com/Canada/Jarvis/examination/.**

ABNORMAL FINDINGS
FOR ADVANCED PRACTICE

TABLE 22-2	Abnormalities Affecting Multiple Joints

INFLAMMATORY CONDITIONS

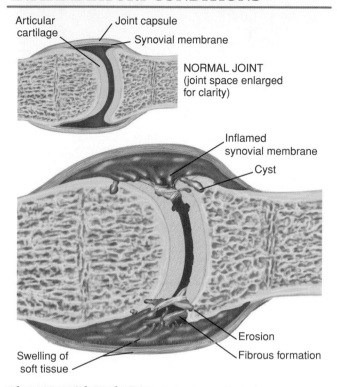

Rheumatoid Arthritis

This is a chronic, systemic inflammatory disease of joints and surrounding connective tissue. Inflammation of synovial membrane leads to thickening; then to fibrosis, which limits motion, and finally to bony ankylosis. The disorder is symmetrical and bilateral and is characterized by heat, redness, swelling, and painful motion of the affected joints. Rheumatoid arthritis (RA) is associated with fatigue, weakness, anorexia, weight loss, low-grade fever, and lymphadenopathy. Associated signs are described in the following tables, especially Table 22-5, p. 644.

Ankylosing Spondylitis (not illustrated)

Chronic progressive inflammation of spine, sacroiliac, and larger joints of the extremities, leading to bony ankylosis and deformity. A form of RA, this affects primarily men by a 10:1 ratio, in late adolescence or early adulthood. Spasm of paraspinal muscles pulls spine into forward flexion, obliterating cervical and lumbar curves. Thoracic curve exaggerated into single kyphotic rounding. Also includes flexion deformities of hips and knees.

DEGENERATIVE CONDITIONS

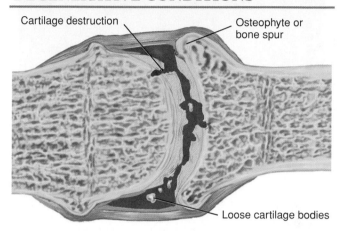

Osteoarthritis (Degenerative Joint Disease)

Noninflammatory, localized, progressive disorder involving deterioration of articular cartilages and subchondral bone and formation of new bone (osteophytes) at joint surfaces. Aging increases incidence; nearly all adults over 60 years old show some signs of osteoarthritis on X-ray. Asymmetrical joint involvement commonly affects hands, knees, hips, and lumbar and cervical segments of the spine. Affected joints have stiffness, swelling with hard, bony protuberances, pain with motion, and limitation of motion (see Table 22-5, p. 644).

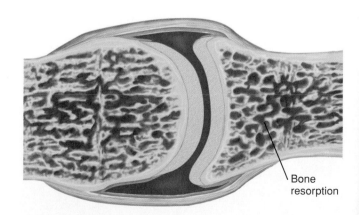

Osteoporosis

Decrease in skeletal bone mass occurring when rate of bone resorption is greater than that of bone formation. The weakened bone state increases risk for stress fractures, especially at wrist, hip, and vertebrae. Occurs primarily in postmenopausal White women. Osteoporosis risk also is associated with smaller height and weight, younger age at menopause, lack of physical activity, and lack of estrogen replacement therapy.

TABLE 22-3	Abnormalities of the Shoulder

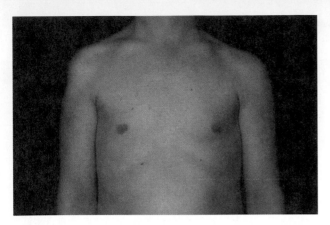

Atrophy

Loss of muscle mass is exhibited as a lack of fullness surrounding the deltoid muscle. In this case, atrophy is due to axillary nerve palsy. Atrophy also occurs from disuse, muscle tissue damage, or motor nerve damage.

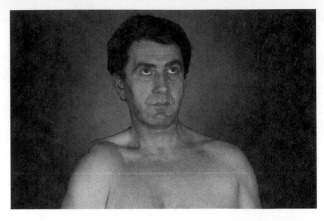

Dislocated Shoulder

Anterior dislocation (95%) is exhibited when hunching the shoulder forward and the tip of the clavicle dislocates. It occurs with trauma involving abduction, extension, and rotation (e.g., falling on an outstretched arm or diving into a pool).

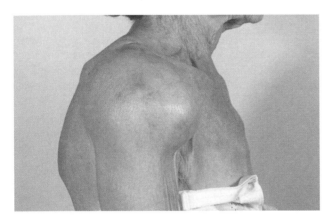

Joint Effusion

Swelling from excess fluid in the joint capsule, here from rheumatoid arthritis. Best observed anteriorly. Fluctuant on palpation. Considerable fluid must be present to cause a visible distension because the capsule normally is loose.

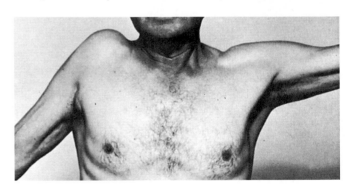

Tear of Rotator Cuff

Characteristic "hunched" position and limited abduction of arm. Occurs from traumatic adduction while arm is held in abduction, or from fall on shoulder, throwing, or heavy lifting. Positive drop arm test: if the arm is passively abducted at the shoulder, the person is unable to sustain the position and the arm falls to the side.

◀ Frozen Shoulder—Adhesive Capsulitis

Fibrous tissues form in the joint capsule, causing stiffness, progressive limitation of motion, and pain. Motion limited in abduction and external rotation; unable to reach overhead. It may lead to atrophy of shoulder girdle muscles. Gradual onset; unknown cause. It is associated with prolonged bed rest or shoulder immobility. May resolve spontaneously.

Subacromial Bursitis (not illustrated)

Inflammation and swelling of subacromial bursa over the shoulder cause limited range of motion and pain with motion. Localized swelling under deltoid muscle may increase by partial passive abduction of the arm. Caused by direct trauma, strain during sports, local or systemic inflammatory process, or repetitive motion injury.

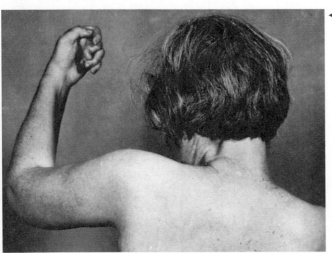

TABLE 22-4 | Abnormalities of the Elbow

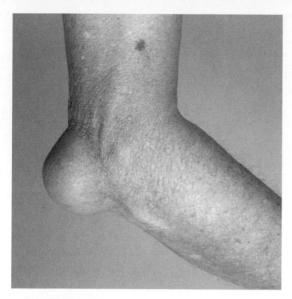

Olecranon Bursitis

Large soft knob, or "goose egg," and redness from inflammation of olecranon bursa. Localized and easy to see because bursa lies just under skin.

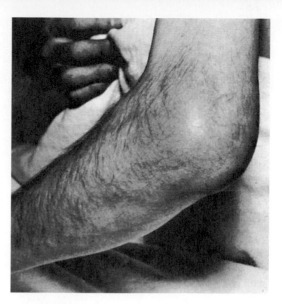

Gouty Arthritis

Joint effusion or synovial thickening, seen first as bulge or fullness in grooves on either side of olecranon process. Redness and heat can extend beyond area of synovial membrane. Soft, boggy, or fluctuant fullness to palpation. Limited extension of elbow.

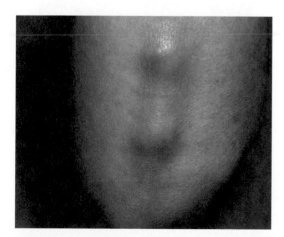

Subcutaneous Nodules

Raised, firm, nontender nodules that occur with rheumatoid arthritis. Common sites are in the olecranon bursa and along extensor surface of arm. The skin slides freely over the nodules.

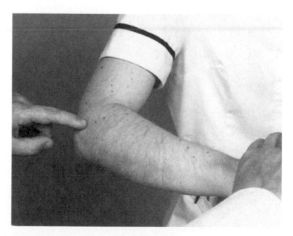

Epicondylitis—Tennis Elbow

Chronic disabling pain at lateral epicondyle of humerus, radiates down extensor surface of forearm. Pain can be located by touching with one finger. Resisting extension of the hand will increase the pain. Occurs with activities combining excessive pronation and supination of forearm with an extended wrist (e.g., racket sports or using a screwdriver).

Medial epicondylitis is rarer and is due to activity of forced palmar flexion of wrist against resistance.

TABLE 22-5	Abnormalities of the Wrist and Hand

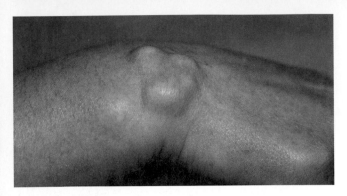

Ganglion Cyst

Round, cystic, nontender nodule overlying a tendon sheath or joint capsule, usually on dorsum of wrist. Flexion makes it more prominent. A common benign tumour; it does not become malignant.

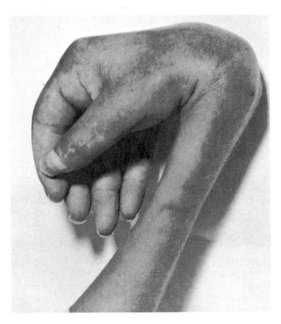

Ankylosis

Wrist in extreme flexion, due to severe rheumatoid arthritis. This is a functionally useless hand because when the wrist is palmar flexed, a good deal of power is lost from the fingers, and the thumb cannot oppose the fingers.

Colles' Fracture (not illustrated)

Nonarticular fracture of distal radius, with or without fracture of ulna at styloid process. Usually from a fall on an outstretched hand; occurs more often in older women. Wrist looks puffy, with "silver fork" deformity, a characteristic hump when viewed from the side.

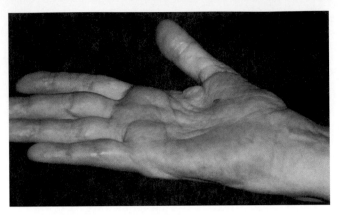

Carpal Tunnel Syndrome with Atrophy of Thenar Eminence

Atrophy occurs from interference with motor function due to compression of the median nerve inside the carpal tunnel. Caused by chronic repetitive motion; occurs between 30 and 60 years of age and is five times more common in women than in men. Symptoms of carpal tunnel syndrome include pain, burning and numbness, positive findings on Phalen's test, positive indication of Tinel's sign, and often atrophy of thenar muscles.

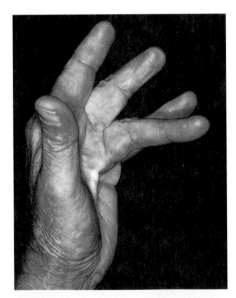

Dupuytren's Contracture

Chronic hyperplasia of the palmar fascia causes flexion contractures of the digits, first in the fourth digit, then the fifth digit, and then the third digit. Note the bands that extend from the midpalm to the digits and the puckering of palmar skin. The condition occurs commonly in men past 40 years of age and is usually bilateral. It occurs with diabetes, epilepsy, and alcoholic liver disease and as an inherited trait. The contracture is painless but impairs hand function.

TABLE 22-5 | Abnormalities of the Wrist and Hand—cont'd

CONDITIONS CAUSED BY CHRONIC RHEUMATOID ARTHRITIS

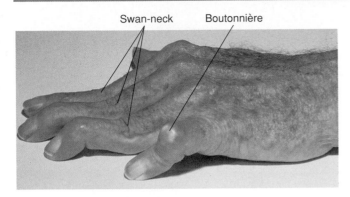

Swan-neck   Boutonnière

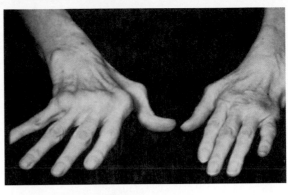

Swan-Neck and Boutonnière Deformity

Flexion contracture resembles curve of a **swan's neck.** Note flexion contracture of metacarpophalangeal joint, then hyperextension of the proximal interphalangeal joint, and flexion of the distal interphalangeal joint. It occurs with chronic rheumatoid arthritis and is often accompanied by ulnar drift of the fingers.

In **boutonnière deformity**, the knuckle looks as if it is being pushed through a buttonhole. It is a relatively common deformity and includes flexion of proximal interphalangeal joint with compensatory hyperextension of distal interphalangeal joint.

Reprinted from the Clinical Slide Collection on the Rheumatic Diseases, © 1991, 1995, 1997. Used by permission of the American College of Rheumatology.

Ulnar Deviation or Drift

Fingers drift to the ulnar side because of stretching of the articular capsule and muscle imbalance. Also note subluxation and swelling in the joints and muscle atrophy on the dorsa of the hands. This is caused by chronic rheumatoid arthritis.

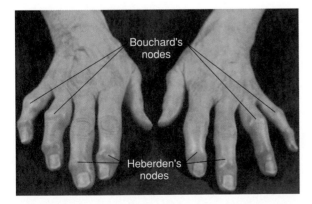

Bouchard's nodes

Heberden's nodes

Degenerative Joint Disease or Osteoarthritis

Osteoarthritis is characterized by hard, nontender nodules, 2 to 3 mm or more. These osteophytes (bony overgrowths) of the distal interphalangeal joints are called Heberden's nodes, and those of the proximal interphalangeal joints are called Bouchard's nodes.

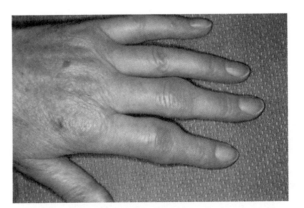

Acute Rheumatoid Arthritis

Painful swelling and stiffness of joints, with fusiform or spindle-shaped swelling of the soft tissue of proximal interphalangeal joints. Fusiform swelling is usually symmetrical, the hands are warm, and the veins are engorged. The inflamed joints have a limited range of motion.

Continued

Abnormal Findings

TABLE 22-5	Abnormalities of the Wrist and Hand—cont'd

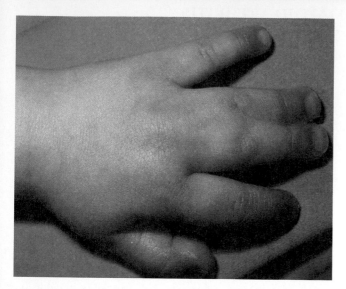

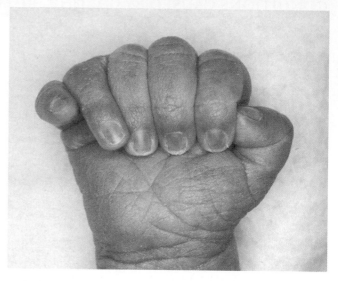

Syndactyly

Webbed fingers are a congenital deformity, usually requiring surgical separation. The metacarpals and phalanges of the webbed fingers are different lengths, and the joints do not line up. Not correcting fused fingers would therefore limit their flexion and extension.

Polydactyly

Extra digits are a congenital deformity, usually occurring at the fifth finger or the thumb. Surgical removal is considered for cosmetic reasons. The sixth finger shown here was not removed because it had full ROM and sensation and a normal appearance.

TABLE 22-6   Abnormalities of the Knee

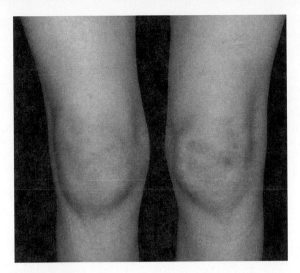

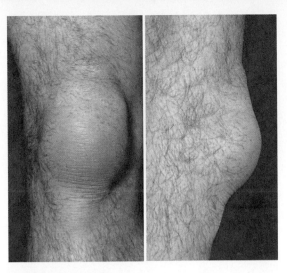

Mild Synovitis

Loss of normal hollows on either side of the patella, which are replaced by mild distension. Occurs with synovial thickening or effusion (excess fluid). Also note mild distension of the suprapatellar pouch.

Prepatellar Bursitis

Localized swelling on anterior knee between patella and skin. A tender fluctuant mass indicates swelling; in some cases, infection spreads to surrounding soft tissue. The condition is limited to the bursa, and the knee joint itself is not involved. Overlying skin may be red, shiny, atrophic, or coarse and thickened.

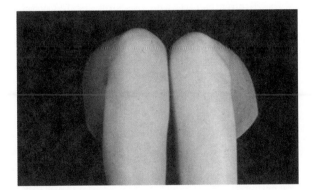

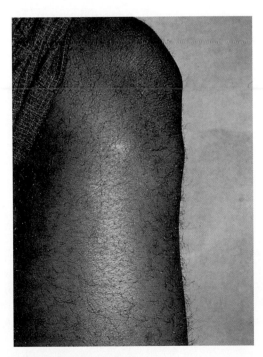

Swelling of Menisci

Localized soft swelling from cyst in lateral meniscus shows at the midpoint of the anterolateral joint line. Semiflexion of the knee makes swelling more prominent.

Osgood-Schlatter Disease

Painful swelling of the tibial tubercle just below the knee, probably from repeated stress on the patellar tendon. Occurs mostly in puberty during rapid growth and most often in males. Pain increases with kicking, running, bicycling, stair climbing, or kneeling. The condition is usually self-limited, and symptoms resolve with rest.

Chondromalacia Patellae (not illustrated)

Degeneration of articular surface of patellae. The condition occurs most often in females, and its cause is unknown. May produce mild effusion. Joint motion is painless, but crepitus may be present. Kneeling causes onset of pain.

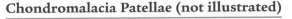

TABLE 22-7   **Abnormalities of the Ankle and Foot**

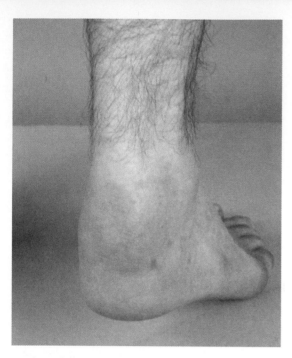

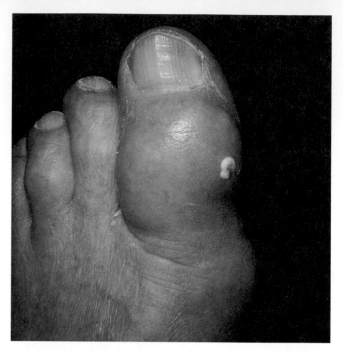

Achilles Tenosynovitis

Inflammation of a tendon sheath near the ankle (here, the Achilles tendon) produces a superficial linear swelling and a localized tenderness along the route of the sheath. Movement of the involved tendon usually causes pain.

Tophi With Chronic Gout

Hard, painless nodule (tophi) over metatarsophalangeal joint of first toe. Tophi are collections of sodium urate crystals due to chronic gout in and around the joint that cause extreme swelling and joint deformity. They sometimes burst with a chalky discharge.

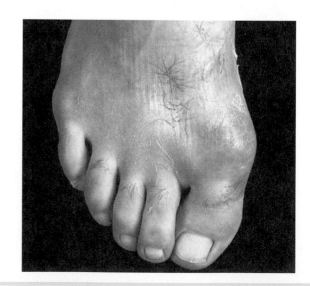

Acute Gout   ▶

Acute episode of gout usually involves first the metatarsophalangeal joint. Clinical findings consist of redness, swelling, heat, and extreme tenderness. Gout is a metabolic disorder of disturbed purine metabolism, associated with elevated serum uric acid. It occurs primarily in men over 40 years of age.

TABLE 22-7	Abnormalities of the Ankle and Foot—cont'd

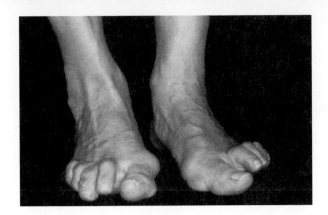

◄ Hallux Valgus With Bunion and Hammertoes

Hallux valgus is a common deformity from rheumatoid arthritis. It is a lateral or outward deviation of the great toe with medial prominence of the head of the first metatarsal. The **bunion** is the inflamed bursa that forms at the pressure point. The great toe loses power to push off while walking; this stresses the second and third metatarsal heads, and they develop calluses and pain. Chronic sequelae include corns, calluses, hammertoes, and joint subluxation.

Note the **hammertoe** deformities in the second, third, fourth, and fifth toes. Often associated with hallux valgus, hammertoe includes hyperextension of the metatarsophalangeal joint and flexion of the proximal interphalangeal joint.

Corns (thickening of soft tissue) develop on the dorsum over the bony prominence from prolonged pressure from shoes.

Callus (not illustrated)

Hypertrophy of the epithelium develops because of prolonged pressure, commonly on the plantar surface of the first metatarsal head in the hallux valgus deformity. The condition is not painful.

Plantar Wart (not illustrated)

Vascular papillomatous growth is probably due to a virus and occurs on the sole of the foot, commonly at the ball. The condition is extremely painful.

Ingrown Toenail (not illustrated)

A misnomer; the nail does not grow in, but the soft tissue grows over the nail and obliterates the groove. It occurs almost always on the great toe on the medial or lateral side. It is due to trimming the nail too short or toe-crowding in tight shoes. The area becomes infected when the nail grows and its corner penetrates the soft tissue.

Abnormal Findings

TABLE 22-8	Abnormalities of the Spine

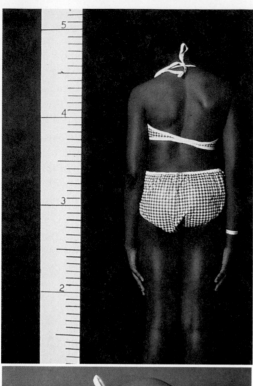

◀ **Scoliosis**

Lateral curvature of thoracic and lumbar segments of the spine, usually with some rotation of involved vertebral bodies.

Functional scoliosis is flexible; it is apparent on standing and disappears on forward bending. It may be compensatory for other abnormalities such as leg length discrepancy.

Structural scoliosis is fixed; the curvature shows both on standing and on bending forward. Note rib hump with forward flexion. When the person is standing, note unequal shoulder elevation, unequal scapulae, obvious curvature, and unequal hip level. At greatest risk are females 10 years of age through adolescence, during the peak of the growth spurt.

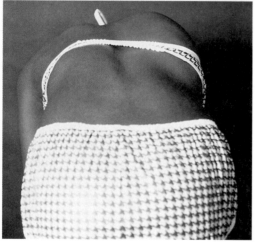

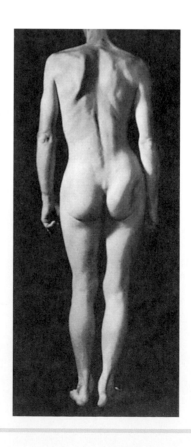

Herniated Nucleus Pulposus   ▶

The nucleus pulposus (at the centre of the intervertebral disc) ruptures into the spinal canal and puts pressure on the local spinal nerve root. Usually occurs from stress, such as lifting, twisting, continuous flexion with lifting, or fall on buttocks. Occurs mostly in men 20 to 45 years of age. Lumbar herniations occur mainly in interspaces L4 to L5 and L5 to S1. Note sciatic pain, numbness, and paresthesia of involved dermatome; listing away from affected side; decreased mobility; low back tenderness; and decreased motor and sensory function in leg. Straight leg raising tests reproduce sciatic pain.

TABLE 22-9 | **Common Congenital or Pediatric Abnormalities**

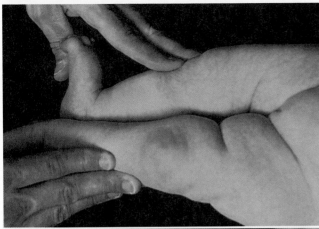

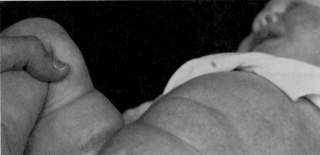

◄ Congenital Dislocated Hip

Head of the femur is displaced out of the cup-shaped acetabulum.

The degree of the condition varies; subluxation may occur as stretched ligaments allow partial displacement of femoral head, and acetabular dysplasia may develop because of excessive laxity of hip joint capsule.

Occurrence is 1:500 to 1:1000 births; common in girls at 7:1 ratio. Signs include limited abduction of flexed thigh, positive indications of Ortolani and Barlow's signs, asymmetrical skin creases or gluteal folds, limb length discrepancy, and positive indication of Trendelenburg's sign in older children.

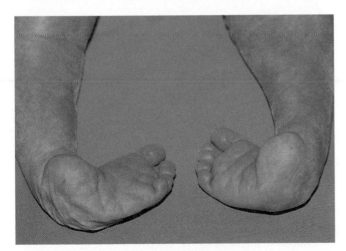

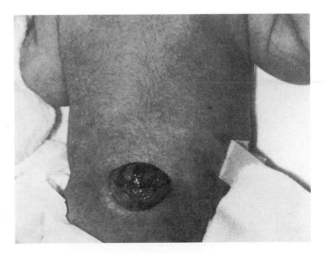

Talipes Equinovarus (Clubfoot)

Congenital, rigid, and fixed malposition of foot, including (1) inversion, (2) forefoot adduction, and (3) foot pointing downward (equinus). A common birth defect, with an incidence of 1:1000 to 3:1000 live births. Males are affected twice as frequently as females.

Spina Bifida

Incomplete closure of posterior part of vertebrae results in a neural tube defect. Seriousness varies from skin defect along the spine to protrusion of the sac containing meninges, spinal fluid, or malformed spinal cord. The most serious type is myelomeningocele (shown here), in which the meninges and neural tissue protrude. In these cases, the child is usually paralyzed below the level of the lesion.

Coxa Plana (Legg-Calvé-Perthes Syndrome) (not illustrated)

Avascular necrosis of the femoral head, occurring primarily in males between 3 and 12 years of age, peaking at age 6 years. In the initial inflammatory stage, interruption of blood supply to femoral epiphysis occurs, halting growth. Revascularization and healing occur later, but significant residual deformity and dysfunction may be present.

Abnormal Findings

BIBLIOGRAPHY

Arthritis Society. *Types of arthritis.* Retrieved January 10, 2008, from http://www.arthritis.ca/types%20of%20arthritis/default.asp?s=1

Austermuehle, P. (2001). Common knee injuries in primary care. *Nurse Practitioner, 26,* 26–47.

Beaupre, L. A., Johnston, D. B., Jones, C. A., Majumdar, S. R., Buckingham, J., & Saunders, D. L. *Integration of services for treatment of elderly patients with hip fracture.* Retrieved April 6, 2008, from http://www.ahfmr.ab.ca/grants/docs/state_of_science_reviews/Saunders_ES.pdf

Benton, M. J. & White, A. (2006). Osteoporosis: Recommendations for resistance exercise and supplementation with calcium and vitamin D to promote bone health. *Journal of Community Health Nursing, 23,* 201–211.

Brown, J. P., & Fortier, M. (2006). Canadian Consensus Conference on Osteoporosis, 2006 update. *Journal of Obstetrics and Gynaecology Canada, 172,* S95–S112.

Brown, J. P., & Josse, R. G., for the Scientific Advisory Council of the Osteoporosis Society of Canada. (2002). 2002 clinical practice guidelines for the diagnosis and management of osteoporosis in Canada. *Canadian Medical Association Journal, 167*(10 Suppl.), S1–S36.

Bruce, M., & Peck, B. (2005). New rheumatoid arthritis treatments. *Nurse Practitioner, 30,* 29–41.

Buckwalter, J. (2006). Arthralgia in women: Strategies for early diagnosis. *Journal of Musculoskeletal Medicine, 23,* 802–808.

Burton, S., & Lloyd, M. (2006). An overview of rheumatoid arthritis. *Nursing Standards, 20,* 46–49.

Buttke, J. (2005). Stepping up foot injury diagnosis. *Nurse Practitioner, 30,* 46–52.

Canadian Institute for Health Information. (2006). *Number of hip and knee replacements by age, Canada, 1994–1995 and 2004–2005.* Retrieved January 19, 2008, from http://secure.cihi.ca/cihiweb/dispPage.jsp?cw_page=indicators_e

Canadian Medical Association. (2008). *The economic cost of wait times in Canada.* Retrieved April 6, 2008, from http://www.cma.ca/multimedia/CMA/Content_Images/Inside_cma/Media_Release/pdf/2008/EconomicReport.pdf

Cline, M. G., Meredith, K. E., Boyer, J. T., & Burrows, B. (1989). Decline of height with age in adults in a general population sample: Estimating maximum height and distinguishing birth cohort effects from actual loss of stature with aging. *Human Biology, 61,* 415–425.

D'Arcy, Y. (2006). Treatment strategies for low back pain relief. *Nurse Practitioner, 31,* 16–27.

De Coster, C., McMillan, S., Brant, R., McGurran, J., & Noseworthy. (2007). The Western Canada Waiting List Project: Development of a priority referral score for hip and knee arthroplasty. *Journal of Evaluation in Clinical Practice, 13,* 192–197.

Dyer, E., & Heflin, M. (2005). Osteoarthritis: Its course in older patients and current treatment methods. *Clinical Geriatrics, 13,* 18–26.

Ebrahim, S., Thompson, P. W., Baskaran, V., & Evans, K. (1997). Randomized placebo-controlled trial of brisk walking in the prevention of postmenopausal osteoporosis. *Age and Aging, 26,* 253–260.

El Miedany, Y. (2006a). Rheumatoid arthritis: A challenge to the geriatrician, part one. *Geriatric Medicine, 36,* 37–42.

El Miedany, Y. (2006b). Rheumatoid arthritis: A challenge to the geriatrician, part two. *Geriatric Medicine, 36,* 83–87.

Evans, A., & Scutter, S. (2004). Prevalence of "growing pains" in young children. *Journal of Pediatrics, 145,* 255–258.

Felson, D. (2006). Osteoarthritis of the knee. *New England Journal of Medicine, 354,* 841–848.

Goldbloom, R. B. (1994). Screening for idiopathic adolescent scoliosis. In Canadian Task Force on the Periodic Health Examination (Eds.), *Canadian Guide to Clinical Preventive Health Care* (pp. 346–354). Ottawa, ON: Health Canada.

Gregg, E. W., Cauley, J. A., Seeley, D. G., Ensrud, K. E., & Bauer, D. C. (1998). Physical activity and osteoporotic fracture risk in older women. *Annals of Internal Medicine, 129,* 81–88.

Hallegua, D., & Wallace, D. (2005). Managing fibromyalgia: A comprehensive approach. *Journal of Musculoskeletal Medicine, 22,* 382–390.

Hanley, D. A., & Josse, R. G. (1996). Prevention and management of osteoporosis: Consensus statements from the Scientific Advisory Board of the Osteoporosis Society of Canada. *Canadian Medical Association Journal, 155,* 921–923.

Hart, L. (2005). Primary care for patients with neurofibromatosis 1. *Nurse Practitioner, 30,* 38–43.

Health Canada. (2003). *Arthritis in Canada: An ongoing challenge.* Ottawa, ON: Author.

Jackson, S. A., Tenenhouse, A., & Robertson, L., and the CaMos Study Group. (2000). Vertebral fracture definition from population-based data: preliminary results from the Canadian Multicentre Osteoporosis Study (CaMos). *Osteoporosis International, 11,* 680–687.

Katz, J., & Simmons, B. (2002). Carpal tunnel syndrome. *New England Journal of Medicine, 346,* 1807–1812.

Khan, A. A., Brown, J. P., Kendler, D. L., Leslie, W. D., Lentle, B. C., Lewiecki, E. M., et al. (2002). The 2002 Canadian bone densitometry recommendations: Take-home messages. *Canadian Medical Association Journal, 167,* 1141–1145.

Lentle, B. C., Brown, J. P., Khan, A., Leslie, W. D., Levesque, J., Lyons, D. J., et al. (2007). Recognizing and reporting vertebral fractures: Reducing the risk of future osteoporotic fractures. *Canadian Association of Radiologists Journal, 58*(1), 27–36.

McFarland, E., Sanguanjit, P., Tasaki, A., & Freehill, M. T. (2006). Common shoulder problems: A "hands-on" approach. *Consultant, 46,* 437–446.

Mochan, E. (2005). Rheumatoid arthritis: Clues to early diagnosis. *Consultant, 45,* 545–552.

Morehead, K., & Fye, K. (2005). Early diagnosis of RA: The therapeutic implications. *Journal of Musculoskeletal Medicine, 22,* 599–606.

Nelson, A., Fragala, G., & Menzel, N. (2003). Myths and facts about back injuries in nursing. *American Journal of Nursing, 103,* 32–41.

Olszynski, W. P., Davison, S., Adachi, J. D., Brown, J. P., Cummings, S. R., Hanley, D. A., et al. (2004). Osteoporosis in men: Epidemiology, diagnosis, prevention, and treatment. *Clinical Therapeutics, 26,* 1, 15–28.

Osteoporosis Canada. (2006). *Physical activity: An important factor in preventing osteoporosis.* Toronto, ON: Author.

Osteoporosis Canada. (2007a). *Men and osteoporosis: Not just a women's disease.* Toronto, ON: Author.

Osteoporosis Canada. (2007b). *Osteoporosis and osteoarthritis.* Toronto, ON: Author.

Papaioannou, A., Joseph, L., Ioannidis, G., Berger, C., Anastassiades, Brown, J. P., et al. (2005). Risk fractures associated with incident clinical vertebral and nonvertebral fractures in postmenopausal women: The Canadian Multicentre Osteoporosis Study (CaMos). *Osteoporosis International, 16,* 568–578.

Patel, H., with the Canadian Task Force on Preventive Health Care. (2001). Preventive health care, 2001 update: Screening and management of developmental dysplasia of the hip in newborns. *Canadian Medical Association Journal, 164,* 1669–1677.

Peschken, C. A., & Esdaile, J. M. (1999). Rheumatic diseases in North America's indigenous peoples. *Seminars in Arthritis and Rheumatism, 28,* 368–391.

Peterson, J. (2005). Fibromyalgia: Understanding and its treatment options. *Nurse Practitioner, 30,* 48–57.

Roodman, G. D. (2003). Recent developments in Paget's disease. *Advances in the Study of Medicine, 3,* 286–292.

Siminoski, K., Leslie, W. D., Frame, H., Hodsman, A., Josse, R. G., Khan, A., et al. (2005). Recommendations for bone mineral density reporting in Canada. *Canadian Association of Radiologists Journal, 56,* 178–188.

Taft, E., & Francis, R. (2003). Evaluation and management of scoliosis. *Journal of Pediatric Health Care, 17,* 42–44.

Tracey, E., Forte, T., Fagbemi, J., & Chaudhary, Z. (2007) Wait time for hip fracture surgery in Canada. *Healthcare Quarterly, 10,* 24–27.

U.S. Preventive Services Task Force. (2003). Screening for osteoporosis in postmenopausal women: Recommendations and rationale. *American Journal of Nursing, 103,* 73–81.

U.S. Preventive Services Task Force. (2005). Screening for idiopathic scoliosis in adolescents: Recommendation statement. *American Family Physician, 71,* 1975–1976.

Vallerand, A. (2003). Treating osteoarthritis pain. *Nurse Practitioner, 28,* 7–17.

Wilson, C. (2005). Rotator cuff versus cervical spine: Making the diagnosis. *Nurse Practitioner, 30,* 45–50.

Neurological System

Written by **Carolyn Jarvis**, PhD, APN, CNP
Adapted by **Annette J. Browne**, PhD, RN

Electronic Resources

On Evolve *evolve*

http://evolve.elsevier.com/Canada/Jarvis/examination
- Interactive Case Studies
- Physical Examination Audio and Printable Summaries
- Bedside Assessment Summary Checklists
- Complete Physical Examination Form
- Nursing Diagnoses Boxes
- Health Promotion Guides
- Quick Assessments for 20 Common Conditions
- Multiple Choice Review Questions
- Chapter Objectives
- Appendices
- Weblinks

On the Companion CD

- Interactive Case Studies with Heart and Lung Sounds
- Health Promotion Guides
- Quick Assessments for 20 Common Conditions
- Head-to-Toe Physical Examination Video Clips

STRUCTURE AND FUNCTION

The nervous system can be divided into two parts—central and peripheral. The **central nervous system** (CNS) includes the brain and spinal cord. The **peripheral nervous system** includes the 12 pairs of cranial nerves, the 31 pairs of spinal nerves, and all their branches. The peripheral nervous system carries sensory (**a**fferent) messages *to* the CNS from sensory receptors, motor (**e**fferent) messages *from* the CNS out to muscles and glands, and autonomic messages that govern the internal organs and blood vessels.

THE CENTRAL NERVOUS SYSTEM

Cerebral Cortex. The cerebral cortex is the cerebrum's outer layer of nerve cell bodies, which looks like "grey matter" because it lacks myelin. Myelin is the white insulation on the axon that increases the conduction velocity of nerve impulses.

The cerebral cortex is the centre for humans' highest functions, governing thought, memory, reasoning, sensation, and voluntary movement (Fig. 23-1). Each half of the cerebrum is a **hemisphere;** the left hemisphere is dominant in most (95%) people, including those who are left-handed.

Each hemisphere is divided into four **lobes:** frontal, parietal, temporal, and occipital. The lobes have certain areas that mediate specific functions.

- The **frontal** lobe has areas concerned with personality, behaviour, emotions, and intellectual function.
- The precentral gyrus of the frontal lobe initiates voluntary movement.
- The **parietal** lobe's postcentral gyrus is the primary centre for sensation.
- The **occipital** lobe is the primary visual receptor centre.
- The **temporal** lobe behind the ear has the primary auditory reception centre.
- **Wernicke's area** in the temporal lobe is associated with language comprehension. When damaged in the person's dominant hemisphere, *receptive aphasia* results. The person hears sound, but it has no meaning, like hearing a foreign language.
- **Broca's area** in the frontal lobe mediates motor speech. When injured in the dominant hemisphere, *expressive aphasia* results; the person cannot talk. The person can understand language and knows what he or she wants to say but can produce only a garbled sound.

Damage to any of these specific cortical areas produces a corresponding loss of function: motor weakness, paralysis, loss of sensation, or impaired ability to understand and process language. Damage occurs when the highly specialized neurological cells are deprived of their blood supply, such as

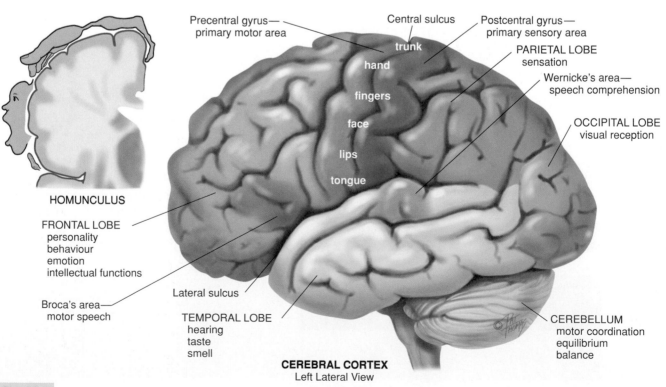

Precentral gyrus—
primary motor area

Central sulcus

Postcentral gyrus—
primary sensory area

trunk

hand

fingers

face

lips

tongue

PARIETAL LOBE
sensation

Wernicke's area—
speech comprehension

OCCIPITAL LOBE
visual reception

HOMUNCULUS

FRONTAL LOBE
personality
behaviour
emotion
intellectual functions

Broca's area—
motor speech

Lateral sulcus

TEMPORAL LOBE
hearing
taste
smell

CEREBELLUM
motor coordination
equilibrium
balance

CEREBRAL CORTEX
Left Lateral View

Fig. 23-1

© Pat Thomas, 2006.

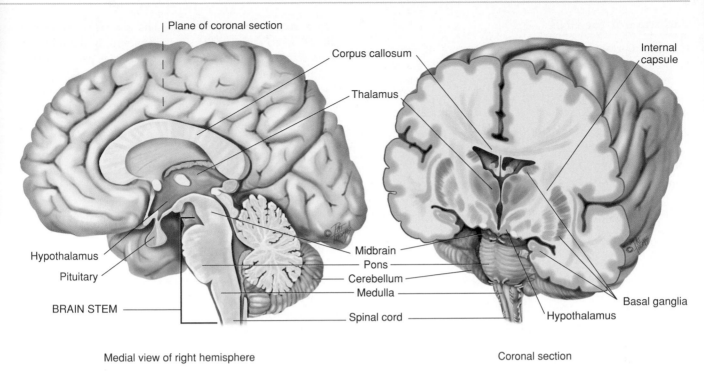

Medial view of right hemisphere

Coronal section

COMPONENTS OF THE CENTRAL NERVOUS SYSTEM

Fig. 23-2

© Pat Thomas, 2006.

when a cerebral artery becomes occluded or when vascular bleeding or vasospasm occurs.

Basal Ganglia. The basal ganglia are additional bands of grey matter buried deep within the two cerebral hemispheres that form the subcortical associated motor system (the extra-pyramidal system) (Fig. 23-2). They control automatic associated movements of the body, such as the arm swing alternating with the leg movement during walking.

Thalamus. The thalamus is the main relay station for the nervous system. Sensory pathways of the spinal cord and brain stem form **synapses** (sites of contact between two neurons) on their way to the cerebral cortex.

Hypothalamus. The hypothalamus is a major control centre with many vital functions: temperature, heart rate, and blood pressure controller; sleep centre, anterior and posterior pituitary gland regulator; and coordinator of autonomic nervous system activity and emotional status.

Cerebellum. The cerebellum is a coiled structure located under the occipital lobe that is concerned with motor coordination of voluntary movements, equilibrium (i.e., the postural balance of the body), and muscle tone. It does not initiate movement but coordinates and smooths it, such as the complex and quick coordination of many different muscles needed in playing the piano, swimming, or juggling. It is

like the "automatic pilot" on an airplane in that it adjusts and corrects the voluntary movements but operates entirely below the conscious level.

Brain Stem. The brain stem is the central core of the brain consisting of mostly nerve fibres. It has three areas:
1. **Midbrain**—the most anterior part of the brain stem that still has the basic tubular structure of the spinal cord. It merges into the thalamus and hypothalamus. It contains many motor neurons and tracts.
2. **Pons**—the enlarged area containing ascending and descending fibre tracts.
3. **Medulla**—the continuation of the spinal cord in the brain that contains all ascending and descending fibre tracts connecting the brain and spinal cord. It has vital autonomic centres (respiratory, cardiac, gastrointestinal functions), as well as nuclei for cranial nerves VIII through XII. Pyramidal decussation (crossing of the motor fibres) occurs here (see p. 657).

Spinal Cord. The spinal cord is the long cylindrical structure of nervous tissue about as big around as the little finger. It occupies the upper two thirds of the vertebral canal from the medulla to lumbar vertebrae L1 and L2. It is the main highway for ascending and descending fibre tracts that connect the brain to the spinal nerves, and it mediates reflexes. Its nerve cell bodies, or grey matter, are arranged in a butterfly shape with anterior and posterior "horns."

Pathways of the CNS

Crossed representation is a notable feature of the nerve tracts; the *left* cerebral cortex receives sensory information from and controls motor function to the *right* side of the body, whereas the *right* cerebral cortex interacts with the *left* side of the body. Knowledge of where the fibres cross the midline will help you interpret clinical findings.

Sensory Pathways

Millions of sensory receptors are embroidered into the skin, mucous membranes, muscles, tendons, and viscera. They monitor conscious sensations, internal organ functions, body positions, and reflexes. Sensation travels in the afferent fibres in the peripheral nerve, then through the posterior (dorsal) root, and then into the spinal cord. There, it may take one of two routes—the spinothalamic tract or the posterior (dorsal) columns (Fig. 23-3).

Spinothalamic Tract. The spinothalamic tract contains sensory fibres that transmit the sensations of pain, temperature, and crude or light touch (i.e., not precisely localized). The fibres enter the dorsal root of the spinal cord and synapse with a second sensory neuron. The second-order neuron fibres cross to the opposite side and ascend up the spinothalamic tract to the thalamus. Fibres carrying pain and temperature sensations ascend the *lateral* spinothalamic tract, whereas those of crude touch form the *anterior* spinothalamic tract. At the thalamus, the fibres synapse with a third sensory neuron, which carries the message to the sensory cortex for full interpretation.

Posterior (Dorsal) Columns. These fibres conduct the sensations of position, vibration, and finely localized touch.
- **Position** (proprioception)—without looking, you know where your body parts are in space and in relation to each other
- **Vibration**—feeling vibrating objects
- **Finely localized touch** (stereognosis)—without looking, you can identify familiar objects by touch

These fibres enter the dorsal root and proceed immediately up the same side of the spinal cord to the brain stem. At the medulla, they synapse with a second sensory neuron and then cross. They travel to the **thalamus**, synapse again, and proceed to the sensory cortex, which localizes the sensation and makes full discrimination.

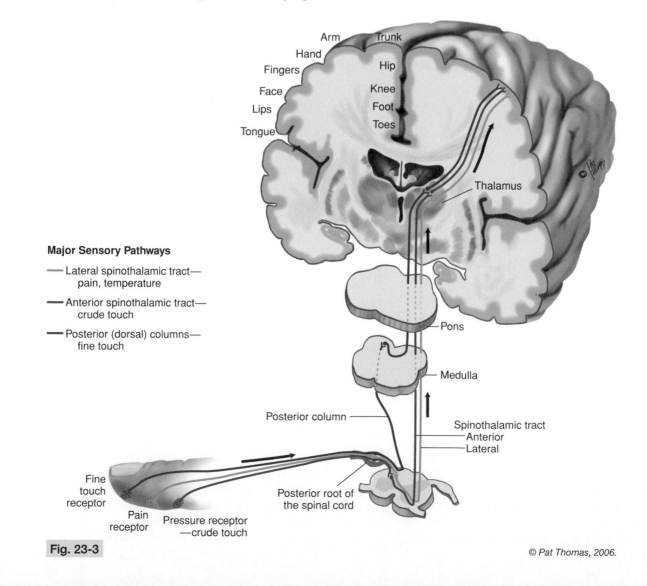

Major Sensory Pathways

— Lateral spinothalamic tract—
pain, temperature

— Anterior spinothalamic tract—
crude touch

— Posterior (dorsal) columns—
fine touch

Fig. 23-3

© Pat Thomas, 2006.

The sensory cortex is arranged in a specific pattern forming a corresponding "map" of the body (see the homunculus in Fig. 23-1). Pain in the right hand is perceived at its specific spot on the left cortex map. Some organs are absent from the brain map, such as the heart, liver, and spleen. You know you have one, but you have no "felt image" of it. Pain originating in these organs is referred because no felt image exists in which to have pain. Pain is felt "by proxy" by another body part that does have a felt image. For example, pain in the heart is referred to the chest, shoulder, and left arm, which were its neighbours during fetal development. Pain originating in the spleen is felt on the top of the left shoulder.

Motor Pathways

Corticospinal or Pyramidal Tract. The area has been named "pyramidal" because it originates in pyramid-shaped cells in the motor cortex (Fig. 23-4). Motor nerve fibres originate in the motor cortex and travel to the brain stem, where they cross to the opposite or contralateral side *(pyramidal decussation)* and then pass down in the lateral column of the spinal cord. At each cord level, they synapse with a lower motor neuron contained in the anterior horn of the spinal cord. Ten percent of corticospinal fibres do *not* cross, and these descend in the anterior column of the spinal cord. Corticospinal fibres mediate voluntary movement, particularly very skilled, discrete, purposeful movements, such as writing.

The corticospinal tract is a newer, "higher" motor system in humans that permits very skilled and purposeful movements. The tract's origin in the motor cortex is arranged in a specific pattern called *somatotopic organization.* It is another body map, this one of a person, or *homunculus,* hanging "upside down" (see Fig. 23-1). Body parts are not equally represented on the map, and the homunculus looks distorted. To use political terms, it is more like an electoral map than a geographical map. That is, body parts whose movements are relatively more important to humans (e.g., the hand) occupy proportionally more space on the brain map.

Extrapyramidal Tracts. The extrapyramidal tracts include all the motor nerve fibres originating in the motor cortex, basal ganglia, brain stem, and spinal cord that are *outside* the pyramidal tract. This is a phylogenetically older, "lower," more primitive motor system. These subcortical motor fibres maintain muscle tone and control body movements, especially gross automatic movements, such as walking.

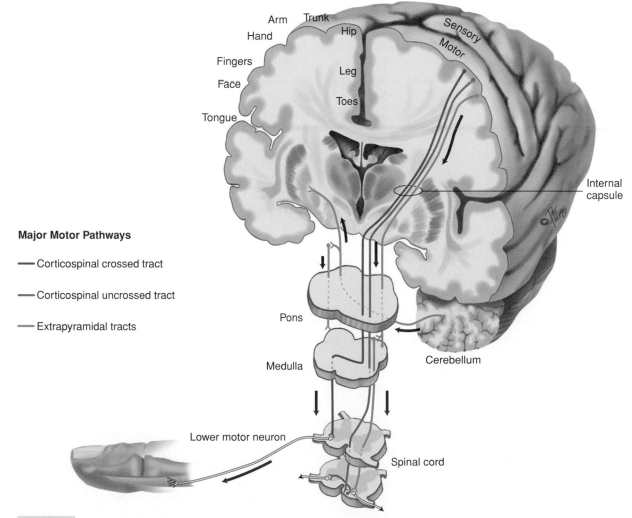

Major Motor Pathways

— Corticospinal crossed tract

— Corticospinal uncrossed tract

— Extrapyramidal tracts

Fig. 23-4

© Pat Thomas, 2006.

Cerebellar System. This complex motor system coordinates movement, maintains equilibrium, and helps maintain posture. The cerebellum receives information about the position of muscles and joints—the body's equilibrium—and the kind of motor messages are being sent from the cortex to the muscles. The information is integrated, and the cerebellum uses feedback pathways to exert its control back on the cortex or down to lower motor neurons in the spinal cord. This entire process occurs on a subconscious level.

Upper and Lower Motor Neurons

Upper motor neurons (UMNs) are a complex of all the descending motor fibres that can influence or modify the lower motor neurons. Upper motor neurons are located completely within the CNS. The neurons convey impulses from the motor areas of the cerebral cortex to the lower motor neurons in the anterior horn cells of the spinal cord. Examples of upper motor neurons are corticospinal, corticobulbar, and extrapyramidal tracts. Examples of upper motor neuron diseases are cerebrovascular accident, cerebral palsy, and multiple sclerosis.

Lower motor neurons (LMNs) are located mostly in the peripheral nervous system. The cell body of the lower motor neuron is located in the anterior grey column of the spinal cord, but the nerve fibre extends from here to the muscle. The lower motor neuron is the "final common pathway" because it funnels many neural signals here, and it provides the final direct contact with the muscles. Any movement must be translated into action by lower motor neuron fibres. Examples of lower motor neurons are cranial nerves and spinal nerves of the peripheral nervous system. Examples of lower motor neuron diseases are spinal cord lesions, poliomyelitis, and amyotrophic lateral sclerosis.

THE PERIPHERAL NERVOUS SYSTEM

A **nerve** is a bundle of fibres *outside* the CNS. The peripheral nerves carry input to the CNS via their sensory afferent fibres and deliver output from the CNS via the efferent fibres.

Reflex Arc

Reflexes are basic defence mechanisms of the nervous system. They are involuntary, operating below the level of conscious control and permitting a quick reaction to potentially painful or damaging events. Reflexes also help the body maintain balance and appropriate muscle tone. There are four types of reflexes: (1) **deep tendon reflexes** (myotatic), such as patellar or knee jerk; (2) **superficial,** such as corneal reflex, abdominal reflex; (3) **visceral** (organic), such as pupillary response to light and accommodation; and (4) **pathological** (abnormal), such as Babinski's or extensor plantar reflex.

The fibres that mediate the reflex are carried by a specific spinal nerve. In the most simple reflex, tapping the tendon stretches the muscle spindles in the muscle, which activates the sensory afferent nerve. The sensory afferent fibres carry the message from the receptor and travel through the dorsal

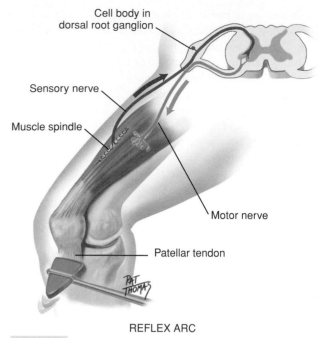

REFLEX ARC

Fig. 23-5

root into the spinal cord (Fig. 23-5). They synapse directly in the cord with the motor neuron in the anterior horn. Motor efferent fibres leave via the ventral root and travel to the muscle, stimulating a sudden contraction.

The deep tendon (myotatic or stretch) reflex (DTR) has five components: (1) an intact sensory nerve (afferent); (2) a functional synapse in the cord; (3) an intact motor nerve fibre (efferent); (4) the neuromuscular junction; and (5) a competent muscle.

Cranial Nerves

Cranial nerves enter and exit the brain rather than the spinal cord (Fig. 23-6). Cranial nerves I and II extend from the cerebrum; cranial nerves III to XII extend from the lower diencephalon and brain stem. The 12 pairs of cranial nerves supply primarily the head and neck, except the vagus nerve (Lat. *vagus,* or wanderer, as in "vagabond"), which travels to the heart, respiratory muscles, stomach, and gallbladder.

Spinal Nerves

The 31 pairs of **spinal nerves** arise from the length of the spinal cord and supply the rest of the body. They are named for the region of the spine from which they exit: 8 cervical, 12 thoracic, 5 lumbar, 5 sacral, and 1 coccygeal. They are "mixed" nerves because they contain both sensory and motor fibres. The nerves enter and exit the cord through roots—sensory afferent fibres through the posterior or dorsal roots, and motor efferent fibres through the anterior or ventral roots.

The nerves exit the spinal cord in an orderly ladder shape. Each nerve innervates a particular segment of the body. **Dermal segmentation** is the cutaneous distribution of the various spinal nerves.

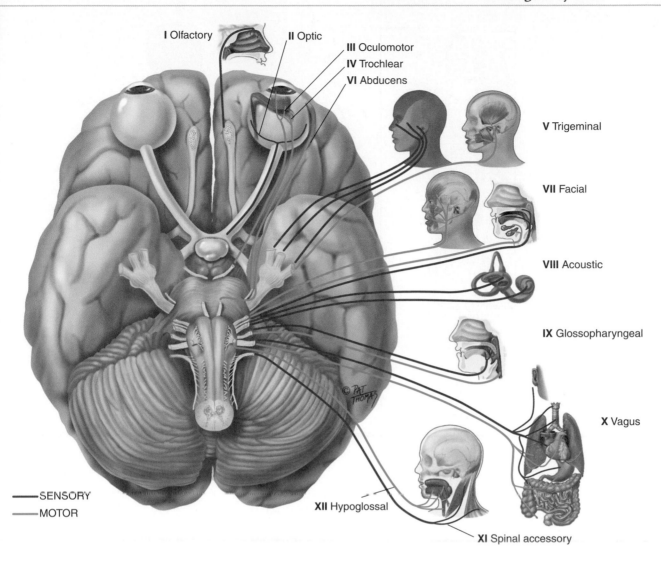

CRANIAL NERVES

Cranial Nerve	Type	Function
I: Olfactory	Sensory	Smell
II: Optic	Sensory	Vision
III: Oculomotor	Mixed*	Motor—most EOM movement, opening of eyelids
		Parasympathetic—pupil constriction, lens shape
IV: Trochlear	Motor	Down and inward movement of eye
V: Trigeminal	Mixed	Motor—muscles of mastication
		Sensory—sensation of face and scalp, cornea, mucous membranes of mouth and nose
VI: Abducens	Motor	Lateral movement of eye
VII: Facial	Mixed	Motor—facial muscles, close eye, labial speech, close mouth
		Sensory—taste (sweet, salty, sour, bitter) on anterior two thirds of tongue
		Parasympathetic—saliva and tear secretion
VIII: Acoustic	Sensory	Hearing and equilibrium
IX: Glossopharyngeal	Mixed	Motor—pharynx (phonation and swallowing)
		Sensory—taste on posterior one third of tongue, pharynx (gag reflex)
		Parasympathetic—parotid gland, carotid reflex
X: Vagus	Mixed	Motor—pharynx and larynx (talking and swallowing)
		Sensory—general sensation from carotid body, carotid sinus, pharynx, viscera
		Parasympathetic—carotid reflex
XI: Spinal accessory	Motor	Movement of trapezius and sternomastoid muscles
XII: Hypoglossal	Motor	Movement of tongue

*Mixed refers to a nerve carrying a combination of fibres: motor + sensory; motor + parasympathetic; or motor + sensory + parasympathetic.

Fig. 23-6

© Pat Thomas, 2006.

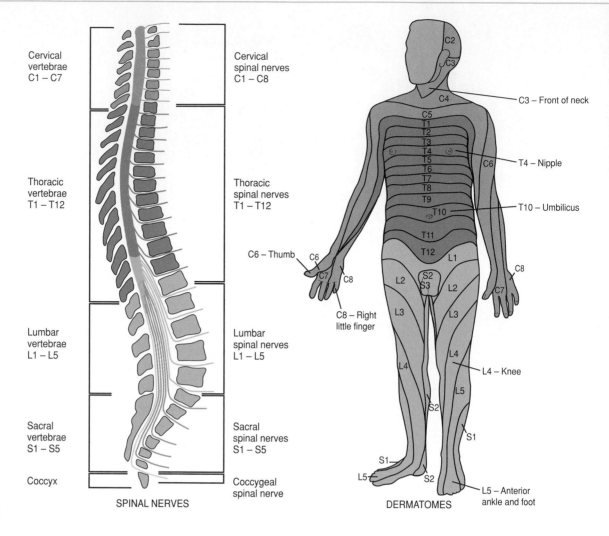

Fig. 23-7

SPINAL NERVES

DERMATOMES

A **dermatome** is a circumscribed skin area that is supplied mainly from one spinal cord segment through a particular spinal nerve (Fig. 23-7). The dermatomes overlap, which is a form of biological insurance. That is, if one nerve is severed, most of the sensations will continue to be transmitted by the one above and the one below. Do not attempt to memorize all dermatome segments; just focus on the following as useful landmarks:

- The **thumb, middle finger,** and **fifth finger** are each in the dermatomes of **C6, C7,** and **C8.**
- The **axilla** is at the level of **T1.**
- The **nipple** is at the level of **T4.**
- The **umbilicus** is at the level of **T10.**
- The **groin** is in the region of **L1.**
- The **knee** is at the level of **L4.**

Autonomic Nervous System

The peripheral nervous system is composed of cranial nerves and spinal nerves. These nerves carry fibres that can be divided functionally into two parts—somatic and autonomic. The somatic fibres innervate the skeletal (voluntary) muscles; the autonomic fibres innervate smooth (involuntary) muscles, cardiac muscle, and glands. The autonomic system mediates unconscious activity. Although a description of the autonomic system is beyond the scope of this book, its overall function is to maintain homeostasis of the body.

DEVELOPMENTAL CARE

Infants

The neurological system is not completely developed at birth. Motor activity in the newborn is under the control of the spinal cord and medulla. Very little cortical control exists, and the neurons are not yet myelinated. Movements are directed primarily by primitive reflexes. As the cerebral cortex develops during the first year, it inhibits these reflexes, and they disappear at predictable times. Persistence of the primitive reflexes is an indication of CNS dysfunction.

The infant's sensory and motor development proceeds along with the gradual acquisition of myelin because myelin is needed to conduct most impulses. The process of myelinization follows a cephalocaudal and proximodistal order (head, neck, trunk, and extremities). This is just the order we observe in the infant gaining motor control (lifts head, lifts head and shoulders, rolls over, moves whole arm, uses hands, walks). As the milestones are achieved, each movement is more complex and coordinated. Milestones occur in an orderly sequence, although the exact age of occurrence may vary.

Sensation also is rudimentary at birth. The newborn needs a strong stimulus and then responds by crying and with whole body movements. As myelinization develops, the infant is able to localize the stimulus more precisely and to make a more accurate motor response.

The Aging Adult

The aging process causes a general atrophy with a steady loss of neurons in the brain and spinal cord. The loss of neurons causes a decrease in weight and volume so that by 80 years, the brain has decreased in weight by 15% (Waxman, 2000). Neuron loss leads many people over 65 to show signs that would be considered abnormal in the younger adult, such as general loss of muscle bulk, loss of muscle tone in the face, in the neck, and around the spine, decreased muscle strength, impaired fine coordination and agility, loss of vibratory sense at the ankle, decreased or absent Achilles reflex, loss of position sense at the big toe, pupillary miosis, irregular pupil shape, and decreased pupillary reflexes.

The velocity of nerve conduction decreases between 5 and 10% with aging, making the reaction time slower in some older persons. An increased delay at the synapse also occurs, so the impulse takes longer to travel. As a result, touch and pain sensation, taste, and smell may be diminished.

The motor system may show a general slowing down of movement. Muscle strength and agility decrease. A generalized decrease occurs in muscle bulk, which is most apparent in the dorsal hand muscles. Muscle tremors may occur in the hands, head, and jaw, along with possible repetitive facial grimacing (dyskinesias).

Aging involves a progressive decrease in cerebral blood flow and oxygen consumption. In some people, this causes dizziness and a loss of balance with position change. Older people need to be taught to get up slowly. Otherwise, they have an increased risk for falls and resulting injuries. Additionally, older people may forget that they fell, which makes it hard to diagnose the cause of an injury.

When they are in good health, older people walk about as well as they did during their middle and younger years, except more slowly and more deliberately. Some survey the ground for obstacles or uneven terrain. Some show hesitation and take a slightly wayward path.

CULTURAL AND SOCIAL CONSIDERATIONS

According to the Heart and Stroke Foundation of Canada (2008a), research has shown that people of Aboriginal, African, or South Asian descent are more likely to have high blood pressure and diabetes and are at greater risk of heart disease and stroke than are the general population. The foundation has translated and culturally adapted some health education resources to help patients who read or understand Ojibwe, Oji-cree, Punjabi, Hindi, Mandarin, or Cantonese, among other languages, to learn the risk factors and warning signs for heart disease and stroke.

People's social circumstances influence their ability to manage after a stroke. Social resources have been found to have a buffering effect in survivors, serving to reduce the adverse effects of physical disability on subjective well-being after stroke (Clarke et al., 2002). Stroke survivors with higher levels of education have been found to report a greater sense of personal growth, purpose in life, and environmental mastery than survivors with fewer years of education. Compared with men, women who had stroke are more likely to live alone and less likely to have social supports (Heart and Stroke Foundation, 2008b).

SUBJECTIVE DATA

1. Headache
2. Head injury
3. Dizziness or vertigo
4. Seizures
5. Tremors
6. Weakness
7. Incoordination
8. Numbness or tingling
9. Difficulty swallowing
10. Difficulty speaking
11. Significant past history
12. Environmental and occupational hazards

Examiner Asks	Rationale
1. Headache. Any unusually frequent or severe headaches? • When did this start? How often does it occur? • Where in your head do you feel the headaches? Do the headaches seem to be associated with anything? (Headache history is fully discussed in Chapter 13.)	
2. Head injury. Ever had any **head injury?** Please describe. • What part of your head was hit? • Did you experience loss of consciousness? For how long?	
3. Dizziness/vertigo. Ever feel lightheaded, a swimming sensation, like feeling faint? • When have you noticed this? How often does it occur? Does it occur with activity, change in position?	**Syncope** is a sudden loss of strength, a temporary loss of consciousness (a faint) due to lack of cerebral blood flow, such as low blood pressure.

Examiner Asks	Rationale
• Do you ever feel a sensation called **vertigo,** a rotational spinning sensation? (Note: Distinguish vertigo from dizziness.) Do you feel as if the room spins (objective vertigo)? Or do you feel that you are spinning (subjective vertigo)? Did this come on suddenly or gradually?	True **vertigo** is rotational spinning caused by neurological disease in the vestibular apparatus in the ear, or in the vestibular nuclei in the brain stem.
4. Seizures. Ever had any convulsions? When did they start? How often do they occur?	**Seizures** occur with epilepsy, a paroxysmal disease characterized by altered or loss of consciousness, involuntary muscle movements, and sensory disturbances.
• Course and duration—When a seizure starts, do you have any warning sign? What type of sign?	*Aura* is a subjective sensation that precedes a seizure; it could be auditory, visual, or motor.
• Motor activity—Where in your body do the seizures begin? Do the seizures travel through your body? On one side or both? Does your muscle tone seem tense or limp?	
• Any associated signs—Colour change in face or lips, loss of consciousness, for how long, automatisms (eyelid-fluttering, eye-rolling, lip-smacking), incontinence?	
• Postictal phase—After the seizure, are you told that you spend time sleeping or have any confusion, weakness, headache, or muscle ache?	
• Precipitating factors—Does anything seem to bring on the seizures: activity, discontinuing medication, fatigue, stress?	
• Are you on any medication?	
• Coping strategies—How have the seizures affected daily life, occupation?	
5. Tremors. Any shakes or **tremors** in the hands or face? When did these start?	*Tremor* is an involuntary shaking, vibrating, or trembling.
• Do they seem to grow worse with anxiety, intention, or rest?	
• Are they relieved with rest, activity, alcohol? Do they affect daily activities?	
6. Weakness. Any **weakness** or problem moving any body part? Is this generalized or local? Does weakness occur with any particular movement? (e.g., with proximal or large muscle weakness, it is hard to get up out of a chair or reach for an object; with distal or small muscle weakness, it is hard to open a jar, write, use scissors, or walk without tripping)	*Paresis* is a partial or incomplete paralysis. *Paralysis* is a loss of motor function due to a lesion in the neurological or muscular system or loss of sensory innervation.
7. Incoordination. Any problem with **coordination?** Any problem with balance when walking? Do you list to one side? Any falling? Which way? Do your legs seem to give way? Any clumsy movement?	*Dysmetria* is the inability to control range of motion of muscles.
8. Numbness or tingling. Any **numbness or tingling** in any body part? Does it feel like pins and needles? When did this start? Where do you feel it? Does it occur with activity?	*Paresthesia* is an abnormal sensation, such as burning, tingling.
9. Difficulty swallowing. Any problem **swallowing?** Occur with solids or liquids? Have you experienced excessive salivation, drooling?	
10. Difficulty speaking. Any problem **speaking:** with forming words or with saying what you intended to say? When did you first notice this? How long did it last?	*Dysarthria* is difficulty forming words; *dysphasia* is difficulty with language comprehension or expression (see Table 6-4, p. 109).
11. Significant past history. Past history of stroke (cerebrovascular accident), spinal cord injury, meningitis or encephalitis, congenital defect, or alcoholism?	

Examiner Asks	Rationale

12. Environmental and occupational hazards. Are you exposed to any environmental or occupational hazards: insecticides, organic solvents, lead?
- Are you taking any medications now?
- How much alcohol do you drink? Each week? Each day?
- How about other mood-altering drugs: marijuana, cocaine, barbiturates, tranquilizers?

Review anticonvulsant, antitremor, antivertigo, pain medications.

Additional History for Infants and Children

1. Did you (the mother) have any health problems during the pregnancy: any infections or illnesses, medications taken, toxemia, hypertension, alcohol or drug use, diabetes?

Prenatal history may affect infant's neurological development.

2. Please tell me about this baby's birth. Was the baby at term or premature? Birth weight?
- Any birth trauma? Did the baby breathe immediately?
- Were you told the baby's Apgar scores?
- Any congenital defects?

3. Reflexes—What have you noticed about the baby's behaviour? Do the baby's sucking and swallowing seem coordinated? When you touch the cheek, does the baby turn his or her head toward the touch? Is the baby startled by a loud noise or shake of crib? Does the baby grasp your finger?

4. Does the child seem to have any problem with balance? Have you noted any unexplained falling, clumsy or unsteady gait, progressive muscular weakness, problem with going up or down stairs, problem with getting up from lying position?

If occurs, may not be noticed until starts to walk in late infancy.
Screen for muscular dystrophy.

5. Has this child had any seizures? Please describe. Did the seizure occur with a high fever? Did any loss of consciousness occur—how long? How many seizures occurred with this same illness (if occurred with high fever)?

Seizures may occur with high fever in infants and toddlers. Or seizures may be sign of neurological disease.

6. Did this child's motor or developmental milestones seem to occur at about the right age? Does this child seem to be growing and maturing normally to you? How does this child's development compare with siblings or that of age-mates?

7. Do you know if your child has had any environmental exposure to lead?

Chronically elevated lead levels may cause developmental delay, loss of a newly acquired skill, or no clinical signs may be present.

8. Have you been told about any learning problems in school: has problems with attention span, cannot concentrate, is hyperactive?

9. Any family history of seizure disorder, cerebral palsy, muscular dystrophy?

Additional History for the Aging Adult

1. Any problem with dizziness? Does this occur when you first sit or stand up, when you move your head, when you get up and walk just after eating? Does this occur with any of your medications?

Diminished cerebral blood flow and diminished vestibular response may produce staggering with position change, which increases risk of falls.

Subjective Data

Examiner Asks	Rationale
• (For men) Do you ever get up at night and then feel faint while standing to urinate?	Micturition syncope.
• How does dizziness affect your daily activities? Are you able to drive safely and to manoeuvre within your house safely?	
• What safety modifications have you applied at home?	
2. Have you noticed any decrease in memory, changes in mental function? Have you felt any confusion? Did this seem to come on suddenly or gradually?	
3. Have you ever noticed any tremor? Is this in your hands or face? Is this worse with anxiety, activity, rest? Does the tremor seem to be relieved with alcohol, activity, rest? Does the tremor interfere with daily or social activities?	Senile tremor is relieved by alcohol, although this is not a recommended treatment. Assess if the person is abusing alcohol in effort to relieve tremor.
4. Have you ever had any sudden vision change, fleeting blindness? Did this occur along with weakness? Did you have any loss of consciousness?	Screen for symptoms of stroke.

OBJECTIVE DATA

PREPARATION

Perform a **screening neurological examination** (items identified in following sections) on seemingly well persons who have no significant subjective findings from the history.

Perform a **complete neurological examination** on persons who have neurological concerns (e.g., headache, weakness, loss of coordination) or who have shown signs of neurological dysfunction.

Perform a **neurological recheck** examination on persons with demonstrated neurological deficits who require periodic assessments (e.g., hospitalized persons or those in extended care), using the examination sequence beginning on p. 692.

Integrate the steps of the neurological examination with the examination of each particular part of the body, as much as you are able. For example, test cranial nerves while assessing the head and neck (recall Chapters 13 through 16) and superficial abdominal reflexes while assessing the abdomen (Chapter 21). When recording your findings, however, consider all neurological data as a functional unit, and record them all together.

Use the following sequence for the complete neurological examination:
1. Mental status (see Chapter 6)
2. Cranial nerves
3. Motor system
4. Sensory system
5. Reflexes

Ask the person to sit up with the head at your eye level.

EQUIPMENT NEEDED
Penlight
Tongue blade
Cotton swab
Cotton ball
Tuning fork (128 Hz or 256 Hz)
Percussion hammer
(Possibly) familiar aromatic substances, such as peppermint, coffee, vanilla

Normal Range of Findings	Abnormal Findings

TEST CRANIAL NERVES

Cranial Nerve I: Olfactory Nerve

Do not test routinely. Test the sense of smell in those who report loss of smell, those with head trauma, and those with abnormal mental status, and when the presence of an intracranial lesion is suspected. First, assess patency by occluding one nostril at a time and asking the person to sniff. Then, with the person's eyes closed, occlude one nostril and present an aromatic substance. Use familiar,

Smell cannot be tested when air passages are occluded with upper respiratory infection or with sinusitis.

Normal Range of Findings	Abnormal Findings
conveniently obtainable, and non-noxious smells, such as coffee, toothpaste, orange, vanilla, soap, or peppermint. Alcohol wipes smell familiar and are easy to find but are irritating. Normally, a person can identify an odour through each side of the nose. The sense of smell normally decreases bilaterally with aging. Any asymmetry in the sense of smell is important.	Anosmia—decrease or loss of smell occurs bilaterally with tobacco smoking, allergic rhinitis, and cocaine use. Unilateral loss of smell in the absence of nasal disease is *neurogenic anosmia* (see Table 23-2 on p. 699).

Cranial Nerve II: Optic Nerve

Test visual acuity and test visual fields by confrontation (see Chapter 14). Using the ophthalmoscope, examine the ocular fundus to determine the colour, size, and shape of the optic disc (see Chapter 14).	Visual field loss (see Table 14-5, p. 335). Papilledema with increased intracranial pressure; optic atrophy (see Table 14-9, p. 338).

Cranial Nerves III, IV, and VI: Oculomotor, Trochlear, and Abducens Nerves

Palpebral fissures are usually equal in width or nearly so. Check pupils for size, regularity, equality, direct and consensual light reactions, and accommodation (see Chapter 14). Assess extraocular movements by the cardinal positions of gaze (see Chapter 14). Nystagmus is a back-and-forth oscillation of the eyes. End-point nystagmus, a few beats of horizontal nystagmus at extreme lateral gaze, occurs normally. Assess any other nystagmus carefully, noting: • Presence of nystagmus in one or both eyes. • *Pendular* movement (oscillations move equally left to right) or *jerk* (a quick phase in one direction, then a slow phase in the other). Classify the jerk nystagmus in the direction of the quick phase. • Amplitude. Judge whether the degree of movement is fine, medium, or coarse. • Frequency. Is it constant, or does it fade after a few beats? • Plane of movement: horizontal, vertical, rotary, or a combination.	Ptosis (drooping) occurs with myasthenia gravis, dysfunction of cranial nerve III, or Horner syndrome (see Table 14-2, p. 331). Increasing intracranial pressure causes a sudden, unilateral, dilated and nonreactive pupil. Strabismus (deviated gaze) or limited movement (see Table 14-1, p. 330). Nystagmus occurs with disease of the vestibular system, cerebellum, or brain stem.

Cranial Nerve V: Trigeminal Nerve

Motor Function. Assess the muscles of mastication by palpating the temporal and masseter muscles as the person clenches the teeth (Fig. 23-8). Muscles should feel equally strong on both sides. Next, try to separate the jaws by pushing down on the chin; normally you cannot.	Decreased strength on one or both sides. Asymmetry in jaw movement. Pain with clenching of teeth.

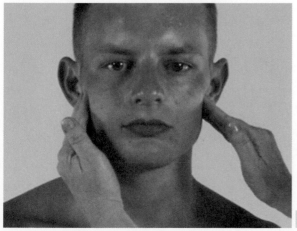

Fig. 23-8

Normal Range of Findings	Abnormal Findings

Sensory Function. With the person's eyes closed, test light touch sensation by touching a cotton wisp to these designated areas on person's face: forehead, cheeks, and chin (Fig. 23-9). Ask the person to say "Now," whenever the touch is felt. This tests all three divisions of the nerve: (1) ophthalmic, (2) maxillary, and (3) mandibular.

Decreased or unequal sensation.

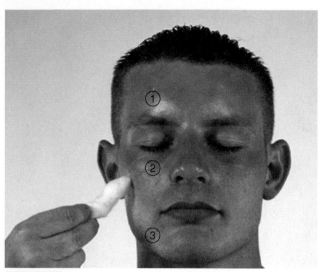

Fig. 23-9

Corneal Reflex. (Omit this test, unless the person has abnormal facial sensation or abnormalities of facial movement.) Ask the person to remove any contact lenses. With the person looking forward, bring a wisp of cotton in from the side (to minimize defensive blinking) and lightly touch the cornea, not the conjunctiva (Fig. 23-10). Normally, the person will blink bilaterally. The corneal reflex may be decreased or absent in those who have worn contact lenses. This procedure tests the sensory afferent in cranial nerve V and the motor efferent in cranial nerve VII (muscles that close the eye).

No blink occurs with a lesion of cranial nerve V or cranial nerve VII paralysis.

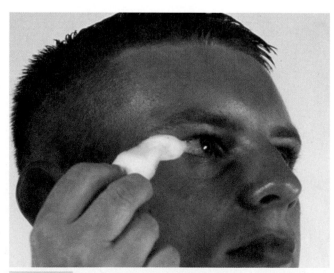

Fig. 23-10

Normal Range of Findings	Abnormal Findings

Cranial Nerve VII: Facial Nerve

Motor Function. Note mobility and facial symmetry as the person responds to these requests: smile (Fig. 23-11), frown, close eyes tightly (against your attempt to open them), lift eyebrows, show teeth, and puff cheeks (Fig. 23-12). Then, press the person's puffed cheeks in, and note if the air escapes equally from both sides.

Muscle weakness is shown by flattening of the nasolabial fold, drooping of one side of the face, lower eyelid sagging, and escape of air from only one cheek that is pressed in.

Loss of movement and asymmetry of movement occur with both central nervous system lesions (e.g., brain attack or stroke that affects the lower face on one side) and peripheral nervous system lesions (e.g., Bell's palsy that affects the upper *and* lower face on one side).

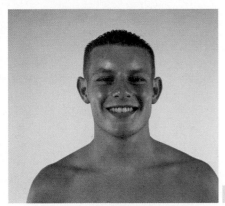

Fig. 23-11

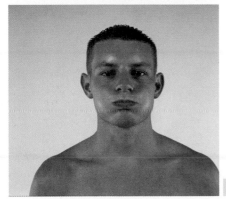

Fig. 23-12

Sensory Function. Do not test routinely. Test only when you suspect facial nerve injury. When indicated, test sense of taste by applying to the tongue a cotton applicator soaked in a solution of sugar, salt, or lemon juice (sour). Ask the person to identify the taste.

Cranial Nerve VIII: Acoustic (Vestibulocochlear) Nerve

Test hearing acuity by the ability to hear normal conversation, by the whispered voice test, and by Weber and Rinne tuning fork tests (see Chapter 15).

Cranial Nerves IX and X: Glossopharyngeal and Vagus Nerves

Motor Function. Depress the tongue with a tongue blade, and note pharyngeal movement as the person says "ahhh" or yawns; the uvula and soft palate should rise in the midline, and the tonsillar pillars should move medially.

Absence or asymmetry of soft palate movement.
Uvula deviates to side.
Asymmetry of tonsillar pillar movement.

Touch the posterior pharyngeal wall with a tongue blade, and note the gag reflex. Also note that the voice sounds smooth and not strained.

Hoarse or brassy voice occurs with vocal cord dysfunction; nasal twang occurs with weakness of soft palate.

Sensory Function. Cranial nerve IX does mediate taste on the posterior one third of the tongue, but technically this sensation is too difficult to test.

Objective Data

Normal Range of Findings	Abnormal Findings

Objective Data

Cranial Nerve XI: Spinal Accessory Nerve

Examine the sternomastoid and trapezius muscles for equal size. Check equal strength by asking the person to rotate the head forcibly against resistance applied to the side of the chin (Fig. 23-13). Then ask the person to shrug the shoulders against resistance (Fig. 23-14). These movements should feel equally strong on both sides.

Atrophy.
Muscle weakness or paralysis.

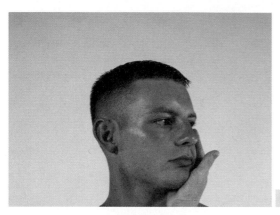

Fig. 23-13

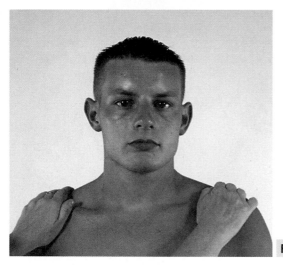

Fig. 23-14

Cranial Nerve XII: Hypoglossal Nerve

Inspect the tongue. No wasting or tremors should be present. Note the forward thrust in the midline as the person protrudes the tongue. Also ask the person to say "light, tight, dynamite," and note that lingual speech (sounds of letters l, t, d, n) is clear and distinct.

Atrophy. Fasciculations.
Tongue deviates to side with lesions of the hypoglossal nerve. (When this occurs, deviation is toward the paralyzed side.)

INSPECT AND PALPATE THE MOTOR SYSTEM

Muscles

Size. As you proceed through the examination, inspect all muscle groups for size. Compare the right side with the left. Muscle groups should be within the normal size limits for age and should be symmetric bilaterally. When muscles in the extremities look asymmetrical, measure each in centimetres, and record the difference. A difference of 1 cm or less is not significant. Note that it is difficult to assess muscle mass in very obese people.

Atrophy—abnormally small muscle with a wasted appearance; occurs with disuse, injury, lower motor neuron disease such as polio, diabetic neuropathy.
Hypertrophy—increased size and strength; occurs with isometric exercise.

Normal Range of Findings	Abnormal Findings
Strength. (See Chapter 22.) Test the power of homologous muscles simultaneously. Test muscle groups of the extremities, neck, and trunk.	Paresis or weakness is diminished strength; paralysis or plegia is absence of strength.
Tone. Tone is the normal degree of tension (contraction) in voluntarily relaxed muscles. It shows as a mild resistance to passive stretch. To test muscle tone, move the extremities through a passive range of motion. First, persuade the person to relax completely, to "go loose like a rag doll." Move each extremity smoothly through a full range of motion. Support the arm at the elbow and the leg at the knee (Fig. 23-15). Normally, you will note a mild, even resistance to movement.	Limited range of motion. Pain with motion. Flaccidity—decreased resistance, hypotonicity. Spasticity and rigidity—types of increased resistance (see Table 23-3, p. 700).

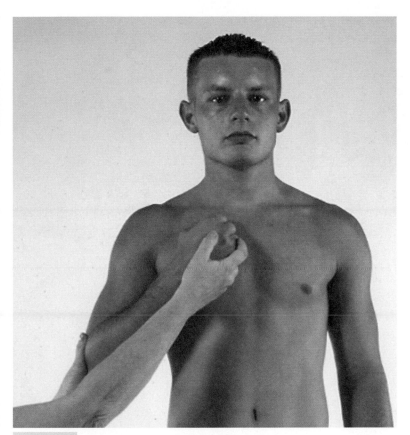

Fig. 23-15

Involuntary Movements. Normally, no involuntary movements occur. If they are present, note their location, frequency, rate, and amplitude. Note if the movements can be controlled at will.	Tic, tremor, fasciculation, myoclonus, chorea, and athetosis (see Table 23-4, p. 701).

Cerebellar Function

Balance Tests

Gait. Observe as the person walks 3 to 6 m, turns, and returns to the starting point. Normally, the person moves with a sense of freedom. The gait is smooth, rhythmic, and effortless; the opposing arm swing is coordinated; the turns are smooth. The step length is about 30 cm from heel to heel.	Stiff, immobile posture. Staggering or reeling. Wide base of support. Lack of arm swing or rigid arms. Unequal rhythm of steps. Slapping of foot. Scraping of toe of shoe. Ataxia—uncoordinated or unsteady gait (see Table 23-5, p. 703).

Objective Data

Normal Range of Findings	**Abnormal Findings**

Ask the person to walk a straight line in a heel-to-toe fashion (tandem walking) (Fig. 23-16). This decreases the base of support and will accentuate any problem with coordination. Normally, the person can walk straight and stay balanced.

Crooked line of walk.
Widens base to maintain balance.
Staggering, reeling, loss of balance.
An ataxia that did not appear with regular gait may appear now. Inability to tandem walk is indicative of an upper motor neuron lesion such as multiple sclerosis acute cerebellar dysfunction such as alcohol intoxication.

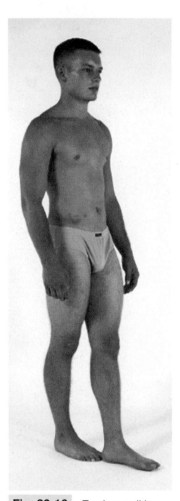

Fig. 23-16   Tandem walking.

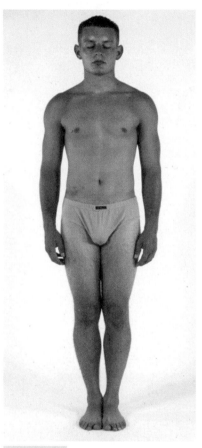

Fig. 23-17   Romberg test.

You may also test for balance by asking the person to walk on his toes, then on his heels for a few steps.

Muscle weakness in the legs makes this difficult.

The Romberg Test. Ask the person to stand up with feet together and arms at the sides. Once in a stable position, ask the person to close the eyes and to hold the position (Fig. 23-17). Wait about 20 seconds. Normally, a person can maintain posture and balance even with the visual orienting information blocked, although slight swaying may occur. (Stand close to catch the person in case he or she falls.)

Sways, falls, widens base of feet to avoid falling.
Positive Romberg sign is loss of balance that occurs when closing the eyes. You eliminate the advantage of orientation with the eyes, which had compensated for sensory loss. A positive Romberg sign occurs with cerebellar ataxia (multiple sclerosis, alcohol intoxication), loss of proprioception, and loss of vestibular function.

Normal Range of Findings	**Abnormal Findings**

Ask the person to perform a shallow knee bend or to hop in place, first on one leg, then the other (Fig. 23-18). This demonstrates normal position sense, muscle strength, and cerebellar function. Note that some individuals cannot hop because of aging or obesity.

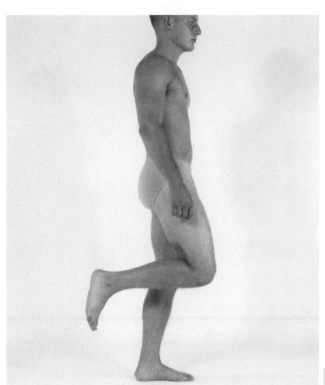

Fig. 23-18

Unable to perform knee bend because of weakness in quadriceps muscle or hip extensors.

Coordination and Skilled Movements

Rapid Alternating Movements (RAM). Ask the person to pat the knees with both hands, lift up, turn hands over, and pat the knees with the backs of the hands (Fig. 23-19). Then ask the person to do this faster. Normally, this is done with equal turning and a quick rhythmic pace.

Alternatively, ask the person to touch the thumb to each finger on the same hand, starting with the index finger, then reverse direction (Fig. 23-20). Normally, this can be done quickly and accurately.

Lack of coordination.
Slow, clumsy, and sloppy response is termed *dysdiadochokinesia* and occurs with cerebellar disease.
Lack of coordination.

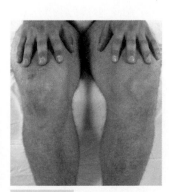

Fig. 23-19

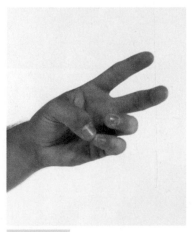

Fig. 23-20

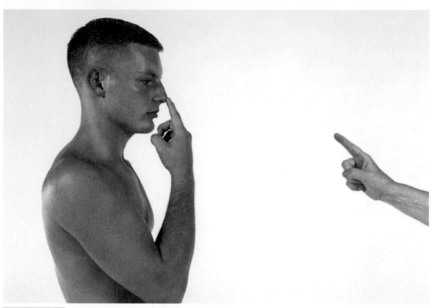

Fig. 23-21

<table>
<tr><td>

Normal Range of Findings

Finger-to-Finger Test. With the person's eyes open, ask that he or she use the index finger to touch your finger, then his or her own nose (Fig. 23-21). After a few times move your finger to a different spot. The person's movement should be smooth and accurate.

</td><td>

Abnormal Findings

Dysmetria is clumsy movement with overshooting the mark and occurs with cerebellar disorders or acute alcohol intoxication.

Past-pointing is a constant deviation to one side.

</td></tr>
<tr><td>

Finger-to-Nose Test. Ask the person to close the eyes and to stretch out the arms. Ask the person to touch the tip of his or her nose with each index finger, alternating hands and increasing speed. Normally this is done with an accurate and smooth movement.

</td><td>

Misses nose. Worsening of coordination when the eyes are closed occurs with cerebellar disease or alcohol intoxication.

</td></tr>
<tr><td>

Heel-to-Shin Test. Test lower extremity coordination by asking the person, who is in a supine position, to place the heel on the opposite knee, and run it down the shin from the knee to the ankle (Fig. 23-22). Normally, the person moves the heel in a straight line down the shin.

</td><td>

Lack of coordination, heel falls off shin, occurs with cerebellar disease.

</td></tr>
</table>

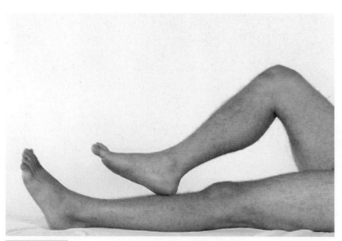

Fig. 23-22

Objective Data

Normal Range of Findings	Abnormal Findings

ASSESS THE SENSORY SYSTEM

Ask the person to identify various sensory stimuli in order to test the intactness of the peripheral nerve fibres, the sensory tracts, and higher cortical discrimination.

Ensure the validity of sensory system testing by making sure the person is alert, co-operative, comfortable, and has an adequate attention span. Otherwise, you may get misleading and invalid results. Testing of the sensory system can be fatiguing. You may need to repeat the examination later or to break it into parts when the person is tired.

You do not need to test the entire skin surface for every sensation. Routine screening procedures include testing superficial pain, light touch, and vibration in a few distal locations, and testing stereognosis. This will suffice for all who have not demonstrated any neurological symptoms or signs. Complete testing of the sensory system is warranted in those with neurological symptoms (e.g., localized pain, numbness, and tingling) or when you discover abnormalities (e.g., motor deficit). Then, test all sensory modalities and cover most dermatomes of the body.

Compare sensations on symmetrical parts of the body. When you find a definite decrease in sensation, map it out by systematic testing in that area. Proceed from the point of decreased sensation toward the sensitive area. By asking the person to tell you where the sensation changes, you can map the exact borders of the deficient area. Note your results on a diagram.

Avoid asking leading questions, "Can you feel this pinprick?" This creates an expectation of how the person should feel the sensation, which is called *suggestion*. Instead, use unbiased directions.

The person's eyes should be closed during each of the tests. Take time to explain what will be happening and exactly how you expect the person to respond.

Note if the topographical pattern of sensory loss is distal, that is, over the hands and feet in a "glove and stocking" distribution, or if it is over a specific dermatome.

Spinothalamic Tract

Pain. Pain is tested by the person's ability to perceive a pinprick. Break a tongue blade lengthwise, forming a sharp point at the fractured end and a dull spot at the rounded end. Lightly apply the sharp point or the dull end to the person's body in a random, unpredictable order (Fig. 23-23). Ask the person to say "sharp" or "dull," depending on the sensation felt. (Note that the sharp edge is used to test for pain; the dull edge is used as a general test of the person's responses.)

Let at least 2 seconds elapse after each stimulus to avoid *summation*. With summation, frequent consecutive stimuli are perceived as one strong stimulus. Discard tongue blade.

Hypoalgesia—decreased pain sensation.
Analgesia—absent pain sensation.
Hyperalgesia—increased pain sensation.

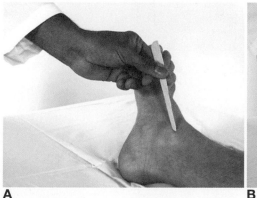
A

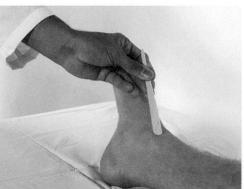
B

Fig. 23-23

Normal Range of Findings	Abnormal Findings

Temperature. Test temperature sensation only when pain sensation is abnormal; otherwise, you may omit it because the fibre tracts are much the same. Fill two test tubes, one with hot water and one with cold water, and apply the bottom ends to the person's skin in a random order. Ask the person to say which temperature is felt. Alternatively, you could place the flat side of the tuning fork on the skin; its metal always feels cool.

Light Touch. Apply a wisp of cotton to the skin. Stretch a cotton ball to make a long end and brush it over the skin in a random order of sites and at irregular intervals (Fig. 23-24). This prevents the person from responding just from repetition. Include the arms, forearms, hands, chest, thighs, and legs. Ask the person to say "now" or "yes" when touch is felt. Compare symmetrical points.

Hypoesthesia—decreased touch sensation.
Anesthesia—absent touch sensation.
Hyperesthesia—increased touch sensation.

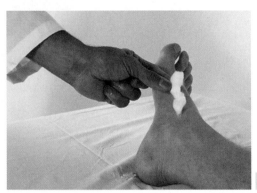

Fig. 23-24

Posterior Column Tract

Vibration. Test the person's ability to feel vibrations of a tuning fork over bony prominences. Use a low-pitch tuning fork (128 Hz or 256 Hz) because its vibration has a slower decay. Strike the tuning fork on the heel of your hand, and hold the base on a bony surface of the fingers and great toe (Fig. 23-25). Ask the person to indicate when the vibration starts and stops. If the person feels the normal vibration or buzzing sensation on these distal areas, you may assume proximal spots are normal and proceed no further. If no vibrations are felt, move proximally and test ulnar processes, and ankles, patellae, and iliac crests. Compare the right side with the left side. If you find a deficit, note whether it is gradual or abrupt.

Unable to feel vibration. Loss of vibration sense occurs in peripheral neuropathy such as diabetes and alcoholism. Often, this is the first sensation lost.

Peripheral neuropathy is worse at the feet and gradually improves as you move up the leg, as opposed to a specific nerve lesion, which has a clear zone of deficit for its dermatome.

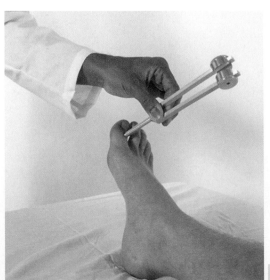

Fig. 23-25

Objective Data

Normal Range of Findings	Abnormal Findings

Position (Kinesthesia). Test the person's ability to perceive passive movements of the extremities. Move a finger or the big toe up and down, and ask the person to tell you which way it is moved (Fig. 23-26). The test is done with the person's eyes closed, but to be sure it is understood, have the person watch a few trials first. Vary the order of movement up or down. Hold the digit by the sides, since upward or downward pressure on the skin may provide a clue as to how it has been moved. Normally, a person can detect movement of a few millimetres.

Loss of position sense.

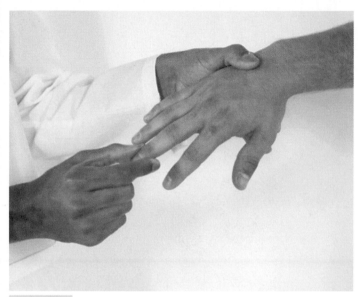

Fig. 23-26

Tactile Discrimination (Fine Touch). The following tests also measure the discrimination ability of the sensory cortex. As a prerequisite, the person needs a normal or near-normal sense of touch and position sense.

Problems with tactile discrimination occur with lesions of the sensory cortex or posterior column.

Stereognosis. Test the person's ability to recognize objects by feeling their forms, sizes, and weights. With the eyes closed, place a familiar object (paper clip, key, coin, cotton ball, or pencil) in the person's hand, and ask the person to identify it (Fig. 23-27). Normally, a person will explore it with the fingers and correctly name it. Test a different object in each hand; testing the left hand assesses right parietal lobe functioning.

Astereognosis—inability to identify object correctly. Occurs with sensory cortex lesions such as brain attack (stroke).

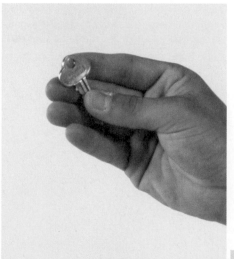

Fig. 23-27   Stereognosis.

Objective Data

Objective Data

Normal Range of Findings	Abnormal Findings

Graphesthesia. Graphesthesia is the ability to "read" a number by having it traced on the skin. Ask the person to close the eyes, and, use a blunt instrument to trace a single digit number or a letter on the palm (Fig. 23-28). Ask the person to tell you what it is. Graphesthesia is a good measure of sensory loss if the person cannot make the hand movements needed for stereognosis, as occurs in arthritis.

Inability to distinguish number occurs with lesions of the sensory cortex.

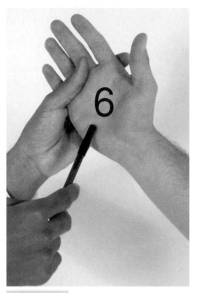

Fig. 23-28   Graphesthesia.

Two-Point Discrimination. Test the person's ability to distinguish the separation of two simultaneous pin points on the skin. Apply the two points of an opened paper clip lightly to the skin in ever-closing distances. Note the distance at which the person no longer perceives two separate points. The level of perception varies considerably with the region tested; it is most sensitive in the fingertips (2 to 8 mm) and least sensitive on the upper arms, thighs, and back (40 to 75 mm).

An increase in the distance it normally takes to identify two separate points occurs with sensory cortex lesions.

Extinction. Simultaneously touch both sides of the body at the same point. Ask the person to state how many sensations are felt and where they are. Normally, both sensations are felt.

The ability to recognize only one of the stimuli occurs with sensory cortex lesion; the stimulus is extinguished on the side *opposite* the cortex lesion.

Point Location. Touch the skin, and withdraw the stimulus promptly. Tell the person, "Put your finger where I touched you." You can perform this test simultaneously with light touch sensation.

With a sensory cortex lesion, the person cannot localize the sensation accurately, even though light touch sensation may be retained.

TEST THE REFLEXES

Stretch, or Deep Tendon Reflexes

Measurement of the stretch reflexes reveals the intactness of the reflex arc at specific spinal levels as well as the normal override on the reflex of the higher cortical levels.

For an adequate response, the limb should be relaxed and the muscle partially stretched. Stimulate the reflex by directing a short, snappy blow of the reflex hammer onto the muscle's insertion tendon. Use a relaxed hold on the hammer.

Normal Range of Findings

As with the percussion technique, the action takes place at the wrist. Strike a brief, well-aimed blow, and bounce up promptly; do not let the hammer rest on the tendon. Use the pointed end of the reflex hammer when aiming at a smaller target, such as your thumb, on the tendon site; use the flat end when the target is wider or to diffuse the impact and prevent pain.

Use just enough force to get a response. Compare right and left sides—The responses should be equal. The reflex response is graded on a four-point scale:

4+ Very brisk, hyperactive with clonus, indicative of disease
3+ Brisker than average, may indicate disease
2+ Average, normal
1+ Diminished, low normal
0   No response

This is a subjective scale and requires some clinical practice. Even then the scale is not completely reliable because no standard exists to say *how* brisk a reflex should be to warrant a grade of 3+. Also, a wide range of normal exists in reflex responses. Healthy people may have diminished or brisk reflexes. Your best plan is to interpret the DTRs *only* within the context of the rest of the neurological examination.

Sometimes the reflex response fails to appear. Try further encouragement of relaxation, varying the person's position, or increasing the strength of the blow. **Reinforcement** is another technique to relax the muscles and enhance the response (Fig. 23-29). Ask the person to perform an isometric exercise in a muscle group somewhat away from the one being tested. For example, to enhance a patellar reflex, ask the person to lock the fingers together and "pull." Then strike the tendon. To enhance a biceps response, ask the person to clench the teeth or to grasp the thigh with the opposite hand.

Abnormal Findings

Clonus is a set of rapid, rhythmic contractions of the same muscle.

Hyperreflexia is the exaggerated reflex seen when the monosynaptic reflex arc is released from the usually inhibiting influence of higher cortical levels. This occurs with upper motor neuron lesions, for example, a brain attack.

Hyporeflexia, which is the absence of a reflex, is a lower motor neuron problem. It occurs due to interruption of sensory afferents or destruction of motor efferents and anterior horn cells, as in spinal cord injury.

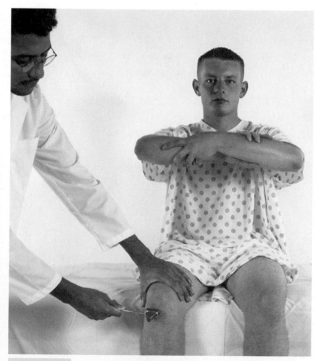

Fig. 23-29 Reinforcement.

Objective Data

Normal Range of Findings	Abnormal Findings

Biceps Reflex (C5 to C6). Support the person's forearm on yours; this position relaxes, as well as partially flexes, the person's arm. Place your thumb on the biceps tendon and strike a blow on your thumb. You can feel as well as see the normal response, which is contraction of the biceps muscle and flexion of the forearm (Fig. 23-30).

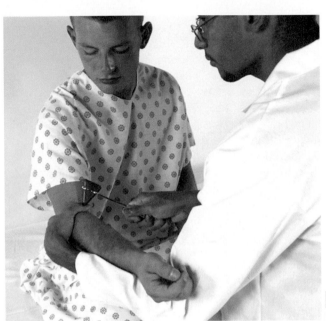

Fig. 23-30
Biceps reflex.

Triceps Reflex (C7 to C8). Tell the person to let the arm "just go dead" as you suspend it by holding the upper arm. Strike the triceps tendon directly just above the elbow (Fig. 23-31). The normal response is extension of the forearm. Alternatively, hold the person's wrist across the chest to flex the arm at the elbow, and tap the tendon.

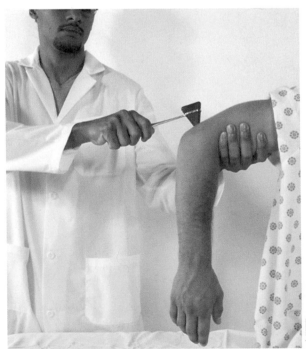

Fig. 23-31
Triceps reflex.

Normal Range of Findings	**Abnormal Findings**

Brachioradialis Reflex (C5 to C6). Hold the person's thumbs to suspend the forearms in relaxation. Strike the forearm directly, about 2 to 3 cm above the radial styloid process (Fig. 23-32). The normal response is flexion and supination of the forearm.

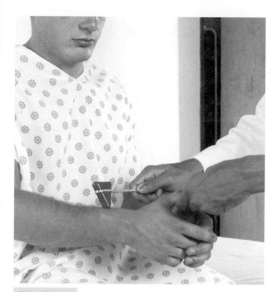

Fig. 23-32   Brachioradialis reflex.

Quadriceps Reflex ("Knee Jerk") (L2 to L4). Let the lower legs dangle freely to flex the knee and stretch the tendons. Strike the tendon directly just below the patella (Fig. 23-33). Extension of the lower leg is the expected response. You also will palpate contraction of the quadriceps.

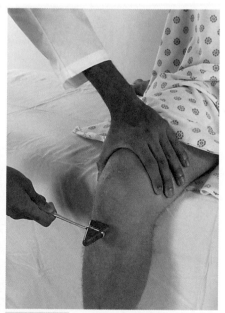

Fig. 23-33   Quadriceps reflex.

Objective Data

Normal Range of Findings	Abnormal Findings

For the person in the supine position, use your own arm as a lever to support the weight of one leg against the other leg (Fig. 23-34). This manoeuvre also flexes the knee.

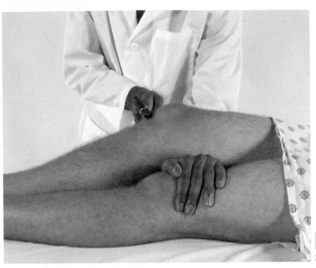

Fig. 23-34
Supine quadriceps reflex.

Achilles Reflex ("Ankle Jerk") (L5 to S2). Position the person with the knee flexed and the hip externally rotated. Hold the foot in dorsiflexion, and strike the Achilles tendon directly (Fig. 23-35). Feel the normal response as the foot plantar flexes against your hand.

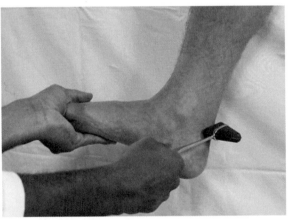

Fig. 23-35
Achilles reflex.

For the person in the supine position, flex one knee and support that lower leg against the other leg so that it falls "open." Dorsiflex the foot and tap the tendon (Fig. 23-36).

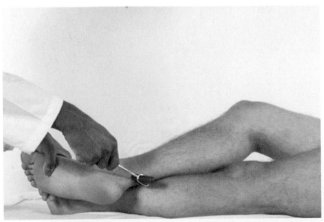

Fig. 23-36
Supine Achilles reflex.

Objective Data

Normal Range of Findings	Abnormal Findings

Clonus. Test for clonus, particularly when the reflexes are hyperactive. Support the lower leg in one hand. With your other hand, move the foot up and down a few times to relax the muscle. Then stretch the muscle by briskly dorsiflexing the foot. Hold the stretch (Fig. 23-37). With a normal response, you feel no further movement. When clonus is present, you will feel and see rapid rhythmic contractions of the calf muscle and movement of the foot.

Clonus is repeated reflex muscular movements. A hyperactive reflex with sustained clonus (lasting as long as the stretch is held) occurs with upper motor neuron disease.

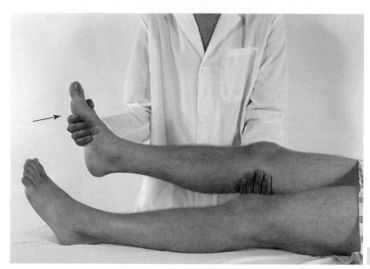

Fig. 23-37

Superficial (Cutaneous) Reflexes

Here, the sensory receptors are in the skin rather than in the muscles. The motor response is a localized muscle contraction.

Abdominal Reflexes: Upper (T8 to T10), Lower (T10 to T12). Have the person assume a supine position, with the knees slightly bent. Use the handle end of the reflex hammer, a wood applicator tip, or the end of a split tongue blade to stroke the skin. Move from the side of the abdomen toward the midline at both the upper and lower abdominal levels (Fig. 23-38). The normal response is ipsilateral contraction of the abdominal muscle, with an observed deviation of the umbilicus toward the stroke. When the abdominal wall is very thick, pull the skin to the opposite side, and feel it contract toward the stimulus.

Superficial reflexes are absent with diseases of the pyramidal tract (e.g., they are absent on the contralateral side with brain attack).

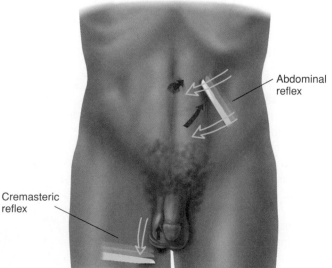

Abdominal reflex

Cremasteric reflex

Fig. 23-38

Normal Range of Findings	Abnormal Findings

Cremasteric Reflex (L1 to L2). This is not routinely done. On the male, lightly stroke the inner aspect of the thigh with the reflex hammer or tongue blade (see Fig. 23-38). Note the elevation of the ipsilateral testicle.

Absent in both UMN and LMN lesions.

Plantar Reflex (L4 to S2). Position the thigh in slight external rotation. With the reflex hammer, draw a light stroke up the lateral side of the sole of the foot and inward across the ball of the foot, like an upside-down **J** (Fig. 23-39, *A*). The normal response is plantar flexion of the toes and inversion and flexion of the forefoot.

Except in infancy, the abnormal response is dorsiflexion of the big toe and fanning of all toes, which is a positive Babinski sign, also called "upgoing toes" (Fig. 23-39, *B*). This occurs with upper motor neuron disease of the corticospinal (or pyramidal) tract.

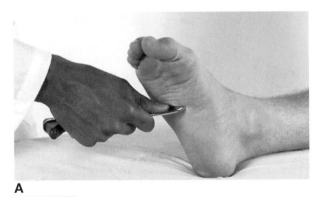

A

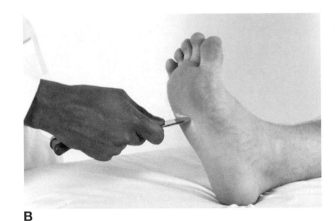

B

Fig. 23-39   **A**, Plantar reflex. **B**, Babinski sign.

⚜ DEVELOPMENTAL CARE

Infants (Birth to 12 Months)

The neurological system shows dramatic growth and development during the first year of life. Assessment includes noting that milestones you normally would expect for each month have indeed been achieved, and that the early, more primitive reflexes are eliminated from the baby's repertory when they are supposed to be.

At birth, the newborn is very alert, with the eyes open, and demonstrates strong, urgent sucking. The normal cry is loud, lusty, and even angry. The next 2 or 3 days may be spent mostly sleeping as the baby recovers from the birth process. After that, the pattern of sleep and waking activity is highly variable; it depends on the baby's individual body rhythm as well as external stimuli.

The behavioural assessment should include your observations of the infant's spontaneous waking activity, responses to environmental stimuli, and social interaction with the parents and others.

By 2 months of age, the baby smiles responsively and recognizes the parent's face. Babbling occurs at 4 months, and one or two words (mama, dada) are used nonspecifically after 9 months.

Failure to attain a skill by expected time.
Persistence of reflex behaviour beyond the normal time.

A high-pitched, shrill cry or feline screech occurs with CNS damage.
A weak, groaning cry or expiratory grunt occurs with respiratory distress.
Lethargy, hyporeactivity, hyperirritability, and parent's report of significant change in behaviour all warrant referral.

Normal Range of Findings	Abnormal Findings

The cranial nerves cannot be tested directly, but you can infer their proper functioning by the manoeuvres shown in Table 23-1.

TABLE 23-1	Testing Cranial Nerve Function of Infants
Cranial Nerve	**Response**
II, III, IV, VI	Optical blink reflex—shine light in open eyes, note rapid closure
	Size, shape, equal-sized pupils
	Regards face or close object
	Eyes follow movement
V	Rooting reflex, sucking reflex
VII	Facial movements (e.g., wrinkling forehead and nasolabial folds) symmetrical when crying or smiling
VIII	Loud noise yields Moro reflex (until 4 mo)
	Acoustic blink reflex—infant blinks in response to a loud hand clap 30 cm (12 in.) from head (avoid creating air current)
	Eyes follow direction of sound
IX, X	Swallowing, gag reflex
	Coordinated sucking and swallowing
XII	Pinch nose, infant's mouth will open and tongue rise in midline

The Motor System

Observe spontaneous motor activity for smoothness and symmetry. Smoothness of movement suggests proper cerebellar function, as does the coordination involved in sucking and swallowing. To screen gross and fine motor coordination, use the Denver II test with its age-specific developmental milestones. You also can assess movement by testing the reflexes listed in the following section. Note their smoothness of response and symmetry. Also, note whether their presence or absence is appropriate for the infant's age.

Assess muscle tone by first observing resting posture. The newborn favours a flexed position; extremities are symmetrically folded inward, the hips are slightly abducted, and the fists are tightly flexed (Fig. 23-40). Infants born by breech delivery, however, do not have flexion in the lower extremities.

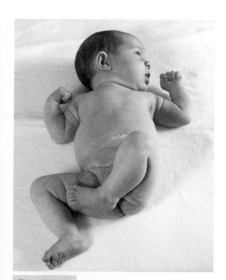

Fig. 23-40

Delay in motor activity occurs with brain damage, intellectual disability, peripheral neuromuscular damage, prolonged illness, and parental neglect.

Abnormal postures:

Frog position—hips abducted and almost flat against the table, externally rotated (only normal after breech delivery).

Opisthotonos—head arched back, stiffness of neck, and extension of arms and legs; occurs with meningeal or brain stem irritation and kernicterus (see Table 23-9, p. 708).

Extension of limbs may occur with intracranial hemorrhage.

Any type of continual asymmetry (e.g., asymmetry of upper limbs occurs with brachial plexus palsy).

Normal Range of Findings	Abnormal Findings

After 2 months of age, flexion gives way to gradual extension, beginning with the head and continuing in a cephalocaudal direction. Now is the time to check for spasticity; none should be present. Test for spasticity by flexing the infant's knees onto the abdomen and then quickly releasing them. They will unfold but not too quickly. Also, gently push the head forward—the baby should comply.

Spasticity is an early sign of cerebral palsy. After releasing flexed knees, legs will quickly extend and adduct, even to a "scissoring" motion when spasticity is present. Also, the baby often resists head flexion and extends back against your hand when spasticity is present.

The fists normally are held in tight flexion for the first 3 months. Then the fists open for part of the time. A purposeful reach for an object with both hands occurs around 4 months of age, a transfer of an object from hand to hand at 7 months of age, a grasp using fingers and opposing thumb at 9 months of age, and a purposeful release at 10 months of age. Babies are normally ambidextrous for the first 18 months.

Note persistent one-hand preference in baby younger than 18 months of age, which may indicate a motor deficit on the opposite side.

Head control is an important milestone in motor development. You can incorporate the following two movements into every infant assessment to check the muscle tone necessary for head control.

First, holding the wrists, pull the baby up to the sitting position, and note head control (Fig. 23-41). The newborn will hold the head almost in the same plane as the body; the head will balance briefly when the baby reaches the sitting position and then flop forward. (Even a premature infant shows some head flexion.) At 4 months of age, the head stays in line with the body and does not flop.

Because development progresses in a cephalocaudal direction, head lag is an early sign of brain damage.

After 6 months of age, refer any baby with failure to hold head in midline when sitting.

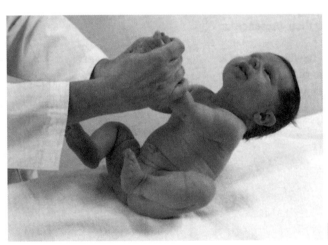

Fig. 23-41

Second, lift up the baby in a prone position, with one hand supporting the chest (Fig. 23-42). The term newborn holds the head at an angle of 45 degrees or less from horizontal, the back is straight or slightly arched, and the elbows and knees are partly flexed.

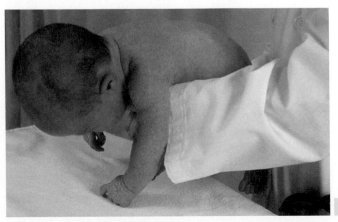

Fig. 23-42

Normal Range of Findings	**Abnormal Findings**

At 3 months of age, the baby raises the head and arches the back, as in a swan dive. This is the *Landau reflex,* which persists until 1½ years of age (Fig. 23-43).

Head lag, a limp floppy trunk, and dangling arms and legs.

Absence of the reflex indicates motor weakness, upper motor neuron disease, or intellectual disability.

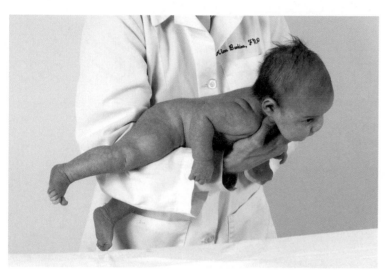

Fig. 23-43

Assess muscle strength by noting the strength of sucking and of spontaneous motor activity. Normally, no tremors are present, and no continual overshooting of the mark occurs when reaching.

The Sensory System

You will perform very little sensory testing with infants and toddlers. The newborn normally has hypoesthesia and requires a strong stimulus to elicit a response. The baby responds to pain by crying and a general reflex withdrawal of all limbs. By 7 to 9 months of age, the infant can localize the stimulus and shows more specific signs of withdrawal. Other sensory modalities are not tested.

Unusually rapid withdrawal is *hyperesthesia,* which occurs with spinal cord lesions, CNS infections, increased intracranial pressure, peritonitis.

No withdrawal is decreased sensation, which occurs with decreased consciousness, mental disability, spinal cord or peripheral nerve lesions.

Reflexes

Infantile automatisms are reflexes that have a predictable timetable of appearance and departure. The reflexes most commonly tested are listed in the following section. For the screening examination, you can just check the rooting, grasp, tonic neck, and Moro reflexes.

Objective Data

Objective Data

Normal Range of Findings	Abnormal Findings

Rooting Reflex. Brush the infant's cheek near the mouth. Note whether the infant turns the head toward that side and opens the mouth (Fig. 23-44). Appears at birth and disappears at 3 to 4 months.

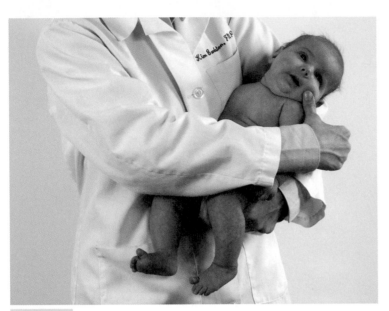

Fig. 23-44

Sucking Reflex. Touch the lips and offer your gloved little finger to suck. Note strong sucking reflex. The reflex is present at birth and disappears at 10 to 12 months.

Palmar Grasp. Place the baby's head midline to ensure symmetrical response. Offer your finger from the baby's ulnar side, away from the thumb. Note tight grasp of all the baby's fingers (Fig. 23-45). Sucking enhances grasp. Often, you can pull the baby to a sit from grasp. The reflex is present at birth, is strongest at 1 to 2 months, and disappears at 3 to 4 months.

The palmar grasp reflex is absent with brain damage and with local muscle or nerve injury.

Persistence of palmar grasp reflex after 4 months of age occurs with frontal lobe lesion.

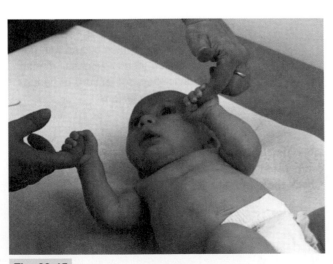

Fig. 23-45

Normal Range of Findings

Plantar Grasp. Touch your thumb at the ball of the baby's foot. Note that the toes curl down tightly (Fig. 23-46). The reflex is present at birth and disappears at 8 to 10 months.

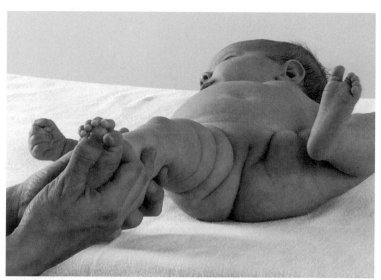

Fig. 23-46

Babinski's Reflex. Stroke your finger up the lateral edge and across the ball of the infant's foot. Note fanning of toes (positive Babinski's reflex) (Fig. 23-47). The reflex is present at birth and disappears (changes to the adult response) by 24 months of age (variable).

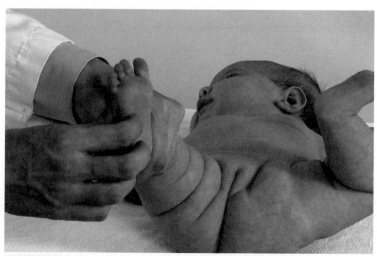

Fig. 23-47

Abnormal Findings

Positive Babinski's reflex after 2 or 2½ years of age occurs in pyramidal tract disease.

Objective Data

Normal Range of Findings	Abnormal Findings

Tonic Neck Reflex. With the baby supine, relaxed, or sleeping, turn the head to one side with the chin over shoulder. Note ipsilateral extension of the arm and leg, and flexion of the opposite arm and leg; this is the "fencing" position. If you turn the infant's head to the opposite side, positions will be reversed (Fig. 23-48). The reflex appears by 2 to 3 months, decreases at 3 to 4 months, and disappears by 4 to 6 months.

Persistence in later infancy occurs with brain damage.

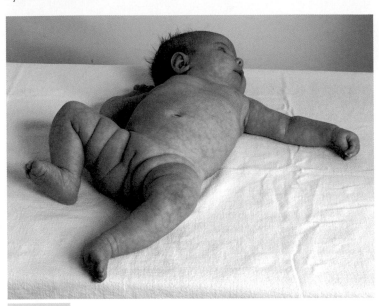

Fig. 23-48 Tonic neck reflex.

Moro Reflex. Startle the infant by jarring the crib, making a loud noise, or supporting the head and back in a semi-sitting position and quickly lowering the infant to 30 degrees. The baby looks as if he or she is hugging a tree. That is, symmetrical abduction and extension of the arms and legs, fanning fingers, and curling of the index finger and thumb to C position occur. The infant then brings in both arms and legs (Fig. 23-49). The reflex is present at birth and disappears at 1 to 4 months.

Absence of the Moro reflex in the newborn or persistence after 5 months of age indicates severe CNS injury.

Absence of movement in just one arm occurs with fracture of the humerus or clavicle and with brachial nerve palsy.

Absence in one leg occurs with a lower spinal cord problem or a dislocated hip.

A hyperactive Moro reflex occurs with tetany or CNS infection.

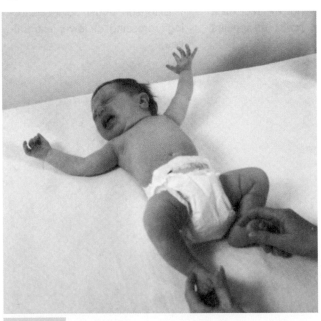

Fig. 23-49 Moro reflex.

Normal Range of Findings	Abnormal Findings

Placing Reflex. Hold the infant upright under the arms, close to a table. Let the dorsal "top" of foot touch the underside of table. Note flexing of hip and knee, followed by extension at the hip, to place foot on table (Fig. 23-50). Reflex appears at 4 days after birth.

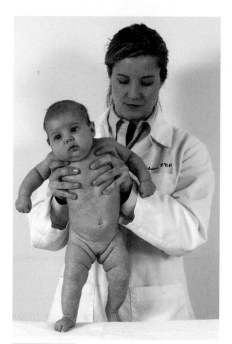

Fig. 23-50   Placing reflex.

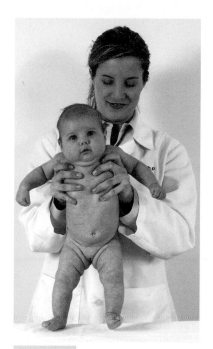

Fig. 23-51   Stepping reflex.

Stepping Reflex. Hold the infant upright under the arms, with the feet on a flat surface. Note regular alternating steps (Fig. 23-51). The reflex disappears before voluntary walking.

Extensor thrust, or "scissoring"; crossing of lower extremities.

Preschool- and School-Age Children

Use the same sequence of neurological assessment as with the adult, with the omissions or modifications mentioned in the following section.

Assess the child's general behaviour during play activities, reaction to parent, and co-operation with parent and with you. Complete details are described in Chapter 6.

Smell and taste are almost never tested, but if you need to test the child's sense of smell (cranial nerve I), use a scent familiar to the child such as orange peel. When testing visual fields (cranial nerve II) and cardinal positions of gaze (cranial nerves III, IV, VI), you often need to gently immobilize the head, or the child will track with the whole head. Make a game out of asking the child to imitate your "funny faces" (cranial nerve VII); thus, the child has fun, and you have won a friend.

Objective Data

Objective Data

Normal Range of Findings	Abnormal Findings

Normal Range of Findings

Much of the motor assessment can be derived from watching the child undress and dress and manipulate buttons. This indicates muscle strength, symmetry, joint range of motion, and fine motor skills. Use the Denver II to screen gross and fine motor skills that are appropriate for the child's specific age. Be familiar with developmental milestones described in Chapter 2 for each age.

Note the child's gait during both walking and running. Allow for the normal wide-based gate of the toddler and the normal knock-kneed walk of the preschooler. Normally, the child can balance on one foot for about 5 seconds by 4 years of age, can balance for 8 to 10 seconds at 5 years of age, and can hop at 4 years. Children enjoy participating these tests (Fig. 23-52).

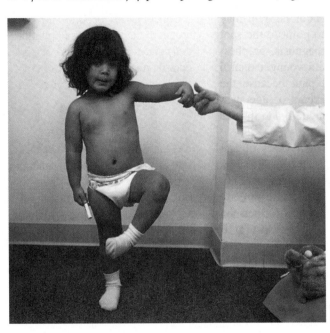

Fig. 23-52

Observe the child as he or she rises from the supine position on the floor to the sitting position, and then to the standing position. Note the muscles of the neck, abdomen, arms, and legs. Normally, the child curls up in the midline to sit up, then pushes off with both hands against the floor to stand (Fig. 23-53, *A*).

Abnormal Findings

Muscle hypertrophy or atrophy occurs with muscular dystrophy.

Muscle weakness.

Incoordination.

Causes of motor delay are listed earlier in the infant section.

Staggering, falling.

Weakness climbing up or down stairs occurs with muscular dystrophy.

Broad-based gait beyond toddlerhood, scissor gait (see Table 23-5, p. 703).

Failure to hop after 5 years of age indicates incoordination of gross motor skill.

Weak pelvic muscles are a sign of muscular dystrophy; from the supine position, the child will roll to one side, bend forward to all four extremities, plant hands on legs, and literally "climb" up himself or herself. This is *Gower's sign* (Fig. 23-53, *B*).

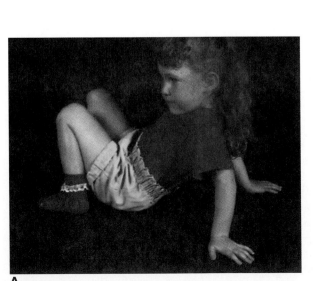

A

Fig. 23-53

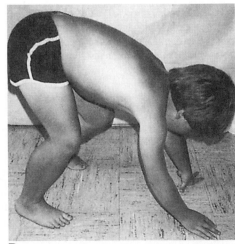

B

Normal Range of Findings	Abnormal Findings

Assess fine coordination by using the finger-to-nose test if you can be sure the young child understands your directions. Demonstrate the procedure first, then ask the child to do the test with the eyes open, then with the eyes closed. Fine coordination is not fully developed until the child has reached 4 or 6 years of age. Consider it normal if a younger child can bring the finger to within 2 to 5 cm of the nose.

Testing sensation is very unreliable in toddlers and preschoolers. You may test light touch by asking the child to close the eyes and then to point to the spot where you touch or tickle. Testing of vibration, position, stereognosis, graphesthesia, or two-point discrimination usually is not done on a child younger than 6 years of age. Also, do not test for perception of superficial pain. In children older than 6 years of age, you may perform sensory testing as with adults. Use a broken tongue blade if you need to test superficial pain.

The DTRs usually are not tested in children younger than 5 years of age due to lack of co-operation in relaxation. When you need to test DTRs in a young child, use your finger to percuss the tendon. Use a reflex hammer only with an older child. Coax the child to relax, or distract and percuss discreetly when the child is not paying attention. The knee jerk is present at birth, then the ankle jerk and brachial reflex appear, and the triceps reflex is present at 6 months.

Failure of the finger-to-nose test with the eyes open indicates gross incoordination; failure of the test with the eyes closed indicates minor incoordination or lack of position sense.

Sensory loss occurs with decreased consciousness, mental deficiency, or spinal cord or peripheral nerve dysfunction.

Hyperactivity of DTRs occurs with upper motor neuron lesion, hypocalcemia, and hyperthyroidism, and with muscle spasm associated with early poliomyelitis.

Decreased or absent reflexes occur with a lower motor neuron lesion, muscular dystrophy, and flaccidity or flaccid paralysis.

Clonus may occur with fatigue, but it usually indicates hyperreflexia.

The Aging Adult

Use the same examination as used with the younger adult. Be aware that some aging adults show a slower response to your requests, especially to those calling for coordination of movements. The conditions discussed in the following sections are normal variants related to aging.

Although the cranial nerves mediating taste and smell are not usually tested, they may show some decline in function.

Any decrease in muscle bulk is most apparent in the hand, as seen by guttering between the metacarpals. These dorsal hand muscles often look wasted, even with no apparent arthropathy. The grip strength remains relatively good.

Senile tremors occasionally occur. These benign tremors include an intention tremor of the hands, head nodding (as if saying yes or no), and tongue protrusion. *Dyskinesias* are the repetitive stereotyped movements in the jaw, lips, or tongue that may accompany senile tremors. No associated rigidity is present.

The gait may be slower and more deliberate than that in the younger person, and it may deviate slightly from a midline path.

The rapid alternating movements, such as pronating and supinating the hands on the thigh, may be more difficult to perform by the aging adult.

After 65 years of age, loss of the sensation of vibration at the ankle malleolus is common and is usually accompanied by loss of the ankle jerk. Position sense in the big toe may be lost, although this is less common than vibration loss. Tactile sensation may be impaired. The aging person may need stronger stimuli for light touch and especially for pain.

The DTRs are less brisk. Those in the upper extremities are usually present, but the ankle jerks are commonly lost. Knee jerks may be lost, but this occurs less often. Because aging people find it difficult to relax their limbs, always use reinforcement when eliciting the DTRs.

Hand muscle atrophy is worsened with disuse and degenerative arthropathy.

Distinguish senile tremors from tremors of parkinsonism. The latter includes rigidity and slowness and weakness of voluntary movement.

Absence of a rhythmic reciprocal gait pattern is seen in parkinsonism and hemiparesis (see Table 23-5, p. 703).

Note any difference in sensation between right and left sides, which may indicate a neurological deficit.

Objective Data

Objective Data

Normal Range of Findings	Abnormal Findings

The plantar reflex may be absent or difficult to interpret. Often, you will not see a definite normal flexor response. However, you still should consider a definite extensor response to be abnormal.

The superficial abdominal reflexes may be absent, probably because of stretching of the musculature through pregnancy or obesity.

NEUROLOGICAL RECHECK

Some hospitalized persons have head trauma or a neurological deficit due to a systemic disease process. These people must be monitored closely for any improvement or deterioration in neurological status and for any indication of increasing intracranial pressure. Signs of increasing intracranial pressure signal impending cerebral disaster and death and require early and prompt intervention.

Use an abbreviation of the neurological examination in the following sequence:
1. Level of consciousness
2. Motor function
3. Pupillary response
4. Vital signs

Level of Consciousness. A *change* in the level of consciousness is the single most important factor in this examination. It is the earliest and most sensitive index of change in neurological status. Note the ease of *arousal* and the state of awareness, or *orientation*. Assess orientation by asking questions about:
- Person—own name, occupation, names of workers around person, their occupations
- Place—where person is, nature of building, city, province
- Time—day of week, month, year

Vary the questions during repeat assessments to ensure that the person is not merely memorizing and recalling answers. Note the quality and the content of the verbal response; articulation, fluency, manner of thinking; and any deficit in language comprehension or production (see Chapter 6).

When the person is intubated and cannot speak, you will have to ask questions that require a nod or shake of the head, "Is this a hospital?" "Are you at home?" "Are we in Alberta?"

A person is fully alert when his or her eyes open at your approach or spontaneously; when he or she is oriented to person, place, and time; and when he or she is able to follow verbal commands appropriately.

If the person is not fully alert, increase the amount of stimulus used in this order:
1. Name called
2. Light touch on person's arm
3. Vigorous shake of shoulder
4. Pain applied (pinch nail bed, pinch trapezius muscle, rub your knuckles on the person's sternum)
Record the stimulus used as well as the person's response to it.

Motor Function. Check the voluntary movement of each extremity by giving the person specific commands. (This procedure also tests level of consciousness by noting the person's ability to follow commands.)

Ask the person to lift the eyebrows, frown, bare teeth. Note symmetrical facial movements and bilateral nasolabial folds (cranial nerve VII).

A change in consciousness may be subtle. Note any decreasing level of consciousness, disorientation, memory loss, uncooperative behaviour, or even complacency in a previously combative person.

Review Table 6-3, p. 106.

Normal Range of Findings	**Abnormal Findings**

You can check upper arm strength by checking hand grasps. Ask the person to squeeze your fingers. Offer your two fingers, one on top of the other, so that a strong hand grasp does not hurt your knuckles (Fig. 23-54). Be judicious about asking the person to squeeze your hands; some persons with diffuse brain damage, especially frontal lobe injury, have a grasp that is a reflex only.

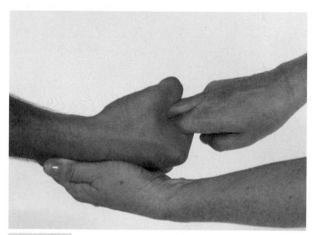

Fig. 23-54

Alternatively, ask the person to lift each hand or to hold up one finger. You also can check upper extremity strength by palmar drift. Ask the person to extend both arms forward or halfway up, palms up, eyes closed, and hold for 10 to 20 seconds (Fig. 23-55). Normally, the arms stay steady with no downward drift.

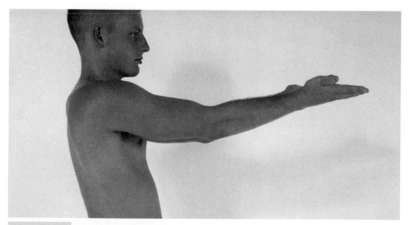

Fig. 23-55

Check lower extremities by asking the person to do straight leg raises. Ask the person to lift one leg at a time straight up off the bed (Fig. 23-56). Full strength allows the leg to be lifted 90 degrees. If multiple trauma, pain, or equipment preclude this motion, ask the person to push one foot at a time against your hand's resistance, "like putting your foot on the gas pedal of your car" (Fig. 23-57).

Objective Data

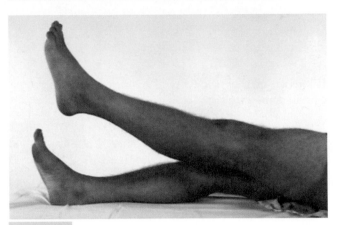

Fig. 23-56

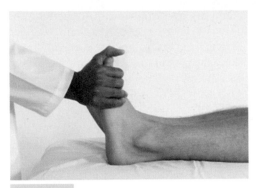

Fig. 23-57

Objective Data

Normal Range of Findings

In the person with decreased level of consciousness, note if movement occurs spontaneously and as a result of noxious stimuli such as pain or suctioning. An attempt to push away your hand after such stimuli is called *localizing* and is characterized as purposeful movement.

Pupillary Response. Note the size, shape, and symmetry of both pupils. Shine a light into each pupil and note the direct and consensual light reflex. Both pupils should constrict briskly. (Allow for the effects of any medication that could affect pupil size and reactivity.) When recording, pupil size is best expressed in millimetres. Tape a millimetre scale onto a tongue blade and hold it next to the person's eyes for the most accurate measurement (Fig. 23-58).

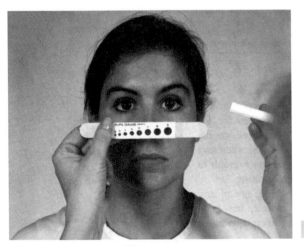

Fig. 23-58

Vital Signs. Measure the temperature, pulse, respiration, and blood pressure as often as the person's condition warrants. Although they are vital to the overall assessment of the critically ill person, pulse and blood pressure are notoriously unreliable parameters of CNS deficit. Any changes are late consequences of rising intracranial pressure.

The Glasgow Coma Scale. Since the terms describing levels of consciousness are ambiguous, the Glasgow Coma Scale (GCS) was developed as an accurate and reliable *quantitative* tool (Fig. 23-59). The GCS is a standardized, objective assessment that defines the level of consciousness by giving it a numerical value. The scale is divided into three areas: eye opening, verbal response, and motor response. Each area is rated separately, and a number is given for the person's best response. The three numbers are added; the total score reflects the brain's

Abnormal Findings

Any abnormal posturing, decorticate rigidity, or decerebrate rigidity indicates diffuse brain injury (see Table 23-9, p. 708).

In a brain-injured person, a sudden, unilateral, dilated and nonreactive pupil is ominous. Cranial nerve III runs parallel to the brain stem. When increasing intracranial pressure pushes the brain stem down (uncal herniation), it puts pressure on cranial nerve III, causing pupil dilatation.

The Cushing reflex shows signs of increasing intracranial pressure: blood pressure—sudden elevation with widening pulse pressure; pulse—decreased rate, slow and bounding.

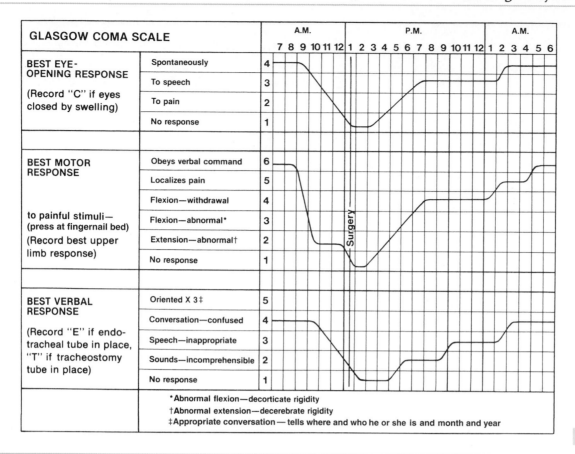

GLASGOW COMA SCALE			A.M.	P.M.	A.M.
			7 8 9 10 11 12	1 2 3 4 5 6 7 8 9 10 11 12	1 2 3 4 5 6
BEST EYE-OPENING RESPONSE (Record "C" if eyes closed by swelling)	Spontaneously	4			
	To speech	3			
	To pain	2			
	No response	1			
BEST MOTOR RESPONSE to painful stimuli— (press at fingernail bed) (Record best upper limb response)	Obeys verbal command	6			
	Localizes pain	5			
	Flexion—withdrawal	4			
	Flexion—abnormal*	3		Surgery	
	Extension—abnormal†	2			
	No response	1			
BEST VERBAL RESPONSE (Record "E" if endo-tracheal tube in place, "T" if tracheostomy tube in place)	Oriented X 3‡	5			
	Conversation—confused	4			
	Speech—inappropriate	3			
	Sounds—incomprehensible	2			
	No response	1			

*Abnormal flexion—decorticate rigidity
†Abnormal extension—decerebrate rigidity
‡Appropriate conversation—tells where and who he or she is and month and year

Fig. 23-59

Normal Range of Findings	**Abnormal Findings**

functional level. A fully alert, normal person has a score of 15, whereas a score of 7 or less reflects coma. Serial assessments can be plotted on a graph to illustrate visually whether the person is stable, improving, or deteriorating.

The GCS assesses the functional state of the brain as a whole, not of any particular site in the brain. The scale is easy to learn and master, has good inter-rater reliability (Juarez & Lyons, 1995), and enhances interprofessional communication by providing a common language.

The Canadian Neurological Scale (CNS) is also a valid and reliable tool that is used to monitor mentation and motor functions in stroke patients. The CNS Reference Card is available in Appendix E.

Summary Checklist: Neurological Examination

 For a PDA-downloadable version, go to http://evolve.elsevier.com/Canada/Jarvis/examination/.

Neurological Screening Examination
1. Mental status
2. Cranial nerves
   II: Optic
   III, IV, VI: Extraocular muscles
   V: Trigeminal
   VII: Facial mobility
3. Motor function
   Gait and balance
   Knee flexion—hop or shallow knee bend
4. Sensory function
   Superficial pain and light touch—arms and legs
   Vibration—arms and legs

5. Reflexes
   Biceps
   Triceps
   Patellar
   Achilles

Neurological Complete Examination
1. Mental status
2. Cranial nerves II through XII
3. Motor system
   Muscle size, strength, tone
   Gait and balance
   Rapid alternating movements

4. Sensory function
   Superficial pain and light touch
   Vibration
   Position sense
   Stereognosis, graphesthesia, two-point discrimination
5. Reflexes
   DTRs: biceps, triceps, brachioradialis, patellar, Achilles
   Superficial: abdominal, plantar

Promoting Health: Stroke Prevention

Symptoms and Risk Factors (Nonmodifiable, and Well-Documented Modifiable) for Stroke

Almost 50,000 new cases of stroke occur in Canada each year, and the associated short-term mortality is about 20 to 25% (Côté et al., 2007). The prevalence of stroke increases with age and other risk factors, such as hypertension, smoking, and associated cardiac conditions such as atrial fibrillation. A stroke, or cerebrovascular accident (CVA), occurs when the blood flow is interrupted to a part of the brain, which is why it is often referred to as a "brain attack." The most common type is an ischemic stroke, occurring when a blood clot blocks a blood vessel in the brain. Less common is a hemorrhagic stroke, which occurs when a blood vessel in the brain ruptures and causes bleeding. The symptoms and after-effects of a stroke depend on which area of the brain is affected and to what extent. This can make a stroke difficult to diagnose. However, early recognition of symptoms and prompt treatment are essential.

The **most common** symptoms of stroke include:
1. Sudden weakness or numbness in the face, arms, or legs, especially when it is on one side of the body
2. Sudden confusion, trouble speaking or understanding speech
3. Sudden changes in vision, such as blurry vision or partial or complete loss of vision in one or both eyes
4. Sudden trouble walking, dizziness, or loss of balance or coordination
5. Sudden severe headache with no reason or explanation

Less common symptoms of stroke include:
1. Sudden nausea or vomiting
2. Brief loss of consciousness, including fainting

Stroke symptoms usually do not hurt, which is why many people ignore them or delay seeking medical attention. Sometimes, people can have a "mini-stroke," or transient ischemic attack (TIA). In these cases, the stroke symptoms are only temporary and then disappear, often within an hour. Because the symptoms "go away," people too often do not report them or seek medical attention. However, a TIA is a warning sign that should not be ignored. The risk of experiencing an ischemic stroke after an initial stroke or after a TIA is approximately 10 to 20% in the first year (Côté et al., 2007). When people experience chest pain, they should seek medical attention to rule out a heart attack. Having a TIA should also prompt people to seek medical attention to rule out the possibility of a future "brain attack."

Stroke can strike anyone without any warning. Preventing a stroke is still the best medicine. People need to be aware of their stroke risk and take steps to change the risk factors they can control.

Most risk factors for stroke, such as high blood pressure, diabetes, smoking, inactivity, and high cholesterol are equivalent for men and women and are potentially modifiable depending on peoples' personal and social contexts. Gender, however, is an important risk factor. In Canada, the mortality rate due to stroke is 45% greater for women than for men (Heart and Stroke Foundation, 2008b). At all ages, men have higher risks for having a stroke than women, but the mortality rate is higher for women and the gap is widening. In part, this is due to women living longer on average than men, but new research suggests that there may be some risk factors that are uniquely important for women. For example, women who have migraines with visual disturbances such as flashing dots or blind spots can be up to 10 times more likely to have a stroke; women who develop pre-eclampsia in pregnancy may have a 60% greater risk of non–pregnancy-related ischemic stroke; and women who smoke and who are taking oral contraceptives or have high blood pressure, migraines, or blood clotting disorders have an increased risk of stoke.

Well-documented modifiable risk factors for stroke include:
1. History of cardiovascular disease
   a. Coronary heart disease
   b. Cardiac failure
   c. Symptomatic peripheral artery disease (PAD)
2. Hypertension
3. Cigarette smoking or exposure to secondhand smoke
4. Diabetes
5. Atrial fibrillation
6. Other cardiac conditions
   a. Dilated cardiomyopathy
   b. Valvular heart disease (e.g., mitral valve prolapse, endocarditis, and prosthetic cardiac valves)
   c. Intracardiac congenital defects (e.g., patent foraman ovale, atrial septal defect, and atrial septal aneurysm)
7. Dyslipidemia
8. Asymptomatic carotid stenosis
9. Sickle cell disease
10. Postmenopausal hormone therapy
11. Diet and nutrition
12. Physical inactivity
13. Obesity and fat distribution
14. History of TIA

Nonmodifiable risk factors for stroke may still help identify those who, in conjunction with well-documented modifiable risks, are at highest risk of stroke and who may benefit from more rigorous treatment of modifiable risk factors.

Nonmodifiable risk factors for stroke include:
1. Age
2. Gender—strokes are generally more prevalent in men than in women. However, the mortality rate for women is higher.
3. Low birth weight
4. Ethnocultural background—Aboriginial people and those of African or South Asian descent are more likely to have high blood pressure and diabetes and are therefore at greater risk of heart disease and stroke than the general population
5. Genetic factors, disorders (e.g., Marfan syndrome, Fabry disease, Cerebral autosomal dominant arteriopathy with subcortical infarcts, and leukoencephalopathy (CADASIL)

American Stroke Association; Goldstein, et al., 2006; Institute of Neurological Disorders and Stroke.
Heart and Stroke Foundation of Canada. (2008). Stroke. Retrieved on February 12, 2008, from http://www.heartandstroke.com/site/c.iklQLcMWJtE/b.3483933/

Objective Data

DOCUMENTATION AND CRITICAL THINKING

Sample Charting

SUBJECTIVE

No unusually frequent or severe headaches, no head injury, dizziness or vertigo, seizures or tremors. No weakness, numbness or tingling, difficulty swallowing or speaking. Has no past history of stroke, spinal cord injury, meningitis, or alcoholism.

OBJECTIVE

Mental Status: Appearance, behaviour, and speech appropriate; alert and oriented to person, place, and time; recent and remote memory intact.

Cranial Nerves:

I: Identifies coffee and peppermint.

II: Vision 20/20 OS, 20/20 OD, peripheral fields intact by confrontation, fundi normal.

III, IV, VI: EOMs intact, no ptosis or nystagmus; pupils equal, round, react to light and accommodation (PERRLA).

V: Sensation intact and equal bilaterally, jaw strength equal bilaterally.

VII: Facial muscles intact and symmetrical.

VIII: Hearing—whispered words heard bilaterally, Weber test—tone is heard midline without lateralization.

IX, X: Swallowing intact, gag reflex present, uvula rises in midline on phonation.

XI: Shoulder shrug, head movement intact and equal bilaterally.

XII: Tongue protrudes midline, no tremors.

Motor: No atrophy, weakness, or tremors. Gait smooth and coordinated, able to tandem walk, negative Romberg. Rapid alternating movements (RAM)—finger-to-nose smoothly intact.

Sensory: Pinprick, light touch, vibration intact. Stereognosis—able to identify key.

Reflexes: Normal abdominal, no Babinski's sign, DTRs 2+ and = bilaterally with downgoing toes, see drawing below:

ASSESSMENT

Neurological system intact, normal function

Focused Assessment: Clinical Case Study

J.T. is a 61-year-old male carpenter at a large building firm; he is admitted to the Rehabilitation Institute with a diagnosis of right hemiplegia and aphasia following a brain attack (CVA) 4 weeks PTA.

SUBJECTIVE

- Because of J.T.'s speech dysfunction, history provided by wife.
- 4 weeks PTA—complaint of severe headache, then sudden onset of collapse and loss of consciousness while at work. Did not strike head as fell. Transported by ambulance to Memorial Hospital where admitting physician said J.T. "probably had a stroke." Right arm and leg were limp, and he remained unconscious. Admitted to critical care unit. Regained consciousness

Continued

day 3 after admission, unable to move right side, unable to speak clearly or write. Remained in ICU 4 more days until "doctors were sure heart and breathing were steady."

- 3 weeks PTA—transferred to medical floor where care included physical therapy twice per day, and passive ROM 4 X/day.
- Now—some improvement in right motor function. Bowel control achieved with use of commode same time each day (after breakfast). Bladder control improved. Some occasional incontinence, usually when unable to tell people he needs to urinate.

OBJECTIVE

Mental Status: Dressed in jogging suit, sitting in wheelchair, appears alert with appropriate eye contact, listening intently to history. Speech is slow, requires great effort, able to give one-word answers that are appropriate but lack normal tone. Seems to understand all language spoken to him. Follows requests appropriately, within limits of motor weakness.

Cranial Nerves:

II: Acuity normal, fields by confrontation—right homonymous hemianopsia, fundi normal.

III, IV, VI: EOMs intact, no ptosis or nystagmus, PERRLA.

V: Sensation intact to pinprick and light touch. Jaw strength weak on right.

VII: Flat nasolabial fold on right, motor weakness on right lower face. Able to wrinkle forehead bilaterally, but unable to smile or bare teeth on right.

VIII: Hearing intact.

IX, X: Swallowing intact, gag reflex present, uvula rises midline on phonation.

XI: Shoulder shrug, head movement weaker on right.

XII: Tongue protrudes midline, no tremors.

Sensory: Pinprick and light touch present but diminished on right arm and leg. Vibration intact. Position sense impaired on right side. Stereognosis intact.

Motor: Right hand grip weak, right arm drifts, right leg weak, unable to support weight. Spasticity in right arm and leg muscles, limited range of motion on passive motion. Unable to stand up and walk unassisted. Unable to perform finger-to-nose or heel-to-shin on right side, left side smoothly intact.

Reflexes: Hyperactive 4+ with clonus, and upgoing toes in right leg. Abdominal and cremasteric reflexes absent on right.

ASSESSMENT

Impaired verbal communication R/T effects of CVA
Impaired physical mobility R/T neuromuscular impairment
Disturbed body image R/T effects of loss of body function
Self-care deficits: feeding, bathing, toileting, dressing/grooming R/T muscular weakness
Disturbed sensory perception (absent right visual fields) R/T neurological impairment
Risk for injury R/T visual field deficit

Nursing Diagnoses Commonly Associated With Neurological Disorders

All nursing diagnoses can be found on the Evolve Web site at **http://evolve.elsevier.com/Canada/Jarvis/examination/.**

ABNORMAL FINDINGS

TABLE 23-2	**Abnormalities in Cranial Nerves**		
Nerve	Test	Abnormal Findings	Possible Causes
I: Olfactory	Identify familiar odours	Anosmia	Upper respiratory infection (temporary); tobacco or cocaine use; fracture of cribriform plate or ethmoid area; frontal lobe lesion; tumour in olfactory bulb or tract
II: Optic	Visual acuity	Defect or absent central vision	Congenital blindness, refractive error, acquired vision loss from numerous diseases (e.g., cerebrovascular accident, diabetes), trauma to globe or orbit (see discussion of cranial nerve III)
	Visual fields	Defect in peripheral vision, hemianopsia	
	Shine light in eye	Absent light reflex	
	Direct inspection	Papilledema	Increased intracranial pressure
		Optic atrophy	Glaucoma
		Retinal lesions	Diabetes
III: Oculomotor	Inspection	Dilated pupil, ptosis, eye turns out and slightly down	Paralysis in cranial nerve III from internal carotid aneurysm, tumour, inflammatory lesions, uncal herniation with increased intracranial pressure
	Extraocular muscle movement	Failure to move eye up, in, down	Ptosis from myasthenia gravis, oculomotor nerve palsy, Horner syndrome
	Shine light in eye	Absent light reflex	Blindness, drug influence, increased intracranial pressure, CNS injury, circulatory arrest, CNS syphilis
IV: Trochlear	Extraocular muscle movement	Failure to turn eye down or out	Fracture of orbit, brain stem tumour
V: Trigeminal	Superficial touch—three divisions	Absent touch and pain, paresthesias	Trauma, tumor, pressure from aneurysm, inflammation, sequelae of alcohol injection for trigeminal neuralgia
	Corneal reflex	No blink	
	Clench teeth	Weakness of masseter or temporalis muscles	Unilateral weakness with cranial nerve V lesion; bilateral weakness with upper or lower motor neuron disorder
VI: Abducens	Extraocular muscle movement to right and left sides	Failure to move laterally, diplopia on lateral gaze	Brain stem tumour or trauma, fracture of orbit

Continued

TABLE 23-2	Abnormalities in Cranial Nerves—cont'd		
Nerve	Test	Abnormal Findings	Possible Causes
VII: Facial	Wrinkle forehead, close eyes tightly	Absent or asymmetrical facial movement	Bell's palsy (lower motor neuron lesion) causes paralysis of entire half of face
	Smile, puff cheeks Identify tastes	Loss of taste	Upper motor neuron lesions (cerebrovascular accident, tumour, inflammatory) cause paralysis of lower half of face, leaving forehead intact Other lower motor neuron causes of paralysis: swelling from ear or meningeal infections
VIII: Acoustic	Hearing acuity	Decrease or loss of hearing	Inflammation, occluded ear canal, otosclerosis, presbycusis, drug toxicity, tumour
IX: Glossopharyngeal	Gag reflex	See cranial nerve X	
X: Vagus	Phonates "ahh"	Uvula deviates to side	Brain stem tumour, neck injury, cranial nerve X lesion
	Gag reflex Note voice quality	No gag reflex Hoarse or brassy Nasal twang Husky	Vocal cord weakness Soft palate weakness Unilateral cranial nerve X lesion
	Note swallowing	Dysphagia, fluids regurgitate through nose	Bilateral cranial nerve X lesion
XI: Spinal accessory	Turn head, shrug shoulders against resistance	Absent movement of sternomastoid or trapezius muscles	Neck injury, torticollis
XII: Hypoglossal	Protrude tongue Wiggle tongue from side to side	Deviates to side Slowed rate of movement	Lower motor neuron lesion Bilateral upper motor neuron lesion

TABLE 23-3	Abnormalities in Muscle Tone	
Condition	Description	Associated With
Flaccidity	Decreased muscle tone or *hypotonia;* muscle feels limp, soft, and flabby; muscle is weak and easily fatigued	Lower motor neuron injury anywhere from the anterior horn cell in the spinal cord to the peripheral nerve (peripheral neuritis, poliomyelitis, Guillain-Barré syndrome). Early cerebrovascular accident and spinal cord injury are flaccid at first.
Spasticity	Increased tone or *hypertonia;* increased resistance to passive lengthening; then may suddenly give way (clasp-knife phenomenon)	Upper motor neuron injury to corticospinal motor tract, such as paralysis with cerebrovascular accident (chronic stage)
Rigidity	Constant state of resistance (lead-pipe rigidity); resists passive movement in any direction; dystonia	Injury to extrapyramidal motor tracts, for example, basal ganglia with parkinsonism
Cogwheel rigidity	Type of rigidity in which the increased tone is released by degrees during passive range of motion so it feels like small regular jerks	Parkinsonism

| TABLE 23-4 | Abnormalities in Muscle Movement |

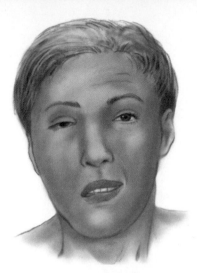

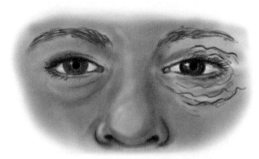

Paralysis

Decreased or loss of motor power due to problem with motor nerve or muscle fibres. Causes: acute—trauma, spinal cord injury, brain attack, poliomyelitis, polyneuritis, Bell's palsy; chronic—muscular dystrophy, diabetic neuropathy, multiple sclerosis; episodic—myasthenia gravis.

Patterns of paralysis: *hemiplegia*—spastic or flaccid paralysis of one side (right or left) of body and extremities; *paraplegia*—symmetrical paralysis of both lower extremities; *quadriplegia*—paralysis in all four extremities; *paresis*—weakness of muscles rather than paralysis.

Fasciculation

Rapid, continuous twitching of resting muscle or part of muscle, without movement of limb, that can be seen or palpated. Types: fine—occurs with lower motor neuron disease, associated with atrophy and weakness; coarse—occurs with cold exposure or fatigue and is not significant.

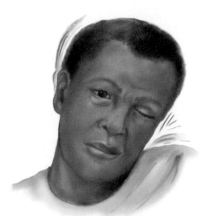

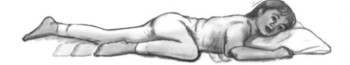

Tic

Involuntary, compulsive, repetitive twitching of a muscle group, such as wink, grimace, head movement, shoulder shrug; due to a neurological cause, such as tardive dyskinesias, Tourette's syndrome, or psychogenic cause (habit tic).

Myoclonus

Rapid, sudden jerk or a short series of jerks at fairly regular intervals. A hiccup is a myoclonus of diaphragm. Single myoclonic arm or leg jerk is normal when the person is falling asleep; myoclonic jerks are severe with grand mal seizures.

Continued

TABLE 23-4	Abnormalities in Muscle Movement—cont'd

Tremor

Involuntary contraction of opposing muscle groups. Results in rhythmic, back-and-forth movement of one or more joints. May occur at rest or with voluntary movement. All tremors disappear while sleeping. Tremors may be slow (3 to 6 per second) or rapid (10 to 20 per second).

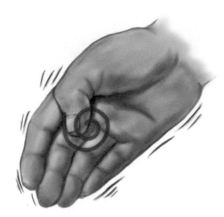

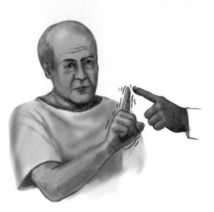

Rest Tremor

Coarse and slow (3 to 6 per second); partly or completely disappears with voluntary movement (e.g., "pill rolling" tremor of parkinsonism, with thumb and opposing fingers).

Intention Tremor

Rate varies; worse with voluntary movement. Occurs with cerebellar disease and multiple sclerosis.

Essential tremor (familial)—a type of intention tremor; most common tremor with older people. Benign (no associated disease) but causes emotional stress in work or social situations. Improves with the administration of sedatives, propranolol, alcohol, but use of alcohol is discouraged because of the risk of addiction.

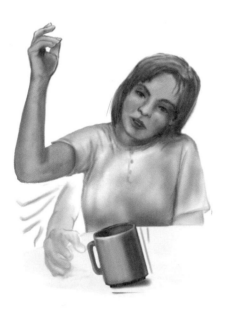

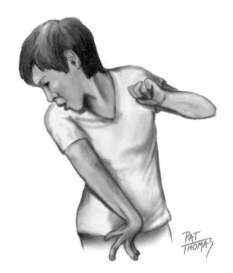

Chorea

Sudden, rapid, jerky, purposeless movement involving limbs, trunk, or face.

Occurs at irregular intervals, not rhythmic or repetitive, more convulsive than a tic. Some are spontaneous, and some are initiated; all are accentuated by voluntary acts. Disappears with sleep. Common with Sydenham's chorea and Huntington's disease.

Athetosis

Slow, twisting, writhing, continuous movement, resembling a snake or worm. Involves distal part of limb more than the proximal part. Occurs with cerebral palsy. Disappears with sleep. "Athetoid" hand—some fingers are flexed and some are extended.

ABNORMAL FINDINGS
FOR ADVANCED PRACTICE

TABLE 23-5	Abnormal Gaits	
Type	Characteristic Appearance	Possible Causes
Spastic Hemiparesis 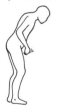	Arm is immobile against the body, with flexion of the shoulder, elbow, wrist, fingers, and adduction of shoulder. The leg is stiff and extended and circumducts with each step (drags toe in a semi-circle)	Upper motor neuron lesion of the corticospinal tract, such as cerebrovascular accident, trauma
Cerebellar Ataxia 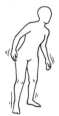	Staggering, wide-based gait; difficulty with turns; uncoordinated movement with positive Romberg sign	Alcohol or barbiturate effect on cerebellum; cerebellar tumour; multiple sclerosis
Parkinsonian (Festinating)	Posture is stooped; trunk is pitched forward; elbows, hips, and knees are flexed. Steps are short and shuffling. Hesitation to begin walking, and difficult to stop suddenly. The person holds the body rigid. Walks and turns body as one fixed unit. Difficulty with any change in direction	Parkinsonism
Scissors 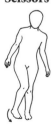	Knees cross or are in contact, like holding an orange between the thighs. The person uses short steps, and walking requires effort	Paraparesis of legs, multiple sclerosis
Steppage or Footdrop 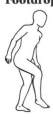	Slapping quality—looks as if walking up stairs and finds no stair there. Lifts knee and foot high and slaps it down hard and flat to compensate for footdrop	Weakness of peroneal and anterior tibial muscles; due to lower motor neuron lesion at the spinal cord, such as poliomyelitis, Charcot-Marie-Tooth disease (an inherited peripheral neuropathy)

Continued

TABLE 23-5	Abnormal Gaits—cont'd	
Type	Characteristic Appearance	Possible Causes
Waddling	Weak hip muscles—when the person takes a step, the opposite hip drops, which allows compensatory lateral movement of pelvis. Often, the person also has marked lumbar lordosis and a protruding abdomen	Hip girdle muscle weakness due to muscular dystrophy, dislocation of hips
Short Leg	Leg length discrepancy >2.5 cm. Vertical telescoping of affected side, which dips as the person walks. Appearance of gait varies depending on amount of accompanying muscle dysfunction	Congenital dislocated hip; acquired shortening due to disease, trauma

TABLE 23-6	Characteristics of Upper and Lower Motor Neuron Lesions	
	Upper Motor Neuron Lesion	Lower Motor Neuron Lesion
Weakness or paralysis	In muscles corresponding to distribution of damage in pyramidal tract lesion; usually in hand grip, arm extensors, leg flexors	In specific muscles served by damaged spinal segment, ventral root, or peripheral nerve
Location	Descending motor pathways that originate in the motor areas of cerebral cortex and carry impulses to the anterior horn cells of the spinal cord	Nerve cells that originate in the anterior horn of spinal cord or in brain stem, and carry impulses by the spinal nerves or cranial nerves to the muscles, the "final common pathway"
Example	Brain attack or cerebrovascular accident	Poliomyelitis, herniated intervertebral disc
Muscle tone	Increased tone; spasticity	Loss of tone, flaccidity
Bulk	May have some atrophy from disuse; otherwise normal	Atrophy (wasting), may be marked
Abnormal movements	None	Fasciculations
Reflexes	Hyperreflexia, ankle clonus; diminished or absent superficial abdominal reflexes; positive Babinski's sign	Hyporeflexia or areflexia; no Babinski's sign, no pathological reflexes
Possible nursing diagnoses	Risk for contractures; impaired physical mobility	Impaired physical mobility

Abnormal Findings

TABLE 23-7 | Common Patterns of Motor System Dysfunction

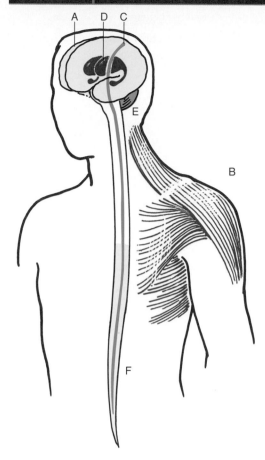

A—Cerebral palsy. Mixed group of paralytic neuromotor disorders of infancy and childhood; due to damage to cerebral cortex caused by a developmental defect, intrauterine meningitis or encephalitis, birth trauma, anoxia, or kernicterus.

B—Muscular dystrophy. Chronic, progressive wasting of skeletal musculature, which produces weakness, contractures, and in severe cases, respiratory dysfunction and death. Onset of symptoms occurs in childhood. Many types exist; the most severe is Duchenne's dystrophy, characterized by the waddling gait described in Table 23-5.

C—Hemiplegia. Damage to corticospinal tract (e.g., CVA or stroke). Upper motor neuron damage occurs above the pyramidal decussation crossover, so motor impairment is on contralateral (opposite) side. Initially flaccid when the lesion is acute; later, the muscles become spastic, and abnormal reflexes appear. Characteristic posture: arm—shoulder adducted, elbow flexed, wrist pronated, leg extended; face—weakness only in lower muscles. Hyperreflexia and possible clonus occur on the involved side; loss of corneal, abdominal, and cremasteric reflexes; positive Babinski's and Hoffman's reflexes.

D—Parkinsonism. Defect of extrapyramidal tracts, in the region of the basal ganglia, with loss of the neurotransmitter dopamine. Classic triad of symptoms: tremor, rigidity, akinesia. Also slower monotonous speech and diminutive writing. Body tends to stay immobile; facial expression is flat, staring, expressionless; excessive salivation occurs; reduced eye blinking. Posture is stooped; equilibrium is impaired; loses balance easily; gait is described in Table 23-5. Parkinsonian tremor; cogwheel rigidity on passive range of motion.

E—Cerebellar. A lesion in one hemisphere produces motor abnormalities on the ipsilateral side. Characterized by ataxia, lurching forward of affected side while walking, rapid alternating movements are slow and arrhythmic, finger-to-nose test reveals ataxia and tremor with overshoot or undershoot, and eyes display coarse nystagmus.

F—Paraplegia. Lower motor neuron damage caused by spinal cord injury. A severe injury or complete transection initially produces "spinal shock," which is defined as no movement or reflex activity below the level of the lesion. Gradually, deep tendon reflexes reappear and become increased, flexor spasms of legs occur, and finally, extensor spasms of legs occur; these spasms lead to prevailing extensor tone.

TABLE 23-8	Common Patterns of Sensory Loss	
Type	Characteristics	Possible Causes
Peripheral Neuropathy 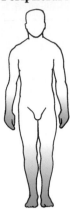	Loss of sensation involves all modalities. Loss is most severe distally (feet and hands); response improves as stimulus is moved proximally (glove-and-stocking anaesthesia). Anaesthesia zone gradually merges into a hypoesthesia zone, then gradually becomes normal.	Diabetes, chronic alcoholism, nutritional deficiency
Individual Nerves or Roots 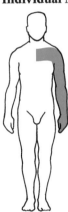	Decrease or loss of all sensory modalities. Area of sensory loss corresponds to distribution of the involved nerve.	Trauma, vascular occlusion
Spinal Cord Hemisection (Brown-Séquard Syndrome) 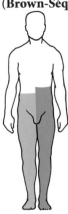	Loss of pain and temperature, contralateral side, starting one to two segments below the level of the lesion. Loss of vibration and position discrimination on the ipsilateral side, below the level of the lesion.	Meningioma, neurofibroma, cervical spondylosis, multiple sclerosis

TABLE 23-8	Common Patterns of Sensory Loss—cont'd	
Type	Characteristics	Possible Causes
Complete Transection of the Spinal Cord 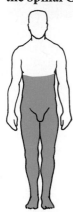	Complete loss of *all* sensory modalities below the level of the lesion. Condition is associated with motor paralysis and loss of sphincter control.	Spinal cord trauma, demyelinating disorders, tumour
Thalamus 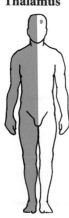	Loss of *all* sensory modalities on the face, arm, and leg on the side contralateral to the lesion.	Vascular occlusion
Cortex 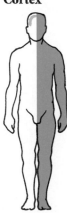	Since pain, vibration, and crude touch are mediated by thalamus, little loss of these sensory functions occurs with a cortex lesion. Loss of discrimination occurs on the contralateral side. Loss of graphesthesia, stereognosis, recognition of shapes and weights, finger finding.	Cerebral cortex, parietal lobe lesion (e.g., CVA or stroke)

TABLE 23-9 | Abnormal Postures

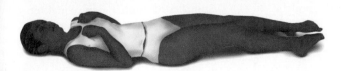

Decorticate Rigidity

Upper extremities—flexion of arm, wrist, and fingers; adduction of arm (i.e., tight against thorax). Lower extremities—extension, internal rotation, plantar flexion. This indicates hemispheric lesion of cerebral cortex.

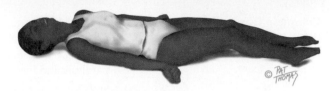

Decerebrate Rigidity

Upper extremities stiffly extended, adducted, internal rotation, palms pronated. Lower extremities stiffly extended, plantar flexion; teeth clenched; hyperextended back. More ominous than decorticate rigidity; indicates lesion in brain stem at midbrain or upper pons.

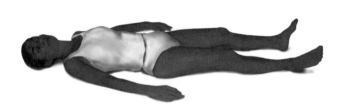

Flaccid Quadriplegia

Complete loss of muscle tone and paralysis of all four extremities, indicating completely nonfunctional brain stem.

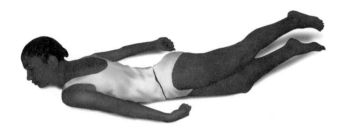

Opisthotonos

Prolonged arching of the back, with head and heels bent backward. This indicates meningeal irritation.

Images © Pat Thomas, 2006.

TABLE 23-10 | Pathological Reflexes

Reflex	Method of Testing	Abnormal Response (Reflex Is Present)	Indications
Babinski	Stroke lateral aspect and across ball of foot	Extension of great toe, fanning of toes	Corticospinal (pyramidal) tract disease (e.g., stroke, trauma)
Oppenheim	Using heavy pressure with your thumb and index finger, stroke anterior medial tibial muscle	Same as above	Same
Gordon	Firmly squeeze calf muscles	Same as above	Same
Hoffman	With patient's hand relaxed, wrist dorsified, fingers slightly flexed, sharply flick nail of distal phalanx of middle or index finger	Clawing of fingers and thumb	Same
Kernig	In flat-lying supine position, raise leg straight or flex thigh on abdomen, then extend knee	Resistance to straightening (because of hamstring spasm), pain down posterior thigh	Meningeal irritation (e.g., meningitis, infections)
Brudzinski	With one hand under the neck and other hand on person's chest, sharply flex chin on chest, watch hips and knees	Resistance and pain in neck, with flexion of hips and knees	Meningeal irritation (e.g., meningitis, infections)

TABLE 23-11	**Frontal Release Signs**

Reflex

Snout

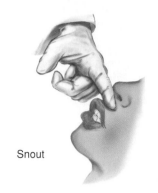

Snout

Method of Testing
Gently percuss oral region
Abnormal Response (Reflex Is Present)
Puckers lips
Indications
Frontal lobe disease, cerebral degenerative disease (Alzheimer's), amyotrophic sclerosis, corticobulbar lesions

Sucking

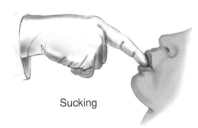

Sucking

Method of Testing
Touch oral region
Abnormal Response (Reflex Is Present)
Sucking movement of lips, tongue, jaw, swallowing
Indications
Same as for snout reflex

Grasp

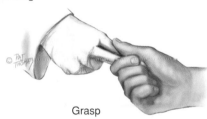

Grasp

Method of Testing
Touch palm with your finger
Abnormal Response (Reflex Is Present)
Uncontrolled, forced grasping (grasp is usually last of these signs to appear, so its presence indicates severe disease)
Indications
When unilateral, frontal lobe lesion on contralateral side; when bilateral, diffuse bifrontal lobe disease

Images © Pat Thomas, 2006.

Abnormal Findings

BIBLIOGRAPHY

American Stroke Association. Retrieved from http://www.strokeassociation.org

Bateman, D. (2001). Neurological assessment of coma [Electronic version]. *Journal of Neurology and Neurosurgical Psychiatry, 71*(Suppl. 1), 13–17.

Budson, A., & Price, B. (2005). Memory dysfunction [Electronic version]. *New England Journal of Medicine, 352,* 692–699.

Byrd, C. (2006). Normal pressure hydrocephalus: Dementia's cause. *Nurse Practitioner, 31*(7), 28–37.

Chasens, E. R., & Umlauf, M. G. (2000). Post-polio syndrome. *American Journal of Nursing, 100*(12), 60–66.

Clarke, P., Marshall, V., Black, S., & Colantonio, A. (2002). Well-being after stroke in Canadian seniors: Findings from the Canadian study of health and aging. *Stroke, 33,* 1016–1021.

Côté, R., Battista, R. N., et al. (1989). The Canadian Neurological Scale: Validation and reliability assessment. *Neurology, 39,* 638–643.

Côté, R., David, M., Deveber, G., Teal, P., Roussin, A., Sharma, M. (2007). *Stroke prevention.* The Thrombosis Interest Group of Canada. Retrieved February 11, 2008, from http://www.tigc.org/eguidelines/previschemstroke05.htm

Côté, R., Hachinski, V. C., Shurvell, B. L., Norris, J. W., & Wolfson, C. (1986). The Canadian Neurological Scale: A preliminary study in acute stroke. *Stroke, 17,* 731–737.

Fenichel, G. M. (2005). *Clinical pediatric neurology* (5th ed.). Philadelphia, PA: W.B. Saunders.

Fischer, J., & Mathieson, C. (2001). The history of the Glasgow Coma Scale: Implications for practice. *Critical Care Nursing Quarterly, 23*(4), 52–58.

Franges, E. Z. (2006). When a headache is really a brain tumor. *Nurse Practitioner, 31*(4), 47–51.

Gavin, C., & Gray, J. (2005). Assessment and management of neurological problems (2) [Electronic version]. *Emergency Medicine Journal, 22,* 564–571.

Gilden, D. (2004). Bell's palsy [Electronic version]. *New England Journal of Medicine, 351,* 1323–1331.

Goldstein, L. B., Appel, L. J., Culebras, A., Gorelick, P. B., Howard, G., & Sacco, R. L. (2006). Primary prevention of ischemic stroke: A guideline from the American Heart Association/American Stroke Association Stroke Council. *Stroke, 37,* 1583–1633.

Gouzd, B. (2000). Whiplash injury: symptoms are variable, and the road to recovery may be long and difficult. *American Journal of Nursing, 100*(3), 41–42.

Heart and Stroke Foundation of Canada. (2008a). *Multilingual and multicultural resources.* Retrieved on February 12, 2008, from http://www.heartandstroke.com/site/c.ikIQLcMWJtE/b.3532103/apps/s/content.asp?ct=4512409

Heart and Stroke Foundation of Canada. (2008b). *Women and stroke special risks, worse prognosis.* Retrieved on February 12, 2008, from http://www.heartandstroke.com/site/c.ikIQLcMWJtE/b.3532103/apps/s/content.asp?ct=4512777

Hess, D., & Hughes, M. (2005). Multiple sclerosis: when to suspect-keys to diagnosis. *Consultant, 45,* 844–852.

Hilton, G. (2001). Acute head injury. *American Journal of Nursing, 101*(9), 51–52.

Hobdell, E. (2001). Infant neurologic assessment. *Journal of Neuroscience Nursing, 33*(4), 190. Retrieved February 7, 2006, from http://galenet.galegroup.com.proxy.lib.umich.edu/servlet/HWRC

Jagoda, A., & Riggio, S. (2004). What you forgot about the neurologic exam, part 1: History, mental status, cranial nerves. *Consultant, 44,* 1773–1780.

Juarez, V. J., & Lyons, M. (1995). Interrater reliability of the Glasgow Coma Scale. *Journal of Neuroscience Nursing, 27,* 283–286.

Lehman, C. A, Hayes, J. M., LaCroix, J. M., Owen, M., Nauta, S. V. (2003). Development and implementation of a problem-focused neurological assessment system. *Journal of Neuroscience Nursing, 35,* 185–188. Retrieved February 6, 2006, from http://infotrac.galegroup.com/default

LeJeune, G., & Howard-Fain, T. (2002). Nursing assessment and management of patients with head injuries. *Dimensions in Critical Care Nursing, 21,* 226–229. Retrieved February 13, 2006, from http://gateway.ut.ovid.com/gw1/ovidweb.cgi

Lower, J. (2002). Facing neuro assessment fearlessly. *Nursing, 32*(2), 58–65.

Marjama-Lyons, J., & Koller, W. (2001). Parkinson's disease: update in diagnosis and symptom management. *Geriatrics, 56*(8), 24–35.

McNarry, A., & Goldhill, D. (2004). Simple bedside assessment of level of consciousness: Comparison of two simple assessment scales with the Glasgow Coma Scale. *Anaesthesia, 59,* 34–37.

National Institute of Neurological Disorders and Stroke. (2006). Retrieved February 2006 from http://www.ninds.nih.gov

Orfanelli, L. (2001). Neurologic examination of the toddler: How to assess for increased intracranial pressure following head trauma. *American Journal of Nursing, 101*(12), 24CC–FF.

Pena, C. (2003). Seizure: A calm response and careful observation are crucial. *American Journal of Nursing, 103*(11), 73–81.

Raup, G. (2002). Assessment of the patient who is neurologically impaired. *Journal of Infusion Nursing, 25,* 172–175. Retrieved February 13, 2006, from http://gateway.ut.ovid.com/gw1/ovidweb.cgi

Riggio, S., & Jagoda, A. (2005). What you forgot about the neurologic exam, part 2: Movement, reflexes, sensation, balance. *Consultant, 45*(1), 53–61.

Schutte, D. L. (2006). Alzheimer disease and genetics. *American Journal of Nursing, 106*(12), 40–48.

Sejvar, J. J, Haddad, M. B., Tierney, B. C., Campbell, G. L., Marfin, A. A., Van Gerpen, J. A., et al. (2003). Neurologic manifestations and outcome of West Nile virus infection [Electronic version]. *Journal of the American Medical Association, 290,* 511–515.

Siderowf, A., & Stern, M. (2003). Update on Parkinson disease. *Annals of Internal Medicine, 138,* 651–658.

Smith, M., & Buckwalter, K. (2005). Behaviors associated with dementia. *American Journal of Nursing, 105*(7), 40–53.

Waxman, S. G. (2000). *Correlative neuroanatomy* (24th ed.). Stamford, CT: Appleton & Lange.

Whyte, J. (2003). Guillain-Barre: A case of muscular weakness and ambulatory difficulty. *Nurse Practitioner, 28*(3), 58–64.

Chapter Twenty-Four

Male Genitourinary System

Written by **Carolyn Jarvis**, PhD, APN, CNP
Adapted by **Marian Luctkar-Flude**, RN, MScN

Electronic Resources ———❧

On Evolve *evolve*

http://evolve.elsevier.com/Canada/Jarvis/examination/
- Interactive Case Studies
- Physical Examination Audio and Printable Summaries
- Bedside Assessment Summary Checklists
- Complete Physical Examination Form
- Nursing Diagnoses Boxes
- Health Promotion Guides
- Quick Assessments for 20 Common Conditions
- Multiple Choice Review Questions
- Chapter Objectives
- Appendices
- Weblinks

On the Companion CD
- Interactive Case Studies with Heart and Lung Sounds
- Health Promotion Guides
- Quick Assessments for 20 Common Conditions
- Head-to-Toe Physical Examination Video Clips

STRUCTURE AND FUNCTION

THE MALE GENITALIA

The male genital structures include the penis and scrotum externally and the testis, epididymis, and vas deferens internally. Glandular structures accessory to the genital organs (the prostate, seminal vesicles, and bulbourethral glands) are discussed in Chapter 25.

Penis

The **penis** is composed of three cylindrical columns of erectile tissue: the two corpora cavernosa on the dorsal side and the corpus spongiosum ventrally (Fig. 24-1). At the distal end of the shaft, the corpus spongiosum expands into a cone of erectile tissue, the **glans.** The shoulder where the glans joins the shaft is the **corona.** The **urethra** transverses the corpus spongiosum, and its meatus forms a slit at the glans tip. Over the glans, the skin folds in and back on itself forming a hood or flap. This is the **foreskin** or **prepuce.** Sometimes, it is surgically removed shortly after birth by circumcision. The **frenulum** is a fold of the foreskin extending from the urethral meatus ventrally.

Scrotum

The **scrotum** is a loose protective sac, which is a continuation of the abdominal wall (Fig. 24-2). After adolescence, the scrotal skin is deeply pigmented and has large sebaceous follicles. The scrotal wall consists of thin skin lying in folds, or **rugae,** and the underlying cremaster muscle. The **cremaster muscle** controls the size of the scrotum by responding to ambient temperature. This is to keep the testes at 3°C below abdominal temperature, the best temperature for producing sperm. When it is cold, the muscle contracts, raising the sac and bringing the testes closer to the body to absorb heat necessary for sperm viability. As a result, the scrotal skin looks corrugated. When it is warmer, the muscle relaxes, the scrotum lowers, and the skin looks smoother.

Inside, a septum separates the sac into two halves. In each scrotal half is a **testis,** which produces sperm. The testis has a solid oval shape, which is compressed laterally and measures 4 to 5 cm long by 3 cm wide in the adult. The testis is suspended vertically by the spermatic cord. The left testis is lower than the right because the left spermatic cord is longer. Each testis is covered by a double-layered membrane, the tunica vaginalis, which separates it from the scrotal wall. The two layers are lubricated by fluid so that the testis can slide a little within the scrotum; this helps prevent injury.

Sperm are transported along a series of ducts. First, the testis is capped by the **epididymis,** which is a markedly coiled duct system and the main storage site of sperm. It is a comma-shaped structure, curved over the top and the posterior surface of the testis. Occasionally (in 6 to 7% of males), the epididymis is anterior to the testis.

The lower part of the epididymis is continuous with a muscular duct, the **vas deferens.** This duct approximates with other vessels (arteries and veins, lymphatics, nerves) to form the **spermatic cord.** The spermatic cord ascends along the posterior border of the testis and runs through the tunnel of the inguinal canal into the abdomen. Here, the vas deferens continues back and down behind the bladder, where it

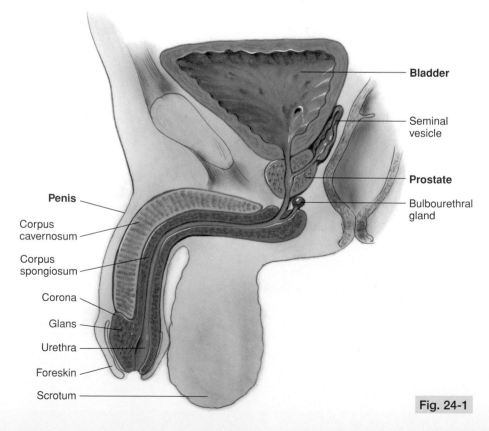

Penis
Corpus cavernosum
Corpus spongiosum
Corona
Glans
Urethra
Foreskin
Scrotum

Bladder
Seminal vesicle
Prostate
Bulbourethral gland

Fig. 24-1

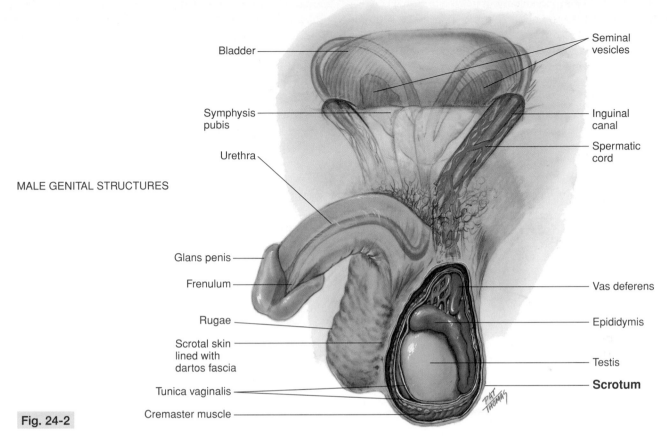

MALE GENITAL STRUCTURES

Labels: Bladder, Symphysis pubis, Urethra, Glans penis, Frenulum, Rugae, Scrotal skin lined with dartos fascia, Tunica vaginalis, Cremaster muscle, Seminal vesicles, Inguinal canal, Spermatic cord, Vas deferens, Epididymis, Testis, **Scrotum**

Fig. 24-2

joins the duct of the seminal vesicle to form the **ejaculatory duct.** This duct empties into the urethra.

The **lymphatics** of the penis and scrotal surface drain into the inguinal lymph nodes, whereas those of the testes drain into the abdomen. Abdominal lymph nodes are not accessible to clinical examination.

Inguinal Area

The **inguinal area,** or groin, is the juncture of the lower abdominal wall and the thigh (Fig. 24-3). Its diagonal borders are the anterior superior iliac spine and the symphysis pubis. Between these landmarks lies the **inguinal ligament** (Poupart's

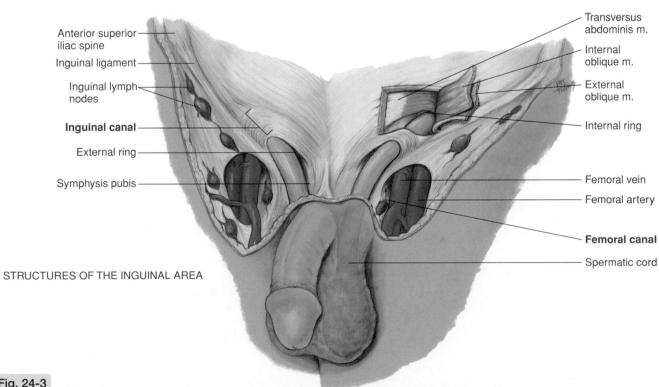

STRUCTURES OF THE INGUINAL AREA

Labels: Anterior superior iliac spine, Inguinal ligament, Inguinal lymph nodes, **Inguinal canal**, External ring, Symphysis pubis, Transversus abdominis m., Internal oblique m., External oblique m., Internal ring, Femoral vein, Femoral artery, **Femoral canal**, Spermatic cord

Fig. 24-3

ligament). Superior to the ligament lies the **inguinal canal,** a narrow tunnel passing obliquely between layers of abdominal muscle. It is 4 to 6 cm long in the adult. Its openings are an internal ring, located 1 to 2 cm above the midpoint of the inguinal ligament, and an external ring, located just above and lateral to the pubis.

Inferior to the inguinal ligament is the **femoral canal.** It is a potential space located 3 cm medial to and parallel with the femoral artery. You can use the artery as a landmark to find this space.

Knowledge of these anatomical areas in the groin is useful because they are potential sites for a hernia, which is a loop of bowel protruding through a weak spot in the musculature.

❖ DEVELOPMENTAL CARE

Infants

Prenatally, the testes develop in the abdominal cavity near the kidneys. During the later months of gestation the testes migrate, pushing the abdominal wall in front of them and dragging the vas deferens, the blood vessels, and nerves behind. The testes descend along the inguinal canal into the scrotum before birth. At birth, each testis measures 1.5 to 2 cm long and 1 cm wide. Only a slight increase in size occurs during the prepubertal years.

Adolescents

Puberty begins sometime between the ages of 9½ and 13½. The first sign is enlargement of the testes. Next, pubic hair appears, then penis size increases. The stages of development are documented in Tanner's sexual maturity rating (SMR) (Table 24-1).

The complete change in development from a preadolescent to an adult takes around 3 years, although the normal

range is 2 to 5 years (Fig. 24-4). The chart shown in Figure 24-4 is useful in teaching a boy the expected sequence of events and in reassuring him about the wide range of normal ages when these events are experienced.

Adults and Aging Adults

The level of sexual development at the end of puberty remains constant through young and middle adulthood, with no further genital growth and no change in circulating sex hormone.

The male does not experience a definite end to fertility as the female does. Around age 40 years, the production of sperm begins to decrease, although it continues into the 80s and 90s. After age 55 to 60 years, testosterone production declines. This decline proceeds very gradually so that resulting physical changes are not evident until later in life. Aging changes also are due to decreased muscle tone, decreased subcutaneous fat, and decreased cellular metabolism.

In the older male, the amount of pubic hair decreases, and the remaining hair turns grey. Penis size decreases. Due to decreased tone of the dartos muscle, the scrotal contents hang lower, the rugae decrease, and the scrotum looks pendulous. The testes decrease in size and are less firm to palpation. Increased connective tissue is present in the tubules, so these become thickened and produce less sperm.

In general, declining testosterone production leaves the older male with a slower and less intense sexual response. Although a wide range of individual differences can occur, the older male may find that an erection takes longer to develop and that it is less full or firm. Once obtained, the erection may be maintained for longer periods without ejaculation. Ejaculation is shorter and less forceful, and the volume of seminal fluid is less than when the man was younger. After ejaculation, rapid detumescence (return to the flaccid state) occurs, especially after 60 years of age. This occurs in a few seconds as compared with minutes or hours in the younger male. The refractory state (when the male is physiologically unable to ejaculate) lasts longer, from 12 to 24 hours as compared with 2 minutes in the younger male.

Sexual Expression in Later Life. Chronological age by itself should not mean a halt in sexual activity. The above-mentioned physical changes need not interfere with the libido or pleasure from sexual intercourse. The older male is capable of sexual function as long as he is in reasonably good health and has an interested, willing partner. Even chronic illness does not mean a complete end to sexual desire or activity.

The danger is in the male misinterpreting normal age changes as a sexual failure. Once this idea occurs, it may demoralize the man and place undue emphasis on performance rather than on pleasure. In the absence of disease, a withdrawal from sexual activity may be due to:

- Loss of spouse
- Depression
- Preoccupation with work

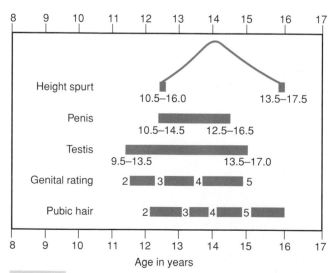

Fig. 24-4

TABLE 24-1	Sexual Maturity Rating in Boys			
Developmental Stage	Pubic Hair	Penis	Scrotum	
1	No pubic hair. Fine body hair on abdomen (vellus hair) continues over pubic area	Preadolescent, size and proportion the same as during childhood	Preadolescent, size and proportion the same as during childhood	
2	Few straight slightly darker hairs at base of penis. Hair is long and downy	Little or no enlargement	Testes and scrotum begin to enlarge. Scrotal skin reddens and changes in texture	
3	Sparse growth over entire pubis. Hair darker, coarser, and curly	Penis begins to enlarge, especially in length	Further enlarged	
4	Thick growth over pubic area but not on thighs. Hair coarse and curly as in adult	Penis grows in length and diameter, with development of glans	Testes almost fully grown, scrotum darker	
5	Growth spread over medial thighs, although not yet up toward umbilicus. After puberty, pubic hair growth continues until the mid-20s, extending up the abdomen toward the umbilicus	Adult size and shape	Adult size and shape	

Adapted from Tanner, J.M. (1962). *Growth at adolescence.* Oxford, England: Blackwell Scientific Publications.

- Marital or family conflict
- Side effects of medications such as antihypertensives, psychotropics, antidepressants, antispasmodics, sedatives, tranquilizers or narcotics, and estrogens
- Heavy use of alcohol
- Lack of privacy (living with adult children or in a nursing home)
- Economic or emotional stress
- Poor nutrition
- Fatigue

CULTURAL AND SOCIAL CONSIDERATIONS

Circumcision. Occasionally, during pregnancy or the immediate neonatal period, parents will ask you about whether or not to circumcise the male infant. Common reasons given in favour of circumcision are hygiene, avoidance of later circumcision, medical indications, the father's circumcision status, and religious and cultural values. Since 1975 the Canadian Paediatric Society (CPS) has held the policy that there is no medical indication for male neonatal circumcision. A CPS statement issued in 1996 and reaffirmed in 2002 strongly recommended that circumcision of newborns should not be routinely performed, and nontherapeutic male neonatal circumcision is no longer covered by provincial health insurance plans. Neonatal circumcision rates in Canada have declined from about 47% in 1973 to about 9% in 2005.

For the uncircumcised newborn, assess the parents' knowledge about care of the uncircumcised penis. The infant's penis should be cleansed with soap and water, but the foreskin should not be forcibly retracted. When the foreskin retracts easily, the area under the foreskin should be cleansed occasionally. By the age of 3 or 4 years, a boy can be taught to clean under his foreskin. When a boy reaches puberty, he needs to clean under his foreskin daily.

Circumcision carries a very small but possible risk of complications, such as sepsis, amputation of the distal edge of the glans, removal of an excessive amount of foreskin, urethrocutaneous fistula (Behrman, 2003), and significant pain, about which the parents should know. Parents should feel free to discuss pain management measures for their infant. These include oral and transdermal pain medication for the infant, dorsal penile nerve block, and comfort measures such as oral sucrose pacifier, stroking the infant, talking, and rocking (Stratman-Lucey & Caldwell, 2006).

SUBJECTIVE DATA

1. Frequency, urgency, and nocturia
2. Dysuria
3. Hesitancy and straining
4. Urine colour

5. Genitourinary history
6. Penis—pain, lesion, discharge
7. Scrotum, self-care behaviours, lump

8. Sexual activity and contraceptive use
9. STI contact

Examiner Asks	Rationale
1. Frequency, urgency, and nocturia. Urinating more often than usual?	**Frequency.** Average adult voids five to six times per day, varying with fluid intake, individual habits.
	Polyuria—excessive quantity.
	Oliguria—diminished quantity, <400 mL/24 hr.
• Feel as if you cannot wait to urinate?	**Urgency.**
• Awaken during the night because you need to urinate? How often? Is this a recent change?	**Nocturia** occurs together with frequency and urgency in urinary tract disorders. Other origins: cardiovascular, habitual, diuretic medication.
2. Dysuria. Any pain or burning with urinating?	**Dysuria.** Burning is common with acute cystitis, prostatitis, urethritis.
3. Hesitancy and straining. Any trouble starting the urine stream?	**Hesitancy.**
• Need to strain to start or maintain stream?	Straining.
• Any change in force of stream: narrowing, becoming weaker?	Loss of force and decreased calibre.
• Dribbling, such that you must stand closer to the toilet?	Terminal dribbling.
• Afterward, do you still feel you need to urinate?	Sense of residual urine.
• Ever had any urinary tract infections?	Recurrent episodes of acute cystitis.
	Above-mentioned symptoms (i.e., hesitancy, and so on) suggest progressive prostatic obstruction.

Examiner Asks	Rationale

4. Urine colour. Is the usual **urine** clear or discolored, cloudy, foul-smelling, bloody (Fig. 24-5)?

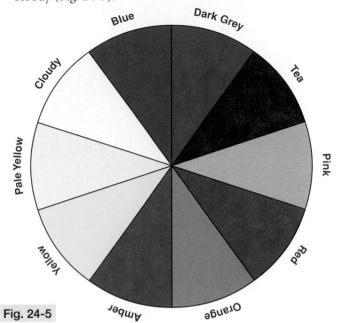

Fig. 24-5

Cloudy in urinary tract infection.

Hematuria—a danger sign that warrants further workup.

Some colour changes are temporary or harmless. However, for blood in urine or for a colour change lasting >1 day, the person should seek health care. For a complete description, see Table 24-2, p. 730.

5. Genitourinary history. Any difficulty controlling your urine?

- Accidentally urinate when you sneeze, laugh, cough, or bear down?

- Any **history** of kidney disease, kidney stones, flank pain, urinary tract infections, prostate trouble?

True incontinence—loss of urine without warning.

Urgency incontinence—sudden loss, as with acute cystitis.

Stress incontinence—loss of urine with physical strain due to weakness of sphincters.

6. Penis—pain, lesion, discharge. Any problem with penis—**pain, lesions?**
- Any **discharge?** How much? Has that increased or decreased since start?
- The colour? Any odour? Discharge associated with pain or with urination?

Urethral discharge occurs with infection.

7. Scrotum, self-care behaviours, lump. Any problem with the scrotum or testicles?
- Do you perform testicular self-examination (TSE)?
- Noticed any **lump** or **swelling** on testes?
- Noted any change in size of the scrotum?
- Noted any bulge or swelling in the scrotum? For how long? Ever been told you have a hernia? Any dragging, heavy feeling in scrotum?

Self-care behaviours.

Possible hernia.

8. Sexual activity and contraceptive use. Are you now in a relationship involving sexual intercourse?
- Are aspects of sex satisfactory to you and your partner?
- Are you satisfied with the way you and your partner communicate about sex?
- Occasionally a man notices a change in ability to have an erection when aroused. Have you noticed any changes?*
- Do you and your partner use a contraceptive? Which method? Is this satisfactory? Any questions about this method?

Questions about **sexual activity** should be routine in review of body systems for these reasons:
- Communicates that you accept individual's sexual activity and believe it is important
- Your comfort with discussion prompts person's interest and possibly relief that topic has been introduced

*Phrase your questions so the person is comfortable acknowledging a problem.

Subjective Data

Examiner Asks	Rationale

• How many sexual partners have you had in the last 6 months?

• Establishes a database for comparisons with any future sexual activities
• Provides opportunity to screen sexual problems

Your questions should be objective and matter-of-fact.

• What is your sexual preference—relationship with a woman, a man, both?

Gay and bisexual men need to feel acceptance to discuss their health concerns.

9. STI contact. Any sexual contact with a partner having a sexually transmitted infection, such as gonorrhea, herpes, acquired immunodeficiency syndrome (AIDS), *Chlamydia*, venereal warts, syphilis?
• When was this contact? Did you become infected?
• How was it treated? Any complications?
• Do you use condoms to help prevent STIs?
• Any questions or concerns about any of these infections?

Additional History for Infants and Children

1. Does your child have any problem urinating? Urine stream look straight?
• Any pain with urinating, crying, or holding the genitals?
• Any urinary tract infection?

2. (If child older than 2 to 2½ years of age) Has toilet training started? How is it progressing?
(If child 5 years or older) Wet the bed at night? Is this a problem for child or for you (parents)? What have you done? How does the child feel about it?

Nocturnal enuresis—involuntary passing of urine after an age at which continence is expected.

3. Any problem with child's penis or scrotum: sores, swelling, discoloration?
• Told if his testes are descended?
• Ever had a hernia or hydrocele?
• Swelling in his scrotum during crying or coughing?

4. (Ask directly to preschooler or young school-age child) "Has anyone ever touched your penis or in between your legs and you did not want them to? Sometimes that happens to children and it's not OK." They should remember that they have not been bad. They should try to tell an adult about it. "Can you tell me three different big people you trust who you could talk to?"

Screen for sexual abuse. For prevention, teach the child that it's not OK for someone to look at or touch their private parts while telling them it's a secret. Naming three trusted adults will include someone outside the family—important, since most molestation is by a parent.

Additional History for Preadolescents and Adolescents

Use the following questions regarding sexual growth and development and sexual behaviour. First:
• Ask questions that seem appropriate for a boy's age but be aware that norms vary widely. When you are in doubt, it is better to ask too many questions than to omit something. Children obtain information, often misinformation, from the media and from peers at surprisingly early ages. You may be sure your information will be more thoughtful and accurate.
• Ask direct, matter-of-fact questions. Avoid sounding judgemental.
• Start with a *permission statement.* "Often boys your age experience . . ." This conveys that it is normal and all right to think or feel a certain way.

Examiner Asks	Rationale

- Try the *ubiquity approach.* "When did you . . . " rather than "Do you . . . " This method is less threatening because it implies that the topic is normal and unexceptional.
- Do not be concerned if a boy will not discuss sexuality with you or respond to offers for information. He may not wish to let on that he needs or wants more information. You do well to "open the door." The adolescent may come back at a future time.

1. Around age 12 to 13 years, but sometimes earlier, boys start to change and grow around the penis and scrotum. What changes have you noticed? Have you ever seen charts and pictures of normal growth patterns for boys? Let us go over these now.

   Who can you talk to about your body changes and about sex information? How do these talks go? Do you think you get enough information? What about sex education classes at school? How about your parents? Is there a favourite teacher, nurse, doctor, minister, or counsellor to whom you can talk?

2. Boys around age 12 to 13 years (SMR3) have a normal experience of fluid coming out of the penis at night, called a nocturnal emission, or "wet dream." Have you had this?

   Occasionally a boy confuses this with a sign of STI or feels guilty.

3. Teenage boys have other normal experiences and wonder if they are the only ones who ever had them, like having an erection at embarrassing times, having sexual fantasies, or masturbating. Also, a boy might have a thought about touching another boy's genitals and wonder if this means he might be homosexual. Would you like to talk about any of these things?

   A boy may feel guilty about experiencing these things if not informed that they are normal.

4. Often boys your age have questions about sexual activity. What questions do you have? How about things like birth control, or STIs such as gonorrhea or herpes? Any questions about these?

   Assess level of knowledge. Many boys will not admit they need more knowledge.

   - Are you dating? Someone steady? Have you had intercourse? Are you using birth control? What kind?

   Avoid the term "having sex." It is ambiguous, and teens can take it to mean anything from foreplay to intercourse.

   - What kind of birth control did you use the *last* time you had intercourse?

   This particular question often reveals that the teen is not using any method of birth control.

5. Has a nurse or doctor ever taught you how to examine your own testicles to make sure they are healthy?

   Assess knowledge of TSE.

6. Has anyone ever touched your genitals when you did not want them to? Another boy, or an adult, even a relative? Sometimes that happens to teenagers. They should remember it is not their fault. They should tell another adult about it.

Additional History for the Aging Adult

1. Any difficulty urinating? Any hesitancy and straining? A weakened force of stream? Any dribbling? Or any incomplete emptying?

   Early symptoms of enlarging prostate may be tolerated or ignored. Later symptoms are more dramatic: hematuria, urinary tract infection.

2. Do you ever leak water/urine when you don't want to? Do you use pads or tissue to catch urine in your underwear?

   Incontinence is any involuntary leaking of urine.

3. Do you need to get up at night to urinate? What medications are you taking? What fluids do you drink in the evening?

   Nocturia may be due to diuretic medication, habit, or fluid ingestion 3 hours before bedtime, especially coffee and alcohol

Examiner Asks	Rationale
	have a diuretic effect. Also, fluid retention from mild heart failure or varicose veins produces nocturia because recumbency at night mobilizes fluid.
4. A man in his 70s, 80s, or 90s may notice changes in his sexual relationship or in his sexual response and wonder if it is normal. For example, it is normal for an erection to develop slowly at this age. This is not a sign of impotence, but a man might wonder if it is.	Excluding physical illness, an older man is fully capable of sexual function. But some assume normal changes mean that they are "old men" and withdraw from sexual activity. The older person is not reluctant to discuss sexual activity, and most welcome the opportunity.
	Depressants to sexual desire and function include antihypertensives, sedatives, tranquilizers, estrogens, and alcohol. Alcohol decreases the sexual response even more dramatically in the older person.

OBJECTIVE DATA

PREPARATION

Position the male standing with undershorts down. Appropriate draping protects the modesty of the patient. This is important for males of all ethnocultural backgrounds. The examiner should be sitting. Alternatively, the male may be supine for the first part of the examination and stand to be checked for a hernia.

It is normal for a male to feel apprehensive about having his genitalia examined, especially by a female examiner. Younger adolescents usually have more anxiety than older adolescents. But any male may have difficulty dissociating a necessary, matter-of-fact step in the physical examination from the feeling this is an invasion of his privacy. His concerns are similar to those experienced by the female during the examination of the genitalia: modesty, fear of pain, cold hands, negative judgement, or memory of previously uncomfortable examinations. Additionally, he may fear comparison to others, or fear having an erection during the examination and that this would be misinterpreted by the examiner.

This normal apprehension becomes manifested in different behaviors. Many act resigned and embarrassed and avoid eye contact. Occasionally a man will laugh and make jokes to cover embarrassment. Also, a man may refuse examination by a female and insist on a male examiner.

Take time to consider these feelings, as well as to explore your own. It is normal for you to feel embarrassed and apprehensive, too. You may worry about your age, lack of clinical experience, causing pain, or even that your movements might "cause" an erection. Some examiners feel guilty when this occurs. You need to accept these feelings and work through them so that you can examine the male in a professional way. Discuss these concerns with an experienced examiner. Your demeanour is important. Your unresolved discomfort magnifies any discomfort the man may have.

Your demeanour should be *confident* and relaxed, unhurried yet business-like. Do not discuss genitourinary history or sexual practices while you are performing the examination. This may be perceived as judgemental. Use a firm deliberate touch, not a soft, stroking one. If an erection does occur, do *not* stop the examination or leave the room. This only focuses more attention on the erection and increases embarrassment. Reassure the male that this is only a normal physiological response to touch, just as when the pupil constricts in response to bright light. Proceed with the rest of the examination.

EQUIPMENT NEEDED

Gloves—wear gloves during every male genitalia examination
Occasionally: glass slide for urethral specimen
Materials for cytology
Flashlight

Objective Data

Normal Range of Findings	Abnormal Findings

INSPECT AND PALPATE THE PENIS

The skin normally looks wrinkled, hairless, and without lesions. The dorsal vein may be apparent (Fig. 24-6).

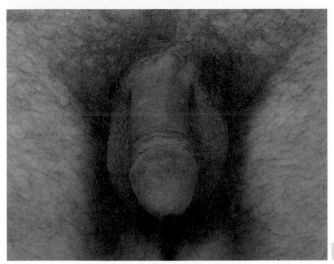

Fig. 24-6

The glans looks smooth and without lesions. Ask the uncircumcised male to retract the foreskin, or you retract it. It should move easily. Some cheesy smegma may have collected under the foreskin. After inspection, slide the foreskin back to the original position.

The urethral meatus is positioned just about centrally.

At the base of the penis, pubic hair distribution is consistent with age. Hair is without infestations.

Compress the glans anteroposteriorly between your thumb and forefinger (Fig. 24-7). The meatus edge should appear pink, smooth, and without discharge.

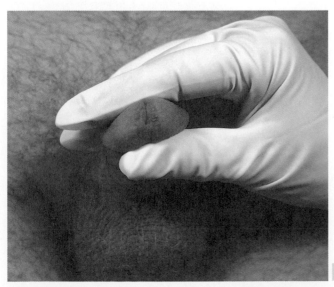

Fig. 24-7

Abnormal Findings

Inflammation.
Lesions: nodules, solitary ulcer (chancre), grouped vesicles or superficial ulcers, wartlike papules (Table 24-3, p. 731).

Inflammation. Lesions on glans or corona.
Phimosis—unable to retract the foreskin.
Paraphimosis—unable to return foreskin to original position.

Hypospadias—ventral location of meatus.
Epispadias—dorsal location of meatus (Table 24-4, p. 732).
Pubic lice or nits can be seen with the unaided eye. Excoriated skin usually accompanies.
Stricture—narrowed opening.
Edges that are red, everted, edematous, along with purulent discharge, suggest urethritis (see Table 24-3, p. 731).

Objective Data

Normal Range of Findings	Abnormal Findings

Objective Data

If you note urethral discharge, collect a smear for microscopic examination and a culture. If no discharge shows but the person gives a history of it, ask him to milk the shaft of the penis. This should produce a drop of discharge.

Palpate the shaft of the penis between your thumb and first two fingers. Normally, the penis feels smooth, semifirm, and nontender.

Nodule or induration.
Tenderness.

INSPECT AND PALPATE THE SCROTUM

Inspect the scrotum as male holds the penis out of the way. Alternatively, you hold the penis out of the way with the back of your hand (Fig. 24-8). Scrotal size varies with ambient room temperature. Asymmetry is normal, with the left scrotal half usually lower than the right.

Scrotal swelling (edema) may be taut and pitting. This occurs with heart failure, renal failure, or local inflammation.
Lesions.

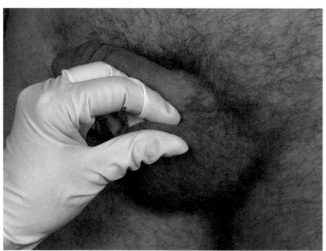
Fig. 24-8

Spread rugae out between your fingers. Lift the sac to inspect the posterior surface. Normally, no scrotal lesions are present, except for the commonly found sebaceous cysts. These are yellowish, 1-cm nodules and are firm, nontender, and often multiple.

Palpate gently each scrotal half between your thumb and first two fingers (Fig. 24-9). The scrotal contents should slide easily. Testes normally feel oval, firm and rubbery, smooth, and equal bilaterally, and are freely movable and slightly tender to moderate pressure. Each epididymis normally feels discrete, softer than the testis, smooth, and nontender.

Inflammation.

Absent testis—may be a temporary migration or true cryptorchidism (Table 24-5, p. 734).
Atrophied testes—small and soft.
Fixed testes.
Nodules on testes or epididymides.
Marked tenderness.
An indurated, swollen, and tender epididymis indicates epididymitis.

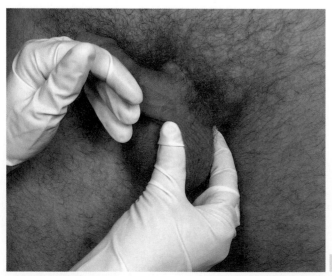
Fig. 24-9

Normal Range of Findings	Abnormal Findings
Palpate each spermatic cord between your thumb and forefinger, along its length from the epididymis up to the external inguinal ring (Fig. 24-10). You should feel a smooth, nontender cord.	Thickened cord. Soft, swollen, and tortuous cord—see the discussion of varicocele, Table 24-5, p. 734.

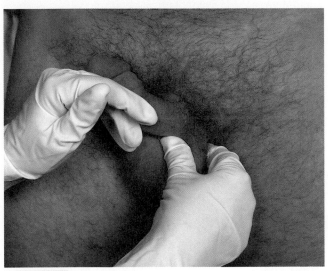

Fig. 24-10

Normally, no other scrotal contents are present. If you do find a mass, note: • Is there any tenderness? • Is the mass distal or proximal to testis? • Can you place your fingers over it? • Does it reduce when person lies down? • Can you auscultate bowel sounds over it?	Abnormalities in the scrotum: hernia, tumour, orchitis, epididymitis, hydrocele, spermatocele, varicocele (see Table 24-4, p. 734).
Transillumination. Perform this manoeuvre if you note a swelling or mass. Darken the room. Shine a strong flashlight from behind the scrotal contents. Normal scrotal contents do not transilluminate.	Serous fluid does transilluminate and shows as a red glow, such as hydrocele or spermatocele. Solid tissue and blood do not transilluminate, such as hernia, epididymitis, or tumour (see Table 24-5, p. 734).

INSPECT AND PALPATE FOR HERNIA

Inspect the inguinal region for a bulge as the person stands and as he strains down. Normally, none is present.	Bulge at external inguinal ring or at femoral canal. (A hernia may be present but easily reduced and may appear only intermittently with an increase in intra-abdominal pressure.)

Objective Data

Normal Range of Findings	Abnormal Findings

Palpate the inguinal canal (Fig. 24-11). For the right side, ask the male to shift his weight onto the left (unexamined) leg. Place your right index finger low on the right scrotal half. Palpate up the length of the spermatic cord, invaginating the scrotal skin as you go, to the external inguinal ring. It feels like a triangular slit-like opening, and it may or may not admit your finger. If it will admit your finger, gently insert it into the canal and ask the person to "bear down."* Normally, you feel no change. Repeat the procedure on the left side.

Palpate the femoral area for a bulge. Normally you feel none.

Palpable herniating mass bumps your fingertip or pushes against the side of your finger (Table 24-6, p. 737).

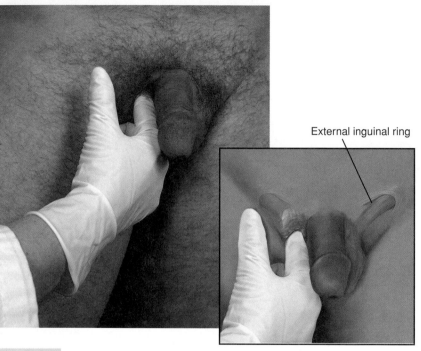

External inguinal ring

Fig. 24-11

PALPATE THE INGUINAL LYMPH NODES

Palpate the horizontal chain along the groin inferior to the inguinal ligament and the vertical chain along the upper inner thigh.

It is normal to palpate an isolated node on occasion; it then feels small (<1 cm), soft, discrete, and movable (Fig. 24-12).

Enlarged, hard, matted, fixed nodes.

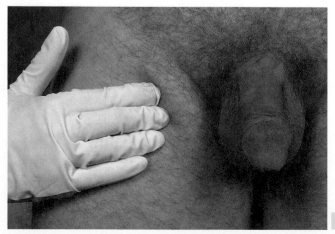

Fig. 24-12

*Avoid the old instruction, "turn your head and cough." For one thing, a brief cough does not give the steady, increased intra-abdominal pressure you need. For another, the person is likely to cough right in your face.

Objective Data

Normal Range of Findings	Abnormal Findings

SELF-CARE: TESTICULAR SELF-EXAMINATION (TSE)

Encourage self-care by teaching every male (from 13 to 14 years old through adulthood) how to examine his own testicles every month. The overall incidence of testicular cancer is still rare, but testicular cancer most commonly occurs in young men aged 15 to 49. Other risk factors include a delayed descent of the testicles (if not corrected early), a family or personal history of testicular cancer, and abnormal development of the testicle. Some men develop testicular cancer without having any of these risk factors. The most common early symptoms of testicular cancer are lumps or swelling on a testicle. The lumps may be painless or slightly uncomfortable. A sense of heaviness or discomfort in the lower abdomen or scrotum is also common (Canadian Cancer Society, 2006). If detected early by palpation and treated, the cure rate is almost 100%.

Early detection is enhanced if the male is familiar with his normal consistency. Points to include during health teaching are:

- **T** = timing, once a month
- **S** = shower, warm water relaxes scrotal sac
- **E** = examine, check for changes, report changes immediately

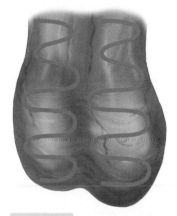

Fig. 24-13   Instruct patients to check each testicle by feeling it in a systematic pattern such as the one shown.

Phrase your teaching something like this (Fig. 24-13):

A good time to examine the testicles is during the shower or bath, when your hands are warm and soapy and the scrotum is warm. Cold hands stimulate a muscle (cremasteric) reflex, retracting the scrotal contents. The procedure is simple. Hold the scrotum in the palm of your hand and gently feel each testicle using your thumb and first two fingers. If it hurts, you are using too much pressure. The testicle is egg-shaped and movable. It feels rubbery with a smooth surface, like a peeled hard-boiled egg. The epididymis is on top and behind the testicle; it feels a bit softer. If you ever notice a firm, painless lump, a hard area, or an overall enlarged testicle, call your physician for a further check.

DEVELOPMENTAL CARE

Infants and Children

For an infant or toddler, perform this procedure right after the abdominal examination. In a preschool-age to young school-age child (3 to 8 years of age), leave underpants on until just before the examination. In an older school-age child or adolescent, offer an extra drape, as with the adult. Reassure child and parents of normal findings.

Normal Range of Findings	Abnormal Findings

Inspect the penis and scrotum. Penis size is usually small in infants (2 to 3 cm) (Fig. 24-14) and in young boys until puberty. In the obese boy, the penis looks even smaller because of folds of skin covering the base.

Rarely, a very small penis may be an enlarged clitoris in a genetically female infant.

Enlarged penis—precocious puberty.

Redness, swelling, lesions.

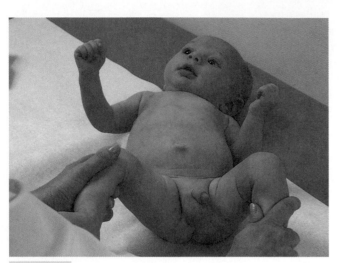

Fig. 24-14

In the circumcised infant, the glans looks smooth with the meatus centred at the tip. During the diaper-wearing stage, the meatus may become ulcerated from ammonia irritation. This is more common in circumcised infants.

Hypospadias, epispadias (see Table 24-4, p. 732).

Stricture—narrowed opening.

Discharge.

Occasionally, ulceration may produce a stricture, shown by a pinpoint meatus and a narrow stream. This increases the risk of urine obstruction.

If possible, observe the newborn's first voiding to assess strength and direction of stream.

Poor stream is significant, because it may indicate a stricture or neurogenic bladder.

If uncircumcised, the foreskin is normally tight during the first 3 months and should not be retracted because of the risk of tearing the membrane attaching the foreskin to the shaft. This leads to scarring and, possibly, to adhesions later in life. In infants older than 3 months of age, retract the foreskin gently to check the glans and meatus. It should return to its original position easily.

Phimosis—the foreskin is tight and cannot be retracted.

Paraphimosis—the foreskin cannot be slipped forward once it is retracted.

Dirt and smegma collecting under foreskin.

The scrotum looks pink in light-skinned infants and dark brown in dark-skinned infants. Rugae are well formed in the full-term infant. Size varies with ambient temperature, but overall, the infant's scrotum looks large in relation to the penis. No bulges, either constant or intermittent, are present.

Palpate the scrotum and testes. The cremasteric reflex is strong in the infant, pulling the testes up into the inguinal canal and abdomen from exposure to cold, touch, exercise, or emotion. Take care not to elicit the reflexing by: (1) keeping your hands warm and palpating from the external inguinal ring down; (2) blocking the inguinal canals with the thumb and forefinger of your other hand to prevent the testes from retracting (Fig. 24-15).

Normal Range of Findings	Abnormal Findings

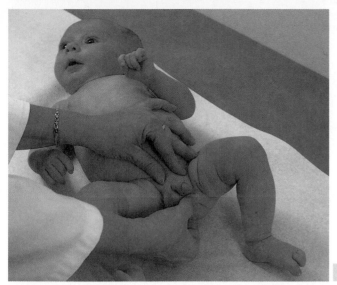

Fig. 24-15

Normally, the testes are descended and are equal in size bilaterally (1.5 to 2 cm until puberty). It is important to document that you have palpated the testes. Once palpated, they are considered descended, even if they have retracted momentarily at the next visit.

If the scrotal half feels empty, search for the testes along the inguinal canal and try to milk them down. Ask the toddler or child to squat with the knees flexed up; this pressure may force the testes down. Or, have the young child sit cross-legged to relax the reflex (Fig. 24-16).

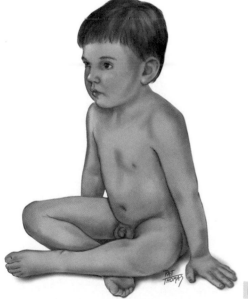

Fig. 24-16

Migratory testes (physiological cryptorchidism) are common because of the strength of the cremasteric reflex and the small mass of the prepubertal testes. Note that the affected side has a normally developed scrotum (with true cryptorchidism, the scrotum is atrophic) and that the testis can be milked down. These testes descend at puberty and are normal.

Palpate the epididymis and spermatic cord as described in the adult section. A common scrotal finding in the boy under 2 years of age is a **hydrocele,** or fluid in the scrotum. It appears as a large scrotum and transilluminates as a faint pink glow. It usually disappears spontaneously.

Cryptorchidism: undescended testes (those that have never descended). Undescended testes are common in premature infants. They occur in 3 to 4% of term infants, although most have descended by 3 months of age. Physicians' opinions differ concerning the age at which child should be referred (see Table 24-5, p. 734).

A hydrocele is a cystic collection of serous fluid in the tunica vaginalis, surrounding the testis (see Table 24-5, p. 734).

Normal Range of Findings	Abnormal Findings

Inspect the inguinal area for a bulge. If you do not see a bulge but the parent gives a positive history of one, try to elicit it by increasing intra-abdominal pressure. Ask the boy to hold his breath and strain down or have him blow up a balloon.

If a hernia is suspected, palpate the inguinal area. Use your little finger to reach the external inguinal ring.

The Adolescent

The adolescent shows a wide variation in normal development of the genitals. Using the SMR charts, note: (1) enlargement of the testes and scrotum; (2) pubic hair growth; (3) darkening of scrotal colour; (4) roughening of scrotal skin; (5) increase in penis length and width; and (6) axillary hair growth.

Be familiar with the normal sequence of growth.

The Aging Adult

In the older male, you may note thinner, greying pubic hair and the decreased size of the penis. The size of the testes may be decreased and may feel less firm. The scrotal sac is pendulous with fewer rugae. The scrotal skin may become excoriated if the man continually sits on it.

Summary Checklist: Male Genitalia Examination

 For a PDA-downloadable version, go to http://evolve.elsevier.com/Canada/Jarvis/examination/.

1. Inspect and palpate **the penis**
2. Inspect and palpate **the scrotum**
3. If a mass exists, **transilluminate it**
4. Palpate for an **inguinal hernia**
5. Palpate the **inguinal lymph nodes**

Objective Data

DOCUMENTATION AND CRITICAL THINKING

Sample Charting

SUBJECTIVE

Urinates four to five times per day, clear, straw-coloured. No nocturia, dysuria, or hesitancy. No pain, lesions, or discharge from penis. Does not do testicular self-examination. No history of genitourinary disease. Sexually active in a monogamous relationship. Sexual life satisfactory to self and partner. Uses birth control via barrier method (partner uses diaphragm). No known STI contact.

OBJECTIVE

No lesions, inflammation, or discharge from penis. Scrotum—testes descended, symmetrical, no masses. No inguinal hernia.

ASSESSMENT

Genital structures normal

Focused Assessment: Clinical Case Study

SUBJECTIVE

- R.C. is a 19-year-old student who 2 days PTA noted acute onset of painful urination, frequency, and urgency. Noted some thick penile discharge. States has no side pain, no abdominal pain, no fever, no genital skin rash. R.C. is concerned he has an STI because of episode of unprotected intercourse with a new partner 6 days PTA. Has no known allergies.

OBJECTIVE

Vital signs 37°C-72-16. No lesions or inflammation around penis or scrotum. Urethral meatus has mild edema with purulent urethral discharge. No pain on palpation of genitalia. Testes symmetrical with no masses. No lymphadenopathy.

ASSESSMENT

Urethral discharge
Deficient knowledge about STI prevention R/T lack of information recall

Nursing Diagnoses Commonly Associated With the Male Genitalia and Related Disorders

All nursing diagnoses can be found on the Evolve Web site at **http://evolve.elsevier.com/Canada/Jarvis/examination/.**

Documentation
and Critical Thinking

⊷ ABNORMAL FINDINGS ⊶

TABLE 24-2	**Urine Colour and Discolorations**

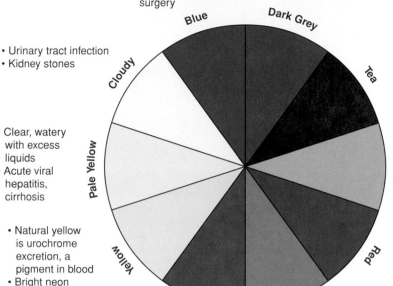

- Medication side effect: amitriptyline, indomethacin (Indocin)
- Foods: asparagus
- Dye after prostate surgery

- Urine contains melanin, melaninuria

- Liver disease, especially with pale stools, jaundice
- Myoglobinuria
- Some medications or food dyes
- Blood in urine

- Urinary tract infection
- Kidney stones

Blue   **Dark Grey**   **Tea**

Cloudy

- Clear, watery with excess liquids
- Acute viral hepatitis, cirrhosis

Pale Yellow

- Some foods: beets, berries, food dyes
- Some laxatives
- Kidney stones
- Urinary tract infection

Pink

- Natural yellow is urochrome excretion, a pigment in blood
- Bright neon yellow with vitamin supplements

Yellow

Red

- Blood in urine
- Nephritis, cystitis
- Cancer
- Following prostate surgery

Amber   **Orange**

- Gold coloured or concentrated with dehydration
- Some laxatives
- Food or supplements with B-complex vitamins

- Medication side effect: rifampin for meningitis, phenazopyridine (Pyridium), warfarin (Coumadin)
- Some foods, food dyes, laxatives
- Dehydration
- Jaundice (bilirubinemia)

ABNORMAL FINDINGS
FOR ADVANCED PRACTICE

TABLE 24-3	Male Genital Lesions

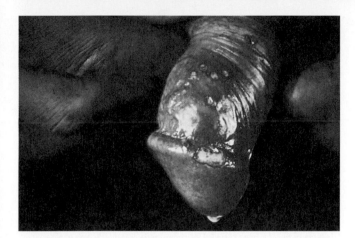

Genital Herpes—HSV-2 Infection

Clusters of small vesicles with surrounding erythema, which are often painful, erupt on the glans or foreskin. These rupture to form superficial ulcers. A sexually transmitted infection (STI), the initial infection lasts 7 to 10 days. The virus remains dormant indefinitely; recurrent infections last 3 to 10 days with milder symptoms.

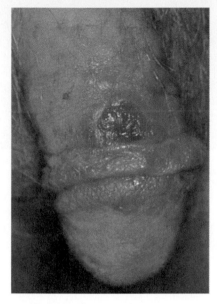

Syphilitic Chancre

Begins within 2 to 4 weeks of infection, as a small, solitary, silvery papule that erodes to a red, round or oval, superficial ulcer with a yellowish serous discharge. Palpation reveals a nontender indurated base that can be lifted like a button between the thumb and the finger. Lymph nodes enlarge early but are nontender. This is an STI.

Reprinted from Emond, R. (1995). Colour atlas of infectious diseases (3rd ed. p. 173), by permission of the publisher Mosby.

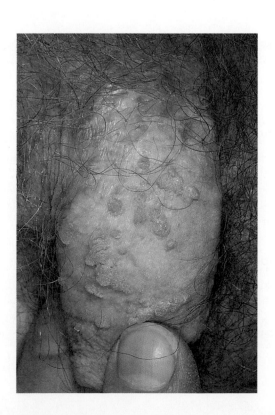

◀ Genital Warts

Soft, pointed, moist, fleshy, painless papules may be single or multiple in a cauliflowerlike patch. Colour may be grey, pale yellow, or pink in White males, and black or translucent grey-black in Black males. They occur on shaft of penis, behind corona, or around the anus where they may grow into large grapelike clusters.

These are caused by the human papillomavirus (HPV) and are one of the most common STIs. The HPV infection is correlated with early onset of sexual activity, infrequent use of contraception, and multiple sexual partners.

Continued

TABLE 24-3	Male Genital Lesions—cont'd

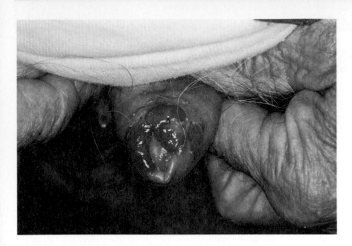

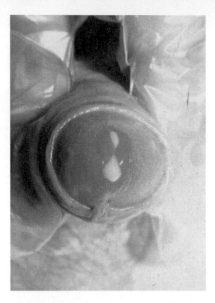

Carcinoma

Begins as red, raised warty growth or as an ulcer, with watery discharge. As it grows, may necrose and slough. Usually painless. Almost always on glans or inner lip of foreskin and following chronic inflammation. Enlarged lymph nodes are common.

Urethritis (Urethral Discharge and Dysuria)

Infection of urethra causes painful burning urination. Meatus edges are reddened, everted, and swollen. Purulent urethral discharge is present. Urine is cloudy with discharge and mucous shreds. Cause determined by culture: (1) gonococcal urethritis has thick, profuse, yellow or grey-brown discharge; (2) nonspecific urethritis (NSU) may have similar discharge but often has scanty, mucoid discharge. Of these, about 50% are caused by *Chlamydia* infection. This is important to differentiate because antibiotic treatment is different.

Reprinted from Emond, R. (1995). Colour atlas of infectious diseases (3rd ed., p. 161), by permission of the publisher, Mosby.

TABLE 24-4	Abnormalities of the Penis

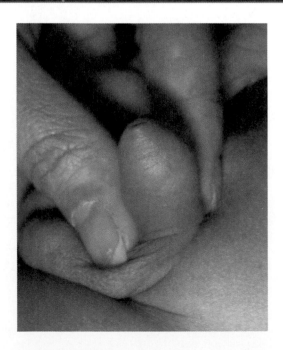

◀ Phimosis

Foreskin is advanced and fixed so tight it is impossible to retract over glans. May be congenital or acquired from adhesions secondary to infection. Poor hygiene leads to retained dirt and smegma, which increases risk of inflammation or calculus formation.

Paraphimosis (not illustrated)

Foreskin is retracted and fixed. Once retracted behind glans, a tight or inflamed foreskin cannot return to its original position. Constriction impedes circulation, so glans swells. If untreated, it may compromise arterial circulation.

TABLE 24-4 | Abnormalities of the Penis—cont'd

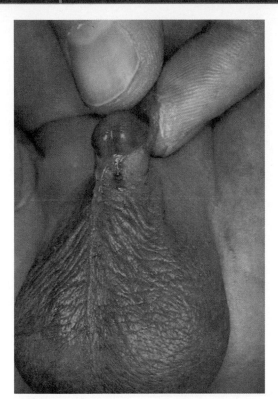

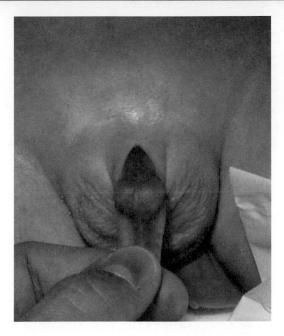

Hypospadias

Urethral meatus opens on the ventral (under-) side of glans, shaft, or at the penoscrotal junction. A groove extends from the meatus to the normal location at the tip. This is a congenital defect that is important to recognize at birth. The newborn should not be circumcised because surgical correction may use foreskin tissue to extend urethral length.

Epispadias

Meatus opens on the dorsal (upper) side of glans or shaft above a broad, spadelike penis. Rare; less common than hypospadias but more disabling because of associated urinary incontinence and separation of pubic bones.

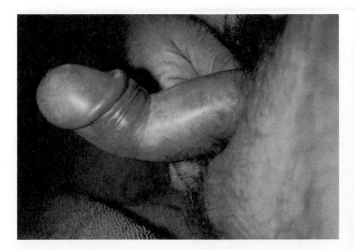

Urethral Stricture (not illustrated)

Pinpoint, constricted opening at meatus or inside along urethra. Occurs congenitally or secondary to urethral injury. Gradual decrease in force and calibre of urine stream is most common symptom. Shaft feels indurated along ventral aspect at the site of the stricture.

Priapism (not illustrated)

Prolonged painful erection of penis without sexual desire. Rare condition occurs with sickle-cell trait or disease; leukemia where increased numbers of white blood cells produce engorgement; malignancy; or local trauma or spinal cord injuries with autonomic nervous system dysfunction.

Peyronie's Disease

Hard, nontender, subcutaneous plaques palpated on dorsal or lateral surface of penis. May be single or multiple and asymmetrical. They are associated with painful bending of the penis during erection. Plaques are fibrosis of covering of corpora cavernosa. Usually occurs after 45 years. Its cause is trauma to the erect penis, such as an unexpected change in angle during intercourse. More common in men with diabetes, gout, and Dupuytren's contracture of the palm.

TABLE 24-5	Abnormalities in the Scrotum	
Disorder	Clinical Findings	Discussion

Absent Testis Cryptorchidism

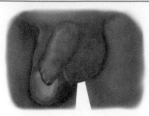

S: Empty scrotal half
O: Inspection—in true maldescent, atrophic scrotum on affected side
Palpation—no testis
A: Absent testis

True cryptorchidism—testes that have never descended. Incidence at birth is 3 to 4%; one-half of these descend in first month. Incidence with premature infants is 30%; in the adult 0.7 to 0.8%. True undescended testes have a histological change by 6 years, causing decreased spermatogenesis and infertility.

Small Testis

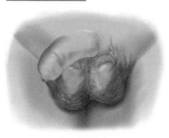

S: (None)
O: Palpation—small and soft (rarely may be firm)
A: Small testis

Small and soft (<3.5 cm) indicates atrophy as with cirrhosis, hypopituitarism, following estrogen therapy, or as a sequelae of orchitis. Small and firm (<2 cm) occurs with Klinefelter's syndrome (hypogonadism).

Testicular Torsion

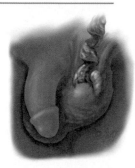

S: Excruciating pain in testicle of sudden onset, often during sleep or following trauma. May also have lower abdominal pain, nausea and vomiting, no fever
O: Inspection—red, swollen scrotum, one testis (usually left) higher owing to rotation and shortening
Palpation—cord feels thick, swollen, tender, epididymis may be anterior, cremasteric reflex is absent on side of torsion
A: Acute, painful swelling of spermatic cord, with elevation of one testis

Sudden twisting of spermatic cord. Occurs in late childhood, early adolescence, rare after age of 20 years. Torsion occurs usually on the left side. Faulty anchoring of testis on wall of scrotum allows testis to rotate. The anterior part of the testis rotates medially toward the other testis. Blood supply is cut off, resulting in ischemia and engorgement. This is an emergency requiring surgery; testis can become gangrenous in a few hours.

Epididymitis

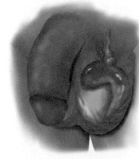

S: Severe pain of sudden onset in scrotum, somewhat relieved by elevation (a positive Phren's sign); also rapid swelling, fever
O: Inspection—enlarged scrotum; reddened
Palpation—exquisitely tender; epididymis enlarged, indurated; may be hard to distinguish from testis. Overlying scrotal skin may be thick and edematous
Laboratory—white blood cells and bacteria in urine
A: Tender swelling of epididymis

Acute infection of epididymis commonly caused by prostatitis, after prostatectomy because of trauma of urethral instrumentation, or due to *Chlamydia*, gonorrhea, or other bacterial infection. Often difficult to distinguish between epididymitis and testicular torsion.

S, Subjective data; O, objective data; A, assessment.

Abnormal Findings

TABLE 24-5	Abnormalities in the Scrotum—cont'd		
Disorder	**Clinical Findings**		**Discussion**

Spermatic Cord Varicocele

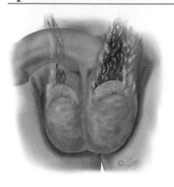

S: Dull pain; constant pulling or dragging feeling; or may be asymptomatic

O: Inspection—usually no sign. May show bluish colour through light scrotal skin
Palpation—when standing, feel soft, irregular mass posterior to and above testis; collapses when supine, refills when upright. Feels distinctive, like a "bag of worms"
The testis on the side of the varicocele may be smaller owing to impaired circulation

A: Soft mass on spermatic cord

A varicocele is dilated, tortuous varicose veins in the spermatic cord due to incompetent valves within the vein, which permit reflux of blood. Most often on left side, perhaps because left spermatic vein is longer and inserts at a right angle into left renal vein. Common in young males. Screen at early adolescence; early treatment important to prevent potential infertility when an adult.

Spermatocele

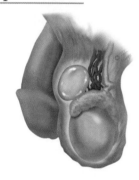

S: Painless, usually found on examination

O: Inspection—does transilluminate higher in the scrotum than a hydrocele, and the sperm may fluoresce
Palpation—round, freely movable mass lying above and behind testis. If large, feels like a third testis

A: Free cystic mass on epididymis

Retention cyst in epididymis. Cause unclear but may be obstruction of tubules. Filled with thin, milky fluid that contains sperm. Most spermatoceles are small (<1 cm); occasionally, they may be larger and then mistaken for hydrocele.

Early Testicular Tumour

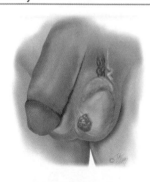

S: Painless, found on examination

O: Palpation—firm nodule or harder than normal section of testicle

A: Solitary nodule

Most testicular tumours occur in men between the ages of 18 and 35. Practically all are malignant. Occur in Whites; relatively rare in Blacks, Mexican Americans, and Asians. Must biopsy to confirm. Most important risk factor is undescended testis, even those surgically corrected. Early detection important in prognosis, but practice of testicular self-examination is currently low.

Diffuse Tumour

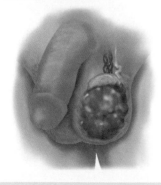

S: Enlarging testis (most common symptom). When enlarges, has feel of increased weight

O: Inspection—enlarged, does not transilluminate
Palpation—enlarged, smooth, ovoid, firm
Important—firm palpation does *not* cause usual sickening discomfort as with normal testis

A: Nontender swelling of testis

Diffuse tumour maintains shape of testis.

Images © Pat Thomas, 2006.
Continued

TABLE 24-5	Abnormalities in the Scrotum—cont'd	
Disorder	**Clinical Findings**	**Discussion**
Hydrocele 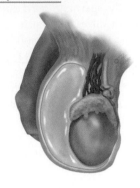	S: Painless swelling, although person may complain of weight and bulk in scrotum O: Inspection—enlarged, mass does transilluminate with a pink or red glow (in contrast to a hernia) Palpation—nontender mass, able to get fingers above mass (in contrast to scrotal hernia) A: Nontender swelling of testis	Cystic. Circumscribed collection of serous fluid in tunica vaginalis, surrounding testis. May occur following epididymitis, trauma, hernia, tumour of testis, or spontaneously in the newborn.
Scrotal Hernia 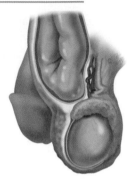	S: Swelling, may have pain with straining O: Inspection—enlarged, may reduce when supine, does not transilluminate Palpation—soft mushy mass, palpating fingers cannot get above mass; mass is distinct from testicle that is normal A: Nontender swelling of scrotum	Scrotal hernia usually due to indirect inguinal hernia (see Table 24-6).
Orchitis 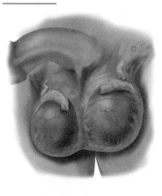	S: Acute or moderate pain of sudden onset, swollen testis, feeling of weight, fever O: Inspection—enlarged, edematous, reddened; does not transilluminate Palpation—swollen, congested, tense, and tender; hard to distinguish testis from epididymis A: Tender swelling of testis	Acute inflammation of testis. Most common cause is mumps; can occur with any infectious disease. May have associated hydrocele that does transilluminate.
Scrotal Edema 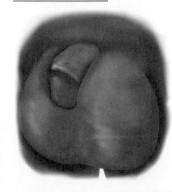	S: Tenderness O: Inspection—enlarged, may be reddened (with local irritation) Palpation—taut with pitting; probably unable to feel scrotal contents A: Scrotal edema	Accompanies marked edema in lower half of body, such as congestive heart failure, renal failure, and portal vein obstruction. Occurs with local inflammation: epididymitis, torsion of spermatic cord. Also obstruction of inguinal lymphatics produces lymphedema of scrotum.

TABLE 24-6 | Inguinal and Femoral Hernias

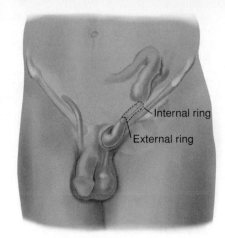
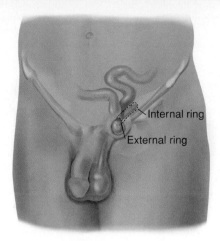
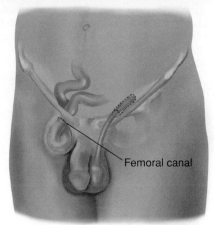

© Pat Thomas, 2006.

	Indirect Inguinal	Direct Inguinal	Femoral
Course	Sac herniates through internal inguinal ring; can remain in canal or pass into scrotum	Directly behind and through external inguinal ring, above inguinal ligament; rarely enters scrotum	Through femoral ring and canal, below inguinal ligament, more often on right side
Clinical Symptoms and Signs	Pain with straining; soft swelling that increases with increased intra-abdominal pressure; may decrease when lying down	Usually painless; round swelling close to the pubis in area of internal inguinal ring; easily reduced when supine[1]	Pain may be severe; hernia may become strangulated
Frequency	Most common; 60% of all hernias. More common in infants <1 year and in males 16 to 20 years of age	Less common, occurs most often in men >40, rare in women	Least common, 4% of all hernias; more common in women
Cause	Congenital or acquired	Acquired weakness; brought on by heavy lifting, muscle atrophy, obesity, chronic cough, or ascites	Acquired; due to increased abdominal pressure, muscle weakness, or frequent stooping

[1]**Reducible**—contents will return to abdominal cavity by gentle pressure or when patient is supine. **Incarcerated**—herniated bowel cannot be returned to abdominal cavity. **Strangulated**—blood supply to hernia is shut off. Accompanied by nausea, vomiting, and tenderness.

BIBLIOGRAPHY

Adelman, W., & Joffe, A. (2004). Controversies in male adolescent health: Varicocele, circumcision, and testicular self-examination. *Current Opinion in Pediatrics, 16*, 363–367.

Adelman, W. P., & Joffe, A. (2000). Revisiting the adolescent male genital examination. *Patient Care, 34*(4), 83–93.

Albaugh, J., & Kellogg-Spadt, S. (2003). Genital and dermatologic examination part II: The male patient. *Urologic Nursing, 23*, 366–367.

Behrman, R. E. (2003). *Nelson textbook of pediatrics* (17th ed.). Philadelphia, PA: W.B. Saunders.

Berry, A. (2006). Helping children with nocturnal enuresis. *American Journal of Nursing, 106*(8), 56–64.

Bickford, J. (2006). Sexual history taking and genital examination. *Primary Health Care, 16*(2), 33–35.

British Medical Association. (2004). The law and ethics of male circumcision. *Journal of Medical Ethics, 30*, 259–263.

Canadian Cancer Society. (2006). *Testicular cancer: Understanding your diagnosis.* Vancouver, BC: Author. Also available at http://www.ontario.cancer.ca/ccs/internet/publication/o,,3278_286016785_1491857775_langId-en.html

Canadian Cancer Society. (2007). *Prostate cancer: Understanding your diagnosis.* Vancouver, BC: Author. Also available at http://cancer.ca/ccs/internet/publicationlist/0,,3278_286016785_292304666_langId-en.html

Circumcision Information and Resource Pages. (2006). Canada circumcision statistics. Retrieved January 20, 2008, from http://www.cirp.org/library/statistics/Canada/

Elford, R. W. (1994). Screening for testicular cancer. In Canadian Task Force on the Periodic Health Examination (Eds.), *Canadian guide to clinical preventive health care* (pp. 891–898). Ottawa, ON: Health Canada.

Fackler, A., & Henley, C. (2006). *Caring for your young son's uncircumcised penis.* Retrieved April 10, 2008, from http://www.bchealthguide.org/kbase/topic/special/hw142263spec/sec1.htm

Feightner, J. W. (1994). Screening for prostate cancer. In Canadian Task Force on the Periodic Health Examination (Eds.), *Canadian guide to clinical preventive health care* (pp. 811–823). Ottawa, ON: Health Canada.

Fetus and Newborn Committee, Canadian Pediatric Society. (1996—reaffirmed 2002). Neonatal circumcision revisited. *Canadian Medical Association Journal, 154*, 769–780.

Fracchia, M., Pareek, G., & Armenakas, N. (2004). Scrotal pathology in children: Benign or serious? *Consultant, 44*, 1114–1120.

Gilmour, C. (2005). Assessing and recording a patient's sexual history. *Nursing Times, 101*(44), 28–30.

Gray, M. (2005). Assessment and management of urinary incontinence. *Nurse Practitioner 30*(7), 33–45.

Joseph, A. (2003). Continence: the sixth vital sign? Let's not ignore urinary incontinence [Electronic version]. *American Journal of Nursing, 103*(7), 11.

Kleier, J. (2004). Nurse practitioners' behavior regarding teaching testicular self-examination. *Journal of the American Academy of Nurse Practitioners, 16*, 206–218.

Legg, V. (2005). Complications of chronic kidney disease: A close look at renal osteodystrophy, nutritional disturbances, and inflammation. *American Journal of Nursing, 105*(6), 40–50.

Lewis, J., Rosen, R., & Goldstein, I. (2004). Erectile dysfunction in primary care. *Nurse Practitioner, 29*(12), 42–57.

Marshall, W., & Tanner, J. (1970). Variations in the pattern of pubertal changes in boys. *Archives of Disease in Childhood, 45*, 13.

Ritchie, B., & Archer, A. (2004). Circumcision: Issues and education. *University of Toronto Medical Journal, 81*(2), 90–94.

Stratman-Lucey, D., & Caldwell, D. (2006, August–September). Pain management protocol with infant circumcision. *The Illinois Nurse, 13.*

Taylor, J. S., Dubé, C. E., Pipas, C. F., Fuller, B. K., Lavallee, L. K., & Rosen, R. (2004). Teaching the testicular exam: a model curriculum from "A" to "Zack." *Family Medicine, 36*, 209–213.

Warnock, F., & Sandrin, D. (2004). Comprehensive description of newborn distress behavior in response to acute pain (newborn male circumcision). *Pain, 107*, 242–255.

Wirth, J. L. (1980). Current circumcision practices: Canada. *Pediatrics, 66*, 705–708.

Wynd, C. (2002). Testicular self-examination in young adult men. *Journal of Nursing Scholarship, 34*, 251–255.

Anus, Rectum, and Prostate

Written by **Carolyn Jarvis**, PhD, APN, CNP
Adapted by **Marian Luctkar-Flude**, RN, MScN

Electronic Resources

On Evolve *evolve*

http://evolve.elsevier.com/Canada/Jarvis/examination/

- Interactive Case Studies
- Physical Examination Audio and Printable Summaries
- Bedside Assessment Summary Checklists
- Complete Physical Examination Form
- Nursing Diagnoses Boxes
- Health Promotion Guides
- Quick Assessments for 20 Common Conditions
- Multiple Choice Review Questions
- Chapter Objectives
- Appendices
- Weblinks

On the Companion CD

- Interactive Case Studies with Heart and Lung Sounds
- Health Promotion Guides
- Quick Assessments for 20 Common Conditions
- Head-to-Toe Physical Examination Video Clips

Structure and Function

STRUCTURE AND FUNCTION

ANUS AND RECTUM

The **anal canal** is the outlet of the gastrointestinal tract, and it is about 3.8 cm long in the adult. It is lined with modified skin (having no hair or sebaceous glands) that merges with rectal mucosa at the anorectal junction. The canal slants forward toward the umbilicus, forming a distinct right angle with the rectum, which rests back in the hollow of the sacrum. Although the rectum contains only autonomic nerves, numerous somatic sensory nerves are present in the anal canal and external skin, so a person feels sharp pain from any trauma to the anal area.

The anal canal is surrounded by two concentric layers of muscle, the **sphincters** (Fig. 25-1). The internal sphincter is under involuntary control by the autonomic nervous system. The external sphincter surrounds the internal sphincter but also has a small section overriding the tip of the internal sphincter at the opening. It is under voluntary control. Except for the passing of feces and gas, the sphincters keep the anal canal tightly closed. The **intersphincteric groove** separates the internal and external sphincters and is palpable.

The **anal columns** (or columns of Morgagni) are folds of mucosa. These extend vertically down from the rectum and end in the **anorectal junction** (also called the mucocutaneous junction, pectinate, or dentate line). This junction is not palpable, but it is visible on proctoscopy. Each anal column contains an artery and a vein. Under conditions of chronic increased venous pressure, the vein may enlarge, forming a hemorrhoid. At the lower end of each column is a small crescent fold of mucous membrane, the **anal valve.** The space above the anal valve (between the columns) is a small recess, the **anal crypt.**

The **rectum,** which is 12 cm long, is the distal portion of the large intestine. It extends from the sigmoid colon, at the level of the third sacral vertebra, and ends at the anal canal. Just above the anal canal, the rectum dilates and turns posteriorly, forming the rectal ampulla. The rectal interior has three semilunar transverse folds called the **valves of Houston.** These cross one half of the circumference of the rectal lumen. Their function is unclear, but they may serve to hold feces as the flatus passes. The lowest is within reach of palpation,

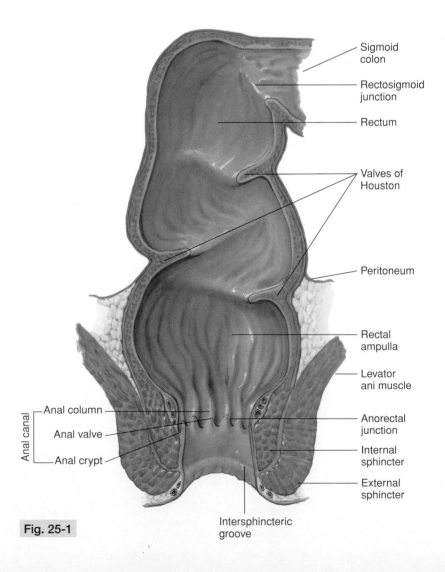

Sigmoid colon

Rectosigmoid junction

Rectum

Valves of Houston

Peritoneum

Rectal ampulla

Levator ani muscle

Anorectal junction

Internal sphincter

External sphincter

Anal canal
Anal column
Anal valve
Anal crypt

Intersphincteric groove

Fig. 25-1

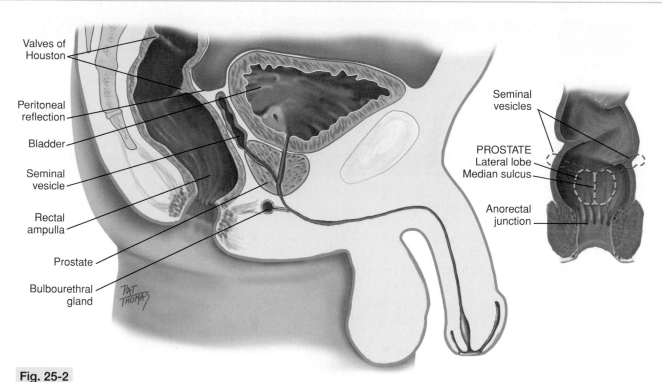

Valves of
Houston

Peritoneal
reflection

Bladder

Seminal
vesicle

Rectal
ampulla

Prostate

Bulbourethral
gland

Seminal
vesicles

PROSTATE
Lateral lobe
Median sulcus

Anorectal
junction

Fig. 25-2

usually on the person's left side, and must not be mistaken for an intrarectal mass.

Peritoneal Reflection. The peritoneum covers only the upper two thirds of the rectum. In the male, the anterior part of the peritoneum reflects down to within 7.5 cm of the anal opening, forming the **rectovesical pouch** (Fig. 25-2) and then covers the bladder. In the female, this is termed the **rectouterine pouch,** and extends down to within 5.5 cm of the anal opening.

PROSTATE

In the male, the **prostate gland** lies in front of the anterior wall of the rectum and 2 cm behind the symphysis pubis. It surrounds the bladder neck and the urethra and has 15 to 30 ducts that open into the urethra. The prostate secretes a thin, milky alkaline fluid that helps sperm viability. It is a bilobed structure with a round or heart shape. It measures 2.5 cm long and 4 cm in diameter. The two lateral lobes are separated by a shallow groove called the **median sulcus.**

The two **seminal vesicles** project like rabbit ears above the prostate. The seminal vesicles secrete a fluid that is rich in fructose, which nourishes the sperm, and contains prostaglandins. The two **bulbourethral** (Cowper's) glands are each the size of a pea and are located inferior to the prostate on either side of the urethra (see Fig. 25-5 on page 745). They secrete a clear, viscid mucus.

REGIONAL STRUCTURES

In the female, the uterine cervix lies in front of the anterior rectal wall and may be palpated through it.

The combined length of the anal canal and the rectum is about 16 cm in the adult. The average length of the examin-

ing finger is 6 to 10 cm, bringing many rectal structures within reach.

The sigmoid colon is named from its S-shaped course in the pelvic cavity. It extends from the iliac flexure of the descending colon and ends at the rectum. It is 40 cm long and is accessible to examination only through the colonoscope. The flexible fibreoptic scope in current use provides a view of the entire mucosal surface of the sigmoid, as well as the colon.

🌱 DEVELOPMENTAL CARE

The first stool passed by the newborn is dark green meconium and occurs within 24 to 48 hours of birth, indicating anal patency. From that time on, the infant usually has a stool after each feeding. This response to eating is a wave of peristalsis called the gastrocolic reflex. It continues throughout life, although children and adults usually produce no more than one or two stools per day.

The infant passes stools by reflex. Voluntary control of the external anal sphincter cannot occur until the nerves supplying the area have become fully myelinated, usually around $1\frac{1}{2}$ to 2 years of age. Toilet training usually starts after age 2 years.

At male puberty, the prostate gland undergoes a very rapid increase to more than twice its prepubertal size. During young adulthood its size remains fairly constant.

The prostate gland commonly starts to enlarge during the middle adult years. This **benign prostatic hypertrophy (BPH)** is present in one of 10 males at the age of 40 years and increases with age. It is thought that the hypertrophy is caused by a hormonal imbalance that leads to the proliferation of benign adenomas. These gradually impede urine output because they obstruct the urethra.

SUBJECTIVE DATA

1. Usual bowel routine
2. Change in bowel habits
3. Rectal bleeding, blood in the stool

4. Medications (laxatives, stool softeners, iron)
5. Rectal conditions (pruritus, hemorrhoids, fissure, fistula)

6. Family history
7. Self-care behaviours (diet of high-fibre foods, most recent examinations)

Examiner Asks	Rationale
1. **Usual bowel routine.** Defecate regularly? How often? Usual colour? Hard or soft? Pain while passing a bowel movement?	Assess usual bowel routine. **Dyschezia.** Pain may be due to a local condition (hemorrhoid, fissure) or constipation.
2. **Change in bowel habits.** Any **change** in usual **bowel habits?** Loose stools, or diarrhea? When did this start? Is the diarrhea associated with nausea and vomiting, abdominal pain, something you ate recently? • Eaten at a restaurant recently? Anyone else in your group or family have the same symptoms? • Travelled to a foreign country during the past 6 months? • Stools have a hard consistency? When did this start?	Diarrhea occurs with gastroenteritis, colitis, irritable colon syndrome. Consider food poisoning. Consider parasitic infection. Constipation.
3. **Rectal bleeding, blood in the stool.** Ever had black or bloody stools? When did you first notice blood in the stools? What is the colour: bright red or dark red-black? How much blood: spotting on the toilet paper or outright passing of blood with the stool? Do the bloody stools have a particular smell? • Ever had clay-coloured stools? • Ever had mucus or pus in stool? • Frothy stool? • Need to pass gas frequently?	**Melena.** Black stools may be tarry due to occult blood (melena) from gastrointestinal bleeding, or nontarry from ingestion of iron medications. Red blood in stools occurs with gastrointestinal bleeding or localized bleeding around the anus, and also with colon and rectal cancer. Clay colour indicates absent bile pigment. **Steatorrhea** is excessive fat in the stool as in malabsorption of fat. Flatulence.
4. **Medications.** What **medications** do you take—prescription and over-the-counter? Laxatives or stool softeners? Which ones? How often? Iron pills? Do you ever use enemas to move your bowels? How often?	
5. **Rectal conditions.** Any problems in rectal area: itching, pain or burning, hemorrhoids? How do you treat these? Any hemorrhoid preparations? Ever had a fissure, or fistula? How was this treated? • Ever had a problem controlling your bowels?	Pruritus. Fecal incontinence. Mucoid discharge and soiled underwear occur with prolapsed hemorrhoids.
6. **Family history.** Any **family history:** polyps or cancer in colon or rectum, inflammatory bowel disease, prostate cancer?	Risk factors for colon cancer, rectal cancer, prostate cancer.

Examiner Asks	Rationale
7. Self-care behaviours. What is the usual amount of **high-fibre foods** in your daily diet: cereals, apples or other fruits, vegetables, whole-grain breads? How many glasses of water do you drink each day?	High-fibre foods of the soluble type (beans, prunes, barley, carrots, broccoli, cabbage) have been shown to lower cholesterol, while insoluble-fibre foods (cereals, wheat germ) reduce the risk of colon cancer. Also, fibre foods fight obesity, stabilize blood sugar, and help certain gastrointestinal disorders.
• Date last: DRE, stool blood test, colonoscopy (for men), PSA blood test.	Early detection for cancer: refer to Table 25-1 on p. 749 and the Promoting Health boxes on p. 748 for colon and prostate cancer screening guidelines.

Additional History for Infants and Children

1. Have you ever noticed any irritation in your child's anal area: redness, raised skin, frequent itching?	In children, pinworms are a common cause of intense itching and irritated anal skin.
2. How are your child's bowel movements (BMs)? Frequency? Any problems? Any pain or straining with BM?	Assess usual stooling pattern. Constipation is a decrease in BM frequency, with difficult passing of very hard, dry stools. **Encopresis** is persistent passing of stools into clothing in a child older than age 4 years, at which age continence would be expected.

— **OBJECTIVE DATA** —

PREPARATION

Perform a rectal examination on all adults and particularly for those in middle and late years. Help the person assume one of the following positions (Fig. 25-3): Examine the male in the left lateral decubitus or standing position. Instruct the standing male to point his toes together; this relaxes the regional muscles, making it easier to spread the buttocks.

Place the female in the lithotomy position if examining genitalia as well; use the left lateral decubitus position for the rectal area alone.

EQUIPMENT NEEDED

Penlight
Lubricating jelly
Glove
Guaiac test container

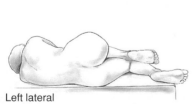
Left lateral

Lithotomy

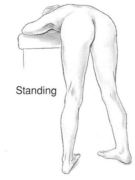
Standing

Fig. 25-3   Positions for rectal examination.

Normal Range of Findings	Abnormal Findings

INSPECT THE PERIANAL AREA

Spread the buttocks wide apart and observe the perianal region. The anus normally looks moist and hairless, with coarse folded skin that is more pigmented than the perianal skin. The anal opening is tightly closed. No lesions are present.

Inflammation. Lesions or scars. Linear split—fissure.

Flabby skin sac—hemorrhoid. Shiny blue skin sac—thrombosed hemorrhoid.

Small round opening in anal area —fistula (see Table 25-2 on p. 750).

Inspect the sacrococcygeal area. Normally, it appears smooth and even.

Inflammation or tenderness, swelling, tuft of hair, or dimple at tip of coccyx may indicate pilonidal cyst (see Table 25-2, p. 750).

Instruct the person to hold the breath and bear down by performing a Valsalva manoeuvre. No break in skin integrity or protrusion through the anal opening should be present. Describe any abnormality in clock-face terms, with 12:00 as the anterior point toward the symphysis pubis and 6:00 toward the coccyx.

Appearance of fissure, or hemorrhoids. Circular red doughnut of tissue—rectal prolapse.

PALPATE THE ANUS AND RECTUM

Drop lubricating jelly onto your gloved index finger. Instruct the person that palpation is not painful but may feel like needing to move the bowels. Place the pad of your index finger gently against the anal verge (Fig. 25-4). You will feel the sphincter tighten, then relax. As it relaxes, flex the tip of your finger and slowly insert it into the anal canal in a direction toward the umbilicus. *Never* approach the anus at right angles with your index finger extended. Such a jabbing motion does not promote sphincter relaxation and is painful.

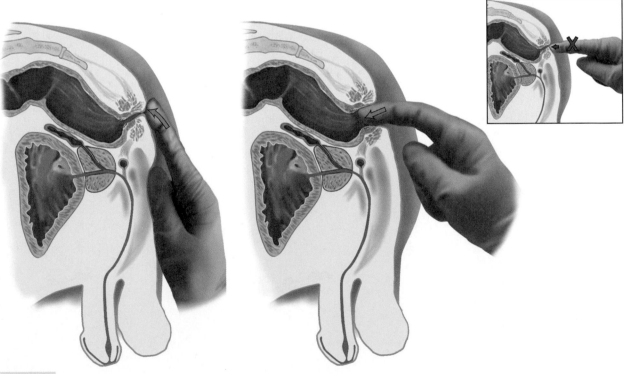

Fig. 25-4

Objective Data

Normal Range of Findings	Abnormal Findings

Rotate your examining finger to palpate the entire muscular ring. The canal should feel smooth and even. Note the intersphincteric groove circling the canal wall. To assess tone, ask the person to tighten the muscle. The sphincter should tighten evenly around your finger with no pain to the person.

Use a bidigital palpation with your thumb against the perianal tissue (Fig. 25-5). Press your examining finger toward it. This manoeuvre highlights any swelling or tenderness and helps assess the bulbourethral glands.

Decreased tone.
Increased tone occurs with inflammation and anxiety.

Tenderness.

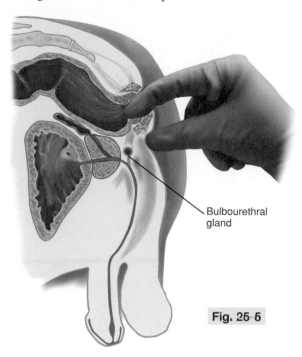

Bulbourethral gland

Fig. 25-5

Above the anal canal, the rectum turns posteriorly, following the curve of the coccyx and sacrum. Insert your finger farther and explore all around the rectal wall. It normally feels smooth with no nodularity. Promptly report any mass you discover for further examination.

Internal hemorrhoid above anorectal junction is not palpable unless thrombosed.
A soft, slightly movable mass may be a polyp.
A firm or hard mass with irregular shape or rolled edges may signify carcinoma (see Table 25-2, p. 750).

Prostate Gland. On the anterior wall in the male, note the elastic, bulging prostate gland (Fig. 25-6). Palpate the entire prostate in a systematic manner, but note that only the superior and part of the lateral surfaces are accessible to examination. Press *into* the gland at each location, because when a nodule occurs, it will not project into the rectal lumen. The surface should feel smooth and muscular; search for any distinct nodule or diffuse firmness. Note these characteristics:

Size—2.5 cm long by 4 cm wide; should not protrude more than 1 cm into the rectum
Shape—heart shape, with palpable central groove
Surface—smooth
Consistency—elastic, rubbery
Mobility—slightly movable
Sensitivity—nontender to palpation

Enlarged, or atrophied gland.

Flat with no groove.
Nodular.
Hard; or boggy, soft, fluctuant.
Fixed.
Tender.
Enlarged, firm smooth gland with central groove obliterated suggests BPH.
Swollen, exquisitely tender gland accompanies prostatitis.
Any stone-hard, irregular, fixed nodule indicates carcinoma (see Table 25-4 on p. 753).

Objective Data

| Normal Range of Findings | Abnormal Findings |

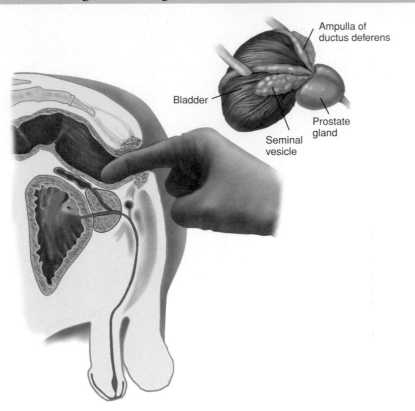

Ampulla of
ductus deferens

Bladder

Prostate
gland

Seminal
vesicle

Fig. 25-6

In the female, palpate the cervix through the anterior rectal wall. It normally feels like a small round mass. You also may palpate a retroverted uterus or a tampon in the vagina. Do not mistake the cervix or a tampon for a tumour.

Withdraw your examining finger; normally, no bright red blood or mucus is on the glove. To complete the examination, offer the person tissues to remove the lubricant and help the person to a more comfortable position.

Examination of Stool. Inspect any feces remaining on the glove. Normally, the colour is brown and the consistency is soft.

Jellylike mucus shreds mixed in stool indicate inflammation.

Bright red blood on stool surface indicates rectal bleeding. Bright red blood mixed with feces indicates possible colonic bleeding.

Test any stool on the glove for **occult blood** using the specimen container that your agency directs. A negative response is normal. If the stool is *hematest* positive, it indicates occult blood. Note that a false-positive finding may occur if the person has ingested significant amounts of red meat within 3 days of the test.

Black tarry stool with distinct malodour indicates upper gastrointestinal bleeding with blood partially digested. (Must lose more than 50 cc from upper gastrointestinal tract to be considered melena.)

Black stool—also occurs with ingesting iron or bismuth preparations.

Grey, tan stool—absent bile pigment, such as obstructive jaundice.

Pale yellow, greasy stool—increased fat content (steatorrhea), as occurs with malabsorption syndrome.

Occult bleeding usually indicates cancer of colon.

Normal Range of Findings	Abnormal Findings

 DEVELOPMENTAL CARE

Infants and Children

For the newborn, hold the feet with one hand and flex the knees up onto the abdomen. Note the presence of the anus. Confirm a patent rectum and anus by noting the first meconium stool passed within 24 to 48 hours of birth. To assess sphincter tone, check the *anal reflex*. Gently stroke the anal area and note a quick contraction of the sphincter.

Imperforate anus.

For each infant and child, note that the buttocks are firm and rounded with no masses or lesions. Recall that the *mongolian spot* is a common variation of hyperpigmentation in newborns of African, Asian, Mediterranean, or Aboriginal descent (see Chapter 12).

Flattened buttocks in cystic fibrosis or celiac syndrome.

Coccygeal mass.

Meningocele (sac containing meninges that protrude through a defect in the bony spine).

Tuft of hair or pilonidal dimple.

The perianal skin is free of lesions. However, diaper rash is common in children younger than 1 year of age and is exhibited as a generalized reddened area with papules or vesicles.

Pustules indicate secondary infection of diaper rash.

Signs of physical or sexual abuse, such as anal abrasions, perianal tears.

Fissure—common cause of constipation or rectal bleeding in child. (Painful, so the child does not defecate.)

Omit palpation unless the history or symptoms warrant. When internal palpation is needed, position the infant or child on the back with the legs flexed, and gently insert a gloved, well-lubricated finger into the rectum. Your fifth finger usually is long enough, and its smaller size is more comfortable for the infant or child. However, you may need to use the index finger because of its better control and increased tactile sensitivity. On withdrawing the finger, scant bleeding or protruding rectal mucosa may occur.

Inspect the perianal region of the school-age child and adolescent during examination of the genitalia. Internal palpation is not performed routinely.

The Aging Adult

As an aging person performs the Valsalva manoeuvre, you may note relaxation of the perianal musculature and decreased sphincter control. Otherwise, the full examination proceeds as that described earlier for the younger adult.

Summary Checklist: Anus, Rectum, and Prostate Examination

 For a PDA-downloadable version, go to http://evolve.elsevier.com/Canada/Jarvis/examination/.

1. **Inspect anus** and perianal area
2. Inspect during **Valsalva manoeuvre**
3. **Palpate anal canal** and rectum on all adults
4. **Test stool** for occult blood

Promoting Health: Colorectal Cancer Screening

Screening for Life

Colorectal cancer is the third most common cancer in Canadian men and women. Some factors that appear to increase the risk of developing it are being of older age, particularly >50 years; having polyps; having a family history of colorectal cancer, especially a parent, sibling, or child who developed it before the age of 45; having familial adenomatous polyposis (FAP) or hereditary nonpolyposis colon cancer (HNPCC); having inflammatory bowel disease (ulcerative colitis or Crohn's disease); eating a high-fat diet; consuming alcohol; smoking; being physically inactive; being obese; and having Ashkenazi (Eastern European Jewish) ancestry. Some people develop colorectal cancer without any of these risk factors. A diet high in vegetables and fruit is known to lower the risk, and research also suggests that a diet high in fibre and low in animal fats may also decrease the risk.

Colorectal cancer may not cause any symptoms in its early stages. Symptoms often appear once the tumour causes bleeding or blocks the bowel. Possible symptoms include a change in bowel habits, such as diarrhea or constipation; general abdominal discomfort (bloating, fullness, cramps); blood in the stool (either bright red or very dark); stools that are narrower than usual; an urgent need to have a bowel movement; a feeling that the bowel has not completely emptied; nausea or vomiting; fatigue; and weight loss.

The Canadian Cancer Society (2007a) recommends that men and women aged 50 and older should be screened for colorectal cancer. People at higher risk can be screened at an earlier age. Recommendations include a fecal occult blood test (FOBT) at least every 2 years to test for blood in the stool. A positive FOBT may be followed up by a colonoscopy, sigmoidoscopy, a double-contrast barium enema, or all three.

Promoting Health: Screening for Prostrate Cancer

Understanding Prostate Changes

Prostate cancer is the most common cancer in Canadian men. Some factors that appear to increase the risk of developing it are being of older age, particularly >65 years; a family history of prostate cancer; a diet high in fat; and African ancestry. Obesity, physical inactivity, and exposure to cadmium are being studied as possible risk factors. Some men develop prostate cancer without any of these risk factors. Prostate cancer may not cause signs or symptoms, especially in the early stages. Symptoms may appear if the tumour enlarges the prostate and starts to press on the urethra, making it difficult or painful to pass urine, or increasing the frequency of urination.

Through much of a man's life, the prostate gland is typically the size of a walnut. However, by the time a man is 40, it may grow slightly larger, to the size of an apricot. By age 60, it may be the size of a lemon. Although this varies between individuals, this gradual enlargement is considered to be a normal part of aging. This enlargement is termed *benign prostatic hypertrophy,* or BPH. It does not increase an individual's risk for prostate cancer, yet the symptoms for BPH and prostate cancer can be very similar.

The risks and benefits of testing for prostate cancer should be discussed with men aged 50 years and older. Men who are at higher risk for prostate cancer because of family history or African ancestry should discuss the possibility of starting testing at a younger age. The digital rectal examination (DRE) and the prostate-specific antigen (PSA) blood test can help detect prostate cancer early, but they can also cause "false alarms" or miss prostate cancer that is present. In some cases these tests can detect prostate cancer that may not pose a serious threat to a man's health. It is important to talk to men about their personal risk of developing prostate cancer and about the benefits and risks of testing.

PSA is a substance made by the normal prostate gland. However, when prostate cancer develops, the PSA level increases. However, benign or noncancerous enlargement of the prostate (BPH), age, and prostatitis can also cause PSA levels to increase. Ejaculation causes a temporary increase in PSA levels, and men need to be instructed to abstain from ejaculation for 2 days before having their PSA level tested. In addition, there are some medications that falsely lower PSA levels, such as finasteride (Proscar) or dutasteride (Avodart). If the PSA level is elevated, further laboratory work or transrectal ultrasonography (TRUS) and biopsy may be recommended.

The DRE involves a gloved, lubricated finger being inserted into the rectum. The prostate gland is located just in front of the rectum, making it possible to palpate the surface of the gland manually for bumps or hard areas that may represent developing cancer. Although the DRE is less effective than the PSA blood test in finding prostate cancer, it can sometimes find cancers in men who have normal PSA levels. For this reason, PSA and DRE are recommended to be done together when screening for prostate cancer.

TABLE 25-1	Colon Cancer Screening Guidelines
Level of Risk[1]	Recommendations for Screening
No affected family member	Begin screening at age 50. Could include FOBT every 2 years, radiography, endoscopy, or a combination, every 5 years
One first-degree relative with cancer or polyp at age <60, or 2 or more first-degree relatives affected with polyp or colon cancer at any age	Colonoscopy every 5 years beginning at age 40 years or 10 years younger than the youngest diagnosis of polyp or cancer in the family, whichever comes first
One first-degree relative affected at age >60, or 2 or more second-degree relatives with cancer	Average-risk screening but beginning at age 40. Could include FOBT, radiography, endoscopy, or a combination
One second-degree relative or third-degree relative affected	Average-risk screening beginning at age 50. Could include FOBT, radiography, endoscopy, or a combination

[1]Note: First-degree relative = parent, child, or sibling; second-degree relative = grandparent, aunt, uncle, nephew, or niece; third-degree relative = cousin, great-grandparent, or great-grandchild.
FOBT, fecal occult blood test.

DOCUMENTATION AND CRITICAL THINKING

Sample Charting

SUBJECTIVE

Has one BM daily, soft, brown, no pain, no change in bowel routine. Taking no medications. Has no history of pruritus, hemorrhoids, fissure, or fistula. Diet includes one to two servings daily each of fresh fruits and vegetables but no whole-grain cereals or breads.

OBJECTIVE

No fissure, hemorrhoids, fistula, or skin lesions in perianal area. Sphincter tone good, no prolapse. Rectal walls smooth, no masses or tenderness. Prostate not enlarged, no masses or tenderness. Stool brown, hematest negative.

ASSESSMENT

Rectal structures intact, no palpable lesions

Focused Assessment: Clinical Case Study

SUBJECTIVE

- C.M. is a 62-year-old male with chronic obstructive pulmonary disease for 15 years, who today has "diarrhea for 3 days."
- 7 days PTA: C.M. seen at this agency for acute respiratory infection that was diagnosed as acute bronchitis and treated with oral ampicillin. Took medication as directed.
- 3 days PTA: symptoms of respiratory infection improved. Ingesting usual diet. Onset of four to five loose, unformed, brown stools a day. No abdominal pain or cramping. No nausea.
- Now: diarrhea continues. No blood or mucus noticed in stool. No new foods or restaurant food in past 3 days. Wife not ill.

OBJECTIVE

Vital signs: 37°C-88-18. B/P 142/82.
Respiratory: Respirations unlaboured. Barrel chest. Hyperresonant to percussion. Lung sounds clear but diminished. No crackles or rhonchi today.
Abdomen: Flat. Bowel sounds present. No organomegaly or tenderness to palpation.
Rectal: No lesions in perianal area. Sphincter tone good. Rectal walls smooth, no mass or tenderness. Prostate smooth and firm, no median sulcus palpable, no masses or tenderness. Stool brown, hematest negative.

ASSESSMENT

Diarrhea R/T effects of antibiotic medication

Nursing Diagnoses Commonly Associated With Anal and Rectal Disorders

All nursing diagnoses can be found on the Evolve Web site at **http://evolve.elsevier.com/Canada/Jarvis/examination/.**

ABNORMAL FINDINGS

TABLE 25-2	Abnormalities of the Anus and Perianal Region

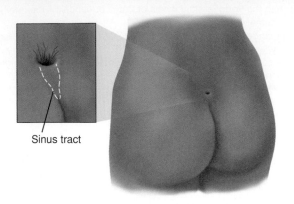

Sinus tract

Pilonidal Cyst or Sinus

A hair-containing cyst or sinus located in the midline over the coccyx or lower sacrum. Often opens as a dimple with visible tuft of hair and, possibly, an erythematous halo. Or, may appear as a palpable cyst. When advanced, has a palpable sinus tract. Although it is a congenital disorder, the lesion is first diagnosed between the ages of 15 and 30 years.

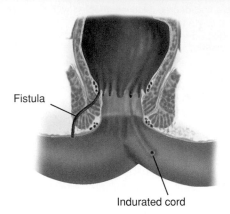

Fistula

Indurated cord

Anorectal Fistula

A chronically inflamed gastrointestinal tract creates an abnormal passage from inner anus or rectum out to skin surrounding anus. Usually originates from a local abscess. The red, raised tract opening may drain serosanguineous or purulent matter when pressure is applied. Bidigital palpation may reveal an indurated cord.

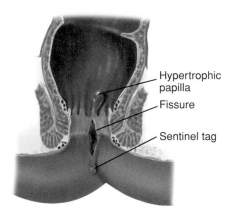

Hypertrophic papilla

Fissure

Sentinel tag

Fissure

A painful longitudinal tear in the superficial mucosa at the anal margin. Most fissures (>90%) occur in the posterior midline area. They are frequently accompanied by a papule of hyperplastic skin, called a *sentinel tag,* on the anal margin below. Fissures often result from trauma, for example from passing a large, hard stool or from irritant diarrheal stools. The person has itching, bleeding, and exquisite pain. A resulting spasm in the sphincters makes the area painful to examine; local anaesthesia may be indicated.

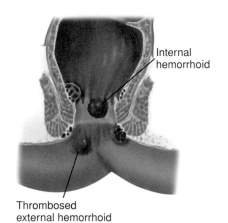

Internal hemorrhoid

Thrombosed external hemorrhoid

Hemorrhoids

These painless, flabby papules are due to a varicose vein of the hemorrhoidal plexus. An *external hemorrhoid* originates below the anorectal junction and is covered by anal skin. When *thrombosed,* it contains clotted blood and becomes a painful, swollen, shiny blue mass that itches and bleeds with defecation. When it resolves, it leaves a painless, flabby skin sac around the anal orifice. An *internal hemorrhoid* originates above the anorectal junction and is covered by mucous membrane. When the person performs a Valsalva manoeuvre, it may appear as a red mucosal mass. It is not palpable. All hemorrhoids result from increased portal venous pressure, as occurs with straining at stool, chronic constipation, pregnancy, obesity, chronic liver disease, or the low-fibre diet common in Western society.

TABLE 25-2 | **Abnormalities of the Anus and Perianal Region—cont'd**

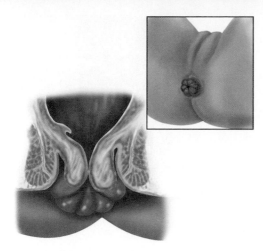

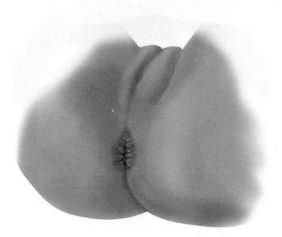

Rectal Prolapse

The rectal mucous membrane protrudes through the anus, appearing as a moist red doughnut with radiating lines. When prolapse is incomplete, only the mucosa bulges. When complete, it includes the anal sphincters. Occurs following a Valsalva manoeuvre, such as straining at stool, or with exercise.

Pruritus Ani

Intense perianal itching is manifested by red, raised, thickened, excoriated skin around the anus. Common causes are pinworms in children and fungal infections in adults. The area is swollen and moist, and with a fungal infection, it appears dull greyish pink. The skin is dry and brittle with psychosomatic itching.

TABLE 25-3	Abnormalities of the Rectum

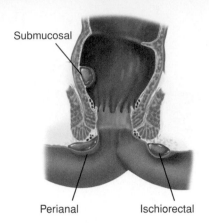

Abscess

A localized cavity of pus from infection in a pararectal space. Infection usually extends from an anal crypt. Characterized by persistent throbbing rectal pain. Termed by the space it occupies, for example, a perianal abscess is superficial around the anal skin, and appears red, hot, swollen, indurated, and tender. An ischiorectal abscess is deep and tender to bidigital palpation. It occurs laterally between the anus and ischial tuberosity and is uncommon.

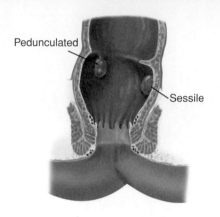

Rectal Polyp

A protruding growth from the rectal mucous membrane that is fairly common. The polyp may be *pedunculated* (on a stalk) or *sessile* (a mound on the surface, close to the mucosal wall). The soft nodule is difficult to palpate. Proctoscopy is needed as well as biopsy to screen for a malignant growth.

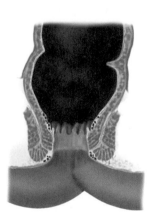

Fecal Impaction

A collection of hard, desiccated feces in the rectum. The obstruction often results from decreased bowel motility, in which more water is reabsorbed from the stool. Also occurs with retained barium from gastrointestinal X-ray examination. The person may complain of constipation or of diarrhea as a fecal stream passes around the impaction.

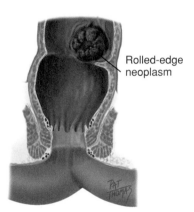

Carcinoma

A malignant neoplasm in the rectum is asymptomatic, thus the importance of routine rectal palpation. An early lesion may be a single firm nodule. You may palpate an ulcerated centre with rolled edges. As the lesion grows, it has an irregular cauliflower shape and is fixed and stone hard. Refer a person with any rectal lesion for further study because about half are malignant.

ABNORMAL FINDINGS
FOR ADVANCED PRACTICE

| TABLE 25-4 | Abnormalities of the Prostate Gland |

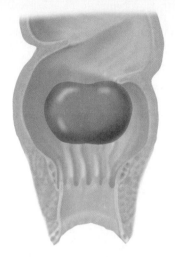

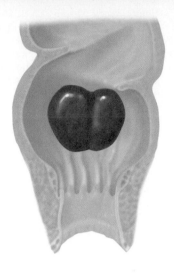

Benign Prostatic Hypertrophy

S: Urinary frequency, urgency, hesitancy, straining to urinate, weak stream, intermittent stream, sensation of incomplete emptying, nocturia.

O: A symmetrical nontender enlargement, commonly occurs in males beginning in the middle years. The prostate surface feels smooth, rubbery, or firm (like the consistency of the nose), with the median sulcus obliterated.

Prostatitis

S: Fever, chills, malaise, urinary frequency and urgency, dysuria, urethral discharge, dull, aching pain in perineal and rectal area.

O: An exquisitely tender enlargement is *acute* inflammation of the prostate gland yielding a swollen, slightly asymmetrical gland that is quite tender to palpation.

With a chronic inflammation the signs can vary from tender enlargement with a boggy feel to isolated firm areas due to fibrosis. Or the gland may feel normal.

Carcinoma ▶

S: Frequency, nocturia, hematuria, weak stream, hesitancy, pain or burning on urination, continuous pain in lower back, pelvis, thighs.

O: A malignant neoplasm often starts as a single hard nodule on the posterior surface, producing asymmetry and a change in consistency. As it invades normal tissue, multiple hard nodules appear, or the entire gland feels stone-hard and fixed. The median sulcus is obliterated.

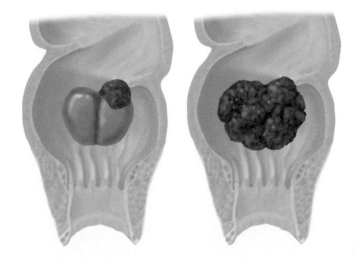

S, Subjective data; *O*, objective data.

BIBLIOGRAPHY

Ahmed, D. S. (2000). Hidden factors in occult blood testing. *American Journal of Nursing, 100*(12), 25.

Albright, L., Schwab, A., Camp, N. J., Farnham, J. S., & Thomas, A. (2005). Population-based risk assessment for other cancers in relatives of hereditary prostate cancer cases. *Prostate, 64*, 347–355.

Bodell, A. (2002). Prostate cancer screening in asymptomatic men in a community setting. *Urologic Nursing, 22*(1), 31–37.

Boyd-Carson, W. (2003). Faecal incontinence in adults. *Nursing Standard, 18*(8), 45–51.

Canadian Cancer Society. (2007a). *Colorectal cancer: Understanding your diagnosis.* Retrieved May 19, 2008, from www.cancer.ca

Canadian Cancer Society. (2007b). *Early detection and screening: Facts for men.* Retrieved May 19, 2008, from www.cancer.ca

Canadian Cancer Society. (2007c). *Prostate cancer: Understanding your diagnosis.* Retrieved May 19, 2008, from www.cancer.ca

Canadian Task Force on Preventive Health Care. (2001). Colorectal cancer screening: Recommendation statement from the Canadian Task Force on Preventive Health Care. *Canadian Medical Association Journal, 165*(2), 206–208.

Cydulka, R. K. (2002). Digital rectal examination for trauma: Does every patient need one? *Annals of Emergency Medicine, 39*, 462.

Duncan, M. K., & Sanger, M. (2004). Coping with the pediatric anogenital exam. *Journal of Child and Adolescent Psychiatric Nursing, 17*, 126–136.

Gilchrist, K. (2004). Benign prostatic hyperplasia: Is it a precursor to prostatic cancer? *Nurse Practitioner, 29*(6), 30–39.

Grumet, S., & Bruner, D. (2000). The identification and screening of men at high risk for developing prostate cancer. *Urologic Nursing, 20*(1), 15.

Heppenstall-Heger, A., McConnell, G., Ticson, L., Guerra, L., Lister, J., & Zaragoza, T. (2003). Healing patterns in anogenital injuries: A longitudinal study of injuries associated with sexual abuse, accidental injuries, or genital surgery in the preadolescent child. *Pediatrics, 112*, 829–837.

Knight, D. (2004). Health care screening for men who have sex with men. *American Family Physician, 69*, 2149–2156.

Kong, A. P., & Stamos, M. J. (2005a). Anorectal complications: Office diagnosis and treatment, part 1. *Consultant, 45*, 731–734.

Kong, A. P., & Stamos, M. J. (2005b). Anorectal complications: Office diagnosis and treatment, part 2. *Consultant, 45*, 735–738.

Leddin, D., Hunt, R., Champion, M., Cockeram, A., Flook, N., Gould, M., et al. (2004). Canadian Association of Gastroenterology and the Canadian Digestive Health Foundation: Guidelines on colon cancer screening. *Canadian Journal of Gastroenterology, 18*(2), 93–99.

McLeod, R., with the Canadian Task Force on Preventive Health Care. (2001). *Screening strategies for colorectal cancer: Systematic review and recommendations* (CHFPHC Technical Report #01-2). London, ON: Canadian Task Force.

Mason, D., Tobias, N., Lutkenhoff, M., Stoops, M., & Ferguson, D. (2004). The APN's guide to pediatric constipation management. *Nurse Practitioner, 29*(7), 13–22.

Mennie, G., & Bejinez-Eastman, A. (2004). Colorectal cancer screening: old obstacles, new tests. *Consultant, 44*(1), 120–127.

Powel, L. L. (2003). Commentary on screening for prostate cancer: Recommendations and rationale. *American Journal of Nursing, 103*(3), 111.

Solomon, M. J., & McLeod, R. S. (1994). Screening for colorectal cancer. In Canadian Task Force on the Periodic Health Examination (Eds.), *Canadian guide to clinical preventive health care* (pp. 798–809). Ottawa, ON: Health Canada.

Zarychanski, R., Chen, Y., Bernstein, C. N., & Hebert, P. C. (2007). Frequency of colorectal cancer screening and the impact of family physicians on screening behaviour. *Canadian Medical Association Journal, 177*, 593–597.

Female Genitourinary System

Written by **Carolyn Jarvis**, PhD, APN, CNP
Adapted by **Marian Luctkar-Flude**, RN, MScN

Electronic Resources

On Evolve *evolve*

http://evolve.elsevier.com/Canada/Jarvis/examination/
- Interactive Case Studies
- Physical Examination Audio and Printable Summaries
- Bedside Assessment Summary Checklists
- Complete Physical Examination Form
- Nursing Diagnoses Boxes
- Health Promotion Guides
- Quick Assessments for 20 Common Conditions
- Multiple Choice Review Questions
- Chapter Objectives
- Appendices
- Weblinks

On the Companion CD

- Interactive Case Studies with Heart and Lung Sounds
- Health Promotion Guides
- Quick Assessments for 20 Common Conditions
- Head-to-Toe Physical Examination Video Clips

STRUCTURE AND FUNCTION

EXTERNAL GENITALIA

The external genitalia are called the **vulva,** or pudendum (Fig. 26-1). The **mons pubis** is a round, firm pad of adipose tissue covering the symphysis pubis. After puberty, it is covered with hair in the pattern of an inverted triangle. The **labia majora** are two rounded folds of adipose tissue extending from the mons pubis down and around to the perineum. After puberty, hair covers the outer surfaces of the labia, whereas the inner folds are smooth and moist and contain sebaceous follicles.

Inside the labia majora are two smaller, darker folds of skin, the **labia minora.** These are joined anteriorly at the clitoris where they form a hood, or prepuce. The labia minora are joined posteriorly by a transverse fold, the **frenulum** or fourchette. The **clitoris** is a small, pea-shaped erectile body, homologous with the male penis and highly sensitive to tactile stimulation.

The labial structures encircle a boat-shaped space, or cleft, termed the **vestibule.** Within it are numerous openings. The **urethral meatus** appears as a dimple 2.5 cm posterior to the clitoris. Surrounding the urethral meatus are the tiny, multiple **paraurethral (Skene's) glands.** Their ducts are not visible but open posterior to the urethra at the 5:00 and 7:00 positions.

The **vaginal orifice** is posterior to the urethral meatus. It appears either as a thin median slit or as a large opening with irregular edges, depending on the presentation of the membranous **hymen.** The hymen is a thin, circular or crescent-shaped fold that may cover part of the vaginal orifice or may be absent completely. On either side and posterior to the vaginal orifice are two **vestibular (Bartholin's) glands,** which secrete a clear lubricating mucus during intercourse. Their ducts are not visible but open in the groove between the labia minora and the hymen.

INTERNAL GENITALIA

The internal genitalia include the **vagina,** a flattened, tubular canal extending from the orifice up and backward into the pelvis (Fig. 26-2). It is 9 cm long and sits between the rectum posteriorly and the bladder and urethra anteriorly. Its walls are in thick transverse folds, or **rugae,** enabling the vagina to dilate widely during childbirth.

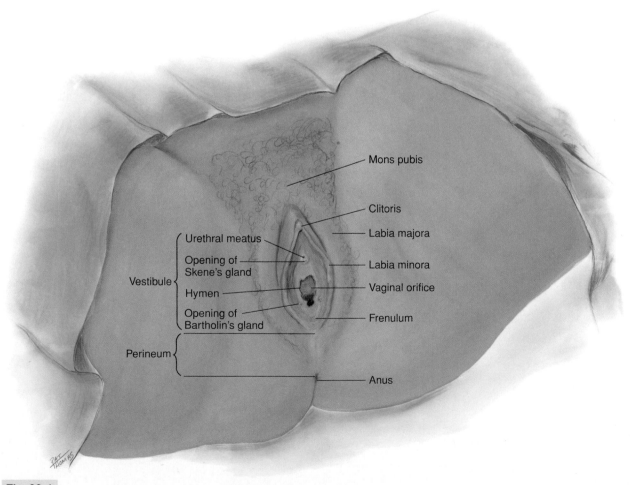

Mons pubis

Clitoris

Labia majora

Labia minora

Vaginal orifice

Frenulum

Anus

Urethral meatus

Opening of Skene's gland

Hymen

Opening of Bartholin's gland

Vestibule

Perineum

Fig. 26-1

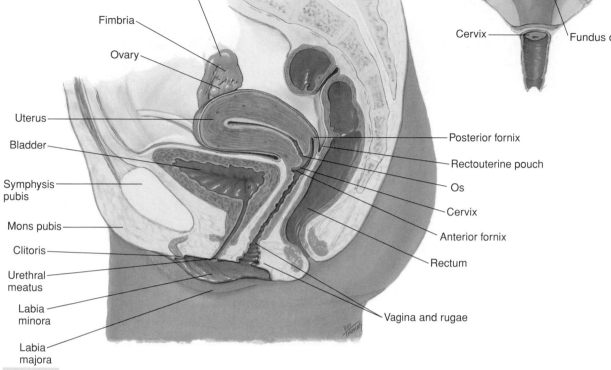

ANTERIOR VIEW OF ADNEXA

Cervix ——— ——— Fundus of uterus

Fallopian tube

Fimbria

Ovary

Uterus ——

Bladder ——

Symphysis
pubis

Mons pubis ——

Clitoris ——

Urethral
meatus

Labia
minora

Labia
majora

——— Posterior fornix

——— Rectouterine pouch

——— Os

——— Cervix

——— Anterior fornix

——— Rectum

——— Vagina and rugae

Fig. 26-2

At the end of the canal, the uterine **cervix** projects into the vagina. In the nulliparous female, the cervix appears as a smooth doughnut-shaped area with a small circular hole, or **os.** After childbirth, the os is slightly enlarged and irregular. The cervical epithelium is of two distinct types. The vagina and cervix are covered with smooth, pink, stratified squamous epithelium. Inside the os, the endocervical canal is lined with columnar epithelium that looks red and rough. The point where these two tissues meet is the **squamocolumnar junction** and is not visible.

A continuous recess is present around the cervix, termed the **anterior fornix** in front and the **posterior fornix** in back. Behind the posterior fornix, another deep recess is formed by the peritoneum. It dips down between the rectum and cervix to form the **rectouterine pouch,** or **cul-de-sac of Douglas.**

The **uterus** is a pear-shaped, thick-walled, muscular organ. It is flattened anteroposteriorly, measuring 5.5 to 8 cm long by 3.5 to 4 cm wide and 2 to 2.5 cm thick. It is freely movable, not fixed, and usually tilts forward and superior to the bladder (a position labelled as anteverted and anteflexed, see p. 775).

The **fallopian tubes** are two pliable, trumpet-shaped tubes, 10 cm in length, extending from the uterine fundus laterally to the brim of the pelvis. There they curve posteriorly, their fimbriated ends located near the **ovaries.** The two ovaries are located one on each side of the uterus at the level of the anterior superior iliac spine. Each is oval shaped, 3 cm long by 2 cm wide by 1 cm thick and serves to develop ova (eggs) and the female hormones.

🌷 DEVELOPMENTAL CARE

Infants and Adolescents

At birth, the external genitalia are engorged because of the presence of maternal estrogen. The structures recede in a few weeks, remaining small until puberty. The ovaries are located in the abdomen during childhood. The uterus is small with a straight axis and no anteflexion.

At puberty, estrogens stimulate the growth of cells in the reproductive tract and the development of secondary sex characteristics. The first signs of puberty are breast and pubic hair development, beginning between the ages of 8½ and 13 years. These signs are usually concurrent, but it is not abnormal if they do not develop together. They take about 3 years to complete.

Menarche occurs during the latter half of this sequence, just after the peak of growth velocity. Irregularity of the menstrual cycle is common during adolescence because of the girl's occasional failure to ovulate. With menarche, the uterine body flexes on the cervix. The ovaries now are in the pelvic cavity.

TABLE 26-1	Sexual Maturity Ratings in Girls

Stage 1 Preadolescent. No pubic hair. Mons and labia covered with fine vellus hair as on abdomen.

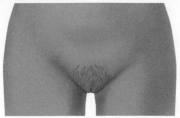

Stage 2 Growth sparse and mostly on labia. Long, downy hair, slightly pigmented, straight or only slightly curly.

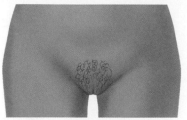

Stage 3 Growth sparse and spreading over mons pubis. Hair is darker, coarser, curlier.

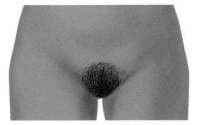

Stage 4 Hair is adult in type but over smaller area; none on medial thigh.

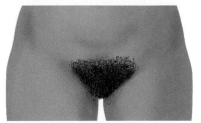

Stage 5 Adult in type and pattern; inverse triangle. Also on medial thigh surface.

Adapted from Tanner, J.M. (1962). *Growth at adolescence.* Oxford, England: Blackwell Scientific.

Tanner's table on the five stages of pubic hair development (sexual maturity rating [SMR]) is helpful in teaching girls the expected sequence of sexual development (Table 26-1).

The Pregnant Female

A complete discussion of pregnancy is presented in Chapter 29. In summary, shortly after the first missed menstrual period, the genitalia show signs of the growing fetus. The cervix softens *(Goodell's sign)* at 4 to 6 weeks, and the vaginal mucosa and cervix look cyanotic *(Chadwick's sign)* at 8 to 12 weeks. These changes occur because of increased vascularity and edema of the cervix and hypertrophy and hyperplasia of the cervical glands. The isthmus of the uterus softens *(Hegar's sign)* at 6 to 8 weeks.

The greatest change is in the uterus itself. It increases in capacity by 500 to 1000 times its nonpregnant state, at first because of hormone stimulation and then because of the increasing size of its contents (Cunningham et al., 2005). The nonpregnant uterus has a flattened pear shape. Its early growth encroaches on the space occupied by the bladder, producing the symptom of urinary frequency. By 10 to 12 weeks' gestation, the uterus becomes globular in shape and is too large to stay in the pelvis. At 20 to 24 weeks, the uterus has an oval shape. It rises almost to the liver, displacing the intestines superiorly and laterally.

A clot of thick, tenacious mucus forms in the spaces of the cervical canal (the mucus plug), which protects the fetus from infection. The mucus plug dislodges when labour begins at the end of term, producing a sign of labour called "bloody show." Cervical and vaginal secretions increase during pregnancy and are thick, white, and more acidic. The increased acidity occurs because of the action of *Lactobacillus acidophilus,* which changes glycogen into lactic acid. The acidic pH keeps pathogenic bacteria from multiplying in the vagina, but the increase in glycogen increases the risk of candidiasis (commonly called a yeast infection) during pregnancy.

The Aging Female

In contrast to the slowly declining hormones in the aging male, the female's hormonal milieu decreases rapidly. *Menopause* is cessation of the menses. Usually this occurs around 48 to 51 years, although a wide variation of ages from 35 to 60 years exists. The stage of menopause includes the preceding 1 to 2 years of decline in ovarian function, shown by irregular menses that gradually become farther apart and produce a lighter flow. Ovaries stop producing progesterone and estrogen. Because cells in the reproductive tract are estrogen dependent, decreased estrogen levels during menopause bring dramatic physical changes.

The uterus shrinks in size because of decreased myometrium. The ovaries atrophy to 1 to 2 cm and are not palpable after menopause. Ovulation still may occur sporadically after menopause. The sacral ligaments relax and the pelvic musculature weakens, so the uterus droops. Sometimes it may protrude, or prolapse, into the vagina. The cervix shrinks and looks paler with a thick, glistening epithelium.

The vagina becomes shorter, narrower, and less elastic because of increased connective tissue. Without sexual activity, the vagina atrophies to one half of its former length and width. The vaginal epithelium atrophies, becoming thinner, drier, and itchy. This results in a fragile mucosal surface that is at risk for bleeding and vaginitis. Decreased vaginal secretions leave the vagina dry and at risk for irritation and pain with intercourse (dyspareunia). The vaginal pH becomes more alkaline, and a decreased glycogen content occurs from the decreased estrogen. These factors also increase the risk of vaginitis because they create a suitable medium for pathogens.

Externally, the mons pubis looks smaller because the fat pad atrophies. The labia and clitoris gradually decrease in size. Pubic hair becomes thin and sparse.

Declining estrogen levels produce some physiological changes in the female sexual response cycle:

PHASE	PHYSIOLOGICAL CHANGE
Excitement	Reduced amount of vaginal secretion and lubrication
Plateau	Less expansion of vagina
	Labia majora do not elevate against perineum
	No colour change in labia minora (was from pink to cardinal-red or dark red)
	Size of clitoris decreases after age 60
Orgasm	Shorter duration
Resolution	Occurs more rapidly

Data from Masters, W.H., & Johnson, V.E. (1966). *Human sexual response.* Boston, MA: Little, Brown, and Company.

However, these changes do not affect sexual pleasure and function. Sexual desire and the need for full sexual expression continue. As with the male, the older female is capable of sexual function given reasonably good health and an interested partner. The problem for many older women is finding a socially acceptable sexual partner. Aging women greatly outnumber their male counterparts, and aging women are more likely to be single, whereas males their same age are more likely to be married.

CULTURAL AND SOCIAL CONSIDERATIONS

Female circumcision or *female genital mutilation* (FGM) is the ritual removal of part or all of the external female genitalia, usually performed on prepubertal girls. FGM is an ancient cultural practice, most common in Africa, but also practised in parts of southeast Asia, the Middle East, and Central and South America; an estimated 120 to 140 million girls have undergone the procedure. The health implications of FGM include both immediate effects, such as severe pain, hemorrhage, urinary retention, infection, sepsis, and death, and long-term effects, such as urinary tract and genital tract dysfunction, painful menstruation, sexual and birth-control difficulties, infertility, difficulties during pregnancy and childbirth, and psychological difficulties. FGM is illegal in Canada and most Western countries; however, an increasing number of immigrant women who have undergone these procedures are now living in Canada. Affected women may be reluctant to seek health care, and when they do they may find it difficult and at times traumatic. Healthcare professionals may be in a position to educate immigrants from practicing communities about the health considerations and legal consequences of FGM.

SUBJECTIVE DATA

1. Menstrual history	5. Urinary symptoms	9. Contraceptive use
2. Obstetrical history	6. Vaginal discharge	10. Sexually transmitted infection (STI) contact
3. Menopause	7. History	11. STI risk reduction
4. Self-care behaviours	8. Sexual activity	

Examiner Asks	Rationale

1. Menstrual history. Tell me about your menstrual periods:
 	
• Date of your last menstrual period?
• Age at first period?
 	
• How often are your periods?
 	
• How many days does your period last?
• Usual amount of flow: light, medium, heavy? How many pads or tampons do you use each day or hour?
	Menstrual history is usually non-threatening; thus it is a good place to start history.
	    LMP—last menstrual period.
	    Menarche—mean age at onset at 12 to 13; delayed onset suggests endocrine or underweight problem.
	    Cycle—normally every 18 to 45 days.
	    Amenorrhea—absent menses.
	    Duration—average 3 to 7 days.
	    Menorrhagia—heavy menses.

Examiner Asks	Rationale

- Any clotting?

  Clotting indicates heavy flow or vaginal pooling.
  Dysmenorrhea.

- Any pain or cramps before or during period? How do you treat it? Interfere with daily activities? Any other associated symptoms: bloating, breast tenderness, moodiness? Any spotting between periods?

2. **Obstetrical history.** Have you ever been pregnant?
   - How many times?
   - How many babies have you had?
   - Any miscarriage or abortion?

   Obstetrical history.

   Gravida—number of pregnancies.
   Para—number of births.
   Abortions—interrupted pregnancies, including elective abortions and spontaneous miscarriages.

   - For each pregnancy, describe: duration, any complication, labour and delivery, baby's sex, birth weight, condition.
   - Do you think you may be pregnant now? What symptoms have you noticed?

3. **Menopause.** Have your periods slowed down or stopped?

   Menopause—cessation of menstruation.
   Perimenopausal period from 40 to 55 years has hormone shifts, resulting in vasomotor instability.

   - Any associated symptoms of menopause (e.g., hot flash, numbness and tingling, headache, palpitations, drenching sweats, mood swings, vaginal dryness, itching)? Any treatment?
   - If hormone replacement, how much? How is it working? Any side effects?

   Side effects of hormone therapy include fluid retention, breast pain or enlargement, vaginal bleeding, possibly breast cancer risk.

   - How do you feel about going through menopause?

   Although this is a normal life stage, reaction varies from acceptance to feelings of loss.

4. **Self-care behaviours.** How often do you have a gynecological checkup?
   - Last Papanicolaou (Pap) smear? Results?
   - Has your mother ever mentioned taking hormones while pregnant with you?

   Assess **self-care behaviours.**

   Maternal ingestion of DES (diethylstilbestrol) causes cervical and vaginal abnormalities in female offspring requiring frequent follow-up.

5. **Urinary symptoms.** Any problems with urinating? Frequently and small amounts? Cannot wait to urinate?
   - Any burning or pain on urinating?
   - Awaken during night to urinate?
   - Blood in the urine?
   - Urine dark, cloudy, foul smelling?
   - Any difficulty controlling urine or wetting yourself?

   Urinary symptoms. Frequency. Urgency.

   Dysuria.
   Nocturia.
   Hematuria.
   Bile in urine or urinary tract infection.
   True incontinence—loss of urine without warning.
   Urgency incontinence—sudden loss, as with acute cystitis.

   - Urinate with a sneeze, laugh, cough, bearing down?

   Stress incontinence—loss of urine with physical strain from muscle weakness.

6. **Vaginal discharge.** Any unusual **vaginal discharge?** Increased amount?

   Normal discharge is small, clear or cloudy, and always nonirritating.

   - Character or colour: white, yellow-green, grey, curdlike, foul smelling?

   Suggests vaginal infection; character of discharge often suggests causative organism (see Table 26-5 on p. 786).

Examiner Asks	Rationale

- When did this begin?
- Is the discharge associated with vaginal itching, rash, pain with intercourse?

Acute versus chronic problem.
Occurs as a result of irritation from discharge.
Dyspareunia occurs with vaginitis of any cause.

- Taking any medications?

Factors that increase risk of vaginitis:
- Oral contraceptives increase glycogen content of vaginal epithelium, providing fertile medium for some organisms.
- Broad-spectrum antibiotics alter balance of normal flora.

- Family history of diabetes?
- What part of your menstrual cycle are you in now?

- Diabetes increases glycogen content.
- Menses, postpartum, menopause have a more alkaline vaginal pH.

- Use a vaginal douche? How often?
- Use feminine hygiene spray?
- Wear nonventilating underpants, pantyhose?
- Treated the discharge with anything? Result?

- Frequent douching alters pH.
- Spray has risk of contact dermatitis.
- Local irritation.

7. **History.** Any other problems in the genital area? Sores or lesions—now or in the past? How were these treated?
- Any abdominal pain?
- Any past surgery on uterus, ovaries, vagina?

Assess feelings. Some fear loss of sexual response after hysterectomy, which may cause problems in intimate relationships.

8. **Sexual activity.** Often women have a question about their **sexual relationship** and how it affects their health. Do you?
- Are you in a relationship involving sex now?
- Are aspects of sex satisfactory to you and your partner?
- Satisfied with the way you and partner communicate about sex?
- Satisfied with your ability to respond sexually?
- Do you have more than one sexual partner?

Begin with open ended question to assess individual needs. Include appropriate questions as a routine:
- Communicates that you accept individual's sexual activity and believe it is important.
- Your comfort with discussion prompts person's interest and possibly relief that the topic has been introduced.
- Establishes a database for comparison with any future sexual activities.
- Provides opportunity to screen sexual problems.

- What is your sexual preference: relationship with a man, with a woman, both?

Lesbians and bisexual women need to feel acceptance to discuss their health concerns.

9. **Contraceptive use.** Currently planning a pregnancy, or avoiding pregnancy?
- Do you and your partner use a **contraceptive?** Which method? Is this satisfactory? Do you have any questions about method?
- Which methods have you used in the past? Have you and partner discussed having children?
- Have you ever had any problems becoming pregnant?

Assess smoking history. Oral contraceptives, together with cigarette smoking, increase the risk of vascular problems.

Infertility is considered after 1 year of engaging in unprotected sexual intercourse without conceiving.

Subjective Data

Examiner Asks	Rationale
10. **Sexually transmitted infection (STI) contact.** Any sexual contact with partner having an STI, such as gonorrhea, herpes, acquired immune deficiency syndrome (AIDS), chlamydial infection, venereal warts, syphilis? When? How was this treated? Were there any complications?	An STI includes all conditions that can be transmitted during intercourse or intimate sexual contact with an infected partner.
11. **STI risk reduction.** Any precautions to reduce risk of STIs? Use condoms at each episode of sexual intercourse?	

Additional History for Infants and Children

1. Does your child have any problem urinating? Pain with urinating, crying, holding genitals? Urinary tract infection?
   - (If the child is older than 2 to 2½ years of age) Has toilet training started? How is it progressing?
   - Does the child wet bed at night? Is this a problem for child or you (parents)? What have you (parents) done?

2. Problem with genital area: itching, rash, vaginal discharge?

Occurs with poor perineal hygiene or insertion of foreign body in vagina.

3. (To child) "Has anyone ever touched you in between your legs and you did not want them to? Sometimes that happens to children and it's not OK." They should remember they have not been bad. They should try to tell an adult about it. "Can you tell me three different big people you trust who you could talk to?"

Screen for sexual abuse (see Chapter 7). For prevention, teach the child that it's not okay for someone to look at or touch their private parts while telling them it's a secret. Naming 3 trusted adults will include someone outside the family—important because most molestation is by a parent.

Additional History for Preadolescents and Adolescents

Use the following questions, as appropriate, to assess sexual growth and development and sexual behaviour. First:
- Ask questions that seem appropriate for girl's age but be aware that norms vary widely. When in doubt, it is better to ask too many questions than to omit something. Children obtain information, often misinformation, from the media and from peers at surprisingly early ages. You can be sure your information will be more thoughtful and accurate.
- Ask direct, matter-of-fact questions. Avoid sounding judgemental.
- Start with a *permission statement*. "Often girls your age experience . . ." This conveys that it is normal to think or feel a certain way.
- Try the *open-ended*. "When did you . . ." rather than "Do you . . ." This is less threatening because it implies that the topic is normal and unexceptional.

1. Around age 9 or 10, girls start to develop breasts and pubic hair. Have you ever seen charts and pictures of normal growth patterns for girls? Let us go over these now.

2. Have your periods started? How did you feel? Were you prepared or surprised?

Assess attitude of girl and parents. Note inadequate preparation or attitude of distaste.

3. Who in your family do you talk to about your body changes and about sex information? How do these talks go? Do you think you get enough information? What about sex education classes at school? Is there a teacher, a nurse or doctor, a minister, a counsellor to whom you can talk?
   Often girls your age have questions about sexual activity. Do you have questions? Are you dating? Someone steady?

Examiner Asks	Rationale
Do you and your boyfriend have intercourse? Are you using condoms? What kind of protection did you use the last time you had sex?	Avoid the term "sexually active," which is ambiguous.
4. Has anyone ever talked to you about sexually transmitted infections, such as chlamydia, herpes, gonorrhea, or AIDS?	Teach STI risk reduction.
5. Sometimes a person touches a girl in a way that she does not want them to. Has that ever happened to you? If that happens, the girl should remember it is not her fault. She should tell another adult about it.	Screen for sexual abuse.

Additional History for the Aging Adult

1. After menopause, noted any vaginal bleeding?	Postmenopausal bleeding warrants further workup and referral.
2. Any vaginal itching, discharge, pain with intercourse?	Associated with atrophic vaginitis.
3. Any pressure in genital area, loss of urine with cough or sneeze, back pain, or constipation?	Occurs with weakened pelvic musculature and uterine prolapse.
4. Are you in a relationship involving sex now? Are aspects of sex satisfactory to you and your partner? Is there adequate privacy for a sexual relationship?	

OBJECTIVE DATA

PREPARATION

Assemble the equipment before helping the woman into position. Arrange within easy reach. Familiarize yourself with the vaginal speculum before the examination. Practise opening and closing the blades, locking them into position, and releasing them. Try both metal and plastic types. Note that the plastic speculum locks and unlocks with a resounding click that can be alarming to the uninformed woman.

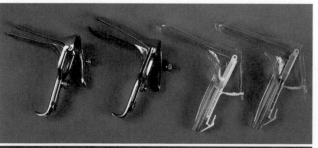
A

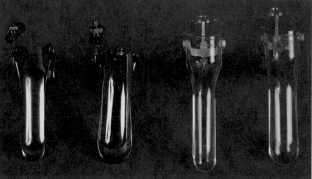
B

Fig. 26-3

EQUIPMENT NEEDED

Gloves
Goose-necked lamp with a strong light
Vaginal speculum of appropriate size (Fig. 26-3)
  Graves' speculum—useful for most adult women, available in varying lengths and widths
  Pederson speculum—narrow blades, useful for young or postmenopausal women with narrowed introitus
Large cotton-tipped applicators (rectal swabs)
Materials for cytological study as specified within your region or facility:
  Glass slide with frosted end
  Specimen container for liquid-based cytology (LBC)
  Sterile Cytobrush or cotton-tipped applicator
  Ayre's spatula
  Spray fixative
  Specimen container for gonorrhea culture (GC)/*Chlamydia*
  Small bottle of normal saline solution, potassium hydroxide (KOH), and acetic acid (white vinegar)
Lubricant

POSITION

Initially, the woman should be sitting up. An equal-status position is important to establish trust and rapport before the vaginal examination.

For the examination, the woman should be placed in the lithotomy position, with the examiner sitting on a stool. Help the woman into lithotomy position, with the body supine, feet in stirrups and knees apart, and buttocks at edge of examining table (Fig. 26-4). Ask the woman to lift her hips as you guide them to the edge of the table. Some women prefer to leave their shoes or socks on. Or, you can place an examination glove over each of the stirrups to warm the stirrups and keep her feet from slipping.

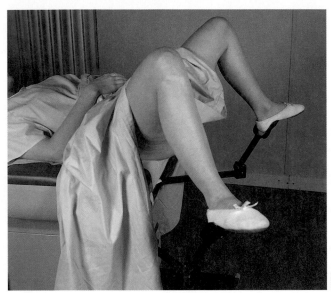

Fig. 26-4

Place her arms at her sides or across the chest, not over the head, because this position only tightens the abdominal muscles. Appropriate draping protects the modesty of the patient. This is important for females of all ethnocultural backgrounds. The traditional mode is to drape the woman fully, covering the stomach and legs, exposing only the vulva to your view. Be sure to push down the drape between the woman's legs and elevate her head so that you can see her face.

The lithotomy position leaves many women feeling helpless and vulnerable. Indeed, many women tolerate the pelvic examination because they consider it basic for health care, yet they find it embarrassing and uncomfortable. Previous examinations may have been painful, or the previous examiner's attitude hurried and patronizing.

The examination need not be this way. You can help the woman relax, decrease her anxiety, and retain a sense of control by using these measures:

- Have her empty the bladder before the examination.
- Position the examination table so that her perineum is not exposed to an inadvertent open door.
- Ask if she would like a friend, family member, or chaperone present. Position this person by the woman's head to maintain privacy.
- Elevate her head and shoulders to a semisitting position to maintain eye contact.
- Place the stirrups so that the legs are not abducted too far.
- Explain each step in the examination before you do it.
- Assure the woman she can stop the examination at any point should she feel any discomfort.
- Use a gentle, firm touch, and gradual movements.
- Communicate throughout the examination. Maintain a dialogue to share information.

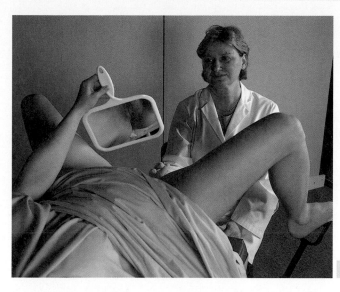

Fig. 26-5

Objective Data

- Use the techniques of the *educational* or *mirror pelvic examination* (Fig. 26-5). This is a routine examination with some modifications in attitude, position, and communication. First, the woman is considered an active participant, one who is interested in learning and in sharing decisions about her own health care. The woman props herself up on one elbow, or the head of the table is raised. Her other hand holds a mirror between her legs, above the examiner's hands. The woman can see all that the examiner is doing and has a full view of her genitalia.

The mirror works well for teaching normal anatomy and its relationship to sexual behaviour. Even women who are in a sexual relationship or who have had children may be surprisingly uninformed about their own anatomy. You will find the woman's enthusiasm on seeing her own cervix is rewarding too.

The mirror pelvic examination also works well when abnormalities arise because the woman can see the rationale for treatment and can monitor progress at the next appointment. She is more willing to comply with treatment when she shares in the decision.

Normal Range of Findings	Abnormal Findings

EXTERNAL GENITALIA

Inspection

Note:
- Skin colour (Fig. 26-6).

Refer any suspicious pigmented lesion for biopsy.

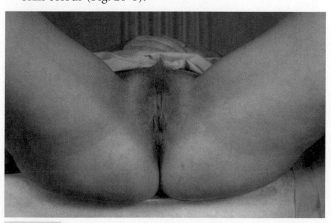

Fig. 26-6

Normal Range of Findings	Abnormal Findings
• Hair distribution is in the usual female pattern of inverted triangle, although it normally may trail up the abdomen toward the umbilicus.	Consider delayed puberty if no pubic hair or breast development has not occurred by age 13 years. Nits or lice at the base of pubic hair. Swelling.
• Labia majora normally are symmetrical, plump, and well formed. In the nulliparous woman, labia meet in the midline; after a vaginal delivery, the labia are gaping and slightly shrivelled.	
• No lesions should be present, except for occasional sebaceous cysts. These are yellowish, 1-cm nodules that are firm, nontender, and often multiple.	
With your gloved hand, separate the labia majora to inspect: • Clitoris (Fig. 26-7).	Excoriation, nodules, rash, or lesions (see Table 26-2, pp. 782).

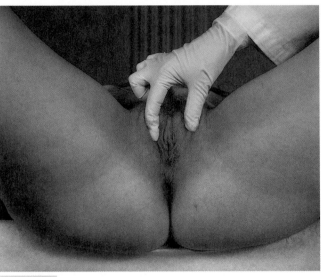

Fig. 26-7

• Labia minora are dark pink and moist, usually symmetrical. • Urethral opening appears stellate or slitlike and is midline. • Vaginal opening, or introitus, may appear as a narrow vertical slit or as a larger opening. • Perineum is smooth. A well-healed episiotomy scar, midline or mediolateral, may be present after a vaginal birth. • Anus has coarse skin of increased pigmentation (see Chapter 25 for assessment).	Inflammation or lesions. Polyp. Foul-smelling, irritating discharge.

Palpation

Assess the urethra and Skene's glands (Fig. 26-8). Dip your gloved finger in a bowl of warm water to lubricate. Then insert your index finger into the vagina, and gently milk the urethra by applying pressure up and out. This procedure should produce no pain. If any discharge appears, culture it.	Tenderness. Induration along urethra. Urethral discharge.

Objective Data

Normal Range of Findings	Abnormal Findings

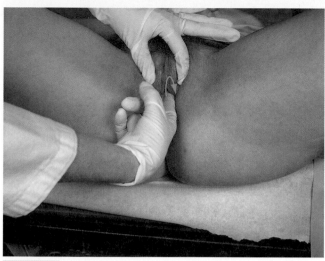

Fig. 26-8

Assess Bartholin's glands. Palpate the posterior parts of the labia majora with your index finger in the vagina and your thumb outside (Fig. 26-9). Normally, the labia feel soft and homogeneous.

Swelling (see Table 26-2, p. 782).
Induration.
Pain with palpation.
Erythema around or discharge from duct opening.

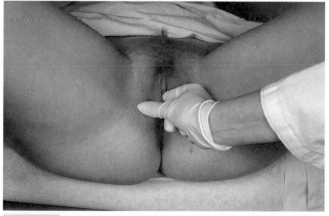

Fig. 26-9

Assess the support of pelvic musculature by using these manoeuvres:
1. Palpate the perineum. Normally, it feels thick, smooth, and muscular in the nulliparous woman, and thin and rigid in the multiparous woman.
2. Ask the woman to squeeze the vaginal opening around your fingers; it should feel tight in the nulliparous woman and have less tone in the multiparous woman.
3. Using your index and middle fingers, separate the vaginal orifice and ask the woman to strain down. Normally, no bulging of vaginal walls or urinary incontinence occurs.

Tenderness.
Paper-thin perineum.
Absent or decreased tone may diminish sexual satisfaction.

Bulging of the vaginal wall indicates cystocele, rectocele, or uterine prolapse (see Table 26-3, p. 784).
Urinary incontinence.

Objective Data

Normal Range of Findings

Abnormal Findings

INTERNAL GENITALIA

Speculum Examination

Select the proper-sized speculum. Warm and lubricate the speculum under warm running water. Avoid gel lubricant at this point because it is bacteriostatic and would distort cells in the cytology specimen you will collect.

A good technique is to dedicate one hand to the patient and the other hand to picking up equipment in the room. For example, hold the speculum in your left hand (the equipment hand), with the index and the middle fingers surrounding the blades and your thumb under the thumbscrew. This prevents the blades from opening painfully during insertion. With your right index and middle fingers (the patient hand), push the introitus down and open to relax the pubococcygeal muscle (Fig. 26-10). Tilt the width of the blades obliquely and insert the speculum past your right fingers, applying any pressure *downward*. This avoids pressure on the sensitive urethra above it.

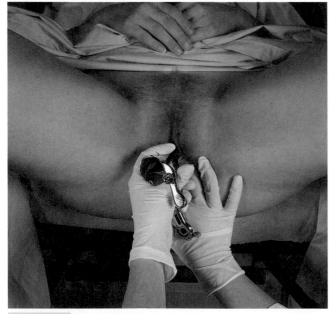

Fig. 26-10

Ease insertion by asking the woman to bear down. This method relaxes the perineal muscles and opens the introitus. (With experience, you can combine speculum insertion with assessing the support of the vaginal muscles.) As the blades pass your right fingers, withdraw your fingers. Now change the hand holding the speculum to your right hand and turn the width of the blades horizontally. Continue to insert in a 45-degree angle *downward* toward the small of the woman's back (Fig. 26-11). This matches the natural slope of the vagina.

Normal Range of Findings	Abnormal Findings

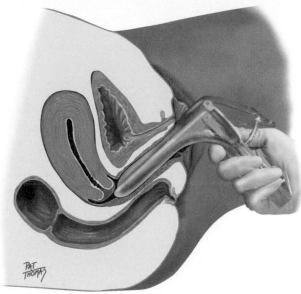

Fig. 26-11

After the blades are fully inserted, open them by squeezing the handles together (Fig. 26-12). The cervix should be in full view. Sometimes this does not occur (especially with beginning examiners), because the blades are angled above the location of the cervix. Try closing the blades, withdrawing about half-way, and reinserting in a more *downward* plane. Then slowly sweep upward. Once you have the cervix in full view, lock the blades open by tightening the thumbscrew.

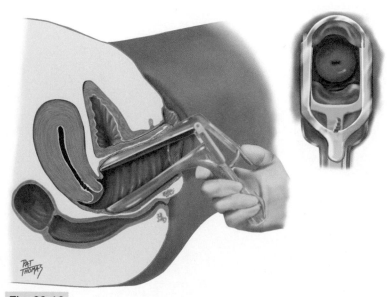

Fig. 26-12

Objective Data

Normal Range of Findings	Abnormal Findings

Inspect the Cervix and Its Os

Note:

- **Colour.** Normally the cervical mucosa is pink and even. During the second month of pregnancy it looks blue (Chadwick's sign), and after menopause it is pale.

- **Position.** Midline, either anterior or posterior. Projects 1 to 3 cm into the vagina.

- **Size.** Diameter is 2.5 cm (1 in).

- **Os.** This is small and round in the nulliparous woman. In the parous woman, it is a horizontal irregular slit and also may show healed lacerations on the sides (Fig. 26-13).

Redness, inflammation.

Pallor with anemia.

Cyanotic other than with pregnancy (see Table 26-4, p. 785).

Lateral position may be due to adhesion or tumour. Projection of more than 3 cm may be a prolapse.

Hypertrophy of more than 4 cm occurs with inflammation or tumour.

NORMAL VARIATIONS OF THE CERVIX

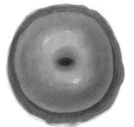

Nulliparous

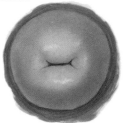

Parous (after childbirth)

LACERATIONS

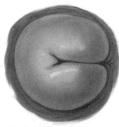

Unilateral transverse

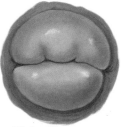

Bilateral transverse

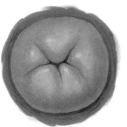

Stellate

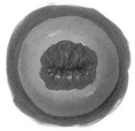

Cervical eversion

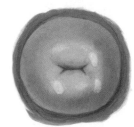

Nabothian cysts

Fig. 26-13

Normal Range of Findings	Abnormal Findings

Normal Range of Findings

- **Surface.** This is normally smooth, but **cervical eversion,** or ectropion, may occur normally after vaginal deliveries. The endocervical canal is everted or "rolled out." It looks like a red, beefy halo inside the pink cervix surrounding the os. It is difficult to distinguish this normal variation from an abnormal condition (e.g., erosion or carcinoma), and biopsy may be needed.

   Nabothian cysts are benign growths that commonly appear on the cervix after childbirth. They are small, smooth, yellow nodules that may be single or multiple. Less than 1 cm, they are retention cysts caused by obstruction of cervical glands.

- **Note the cervical secretions.** Depending on the day of the menstrual cycle, secretions may be clear and thin, or thick, opaque, and stringy. Always they are odourless and nonirritating.

If secretions are copious, swab the area with a thick-tipped rectal swab. This method sponges away secretions, and you have a better view of the structures.

Obtain Cervical Smears and Cultures

The Papanicolaou, or Pap, smear screens for cervical cancer. Do not obtain during the woman's menses or if a heavy infectious discharge is present. Instruct the woman not to douche, have intercourse, or put anything into the vagina within 24 hours before collecting the specimens. Obtain the Pap smear before other specimens so you will not disrupt or remove cells.

   Conventional glass slide cytology remains the most common screening test for cervical cancer available to women in Canada. A single slide is sufficient for the entire specimen. When fixative is to be used, as in most regions in Canada other than British Columbia, it should be applied to the slide immediately after the cells are spread from both sides of the brush or spatula in a thin layer (Murphy, 2007).

   Cervical Scrape. Insert the bifid end of the Ayre spatula into the vagina with the more pointed bump into the cervical os. Rotate it 360 to 720 degrees, using firm pressure (Fig. 26-14). The rounded cervix fits snugly into the spatula's groove. The spatula scrapes the surface of the squamocolumnar junction (SCJ) and cervix as you turn the instrument. Spread the specimen from both sides of the spatula onto a glass slide. Use a single stroke to thin out the specimen, not a back-and-forth motion. Spray with a fixative (or not) according to the procedures required at your agency. This specimen is important for the adolescent whose endocervical cells have not yet migrated into the endocervical canal.

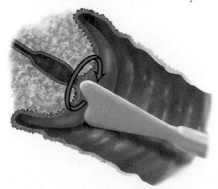

Fig. 26-14

Abnormal Findings

Surface reddened, granular, and asymmetrical, particularly around os.

Friable, bleeds easily.

Any lesions: white patch on cervix; strawberry spot.

Refer any suspicious red, white, or pigmented lesion for biopsy (see erosion, ulceration, and carcinoma, Table 26-4, p. 785).

Cervical polyp—bright red growth protruding from the os (see Table 26-4, p. 785).

Foul-smelling, irritating, with yellow, green, white, or grey discharge (see Table 26-5, p. 786).

Normal Range of Findings	**Abnormal Findings**

Endocervical Specimen. Insert a Cytobrush (instead of a cotton applicator) into the os (Fig. 26-15). A Cytobrush gives a higher yield of endocervical cells at the SCJ and is safe for use during pregnancy (Stillson et al., 1997). The woman may feel a slight pinch with the brush and scant bleeding may occur. For this reason, collect the endocervical specimen last so that bleeding will not obscure cytological evaluation.

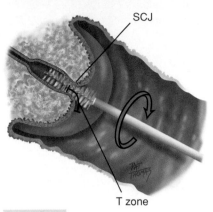

SCJ

T zone

Fig. 26-15

Rotate the brush 720 degrees in ONE direction in the endocervical canal, either clockwise or counterclockwise. Then rotate the brush gently on a slide to deposit all the cells. Rotate in the opposite direction from the one in which you obtained the specimen. Avoid leaving a thick specimen that would be hard to read under the microscope. Immediately (within 2 seconds) spray the slide with fixative to avoid drying, if procedures require this step.

For the woman after hysterectomy whose cervix has been removed, collect a scrape from the end of the vagina and a vaginal pool.

Immediately spray the slides with fixative. The frosted ends of the slides should be labelled with the woman's name. Send these to the laboratory with the following necessary data:

- Date of specimen
- Woman's date of birth
- Date of last menstrual period
- Any hormone medication
- If pregnant, estimated date of delivery
- Known infections
- Prior surgery or radiation
- Prior abnormal cytology
- Abnormal findings on physical examination

These data are important for accurate interpretation; for example, a specimen may be interpreted as positive unless the laboratory technicians know the woman has had prior radiation treatment. Newer methods of cervical screening use a **liquid-based cytology (LBC)**. The sample is collected with a cervical spatula or an endocervical brush but is placed in a vial containing cell-preserving fluid. LBC is currently being used in Ontario and will soon be implemented within cervical cancer screening programs in Newfoundland and British Columbia (Murphy, 2007).

To screen for STIs, and if you note any abnormal vaginal discharge, obtain the **GC/chlamydia** culture. Insert a sterile cotton applicator into the os, rotate it 360 degrees, and leave it in place 10 to 20 seconds for complete saturation. Insert into labelled specimen.

Occasionally you will need the following samples:

Saline Mount, or "Wet Preparation." Spread a sample of the discharge onto a glass slide and add one drop of normal saline solution and a coverslip.

KOH Preparation. To a sample of the discharge on a glass slide, add one drop of potassium hydroxide and a coverslip.

Normal Range of Findings	Abnormal Findings

Anal Culture. Insert a sterile cotton swab into the anal canal about 1 cm. Rotate it, and move it side to side. Leave in place 10 to 20 seconds. If the swab collects feces, discard it and begin again. Insert culture into specimen container.

Acetic Acid Wash. Acetic acid (white vinegar) screens for asymptomatic human papillomavirus (HPV), which causes genital warts. After all other specimens are gathered, soak a thick-tipped cotton rectal swab with acetic acid and "paint" the cervix. Acetic acid dissolves mucus and temporarily causes intracellular dehydration and coagulation of protein. A normal response (indicating no HPV infection) is no change in the cervical epithelium.

Rapid acetowhitening or blanching, especially with irregular borders, suggests HPV infection (see Table 26-2, p. 782).

Inspect the Vaginal Wall

Loosen the thumbscrew but continue to hold the speculum blades open. Slowly withdraw the speculum, rotating it as you go, to fully inspect the vaginal wall. Normally, the wall looks pink, deeply rugated, moist and smooth, and is free of inflammation or lesions. Normal discharge is thin and clear, or opaque and stringy, but always odourless.

Inflammation or lesions.

Leukoplakia, appears as spot of dried white paint.

Vaginal discharge: thick, white, and curdlike with candidiasis; profuse, watery, grey-green, and frothy with trichomoniasis; or any grey, green-yellow, white, or foul-smelling discharge (see Table 26-5, p. 786).

When the blade ends near the vaginal opening, let them close, but be careful not to pinch the mucosa or catch any hairs. Turn the blades obliquely to avoid stretching the opening. Place the metal speculum in a basin to be cleaned later and soaked in a sterilizing and disinfecting solution; discard the plastic variety. Discard your gloves and wash hands.

Bimanual Examination

Rise to a stand, and have the woman remain in lithotomy position. Drop lubricant onto the first two fingers of your gloved intravaginal hand (Fig. 26-16). Assume the "obstetrical" position with the first two fingers extended, the last two flexed onto the palm, and the thumb abducted. Insert your fingers into the vagina, with any pressure directed posteriorly. Wait until the vaginal walls relax, then insert your fingers fully.

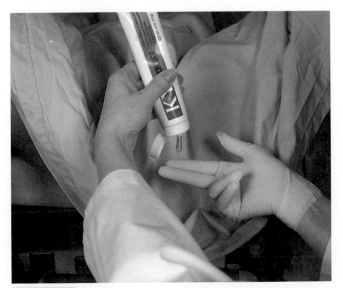

Fig. 26-16

Normal Range of Findings

Abnormal Findings

You will use both hands to palpate the internal genitalia to assess their location, size, and mobility, and to screen for any tenderness or mass. One hand is on the abdomen while the other (often the dominant, more sensitive hand) inserts two fingers into the vagina (Fig. 26-17). It does not matter which you choose as the intravaginal hand; try each way, and settle on the most comfortable method for you.

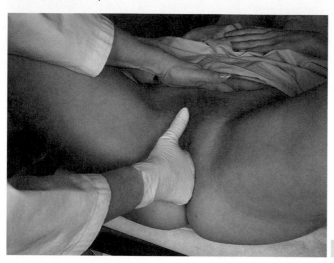

Fig. 26-17

Palpate the vaginal wall. Normally, it feels smooth and has no area of induration or tenderness.

Nodule.
Tenderness.

Cervix. Locate the cervix in the midline, often near the anterior vaginal wall. The cervix points in the opposite direction of the fundus of the uterus. Palpate using the palmar surface of the fingers. Note these characteristics of a normal cervix:

- **Consistency**—feels smooth and firm, as the consistency of the tip of the nose. It softens and feels velvety at 5 to 6 weeks of pregnancy (Goodell's sign).

Hard with malignancy.
Nodular.

- **Contour**—evenly rounded.
- **Mobility**—With a finger on either side, move the cervix gently from side to side. Normally, this produces no pain (Fig. 26-18).

Palpate all around the fornices; the wall should feel smooth.

Irregular.
Immobile with malignancy.

Painful with inflammation or ectopic pregnancy.

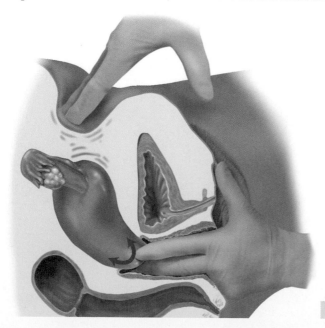

Fig. 26-18

Objective Data

Normal Range of Findings	**Abnormal Findings**

Next, use your abdominal hand to push the pelvic organs closer for your intravaginal fingers to palpate. Place your hand midway between the umbilicus and the symphysis; push down in a slow, firm manner, fingers together and slightly flexed. Brace the elbow of your pelvic arm against your hip, and keep it horizontal. The woman must be relaxed.

Uterus. With your intravaginal fingers in the anterior fornix, assess the uterus. Determine the position, or *version*, of the uterus (Fig. 26-19). This compares the long axis of the uterus with the long axis of the body. In many women, the uterus is anteverted; you palpate it at the level of the pubis with the cervix pointing posteriorly. Two other positions occur normally (midposition and retroverted), as well as two aspects of flexion, where the long axis of the uterus is not straight but is flexed.

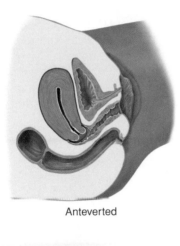
Anteverted

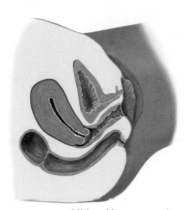
Midposition

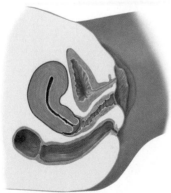
Anteflexed

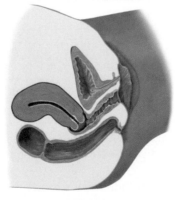
Retroflexed

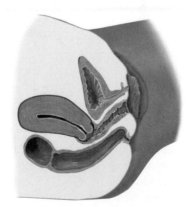
Retroverted

Fig. 26-19

Palpate the uterine wall with your fingers in the fornices. Normally, it feels firm and smooth, with the contour of the fundus rounded. It softens during pregnancy. Bounce the uterus gently between your abdominal and intravaginal hands. It should be freely movable and nontender.

Enlarged uterus (see Table 26-6, p. 788).
Lateral displacement.
Nodular mass. Irregular, asymmetrical uterus.
Fixed and immobile.
Tenderness.

Normal Range of Findings	Abnormal Findings

Adnexa. Move both hands to the right to explore the adnexa. Place your abdominal hand on the lower quadrant just inside the anterior iliac spine and your intravaginal fingers in the lateral fornix (Fig. 26-20). Push the abdominal hand in and try to capture the ovary. Often, you cannot feel the ovary. When you can, it normally feels smooth, firm, and almond shaped, and is highly movable, sliding through the fingers. It is slightly sensitive but not painful. The fallopian tube is not palpable normally. No other mass or pulsation should be felt.

Enlarged adnexa. Nodules or mass in adnexa.

Immobile.
Markedly tender (see Table 26-7, p. 789).

Pulsation or palpable fallopian tube suggests ectopic pregnancy; this warrants immediate referral.

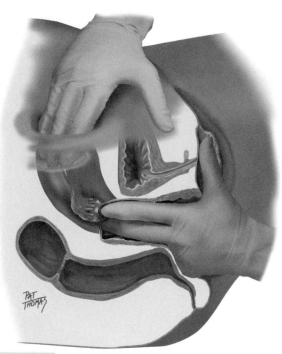

Fig. 26-20

A note of caution: Normal adnexal structures often are not palpable. Be careful not to mistake an abnormality for a normal structure. To be safe, consider abnormal any mass that you cannot *positively* identify, and refer the woman for further study.

Move to the left to palpate the other side. Then, withdraw your hand and check secretions on the fingers before discarding the glove. Normal secretions are clear or cloudy and odourless.

Rectovaginal Examination

Use this technique to assess the rectovaginal septum, posterior uterine wall, cul-de-sac, and rectum. Change gloves to avoid spreading any possible infection. Lubricate the first two fingers. Instruct the woman that this may feel uncomfortable and will mimic the feeling of moving her bowels. Ask her to bear down as you insert your index finger into the vagina and your middle finger gently into the rectum (Fig. 26-21).

Objective Data

Normal Range of Findings   **Abnormal Findings**

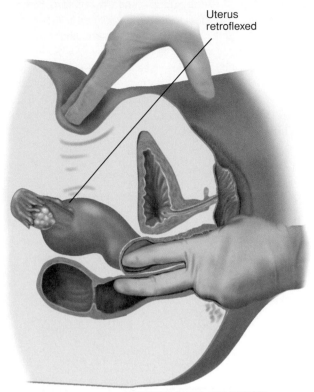

Uterus retroflexed

RECTOVAGINAL PALPATION

Fig. 26-21

While pushing with the abdominal hand, repeat the steps of the bimanual examination. Try to keep the intravaginal finger on the cervix so the intrarectal finger does not mistake the cervix for a mass. Note:

- Rectovaginal septum should feel smooth, thin, firm, and pliable.
- Rectovaginal pouch, or cul-de-sac, is a potential space and usually not palpated.
- Uterine wall and fundus feel firm and smooth.

Rotate the intrarectal finger to check the rectal wall and anal sphincter tone. (See Chapter 25 for assessment of anus and rectum.) Check your gloved finger as you withdraw; test any adherent stool for occult blood.

Give the woman tissues to wipe the area and help her up. Remind her to slide her hips back from the edge before sitting up so she will not fall.

Nodular or thickened.

 DEVELOPMENTAL CARE

Infants and Children

Preparation

- **Infant**—place on examination table.
- **Toddler or preschooler**—place on parent's lap.
  Frog-leg position—hips flexed, soles of feet together and up to bottom.
  Preschool child may want to separate her own labia.
  No drapes—the young girl wants to see what you are doing.
- **School-age child**—place on examination table, frog-leg position, no drapes.

During childhood, a routine screening is limited to inspection of the external genitalia to determine that (1) the structures are intact, (2) the vagina is present, and (3) the hymen is patent.

Normal Range of Findings	Abnormal Findings

Normal Range of Findings

The newborn's genitalia are somewhat engorged. The labia majora are swollen, the labia minora are prominent and protrude beyond the labia majora, the clitoris looks relatively large, and the hymen appears thick. Because of transient engorgement, the vaginal opening is more difficult to see now than it will be later. Place your thumbs on the labia majora. Push laterally while pushing the perineum down, and try to note the vaginal opening above the hymenal ring. Do not palpate the clitoris because it is very sensitive.

A sanguineous vaginal discharge or leukorrhea (mucoid discharge) are normal during the first few weeks because of the maternal estrogen effect. (This also may cause transient breast engorgement and secretion.) During the early weeks, the genital engorgement resolves, and the labia minora atrophy and remain small until puberty (Fig. 26-22).

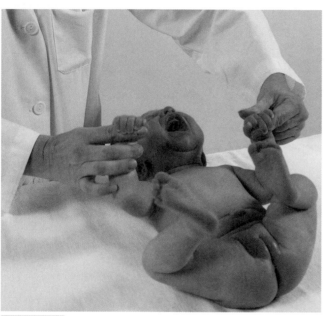

Fig. 26-22

Between the ages of 2 months and 7 years, the labia majora are flat, the labia minora are thin, the clitoris is relatively small, and the hymen is tissue-paper thin. Normally, no irritation or foul-smelling discharge is present.

In the young school-age girl (7 to 10 years), the mons pubis thickens, the labia majora thicken, and the labia minora become slightly rounded. Pubic hair appears beginning around age 11 years, although sparse pubic hair may occur as early as age 8 years. Normally, the hymen is perforate.

Almost always in these age groups, an external examination will suffice. If needed, an internal pelvic examination is best performed by a pediatric gynecologist using specialized instruments.

The Adolescent

The adolescent girl has special needs during the genitalia examination. Examine her alone, without the mother present. Assure her of privacy and confidentiality. Allow plenty of time for health education and discussion of pubertal progress. Assess her growth velocity and menstrual history, and use the SMR charts to teach breast and pubic hair development. Assure her that increased vaginal fluid (physiological *leukorrhea*) is normal because of the estrogen effect.

Abnormal Findings

Ambiguous genitalia are rare but are suggested by a markedly enlarged clitoris, fusion of the labia (resembling scrotum), and palpable mass in fused labia (resembling testes) (see Table 26-8, p. 791).

Imperforate hymen warrants referral.

Lesions, rash.

Poor perineal hygiene.
Pest inhabitants. Excoriations.
During and after toddler age, foul-smelling discharge occurs with lodging of foreign body, pinworms, or infection.

Absence of pubic hair by 13 years indicates delayed puberty.
Amenorrhea in adolescent, together with bluish and bulging hymen, indicates imperforate hymen and warrants referral.

Normal Range of Findings	Abnormal Findings

Perform pelvic examination when contraception is desired, when the girl's sexual activity includes intercourse, or at age 18 years in virgins. Start periodic Pap smears when intercourse begins. Although the techniques of the examination are listed in the adult section, you will need to provide additional time and psychological support for the adolescent having her first pelvic examination.

The experience of the first pelvic examination determines how the adolescent will approach future care. Your accepting attitude and gentle, unhurried approach are important. You have a unique teaching opportunity here. Take the time to teach, using the girl's own body as illustration. Your frank discussion of anatomy and sexual behaviour communicates that these topics are acceptable to discuss and not taboo with healthcare professionals. This affirms the girl's self-concept.

During the bimanual examination, note that the adnexa are not palpable in the adolescent.

Pelvic or adnexal mass.

The Pregnant Female

Depending on the week of gestation of the pregnancy, inspection shows the enlarging abdomen (see Fig. 29-1 on p. 823). The height of the fundus ascends gradually as the fetus grows. At 16 weeks, the fundus is palpable halfway between the symphysis and umbilicus; at 20 weeks, at the lower edge of the umbilicus; at 28 weeks, halfway between the umbilicus and the xiphoid; and at 34 to 36 weeks, almost to the xiphoid. Then close to term, the fundus drops as the fetal head engages in the pelvis.

The external genitalia show hyperemia of the perineum and vulva because of increased vascularity. Varicose veins may be visible in the labia or legs. Hemorrhoids may show around the anus. Both are caused by interruption in venous return from the pressure of the fetus.

Internally, the walls of the vagina appear violet or blue (Chadwick's sign) because of hyperemia. The vaginal walls are deeply rugated and the vaginal mucosa thickens. The cervix looks blue, feels velvety, and feels softer than in the nonpregnant state, making it a bit more difficult to differentiate from the vaginal walls.

During bimanual examination, the isthmus of the uterus feels softer and is more easily compressed between your two hands (Hegar's sign). The fundus balloons between your two hands; it feels connected to, but distinct from, the cervix because the isthmus is so soft.

Search the adnexal area carefully during early pregnancy. Normally, the adnexal structures are not palpable.

An ectopic pregnancy has serious consequences (see Table 26-7, p. 789).

The Aging Adult

Natural lubrication is decreased; to avoid a painful examination, take care to lubricate instruments and the examining hand adequately. Use the Pedersen speculum (rather than the Graves) because its narrower, flatter blades are more comfortable in women with vaginal stenosis or dryness.

Menopause and the resulting decrease in estrogen production cause numerous physical changes. Pubic hair gradually decreases, becoming thin and sparse in later years. The skin is thinner and fat deposits decrease, leaving the mons pubis smaller and the labia flatter. Clitoris size also decreases after age 60 years.

Internally, the rugae of the vaginal walls decrease, and the walls look pale pink because of the thinned epithelium. The cervix shrinks and looks pale and glistening. It may retract, appearing to be flush with the vaginal wall. In some, it is hard to distinguish the cervix from the surrounding vaginal mucosa. Alternately, the cervix may protrude into the vagina if the uterus has prolapsed.

With the bimanual examination, you may need to insert only one gloved finger if vaginal stenosis exists. The uterus feels smaller and firmer, and the ovaries are not palpable normally.

Refer any suspicious red, white, or pigmented lesion for biopsy.

Vaginal atrophy increases the risk of infection and trauma.

Refer any mass for prompt evaluation.

Normal Range of Findings	Abnormal Findings

Cervical cancer screening is not required following total hysterectomy for benign conditions in women who do not have a history of cervical dysplasia and have had a negative and adequate prior screening history (Murphy, 2007); however, recommendations may vary by region. Be aware that older women may have special needs and will appreciate the following plans of care: for those with arthritis, taking a mild analgesic or anti-inflammatory before the appointment may ease joint pain in positioning; schedule appointment times when joint pain or stiffness is at its least; allow extra time for positioning and "unpositioning" after the examination; and be careful to maintain dignity and privacy.

Summary Checklist: Female Genitalia Examination

For a PDA-downloadable version, go to http://evolve.elsevier.com/Canada/Jarvis/examination/.

1. **Inspect external genitalia**
2. **Palpate labia,** Skene's, and Bartholin's glands
3. Using **vaginal speculum,** inspect cervix and vagina
4. Obtain **specimens** for cytological study
5. Perform **bimanual examination:** cervix, uterus, adnexa
6. Perform **rectovaginal** examination
7. **Test stool** for occult blood

Promoting Health: New HPV Vaccine

New Vaccine to Prevent Cervical Cancer: A Breakthrough in Cancer Prevention

Human papillomavirus (HPV) is estimated to be the most prevalent sexually transmitted infection (STI) in Canada, and HPV is responsible for most cases of cervical cancer, the second most common malignancy in women. In 2006 the first HPV vaccine was approved for use in Canada. The National Advisory Committee on Immunization (2007) has recommended the vaccine for (1) females between 9 and 13 years of age, as this is before the onset of sexual intercourse for most Canadian females; (2) females between the ages of 14 and 26 years, even if they are already sexually active, as they may not yet have HPV infection and are very unlikely to have been infected with all four HPV types present in the vaccine; and (3) females between the ages of 14 and 26 who have had previous abnormalities on a Papanicolaou (Pap) smear test, including cervical cancer, or have had genital warts or known HPV, as they are very unlikely to have been infected with all four HPV types in the vaccine. The vaccine is given in three separate injections over a 6-month period. Some Canadian provinces have introduced HPV immunization programs.

Canadian women who are older, immigrant, Aboriginal, or have a lower socioeconomic status are at higher risk for developing cervical cancer, primarily as a result of lower participation rates in regular screening schedules. Reluctance to undergo screening may be due to reasons such as lack of knowledge, lack of access, or failure of the clinician to offer screening. Other factors that appear to increase the risk of developing cervical cancer are becoming sexually active at a young age; having many sexual partners or a sexual partner who has had many partners; being a smoker; having a weakened immune system (e.g., from taking drugs after organ transplantation or having a disease such as acquired immune deficiency syndrome); using oral contraceptives; giving birth to many children; and having taken diethylstilbestrol (DES) or being the daughter of a mother who took DES (Canadian Cancer Society, 2007).

Annual HPV screening with the Pap smear test is recommended within 3 years of first vaginal sexual activity until three negative tests are obtained. The frequency of HPV screening may be reduced to every 3 years until age 70 if tests remain negative (McLachlin et al., 2005). More frequent testing may be considered for women at high risk. Overall, cervical cancer incidence and mortality rates have been declining as a result of widespread Pap test screening. Women who have received the HPV vaccine should still take part in the currently recommended cervical cancer screening programs. As more females receive the vaccine, the recommended type or frequency of screening may be modified.

DOCUMENTATION AND CRITICAL THINKING

Sample Charting

SUBJECTIVE

Menarche age 12 years, cycle usually q28d, duration 5 days, flow moderate, no dysmenorrhea, LMP April 3. Grav 0/Para 0/Ab 0. Gyne checkups yearly. Last Pap test 1 year PTA, negative.

No urinary problems, no irritating or foul-smelling vaginal discharge, no sores or lesions, no history of pelvic surgery. Satisfied with sexual relationship with husband, uses vaginal diaphragm for birth control, no plans for pregnancy at this time. Aware of no contact by self or husband with STIs.

OBJECTIVE

External genitalia: No swelling, lesions, or discharge. No urethral swelling or discharge.
Internal: Vaginal walls have no bulging or lesions, cervix pink with no lesions, scant clear mucoid discharge.
Bimanual: No pain on moving cervix, uterus anteflexed and anteverted, no enlargement or irregularity.
Adnexa: Ovaries not enlarged.
Rectal: No hemorrhoids, fissures, or lesions, no masses or tenderness, stool brown with guaiac test negative.

ASSESSMENT

Genital structures intact and appear healthy

Focused Assessment: Clinical Case Study 1

J.K., 27-year-old, married newspaper reporter, Grav 0/Para 0/Ab 0. Presents at clinic with "urinary burning, vaginal itching, and discharge × 4 days."

SUBJECTIVE

- 3 weeks PTA: treated at clinic for bronchitis with erythromycin. Improved within 5 days.
- 4 to 5 days PTA: noted burning on urination, intense vaginal itching, thick, white, "smelly" discharge. Warm water douche—no relief.
- No previous history vaginal infection, urinary tract infection, or pelvic surgery. Monogamous sexual relationship, has used low-estrogen birth control pills for 3 years with no side effects.

OBJECTIVE

Vulva and vagina erythematous and edematous. Thick, white, curdlike discharge clinging to vaginal walls. Cervix pink, no lesions.
Bimanual examination: No pain on palpating cervix, uterus not enlarged, ovaries not enlarged.
Specimens: Pap smear, GC/chlamydia to lab. KOH prep shows mycelia and spores of *Candida albicans*.

ASSESSMENT

Candida vaginitis
Pain R/T infectious process

Focused Assessment: Clinical Case Study 2

Brenda, 17-year-old, high-school student, comes to clinic for pelvic examination.

SUBJECTIVE

- Menarche 12 years, cycle q30d, duration 6 days, mild cramps relieved by acetaminophen. LMP March 10. No dysuria, vaginal discharge, vaginal itching. Relationship involving intercourse with one boyfriend for 8 months PTA. For birth control, boyfriend uses condoms "sometimes." Wants to start birth control pills. Never had pelvic examination. No knowledge of breast self-examination. No knowledge of STIs except AIDS. Smokes cigarettes, $\frac{1}{2}$ PPD, started age 11 years.

OBJECTIVE

Breasts: Symmetrical, no lesions or discharge, palpation reveals no mass or tenderness.
External genitalia: No redness, lesions, or discharge.
Internal genitalia: Vaginal walls and cervix pink with no lesions or discharge. Specimens obtained. Acetic acid wash shows no acetowhitening.
Bimanual: No tenderness to palpation, uterus anteverted with no enlargement, ovaries not enlarged.
Rectum: No masses, fissure, or tenderness. Stool brown and guaiac test negative.
Specimens: GC, Chlamydia, Pap smear to lab.

ASSESSMENT

Breast and pelvic structures appear healthy
Deficient knowledge regarding: breast self-examination; birth control measures; STI prevention; cigarette smoking R/T lack of exposure

Nursing Diagnoses Commonly Associated With the Female Genitalia and Related Disorders

All nursing diagnoses can be found on the Evolve Web site at **http://evolve.elsevier.com/Canada/Jarvis/examination/.**

ABNORMAL FINDINGS
FOR ADVANCED PRACTICE

| TABLE 26-2 | **Abnormalities of the External Genitalia** |

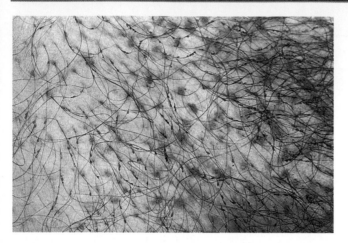

Pediculosis Pubis (Crab Lice)

S: Severe perineal itching.
O: Excoriations and erythematous areas. May see little dark spots (lice are small), nits (eggs) adherent to pubic hair near roots. Usually localized in pubic hair, occasionally in eyebrows or eyelashes.

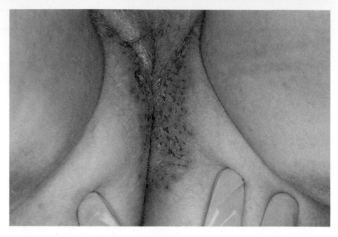

Herpes Simplex Virus Type 2 (Herpes Genitalis)

S: Episodes of local pain, dysuria, fever.
O: Clusters of small, shallow vesicles with surrounding erythema; erupt on genital areas and inner thigh. Also, inguinal adenopathy, edema. Vesicles on labia rupture in 1–3 days, leaving painful ulcers. Initial infection lasts 7–10 days. Virus remains dormant indefinitely; recurrent infections last 3–10 days with milder symptoms.

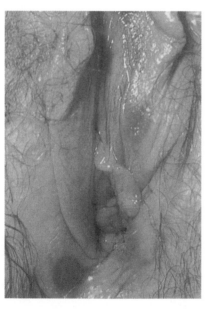

Syphilitic Chancre

O: Begins as a small, solitary silvery papule that erodes to a red, round or oval, superficial ulcer with a yellowish serous discharge. Palpation—nontender indurated base; can be lifted like a button between thumb and finger. Nontender inguinal lymphadenopathy.

Reprinted from Emond, R. (1995). Colour atlas of infectious diseases (3rd ed., p. 173), by permission of the publisher Mosby.

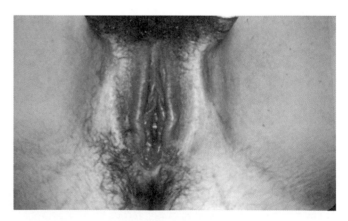

Red Rash—Contact Dermatitis

S: History of skin contact with allergenic substance in environment, intense pruritus.
O: Primary lesion—red, swollen, vesicles. Then may have weeping of lesions, crusts, scales, thickening of skin, excoriations from scratching. May result from reaction to feminine hygiene spray or synthetic underclothing.

S, Subjective data; *O,* objective data.

TABLE 26-2	*Abnormalities of the External Genitalia—cont'd*

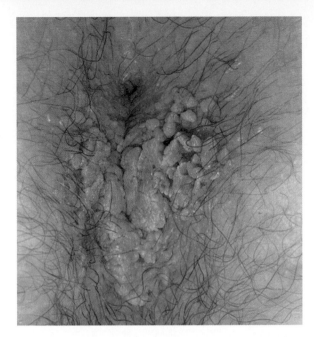

Human Papillomavirus (HPV) Genital Warts

S: Painless warty growths, may be unnoticed by woman.

O: Pink or flesh-coloured, soft, pointed, moist, warty papules. Single or multiple in a cauliflowerlike patch. Occur around vulva, introitus, anus, vagina, cervix.

HPV infection is common among sexually active women, especially adolescents, regardless of ethnicity or socioeconomic status. Risk factors include early age at menarche and multiple sexual partners. The long incubation period (6 weeks–8 months) makes it difficult to establish history of exposure. A strong association of HPV infection and abnormal cervical cytology exists.

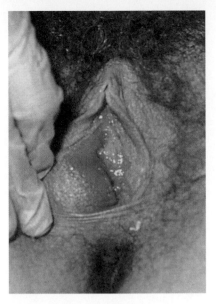

Abscess of Bartholin's Gland

S: Local pain, can be severe.

O: Overlying skin red and hot. Posterior part of labia swollen; palpable fluctuant mass and tenderness. Mucosa shows red spot at site of duct opening; can express purulent discharge. Often secondary to gonococcal infection.

Reprinted from Emond, R. (1995). Colour atlas of infectious diseases (3rd ed., p. 161), by permission of the publisher Mosby.

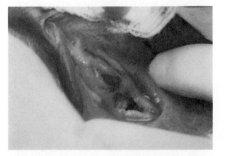

Urethritis (not illustrated)

S: Dysuria.

O: Palpation of anterior vaginal wall shows erythema, tenderness, induration along urethra, purulent discharge from meatus. Caused by *Neisseria gonorrhoeae, Chlamydia,* or *Staphylococcus* infection.

Urethral Caruncle

S: Tender, painful with urination, urinary frequency, hematuria, dyspareunia, or asymptomatic.

O: Small, deep red mass protruding from meatus; usually secondary to urethritis or skenitis; lesion may bleed on contact.

S, Subjective data; *O,* objective data.

TABLE 26-3	Abnormalities of the Pelvic Musculature

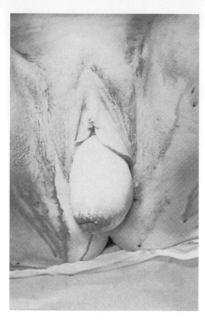

Cystocele (with prolapse)

S: Feeling of pressure in vagina, stress incontinence.

O: With straining or standing, note introitus widening and the presence of a soft, round anterior bulge. The bladder, covered by vaginal mucosa, prolapses into vagina, in this case with an extreme uterine prolapse.

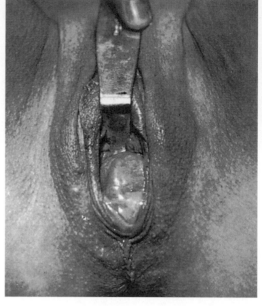

Rectocele

S: Feeling of pressure in vagina, possibly constipation.

O: With straining or standing, note introitus widening and the presence of a soft, round bulge from posterior. Here, part of the rectum, covered by vaginal mucosa, prolapses into vagina.

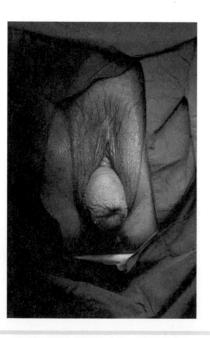

◀ Uterine Prolapse

O: With straining or standing, uterus protrudes into vagina. Prolapse is graded: first degree, cervix appears at introitus with straining; second degree, cervix bulges outside introitus with straining; third degree (in this case), whole uterus protrudes even without straining—essentially, uterus is inside out.

S, Subjective data; *O,* objective data.

TABLE 26-4	Abnormalities of the Cervix

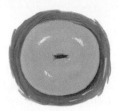

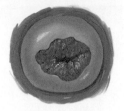

Bluish Cervix—Cyanosis

O: Bluish discoloration of the mucosa occurs normally in pregnancy (Chadwick's sign at 6–8 weeks' gestation) and with any other condition causing hypoxia or venous congestion (e.g., heart failure, pelvic tumour).

Erosion

O: Cervical lips inflamed and eroded. Reddened granular surface is superficial inflammation, with no ulceration (loss of tissue). Usually secondary to purulent or mucopurulent cervical discharge. Biopsy needed to distinguish erosion from carcinoma; cannot rely on inspection.

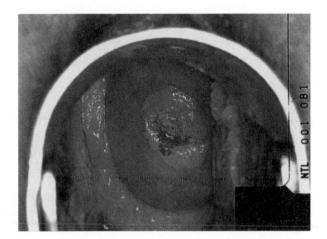

Human Papillomavirus (HPV, Condylomata)

O: Virus can appear in various forms when affecting cervical epithelium. Here warty growth appears as abnormal thickened white epithelium. Visibility of lesion is enhanced by acetic acid (vinegar) wash, which dissolves mucus and temporarily causes intracellular dehydration and coagulation of protein.

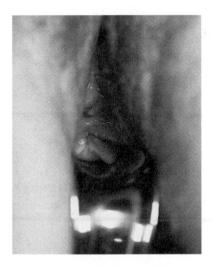

Polyp

S: May have mucoid discharge or bleeding.
O: Bright red, soft, pedunculated growth emerges from os. It is a benign lesion, but this must be determined by biopsy. May be lined with squamous or columnar epithelium.

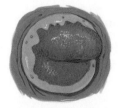

◀ Diethylstilbestrol (DES) Syndrome

S: Prenatal exposure to DES causes cervical and vaginal abnormalities.
O: Red, granular patches of columnar epithelium extend beyond normal squamocolumnar junction onto cervix and into fornices (vaginal adenosis). Also cervical abnormalities: circular groove, transverse ridge, protuberant anterior lip, "cocks-comb" formation. Warrants frequent monitoring.

S, Subjective data; *O,* objective data.   *Continued*

Abnormal Findings

| TABLE 26-4 | Abnormalities of the Cervix—cont'd |

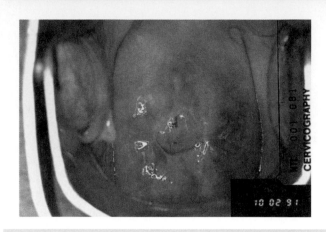

◀ Carcinoma

S: Bleeding between menstrual periods or after menopause, unusual vaginal discharge.

O: Chronic ulcer and induration are early signs of carcinoma, although the lesion may or may not show on the exocervix. (Here, lesion is mostly around the external os.) Diagnosed by Pap smear and biopsy. Risk factors for cervical cancer are early age at first intercourse, multiple sex partners, cigarette smoking, certain sexually transmitted infections.

S, Subjective data; *O,* objective data.

| TABLE 26-5 | Vulvovaginal Inflammations |

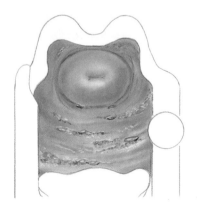

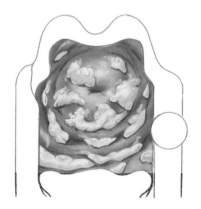

Atrophic Vaginitis

S: Postmenopausal vaginal itching, dryness, burning sensation, dyspareunia, mucoid discharge (may be flecked with blood).

O: Pale mucosa with abraded areas that bleed easily; may have bloody discharge.

An opportunistic infection related to chronic estrogen deficiency.

Candidiasis (Moniliasis)

S: Intense pruritus, thick whitish discharge.

O: Vulva and vagina are erythematous and edematous. Discharge is usually thick, white, curdy, "like cottage cheese." Diagnose by microscopic examination of discharge on potassium hydroxide wet mount.

Predisposing causes—use of oral contraceptives or antibiotics, more alkaline vaginal pH (as with menstrual periods, postpartum, menopause), also pregnancy from increased glycogen and diabetes.

S, Subjective data; *O,* objective data.

TABLE 26-5	Vulvovaginal Inflammations—cont'd

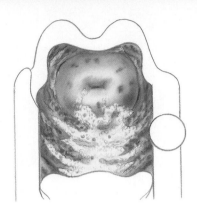

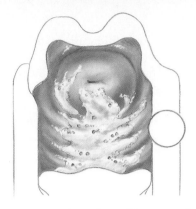

Trichomoniasis

S: Pruritus, watery and often malodorous vaginal discharge, urinary frequency, terminal dysuria. Symptoms are worse during menstruation when the pH becomes optimal for the organism's growth.

O: Vulva may be erythematous. Vagina diffusely red, granular, occasionally with red raised papules and petechiae ("strawberry" appearance). Frothy, yellow-green, foul-smelling discharge. Microscopic examination of saline wet mount specimen shows characteristic flagellated cells.

Bacterial Vaginosis (*Gardnerella vaginalis, Haemophilus vaginalis,* or Nonspecific Vaginitis)

S: Profuse discharge, "constant wetness" with "foul, fishy, rotten" odour.

O: Thin, creamy, grey-white, malodorous discharge. No inflammation on vaginal wall or cervix because this is a surface parasite. Microscopic view of saline wet mount specimen shows typical "clue cells."

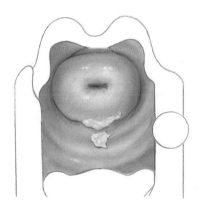

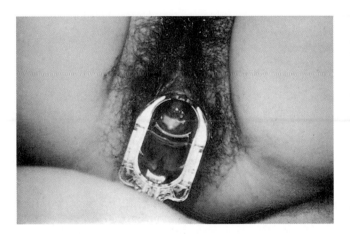

Chlamydia

S: (Mimics gonorrhea.) Three of four infected women have no symptoms. May have urinary frequency, dysuria, or vaginal discharge, postcoital bleeding.

O: May have yellow or green mucopurulent discharge, friable cervix, cervical motion tenderness. Signs are subtle, easily mistaken for gonorrhea. The two are important to distinguish because antibiotic treatment is different; if the wrong drug is given or if the condition is untreated, chlamydia can ascend the reproductive tract to cause pelvic inflammatory disease (PID) and result in infertility. This is the most common STI in the United States; the highest prevalence is among sexually active adolescent girls, with an incidence of almost 30% in some settings (Burstein et al., 1998). Clinicians are urged to screen all sexually active girls every 6 months, regardless of symptoms or risk.

Gonorrhea

S: Variable: vaginal discharge, dysuria, abnormal uterine bleeding, abscess in Bartholin's or Skene's glands; the majority of cases are asymptomatic.

O: Often no signs are apparent. May have purulent vaginal discharge. Diagnose by positive culture of organism. If the condition is untreated, it may progress to acute salpingitis, PID.

S, Subjective data; *O,* objective data.

TABLE 26-6	Uterine Enlargement

Pregnancy

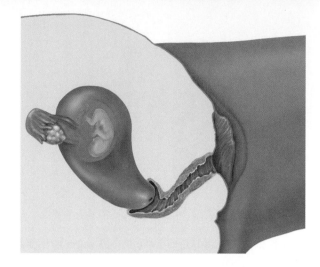

Obviously a normal condition, pregnancy is included here for comparison.

S: Amenorrhea, fatigue, breast engorgement, nausea, change in food tolerance, weight gain.

O: Early signs: cyanosis of vaginal mucosa and cervix (Chadwick's sign). Palpation—soft consistency of cervix, enlarging uterus with compressible fundus and isthmus (Hegar's sign at 10–12 weeks).

Myomas (Leiomyomas, Uterine Fibroids)

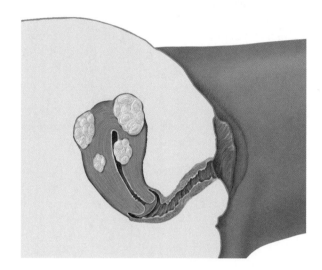

S: Varies, depending on size and location. Often no symptoms. When symptoms do occur, include vague discomfort, bloating, heaviness, pelvic pressure, dyspareunia, urinary frequency, backache, or hypermenorrhea if myoma disturbs endometrium. Heavy bleeding produces anemia.

O: Uterus irregularly enlarged, firm, mobile, and nodular with hard, painless nodules in the uterine wall.

They are usually benign. Highest incidence between the ages of 30 and 45 years and in women of African descent. Myomas are estrogen dependent; after menopause, the lesions usually regress but do not disappear. Surgery may be indicated.

Carcinoma of the Endometrium

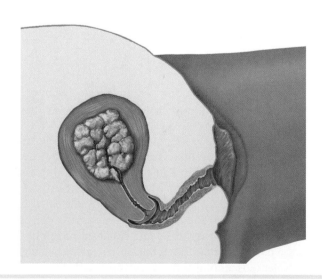

S: Abnormal and intermenstrual bleeding before menopause; postmenopausal bleeding or mucosanguineous discharge. Pain and weight loss occur late in the disease.

O: Uterus may be enlarged.

The Pap smear is rarely effective in detecting endometrial cancer. Women with abnormal vaginal bleeding or at high risk should have an endometrial tissue sample. Risk factors for endometrial cancer are early menarche, late menopause, history of infertility, failure to ovulate, use of tamoxifen, unopposed estrogen therapy (which continually stimulates the endometrium, causing hyperplasia), and obesity (which increases endogenous estrogen).

S, Subjective data; *O,* objective data.

TABLE 26-6	Uterine Enlargement—cont'd

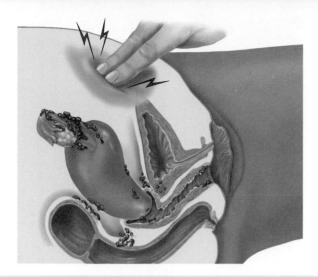

◀ Endometriosis

S: Cyclic or chronic pelvic pain, occurring as dysmenorrhea, or dyspareunia, low backache. Also may have irregular uterine bleeding or hypermenorrhea or may be asymptomatic.

O: Uterus fixed, tender to movement. Small, firm nodular masses tender to palpation on posterior aspect of fundus, uterosacral ligaments, ovaries, sigmoid colon. Ovaries often enlarged.

Masses are aberrant growths of endometrial tissue scattered throughout pelvis as a result of transplantation of tissue by retrograde menstruation. Ectopic tissue responds to hormone stimulation; builds up between periods, sloughs during menstruation. May cause infertility from pelvic adhesions, tubal obstruction, decreased ovarian function.

S, Subjective data; *O,* objective data.

TABLE 26-7	Adnexal Enlargement

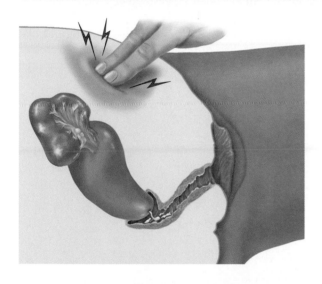

◀ Fallopian Tube Mass—Acute Salpingitis (Pelvic Inflammatory Disease [PID])

S: Sudden fever >38°C, suprapubic pain and tenderness.

O: Acute-rigid boardlike lower abdominal musculature. May have purulent discharge from cervix. Movement of uterus and cervix causes intense pain. Pain in lateral fornices and adnexa. Bilateral adnexal masses difficult to palpate because of pain and muscle spasm. Chronic—bilateral, tender, fixed adnexal masses.

Complications include ectopic pregnancy, infertility, and reinfection. PID usually caused by *Neisseria gonorrhoeae* and *Chlamydia trachomatis.*

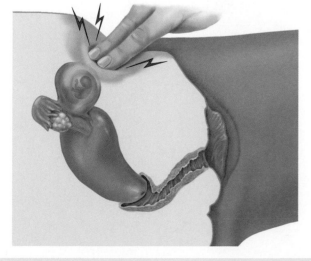

◀ Fallopian Tube Mass—Ectopic Pregnancy

S: Amenorrhea or irregular vaginal bleeding, pelvic pain.

O: Softening of cervix and fundus; movement of cervix and uterus causes pain; palpable tender pelvic mass, which is solid, mobile, unilateral.

This has potential for serious sequelae; seek gynecological consultation immediately before the mass ruptures or shows signs of acute peritonitis.

S, Subjective data; *O,* objective data.

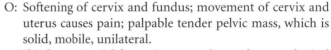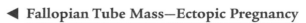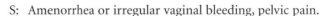

TABLE 26-7 | **Adnexal Enlargement—cont'd**

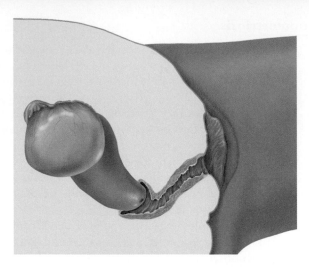

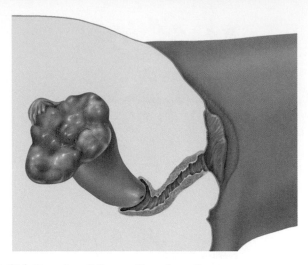

Fluctuant Ovarian Mass—Ovarian Cyst

S: Usually asymptomatic.

O: Smooth, round, fluctuant, mobile, nontender mass on ovary. Some cysts resolve spontaneously within 60 days but must be followed up closely.

Solid Ovarian Mass—Ovarian Cancer

S: Usually asymptomatic. May have abdominal enlargement from fluid accumulation.

O: Solid tumour palpated on ovary. Heavy, solid, fixed, poorly defined mass suggests malignancy; benign mass may feel mobile and solid.

Biopsy necessary to distinguish the two types of masses. The Pap smear does not detect ovarian cancer. Women over age 40 years should have a thorough pelvic examination every year.

S, Subjective data; *O,* objective data.

TABLE 26-8   Abnormalities in Pediatric Genitalia

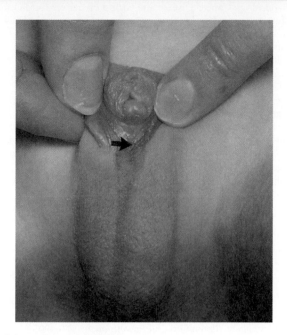

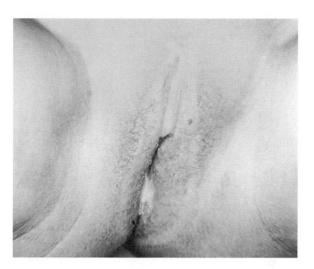

Ambiguous Genitalia

Female pseudohermaphroditism is a congenital anomaly resulting from hyperplasia of the adrenal glands, which exposes the female fetus to excess amounts of androgens. This causes masculinized external genitalia, here shown as enlargement of the clitoris and fusion of the labia. Ambiguous means the enlarged clitoris here may look like a small penis with hypospadias, and the fused labia look like an incompletely formed scrotum with absent testes. Other forms of intersexual conditions occur, and the family must be referred for diagnostic evaluation.

Vulvovaginitis in Child

This infection is caused by *Candida albicans* in a diabetic child. Symptoms include pruritus and burning when urine touches excoriated area. Examination shows red, shiny, edematous vulva, vaginal discharge, excoriated area from scratching.

Other, more common causes of vulvovaginitis in the prepubertal child include infection from a respiratory or bowel pathogen, sexually transmitted infection, or presence of a foreign body.

BIBLIOGRAPHY

Auslander, B., Biro, F., & Rosenthal, S. (2005). Genital herpes in adolescents. *Seminars in Pediatric Infectious Diseases, 16*, 24–30.

Banikarim, C., & Chacko, M. (2005). Pelvic inflammatory disease in adolescents. *Seminars in Pediatric Infectious Diseases, 16*, 175–180.

Bradley, L. (2005). Abnormal uterine bleeding. *Nurse Practitioner, 30*, 38–51.

Canadian Cancer Society. (2007). *Early detection and screening: Facts for women.* Retrieved on May 19, 2008, from www.cancer.ca

Canadian Cancer Society/National Cancer Institute of Canada. (2007). *Canadian cancer statistics 2007.* Toronto, ON: Author.

Canadian Paediatric Society. (2007). Position statement (ID 2007-01): Human papillomavirus vaccine for children and adolescents. *Paediatrics and Child Health, 12*, 599–903.

Champion, J. D, Piper, J., Holden, A., Korte, J., & Shain, R. N. (2004). Abused women and risk for pelvic inflammatory disease. *Western Journal of Nursing Research, 26*, 176–191.

Cunningham, F. G., Leveno, K. J., Bloom, S. L., Hauth, J. C., Gilstrap, L. C., & Wenstrom, K. D. (2005). *Williams' obstetrics* (22nd ed.). New York, NY: McGraw-Hill Professional.

Daley, A. M., & Cromwell, P. F. (2002). How to perform a pelvic exam for the sexually active adolescent. *Nurse Practitioner, 27*, 28–45.

Dawar, M., Deeks, S., & Dobson, S. (2007). Human papillomavirus vaccines launch a new era in cervical cancer protection. *Canadian Medical Association Journal, 177*, 456–461.

Dean, B. B., Borenstein, J. E., Knight, K., & Yonkers, K. (2006). Evaluating the criteria used for identification of PMS. *Journal of Women's Health, 15*, 546–555.

Franco, E. L., Duarte-Franco, E., & Ferenczy, A. (2001). Cervical cancer: Epidemiology, prevention and the role of human papillomavirus infection. *Canadian Medical Association Journal, 164*, 1017–1025.

Freeto, J., & Jay, S. (2006). "What's really going on down there?" A practical approach to the adolescent who has gynecologic complaints. *Pediatric Clinics of North America, 53*, 529–545.

Giudice, L. C. (2004). Endometriosis. *Lancet, 364*, 1789–1799.

Health Canada. (2002). *Cervical cancer screening in Canada: 1998 surveillance report.* Retrieved January 30, 2008, from http://www.phac-aspc.gc.ca/publicat/ccsic-dccuac/index.html

Health Canada, Federal Interdepartmental Working Group on Female Genital Mutilation. (2000). *Female genital mutilation and health care: Current situation and legal status recommendations to improve the health care of affected women.* Retrieved February 3, 2008, from http://www.cwhn.ca/resources/fgm/

Heise, A. (2003). The clinical significance of HPV. *Nurse Practitioner, 28*, 8–21.

Jones, S. (2006). A step-by-step approach to HIV/AIDS. *Nurse Practitioner, 31*, 26–41.

Katz, A. (2005). Sexuality and hysterectomy: Finding the right words. *American Journal of Nursing, 105*, 65–68.

Kimberlin, D. W., & Rouse, D. J. (2004). Genital herpes. *New England Journal of Medicine, 350*, 1970–1977.

Kingsberg, S. (2006). Taking a sexual history. *Obstetrics and Gynecology Clinics of North America, 33*, 535–547.

Kruse, K., Lauver, D., & Hanson, K. (2003). Clinical implications of DES. *Nurse Practitioner, 28*, 26–37.

Lonergan, S., & Hern, G. (2006). Refresher course on sexually transmitted diseases. *Emergency Medicine, 38*, 33–42.

Luce, T., Dow, K., & Holcomb, L. (2003). Early diagnosis key to epithelial ovarian cancer detection. *Nurse Practitioner, 28*, 41–49.

Marcell, D., Ransel, S., Schiau, M., & Duffy, E. G. (2003). Treatment options alleviate female urge incontinence. *Nurse Practitioner, 28*, 48–55.

Mark, H., Hanahan, A., & Stender, S. (2003). Herpes simplex virus type 2: An update. *Nurse Practitioner, 28*, 34–43.

Marshall, W. A., & Tanner, J. M. (1969). Variations in pattern of pubertal changes in girls. *Archives of Disease in Childhood, 44*, 291–303.

McLachlin, C. M., Mai, V., Murphy, J., Fung, M. F. K., Chambers, A., & members of the Cervical Screening Guidelines Development Committee of the Ontario Cervical Screening Program and the Gynecology Cancer Disease Site Group of Cancer Care Ontario. (2005). *Cervical screening: A clinical practice guideline.* Retrieved February 2, 2008, from http://www.cancercare.on.ca/index_cancerScreeningguidelines.htm

Melville, J. L., Katon, W., Delaney, K., & Newton, K. (2005). Urinary incontinence in U.S. women. *Archives of Internal Medicine, 165*, 537–542.

Miller, J., & Holman, J. (2005). Abnormal uterine bleeding: A primary care primer. *Consultant, 45*, 638–645.

Morrison, B. J. (1994). Screening for cervical cancer. In Canadian Task Force on the Periodic Health Examination (Eds.), *Canadian guide to clinical preventive health care* (pp. 883–889). Ottawa, ON: Health Canada.

Murphy, K. J. (2007). Screening for cervical cancer. *Journal of Obstetrics and Gynaecology Canada, 29*(8), S27–S36.

National Advisory Committee on Immunization. (2007). Statement on human papillomavirus vaccine. *Canada Communicable Disease Report, 33*(ACS-2), 1–32.

Noller, K. (2005). Cervical cytology screening and evaluation. *Obstetrics and Gynecology, 106*, 391–397.

Patel, D., & Pearlman, M. (2006). Point-of-care diagnosis of STIs in women. *Contemporary OB/GYN, 51*, 68–74.

Pisani, P., Parkin, M., Munoz, N., & Ferlay, J. (1997). Cancer and infection: Estimates of the attributable fraction in 1990. *Cancer Epidemiology, Biomarkers and Prevention, 6*, 387–400.

Public Health Agency of Canada. (2006). *Canadian guidelines on sexually transmitted infections* (2006 Ed.). Retrieved April 14, 2008, from http://www.phac-aspc.gc.ca/std-mts/sti_2006/sti_intro2006_e.html

Rambourt, L., Hopkins, L., Hutton, B., & Fergusson, D. (2007). Prophylactic vaccination against human papillomavirus infection and disease in women: A systematic review of randomized controlled trials. *Canadian Medical Association Journal, 177*, 469–479.

Robinson, B. A. (2006). *Female genital mutilation in North America and Europe.* Retrieved from http://www.religioustolerance.org/fem_cira.htm

Sellors, J. W., Mahony, J. B., Kaczorowski, J., Lytwyn, A., Bangura, H., Chong, S., et al. (2000). Prevalence and predictors of human papillomavirus infection in women in Ontario, Canada. *Canadian Medical Association Journal, 163*, 503–508.

Shew, M., & Fortenberry, D. (2005). HPV infection in adolescents: Natural history, complications, and indicators for viral typing. *Seminars in Pediatric Infectious Diseases, 16*, 168–174.

Smith, P. (2005). Menopause assessment, treatment, and patient education. *Nurse Practitioner, 30*, 33–45.

Society of Obstetricians and Gynaecologists of Canada. (2007). Canadian consensus guidelines on human papillomavirus. *Journal of Obstetrics and Gynaecology Canada, 29*(8), S1–S56.

Specht, J. (2005). 9 myths of incontinence in older adults. *American Journal of Nursing, 105*, 58–69.

Stillson, T., Knight, A. L., & Elswick, R. K. (1997). The effectiveness and safety of two cervical cytologic techniques during pregnancy. *Journal of Family Practice, 45*, 159–163.

Wasunna, A. (2000). Towards redirecting the female circumcision debate: Legal, ethical and cultural considerations. *McGill Journal of Medicine, 5*(2), 104–110.

Weber, D., & Leone, P. (2005). Understanding human papillomavirus. *Consultant, 45*, S6–S15.

Weir, E. (2000). Female genital mutilation: Epidemiology. *Canadian Medical Association Journal, 162*, 1344.

Woltman, K. J., & Newbold, K. B. (2007). Immigrant women and cervical cancer screening uptake: A multilevel analysis. *Canadian Journal of Public Health, 98*, 470–475.

Women's Health Initiative Steering Committee. (2004). Effects of conjugated equine estrogen in postmenopausal women with hysterectomy. *Journal of the American Medical Association, 291*, 1701–1712.

Xu, F., et al. (2006). Trends in herpes simplex virus type 1 and type 2 sero-prevalence in the United States. *Journal of the American Medical Association, 296*, 964–973.

27

The Complete Health Assessment: Putting It All Together

Written by **Carolyn Jarvis**, PhD, APN, CNP
Adapted by **Marian Luctkar-Flude**, RN, MScN

The choreography of the complete history and physical examination is the art of arranging all the separate steps you have learned so far. Your first examination may seem awkward and contrived; you may have to pause and think of what comes next rather than just gather data. Repeated rehearsals will make the choreography smoother. You will come to the point at which the procedure flows naturally, and even if you forget a step, you will be able to insert it gracefully into the next logical place.

The following examination sequence is one suggested route. It is intended to minimize the number of position changes for the patient and for you. With experience, you may wish to adapt this and arrange a sequence that feels natural for you. Perform all the steps listed here for a complete examination. With experience, you will learn to strike a balance between those steps you must retain to be thorough and those corners you may safely cut when time is pressing.

Have all equipment prepared and accessible before the examination. Review Chapter 8 for the list of necessary equipment, the setting, the patient's emotional state, your demeanour, and the preparation of the patient, considering his or her age.

Sequence	Selected Photos

The patient walks into the room, sits; the examiner sits facing the patient; the patient is in street clothes.

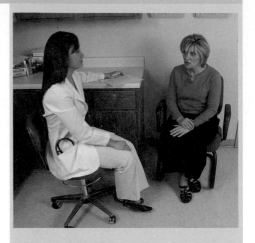

THE HEALTH HISTORY

Collect the history, complete or limited as visit warrants. While obtaining the history and throughout the examination, note data on the person's general appearance.

GENERAL APPEARANCE

1. Appears stated age
2. Level of consciousness
3. Skin colour
4. Nutritional status
5. Posture and position; comfortably erect
6. Obvious physical deformities
7. Mobility
   Gait
   Use of assistive devices
   Range of motion (ROM) of joints
   No involuntary movement
   Able to rise from a seated position easily
8. Facial expression
9. Mood and affect
10. Speech: articulation, pattern, content appropriate, first language
11. Hearing
12. Personal hygiene

MEASUREMENT

1. Weight
2. Height
3. Compute body mass index
4. Vision using Snellen eye chart

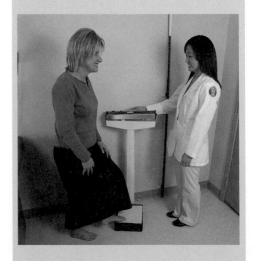

Ask the person to empty the bladder (save specimen, if needed), to disrobe except for underpants, and to put on a gown. The person sits with legs dangling off side of the bed or table; you stand in front of the person.

Sequence	Selected Photos

SKIN

1. Examine both hands and inspect the nails.
2. For the rest of the examination, examine skin with corresponding regional examination.

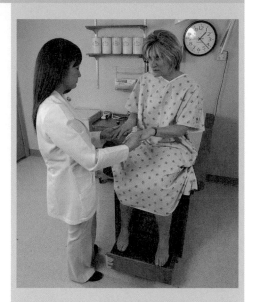

VITAL SIGNS

1. Radial pulse
2. Respirations
3. Blood pressure
4. Temperature (if indicated)

HEAD AND FACE

1. Inspect and palpate scalp, hair, and cranium.
2. Inspect face: expression, symmetry (cranial nerve VII).
3. Palpate the temporal artery, then the temporomandibular joint as the person opens and closes the mouth.
4. Palpate the maxillary sinuses and the frontal sinuses; if tender, transilluminate the sinuses.

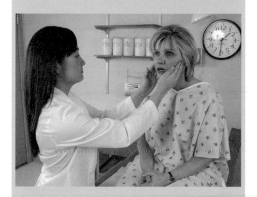

EYE

1. Test visual fields by confrontation (cranial nerve II).
2. Test extraocular muscles: corneal light reflex, six cardinal positions of gaze (cranial nerves III, IV, VI).
3. Inspect external eye structures.
4. Inspect conjunctivae, sclerae, corneas, irides.
5. Test pupil: size, response to light and accommodation.

   Darken room.
6. Using an ophthalmoscope, inspect ocular fundus: red reflex, disc, vessels, and retinal background.

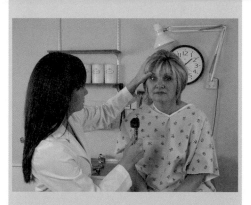

EAR

1. Inspect the external ear: position and alignment, skin condition, and auditory meatus.
2. Move auricle and push tragus for tenderness.
3. With an otoscope, inspect the canal, then the tympanic membrane for colour, position, landmarks, and integrity.
4. Test hearing: voice test; tuning fork tests—Weber and Rinne.

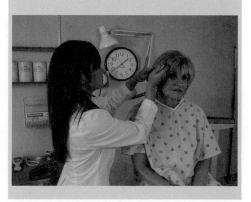

Objective Data

Sequence	Selected Photos

Objective Data

NOSE

1. Inspect the exterior of nose: symmetry, lesions.
2. Inspect facial symmetry (cranial nerve VII).
3. Test the patency of each nostril.
4. With a speculum, inspect the nares: nasal mucosa, septum, and turbinates.

MOUTH AND THROAT

1. With a penlight, inspect the mouth: buccal mucosa, teeth and gums, tongue, floor of mouth, palate, and uvula.
2. Grade tonsils, if present.
3. Note mobility of uvula as the person phonates "ahh," and test gag reflex (cranial nerves IX, X).
4. Ask the person to stick out the tongue (cranial nerve XII).
5. With a gloved hand, bimanually palpate the mouth, if indicated.

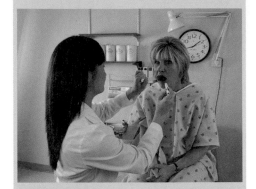

NECK

1. Inspect the neck: symmetry, lumps, and pulsations.
2. Palpate the cervical lymph nodes.
3. Inspect and palpate the carotid pulse, one side at a time. If indicated, listen for carotid bruits.
4. Palpate the trachea in midline.
5. Test ROM and muscle strength against your resistance: head forward and back, head turned to each side, and shoulder shrug (cranial nerve XI).

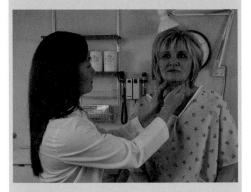

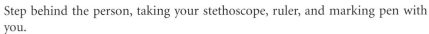

Step behind the person, taking your stethoscope, ruler, and marking pen with you.
6. Palpate thyroid gland, posterior approach.

Open the person's gown to expose all of the back for examination of the thorax, but leave gown on shoulders and anterior chest.

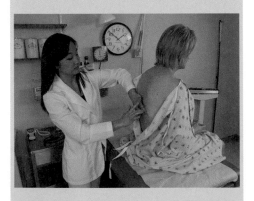

CHEST, POSTERIOR, AND LATERAL

1. Inspect the posterior chest: configuration of the thoracic cage, skin characteristics, and symmetry of shoulders and muscles.
2. Palpate: symmetrical expansion; tactile fremitus; lumps or tenderness.
3. Palpate length of spinous processes.
4. Percuss over all lung fields, percuss diaphragmatic excursion.
5. Percuss costovertebral angle, noting tenderness.
6. Auscultate breath sounds; note any adventitious sounds.

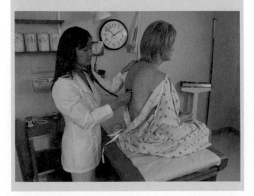

Sequence	Selected Photos

Move around to face the patient; the patient remains sitting. For a female breast examination, ask permission to lift gown to drape on the shoulders, exposing the anterior chest; for a male, lower the gown to the lap.

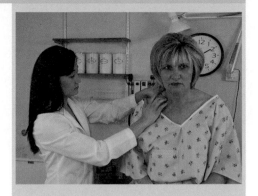

CHEST, ANTERIOR

1. Inspect: respirations and skin characteristics.
2. Palpate: tactile fremitus, lumps, or tenderness.
3. Percuss anterior lung fields.
4. Auscultate breath sounds.

HEART

1. Ask the person to lean forward and exhale briefly; auscultate cardiac base for any murmurs.

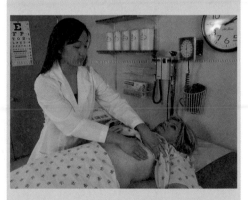

UPPER EXTREMITIES

1. Test ROM and muscle strength of hands, arms, and shoulders.
2. Palpate the epitrochlear nodes.

FEMALE BREASTS

1. Inspect for symmetry, mobility, and dimpling as the woman lifts arms over the head, pushes the hands on the hips, and leans forward.
2. Inspect supraclavicular and infraclavicular areas.

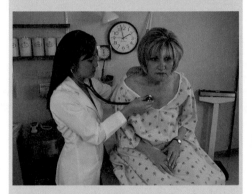

Help the woman to lie supine with head at a flat to 30-degree angle. Stand at the person's *right* side. Drape the gown up across shoulders and place an extra sheet across lower abdomen.

3. Palpate each breast, lifting the same-side arm up over head. Include the tail of Spence and areola.
4. Palpate each nipple for discharge.
5. Support the person's arm and palpate axilla and regional lymph nodes.
6. Teach breast self-examination, if patient requests to learn it.

MALE BREASTS

1. Inspect and palpate while palpating the anterior chest wall.
2. Supporting each arm, palpate the axilla and regional nodes.

NECK VESSELS

1. Inspect each side of neck for a jugular venous pulse, turning the person's head slightly to the other side.
2. Estimate jugular venous pressure, if indicated.

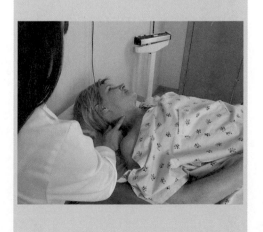

Objective Data

Sequence   **Selected Photos**

HEART

1. Inspect the precordium for any pulsations or heave (lift).
2. Palpate the apical impulse and note the location.
3. Palpate precordium for any abnormal thrill.
4. Auscultate apical rate and rhythm.
5. Auscultate with the diaphragm of the stethoscope to study heart sounds, inching from the apex up to the base, or vice versa.
6. Auscultate the heart sounds with the bell of the stethoscope, again inching through all locations.
7. Turn the person over to left side while again auscultating apex with the bell.

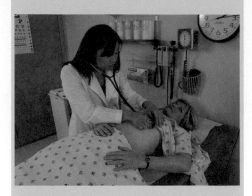

The person should be supine, with the bed or table flat; arrange drapes to expose the abdomen from the chest to the pubis.

ABDOMEN

1. Inspect: contour, symmetry, skin characteristics, umbilicus, and pulsations.
2. Auscultate bowel sounds.
3. Auscultate for vascular sounds over the aorta and renal arteries.
4. Percuss all quadrants.
5. Percuss height of the liver span in right midclavicular line.
6. Percuss the location of the spleen.
7. Palpate: light palpation in all quadrants, then deep palpation in all quadrants.

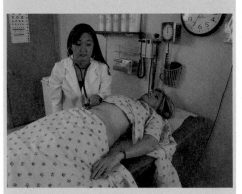

8. Palpate for liver, spleen, kidneys, and aorta.
9. Test the abdominal reflexes, if indicated.

INGUINAL AREA

1. Palpate each groin for the femoral pulse and the inguinal nodes. Lift the drape to expose the legs.

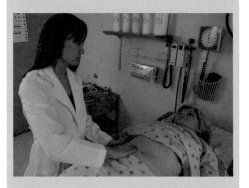

LOWER EXTREMITIES

1. Inspect: symmetry, skin characteristics, and hair distribution.
2. Palpate pulses: popliteal, posterior tibial, dorsalis pedis.
3. Palpate for temperature and pretibial edema.
4. Separate toes and inspect.
5. Test ROM and muscle strength of hips, knees, ankles, and feet.

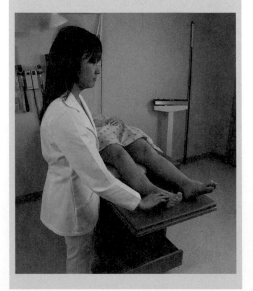

Objective Data

Sequence	Selected Photos

Ask the person to sit up and to dangle the legs off the bed or table. Keep the gown on and the drape over the lap.

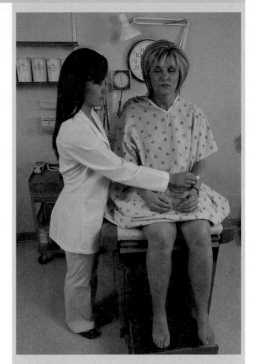

MUSCULOSKELETAL

1. Note muscle strength as person sits up.

NEUROLOGICAL

1. Test sensation in selected areas on face, arms, hands, legs, and feet: superficial pain, light touch, and vibration.
2. Test position sense of finger, one hand.
3. Test stereognosis.

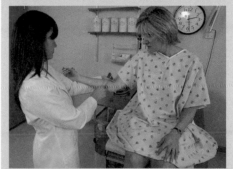

4. Test cerebellar function of the upper extremities using finger-to-nose test or rapid-alternating-movements test.
5. Test the cerebellar function of the lower extremities by asking the person to run each heel down the opposite shin.
6. Elicit deep tendon reflexes: biceps, triceps, brachioradialis, patellar, and Achilles.
7. Test the Babinski reflex.

Sequence	Selected Photos

Ask the person to stand with the gown on. Stand close to the person.

LOWER EXTREMITIES

1. Inspect legs for varicose veins.

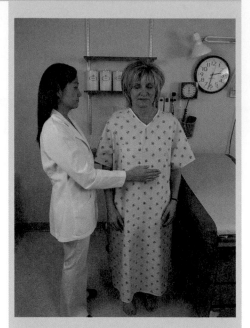

MUSCULOSKELETAL

1. Ask the person to walk across the room in his or her regular walk, turn, then walk back toward you, in heel-to-toe fashion.
2. Ask the person to walk on the toes for a few steps, then to walk on the heels for a few steps.
3. Stand close and check Romberg's sign.

4. Ask the person to hold the edge of the bed and to perform a shallow knee bend, one for each leg.
5. Stand behind and check the spine as the person touches the toes.
6. Stabilize the pelvis and test the ROM of the spine as the person hyperextends, rotates, and laterally bends.

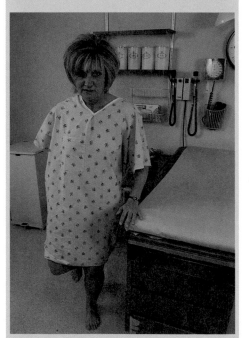

For the male patient, sit on a stool in front of him. The person stands.

MALE GENITALIA

1. Inspect the penis and scrotum.
2. Palpate the scrotal contents. If a mass exists, transilluminate.
3. Check for inguinal hernia.
4. Teach testicular self-examination.

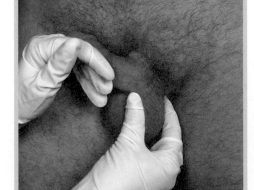

Sequence	Selected Photos

For an adult male, ask him to bend over the examination table, supporting the torso with forearms on the table. Assist the bedridden male to a left lateral position, with the right leg drawn up.

MALE RECTUM

1. Inspect the perianal area.
2. With a gloved lubricated finger, palpate the rectal walls and prostate gland.
3. Save a stool specimen for an occult blood test.

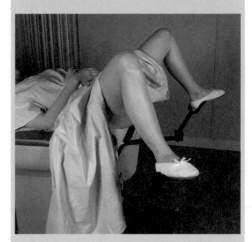

Assist the female back to the examination table, and help her assume the lithotomy position. Drape her appropriately. You sit on a stool at the foot of the table for the speculum examination, then stand for the bimanual examination.

FEMALE GENITALIA

1. Inspect the perineal and perianal areas.
2. With a vaginal speculum, inspect the cervix and vaginal walls.
3. Procure specimens.
4. Perform a bimanual examination; cervix, uterus, and adnexa.
5. Continue the bimanual examination, checking the rectum and rectovaginal walls.
6. Save a stool specimen for an occult blood test.
7. Provide tissues for the female to wipe the perineal area, and help her up to a sitting position.

Tell the patient you are finished with the examination and that you will leave the room as he or she gets dressed. Return to discuss the examination and further plans and to answer any questions. Thank the person for his or her time.

For the hospitalized person, return the bed and any room equipment to the way you found it. Make sure the call bell and telephone are in easy reach.

THE NEONATE AND INFANT

Review Chapter 8 for the steps on preparation and positioning and on developmental principles of the infant. The 1-minute and 5-minute Apgar results will give important data on the neonate's immediate response to extrauterine life. The following sequence will expand these data. You may reorder this sequence as the infant's sleep and wakefulness state or physical condition warrants.

The infant is supine on a warming table or examination table with an overhead heating element. The infant may be nude except for a diaper over a boy.

Vital Signs

Note pulse, respirations, and temperature.

Measurement

Weight, length, and head circumference are measured and plotted on growth curves for the infant's age.

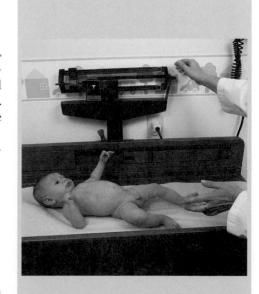

Objective Data

Objective Data

Sequence	Selected Photos

General Appearance

1. Body symmetry, spontaneous position, flexion of head and extremities, and spontaneous movement.
2. Skin colour and characteristics, any obvious deformities.
3. Symmetry and positioning of the facial features.
4. Alert, responsive affect.
5. Strong, lusty cry.

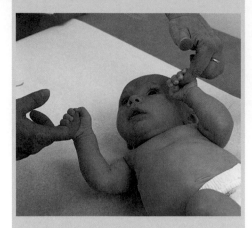

Chest and Heart

1. Inspect the skin condition over the chest and abdomen, chest configuration, and nipples and breast tissue.
2. Note movement of the abdomen with respirations, and any chest retraction.
3. Palpate apical impulse and note its location; chest wall for thrills; tactile fremitus if the infant is crying.
4. Auscultate breath sounds, heart sounds in all locations, and bowel sounds in the abdomen and in the chest.

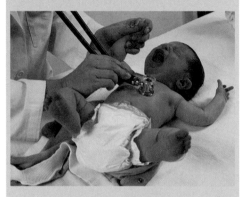

Abdomen

1. Inspect the shape of the abdomen and skin condition.
2. Inspect the umbilicus; count vessels; note condition of cord or stump, any hernia.
3. Palpate skin turgor.
4. Palpate lightly for muscle tone, liver, spleen tip, and bladder.
5. Palpate deeply for kidneys, any mass.
6. Palpate femoral pulses, inguinal lymph nodes.
7. Percuss all quadrants.

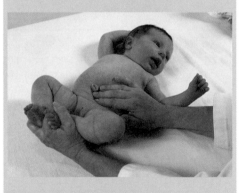

Head and Face

1. Note moulding after delivery, any swelling on cranium, bulging of fontanelle with crying or at rest.
2. Palpate fontanelles, suture lines, and any swellings.
3. Inspect positioning and symmetry of facial features at rest and while the infant is crying.

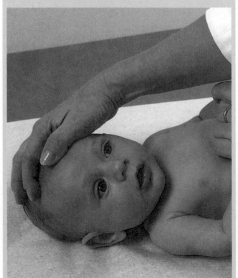

Sequence	Selected Photos

To open the neonate's eyes, support the head and shoulders and gently lower the baby backward, or ask the parent to hold the baby over his or her shoulder while you stand behind the parent.

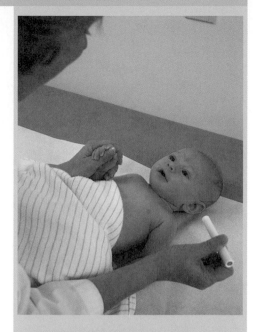

Eyes

1. Inspect the lids (edematous in the neonate), palpebral slant, conjunctivae, any nystagmus, and any discharge.
2. Using a penlight: elicit the pupillary reflex, blink reflex, and corneal light reflex; assess tracking of moving light.
3. Using an ophthalmoscope, elicit the red reflex.

Ears

1. Inspect size, shape, alignment of auricle, patency of auditory canals, any extra skin tags or pits.
2. Note the startle reflex in response to a loud noise.
3. Palpate flexible auricles.
(Defer otoscopic examination until the end of the complete examination.)

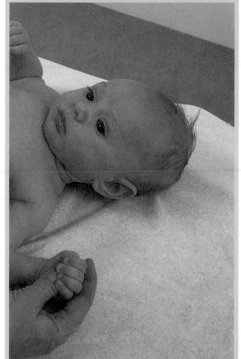

Nose

1. Determine the patency of the nares.
2. Note the nasal discharge, sneezing, and any flaring with respirations.

Mouth and Throat

1. Inspect the lips and gums, high-arched intact palate, buccal mucosa, tongue size, and frenulum of tongue; note absent or minimal salivation in neonate.
2. Note the rooting reflex.
3. Insert a gloved little finger, note the sucking reflex, and palpate palate.

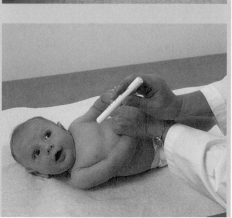

Objective Data

Sequence	Selected Photos

Objective Data

Neck

1. Lift the shoulders and let the head lag to inspect the neck: note midline trachea, any skinfolds, and any lumps.
2. Palpate the lymph nodes, the thyroid, and any masses.
3. While the infant is supine, elicit the tonic neck reflex; note a supple neck with movement.

Upper Extremities

1. Inspect and manipulate, noting ROM, muscle tone, and absence of scarf sign (elbow should not reach midline).
2. Count fingers, count palmar creases, and note colour of hands and nail beds.
3. Place your thumbs in the infant's palms to note the grasp reflex, then wrap your hands around infant's hands to pull up and note the head lag.

Lower Extremities

1. Inspect and manipulate the legs and feet, noting ROM, muscle tone, and skin condition.
2. Note alignment of feet and toes, look for flat soles, and count toes; note any syndactyly.
3. Test Ortolani sign for hip stability.

Genitalia

1. Females. Inspect labia and clitoris (edematous in the newborn), vernix caseosa between labia, and patent vagina.
2. Males. Inspect position of urethral meatus (do not retract foreskin), strength of urine stream if possible, and rugae on scrotum.
3. Palpate the testes in the scrotum.

Lift the infant under the axillae, and hold the infant facing you at eye level.

Neuromuscular

1. Note shoulder muscle tone and the infant's ability to stay in your hands without slipping.
2. Rotate the neonate slowly side to side; note the doll's eye reflex.
3. Turn the infant around so his or her back is to you; elicit the stepping reflex and the placing reflex against the edge of the examination table.

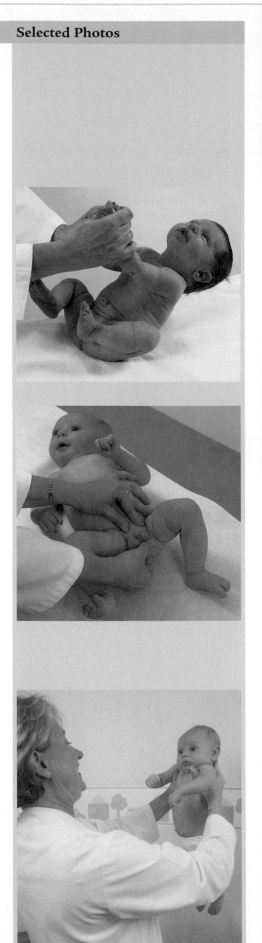

Sequence	Selected Photos

Turn the infant over and hold him or her prone in your hands, or place the infant prone on the examination table.

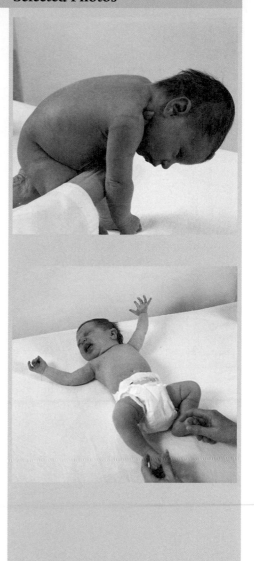

Spine and Rectum

1. Inspect the length of the spine, trunk incurvation reflex, and symmetry of gluteal folds.
2. Inspect intact skin; note any sinus openings, protrusions, or tufts of hair.
3. Note patent anal opening. Check for passage of meconium stool during the first 24 to 48 hours.

Final Procedures

1. With an otoscope, inspect the auditory canal and the tympanic membrane.
2. Elicit the Moro reflex by letting the infant's head and trunk drop back a short way, by jarring crib sides, or by making a loud noise.

THE YOUNG CHILD

Review the developmental considerations in preparing for an examination of the toddler and the young child in Chapter 8. During this time the young child's desire for independence conflicts with his or her basic dependence. Also, the child is aware of and fearful of a new environment, has a fear of invasive procedures, dislikes being restrained, and may be attached to a security object.

Focus on the parent as the child plays with a toy.

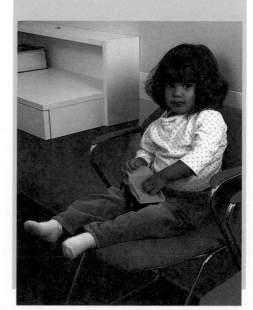

The Health History

1. Collect the history, including developmental data.
   During the history, note data on general appearance.

Objective Data

| **Sequence** | **Selected Photos** |

General Appearance

1. Note child's ability to amuse himself or herself while the parent speaks.
2. Note parent and child interaction.
3. Note gross motor and fine motor skills as the child plays with toys.

Gradually focus on and involve yourself with the child, at first in a "play" period.

4. Evaluate developmental milestones by using the Nipissing Developmental Screen™: gait, jumping, hopping, building a tower, and throwing a ball. (See Appendix F.)
5. Evaluate posture while the child is sitting and standing. Evaluate alignment of the legs and feet while the child is walking.
6. Evaluate speech acquisition.
7. Evaluate vision, hearing ability.
8. Evaluate social interaction.

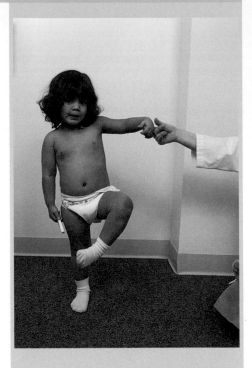

Ask the parent to undress the child to the diaper or the underpants. Position the older infant and young child, 6 months to 2 or 3 years, in the parent's lap. Move your chair to sit knee to knee with the parent. A 4- or 5-year-old child usually feels comfortable on the examination table.

Measurement

Height, weight, head circumference (may need to defer head circumference until later in the examination).

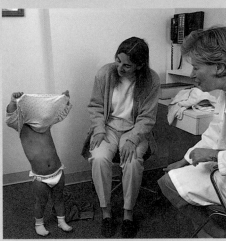

Chest and Heart

1. Auscultate breath sounds and heart sounds in all locations, count respiratory rate, count heart rate, and auscultate bowel sounds.
2. Inspect size, shape, and configuration of chest cage. Assess respiratory movement.
3. Inspect pulsations on the precordium. Note nipple and breast development.
4. Palpate apical impulse and note location, chest wall for thrills, any tactile fremitus.

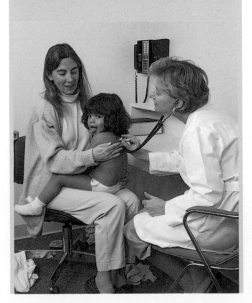

Sequence	Selected Photos

The child should be sitting up in the parent's lap or on the examination table, in diaper or underpants.

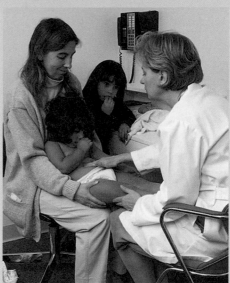

Abdomen

1. Inspect shape of abdomen, skin condition, and periumbilical area.
2. Palpate skin turgor, muscle tone, liver edge, spleen, kidneys, and any masses.
3. Palpate the femoral pulses. Compare strength with radial pulses.
4. Palpate inguinal lymph nodes.

Genitalia

1. Inspect the external genitalia.
2. On males, palpate the scrotum for testes. If masses are present, transilluminate.

Lower Extremities

1. Test Ortolani sign for hip stability.
2. Note skin condition and alignment of legs.
3. Note alignment of feet. Inspect toes and longitudinal arch.
4. Palpate the dorsalis pedis pulse.
5. Gain child's co-operation by allowing him or her to play with the reflex hammer. Elicit plantar, Achilles, and patellar reflexes.

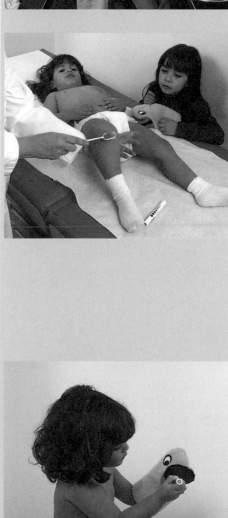

The child should be sitting up in the parent's lap or on the examination table, in diaper or underpants.

Upper Extremities

1. Inspect arms and hands for alignment, skin condition; inspect fingers and note palmar creases.
2. Palpate and count the radial pulse.
3. Test biceps and triceps reflexes with a reflex hammer.
4. Measure blood pressure.

Objective Data

| **Sequence** | **Selected Photos** |

Head and Neck

1. Inspect the size and shape of the head and symmetry of facies.
2. Palpate the fontanelles and cranium. Palpate the cervical lymph nodes, trachea, and thyroid gland.
3. Measure the head circumference.

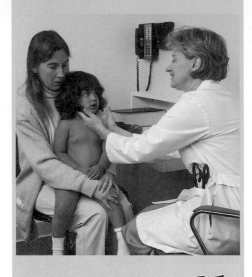

Eyes

1. Inspect the external structures. Note any palpebral slant.
2. With a penlight, test the corneal light and pupillary light reflexes.
3. Direct a moving penlight for cardinal positions of gaze.
4. If indicated, perform the cover test, covering the eye with your thumb in a young child, or use an index card.
5. Inspect conjunctivae and sclerae.
6. With an ophthalmoscope, check the red reflex. Inspect the fundus as much as possible.

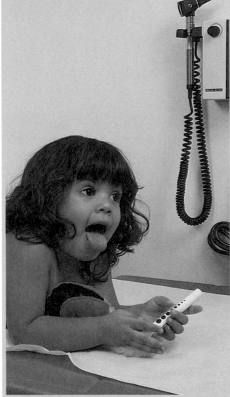

Nose

1. Inspect the skin condition, and the exterior of the nose.
2. With a penlight, inspect the nares for foreign body, mucosa, septum, and turbinates.

Mouth and Throat

1. With a penlight, inspect the mouth, buccal mucosa, teeth and gums, tongue, palate, and uvula in midline. Use a tongue blade as the last resort.

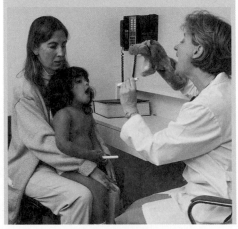

Sequence	Selected Photos

Ears

1. Inspect and palpate the auricle. Note any discharge from the auditory meatus. Check for any foreign body.
2. With an otoscope, inspect the ear canal and tympanic membrane. Gain cooperation through the use of a puppet, encouraging the child to handle the equipment or to look in the parent's ear as you hold the otoscope. You may need to have the parent help restrain the child.

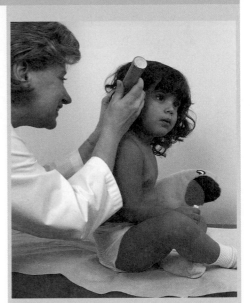

THE SCHOOL-AGE CHILD, THE ADOLESCENT, AND THE AGING ADULT

The sequence of the examination for people in these age groups is the head-to-toe format described in the adult section. However, you should be aware of differences in approach and timing and special developmental considerations. Review Chapter 8 for a full discussion of these factors.

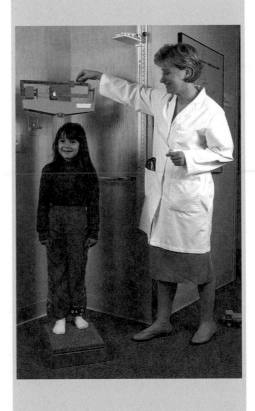

✦— DOCUMENTATION AND CRITICAL THINKING —✦

Recording the Data

Record the data from the history and physical examination as soon after the event as possible. Memory fades as the day develops, especially when you are responsible for the care of more than one person.

It is difficult to strike a balance between recording too much data and recording too little. It is important to remember that, from a legal perspective, if it is not documented, it was not done. Data important for the diagnosis and treatment of the person's health should be recorded, as well as data that contribute to your decision-making process. This includes charting relevant normal or negative findings.

On the other hand, a listing of every assessment parameter described in this text yields an unwieldy, unworkable record. One way to keep your record complete yet succinct is to study your writing style. Use short, clear phrases. Avoid redundant introductory phrases such as, "The patient states that. . . ." Avoid redundant descriptions such as "no inguinal, femoral, or umbilical hernias." Just write "no hernias."

Use simple line drawings to describe your findings. You do not need artistic talent; draw a simple sketch of a tympanic membrane, breast, abdomen, or cervix and mark your findings on it. A clear picture is worth many words.

Study the following complete history and physical examination for a sample write-up. Note that the subject is the same young woman introduced in Chapter 1 of this text.

Health History

BIOGRAPHICAL DATA

Name: Ellen K.

Address: 123 Centre St.

Marital Status: Single

Birth date: 1/18/

Birthplace: Mt. Albert

Ethnocultural background: Euro-Canadian

Ellen K. is a 23-year-old, single, female cashier at a tavern, currently unemployed for 6 months.

Source. Ellen, seems reliable.

Reason for seeking care. "I'm coming in for alcohol treatment."

History of present illness. First alcoholic drink, age 16. First intoxication, age 17, drinking one to two times per week, a six-pack per occasion. Attended high-school classes every day, but grades slipped from A−/B+ average to C− average. At age 20, was drinking two times per week, six to nine beers per occasion. At age 22, was drinking two times per week, a 12-pack per occasion, and occasionally a six-pack the next day to "help with the hangover." During this year, experienced blackouts, failed attempts to cut down on drinking, being physically sick the morning after drinking, and being unable to stop drinking once started. Also, incurred three impaired driving legal offences. Last offence 1 month PTA, last alcohol use just before offence, 18 beers that occasion. Abstinent since that time.

PAST HEALTH

Childhood illnesses. Chicken pox at age 6. No measles, mumps, croup, pertussis. No rheumatic fever, scarlet fever, or polio.

Accidents. 1. Auto accident, age 12, father driving, Ellen thrown from car, right leg crushed. Hospitalized at Memorial, surgery for leg pinning to repair multiple compound fracture. 2. Auto accident, age 21, head hit dashboard, no loss of consciousness, treated and released at Memorial Hospital ED. 3. Auto accident, age 23, "car hit median strip," no injuries, not seen at hospital.

Chronic illnesses. None.

Hospitalizations. Age 12, Memorial Hospital, surgery to repair right leg as described, Dr. M.J. Carlson, surgeon.

Obstetrical history. Gravida 0/Para 0/Abortion 0.

Immunizations. Childhood immunizations up to date. Last tetanus "probably high school." No TB skin test.

Last examinations. Yearly pelvic examinations at health department since age 15, told "normal." High-school sports physical, age 17. Last dental examination, age 15; last vision test for driver's licence, age 16; never had ECG or chest X-ray.

Allergies. No known allergies.

Current medications. Birth control pills, low-estrogen type, 1/day, for 5 years. No other prescription or over-the-counter medications.

FAMILY HISTORY

Ellen is second youngest child, parents divorced 8 years, father has chronic alcoholism. See family genogram below.

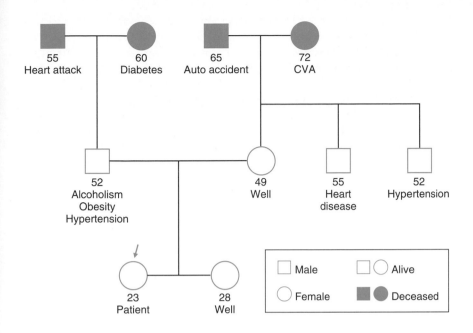

REVIEW OF SYSTEMS

General health. Reports usual health "OK." No recent weight change, no fatigue, weakness, fever, sweats.

Skin. No change in skin colour, pigmentation, or nevi. No pruritus, rash, lesions. Has bruise now over right eye, struck by boyfriend 1 week PTA. No history skin disease. Hair, no loss, change in texture. Nails, no change. Self-care. Stays in sun "as much as I can." No use of sunscreen. Goes to tanning beds at hair salon twice/week during winter.

Head. No unusually frequent or severe headaches, no head injury, dizziness, syncope, or vertigo.

Eyes. No difficulty with vision or double vision. No eye pain, inflammation, discharge, lesions. No history glaucoma or cataracts. Wears no corrective lenses.

Ears. No hearing loss or difficulty. No earaches, infections now or as child, no discharge, tinnitus, or vertigo. Self-care. No exposure to environmental noise, cleans ears with washcloth.

Nose. No discharge, has two to three colds per year, no sinus pain, nasal obstruction, epistaxis, or allergy.

Mouth and throat. No mouth pain, bleeding gums, toothache, sores or lesions in mouth, dysphagia, hoarseness, or sore throat. Has tonsils. Self-care. Brushes teeth twice/day, no flossing.

Neck. No pain, limitation of motion, lumps, or swollen glands.

Breast. No pain, lump, nipple discharge, rash, swelling, or trauma. No history breast disease in self, mother, or sister. No surgery. Self-care. Does not do breast self-examination.

Respiratory. No history of lung disease, no chest pain with breathing, wheezing, shortness of breath. Colds sometimes "go to my chest," treats with over-the-counter cough medicine and aspirin. Occasional early morning cough, nonproductive. Smokes cigarettes 2 PPD × 2 years, prior use 1 PPD × 4 years. Never tried to quit. Works in poorly ventilated tavern, "everybody smokes."

Cardiovascular. No chest pain, palpitation, cyanosis, fatigue, dyspnea with exertion, orthopnea, paroxysmal nocturnal dyspnea, nocturia, edema. No history of heart murmur, hypertension, coronary artery disease, or anemia.

Peripheral vascular. No pain, numbness or tingling, swelling in legs. No coldness, discoloration, varicose veins, infections, or ulcers. Legs are unequal in length as sequelae of accident age 12. Self-care. Usual work as cashier involves standing for 8-hour shifts, no support hose.

Gastrointestinal. Appetite good with no recent change. No food intolerance, heartburn, indigestion, pain in abdomen, nausea, or vomiting. No history of ulcers, liver or gallbladder disease, jaundice, appendicitis, or colitis. Bowel movement 1/day, soft, brown, no rectal bleeding or pain. Self-care. No use of vitamins, antacids, laxatives. Diet recall—see Functional Assessment.

Continued

Urinary. No dysuria, frequency, urgency, nocturia, hesitancy, or straining. No pain in flank, groin, suprapubic region. Urine colour yellow, no history kidney disease.

Genitalia. Menarche age 11. Last menstrual period April 18. Cycle usually q28d, duration 4 to 5 days, flow moderate, no dysmenorrhea. No vaginal itching or discharge, sores or lesions.

Sexual health. In relationship now that includes intercourse. This boyfriend has been her only sexual partner for 2 years, had one other partner before that. Uses birth control pills to prevent pregnancy, partner uses no condoms. Concerned that boyfriend may be having sex with other women but has not confronted him. Aware of no STI contact. Never been tested for AIDS. History of sexual abuse by father from ages 12 to 16 years, abuse did not include intercourse. Ellen is unwilling to discuss further at this time.

Musculoskeletal. No history of arthritis, gout. No joint pain, stiffness, swelling, deformity, limitation of motion. No muscle pain or weakness. Bone trauma at age 12, has sequela of unequal leg lengths, right leg shorter, walks with limp. Self-care. No walking or running for sport or exercise "because of leg." Able to stand as cashier. Uses lift pad in right shoe to equalize leg length.

Neurological. No history of seizure disorder, stroke, fainting. Has had blackouts with alcohol use. No weakness, tremor, paralysis, problems with coordination, difficulty speaking or swallowing. No numbness or tingling. Not aware of memory problem, nervousness or mood change, depression. Had counselling for sexual abuse in the past. Denies any suicidal ideation or intent during adolescent years or now.

Hematological. No bleeding problems in skin, excessive bruising. Not aware of exposure to toxins, never had blood transfusion, never used needles to shoot drugs.

Endocrine. Paternal grandmother with diabetes. No increase in hunger, thirst, or urination; no problems with hot or cold environments; no change in skin, appetite, or nervousness.

FUNCTIONAL ASSESSMENT

Self-concept. Graduated from high school. Trained "on-the-job" as bartender, also worked as cashier in tavern. Unemployed now, on social assistance, does not perceive she has enough money for daily living. Lives with older sister. Raised as Presbyterian, believes in God, does not attend church. Believes self to be "honest, dependable." Believes limitations are "smoking, weight, drinking."

Activity and exercise. Typical day: arises 9 AM, light chores or TV, spends day looking for work, running errands, with friends, bedtime at 11 PM. No sustained physical exercise. Believes self able to perform all ADLs; limp poses no problem in bathing, dressing, cooking, household tasks, mobility, driving a car, or work as cashier. No mobility aids. Hobbies are fishing, boating, snowmobiling, although currently has no finances to engage in most of these.

Sleep and rest. Bedtime 11 PM. Sleeps 8 to 9 hours. No sleep aids.

Nutrition. 24-hour recall: breakfast, none; lunch, bologna sandwich, chips, diet pop; dinner, hamburger, french fries, coffee; snacks, peanuts, pretzels, potato chips, "bar food." This menu is typical of most days. Eats lunch at home alone. Most dinners at fast-food restaurants or in tavern. Shares household grocery expenses and cooking chores with sister. No food intolerances.

Alcohol. See present illness. Denies use of street drugs. Cigarettes, smokes 2 PPD × 2 years, prior use 1 PPD × 4 years. Never tried to quit. Boyfriend smokes cigarettes.

Interpersonal relationships. Describes family life growing up as chaotic. Father physically abusive toward mother and sexually abusive toward Ellen. Parents divorced because of father's continual drinking. Few support systems currently. Estranged from mother, "didn't believe me about my father." Father estranged from entire family. Gets along "OK" with sister. Relationship with boyfriend chaotic, has hit her twice in the past. Ellen has never pressed legal charges. No close women friends. Most friends are "drinking buddies" at tavern.

Coping and stress management. Believes housing adequate, adequate heat and utilities, and neighbourhood safe. Believes home has no safety hazards. Does not use seat belts. No travel outside 100 km of home town.

Identifies current stresses to be drinking, legal problems with impaired driving offences, unemployment, financial worries. Considers her drinking to be problematic.

PERCEPTION OF HEALTH

Identifies alcohol as a health problem for herself, feels motivated for treatment. Never been interested in physical health and own body before, "Now I think it's time I learned." Expects healthcare professionals to "Help me with my drinking. I don't know beyond that." Expects to stay at this agency for 6 weeks, "Then, I don't know what."

MEASUREMENT

Height: 163 cm (5'4'') Weight: 68.6 kg (151 lb)
B/P: 142/100 right arm, sitting
140/96 right arm, lying
138/98 left arm, lying
Temp: 37°C   Pulse: 76, regular   Respirations: 16, unlaboured

General survey. Ellen K. is a 23-year-old female, not currently under the influence of alcohol or other drugs, who articulates clearly, ambulates without difficulty, and is in no distress.

HEAD-TO-TOE EXAMINATION

Skin. Uniformly tan-pink in colour, warm, dry, intact, turgor good. No lesions, birthmarks, edema. Resolving 2-cm yellow-green hematoma present over right eye, no swelling, ocular structures not involved. Hair, normal distribution and texture, no visible infestations. Nails, no clubbing, biting, or discolorations. Nail beds pink and firm with prompt capillary refill.

Head. Normocephalic, no lesions, lumps, scaling, parasites, or tenderness. Face, symmetrical, no weakness, no involuntary movements.

Eyes. Acuity by Snellen chart O.D. 20/20, O.S. 20/20−1. Visual fields full by confrontation. EOMs intact, no nystagmus. No ptosis, lid lag, discharge, or crusting. Corneal light reflex symmetrical, no strabismus. Conjunctivae clear. Sclera white, no lesion or redness. PERRLA. Fundi: discs flat with sharp margins. Vessels present in all quadrants without crossing defects. Background has even colour, no hemorrhage or exudates.

Ears. Pinna no mass, lesions, scaling, discharge, or tenderness to palpation. Canals clear. Tympanic membrane pearly grey, landmarks intact, no perforation. Whispered words heard bilaterally. Weber test—tone heard midline with lateralization. Rinne test—AC > BC and = bilaterally.

Nose. No deformities or tenderness to palpation. Nares patent. Mucosa pink, no lesions. Septum midline, no perforation. No sinus tenderness.

Mouth. Mucosa and gingivae pink, no lesions or bleeding. Right lower first molar missing, multiple dark spots on most teeth, gums receding on lower incisors. Tongue symmetrical, protrudes midline, no tremor. Pharynx pink, no exudate. Uvula rises midline on phonation. Tonsils 1+. Gag reflex present.

Neck. Neck supple with full ROM. Symmetrical, no masses, tenderness, lymphadenopathy. Trachea midline. Thyroid nonpalpable, not tender. Jugular veins flat at 45 degrees. Carotid arteries 2+ and = bilaterally, no bruits.

Spine and back. Normal spinal profile, no scoliosis. No tenderness over spine, no CVA tenderness.

Thorax and lungs. AP < transverse diameter. Chest expansion symmetrical. Tactile fremitus equal bilaterally. Lung fields resonant. Diaphragmatic excursion 4 and 5 cm bilaterally. Breath sounds diminished. Expiratory wheeze in posterior chest at both bases, scattered rhonchi in posterior chest at both bases, do not clear with coughing.

Breasts. Symmetrical; no retraction, discharge, or lesions. Contour and consistency firm and homogeneous. No masses or tenderness, no lymphadenopathy.

Heart. Precordium, no abnormal pulsations, no heaves. Apical impulse at fifth ICS in left MCL, no thrills. S1–S2 are not diminished or accentuated, no S3 or S4. Systolic murmur, grade ii/vi, loudest at left lower sternal border, no radiation, present supine and sitting.

Abdomen. Flat, symmetrical. Skin smooth with no lesions, scars, or striae. Bowel sounds present, no bruits. Tympany predominates in all quadrants. Liver span 7 cm in right MCL. Abdomen soft, no organomegaly, no masses or tenderness, no inguinal lymphadenopathy.

Extremities. Colour tan-pink, no redness, cyanosis, lesions other than surgical scar. Scar right lower leg, anterior, 28 cm × 2 cm wide, well healed. No edema, varicosities. No calf tenderness. All peripheral pulses present, 2+ and = bilaterally. Asymmetrical leg length, right leg 3 cm shorter than left.

Musculoskeletal. Temporomandibular joint no slipping or crepitation. Neck full ROM, no pain. Vertebral column no tenderness, no deformity or curvature. Full extension, lateral bending, rotation. Arms symmetrical, legs measure as above, extremities have full ROM, no pain or crepitation. Muscle strength, able to maintain flexion against resistance and without tenderness.

Continued

Documentation and Critical Thinking

Neurological. Mental status. Appearance, behaviour, speech appropriate. Alert and oriented to person, place, time. Thought coherent. Remote and recent memories intact. Cranial nerves II through XII intact. Sensory: pinprick, light touch, vibration intact. Stereognosis, able to identify key. Motor: no atrophy, weakness, or tremors. Gait has limp, able to tandem walk with shoes on. Negative Romberg's sign. Cerebellar, finger-to-nose smoothly intact. DTRs (see stick gram).

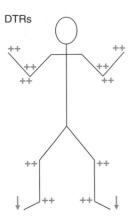

DTRs

Genitalia. External genitalia has no lesion, discharge. Internal genitalia: vaginal walls pink, no lesion. Cervix pink, nulliparous os, no lesions, small amount nonodorous clear discharge. Specimens for Pap test, GC/Chlamydia, trichomoniasis, moniliasis obtained. Swabbing mucosa with acetic acid shows no acetowhitening.

Bimanual, no pain on moving cervix, uterus midline, no enlargement, masses, or tenderness. Adnexa, ovaries not enlarged, no tenderness. Anus, no hemorrhoids, fissures, or lesions. Rectal wall intact, no masses or tenderness. Stool soft, brown; Hematest negative.

ASSESSMENT

Alcohol dependence, severe, with physiological dependence
Nicotine dependence with physiological dependence
Elevated blood pressure
Systolic heart murmur
Ineffective airway clearance R/T tracheobronchial secretions and obstruction
Right orbital contusion (resolving)
Risk for trauma
Self-care deficit: oral hygiene R/T lack of motivation
Deficient knowledge about alcoholism disease process, treatment options, support systems R/T lack of exposure
Deficient knowledge about balanced diet R/T lack of exposure and substance abuse
Dysfunctional family processes: alcoholism
Chronic low self-esteem R/T effects of alcoholism, sexual abuse, physical abuse

Reassessment of the Hospitalized Adult

Written by **Ian M. Camera**, MSN, ND, RN
Adapted by **Marian Luctkar-Flude**, RN, MScN

In a hospital setting, the patient does not require a complete head-to-toe physical examination during every 24-hour stay. The patient *does* require a consistent specialized examination that focuses on certain parameters at least every 8 hours. Note that some measurements, such as daily weights, abdominal girth, or the circumference of a limb, must be taken very carefully. The utility of such measurements depends entirely on the consistency of the procedure from nurse to nurse.

Also remember that many assessments must be conducted frequently throughout the course of a shift. This chapter outlines the initial assessment that will allow you to get to know your patient. As you perform this sequence, take note of anything that will need continuous monitoring, such as a blood pressure or pulse oximetry reading that is not what you expect, or breath sounds that suggest a difficult respiratory effort. If there is no protocol in place for a particular assessment situation, then decide for yourself how often you need to check on the person's status—it is very easy to be distracted by ringing bells and alarms as the shift progresses, but your own judgement about a patient's needs is just as important as any electronic alert or alarm.

The need for multiple assessments of each patient highlights the need for efficiency in the hospital setting. Your assessments must be thorough and accurate, yet you must be able to complete them rapidly without seeming hurried. The only solution to this paradox is practice. Remember that practising in a laboratory setting, with simulated patients or with classmates, may feel artificial but it is the quickest route to feeling confident in the presence of hospitalized patients.

The basic reassessment applies to adults in medical, surgical, and cardiac step-down care areas. Each assessment must then be customized to each adult, and the findings must be integrated into your complete knowledge base regarding the patient. This includes what you read in the chart, what you hear in report, and the results of any laboratory tests and diagnostic imaging that are available.

Sequence	Selected Photos

Assist the person into bed. The patient is in bed with the bed at a comfortable level for the examiner.

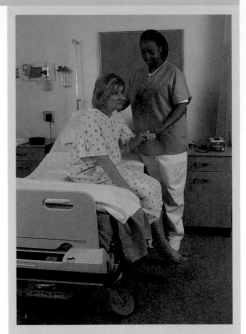

THE HEALTH HISTORY

On your way into the room, verify that any necessary markers or flags are in place at the doorway regarding such conditions as isolation precautions, latex allergies, or fall precautions. Once in the room, introduce yourself as the patient's nurse for the next 8 (or 12) hours. Make direct eye contact and do not allow yourself to be distracted by IV pumps or other equipment as you ask how he or she is feeling, how he or she spent the previous nursing shift, and whether he or she currently is having any pain or discomfort. Refer to what you have heard from the previous shift in the process of your own questioning—this alleviates the person's frustration with answering the same questions every time a new staff member walks through the door.

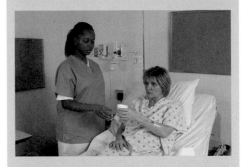

Offer water as a courtesy and note the data this gives you: the person's ability to hear, follow directions, cross the midline, and especially, ability to swallow. As you collect this and subsequent history, note data on general appearance. Complete your initial overview by verifying that the correct name band has been applied to the wrist.

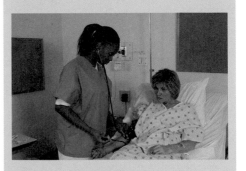

GENERAL APPEARANCE

1. Facial expression, appropriate to the situation
2. Body position, relaxed and comfortable or tense, in pain
3. Level of consciousness, alert and oriented, attentive to your questions, responds appropriately
4. Skin colour, even tone consistent with ethnocultural heritage
5. Nutritional status, weight appears in healthy range, even fat distribution, hydration appears healthy
6. Speech, articulation clear and understandable, pattern fluent and even, content appropriate
7. Hearing, responses and facial expression consistent with what you have said
8. Personal hygiene, ability to attend to hair, makeup, shaving

MEASUREMENT

1. Temperature
2. Pulse
3. Respiration
4. Blood pressure (note to avoid an arm because of surgery or venous access on that side)
5. Pulse oximetry (oxygen saturation)
6. Rate pain level on 0 to 10 scale, and note location of pain
7. Assess pain intensity on scale of 0 to 10 prior to and following administration of analgesics; note response in 15 minutes for IV administration and in 1 hour for oral administration

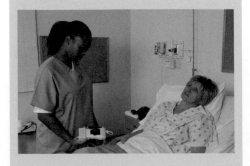

Objective Data

Sequence	Selected Photos

NEUROLOGICAL SYSTEM

1. Eyes open spontaneously to name
2. Motor response
3. Verbal response
4. Pupil size in millimetres and reaction, R and L
5. Muscle strength, R and L upper
6. Muscle strength, R and L lower
7. Any ptosis, facial droop
8. Sensation
9. Communication
10. Ability to swallow

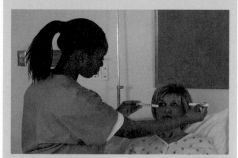

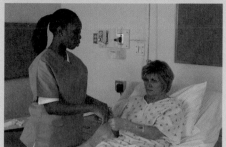

RESPIRATORY SYSTEM

1. Oxygen by mask, nasal prongs, check fitting
2. Note FiO_2
3. Respiratory effort
4. Auscultate breath sounds comparing side to side:
   Posterior lobes: left upper, right upper, left lower, right lower
   Note: If patient not able to sit up, have another nurse hold patient side to side
   Anterior lobes: right upper, left upper, right middle and lower, left lower
5. Cough and deep breathe; any mucus? Check colour and amount

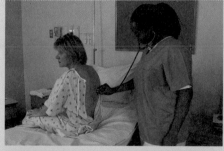

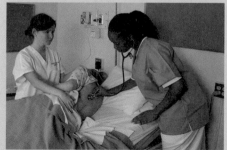

CARDIOVASCULAR SYSTEM

1. Auscultate rhythm at apex: regular, irregular?
2. Check apical pulse against radial pulse, noting perfusion of all beats.

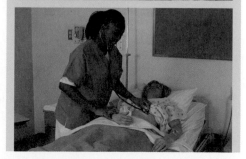

Objective Data

Sequence   **Selected Photos**

CARDIOVASCULAR SYSTEM—cont'd

3. Assess heart sounds in all auscultatory areas: first with diaphragm, repeat with bell.
4. Check capillary refill for prompt return.
5. Check pretibial edema.
6. Palpate posterior tibial pulse, right and left.
7. Palpate dorsalis pedis pulse, right and left.
   Note: Be prepared to assess pulses in the lower extremities by Doppler imaging, if you cannot find them by palpation.
8. Verify that the proper IV solution is hanging and flowing at the proper rate according to the physician's orders and your own assessment of the patient's needs.

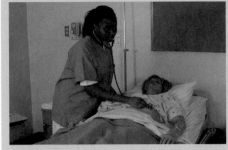

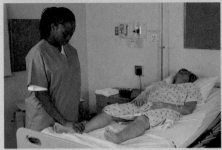

SKIN

1. Note skin colour, consistent with person's ethnocultural heritage.
2. Palpate skin temperature; expect warm and dry.
3. Pinch up a fold of skin under the clavicle or on the forearm to note mobility and turgor.
4. Note skin integrity, any lesions, and the condition of any dressings.
5. Complete any standardized scales used to quantify the risk of skin breakdown (see Braden Risk Assessment Scale in Appendix A).
6. Verify that any air loss or pressure loss surfaces being used are properly applied and operating at the correct settings.

ABDOMEN

1. Assess contour of abdomen: flat, rounded, protuberant.
2. Listen to bowel sounds in all four quadrants.
3. Check any tube placement for drainage and insertion site integrity.
4. Inquire whether passing flatus or stool.

GENITOURINARY

1. Inquire whether voiding regularly.
2. Check urine for colour, clarity.
3. If urine output is below the expected value, perform a bladder scan according to agency protocol. Is the problem associated with the production of urine or its retention?

Sequence	Selected Photos

ACTIVITY

1. Assist patient to sitting position, move to chair.
2. Note any assistance needed, how tolerates movement, distance walked to chair, ability to turn.
3. Note need for any ambulatory aid or equipment.
4. Complete any standardized scales used to quantify the patient's risk for falling.

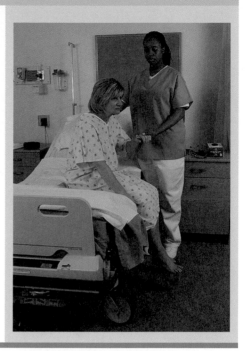

ELECTRONIC CHARTING

Charting in most hospitals is at least partially computerized. Although use of computers for charting can be intimidating at first, it has several advantages. First, for new clinicians, the structure imposed by the computerized database can serve as a prompt to guide them through a complete assessment. Second, it decreases the chances that you will waste time waiting to gain access to a paper chart, or searching for it when it is not in the proper location. Finally, charting in a computer system is rarely dependent on writing or typing in narrative form—check boxes and drop-down menus are much more common. If you avoid the temptation to write everything on paper first and learn to use all the functions programmed into the hospital's system, you will find that computer charting is faster than its paper equivalent.

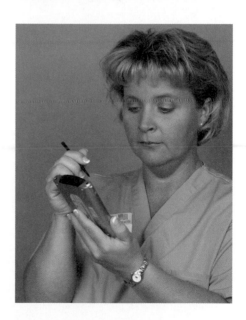

Objective Data

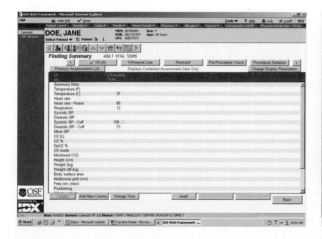

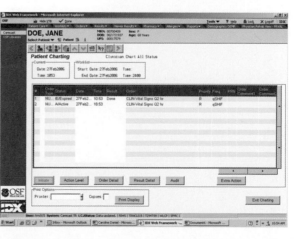

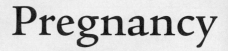

Chapter Twenty-Nine

Pregnancy

Written by **Deborah E. Swenson**, MSN, ARNP
Adapted by **Kim Campbell**, RM, RN, MN

Electronic Resources —————◆

On Evolve *evolve*

http://evolve.elsevier.com/Canada/Jarvis/examination/
- Interactive Case Studies
- Physical Examination Audio and Printable Summaries
- Bedside Assessment Summary Checklists
- Complete Physical Examination Form
- Nursing Diagnoses Boxes
- Health Promotion Guides
- Quick Assessments for 20 Common Conditions
- Multiple Choice Review Questions
- Chapter Objectives
- Appendices
- Weblinks

On the Companion CD

- Interactive Case Studies with Heart and Lung Sounds
- Health Promotion Guides
- Quick Assessments for 20 Common Conditions
- Head-to-Toe Physical Examination Video Clips

STRUCTURE AND FUNCTION

PREGNANCY AND THE ENDOCRINE PLACENTA

The first day of the menses is day 1 of the menstrual cycle. For the first 14 days of the cycle, one or more follicles in the ovary develop and mature. One follicle grows faster than the others, and on day 14 of the menstrual cycle, this dominant follicle ruptures and ovulation occurs. If the ovum meets viable sperm, fertilization occurs somewhere in the oviduct (fallopian tube). The remaining cells in the follicle form the **corpus luteum,** or "yellow body," which makes important hormones. Chief among these is progesterone, which prevents the sloughing of the endometrial wall, ensuring a rich vascular network into which the fertilized ovum will implant itself.

The fertilized ovum, now called the **blastocyst,** continues to divide, differentiate, and grow rapidly. Specialized cells in the blastocyst produce human chorionic gonadotropin (hCG), which stimulates the corpus luteum to continue making progesterone. Between days 20 and 24, the blastocyst implants itself into the wall of the uterus, which may cause a small amount of vaginal bleeding. A specialized layer of cells around the blastocyst becomes the **placenta.** The placenta starts to produce progesterone to support the pregnancy at 7 weeks and takes over this function completely from the corpus luteum at about 10 weeks.

The placenta functions as an endocrine organ and produces several hormones. These hormones help in the growth and maintenance of the fetus, and they direct changes in the woman's body in preparation for birth and lactation. The hCG stimulates the rise in progesterone during pregnancy. Progesterone maintains the endometrium around the fetus, increases the alveoli in the breast, and keeps the uterus in a quiescent state. Estrogen stimulates the duct formation in the breast, increases the weight of the uterus, and increases certain receptors in the uterus that are important at birth.

The average length of pregnancy is 280 days from the first day of the last menstrual period (LMP), which is equal to 40 weeks, 10 lunar months, or 9 calendar months. Note that this includes the 2 weeks when the follicle was maturing but before conception actually occurred. Pregnancy is divided into three trimesters: (1) the first 12 weeks, (2) from 13 to 27 weeks, and (3) from 28 weeks to delivery.

Any woman who has ever been pregnant, regardless of the outcome, is called a gravida (G). In the first pregnancy she is a primigravida. With subsequent pregnancies she becomes a multigravida. Parity (P) refers to a pregnancy that has led to birth at ≥20 weeks' gestation (often referred to as the age of viability). A nulliparous woman is pregnant for the first time (G1 P0). She becomes a primipara after she has given birth at ≥20 weeks' gestation once (G1 P1). A multipara has given birth more than once (G ≥2 P ≥2). Preterm labour (PTL) or preterm birth (PTB) occurs at ≥20 but <37 weeks' gestation. Pregnancy loss at <20 weeks is an abortion (A) that can be spontaneous (miscarriage) or induced (therapeutic). It is common to describe pregnancy history as G (gravida), T (term), P (preterm), A (abortion), L (living children). It may be written G6 T3 P0 A2 L3 if a woman is now pregnant for the sixth time, she has given birth three times at ≥37 weeks' gestation, has had one miscarriage and one therapeutic abortion, and has three living children.

CHANGES DURING NORMAL PREGNANCY

Pregnancy is diagnosed by three types of signs and symptoms. **Presumptive signs** are those the woman experiences, such as amenorrhea, breast tenderness, nausea, fatigue, and increased urinary frequency. **Probable signs** are those detected by the examiner, such as an enlarged uterus. **Positive signs** of pregnancy are those that are direct evidence of the fetus, such as the auscultation of fetal heart tones (FHTs) or positive cardiac activity detected using ultrasound (US).

First Trimester

Conception occurs on approximately the fourteenth day of the menstrual cycle. The blastocyst (developing fertilized ovum) implants itself in the uterus 6 to 10 days after conception, sometimes accompanied by a small amount of painless bleeding, which may be interpreted as a menstrual period (Cunningham et al., 2001). The serum hCG becomes positive after implantation when it is first detectable in maternal serum at approximately 8 to 11 days after conception.

The following menstrual period is missed. At the time of the missed menses, hCG can be detected in the urine. Breast tingling and tenderness begin as the rising estrogen levels promote mammary growth and development of the ductal system; progesterone stimulates the alveolar system as well as the mammary growth. Chorionic somatomammotropin (also called human placental lactogen, or hPL), also produced by the placenta, stimulates breast growth and exerts lactogenic properties (Varney, 2004). More than half of all pregnant women experience nausea and vomiting. The cause is unclear but may involve the hormonal changes of pregnancy, low blood sugar, gastric overloading, slowed peristalsis, an enlarging uterus, and emotional factors. Fatigue is common and may be related to the initial fall in metabolic rate that occurs in early pregnancy (Varney, 2004).

Estrogen, and possibly progesterone, cause hypertrophy of the uterine muscle cells, and uterine blood vessels and lymphatics enlarge. The uterus becomes globular in shape, softens, and flexes easily over the cervix (**Hegar's sign**). This causes compression of the bladder, which results in urinary frequency. Increased vascularity, congestion, and edema cause the cervix to soften (**Goodell's sign**) and become bluish purple (**Chadwick's sign**).

Early first-trimester blood pressures (BPs) reflect pre-pregnancy values. In the seventh gestational week, BP begins to drop until mid-pregnancy as a result of falling peripheral vascular resistance. The BP gradually returns to the nonpregnant baseline by term. Systemic vascular resistance decreases from the vasodilatory effect of progesterone and prostaglandins and possibly because of the low resistance of the placental bed (Creasy and Resnick, 2004).

At the end of 9 weeks, the embryonic period ends, and the fetal period begins, at which time major structures are present (Varney, 2004). FHTs can be heard using Doppler US between 9 and 12 weeks. The uterus may be palpated just above the symphysis pubis at about 12 weeks. See Fig. 29-1 for the growth of the uterine fundus during the first trimester.

Second Trimester

By weeks 12 to 16, the nausea, vomiting, fatigue, and urinary frequency of the first trimester decrease. The woman recognizes fetal movement ("quickening") at approximately 18 to 20 weeks (the multigravida earlier). As breast enlargement continues, the veins of the breast enlarge and are more visible through the skin of light-skinned women. **Colostrum,** or first milk, is yellow and contains more minerals and protein but less sugar and fat than mature milk. Colostrum is rich in antibodies, which protect the newborn during the first weeks of life (Cunningham et al., 2001). Colostrum may be expressed or leak from the breast during pregnancy.

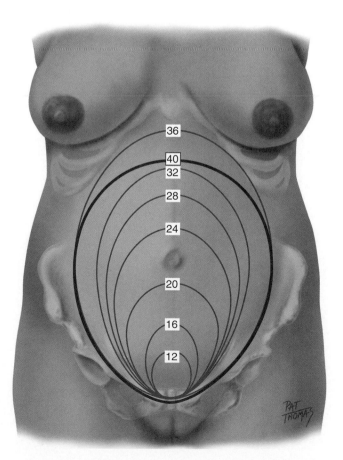

HEIGHT OF FUNDUS AT WEEKS OF GESTATION

Fig. 29-1

The areola and nipples darken, it is thought, because estrogen and progesterone have a melanocyte-stimulating effect, and melanocyte-stimulating hormone levels escalate from the second month of pregnancy until delivery. For the same reason, the midline of the abdominal skin becomes pigmented and is called the **linea nigra.** You may note **striae gravidarum** ("stretch marks") on the breast, abdomen, and areas where weight gain has occured.

During the second trimester, systolic BP may be 2 to 8 mm Hg lower and diastolic BP 5 to 15 mm Hg lower than prepregnancy levels (Cunningham et al., 2001). This drop is most pronounced at 20 weeks and may cause dizziness and faintness, particularly after rising quickly. Stomach displacement due to the enlarging uterus and the altered esophageal sphincter and gastric tone caused by progesterone predispose the woman to heartburn. Intestines are also displaced by the growing uterus, and tone and motility are decreased because of the action of progesterone, often causing constipation. The gallbladder, possibly resulting from the action of progesterone on its smooth muscle, empties sluggishly and may become distended. The stasis of bile, together with the increased cholesterol saturation of pregnancy, predisposes some women to gallstone formation.

Progesterone and, to a lesser degree, estrogen cause increased respiratory effort during pregnancy by increasing tidal volume. Hemoglobin, and therefore oxygen-carrying capacity, also increases. Increased tidal volume causes a slight drop in partial pressure of arterial carbon dioxide ($PaCO_2$), causing the woman to occasionally have dyspnea (Cunningham et al., 2001).

The high level of estrogen during pregnancy causes an increase in the major thyroxine transport protein, thyroxine-binding globulin. Several thyroid-stimulating factors of placental origin are produced. The thyroid gland enlarges as a result of hyperplasia and increased vascularity. Thyroid function plays a vital role in maternal–fetal morbidity and mortality. Maternal hypothyroidism increases the risk of intrauterine fetal death, pre-eclampsia, low birth weight, spontaneous miscarriage, and abruptio placentae (Smallridge, 2001). Even mild maternal hypothyroidism adversely effects the fetus, leading to lower IQ (Haddow et al., 1999).

Cutaneous blood flow is augmented during pregnancy caused by decreased vascular resistance, presumably helping to dissipate heat generated by increased metabolism. Gums may hypertrophy and bleed easily. This condition is called **gingivitis** or **epulis of pregnancy,** and it occurs as a result of growth of the capillaries of the gums (Cunningham et al., 2001). For the same reason, nosebleeds may occur more frequently than usual. Pregnant women with periodontal disease, a chronic local oral infection, are at risk for PTB. Untreated, this may lead to a systemic infection that affects the maternal levels of prostaglandin E_2 (PGE-2) (Boggess, 2003).

FHTs are audible by fetoscope (as opposed to Doppler imaging) at approximately 17 to 19 weeks. The fetal outline is palpable through the abdominal wall at approximately 20 weeks. See Fig. 29-1 for the growth of the uterine fundus during the second trimester.

Third Trimester

Blood volume, which increased rapidly during the second trimester, peaks in the middle of the third trimester at approximately 45% greater than the pre-pregnancy level and plateaus thereafter. This volume is greater in multiple gestations (Creasy and Resnick, 2004). Erythrocyte mass increases by 20 to 30% (caused by an increase in erythropoiesis, mediated by progesterone, estrogen, and placental chorionic somatomammotropin). However, plasma volume increases slightly more, causing a slight hemodilution and a small drop in hematocrit. BP slowly rises again to approximately the pre-pregnant level (Cunningham et al., 2001).

Uterine enlargement causes the diaphragm to rise and the shape of the rib cage to widen at the base. Decreased space for lung expansion may cause a sense of shortness of breath. The rising diaphragm displaces the heart up and to the left. Cardiac output, stroke volume, and force of contraction are increased. The pulse rate rises 15 to 20 beats per minute (Creasy and Resnick, 2004). Because of the increase in blood volume, a functional systolic murmur, grade ii/iv or less, can be heard in more than 95% of pregnant women (Creasy and Resnick, 2004).

Edema of the lower extremities may occur as a result of the enlarging fetus impeding venous return, and from lower colloid osmotic pressure. The edema worsens with dependency, such as prolonged standing. Varicosities, which have a familial tendency, may form or enlarge from progesterone-induced vascular relaxation. Also causing varicosities is the engorgement caused by the weight of the full uterus compressing the inferior vena cava and the vessels of the pelvic area, resulting in venous congestion in the legs, vulva, and rectum. Hemorrhoids are varicosities of the rectum that are worsened by constipation that is caused by relaxation of the large bowel by progesterone.

Progressive lordosis (an inward curvature of the lumbar spine) occurs to compensate for the shifting centre of balance caused by the anteriorly enlarging uterus, predisposing the woman to backaches. Slumping of the shoulders and anterior flexion of the neck from the increasing weight of the breasts may cause aching and numbness of the arms and hands as a result of compression of the median and ulnar nerves in the arm (Varney, 2004), commonly referred to as carpal tunnel syndrome.

Approximately 2 weeks before going into labour, the primigravida experiences engagement (also called "lightening" or "dropping"), when the fetal head moves down into the pelvis. Symptoms include a lower-appearing and smaller-measuring fundus, urinary frequency, increased vaginal secretions from increased pelvic congestion, and increased lung capacity. In the multigravida, the fetus may move down at any time in late pregnancy or often not until labour. The cervix, in preparation for labour, begins to thin (efface) and open (dilate). A thick **mucus plug,** formed in the cervix as a mechanical barrier during pregnancy, is expelled at variable times before or during labour. Between 37 and 42 weeks, the pregnancy is considered full term. After 42 weeks, the pregnancy is considered post-term.

Determining Gestational Age

The expected date of birth, or EDB (also known as expected date of delivery, or EDD), occurs 266 days after conception or 280 days (40 weeks) after the first day of the LMP. The LMP can only be reliable to determine EDB with a history of spontaneous regular 28- to 30-day cycles with normal flow and duration. Implantation of the fertilized egg can cause some light bleeding and may be wrongly noted as the LMP. The due date may be calculated by **Nägele's rule,** by adding 7 days to the LMP and subtracting 3 months. Pregnancy wheels or calculators can also be used (Fig. 29-2). On the wheel, move day 1 of the LMP on the outer wheel to align with the LMP line on the inner wheel. The EDB falls on the 40-week mark at the corresponding date. Gestational age is identified by finding the corresponding date on the wheel. Because Nägele's rule and the pregnancy wheels are based upon regular 28-day cycles, adjustments must be made for longer or shorter menstrual cycles. Accurate history of coitus, ovulation, and fertility treatments, combined with physical findings (pelvic and bimanual, auscultation of the fetal heart rate (FHR), beta human chorionic gonadotropin (β-hCG) levels, and perceived fetal movement) aid in estimation of due date. The most reliable method of dating a pregnancy in the absence of an excellent history is first trimester ultrasound. (See Table 29-4 on p. 850 for notes on inconsistencies between fetal size and dates.)

Weight Gain During Pregnancy

The amount of weight gained by term takes into account fetal weight, amniotic fluid, placenta, increased uterine size, increased blood volume, increased extravascular fluid, maternal fat

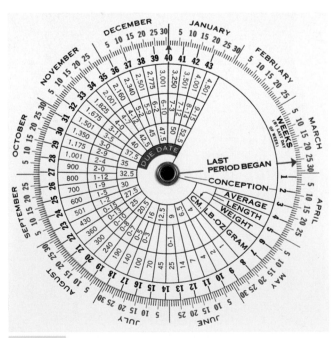

Fig. 29-2

stores, and increased breast size. Weight gain during pregnancy reflects that in both the mother and fetus and is approximately 62% water gain, 30% fat gain, and 8% protein. Approximately 25% of the total gain is attributed to the fetus, 11% to the placenta and amniotic fluid, and the remainder to the mother (Blackburn, 2002). A healthy outcome may be expected within a great range of weight gain (Cunningham et al., 2001), as indicated in Table 29-1.

DEVELOPMENTAL CARE

In industrialized countries, the risks for the pregnant adolescent are largely psychosocial. This young woman is at risk for the downward spiral of poverty beginning with an incomplete education and failure to limit family size and continuing with failure to establish a vocation and become independent. She may be unprepared emotionally to be a mother. Her social situation may be stressful. She may not have the support of her family, her partner, or his family. Medical risks for the pregnant adolescent are generally related to poverty, inadequate nutrition, substance abuse, and sometimes sexually transmitted infections (STIs), poor health before pregnancy, and emotional and physical abuse from her partner.

The adolescent is also at risk for pre-eclampsia and for a low-birth-weight infant, and it is unclear whether this is due to biological or social factors (Cunningham et al., 2001). The adolescent, for social reasons, often seeks health care later, though early prenatal care has been shown to provide optimal management. In developing countries, maternal mortality for pregnant teenagers is a major concern because of hypertension, embolism, ectopic pregnancy, and complications from illegal abortions (Cunningham et al., 2001).

More women are delaying pregnancy. Births among women of "advanced maternal age" of ≥35 years more than doubled between 1978 and 2000 (March of Dimes, 2002). Fertility declines as women age, in part due to a decrease in both viable eggs and ovulation as well as other conditions including endometriosis, early-onset menopause, and an increase in pregnancy loss. Pregnancy in women of advanced maternal age is related to an increase in congenital anomalies. Down syndrome (trisomy 21) increases from one in 1250 at 25 years to one in 365 at 35 years; one in 109 at 40 years; and one in 32 at 45 years (March of Dimes, 2002).

Women of advanced age are more likely to have chronic health conditions such as hypertension, diabetes, and obesity that further complicate any pregnancy (Cunningham et al., 2001). Hypertension and diabetes are associated with intrauterine growth retardation (IUGR) and pre-eclampsia, which, in turn, are associated with oligohydramnios, placental abruption, and premature birth. Older women are also more likely to experience multiple pregnancy and complications including Caesarean delivery and, although rare in Canada, maternal death.

CULTURAL AND SOCIAL CONSIDERATIONS

Pregnancy is a state of health; however, some complications of pregnancy occur more frequently in particular groups. In Canada, immigration has resulted in a complex mix of hereditary and genetic factors that may not always be discernible. Certain population groups are known to have an increased risk for carrying particular genetic disorders (Society of Obstetricians and Gynaecologists of Canada [SOGC], 2001a). For example, mutations for hemoglobinopathies (e.g., sickle cell anemia, β-thalassemia, α-thalassemia) are common among people whose ancestors come from areas where malaria is endemic, including Africa, the Mediterranean basin, the Middle East, the Indian subcontinent, Southeast Asia, and southern China. In practice, it has been recommended that everyone whose ancestors do not come from northern Europe should be considered at high risk for these genetically linked disorders. The carrier frequency for Tay-Sachs disease, another genetic disorder, is one in 30 among Ashkenazi Jews and one in 14 among French Canadians in Eastern Quebec. The frequency outside Eastern Quebec, however, is much lower (one in 41 to one in 98). Pregnancy and breastfeeding outcomes are also significantly affected by the social determinants of health, particularly among women with lower educational levels, low income, and diminished social support systems.

All families, regardless of ethnocultural background, recognize the birth of a child as a unique and significant moment for women, families, and communities. It marks a psychological, social, and spiritual moment in people's lives. Complex and important rituals, customs, and beliefs are integrated into this experience. The spiritual practices and beliefs that are the fabric of women's lives are unique to each woman and her family. Using a relational approach to nursing (see Ch. 1) will enable you to provide compassionate care in a culturally safe way as women deal with emotionally charged issues such as sexuality, relationships, contraception, maternal weight gain, and, in some cases, therapeutic abortion. You may begin by inquiring whether the woman or her significant other have any special requests. Sensitivity and dialogue that communicate respect for people's preferences and differences are essential components of developing a rapport and will enable the woman and her family to share concerns as they develop. Use your skill to understand such preferences within a sociocultural context and accept rather than judge

TABLE 29-1	Guidelines for Gestational Weight Gain Ranges	
BMI Category*	**Recommended Total Gain**	
	Kilograms	Pounds
BMI <20	12.5–18.0	28–40
BMI 20–27	11.5–16.0	25–35
BMI >27	7.0–11.5	15–25

*Canadian body mass index (BMI) categories for healthy weights, established in 1988 by Health Canada, correspond closely, although not exactly, to the BMI categories used by the United States Institute of Medicine (IOM). These guidelines do not apply to multiple gestations.

the person. Whenever safe and possible, respect such wishes. This enhances the success of childbirth in its psychological and social dimensions.

Safe Motherhood: Global Pregnancy Outcomes

The World Health Organization (WHO) defines **maternal death** as any death that occurs in pregnancy or within 42 days after termination of any pregnancy. It must be a direct or indirect result of the pregnancy or any condition aggravated by the pregnancy. It does not include deaths that result from acciden-tal or incidental causes. The **maternal mortality rate** (MMR) is the number of maternal deaths per 100,000 live births. The MMR represents the risk of dying a pregnant woman faces with each pregnancy. In 2005, WHO estimated there were 536,000 maternal deaths in the world. Developing nations account for 99% of these deaths. In 2005, Canada had an MMR of seven per 100,000 (WHO, 2007). In contrast, women in the developed world have a lifetime risk of one in 7300 (WHO, 2007). Over 80% of maternal deaths worldwide are due to hemorrhage, sepsis, unsafe abortion, obstructed labour, and pregnancy-induced hypertension (United Nations Population Fund, 2001).

SUBJECTIVE DATA

1. Menstrual history
2. Gynecological history
3. Obstetrical history

4. Current pregnancy
5. Medical history
6. Family history

7. Review of systems
8. Nutritional history
9. Environment and hazards

Examiner Asks	Rationale
1. Menstrual history • When was the first day of your last menstrual period that was normal in timing? Premenstrual symptoms, length, amount of flow, cramping? • Number of days in cycle? • Age at menarche?	Using Nägele's rule, calculate the EDB with this date. Using a pregnancy wheel, determine the current number of weeks of gestation.
2. Gynecological history • Ever had surgery of the cervix? Uterus?	Cervical surgery may affect the integrity of the cervix during pregnancy and, during labour, may impede cervical dilation. Uterine surgery increases risk for cervical insufficiency and uterine rupture during pregnancy and labour.
• Any known history of or exposure to genital herpes?	Onset during pregnancy is potentially *teratogenic* (i.e., causing physical defects in the developing fetus) and a lesion at time of delivery precludes vaginal birth.
• When your mother was pregnant with you, did she ever take a drug called diethylstilbestrol (DES)? (DES was a synthetic nonsteroidal estrogen given to pregnant women between 1948 and 1971 in an attempt to prevent various pregnancy-related complications.)	Prenatal exposure to DES may cause vaginal, cervical, or uterine abnormalities in the female fetus, which may increase the risk of spontaneous abortion or affect the integrity of the cervix during pregnancy.
• Papanicolaou (Pap) test: When was your last one? Any history of abnormality? If so, when? Have you ever had a colposcopy?	Because more women delay child-bearing, there may be an increase in diagnosing gynecological cancers during pregnancy. Approximately one third of recorded maternal deaths are the result of a coexisting malignancy (Gabbe et al., 2002).

Examiner Asks	Rationale
• Any history of infertility, fibroids, or uterine abnormalities?	May increase risk for ectopic pregnancy, miscarriage, PTL/PTB.
• Any history of gonorrhea, chlamydia, syphilis, trichomoniasis, pelvic inflammatory disease (PID)?	STIs increase the risk of premature rupture of membranes, PTL/PTB, postpartum maternal and fetal infections.
• Do you or your partner have more than one sexual partner?	Increases the risk of STIs and human immunodeficiency virus (HIV) infection.
• Were you a preterm infant?	Women who themselves were preterm infants are at increased risk for PTB.
• Have you had a mammogram, breast biopsy, breast implants, lumpectomy, or mastectomy?	Approximately 2 to 3% of all breast cancers in women under age 40 years occur concurrently with pregnancy or lactation (Gabbe et al., 2004).

3. Obstetrical history

• In earlier pregnancies, any history of hypertension, pre-eclampsia, eclampsia, HELLP (hemolysis, elevated liver enzymes, low platelet count) syndrome, diabetes, β-hemolytic *Streptococcus* infection, IUGR, congenital anomalies, premature labour, postpartum hemorrhage, or postpartum depression?

The woman who has experienced these complications in the past is at increased risk for them in subsequent pregnancies.

• How did you experience previous pregnancies and births?

The subjective quality of previous experiences has an impact on emotions regarding the current pregnancy.

• Ever had a Caesarean section? If so, what was the indication? At how many centimetres of dilation, if any, was the surgery performed? What type of uterine incision was made? (Confirming records of this surgery must be obtained.) Have you ever had a vaginal birth after a Caesarean section (VBAC)?

The woman who has had surgery on her uterus is at risk for uterine rupture during pregnancy and labour. The vertical, or "classic," incision carries a higher risk of rupture and mandates that all subsequent births be by Caesarean section. The "low transverse" or horizontal incision carries a low risk, and subsequent births may be vaginal. Note that the direction of the scar does not indicate how the uterus was incised.

• Number of times pregnant? Number of term or preterm births? Number of spontaneous miscarriages, elective abortions, or ectopic pregnancies? Any fetal or neonatal deaths?

Establishing an obstetrical history is beneficial in providing care during the current pregnancy.

• Any history of infertility? Have you used assisted reproductive technology?

In the case of donor eggs, the age of the egg donor is used in calculating genetic testing.

• Any history of preterm labour or preterm rupture of membranes?

This woman requires close observation during the current pregnancy. Previous PTB is associated with recurrence.

• Have you been told you have cervical insufficiency? Incompetency? Have you had a cervical cerclage placed in previous pregnancies?

• Tell me the gestational ages and weights of your babies at birth.

A small infant may indicate prematurity or IUGR—complications that are repeatable. A large infant may indicate GDM (also repeatable). Conversely, birth weights of other children may indicate a "constitutional size" (e.g., the tendency of a couple to conceive smaller but normal children). Also, the woman's pelvis

Subjective Data

Subjective Data

Examiner Asks	Rationale
	has been "proven" to the weight of the largest baby born vaginally; bear this number in mind as labour begins, estimating and comparing the weight of the baby about to be born.
• Have you breastfed before? How was that experience for you?	The woman's experience and knowledge base will shape your teaching and support.
• Any history of mastitis?	A poor or painful previous experience increases the need for breastfeeding support after this pregnancy.
4. Current pregnancy. (Having calculated the current number of weeks of gestation, you can reassess the probable accuracy of that date when eliciting the following history.)	
• What method of contraceptive did you use most recently, and when did you discontinue it?	Recent use of birth control pills or other hormonal contraceptives may cause delayed ovulation and irregular menses—consider when establishing the EDB. An intrauterine device (IUD) that is still in place requires removal; it threatens the pregnancy. Also, this raises question whether pregnancy was planned.
• Was the pregnancy planned? How do you feel about it?	Even a planned pregnancy represents loss for the woman—perhaps a loss of freedom, compromise of goals, loss of time with other children or partner. The first trimester is known as the "trimester of ambivalence," and encouraging acceptance and expression of these feelings facilitates resolution.
• How does the baby's father feel about the pregnancy? Other family members?	Women may need assistance in gathering support groups. Inviting significant others to future visits affirms their importance and supports involvement.
• Experienced any vaginal bleeding? When? How much? What colour? Accompanied by any pain? Determine Rh status.	Vaginal bleeding may indicate threatened abortion, cervicitis, or other complications and must be investigated. Rh-negative women should receive Rh(D) immune globulin within 72 hrs of an antepartum bleed, unless the father of the baby is Rh-negative.
• Are you experiencing any nausea or vomiting?	Nausea and vomiting are symptoms of pregnancy that usually begin between weeks 4 and 5, peak between weeks 8 and 12, and resolve between weeks 14 and 16.
• Experienced abdominal pain? When? Where in your abdomen? Accompanied by vaginal bleeding?	The most common causes of abdominal pain in early pregnancy are spontaneous abortion, ectopic pregnancy, urinary tract infection (UTI), and round ligament discomfort. Late pregnancy causes are premature labour, placental abruption, and HELLP syndrome (see Table 29-3, p. 849). Also consider other medical and surgical causes for abdominal pain.

Examiner Asks	Rationale
• Experienced any illnesses since being pregnant? Any recent fever(s), unexplained rash, or infections?	Helps establish any possible exposures to infectious agents.
• Had any X-rays? Taken any medications? Used any recreational drugs or alcohol? Do you smoke cigarettes?	Discuss the potential effect of any teratogenic exposure. Refer for expert counselling if necessary.
• Experiencing any vision changes such as the new onset of blurred vision or spots before your eyes?	In the third trimester, this may be a sign of pre-eclampsia. Evaluate for other signs and symptoms of pre-eclampsia (see Table 29-3, p. 849).
• Experiencing any edema? Where, and under what circumstances?	In the third trimester, differentiate the normal weight-dependent edema of pregnancy from the edema of pre-eclampsia.
• Any frequency, or burning with urination? Any blood in your urine? Do you void in small amounts? Any history of UTIs, pyelonephritis, or kidney stones?	Differentiate the normal urinary frequency of the first and third trimesters from UTI, for which pregnant women are at increased risk. Confirm by urinalysis. UTIs increase the rate of PTB.
• Any vaginal burning or itching? Any foul-smelling or coloured discharge?	Rule out vaginal infection. If symptoms exist, add cultures or a wet mount to the pelvic examination. Discuss partner treatment if necessary. Explain the normal increase in vaginal secretions during pregnancy.
• Do you have cats in the home?	Explain toxoplasmosis, a teratogenic disease transmitted through cat feces. To avoid exposure, another person should empty cat litter at frequent intervals.
• What date did you first feel the baby move?	This sign is compared with the EDB to evaluate the accuracy of that date. Tell the woman who has not felt movement to note and report that event at the following prenatal visit.
• How does the baby move on a daily basis?	Fetal movement is an excellent indicator of fetal health. Clinicians assign women to count fetal movements starting at 28 weeks of pregnancy.
• Do you plan to breastfeed this baby?	Arrange for reading materials, classes, and other support for the woman who is breastfeeding for the first time or for the woman with an unsuccessful earlier experience.
5. Medical history	
• Do you have allergies to medications or foods? If so, what type of reaction?	Prevents prescription errors.
• What is your blood group and type?	Rh-negative women should be identified early in pregnancy so that RhD immune globulin can be given to prevent antibody stimulation in the event of an ante, intra-, or postpartum uptake of fetal blood.
• Any personal or family history of cancer?	Advanced maternal age increases risk of breast, ovarian, uterine, and colon cancers.
• Do you have a history of asthma? If yes, have you ever been intubated?	Poor control and frequent exacerbations of asthma during pregnancy may result in maternal hypoxia and decrease in fetal oxygenation.

Subjective Data

Subjective Data

Examiner Asks	Rationale
• Ever had German measles (rubella)?	This mild childhood disease is highly teratogenic, especially during the first trimester. Instruct the woman who has not had rubella to avoid small children who are ill. Check immunity status in the serum prenatal panel. The nonimmune woman will be offered immunization after delivery.
• Ever had chicken pox?	Rarely, varicella causes congenital anomalies. The nonimmune woman should avoid exposure. Offer postpartum immunization.
• Any injury to the back or another weight-bearing part?	The localized and overall weight gain of pregnancy and the joint-softening property of progesterone causes lordosis and will aggravate such injuries with increasing gestational age.
• Have you been tested for HIV? When? What was the result? Ever had a blood transfusion? Used intravenous drugs? Had a sexual partner with HIV risk? Are you and your partner both monogamous?	Address HIV status to promote the health of the gravida and to decrease the risk of transmission of the virus across the placenta to the fetus. Breastfeeding is contraindicated in the HIV-positive mother because the virus is present in the breast milk. Educate the gravida who engages in high-risk activities.
• Do you smoke cigarettes? How many? For how many years? Ever tried to quit? Drink any alcohol? How many times per week? Use any street drugs?	Explain the danger of using these substances during pregnancy. Smoking increases the risk of ectopic pregnancy, spontaneous abortion, low birth weight, prematurity, preterm rupture of membranes, pregnancy-induced hypertension, placental abruption, and sudden infant death syndrome. Alcohol increases the risk to the fetus of fetal alcohol syndrome (see Table 13-3, p. 293). Cocaine use during pregnancy is associated with congenital anomalies, a fourfold increased risk for abruptio placentae and the risk of fetal addiction. Narcotic-addicted infants may have developmental delays or behavioural disturbances (Cunningham et al., 2001). Refer to a counselling or support program and periodic toxicology screening. Refer patient to a smoking cessation program.
• Do you take any prescribed, over-the-counter, or herbal medications?	Screen all medications to establish safety during pregnancy.
• Do you participate in a regular exercise program? What type?	Regular exercise during pregnancy may reduce risk for pregnancy-induced hypertension and will help control weight gain.
6. Family history.	
• Anyone in your family have hypertension?	Increases the risk of chronic hypertension and of pre-eclampsia.
• Diabetes? If so, of juvenile or adult-onset? Insulin dependent?	A first-degree relative with type 2 diabetes increases the risk of GDM. Counsel on risk and offer nutrition and exercise program, plus screening.
• Mental illness?	Increases risk for postpartum depression (Cunningham et al., 2001).

Examiner Asks	Rationale
• Kidney disease?	Increases risk for renal disease, hypertension, and pre-eclampsia.
• Fraternal twins?	The tendency to ovulate twice in one month is familial, and thus the incidence of twinning is increased.
• Anyone in your family, or in the family of the baby's father, had congenital anomalies?	Some anomalies, such as heart conditions, are familial. Offer genetic counselling if needed.
• Are you of Mediterranean descent? Of African descent? Of Ashkenazi Jewish descent? Of Irish descent?	Increased risk for β-thalassemia. Increased risk for sickle-cell anemia. Increased risk for Tay-Sachs disease. Increased risk for spinal malformations.

7. Review of systems

Examiner Asks	Rationale
• Your weight before pregnancy?	Baseline needed to evaluate changes.
• Wear glasses?	A transient change in vision correction may occur during pregnancy.
• When did you last see the dentist? Need any dental work?	Gums may be puffy and bleed easily during pregnancy, predisposing to caries. Poor dental hygiene can lead to PTB, low-birth-weight babies, and neonatal death. Encourage dental hygiene. Suggest that any dental work be done during the second trimester and that the dentist be notified that the patient is pregnant.
• Been exposed to tuberculosis (TB) or had a positive tuberculin test or chest X-ray?	Consider TB screening with the tuberculin skin test.
• Any cardiovascular disease, such as vascular disease, or disease of a heart valve?	The woman with cardiac disease who becomes pregnant must be monitored carefully for signs of cardiac compromise. Blood volume increases by 40%, and the demand on the heart is significantly increased.
• Any anemia? What kind? When? Was it treated? How? Did it improve?	Pregnancy worsens any pre-existing anemia because iron in the mother's body is used up extensively by the fetus. Identify the need for early supplementation. Sickle-cell anemia may worsen during pregnancy, whereas sickle-cell carriers have more UTIs. Screen the latter periodically for bacteriuria.
• Had thrombophlebitis, pulmonary embolus (PE), or deep venous thrombosis (DVT)?	Pregnancy itself is a hypercoagulable state because of increases in coagulation factors I, VII, VIII, IX, and X. This increases the risk of phlebitis (Cunningham et al., 2001).
• Have you had hypertension or kidney disease?	The woman with renal disease or with chronic hypertension is at increased risk for pre-eclampsia. Know the baseline BP and renal function to evaluate any changes.
• Any history of hepatitis B or C?	Confirm this with serum testing. Perinatal transmission usually occurs by the infant being exposed to infected blood and genital secretions during delivery and by cracked and bleeding nipples during breastfeeding.

Subjective Data

Subjective Data

Examiner Asks	Rationale
• Any history of thyroid disease?	Uncontrolled hypothyroidism is associated with increased neonatal morbidity resulting from preterm birth and low birth weight. Uncontrolled hypothyroidism is related to delayed mental development in children.
• Any history of seizures?	Increased incidence of stillbirths and IUGR is associated with seizure disorders.
• Have you had UTI?	The hormonal levels during pregnancy predisposes the woman to UTI, so a history before pregnancy indicates periodic screening. Pregnancy may also mask the symptoms of UTI. Further, a serious UTI may cause irritability of the uterus, posing a risk for preterm labour. Educate the woman in measures to prevent UTI.
• Have you had depression or any other mental illness?	This woman will be at risk for postpartum depression. Assist her to prepare a support network. Counselling may help her navigate the developmental challenges of becoming a mother.
• Do you feel safe in your relationship or home environment?	Interpersonal violence during pregnancy is common. Questioning the safety of the woman is part of prenatal care.
• Are you in a relationship with someone who physically or emotionally abuses or threatens you?	Most women will not freely offer this information. You must ask these questions at the appropriate time and without causing distress.
• Has anyone forced you to perform sexual activities against your will?	Women who have been subjected to incest or other abuse are candidates for dysfunctional labour and subsequent Caesarean delivery.
• Do you have diabetes? Did you have diabetes during a previous pregnancy?	Diabetes is carefully managed during pregnancy to avoid serious complications, such as a macrosomic infant and operative delivery. Consider early screening and nutritional interventions.
8. Nutritional history	
• Are you taking a folic-acid-fortified multivitamin every day?	A daily multivitamin with at least 0.4 mg folic acid is recommended for all women who could become pregnant, for ≥3 months preconception through the first 3 months of pregnancy, to prevent neural tube defects in the baby (Public Health Agency of Canada, 2008).
• Do you follow a special diet?	A special diet may put the woman at nutritional risk. Help achieve adequate nutrition within the confines of her diet.
• Any food intolerance?	A food intolerance might affect the woman's and fetus's nutrition (e.g., lactose intolerance limits calcium intake).
• Do you crave nonfoods such as ice, paint chips, dirt, or clay?	Craving for ice or dirt is called pica and is associated with anemia.

Examiner Asks	Rationale
9. Environment and hazards • What is your occupation? What are the physical demands of the work? Are you exposed to any strong odours, chemicals, radiation, or other harmful substances? • Do you consider your food and housing adequate? • How do you wear your seat belt when driving? • Other questions or concerns?	Hazards? Possible teratogenic exposures? The woman who is rubella nonimmune may be advised not to continue working in a daycare centre. Suitability for pregnancy? The woman whose job requires long hours of standing may be disabled early if signs of PTL occur. If appropriate, refer for provincial and federal programs to assist with food, housing, or other needs. For maternal and fetal safety, instruct the woman to place the lap belt below the abdomen. Encourage the woman to write down questions that may come up between visits.

OBJECTIVE DATA

PREPARATION

The initial examination for pregnancy may be a woman's first pelvic examination, and many women become extremely anxious about it. Or the woman may not know for certain whether she is pregnant and may be anxious about the findings. Before touching the woman, explain to her what will happen during the examination. Save the pelvic examination for last—by that time the woman will have become more comfortable with your gentle, informative approach. Communicate all findings as you proceed, to demonstrate your respectful affirmation of her control and responsibility in her own health and health care and that of her child's.

Ask the woman to empty her bladder before the examination, reserving a specimen for protein and glucose testing, and for urinalysis, if required. Before the examination, ask her to weigh herself on the office scale. Provide the woman with a chaperone if desired. Some clinics require an escort or chaperone during examinations.

Give the woman a gown and a drape. Begin the examination with the woman sitting on the exam table, wearing the gown, her lap covered by a drape. Take and record vital signs, including BP, pulse, temperature, and fetal heart rate. Before beginning the breast examination, help her to lie down. She remains recumbent for the abdominal and extremity examination. She must be placed in the lithotomy position for the pelvic examination (see Chapter 26). Help her to the sitting position. Recheck after the examination if BP was previously elevated.

EQUIPMENT NEEDED

Stethoscope, BP cuff
Centimetre measuring tape
Fetoscope and Doppler sonometer
Reflex hammer
Urine collection containers
Chemostix for checking urine for glucose and protein
Equipment needed for pelvic examination as noted in Chapter 26

Normal Range of Findings	Abnormal Findings
GENERAL SURVEY Observe the woman's state of nourishment, and her grooming, posture, mood, and affect, which reflect her mental state. Throughout the examination, observe her maturity and ability to pay attention and learn in order to plan how to provide the information she needs to successfully complete a healthy pregnancy.	Undernourished; or obesity. Poor grooming, a slumped posture, and a flat affect may be signs of depression and risk for postpartum depression. Poor grooming may reflect a lack of resources and a need for a social service referral.

Normal Range of Findings	Abnormal Findings

A lack of attention may indicate some preoccupation with a concern. The woman who has had learning difficulties may benefit from printed and oral information, special classes, as well as a support person to accompany her. A flat, unfocused affect may indicate depression or the influence of drugs.

SKIN

Note any scars (particularly those of previous Caesarean delivery). Many pregnant women exhibit skin changes, such as acne or skin tags, that may spontaneously resolve after the pregnancy. Vascular spiders may be present on the upper body. Some women have **chloasma,** known as the "mask of pregnancy," which is a butterfly-shaped pigmentation of the face. Note the presence of the **linea nigra,** a hyperpigmented line that begins at the sternal notch and extends down the abdomen through the umbilicus to the pubis (Fig. 29-3). Also note **striae,** or stretch marks, in areas of weight gain, particularly on the abdomen and breasts of multiparous women. These marks are bright red when they first form, but they will shrink and lighten to a silvery colour (in light-skinned women) after the pregnancy (see Fig. 29-3).

Multiple bruises may suggest physical abuse.

Tracks (scars along easily accessed veins) may indicate intravenous drug use.

Complaints of nasal irritation, nasal crusting, nasal stuffiness, or recurrent nosebleeds may indicate drug sniffing.

Palmar erythema in the first trimester may indicate hepatitis but thereafter is not clinically significant (Varney, 2004).

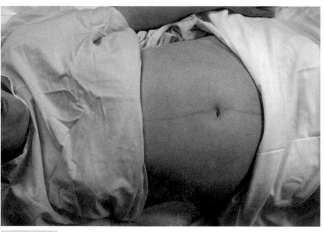

Fig. 29-3

MOUTH

Mucous membranes should be red and moist. Gum hypertrophy (surface looks smooth, and stippling disappears) may occur normally during pregnancy (pregnancy gingivitis). Bleeding gums may be from estrogen stimulation, which causes increased vascularity and fragility.

Pale mucous membranes are indicative of anemia.

Poor dental hygiene during pregnancy may lead to PTB or low-birth-weight infants.

NECK

The thyroid may be palpable and feel full but smooth during the normal pregnancy of a euthyroid woman.

Solitary nodules indicate neoplasm; multiple nodules usually indicate inflammation or a multinodular goitre. Significant diffuse enlargement occurs with hyperthyroidism, thyroiditis, and hypothyroidism.

| **Normal Range of Findings** | **Abnormal Findings** |

BREASTS

The breasts are enlarged (Fig. 29-4), perhaps with resulting striae and may be very tender. The areolae and nipples enlarge and darken in pigmentation, the nipples become more erect, and "secondary areolae" (mottling around the areolae) may develop. The blood vessels of the breast enlarge and may shine blue through a seemingly more translucent than usual chest wall. When auscultating, blood flow through these blood vessels can be heard and may be mistaken for a cardiac murmur. This sound is called the mammary souffle ($\overline{SOO}$-FL). Montgomery's tubercles, located around the areola and responsible for skin integrity of the areola, enlarge. Colostrum, a thick yellow fluid, may be expressed from the nipples.

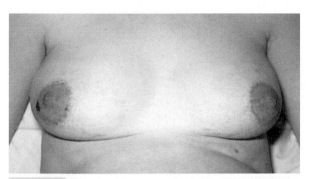

Fig. 29-4

The breast tissue feels nodular as the mammary alveoli hypertrophy. Take this opportunity to teach or reinforce breast self-examination (BSE). For more information on teaching and advising on BSE please review Chapter 17. The woman should expect changes in the breast tissue during pregnancy. Because of the lack of menses, instruct her to perform BSE according to the calendar on a monthly basis, on a date familiar to her such as her birth date.

Recall that some women have an embryological remnant called a supernumerary nipple, which may or may not have breast tissue beneath it. Possibly mistaken previously for moles, these occur under the arm or in a line directly underneath each nipple on the abdominal wall (see Chapter 17). This nipple and breast tissue may show the same changes of pregnancy. Instruct the woman to check these areas as well during BSE.

Refer any unusual breast lump in the patient for further study.

HEART

The pregnant woman often has a functional, soft, blowing, systolic murmur that occurs as a result of increased volume. The murmur requires no treatment and will resolve after pregnancy.

Note any other murmur and refer. Valvular disease may necessitate the use of prophylactic antibiotics at delivery. Pregnancy places a large hemodynamic burden on the heart, and the woman with cardiac disease must be managed closely.

LUNGS

The lungs are clear bilaterally to auscultation with no crackles or wheezing. Shortness of breath is common in the third trimester from pressure on the diaphragm from the enlarged uterus.

Women with asthma exacerbations during pregnancy may have expiratory (and possibly inspiratory) wheeze.

Objective Data

Normal Range of Findings	Abnormal Findings

PERIPHERAL VASCULATURE

The legs may show diffuse, bilateral pitting edema, particularly in the third trimester and if the examination occurs later in the day when the woman has been on her feet. Varicose veins in the legs are common in the third trimester. Non-dependent edema is no longer a criterion for diagnosing pre-eclampsia.

The pregnant woman is at risk for thrombophlebitis. Carefully evaluate any redness, or red, hot, tender swelling to rule out phlebitis. Varicosities increase the risk of thrombophlebitis, and she should not wear restrictive clothing or sit without moving legs for a long period. Varicosities will worsen with the weight and volume of pregnancy, and support hose help to minimize them.

NEUROLOGICAL SYSTEM

Using the reflex hammer, check the biceps, patellar, and ankle deep tendon reflexes (DTRs). Normally these are 1+ to 2+ and equal bilaterally.

Brisk or greater than 2+ DTRs and clonus may be associated with elevated BP and cerebral edema in pre-eclamptic women.

INSPECT AND PALPATE THE ABDOMEN

Observe the shape and contours of the abdomen to discern signs of fetal position. Note linea nigra and any bruises or cuts. As the woman lifts her head, you may see the **diastasis recti,** the separation of the abdominal muscles, which occurs during pregnancy. The muscles return together after pregnancy with abdominal exercise. When palpating, note the abdominal muscle tone, which grows more relaxed with each subsequent pregnancy. Note any tenderness; the uterus is normally nontender.

The fundus should be palpable abdominally from 12 weeks' gestation. Use the side of your hand and begin palpating centrally on the abdomen higher than you expect the uterus to be. Palpate down until you feel the fundus (the top of the uterus). Alternatively, stand at the woman's right side facing her head (Fig. 29-5). Place the palm of your right hand on the curve of the uterus in the left lower quadrant and your left palm on the curve of the uterus in the right lower quadrant. Moving from hand to hand, allowing the curve of the uterus to guide you, "walk" your hands to where they meet centrally at the fundus.

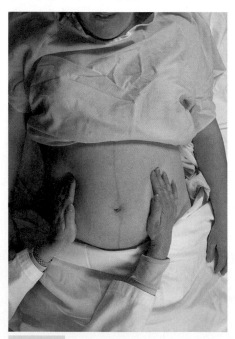

Fig. 29-5

Normal Range of Findings	Abnormal Findings

Note the fundal location by landmarks and fingerbreadths, as described in Fig. 29-1 on p. 823. Note that individual women's variations in location of landmarks and examiner's variations in fingerwidth makes this measurement inexact. From 20 weeks' gestation, it is more accurate to use the centimetre measuring tape and measure the height of the fundus in centimetres from the superior border of the symphysis to the fundus (Fig. 29-6). After 20 weeks, the number of centimetres should approximate the number of weeks of gestation.

A lagging fundal height >2 cm may indicate IUGR, transverse lie, oligohydramnios, inaccurate gestational age, or oblique presentation of the fetus.

An increase in fundal height >2 cm may indicate multiple gestation, macrosomia, polyhydramnios, or inaccurate gestational age.

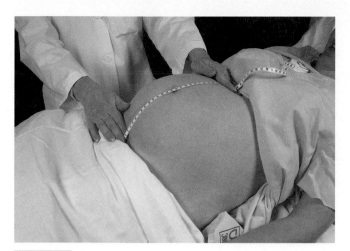

Fig. 29-6

Beginning at 20 weeks, you may feel fetal movement, and the fetus's head can be ballotted. A gentle, quick palpation with the fingertips can locate a head that is not only hard when you push it away, but is hard as it bobs or bounces back against your fingers.

If you suspect the woman to be in labour, palpate for uterine contractions. Palpate the uterus over its entire surface to familiarize yourself with its "indentability." Then rest your hand lightly on the uterine fundus with fingers opened. When the uterus contracts, it rises and pulls together, drawing your fingers closer together.

During the contraction, notice that the uterus is less "indentable." When the uterus relaxes, your fingers relax open again. In this way, contractions can be monitored for frequency (from the beginning of one contraction to the beginning of the next), length, and quality. Note that a mild contraction feels like the firmness of the tip of your nose; a moderate contraction feels like your chin; and a hard contraction feels like a forehead. (Make allowance for the amount of soft tissue between your fingers and the uterus.)

An abnormal uterine contraction is dystonic in nature; the contraction begins in the lower uterine segment and may delay cervical dilation.

An inadequate resting tone can indicate uterine irritability or tachysystole associated with placental abruption. A tender uterus may indicate chorioamnionitis or placental abruption.

Leopold's Manoeuvres

In the third trimester, perform Leopold's manoeuvres to determine fetal lie, presentation, attitude, position, variety, and engagement. **Fetal lie** is the orientation of the fetal spine to the maternal spine and may be longitudinal, transverse, or oblique. **Presentation** describes the part of the fetus that is entering the pelvis first. **Attitude,** the position of fetal parts in relation to each other, may be flexed, military (straight), or extended. **Position** designates the location of a fetal part to the right or left of the maternal pelvis. **Variety** is the location of the fetal back to the anterior, lateral, or posterior part of the maternal pelvis. **Engagement** occurs when the widest diameter of the presenting part has passed through the pelvic inlet. In a term pregnancy, this usually coincides with the leading point of the presenting part being at the level of the ischial spines (Varney, 2004).

Malpresentations are illustrated in Table 29-7 on p. 853.

Objective Data

Normal Range of Findings	Abnormal Findings

Leopold's first manoeuvre is performed by facing the woman's head and placing your fingertips around the top of the fundus (Fig. 29-7). Note its size, consistency, and shape. Imagine what fetal part is in the fundus. The breech feels large and firm. Moving it between the thumb and fingers of the hand, because it is attached to the fetus at the waist, results in moving it slowly and with difficulty. In contrast, the fetal head feels large, round, hard, and mobile. When it is ballotted, it feels hard as you push it away and hard again as it bobs back against your fingers in an "answer." Note that the "bobbing" or "ballotting" sensation of the movement occurs because the head is attached at the neck and moves easily. If there is no part in the fundus, the fetus is in the transverse lie.

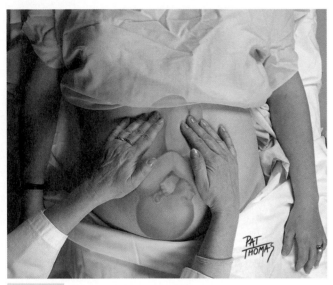

Fig. 29-7   Leopold's first manoeuvre.

For **Leopold's second manoeuvre,** move your hands to the sides of the uterus (Fig. 29-8). Note whether small parts or a long, firm surface are palpable on the woman's left or right side. The long, firm surface is the back. Note whether the back is anterior, lateral, or out of reach (posterior). The small parts, or limbs, indicate a posterior position when they are palpable all over the abdomen.

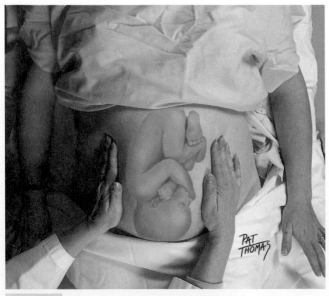

Fig. 29-8   Leopold's second manoeuvre.

Objective Data

Normal Range of Findings

Leopold's third manoeuvre, also called Pawlik's manoeuvre, requires the woman to bend her knees up slightly (Fig. 29-9). Grasp the lower abdomen just above the symphysis pubis between the thumb and fingers of one hand and, as you did at the fundus during the first manoeuvre, to determine what part of the fetus is there. If the presenting part is beginning to engage, it will feel "fixed." With this manoeuvre alone, it may be difficult to differentiate the shoulder from the vertex.

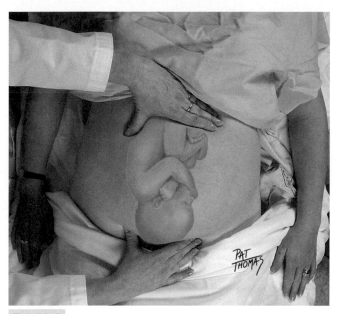

Fig. 29-9   Leopold's third manoeuvre.

The **fourth manoeuvre** assists in determining engagement and, in the vertex presentation, to differentiate shoulder from vertex (Fig. 29-10). The woman's knees are still bent. Facing her feet, place your palms, with fingers pointing toward the feet, on either side of the lower abdomen. Pressing your fingers firmly, move slowly down toward the pelvic inlet. If your fingers meet, the presenting part is not engaged. If your fingers diverge at the pelvic rim meeting a hard prominence on one side, this prominence is the occiput. This indicates the vertex is presenting with a deflexed head (the face presenting). If your fingers meet hard prominences on both sides, the vertex is engaged in either a military or a flexed position. If your fingers come to the pelvic brim diverged but with no prominences palpable, the vertex is "dipping" into the pelvis, or is engaged. In this case, the firm object felt above the symphysis pubis in the third manoeuvre is the shoulder.

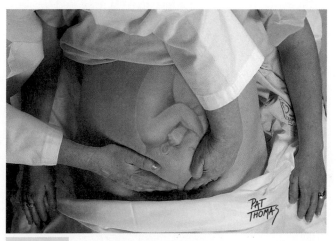

Fig. 29-10   Leopold's fourth manoeuvre.

Abnormal Findings

By 36 weeks the presenting part should be cephalic. If a breech or transverse presentation is detected, referral to an obstetrician is indicated. The woman should be offered external cephalic version in the absence of contraindications.

Normal Range of Findings	Abnormal Findings

See Fig. 29-11 for various fetal positions and where to auscultate the FHTs for each. At the end of pregnancy, 96% of fetal presentations are vertex, 3.5% are breech, 0.3% are face, and 0.4% are shoulder (Cunningham et al., 2001).

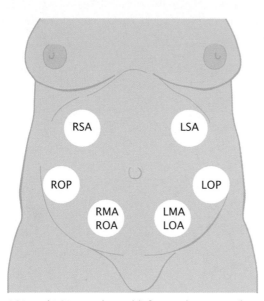

RSA and LSA = right and left sacral anterior (breech)
RMA and LMA = right and left mentum anterior (face)
ROA and LOA = right and left occiput anterior (vertex)
ROP and LOP = right and left occiput posterior (vertex)

Fig. 29-11   Location of FHTs for various fetal positions.

AUSCULTATE THE FETAL HEART TONES

FHTs are a positive sign of pregnancy. A fetal heart should be heard using Doppler US by 12 to 13 weeks' gestation and as early at 8 to 10 weeks in some women. This use of the fetoscope assists in dating the pregnancy. FHTs are auscultated best over the fetal back. After identifying the position of the fetus (see Fig. 29-11), use the heart tones to confirm your findings. Count the FHTs for 15 seconds and multiply by four to obtain the rate (Fig. 29-12). The normal rate is between 110 and 160 beats per minute (SOGC, 2007b). Spontaneous accelerations of FHTs indicate fetal well-being.

If no FHTs are heard, verify fetal cardiac activity with US.

Further investigate any decelerations of FHTs, as they can be an atypical or abnormal finding. Abrupt and brief decelerations are common in the preterm fetus. Decelerations cannot be classified by type unless the fetal heart is assessed by electronic fetal monitoring.

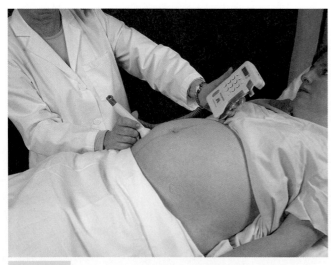

Fig. 29-12

Normal Range of Findings	Abnormal Findings

Differentiate the FHTs from the slower rate of the maternal pulse and the uterine souffle (the soft, swishing sound of the placenta receiving the pulse of maternal arterial blood) by palpating the mother's pulse while you listen. Also, distinguish FHTs from the funic souffle (blood rushing through the umbilical arteries at the same rate as the FHTs). The FHTs are a double sound, like the tick-tock of a watch under a pillow, whereas the funic souffle is a sharp, whistling sound that is heard only 15% of the time (Cunningham et al., 2001).

All the abdominal findings are of interest to the woman. Share them with her. Often she will want to listen to FHTs with her significant other. For the hearing-impaired pregnant woman, place her hand on the fetal monitor to feel the fetal heart vibrating.

PELVIC EXAMINATION

Genitalia

Use the procedure for the pelvic examination described in Chapter 26. Note the following characteristics. The enlargement of the labia minora is common in multiparous women. Labial varicosities may be present. The perineum may be scarred from a previous episiotomy or from lacerations. Note the presence of any hemorrhoids of the rectum.

Speculum Examination

When examining the vagina, you may see **Chadwick's sign,** the bluish purple discoloration and congested look of the vaginal wall and cervix from increased vascularity and engorgement (Fig. 29-13). Note the vaginal discharge. Vaginal discharge in pregnancy may be heavier in amount but should be similar in description to the woman's nonpregnant discharge and should not be associated with itching, burning, or an unusual odour (except that, occasionally, chapping of the vaginal area may be seen due to excessive moisture). Perform a wet mount or culture of the discharge when you are uncertain of its normalcy.

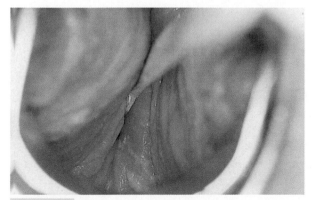

Fig. 29-13

Note whether the cervix appears open. Note whether it is the smooth, round cervix with a dotlike external os of the nulliparous woman or the irregular multiparous cervix with an external os that appears more like a crooked line, the result of cervical dilation and possibly lacerations during a previous pregnancy.

A friable cervix bleeds easily when touched with a cotton swab, Cytobrush, or speculum and may be due to cervicitis. Obtain cultures. Any lesions should be investigated.

Normal Range of Findings	Abnormal Findings

Bimanual Examination

As described in Chapter 26, palpate the uterus between the hand that is performing the internal examination and the hand placed on the abdomen. Note the position of the uterus. The pregnant uterus may be rotated toward the right side as it rises out of the pelvis because of the presence of the descending colon on the left. This is called **dextrorotation.** Irregular enlargement of the uterus may be noted at 8 to 10 weeks and occurs when implantation occurs close to a cornual area of the uterus. This is called **Piskacek's sign.** Also you may note **Hegar's sign,** when the enlarged uterus bends forward on its softened isthmus between the fourth and sixth weeks of pregnancy.

Note the size and consistency of the uterus. The 6-week gestation uterus may seem only slightly enlarged and softened. The 8-week gestation uterus is approximately the size of an avocado, approximately 7 to 8 cm across the fundus. The 10-week gestation uterus is about the size of a grapefruit and may reach to the pelvic brim, but it is narrow and does not fill the pelvis from side to side; the 12-week gestation uterus will fill the pelvis. After 12 weeks, the uterus is sized from the abdomen. The multigravid uterus may be larger initially, and early sizing of this uterus may be less reliable for dating.

Softening of the cervix is called **Goodell's sign.** When examining the cervix, note its position (anterior, midposition, or posterior), degree of effacement (or thinning, expressed in percentages assuming a ≥2-cm long cervix initially), dilation (opening, expressed in centimetres), consistency (soft or firm), and the station of the presenting part (centimetres above or below the ischial plane) (Fig. 29-14).

A shortened cervix is <2 cm.

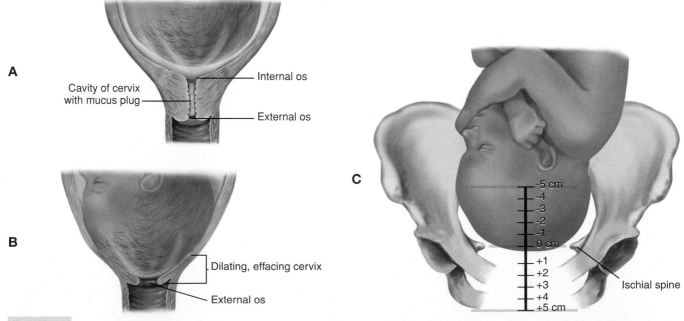

Fig. 29-14 **A,** Cervix before labour. **B,** Cervix begins to efface and dilate. **C,** Station height of presenting part in relation to ischial spines.

The ovaries rise with the growing uterus. Always examine the adnexae to rule out the presence of a mass, such as an ectopic pregnancy.

To determine tone, ask the woman to squeeze your fingers as they rest in the vagina. Take this opportunity to teach Kegel exercise, with the aim to strengthen the pubococcygeus muscles to prevent, reduce, or improve pelvic floor issues such as urinary incontinence, uterine prolapse, and sexual function. Women can identify the muscle by inserting a finger into the vagina. Alternatively, these muscles can be identified by stopping the flow of urine midstream. This should only be done once to help confirm the muscle group. There are several variations

Adnexal enlargement and pain with palpation occurs with ectopic pregnancy or ovarian mass.

Normal Range of Findings	Abnormal Findings

of Kegel exercises, including use of biofeedback. Women should be encouraged to consider a strategy that will work for them. The woman contracts and relaxes the muscle group in sets of 10 or more, several times a day.

Pelvimetry

Assess the bones of the pelvis for shape and size. The dimensions may indicate the favourableness of the bony structure for vaginal delivery but are no longer considered a reliable indicator of pelvic capacity. The relaxation of the pelvic joints, the widening of the pelvis in the squatting position, and the capacity of the fetal head to mould to the shape of the pelvis may enable a vaginal birth despite seemingly unfavourable measurements.

To aid in visualizing the pelvis, imagine three planes: the pelvic inlet (from the sacral promontory to the upper edge of the pubis), the midpelvis, and the pelvic outlet (from the coccyx to the lower edge of the pubis) (Fig. 29-15). Assessment of each of these pelvic planes, as described in the following techniques, allows you to estimate the adequacy of the pelvis for vaginal delivery.

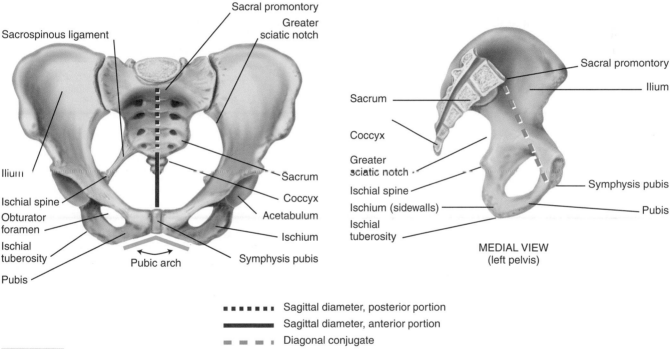

■ ■ ■ ■ ■ ■ Sagittal diameter, posterior portion
━━━━━━ Sagittal diameter, anterior portion
▬ ▬ ▬ ▬ Diagonal conjugate

Fig. 29-15

There are four general types of pelves: gynecoid, anthropoid, android, and platypelloid (Table 29-2). You may postpone examination of the bony pelvis until the third trimester when the vagina is more distensible. With your two fingers still in the vagina, note the shape and width of the pubic arch (a 90-degree arch, or 2 fingerbreadths, is desirable). If you are right-handed, move your hand to the woman's right pelvis. If you are left-handed, move it to the left side of the woman's pelvis. Assess the inclination and curve of the side walls and the prominence of the ischial spine (refer to Fig. 29-15 for location of these landmarks). Move your fingers back and forth between the spines to get an impression of the transverse diameter—10 cm is desirable. Sweep your fingers down the sacrum, noting its shape and inclination (hollow, J-shaped, or straight). Assess the coccyx for prominence and mobility. From the sacrum, locate the sacrospinous ligament. Assess the length of the ligament—2½ to 3 fingerbreadths is adequate. Assess the shape and width of the sacrospinous notch. Shift to the other side of the pelvis and assess it for similarity to the first.

TABLE 29-2 | **The Four Pelvic Types**

The Gynecoid Pelvis

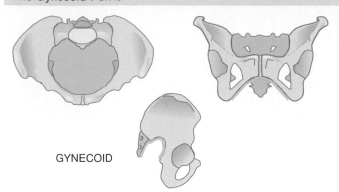

GYNECOID

Inlet round or oval.
Posterior sagittal diameter of inlet only slightly less than anterior sagittal diameter.
Pubic arch wide (90 degrees or more).
Spines are not prominent, allowing a transverse diameter at spines 10 cm or more.
Sacrosciatic notch round and wide.
Straight side walls.
Posterior pelvis is round and wide.

Sacrum is parallel with the symphysis pubis; hollow and concave.

Favours vaginal delivery.
Seen in 50% of all women.

The Android Pelvis

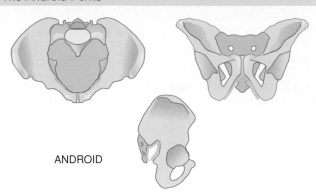

ANDROID

Inlet heart shaped.
Posterior sagittal diameter of inlet less than the anterior sagittal diameter.
Pubic arch narrow (less than 90 degrees).
Spines are prominent, decreasing transverse diameter at spines.

Sacrosciatic notch is narrow and highly arched.
Side walls converge.
Posterior sagittal diameter decreases from inlet to outlet as sacrum inclines forward.
Sacrum is straight and prominent; coccyx may be prominent.
Anterior of pelvis is narrow and triangular.
The "male" pelvis.
Poor prognosis for vaginal delivery.

The Anthropoid Pelvis

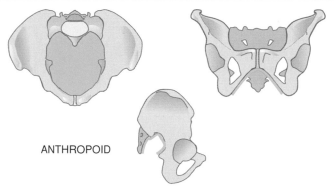

ANTHROPOID

Inlet oval.
Pubic arch may be somewhat narrow.
Spines usually prominent but not encroaching because of the spaciousness of the posterior segment.
Sacrosciatic notch average height but wide (about 4 finger-breadths).
Side walls somewhat convergent.
Sacrum posteriorly inclined, with posterior sagittal diameters long throughout the pelvis.

If pelvis somewhat large, adequate for vaginal delivery because posterior pelvis is generous.

The Platypelloid Pelvis

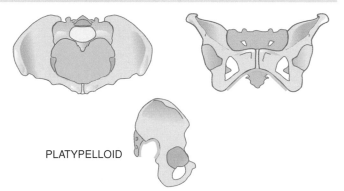

PLATYPELLOID

Inlet shaped like a flattened gynecoid pelvis.
Pubic arch wide.
Spines usually prominent but not encroaching because of the already wide interspinous diameter.
Sacrosciatic notch wide and flat.

Side walls slightly convergent.
Sacrum inclined posteriorly and hollow, making a short and shallow pelvis.
Occurs in less than 3% of all women.
Not conducive to vaginal delivery.

Data from Varney, H. (1997). *Varney's midwifery* (3rd ed.) Sudbury, MA: Jones & Bartlett.

Normal Range of Findings

Abnormal Findings

The pelvic inlet cannot be reached by clinical examination, but you can estimate it by the measure of the **diagonal conjugate,** which indicates the anteroposterior diameter of the pelvic inlet. Having measured the length of the second and third fingers of your examining hand, with your fingers still in the vagina, point these fingers toward the sacral promontory (Fig. 29-16). If you cannot reach the promontory, note the measurement as being greater than the centimetres of length of your examining fingers. A measurement of 11.5 to 12.0 cm is desirable.

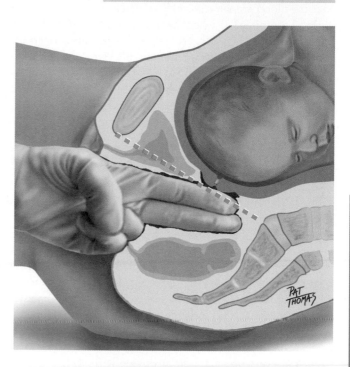

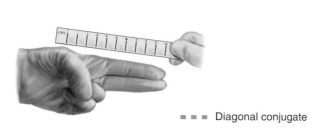

▪ ▪ ▪ Diagonal conjugate

Fig. 29-16   Diagonal conjugate.

Remove your fingers from the vagina. Having previously measured the width of your own hand across the knuckles, form your hand into a closed fist and place it across the perineum between the ischial tuberosities. Estimate this diameter, which is the **bi-ischial diameter** (also known as the intertubous diameter and the transverse diameter of the pelvic outlet). A measurement greater than 8 cm is generally adequate (Fig. 29-17).

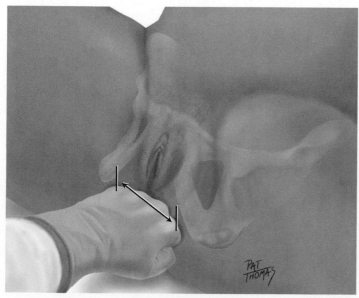

Fig. 29-17
Bi-ischial
diameter.

Normal Range of Findings	Abnormal Findings

When describing pelvimetry, note all the above measurements and state the pelvic type. The pelvis may be described as being "proven" to the number of pounds of the largest vaginally born infant. Alternatively, to describe a small pelvis, you may make the assessment, for example, "adequate for a 3-kg baby."

Blood Pressure

Take the blood pressure after the woman has been sitting quietly, and prior to the physical examination, when the woman is most relaxed. With the woman sitting upright and her arm at heart level, check for an elevated BP. Korotkoff phase 5 should be used to designate diastolic BP. Hypertension in pregnancy is defined by a diastolic BP of ≥90 mm Hg based upon an average of two readings taken in the same arm (SOGC, 2008). "White coat" hypertension is recognized and can be confirmed by a home BP of <135/85 mm Hg.

Chronic hypertension: a documented history of high BP before pregnancy or a persistent elevation of at least 140/90 mm Hg on two occasions more than 24 hours apart before the twentieth week of gestation (Gabbe et al., 2002).

ROUTINE LABORATORY AND RADIOLOGICAL IMAGING STUDIES

At the first prenatal encounter, discuss options for screening and diagnostic tests. In the first trimester or at booking, all women should be offered a complete blood count, rubella antibody titre, blood type, Rhesus factor with antibody screen, syphilis serology, hepatitis B surface antigen, and HIV screen with full counselling and consent. Special populations identified by history can be offered screening for hepatitis C thyroid-stimulating hormone, ferritin, vitamin B_{12}, and TORCH infection.* Screen for sickle cell anemia, β-thalassemia, α-thalassemia, Tay-Sachs disease, and cystic fibrosis in at-risk populations.

A midstream urine culture should be obtained to screen for asymptomatic bacteriuria at 12 to 16 weeks. Whether urinalysis for protein and glucose is needed at every prenatal visit in women without hypertension is debated (British Columbia Perinatal Health Program, 2005; SOGC, 2008).

A pelvic examination should be offered to screen for cervical cancer. Consent should be obtained for a cervical culture for chlamydia and gonorrhea. If the woman has a history of preterm birth or symptoms of infection or bacterial vaginosis, add a vaginal screen for culture and sensitivity. Do a bimanual examination to confirm uterine size for gestational age.

Genetic counselling programs vary across Canada. All women should receive timely counselling and be offered appropriate screening and diagnostic procedures as per regional availability. It is essential that nurses responsible for preconception and prenatal care be aware of screening options and their optimal timing during pregnancy. SOGC recommends that all pregnant women be offered noninvasive screening for Down syndrome, trisomy 18, and open neural tube defects (SOGC, 2007a). Invasive diagnostic procedures should be reserved for those women who screen above the set screen risk cut-off and for women who will be 40 years old by the time of delivery, with counselling provided on the risks of pregnancy

---

*TORCH is an acronym for a special group of infections that can be transmitted to the fetus: **T**oxoplasmosis; **O**ther infections: namely hepatitis B, syphilis, and herpes zoster, the virus that causes chicken pox; **R**ubella (formerly known as German measles); **C**ytomegalovirus; and **H**erpes simplex virus, the cause of genital herpes.

Normal Range of Findings	Abnormal Findings

loss with the procedure. Age alone is no longer recommended as an appropriate risk assessment tool (SOGC, 2007a). Screening programs offer risk assessment based on biochemical and US markers. Noninvasive options include (1) maternal age combined with first trimester serum markers and ultrasound for nuchal translucency, plus second trimester serum testing; (2) second trimester serum screening; and (3) a two-step integrated approach with first and second trimester serum testing with or without an ultrasound for nuchal translucency. Invasive procedures offer diagnosis of a number of chromosomal abnormalities through amniocentesis and chorionic villi sampling.

A screening ultrasound should be offered to all women at 18 to 20 weeks, including a discussion about the risks and benefits, as well as limitations, of US technology. First trimester ultrasound for dating is recommended when the history is unclear or complicated by irregular menstrual cycles. Ultrasounds may also be part of a provincial or regional integrated genetic screening program. Nuchal translucency can be assessed by ultrasonography between 11 and 14 weeks. The single recommended 18- to 20-week ultrasonography provides gestational age assessment within 7 to 10 days, describes fetal number, fetal anatomy (including open neural tube defects, soft markers of fetal aneuploidy), amniotic fluid volume, and placental location including uterine and umbilical arteries blood flow. Ultrasonography can also report on fetal presentation, position, activity, tone, breathing, gender, interval growth, estimated fetal weight, and maternal anatomy, including cervical length and dilation. Additional scans may be indicated at any time for complications such as bleeding, pain, suspected ectopic or molar pregnancy, trauma, fetal concerns, inappropriate fundal height measures, medical complications including hypertension disorders and diabetes, prelabour premature rupture of membranes, and noncephalic presentation.

Additional screening during the second and third trimesters includes an antibody screen for Rh-negative women (at 26 to 28 weeks), hemoglobin (at 28 weeks), gestational diabetic screen (at 24 to 28 weeks), and single vaginal anal swab for group B streptococcus (at 35 to 37 weeks).

Summary Checklist: Pregnancy

 For a PDA-downloadable version, go to http://evolve.elsevier.com/Canada/Jarvis/examination/.

1. **Collect historical information.**
2. **Determine EDD** and current number of weeks of gestation.
3. **Instruct the woman to undress and empty her bladder,** saving her urine for it to be tested for protein and glucose.
4. **Measure weight.**
5. **Perform a physical examination,** starting with general survey.
6. **Inspect skin** for pigment changes, scars.
7. **Check oral mucous membranes.**
8. **Palpate thyroid gland.**
9. **Inspect breast changes** and palpate for masses.
10. **Auscultate** breath sounds, heart sounds, heart rate, and any murmurs.
11. **Check lower extremities** for edema, varicosities, and reflexes.
12. **The abdomen:** measure fundal height, perform Leopold's manoeuvres, auscultate FHTs.
13. **The pelvic examination:** note signs of pregnancy, the condition of the cervix, and the size and position of the uterus.
14. **Perform pelvimetry.**
15. **Measure the BP.**
16. **Obtain appropriate laboratory work.**

DOCUMENTATION AND CRITICAL THINKING

SUBJECTIVE

Rosa G. is a 27-year-old woman, gravida 2/para 1, who presents with her husband and daughter for her first prenatal visit. She is a full-time homemaker who completed 2 years of postsecondary education. Last normal menstrual period (LNMP) was April 4 of this year (certain of date), with an expected date of birth (EDB) of January 11 of next year, making her 10 weeks' gestation today. Her obstetrical history includes a normal spontaneous vaginal delivery (NSVD) 3 years ago of a viable 3.5-kg female infant after an 8-hour labour without anaesthesia, intact perineum. No complications of pregnancy, delivery, or post-partum. She breastfed this daughter, Ana, for 1 year. Present pregnancy was planned, and Rosa and her husband are pleased. Rosa is having breast tenderness, and nausea on occasion, which resolves with crackers. No past medical or surgical conditions are present. She denies allergies. Family history is significant only for diet-controlled adult-onset diabetes in two maternal aunts.

OBJECTIVE

General: Appears well nourished and is carefully groomed. English is second language, and Rosa is fluent.

Skin: Light tan in colour, surface smooth with no lesions, small tattoo noted on left forearm.

Mouth: Good dentition and oral hygiene. Oral mucosa pink, no gum hypertrophy. Thyroid gland small and smooth.

Chest: Expansion equal, respirations effortless. Lung sounds clear bilaterally with no adventitious sounds. No CVA tenderness.

Heart: Rate 76 bpm, regular rhythm, S_1 and S_2 are normal, not accentuated or diminished, with soft, blowing systolic murmur Gr ii/vi at second left interspace.

Breasts: Tender, without masses, with supple, everted nipples. Breast self-examination reviewed.

Abdomen: No masses, bowel sounds present. No hepatosplenomegaly. Uterus nonpalpable. No inguinal lymphadenopathy noted.

Extremities: No varicosities, redness, or edema. DTRs 2+ and equal bilaterally. BP 110/68 sitting.

Pelvic: Bartholin's, urethra, and Skene's glands (BUS) negative for discharge. Vagina: pink, with white, creamy, nonodourous discharge. Cervix: pink, closed, multiparous, 5 cm long, firm.

Uterus: 10-week size, consistent with dates, nontender, dextrorotated. FHTs heard with Doppler, rate 140s.

Pelvis: Pubic arch wide; side walls straight, spines blunt, interspinous diameter >10 cm. Sacrum hollow; coccyx mobile. Sacrospinous ligament 3 fingerbreadths (FBs) wide. Diagonal conjugate >12 cm, bituberous diameter >8 cm. Spacious gynecoid pelvis proven to 3.5 kg.

ASSESSMENT

Intrauterine pregnancy 10 weeks by good dates, size = dates
Rosa and husband happy with pregnancy; she feels well

PLAN

Begin prenatal vitamins.
Prenatal blood screen and urinalysis.
HIV screen offered and accepted.
Reviewed comfort measures for nausea.
Reviewed warning signs—vaginal bleeding and abdominal pain.
Informed of genetic screening options.
Return visit in 4 weeks.

Nursing Diagnoses Commonly Associated With Pregnancy

All nursing diagnoses can be found on the Evolve Web site at **http://evolve.elsevier.com/Canada/Jarvis/examination/.**

ABNORMAL FINDINGS
FOR ADVANCED PRACTICE

TABLE 29-3	Pre-eclampsia

Pre-eclampsia is a condition specific to pregnancy that is rarely seen before 20 weeks gestation except in the presence of a molar (gestational trophoblastic) pregnancy. The etiology remains unknown, but theories include coagulation abnormalities, vascular endothelial damage, cardiovascular maladaptation, immunological phenomena, dietary deficiencies or excess, and genetic predisposition. Predisposing conditions include a family or personal history of pre-eclampsia, nulliparity, obesity, multifetal gestation, pre-existing medical-genetic conditions such as chronic hypertension, renal disease, type 1 (insulin-dependent) diabetes, factor V Leiden, and thrombophelias such as antiphospholipid antibody syndrome (Gabbe et al., 2002).

The classic symptoms of pre-eclampsia are elevated BP and proteinuria. Edema is common in pregnancy, and is no longer considered a part of the diagnosis of pre-eclampsia (Gabbe et al., 2002). However, when edema of the face is of sudden onset and is associated with sudden weight gain, pre-eclampsia should be considered. Proteinuria is a late development in pre-eclampsia and is an indicator of the severity of the disease. The Canadian guidelines for managing hypertension in pregnancy define hypertension as a diastolic BP of >90 mm Hg, by office measurement, with the woman sitting and the arm at the level of the heart using Korotkoff V (SOGC, 2008). The presence of hypertension is necessary for the diagnosis of pre-eclampsia, but pre-eclampsia may be seen without the edema or proteinuria.

Onset and worsening symptoms may be sudden. Subjective signs may include headaches and vision changes (spots, blurring, or flashing lights) caused by cerebral edema or right upper quadrant or epigastric pain from liver enlargement where it becomes enlarged, necrotic, and hemorrhagic. Liver enzyme levels become elevated. Hematocrit usually increases and the platelets drop. Serum creatinine and blood urea

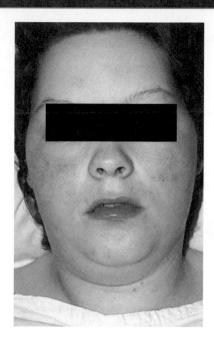

nitrogen elevate. Hemolysis occurs, in part at least, as a result of vasospasm. A serious variant of pre-eclampsia, the **HELLP** syndrome, involves **H**emolysis, **E**levated **L**iver enzymes, and **L**ow **P**latelet count, and represents an ominous clinical picture. Untreated pre-eclampsia may progress to eclampsia, which is manifested by generalized tonic–clonic seizures. Eclampsia may develop as late as 10 days postpartum.

Before the syndrome becomes clinically manifested, it affects the placenta through vasospasm and a series of small infarctions. The placenta's capacity to deliver oxygen and nutrients to the fetus may be seriously diminished, and fetal growth may be restricted.

TABLE 29-4	Fetal Size Inconsistent With Dates
Size Small for Dates	Fundal height measures smaller than expected for dates.
Inaccuracy of Dates	Conception may have occurred later than originally thought. Reconsider the woman's menstrual history, sexual history, contraceptive use, early pregnancy testing, early sizing of the uterus, US results, timing of pregnancy symptoms, including the date of quickening, and the fundal height measurements. If, after this review, the EDB is correct, then further investigation is required.
Preterm Labour and Birth	Preterm birth occurs prior to 37 weeks' gestation; it affected 7.6% of pregnancies in Canada in 2000 (Canadian Perinatal Surveillance System, 2003). The cause of preterm labour is not known, and 50% of PTBs occur in the absence of any known risk factors. The following pre-existing factors are associated with PTB: maternal history of previous PTB, second trimester loss, habitual abortions, uterine anomalies, and cervical conization. Current pregnancy risks include multiple pregnancy, preterm rupture of membranes, polyhydramnios, antepartum hemorrhage, intra-abdominal surgery, urinary tract infection, tobacco or cocaine use, serious maternal infection, and physical or emotional trauma (British Columbia Perinatal Health Program, 2005). Prevention strategies such as bed rest, tocolysis, home uterine monitoring, hydration, and frequent digital cervical examinations have been ineffective. Group prenatal care known as "centring pregnancy" facilitated by midwives has decreased PTB in a high-risk population in the United States (Ickovics et al., 2007). Serial US assessments of cervical effacement and the use of fetal fibronectin sometimes reassures women who present with threatened PTL that they are not likely to give birth; however, the ability to predict who will proceed to have a PTB is not yet possible.
Intrauterine Growth Restriction (IUGR) or Fetal Growth Restriction	IUGR, a syndrome in which the neonate fails to meet its growth potential, is associated with an increase in fetal and neonatal mortality and morbidity. Its origin may be fetoplacental, as with chromosomal abnormalities, genetic syndromes, congenital malformations, infectious diseases, and placental pathology. Or its origin may be maternal, as with decreased uteroplacental blood flow as seen with hypertensive disorders, poor maternal weight gain, poor maternal nutrition, and a previous pregnancy with an IUGR infant. Other contributing factors include infectious diseases (rubella, cytomegalovirus); multiple gestation; and environmental toxins such as cigarette smoke and maternal drug and alcohol use.
Fetal Position	Fetal position varies until about 34 weeks, when the vertex should settle into the pelvis and remain there. The position of the fetus in a transverse lie, or shoulder presentation, results in a widening of the maternal abdomen from side to side and a decrease in fundal height. Fetal malposition may occur with lax maternal abdominal musculature (inability to hold the baby in close), an abnormality in the fetus (e.g., the enlarged head of the hydrocephalic infant), placenta previa (the placenta being implanted over the cervix, blocking fetal descent), or a restricted maternal pelvis.
Oligohydramnios	Oligohydramnios is a reduction in amniotic fluid volume (i.e., an amniotic fluid index (AFI) less than 5 or a single deepest pocket <2 cm).

TABLE 29-4	Fetal Size Inconsistent With Dates—cont'd
Size Large for Dates	Fundal height measures larger than expected for dates.
Inaccuracy of Dates	Review the same findings as listed for "Size Small for Dates."
Hydatidiform Mole	Also termed *gestational trophoblastic neoplasia*, it is a result of abnormal proliferation of trophoblastic tissue associated with pregnancy. In 50% of cases uterine size is excessive; in these cases the gestational age and uterine size do not coincide.
Multiple Fetuses	The frequency of multiple fetuses increases with advanced maternal age and is enhanced by the increasing use of fertility drugs. The uterus enlarges to a point where the fundal height may be beyond the calculated or expected gestational age. US examination confirms the diagnosis.
Polyhydramnios	An amniotic fluid volume is a maximum volume pocket >8.0 cm or an amniotic fluid index (AFI) above the 95th percentile or ≥20 cm. The cause is usually idiopathic but may be due to fetal anomalies, insulin-dependent diabetes, GDM, or multiple fetuses (Creasy et al., 2004).
Leiomyoma (Myoma or "Fibroids")	These are pre-existing benign tumours of the uterine wall, which then are stimulated to enlarge by the estrogen levels of pregnancy. Myomata may be located anywhere in the uterine wall (see Table 26-6). When they grow in the outer uterine wall, the myometrium, they may affect the clinician's judgement of where the fundus of the uterus should be measured. A myoma may grow just underneath the endometrial surface into the uterine cavity, displacing the fetus or preventing its descent into the pelvis.
Fetal macrosomia 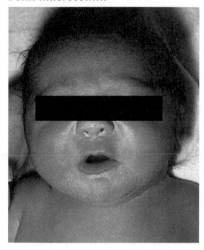	The definition of macrosomia varies between 4000 and 4500 g at birth. Maternal risk factors for macrosomia include a prior history of a macrosomic infant, maternal obesity, increased weight gain during pregnancy, multiparity, male fetus, gestational age >40 weeks, ethnicity, maternal birth weight, maternal height, maternal age <17 years, and gestational diabetes and glucose intolerance. Birth risks to the mother include labour abnormalities, an increased incidence for Caesarean delivery, bladder trauma, and vaginal tissue trauma. Fetal risks include birth trauma such as fractured clavicle and brachial plexus nerve damage from shoulder dystocia, depressed Apgar scores, extended hospitalizations, and possible fetal mortality.

TABLE 29-5	Disorders of Pregnancy
Disorder or Condition	Description
Vaginal Bleeding	Some women will have bright red, pink, or dark brown spotting at some time during the first trimester. This is not always a sign of pending pregnancy loss but may be from a blighted ovum, friable cervix, ectopic pregnancy, perigestational hemorrhage, or cervical lesions. In the second and third trimesters, vaginal bleeding may be indicative of abruptio placentae, placenta previa, uterine rupture, cervical dilation, cervical lesion, or a friable cervix. Risk factors for increased risk of vaginal bleeding include pregnancy-induced hypertension, chronic hypertension, cocaine use, abdominal trauma, uterine anomalies, prolonged premature rupture of membranes, prior placental abruption, and cervical cancer.
Incompetent Cervix	Cervical incompetence is marked by gradual and painless premature dilation and effacement of the cervix that can lead to fetal loss if undetected early enough to have a cervical cerclage placed. Its cause may be congenital, as seen in some women after DES exposure, or it may be acquired after cervical trauma or a cone biopsy.
Hyperemesis Graviderum	Hyperemesis is excessive vomiting in pregnancy that may last well into the second trimester and beyond. It can interfere with electrolytes, acid–base balance, and nutritional status. Dehydration and starvation may ensue and lead to fetal IUGR. Nausea and vomiting are not uncommon in pregnancy and usually resolve between weeks 16 and 20 and may be controlled with dietary and lifestyle changes. Vitamin B_6, ginger, acupuncture, acupressure, or Diclectin can be used with some effectiveness. Diclectin is a delayed release formulation of doxylamine succinate 10 mg with pyridoxine hydrochloride (vitamin B_6) 10 mg. This effective treatment can be offered to alleviate nausea and vomiting. It has a pregnancy risk factor rating of A−. There is no risk to the fetus (Briggs et al., 2008). Risk factors include a previous history of hyperemesis, molar pregnancy, multiple gestation, emotional stress, history of gastrointestinal reflux, uncontrolled thyroid disease, primigravida, and obesity.
Preterm Labour	Preterm labour is labour occurring after 20 weeks and before completion of 37 weeks' gestation. Preterm labour is a major factor for fetal morbidity and mortality. Some risk factors include chronic urinary tract infections, polyhydramnios, multiple gestation, previous PTL or PTB, smoking, substance abuse, poor prenatal care, poor weight gain after 20 weeks' gestation, history of cervical conization, low socioeconomic status, being of non-European descent, uterine infections, and cases where the woman herself was a preterm infant.
Decreased Fetal Movement	Fetal movement is one indicator of fetal well-being. Fetal movement counts should begin from 28 weeks' gestation. Various methods of fetal movement counting have been described in the literature. Evidence supports ensuring maternal awareness of fetal movement during the third trimester, with formal counting occuring with women at risk for adverse perinatal outcome (see Table 29-6).

TABLE 29-6	Fetal Movement Counting Recommendations

1. Daily monitoring of fetal movements starting at 26 to 32 weeks should be done in all pregnancies *with* risk factors for adverse perinatal outcome. (I-A)
2. Healthy pregnant women *without* risk factors for adverse perinatal outcomes should be made aware of the significance of fetal movements in the third trimester and asked to perform a fetal movement count if they perceive decreased movements. (I-B)
3. Women who do not perceive six movements in an interval of two hours require further antenatal testing and should contact their caregivers or the hospital as soon as possible. (III-B)
4. Women who report decreased fetal movements (<6 distinct movements within 2 hours) should have a complete evaluation of maternal and fetal status, including nonstress test or biophysical profile, or both.

TABLE 29-7 | **Malpresentations**

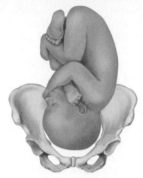

Vertex (for comparison)

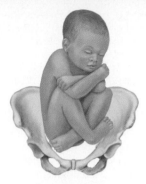

Complete breech

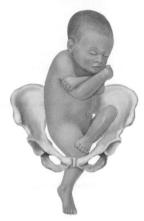

Footling breech

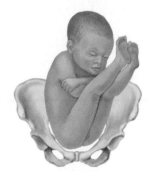

Frank breech

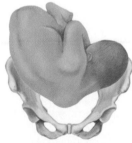

Transverse lie and
shoulder presentation

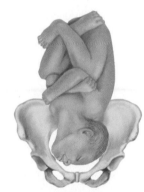

Face presentation

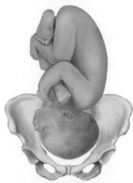

Brow presentation

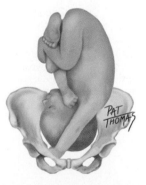

Compound presentation

Malpresentations may be detected by the hands of an experienced examiner, confirmed by the FHT location, and further confirmed by US. Before 34 weeks' gestation, any position is normal. The vertex presentation is desirable thereafter because spontaneous turning becomes less likely as the fetus grows in proportion to the amount of space and fluid available in the uterus and pelvis.

BIBLIOGRAPHY

American College of Obstetricians and Gynecologists. (2000). *Fetal macrosomia* (Technical Bulletin No. 22). Washington, DC: Author.

American College of Obstetricians and Gynecologists. (2001). *Prenatal diagnosis of fetal chromosomal abnormalities* (Practice Bulletin No. 27). Washington, DC: Author.

American College of Obstetricians and Gynecologists. (2002). *Thyroid disease in pregnancy* (Technical Bulletin No. 37). Washington, DC: Author.

American College of Obstetricians and Gynecologists. (2004a). *Prenatal and preconceptional carrier screening for genetic diseases in individuals of eastern European Jewish descent* (Committee Opinion No. 298). Washington, DC: Author.

American College of Obstetricians and Gynecologists. (2004b). *Special problems of multiple gestation* (Educational Bulletin No. 56). Washington, DC: Author.

Beamer, L. C. (2001). Fetal nuchal translucency: A prenatal screening tool. *Journal of Obstetric, Gynecological, and Neonatal Nursing, 30,* 376–385.

Blackburn, S. T., & Loper, D. L. (2002). *Maternal, fetal and neonatal physiology, a clinical perspective* (2nd ed.). Philadelphia, PA: Elsevier Science Health Sciences.

Boggess, K. A. (2003). Is there a link between periodontal disease and preterm birth? *Contemporary OB/GYN, 48,* 79–84.

Briggs, G., Freeman, R., Yaffe, S. (2008). *Drugs in pregnancy and lactation: A reference guide to fetal and neonatal risk* (8th ed.). Baltimore, MD: Lippincott Williams & Wilkins.

British Columbia Perinatal Health Program. (2005a). *Obstetrics guideline 2A: Preterm labour.* Vancouver, BC: Author.

British Columbia Perinatal Health Program. (2005b). *Obstetrics guideline 17: Antenatal screening and diagnostic tests for singleton pregnancies.* Vancouver, BC: Author.

Burrow, G. N., & Duffy, T. P. (Eds.). (2004). *Medical complications during pregnancy* (6th ed.). Philadelphia, PA: W.B. Saunders.

Burton, J., & Reyes, M. (2001). Breath in, breath out: Controlling asthma during pregnancy. *Lifelines, 5,* 25–30.

Canadian Perinatal Surveillance System. (2003). *Canadian perinatal surveillance system report 2003.* Ottawa, ON: Author.

Centers for Disease Control and Prevention. (2001). *Morbidity and Mortality Weekly Reports (MMWR), 50.*

Centers for Disease Control and Prevention. (2006). *National vital statistics reports (NVSS), 54.*

Chin, H. G. (2001). *On call obstetrics and gynecology* (2nd ed.). Philadelphia, PA: W.B. Saunders.

Creasy, R. K., & Resnick, R. (2004). *Maternal–fetal medicine* (5th ed.). Philadelphia, PA: W.B. Saunders.

Cunningham, F. G., Leveno, K. J., Bloom, S. L., Hauth, J. C., Gilstrap, L. C., & Wenstrom, K. D. (2001). *Williams' obstetrics* (21st ed.). Stamford, CT: Appleton & Lange.

Gabbe, S. G., Niebyl, J. R., & Simpson, J. L. (2002). *Obstetrics: Normal and problem pregnancies* (4th ed.). New York, NY: Churchill Livingstone.

Haddow, J. E., Palomaki, G. E., Allan, W. C., Williams, J. R., Knight, G. J., Gagnon, J., et al. (1999). Maternal thyroid deficiency during pregnancy and subsequent neuropsychological development of the child. *New England Journal of Medicine, 341,* 549–555.

Health Canada. (2002). *Guidelines for gestational weight gain ranges.* Retrieved April 26, 2008, from http://www.hc-sc.gc.ca/fn-an/nutrition/prenatal/national_guidelines-lignes_directrices_nationales-06b-table1_e.html

Ickovics, J. R., et al. (2007). Group prenatal care and perinatal outcomes: A randomized controlled trial. *Obstetrics and Gynecology, 110,* 330–339.

March of Dimes. (2002). *Pregnancy after 35.* White Plains, NY: Author.

March of Dimes. (2004). *Weight gain.* White Plains, NY: Author.

March of Dimes. (2006). *Carrier screening for cystic fibrosis.* White Plains, NY: Author.

National Center for Chronic Disease Prevention and Health Promotion. (2001). *CDC report highlights selected racial and ethnic pregnancy-related death rates* [Press release]. Atlanta, GA: Centers for Disease Control and Prevention.

Public Health Agency of Canada. (2008). *Folic acid: Why all women who could become pregnant should be taking folic acid.* Retrieved April 26, 2008, from http://www.phac-aspc.gc.ca/fa-af/index-eng.php

Smallridge, R. C., & Ladenson, P. W. (2001). Hypothyroidism in pregnancy: Consequences to neonatal health. *Journal of Clinical Endocrinology and Metabolism, 86,* 2349–2353.

Society of Obstetricians and Gynaecologists of Canada. (2001a). *Canadian guidelines for prenatal diagnosis: Genetic indications for prenatal diagnosis.* Retrieved April 27, 2008, from http://64.233.167.104/custom?q=cache:-vOFodCKE78J:www.sogc.org/guidelines/public/105E-CPG1-June2001.pdf+sickle+cell&hl=en&ct=clnk&cd=5&client=google-coop-np

Society of Obstetricians and Gynaecologists of Canada. (2001b). Policy statement: A guide for health professionals working with Aboriginal peoples. *Journal of Obstetrics and Gynaecology Canada, 23*(1), 1–15.

Society of Obstetricians and Gynaecologists of Canada. (2007a). Clinical practice guideline: Prenatal screening for fetal aneuploidy. *Journal of Obstetrics and Gynaecology Canada, 29*(2), 146–161.

Society of Obstetricians and Gynaecologists of Canada. (2007b). Fetal health surveillance: Antenatal and intrapartum consensus guideline. *Journal of Obstetrics and Gynaecology Canada, 29* (9 Suppl. 4), S3–S56.

Society of Obstetricians and Gynaecologists of Canada. (2008). Clinical practice guideline: Diagnosis, evaluation and management of the hypertensive disorders of pregnancy. *Journal of Obstetrics and Gynaecology Canada, 30*(3), S1–S48.

Star, W. L., Shannon, M., & Lommel, L. (1999). *Ambulatory obstetrics* (3rd ed.). San Francisco, CA: UCSF Nursing Press.

Swenson, D. (2001). *Telephone triage for the obstetric patient: A nursing guide.* Philadelphia, PA: W.B. Saunders.

United Nations Population Fund. (2001). *Fast facts on maternal health and morbidity.* New York, NY: Author.

Varney, H. (2004). *Varney's midwifery* (4th ed.). Sudbury, MA: Jones and Bartlett.

World Health Organization. (2007). *Maternal mortality in 2005: Estimates developed by WHO, UNICEF, UNFPA and the World Bank.* Geneva, Switzerland: Author.

Functional Assessment of the Older Adult

Written by **Carla Graf**, MS, RN, APRN-BC, and **Melissa A. Lee**, MS, RN, APRN-BC

Adapted by **Dianne Groll**, RN, BA, BScH, MScH, PhD

Canada has a large and growing population of older adults. In 2007, 13.5% of Canadians were 65 years of age or older (Statistics Canada, 2007). Despite being healthier than ever before, seniors remain more likely than younger people to have chronic conditions and to suffer from poor health. In the 2003 Canadian Community Health Survey, 81% of seniors living at home had at least one diagnosed chronic condition, while only 54% of individuals aged 30 to 64 reported a chronic illness (Rapoport et al., 2004).

While seniors make up just 13% of the Canadian population, they account for a third of all acute care hospitalizations and almost half of all hospital days. In 2002–2003 the hospitalization rate of seniors was close to 16,500 per 100,000 population aged 65 or older, compared with about 5000 per 100,000 for people younger than 65 (Rotermann, 2006). The likelihood of being hospitalized was closely tied to chronic conditions, with 27% of community-dwelling seniors with five or more chronic conditions reporting being hospitalized in the previous year, versus 6% of seniors with no chronic conditions. Fifteen percent of seniors living in private households were receiving some form of home care, and 2.7% of seniors were living in residential care facilities (Gilmore et al., 2005).

The comprehensive assessment of an older adult requires not only knowledge of normal aging changes but also the effects of chronic diseases, heredity, and lifestyle. A comprehensive geriatric assessment incorporates not only the physical examination but assessments of the person's mental, functional, social, and economic status, pain, and an examination of the physical environment for safety concerns. Multiple disciplines may participate, including physicians, nurses, physical, occupational and speech therapists, social workers, case managers, nutritionists, and pharmacists. Early recognition of disabilities and treatable conditions is instrumental in preserving function and quality of life for older adults.

The normal process of aging does not necessarily represent pathology, but with the imposition of acute and chronic illnesses, including hospitalization, an older adult may be predisposed to disability. Older adults may arrive not only with an acute illness such as pneumonia but with ongoing chronic "geriatric syndromes," such as urinary incontinence, fragile skin, confusion, problems with eating or feeding, falls, and sleep disorders. If these syndromes are not identified early, an older adult may have functional decline.

Normal aging changes and disease may precipitate transitions from home to settings where nursing-focused assessments are performed. Care may be provided in hospitals, skilled nursing facilities, long-term care, assisted living, acute rehabilitation, hospice, senior centres, home, and clinics. The care setting usually determines the types of assessment and instruments used. However, the goal of the functional assessment remains the same (i.e., to identify an older adult's strengths and any limitations) so that appropriate interventions will promote independence and prevent functional decline.

FUNCTIONAL ABILITY

Functional ability refers to one's ability to perform activities necessary to live in modern society, and can include driving, using the telephone, or performing personal tasks such as bathing and toileting. Functional ability also incorporates an older adult's physiological and psychological status and the physical and social environments (Pearson, 2000). Functional status, as defined by Richmond et al. (2004), is "the individuals' actual performance of activities and tasks associated with their current life roles" and is dependent on motivation, sensory capacity such as vision and hearing, degree of assistance needed to accomplish the tasks, and cognition (Kresevic et al., 2003). For example, the effect that arthritis might have on a person's ability to exercise may affect physical function. A condition such as Alzheimer's disease may affect problem solving, safety concerns, and motivation, which in turn affect function. Lack of social support or a safe physical setting are environmental issues that affect functional status and possibly the ability to live independently. The interaction of these components provides a *snapshot* of an older adult's functional status at a given point (Pearson, 2000). Functional status is not static; older adults may move continuously through varying stages of independence and disability.

The assessment of function is an important geriatric tenet for continuing comparison, predicting prognosis, and assisting the practitioner with objective measures to determine efficacy of treatments. Medical diagnosis is not sufficient to predict functional abilities. Older adults may not experience the usual symptoms of an acute illness. Often a decline in functional status may indicate another process, such as an infection.

A functional assessment of an older adult is the basis for care planning, goal setting, and discharge planning. A functional assessment also is needed for eligibility to obtain many services such as durable medical equipment, home modifications, and inpatient or outpatient rehabilitation services. For the older adult and family, a functional assessment can identify areas for current and future planning, such as the most appropriate living situation.

A functional assessment includes three overarching domains: **activities of daily living (ADLs), instrumental activities of daily living (IADLs),** and **mobility** (Pearson, 2000). A functional evaluation should be systematic, with attention paid to the particular needs of the person, such as the presence of pain, fatigue, shortness of breath, or memory problems. There are two approaches to use for performing a functional assessment: *asking individuals* about their abilities to perform the tasks (using self-reports) or actually *observing* their ability to perform the tasks. For persons with memory problems, the use of surrogate reporters (proxy reports) such as family members or caregivers may be necessary, noting that they may either overestimate or underestimate the actual abilities.

Activities of Daily Living

ADLs are those tasks necessary for self-care. Typically, ADLs measure domains of eating/feeding, bathing, grooming (the individual tasks of washing face, combing hair, shaving, cleaning teeth), dressing (lower body and upper body), toileting (bowel and bladder), walking (including propelling a wheelchair), using stairs (ascending and descending), and transferring (such as bed to chair). The ADL instruments are designed as either self-report, observation of tasks, or proxy/surrogate report.

ADL dependency in both sexes has been related to the presence of chronic disease such as arthritis and rheumatism; diabetes; urinary incontinence; bronchitis, emphysema, chronic obstructive pulmonary disease; the effects of stroke; and Alzheimer's disease (Rotermann, 2006). It is therefore essential to take chronic illness into consideration when assessing ADLs and IADLs, and instruments such as the Functional Comorbidity Index have been designed specifically for this purpose (Groll et al., 2005).

The Katz Index of ADL

The Katz Index of ADL (Katz et al., 1963) is based on the concept of physical disability and was intended to measure physical function in older adults and the chronically ill. It is one of the few functional assessment instruments to provide a theoretical framework for its domains of measurement

(McDowell et al., 1996), and it is the foundation for most of the newer functional assessment instruments (Pearson, 2000). It is widely used in both clinical practice and research to measure performance, evaluate treatment outcomes, and predict the need for continuing supervised care.

The Index of ADL was developed as a hierarchical structure. Katz believed that loss of physical function occurred in the most complex activities first, and these losses were in descending order of complexity, and were regained in ascending order (McDowell et al., 1996). Activities assessed are bathing, dressing, toileting, transferring from bed to chair, continence, and feeding. This instrument has been modified over the years. A simplified scoring method uses a dichotomous rating of independence or dependence in the six activities (Fig. 30-1). One point is given for each independent item. Only those activities that can be performed without help are rated as independent.

The Katz ADL is a useful instrument in many settings. The tool takes approximately 5 minutes to administer, but its use has limitations. In a hospital setting, a patient cannot demonstrate all of the activities and may need to adjust the degree of dependence or independence. Overestimation or underestimation of the activity may occur and small changes in the activities may not be identified.

Remember that the instrument is measuring current function and is valuable for planning specific types of assistance. For example, a person may be unable to bathe independently on hospital discharge but can feed himself or herself and transfer to a commode safely and independently. In this case, plan for a home health aide to go twice weekly to assist the older adult with bathing.

Additional Activity of Daily Living Instruments

Additional tools used to assess ADL ability are the Barthel Index (Mahoney et al., 1965), the Functional Independence Measure (FIM) (Hamilton et al., 1987), and the Rapid Disability Rating Scale-2 (RDS-2) (Linn et al., 1982; Linn, 1988). The Barthel Index includes definitions of each task to facilitate ease of scoring and has a more comprehensive assessment of mobility than the Katz instrument. The Barthel Index is often used to follow progress in rehabilitation settings (Pearson, 2000). The FIM was developed by a consensus panel of physical medicine and rehabilitation staff, has been widely tested on older adults, and has a telephone, an in-person, and a proxy version of the instrument. It is more sensitive to change than the other ADL instruments but takes formal training and is more time consuming (Pearson, 2000). The RDS-2 is completed by a family member or professional caregiver familiar with the abilities of the older adult. It is designed to measure what the person *actually does* versus what he or she may be able to do.

Instrumental Activities of Daily Living

Many IADL instruments have been developed since the 1960s, with the goal of measuring functional abilities necessary for independent community living. Typically IADL tasks include shopping, meal preparation, housekeeping, laundry,

Katz Index of Activities of Daily Living

Activities

Points (1 or 0)

Independence	**Dependence**
(1 Point)	(0 Points)
NO supervision, direction, or personal assistance	WITH supervision, direction, personal assistance, or total care

Bathing

Points _____

(1 Point) Bathes self completely or needs help in bathing only a single part of the body such as the back, genital area, or disabled extremity

(0 Point) Needs help with bathing more than one part of the body or with getting in or out of the tub or shower; requires total bathing

Dressing

Points _____

(1 Point) Gets clothes from closet and drawers and puts on clothes and outer garments complete with fasteners; may have help tying shoes

(0 Point) Needs help with dressing self or needs to be completely dressed

Toileting

Points _____

(1 Point) Gets to toilet, gets on and off, arranges clothes, cleans genital area without help

(0 Point) Needs help transferring to the toilet or cleaning self, or uses bedpan or commode

Transferring

Points _____

(1 Point) Moves into and out of bed or chair unassisted; mechanical transferring aides are acceptable

(0 Point) Needs help in moving from bed to chair or requires a complete transfer

Continence

Points _____

(1 Point) Exercises complete self-control over urination and defecation

(0 Point) Is partially or totally incontinent of bowel or bladder

Feeding

Points _____

(1 Point) Gets food from plate into mouth without help; preparation of food may be done by another person

(0 Point) Needs partial or total help with feeding or requires parenteral feeding

Total Points = _____

6 = High (patient independent)

0 = Low (patient very dependent)

Adapted from Gerontological Society of America. Katz, S., et al. (1970). Progress in the development of the index of ADL. *Gerontologist, 10,* 20–30.

Fig. 30-1

managing finances, taking medications, and using transportation. These instruments may have cultural and gender biases, especially in older cohorts (Pearson, 2000). IADL instruments measure tasks (doing laundry, cooking, housework) historically done by women, and most do not address activities done primarily by men, such as home repairs and working in the yard.

Lawton Instrumental Activities of Daily Living

IADL measures were first developed by Lawton and Brody in 1969 to address higher-order components of the Katz ADL scale and to measure the more complex ADLs required for a person to adapt to the environment (Pearson, 2000). The instrument was originally developed to determine the most suitable living situation for an older adult. The theory was that competence and maintenance of life skills such as shopping, cooking, and managing finances are a meaningful way to assess function because these abilities are a prerequisite for

independent living. As with the Katz Index, the IADL instrument assumes a hierarchical nature of skill acquisition and loss. The Lawton IADL scale contains eight items (Fig. 30-2): use of telephone, shopping, meal preparation, housekeeping, laundry, transportation, self-medication, and management of finances. Women are scored in all eight domains, whereas men are scored on five, omitting laundry, housekeeping, and preparing food.

The Lawton IADL instrument is designed as a self-report measure of performance rather than ability. Direct testing is often not feasible, such as demonstrating the ability to prepare food while a hospital inpatient. Attention to the final score is less important than identifying a person's strengths and areas where assistance is needed. The instrument is useful in acute hospital settings for discharge planning and for ongoing assessment in outpatient settings. It would not be useful for those residing in institutional settings because many of these tasks are already being managed for the resident.

The Lawton Instrumental Activities of Daily Living Scale

A. Ability to Use Telephone	
1. Operates telephone on own initiative; looks up and dials numbers	1
2. Dials a few well-known numbers	1
3. Answers telephone, but does not dial	1
4. Does not use telephone at all	0
B. Shopping	
1. Takes care of all shopping needs independently	1
2. Shops independently for small purchases	0
3. Needs to be accompanied on any shopping trip	0
4. Completely unable to shop	0
C. Food Preparation	
1. Plans, prepares, and serves adequate meals independently	1
2. Prepares adequate meals if supplied with ingredients	0
3. Heats and serves prepared meals or prepares meals, but does not maintain adequate diet	0
4. Needs to have meals prepared and served	0
D. Housekeeping	
1. Maintains house alone with occasional assistance (heavy work)	1
2. Performs light daily tasks such as dishwashing, bed making	1
3. Performs light daily tasks, but cannot maintain acceptable level of cleanliness	1
4. Needs help with all home maintenance tasks	1
5. Does not participate in any housekeeping tasks	0
E. Laundry	
1. Does all personal laundry	1
2. Launders small items, rinses socks, stockings, etc.	1
3. All laundry must be done by others	0
F. Mode of Transportation	
1. Travels independently on public transportation or drives own car	1
2. Arranges own travel via taxi, but does not otherwise use public transportation	1
3. Travels on public transportation when assisted or accompanied by another	1
4. Travel limited to taxi or automobile with assistance of another	0
5. Does not travel at all	0
G. Responsibility for Own Medications	
1. Is responsible for taking medication in correct dosages at correct time	1
2. Takes responsibility if medication is prepared in advance in separate dosages	0
3. Is not capable of dispensing own medication	0
H. Ability to Handle Finances	
1. Manages financial matters independently (budgets, writes cheques, pays rent and bills, goes to bank); collects and keeps track of income	1
2. Manages day-to-day purchases, but needs help with banking, major purchases, etc.	1
3. Incapable of handling money	0

Scoring: For each category, circle the item description that most closely resembles the client's highest functional level (either 0 or 1).

From Lawton, M.P., & Brody E.M. (1969). Assessment of older people: Self-maintaining and instrumental activities of daily living. *Gerontologist, 9*, 179–186. Copyright © The Gerontological Society of America.

Fig. 30-2

Additional IADL Instruments

Other IADL instruments available are the Older Americans Resources and Services Multidimensional Functional Assessment Questionnaire-IADL (OARS-IADL) (Fillenbaum and Smyer, 1981) and the Direct Assessment of Functional Abilities (DAFA) (Karagiozis et al., 1998). The OARS-IADL assesses five areas of personal function: social, economic, mental health, physical health, and self-care capacity; it is administered either as a self-report or trained observer instrument. The questions are the same for men and women. The DAFA is a 10-item observational instrument for use with adults with dementia. It requires the person to demonstrate tasks of money management, shopping, hobbies, meal preparation, awareness, reading, and transportation (Pearson, 2000). The obvious strength of this instrument is the direct observation versus self- or proxy reporting; however, it can take up to an hour and a half to complete, so it would not be feasible to use in an acute hospital setting.

Advanced Activities of Daily Living

Advanced activities of daily living (AADLs) are activities that an older adult performs as a family member and a member of society and community, including occupational and recreational activities (Guse, 2006). Various AADL instruments commonly include self-care, mobility, work (either paid or volunteer), recreational activities/hobbies, and socialization.

A disadvantage of many of the ADL and IADL instruments is the self- or proxy report of functional activities. Incorporating an objective standardized measure of performance prevents overestimation or underestimation of abilities. Many of the physical performance measures also incorporate balance, gait, motor coordination, and endurance. Many of the tests are timed. Although there are clear advantages to directly observing the older adult perform the activities, there are some disadvantages. The instruments can be very time consuming, require training and special equipment, and have the possibility that the individual might fall or sustain an injury during the testing.

The Physical Performance Test (PPT) (Rueben et al., 1990) is appropriate for use with community-dwelling older adults. Administered by a trained observer, the test requires approximately 15 minutes to complete and assesses upper body fine motor and coarse motor activities, balance, mobility, coordination, and endurance. Activities such as eating, dressing, transferring, and stair climbing are simulated and timed.

The performance activities of daily living (PADLs) (Kuriansky et al., 1976) uses a trained observer and specific props. Examples of activities tested are drinking from a cup, combing hair, shaving, lifting food with a spoon and into mouth, putting on and removing slippers, making a phone call, turning a key in a lock. The older adult has 2 minutes to complete each task before moving on to the next one. The instrument has demonstrated high correlations with proxy reports and has a high predictive validity for future hospitalizations and mortality (Pearson, 2000).

The Up and Go Test (Mathias et al., 1986) is a reliable and valid test to quantify functional mobility. The test is quick, requires little training and no special equipment, and is appropriate to use in many settings, including hospitals and clinics. This instrument can predict a person's ability to go outside alone safely. As the practitioner observes, the person rises from a chair, walks 3 m, turns, walks back to chair, and sits down. Factors to note are sitting balance, transferring from sitting to standing (e.g., does the person need to push off the armrest in order to rise), pace and stability of walking, ability to turn without staggering, and sitting back down in the chair. A recent review of 17 functional balance tests recommended the Timed Up and Go Test as valid and reliable for the elderly population (Langley et al., 2007).

Assessment of Cognition

The assessment of cognitive status in older adults is an important part of the functional assessment. Cognitive impairment resulting from disease may be attributed to normal changes with aging and can delay diagnostic workup. In general, a gradual and mild to moderate decline in short-term memory may be attributable to aging; an older adult may need more time to learn new material or a new task or may need a system for reminders. Domains of cognition included in most mental status assessments are attention, memory, orientation, language, visuospatial skills, and higher cognitive functions.

Altered cognition in older adults is commonly attributed to three disorders, **dementia, delirium,** or **depression,** although other disorders, such as normal pressure hydrocephalus, also may be contributory. Depressed persons often complain of memory impairment. Delirium presents as an acute change in cognition, affecting the domain of attention. Delirium is usually attributable to an acute illness such as an infection or a medication side effect, whereas persons with Alzheimer's dementia have alterations in word finding and naming objects in addition to memory problems. These disorders commonly occur simultaneously and can complicate assessments. For example, persons with dementia are at higher risk for delirium and in the early stages of dementia may also be depressed. Nursing guidelines incorporating best practices related to caregiving strategies for adults aged 65 years and older with delirium, dementia, and depression have been developed by the Registered Nurses' Association of Ontario (RNAO) and are available free of charge on the RNAO Web site: http://www.rnao.org (RNAO, 2004).

For nurses in various settings, cognitive assessments provide continuing comparisons to the individual's baseline to detect any acute changes, such as with delirium. The assessments are not diagnostic but are for screening purposes and identify the need for a more comprehensive workup. Cognitive assessments are important for discharge

TABLE 30-1	Common Cognitive Assessment Instruments		
Name of Instrument	Type of Test	Domains Covered	Administration Time
MiniMental State Examination (Folstein et al., 1975)	Mental status	Orientation, immediate and delayed recall, working memory, language, visuospatial ability	10 min
Short Portable Mental Status Questionnaire (Pfeiffer, 1975)	Mental status	Orientation, general/personal information, working memory	5–10 min
Mini-Cog (Borson et al., 2003)	Mental status	Immediate and delayed recall, visuospatial ability	5–10 min
Blessed Orientation-Memory-Concentration Test (BOMC) (Katzman et al., 1983)	Mental status	Orientation, immediate and delayed recall, and working memory	3–6 min
Geriatric Depression Scale, Short Form (Yesavage and Brink, 1983)	Depression	Depression and changes in level of depression	5–10 min
Confusion Assessment Method (Inouye et al., 1990)	Delirium		
Neecham Confusion Scale (Neelon et al., 1996)	Delirium		
Clock Drawing Test (Shulman et al., 1986)	Mental status	Cognitive and adaptive functioning, memory, ability to process information	2–5 min

planning (e.g., will the person remember to take the prescribed medications) and to assess for readiness for learning. As with screening for ADLs and IADLs, assessment of cognition helps with determining the best discharge plan. Common assessment instruments are listed in Table 30-1.

Social Domain

The quality of life an older person experiences is closely linked to the success of social function. The social domain focuses on relationships within family, social groups, and the community, and is composed of multiple dimensions including the sources of formal and informal assistance available from those relationships. Knowledge of the day-to-day routines can give the healthcare professional baseline information and a reference point to detect functional decline during future encounters.

A comprehensive social assessment is typically spread over several evaluation periods. Because more than 80% of all care provided is by family members, the social assessment also addresses assessment of caregivers (Chichin et al., 2001; Stone et al., 1987). Using a multidimensional approach may help to identify potential risks such as elder abuse (Box 30-1).

Social networks consist of informal supports that are accessed by the older adult (Morano et al., 2006). Informal support is based on cultural beliefs regarding who should be providing care, prior relationships, and location and availability of the caregiver. Informal support includes family and close long-time friends and is usually provided free of charge. The value of unpaid, informal caregiving was estimated to be

$50.9 billion in Canada in 1998 (Zukewich, 2003). This includes domestic work such as cooking, cleaning, shopping, and care of other household members.

Formal supports include programs such as social welfare and other social service and healthcare delivery agencies such as home health care. Semiformal supports such as church societies, neighbourhood groups, and senior centres also form an important role in social support (Zarit et al., 1993).

The availability of assistance from family or friends frequently determines whether a functionally dependent older adult remains at home or is institutionalized. Several studies conclude that the presence of a caregiver is the most important factor in the discharge plan of older adults from an acute care hospital (Brown et al., 1990). Knowing who would be available to help the person if he or she becomes ill is important to document even for healthy older adults.

Gather your assessment of social support in a systematic manner. Several standardized assessment instruments are available to provide structured assessment. The Norbeck Social Support Questionnaire (Norbeck et al., 1980, 1983) was developed to measure the multiple components of social support.* It allows the individual to rate his or her own social network and perceived social support from the network. The Norbeck Social Support Questionnaire can also be used to measure social support with caregivers. Primary caregivers (especially spouses and adult children) often face high levels of demand and limitations on personal freedom that can result in increased stress, burden, and impaired physical health.

CAREGIVER ASSESSMENT

Most older adults with functional impairment live in the community with the help of informal support (commonly a spouse or other family member, often a daughter). Many spousal caregivers are as frail as the person they are caring

BOX 30-1	Components of Social Assessment

- Social network (formal, semiformal, informal)
- Caregiver assessment
- Elder abuse
- Environment
- Spiritual

*Norbeck Social Support Questionnaire is available online at http://evolve.elsevier.com/Canada/Jarvis/examination/.

for, or the adult children are themselves over the age of 65 years and may be coping with their own chronic illnesses. Although many caregivers experience satisfaction from providing care, there may also be great mental and physical stressors linked with caregiving (Kramer, 1997). High levels of functional dependency place a burden on the caregiver and may result in caregiver burnout, sleep disturbances, depression, morbidity, and even increased mortality (O'Rourke et al., 2000).

An older person's need for institutionalization often is better predicted from assessment of the caregiver characteristics and stress than from the severity of the patient's illness (Sullivan, 2002). The health and well-being of the patient and caregiver are closely linked. For these reasons, part of caring for a frail elder involves paying attention to the well-being of the caregiver. For the stressed caregiver, a social worker may help identify programs such as caregiver support groups, respite programs, adult daycare, or homecare support workers.

Assessment of Caregiver Burden

All caregivers should be screened for caregiver burden; for individuals caring for a frail elder, or one who may be cognitively impaired elder, the demands can be overwhelming. The level of care the older adult requires may exceed caregiver ability. Caregiver burden is the strain felt by the person who cares for an older, chronically ill, or disabled person, and it is linked to the caregiver's ability to cope and handle stress.

One formal screening tool is the Caregiver Strain Index, which identifies caregivers of any age needing a more comprehensive assessment (Fig. 30-3). It is a brief tool with 13 questions addressing potential strain in employment, financial, physical, social, and time domains (Sullivan, 2002). Caregiver stress can potentially lead to elder abuse; therefore, a thorough assessment may identify opportunities to prevent and stop elder abuse.

Elder Abuse

The World Health Organization (WHO) defines *elder abuse* as "single or repeated acts, or lack of appropriate action, occurring within a relationship where there is an expectation of trust, which causes harm or distress to an older person" (WHO, 2002). Elder abuse is an umbrella term used to describe one or more of the following situations: physical abuse, sexual abuse, emotional or psychological abuse, financial or material exploitation, abandonment, neglect, or a combination of these (Box 30-2).

Caregiver Strain Questionnaire		
I am going to read a list of things that other people have found to be difficult in helping out after somebody comes home from the hospital. ***Would you tell me whether any of these apply to you?*** (GIVE EXAMPLES)		
	Yes = 1	No = 0
Sleep is disturbed (e.g., because . . . is in and out of bed or wanders around at night)		
It is inconvenient (e.g., because helping takes so much time or it's a long drive over to help)		
It is a physical strain (e.g., because of lifting in and out of a chair; effort or concentration is required)		
It is confining (e.g., helping restricts free time or cannot go visiting)		
There have been family adjustments (e.g., because helping has disrupted routine; there has been no privacy)		
There have been changes in personal plans (e.g., had to turn down a job; could not go on vacation)		
There have been emotional adjustments (e.g., because of severe arguments)		
Some behaviour is upsetting (e.g., because of incontinence; . . . has trouble remembering things; or . . . accuses people of taking things)		
It is upsetting to find . . . has changed so much from his/her former self (e.g., he/she is a different person than he/she used to be)		
There have been work adjustments (e.g., because of having to take time off)		
It is a financial strain		
Feeling completely overwhelmed (e.g., because of worry about . . .; concerns about how you will manage)		
Total Score (count yes responses)		

From Sullivan, M.T. (2002). Caregiver strain index (CSI), Try this: Best practice in nursing care to older adults: Issue #14. *Retrieved from http://www. hartfordign.org/publications/trythis/issue14.pdf.*

Fig. 30-3

> **BOX 30-2 | Definitions of the Types of Elder Abuse**
>
> - Psychological abuse—Anything that diminishes a person's sense of dignity, self-worth, or identity
> - Financial or material abuse—Theft or misuse of the older person's money or property
> - Neglect
>   - Active (intentional withholding of basic necessities of life)
>   - Passive (not providing basic necessities due to lack of experience, information, or ability)
> - Physical abuse—Nonaccidental use of force to coerce or harm, does not have to result in injury
> - Sexual abuse—Any nonconsensual sexual behaviour, either physical or psychological
> - Violation of rights—Disregard of basic human and legal rights of the individual
> - Systemic abuse—Rules, regulations, or policies that harm or discriminate against older adults

Most Canadian research indicates that between 4 and 10% of older adults experience one or more forms of abuse or neglect. In the only Canada-wide study, Podnieks et al. (1989) conducted a cross-Canada telephone survey of 2000 randomly chosen elderly persons living in private houses and found that 4% had experienced some form of abuse since their sixty-fifth birthday.

While it is estimated that there are between 168,000 and 421,000 seniors in Canada who are experiencing or have experienced abuse or neglect, most community agencies and government bodies do not collect data involving older adults that come to their attention, and police statistics typically do not identify people's age, making accurate record-keeping very difficult (Canadian Network for the Prevention of Elder Abuse [CNPEA], 2008).

Canada has four major categories of laws to protect older adults from abuse and neglect: family violence laws, the *Criminal Code of Canada*, adult protection laws, and adult guardianship laws.

Family violence laws, which can vary slightly from province to province or territory to territory, focus primarily on physical protection and protecting the person's safety, although some also cover threats or intimidation. The laws tend to come into effect after the fact and usually do not deal with other forms of abuse such as financial abuse. The *Criminal Code of Canada* covers abuses such as physical or sexual assault, intimidation and harassment, and crimes such as theft of property, fraud, or theft by power of attorney. Adult protection laws assign specific provincial health or social service departments the responsibility to respond to the abuse or neglect cases that are brought to their attention. Adult guardianship laws are used when people are mentally incapable of protecting themselves or their property.

It is important to note that older adults may be reluctant to have charges laid or to co-operate with criminal prosecutions if the perpetrator is a friend or relative (often an adult child),

or if they believe they themselves will suffer some form of retribution (CNPEA, 2008).

Assessing for Elder Abuse

When interviewing older adults, a general guideline is to ask direct and simple questions (Box 30-3). Structure your assessment questions in a nonjudgemental and nonthreatening manner. For example, if the person has a physical injury requiring additional assessment, one question could be, "Injuries like this usually do not happen by accident. Was anybody else involved?"

Start with general questions and become progressively more specific if the person's responses indicate elder abuse (Lachs et al., 1995). Arrange time to interview the elder and caregiver together and separately. This is done not only to detect abusive behaviour but to detect disparities in stories or to assess for caregiver stress. Caregivers may be reluctant to discuss their personal problems in the presence of the person who depends on their care.

Although there is not one set marker of abuse, there are several clinical situations that are suggestive of abuse and warrant further assessment (Table 30-2). Clues to elder abuse include observations that the caregiver is reluctant to leave the older adult alone with healthcare professionals, the person defers excessively to the caregiver to answer questions, there are delays between injuries and when treatment is sought, inconsistencies are noted between an observed injury and explanation, there is a lack of appropriate clothing or hygiene, and a history of "doctor shopping" or not having a primary healthcare professional (Beers et al., 2000; Lachs et al., 1995). A positive finding of these clinical situations does not necessarily mean that abuse has occurred. Instead, treat such findings as signs that further assessment is needed.

Risk Factors for Abuse

The typical profile of an elder abuse victim is female, 75 years or older with limited resources, often residing with family (Bonnie et al., 2003). Older adults who are dependent on others for their care are at risk, as are those with physical or mental impairments. An example is someone with cognitive impairment who exhibits disruptive behaviour such as spitting,

> **BOX 30-3 | Canadian Medical Association Screening Questions**
>
> 1. Has anyone ever hurt you?
> 2. Has anyone ever touched you without your consent?
> 3. Has anyone ever made you do things you didn't want to do?
> 4. Has anyone taken anything of yours without asking?
> 5. Has anyone ever scolded or threatened you?
> 6. Have you signed any papers that you didn't understand?
> 7. Is there anyone at home you are fearful of?
> 8. Has anyone ever refused to help you take care of yourself when you needed help?

TABLE 30-2	Elder Abuse: Red Flags		
	Examples	Indicators	Sample Assessment Questions If Abuse Is Suspected
PHYSICAL ABUSE	Slapping, bruising, striking (with or without an object), burning, shaking; inappropriate use of physical restraints; force feeding	Bruised or broken bones, untreated injuries in various stages of healing; laboratory results of medication overdose or underuse; report of being hit, slapped, kicked, or mistreated; a sudden change in behaviour; refusal to allow visitors to see the older adult alone	Are you afraid of anyone at home? Have you been struck, slapped, or kicked? Have you been tied down or locked in a room? Have you been force fed?
SEXUAL ABUSE	Unwanted touching; all sexual assault or battery	Bruises around the breasts or genital area; unexplained genital infections; unexplained vaginal or anal bleeding; torn, stained, or bloody undergarments; an older adult's report	Has anyone touched you in a sexual way without permission?
EMOTIONAL OR PSYCHOLOGICAL ABUSE	Verbal assaults, insults or threats, intimidations or humiliation, treating like an infant, isolating from family, friends, or regular activities, giving "the silent treatment"	Being emotionally upset or agitated, being extremely withdrawn or non-responsive, unusual behaviour usually attributed to cognitive impairment (rocking, biting), an older adult's report	Do you ever feel alone? Have you been threatened with punishment, deprivation, or institutionalization? Have you received "the silent treatment"? Do you receive routine news or information? What happens when you and your caregiver disagree?
ABANDONMENT	Being dropped off at a hospital, nursing facility or institution, or shopping centre	Desertion at home or public location; an older adult's report of being left alone in an unsafe environment for extended periods of time without adequate support	Have you ever been left alone for long periods of time?
FINANCIAL OR MATERIAL EXPLOITATION	Cashing cheques without permission, forging a signature, misusing or stealing money or possessions, coercing or deceiving into signing any document	Excessive cheques made out to "cash," sudden changes in bank account or banking practice, unauthorized withdrawal of funds, unexplained sudden transfer of assets, substandard care being provided or bills unpaid despite the availability of adequate financial resources, an older adult's report	Is money being stolen from you or used inappropriately? Have you been forced to sign a power of attorney, will, or other document against your wishes? Have you been forced to make purchases against your wishes? Does your caregiver depend on you for financial support?
NEGLECT	Failure to provide life necessities such as food, water, clothing, shelter, personal hygiene, medications, comfort, personal safety	Dehydration, malnutrition, untreated pressure ulcers, poor hygiene, dermatitis from urine contact with skin, unsafe living conditions (i.e., no heat or running water), inappropriate use of medications (either under or over), an older adult's report	Do you lack needed items such as eyeglasses, hearing aids, or false teeth? Is your home safe?
SELF-NEGLECT	Older adult's refusal or failure to provide himself/herself with life necessities such as food, water, clothing, shelter, personal hygiene, medications, comfort, personal safety. Self-neglect excludes a situation in which a mentally competent older person makes a conscious and voluntary decision to put oneself in a circumstance that threatens his or her health or safety	Dehydration, malnutrition, untreated pressure ulcers, poor hygiene, dermatitis from urine contact with skin, unsafe living conditions (i.e., no heat or running water)	

Data from National Center on Elder Abuse: *www.elderabusecenter.org*; Administration on Aging: *www.aoa.gov.eldfam.asp*.

screaming, or hitting and poses extra challenges to caregivers (Lachs et al., 1995). Caregivers who are dependent on the older person financially are more likely to mistreat the older person as a way to counteract the feelings of powerlessness (Godkin et al., 1989). Social isolation is another risk factor; no one from the outside is looking in at the situation. Social isolation also makes detection difficult because abuse tends to increase isolation (i.e., the abuser limits visitors, phone calls, and outside interactions) (NCEA, www.elderabusecenter.org). See Box 30-4 for a mnemonic to help identify high-risk situations (SAVED).

Theories and Frameworks of Elder Abuse

A recent study of older adults, as well as formal and informal caregivers, found that gender, ageism, and cultural factors play important roles in elder abuse experiences. Study participants identified that (1) abuse is cyclical and occurs from generation to generation; (2) abuse occurs throughout the lifespan; (3) exposure to multiple forms of elder abuse is common; and (4) spousal abuse continues in older life (Walsh, 2007).

The most common explanations of abuse of older adults focus on the following (Health Canada, 1999):

- **A web of dependent relationships**—Physical, emotional, and financial, between the victim and abuser. Research findings are inconsistent. Not all dependent seniors are abused. Some studies even suggest that abusers are more likely than nonabusers to be dependent on their victims.
- **Traits of the abusive caregiver**—Research has linked mental health problems and social characteristics of caregivers to abuse. One example is that abusers are more likely than nonabusers to have alcohol or other substance abuse problems.
- **Situational stress**—Caregiver stress related to long-term care of an older adult sometimes leads to abuse. The failure of stress-reducing interventions (e.g., home care assistance, respite care) to reduce abuse has led to less emphasis on the singular importance of caregiver stress.
- **Transgenerational family violence**—Children from a long history of family violence "getting back at" a parent. The limited research on this theory suggests that it explains child abuse much more than senior abuse.

BOX 30-4	SAVED: A Mnemonic to Help Identify High-Risk Situations

Social isolation or stressed caregiver
Alcohol or other substance abuse
Violence (previous history; prior interpersonal violence)
Emotions (psychiatric illness)
Dependency and dynamics between caregiver and client

From Benton, D., & Marshall, C. (1991). Elder abuse. *Clinics in Geriatric Medicine, 7,* 831–845.

BOX 30-5	STOP HARM: A Mnemonic to Help Detect, Diagnose, and Manage Elder Abuse

Screen for abuse in all elderly patients
Think about risk factors
Ominous danger signs present?
Physical findings
History
Address issue of elder abuse
Report to adult protective services
Manage with prevention and risk factor modification

From Kruger, R.M., & Moon, C.H. (1999). Can you spot the signs of elder mistreatment? *Postgraduate Medicine, 106,* 169–183.

- **Social isolation**—Isolation has not been established as a cause of abuse, but abused older adults are more likely to have fewer contacts with friends and family members than are nonabused older adults.
- **Pervasive societal power imbalances**—Individual experience is inseparably linked to social forces and institutional practices that may support power imbalances in families (e.g., ageism or sexism).

Documentation

Proper and precise documentation is important in recording suspected cases of elder abuse because medical records may become part of the legal record. If possible, document verbatim descriptions of events and draw or photograph physical findings. See Box 30-5 (STOP HARM) for a mnemonic to help detect, diagnose, and manage elder abuse.

ENVIRONMENTAL ASSESSMENT

The physical environment of the older person includes the home environment and community system and is critical to maintaining independence. Environmental hazards within the home can be a potential constraint on the elder's day-to-day functioning. Common environmental hazards include inadequate lighting, loose throw rugs, curled carpet edges, obstructed hallways, cords in walkways, lack of grab bars in tub and shower, and low and loose toilet seats (Chu, 1998b; Eliopoulis, 1997; Kim and Dyer, 2006). These hazards increase the risk of falls and fractures. Environmental modification can promote mobility and reduce the likelihood of the older adult's falling. The *Inventory of Fall Prevention Initiatives in Canada* (Health Canada, 2005) provides a current overview of fall prevention activities across the country.

The functional assessment should inquire about the safety of the neighbourhood and whether older persons have transportation or transportation services readily available. The older adult needs access to basic services such as food and clothing stores, pharmacists, financial institutions, healthcare

---

BOX 30-6 | The Public Health Agency of Canada's "Keeping Your Home Safe" Checklist

Outside:

- Do all your entrances have an outdoor light?
- Do your outdoor stairs, pathways, or decks have railings and provide good traction (i.e., textured surfaces)?
- Are the front steps and walkways around your house in good repair and free of clutter, snow, and leaves?
- Do the doorways to your balcony or deck have a low sill or threshold?
- Can you reach your mailbox safely and easily?
- Is the number of your house clearly visible from the street and well lit at night?

Inside:

- Are all rooms and hallways in your home well lit?
- Are all throw rugs and scatter mats secured in place to keep them from slipping?
- Have you removed scatter mats from the top of the stairs and high-traffic areas?
- Are your high-traffic areas clear of obstacles?
- Do you always take steps to ensure that your pets are not underfoot?
- If you use floor wax, do you use the nonskid kind?
- Do you have a first aid kit and know where it is?
- Do you have a list of emergency numbers near all phones?

---

facilities, and social service agencies. The environment needs to be safe, and to include street lamps, sidewalks, and police and fire protection (Chu, 1998b). Both the home and community environment affect the safety of the older adult (Carol, 1996). Safety is especially important for older adults dependent in IADLs and still living within the community.

Older persons often have problems not easily detected during an office visit. A home visit can reveal problems in the living situation, such as household and bathing hazards, social isolation, family/caregiver stress, and nutrition issues (Kim et al., 2006). The Canadian Consumer Product Safety Bureau with Health Canada (http://www.hc-sc.gc.ca/cps-spc/index_e.html) provides publications on injury data and the safe handling and design of products. See also Box 30-6.

SPIRITUAL ASSESSMENT

Spirituality provides personal answers about the meaning and purpose of one's own life (Heriot, 1992) and how to interpret life events and regard them as "bigger than oneself." Spiritual health may improve with age, even as physical and mental health deteriorate. The aging process is a part of one's journey, with capability for growth (Berggren-Thomas et al., 1995). Views on spirituality vary greatly from one adult to another and between people of the same faith or belief system. It is important to acknowledge spirituality as a powerful coping mechanism during stressful life events and illness through to the end of life (Moore, 1998).

Spiritual assessment is highly individual and may be delayed until a professional–patient relationship has been developed. Open-ended questions provide a foundation for future dialogue. A sample question posed during the initial assessment may be, "Do you consider yourself to be a spiritual person?" If the person says yes, a follow-up question could be, "How does that spirituality relate to your health or healthcare decisions?" Involving chaplains or clergy members when possible and appropriate can provide the older adult with support and can serve as a resource to the clinician.

SPECIAL CONSIDERATIONS

Assessment of the functional status of an older adult can be more time consuming than for younger adults. It may take longer for the patient to understand and process the questions and to respond. The presence of physical disabilities, anxiety, depression, pain, or fatigue may necessitate several sessions to complete the assessment. The older adult may need assistance with clothing and may prefer that a family member be present for all or parts of the examination. For hospitalized or institutionalized older adults, consider assessing function during normal activities such as grooming, at mealtime, or during toileting.

Understand that a person with multiple medical problems may tire early and easily and that many medications have side effects that contribute to fatigue or affect the attention span. Again, assessments may need to be done incrementally, such as positioning for comfort and clustering similar tasks to prevent fatigue. Having the person use glasses or hearing aids can mitigate communication difficulties resulting from vision or hearing loss. Provide directions in written format if necessary and have hearing amplifiers and page magnifiers available. Face the person as much as possible, speak slowly in a lower-pitched voice, and enunciate words clearly. Be prepared to use interpreters rather than family members for non–English-speaking patients.

Older adults are a heterogeneous group. You must be aware of your own attitudes and beliefs about older adults to ensure that the functional assessment is truly reflecting abilities and not the myth that functional decline is a normal outcome of aging. Demonstrating respect and interest and treating the patient as an individual is imperative. Ask how the older adult would like to be addressed. Maximize communication by using terminology understandable to the person rather than medical jargon. Including the older adult in decision making about how the interview or testing is to be done will establish rapport and promote self-esteem. Be aware of body language and behaviours and be prepared to modify your approach. Touch can also help in establishing rapport and can reduce anxiety.

A functional assessment can be intimidating for older adults. Frustration or embarrassment may arise if some physical manoeuvres cannot be performed or questions cannot be answered during cognitive testing. They may also be fearful about the consequences of functional testing, such as losing independence, or having a caregiver move into the home. Try to provide reassurance that not everyone can complete all of the tasks or answer all of the questions and that, to the extent possible, confidentiality will be honoured.

Ensure adequate space if testing mobility. An older adult may need room to manoeuvre an assistive device. When testing mobility, stand close to him or her to prevent a fall. The environment should be well lit and feature nonskid flooring. Minimize extraneous noise. Warm rooms, access to fluids, close proximity to a bathroom, and privacy are important.

Cultural Considerations

Be aware that culture influences all parts of the person's life (review Chapter 3). Food habits and dietary beliefs may conflict with dietary recommendations made by healthcare professionals. The response to pain, including how it is perceived, how much is considered tolerable, and the reaction to pain experienced, varies among and within different cultures. How the person interprets the symptoms, meaning, and causes of illness can be defined by his or her culture. It also plays a part in when the older adult seeks care and may influence how the illness is treated. He or she may want to try traditional or alternative practices to prevent or treat certain conditions.

Wide differences appear among individuals in every culture. Learn how the person's culture fits together with suggested interventions. Culture influences whether the older adult relies on family for care or the approach to decision making (i.e., involvement of family and friends), disclosure of medical information (i.e., cancer diagnosis), and end-of-life care (i.e., advance directives and resuscitation preferences and nutrition) (Chu, 1998a; Reuben et al., Welch, 1996).

Assessing Those in Pain

Pain is not a normal part of aging. If the older adult is feeling pain or discomfort, the depth of knowledge gathered through the assessments will suffer. Alleviating pain should be a priority over other aspects of the assessment. It may be necessary to administer premedication before portions of the assessment, especially if the assessment requires movement. Another strategy is to use positioning to decrease pain. Ask what position is most comfortable. Providing comfort can help maximize the information gathered. It is paramount to remember that older adults with cognitive impairment do *not* experience less pain.

A variety of pain assessment scales are available to use in cognitively impaired older adults. The "gold standard" continues to be a person's self-report. Several studies have demonstrated that those with cognitive impairment can self-report pain, which must be taken seriously (Pautex et al., 2006).

Assessing Elders With Altered Cognition

Cognitive impairment poses unique challenges. The older adult may not be able to actively participate in the evaluation or provide consistent answers. Cognitive impairment may severely restrict the ability for expression. Gathering information from an older adult firsthand is always best but not always feasible. To ensure the collection of reliable information, one strategy is to interview the caregiver or family to obtain subjective assessment data. Another is to arrange opportunities to assess the patient during different times of the day, when he or she may be more clear-headed. If possible, split the assessment into smaller sections at a time. Be flexible.

Adults with cognitive impairment may need questions or directions broken down into single commands, repeated word for word, ongoing verbal cueing, or a physical cue. For example, after getting the person's attention the interviewer might say "sit here" and pat the chair. Never assume that he or she cannot respond to questions even when there is known cognitive impairment. Using yes or no questions may prevent frustration. Be relaxed and patient because a person with dementia may mirror your emotions. If a family member or caregiver does need to provide collateral information, avoid collecting it in front of the patient.

Assessment at the End of Life

Ideally, all aspects of the social assessment would be completed before the approach to the end of life. If this is not the case, the depth and completeness of the assessment is dependent on the plan of care. If interviewing is not possible, pull all available data together to formulate interventions. Use information from caregivers and other existing sources. Be conscious that caregiver stress may be increased during this time of added strain.

This chapter highlights the importance and components of a functional assessment of older adults in a variety of settings. An additional resource for geriatric assessment tools recommended by the John A. Hartford Foundation and Nurse Competence in Aging initiative is available online at www.geronurseonline.org.

REFERENCES

Administration on Aging. (2006). *Elder abuse prevention*. Retrieved October 14, 2006, from http://www.aoa.gov/eldfam.asp

American Medical Association. (1992). *Diagnostic and treatment guidelines on elder abuse and neglect (1992)*. Retrieved December 4, 2006, from http://www.ama-assn.org/ama1/pub/upload/mm/386/elderabuse.pdfns

Arno, P. S., Levine, C., & Memmott, M. M. (1999). The economic value of informal caregiving. *Health Affairs, 18*, 182–188.

Beers, M. H., & Berkow, R. (Eds.). (2000). *The Merck manual of geriatrics* (3rd ed.). Whitehouse Station, NJ: Merck Research Laboratories.

Berggren-Thomas, P., & Griggs, M. J. (1995). Spirituality in aging: Spiritual need or spiritual journey? *Journal of Gerontological Nursing, 21*(3), 5–10.

Bonnie, R. J., & Wallace, R. B. (Eds.). (2003). *Panel to Review Risk and Prevalence of Elder Abuse and Neglect, National Research Council, Elder mistreatment: Abuse, neglect, and exploitation in an aging America*. Washington, DC: The National Academies Press.

Borson, S., Scanlan, J. M., Chen, P., & Ganguli, M. (2003). The mini cog as a screen for dementia: validation in a population-based sample. *Journal of the American Geriatric Society, 51*, 1451.

Brown, L. J., Potter, J. F., & Foster, B. G. (1990). Caregiver burden should be evaluated during geriatric assessment. *Journal of the American Geriatric Society, 38*, 455–460.

Brownell, P., Berman, J., & Salamone, A. (1999). Mental health and criminal justice issues among perpetrators of elder abuse. *Journal of Elder Abuse and Neglect, 11*, 81–94.

Canadian Network for the Prevention of Elder Abuse. (2008). *What is abuse of seniors?* Retrieved April 18, 2008, from http://www.cnpea.ca/

Carol, W. (1996). Socioeconomic and environmental influences. In A. G. Lueckenotte (Ed.), *Gerontological nursing* (pp. 180–191). St. Louis, MO: C.V. Mosby.

Chichin, E., et al. (2001). Caregiving/mistreatment. In M. Mezey, T. Fulmer, & C. Mariano (Eds.). (2001). *Best nursing practices for older adults: Incorporating essential gerontological content into baccalaureate nursing education and staff development* (3rd ed.). New York, NY: The John A. Hartford Foundation for Geriatric Nursing.

Chu, N. (1998). Environment/home. In A. S. Luggen, S. S. Travis, & S. Meiner (Eds.), *NGNA core curriculum for gerontological advanced practice nurses*. Thousand Oaks, CA: SAGE.

Chu, N. L. (1998). Culture, race, and ethnicity. In A. S. Luggen, S. S. Travis, & S. Meiner (Eds.), *NGNA core curriculum for gerontological advanced practice nurses*. Thousand Oaks, CA: SAGE.

DeFrances, C. J., & Podgornik, M. N. (2006). National hospital discharge survey. *Advance Data, 4*, 1–19.

Eliopoulis, C. (1997). *Gerontological nursing* (4th ed.). Philadelphia, PA: J.B. Lippincott.

Fillenbaum, G. C., & Smyer, M. (1981). The development, validity, and reliability of the ORS, multidimensional functional assessment questionnaire. *Journal of Gerontology, 36*, 428–434.

GeroNurse Online. (2005). *Why gerontological nursing certification?* Retrieved February, 2005 from http://www.geronurseonline.com/

Gilmore, H., & Park, J. (2005). Dependency, chronic conditions and pain in seniors (Statistics Canada Catalogue No. 82-003). *Supplement to Health Reports, 16*.

Godkin, M., Wolf, R., & Pillemer, K. (1989). A case-comparison analysis of elder abuse and neglect. *International Journal of Aging and Human Development, 28*, 207–225.

Groll, D. L., To, T., Bombardier, C., & Wright, J. G. (2005). The development of a comorbidity index with physical function as the outcome. *Journal of Clinical Epidemiology, 58*, 595–602.

Guse, L. W. (2006). Assessment of the older adult. In K. L. Mauk (Ed.), *Gerontological nursing competencies for care* (pp. 265–292). Sudbury, MA: Jones & Bartlett.

Hamilton, B., et al. (1987). A uniform national data system for medical rehabilitation. In M.J. Fuher (Ed.), *Rehabilitation outcomes: Analysis and measurement*. Baltimore, MD: Brooks.

Health Canada. (1999). *Abuse and neglect of older adults. Information from the National Clearinghouse on Family Violence*. Retrieved April 18, 2008, from http://www.phac-aspc.gc.ca/ncfv-cnivf/familyviolence/pdfs/abuseneg98en.pdf

Health Canada. (2005). *Inventory of fall prevention initiatives in Canada*. Retrieved April 18, 2008, from http://hc-sc.gc.ca/seniors-aines/pubs/fall_prevention_initiatives/pdf/fall_prevention_initiatives_e.pdf

Heriot, C. S. (1992). Spirituality and aging. *Holistic Nursing Practice, 7*, 22–31.

Inouye, S. K., van Dyck, C. H., Alessi, C. A., Balkin, S., Siegal, A. P., Horowitz, R. I. (1990). Clarifying confusion: The confusion assessment method. *Annals of Internal Medicine, 113*, 941–948.

Kane, R., & Kane, R. (2000). *Assessing older persons: Measures, meaning, and practical applications*. New York, NY: Oxford University Press.

Karagiozis, H., Gray, S., Sacco, J., Shapiro, M., & Kawas, C. (1998). The direct assessment of functional abilities (DADA): A comparison to an indirect measure of instrumental activities of daily living. *Gerontologist, 38*, 113–121.

Katz, S., Ford, A. B., Moskowitz, R. W., Jackson, B. A., & Jaffe, M. W. (1963). Studies of illness in the aged: The index of ADL, a standardized measure of biological and psychosocial functioning. *Journal of the American Medical Association, 185*, 94–101.

Kim, L. C., & Dyer, C. B. (2006). Assessment of older adults in their homes. In J. J. Gallo (Ed.), *Handbook of geriatric assessment* (4th ed.). Sudbury, MA: Jones & Bartlett.

Kramer, B. (1997). Gain in the caregiving experience: Where are we? What next? *Gerontologist, 37*, 218–232.

Kresevic, D. M., & Mezey, M. (2003). Assessment of function. In M. Mezey et al. (Eds.), *Geriatric nursing protocols for best practice* (2nd ed., pp. 31–46). New York, NY: Springer Publishing Company.

Kruger, R. M., & Moon, C. H. (1999). Can you spot the signs of elder mistreatment? *Postgraduate Medicine, 106*, 169–183.

Kuriansky, J. B., & Gurland, B. (1976). Performance test of activities of daily living. *International Journal of Aging and Human Development, 7*, 343–352.

Lachs, M., & Pillemer, K. (1995). Abuse and neglect of elderly persons. *New England Journal of Medicine, 332*, 437–443.

Langley, F. A., & Mackintosh, S. F. H. (2007). Functional balance assessment of older community dwelling adults: a systematic review of the literature. *Internet Journal of Allied Health Sciences and Practice, 5*(4).

Lawton, M. P., & Brody, E. M. (1969). Assessment of older people: Self-maintaining and instrumental activities of daily living. *Gerontologist, 9*, 179–186.

Linn, M. (1988). Rapid disability: Rating scale-2 (RDRS-2). *Psychopharmacology Bulletin, 24*, 799–800.

Linn, M., & Linn, B. (1982). The rapid disability rating scale-2. *Journal of the American Geriatric Society, 30*, 378–382.

Mahoney, F. I., & Barthel, D. W. (1965). Functional evaluation: The Barthel index. *Maryland State Medical Journal, 14*, 61–65.

Manton, K. G., & Gu, X. (2001). Changes in the prevalence of chronic disability in the United States Black and non-Black population above age 65 from 1982 to 1999. *Proceedings of the National Academy of Science USA, 98*, 6354–6359.

Mathias, S., Nayak, U. S., & Isaacs, B. (1986). Balance in the elderly patient: The "Get Up and Go" test. *Archives of Physical Medicine and Rehabilitation, 67*, 387–389.

Mathieson, K. M., Kronenfeld, J. J., & Keith, V. M. (2002). Maintaining functional independence in elderly adults: The roles of health status and financial resources in predicting home modifications and use of mobility equipment. *Gerontologist, 42,* 24–31.

McDowell, I., & Newell, C. (1996). *Measuring health: A guide to rating scales and questionnaires* (2nd ed., pp. 47–121). New York, NY: Oxford University Press.

Moore, S. (1998). Spirituality. In A. S. Luggen, S. S. Travis, & S. Meiner (Eds.), *NGNA core curriculum for gerontological advanced practice nurses.* Thousand Oaks, CA: SAGE.

Morano, C., & Morano, B. (2006). Social assessment. In J. J. Gallo, H. R. Bogner, T. Fulmer, & G. J. Paveza (Eds.), *Handbook of geriatric assessment* (4th ed). Sudbury, MA: Jones & Bartlett.

National Center on Elder Abuse. (2006). *Is elder abuse a crime? The basics.* Retrieved October 31, 2006, from http://www.elderabusecenter.org

National Center on Elder Abuse at American Public Human Services Association. (1998). *National Elder Abuse Incidence Study.* Retrieved October 30, 2006, from http://www.aoa.gov.eldfam/Elder_Right/Elder_Abuse/AbuseReport_Full.pdf

Norbeck, J. S., Lindsey, A. M., & Carrieri, V. L. (1980). The development of an instrument to measure social support. *Nursing Research, 30,* 264–269.

Norbeck, J. S., Lindsey, A. M., & Carrieri, V. L. (1983). Further development of the Norbeck Social Support Questionnaire: Normative data and validity testing. *Nursing Research, 32,* 4–9.

O'Rourke, N., & Tuokko, H. (2000). The psychological and physical costs of caregiving: The Canadian Study of Health and Aging. *Journal of Applied Gerontology, 19,* 389–404.

Pautex, S., & Gold, G. (2006). Assessing pain intensity in older adults. *Geriatrics and Aging, 9,* 399–402.

Pearson, V. (2000). Assessment of function. In R. Kane & R. Kane (Eds.), *Assessing older persons: Measures, meaning and practical applications* (pp. 17–48). New York, NY: Oxford University Press.

Podnieks, E., Pillemer, K., Nicholson, J., et al. (1989). *National survey on abuse of the elderly in Canada: Preliminary findings.* Toronto, ON: Office of Research and Innovation, Ryerson Polytechnical Institute.

Public Health Agency of Canada. (2005). *The safe living guide— A guide to home safety for seniors* (3rd ed.). Retrieved April 18, 2008, from http://www.hc-sc.gc.ca/seniors-aines/pubs/safelive/index.htm

Rapoport, J., Jacobs, P., Bell, N. R., et al. (2004). Refining the measurement of the economic burden of chronic diseases in Canada. *Chronic Diseases in Canada, 25*(1), 13–21.

Registered Nurses Association of Ontario. (2004). *Caregiving strategies for older adults with delirium, dementia and depression.* Toronto, ON: Author.

Reuben, D. B., Herr, K. A., Pacala, J. T., Pollock, B. G., Potter, J. F., Semla, T. P. (Eds.). 2003. *Geriatrics at your fingertips* (5th ed). Boston: Blackwell/American Geriatrics Society.

Richmond, T., Tang, S. T., Tulman, L., Fawcett, J., & McCorkle, R. (2004). Measuring function. In M. Frank-Stromberg & S. J. Olsen (Eds.), *Instruments for clinical health-care research* (3rd ed.). Sudbury, MA: Jones & Bartlett.

Rosenblatt, D. E., Cho, K. H., & Durance, P. W. (1996). Reporting mistreatment of older adults: The role of physicians. *Journal of the American Geriatric Society, 44,* 65–70.

Rotermann, M. (2006). Seniors' health care use. *Supplement to Health Reports, Volume 16* (Statistics Canada Catalogue No. 82-003).

Rueben, D., & Siu, A. (1990). An objective measure of physical function of elderly outpatients: The physical performance test. *Journal of the American Geriatrics Society, 38,* 1105–1112.

Shulman, K., Shedletsky, R., & Silver, I. (1986). The challenge of time: Clock drawing and cognitive function in the elderly. *International Journal of Geriatric Psychiatry, 1,* 135–140.

Statistics Canada. (2007). Population by sex and age groups, by province and territory (CANSIM, Table 051-0001). Retrieved May 15, 2008, from http://www40.statcan.ca/l01/cst01/demo31a.htm?sdi=population%20age

Stone, R., Cafferate, G. L., & Sangl, J. (1987). Caregivers of the frail elderly: A national profile. *Gerontologist, 27,* 616–626.

Sullivan, M. T. (2002). Caregiver strain index (CSI): Try this. *Best Practice in Nursing Care to Older Adults, 14.* Retrieved from http://www.hartfordign.org/publications/trythis/issue14.pdf

Tatara, T., & Kuzmeskus, L. M. (1999). *Elder abuse information series, No. 1-3.* Washington, DC: National Center on Elder Abuse.

U.S. Consumer Product Safety Commission. (2007). *Older consumers safety checklist.* Retrieved April 13, 2007, from http://www.cpsc.gov/CPSCPUB/PUBS/705.pdf

Walsh, C. A., Ploeg, J., Lohfeld, L., Horne, J., MacMillan, H., & Lai, D. (2007). Violence across the lifespan: Interconnections among forms of abuse as described by marginalized Canadian elders and their caregivers. *British Journal of Social Work, 37,* 491–514.

Welch, A. (1996). Cultural influences. In A. G. Lueckenotte (Ed.), *Gerontological nursing.* St. Louis, MO: C.V. Mosby.

World Health Organization & International Network for the Prevention of Elder Abuse. (2002). Prevention of Elder Abuse. Retrieved May 15, 2008, from http://www.who.int/ageing/projects/elder_abuse/en/

Zarit, S. & Pearlin, L. (1993). Family caregiving: Integrating informal and formal systems for care. In S. Zarit, L. Pearlin, & K. Schaie (Eds.), *Caregiving systems: Informal and formal helpers* (pp. 303–316). Hillsdale, NJ: L. Erlbaum Associates.

Zukewich, N. (2003). Unpaid informal caregiving. Statistics Canada, Catalogue No. 70. 11-008.

APPENDIX A: Braden Risk Assessment Scale

NOTE: Bed and chairbound individuals or those with impaired mobility to reposition should be assessed upon admission for their risk of developing pressure ulcers. Patients with established pressure ulcers should be reassessed periodically.

Patient's Name: _____   Room Number: _____   Date: _____

Sensory Perception	1. Completely Limited	2. Very Limited	3. Slightly Limited	4. No Impairment	Indicate Appropriate Numbers Below
Ability to respond meaningfully to pressure-related discomfort	Unresponsive (does not moan, flinch, grasp) to painful stimuli, due to diminished level of consciousness or sedation. OR limited ability to feel pain over most of body surface.	Responds only to painful stimuli. Cannot communicate discomfort except by moaning or restlessness. OR has a sensory impairment which limits the ability to feel pain or discomfort over 1/2 of body.	Responds to verbal commands, but cannot always communicate discomfort or need to be turned. OR has some sensory impairment which limits ability to feel pain or discomfort in 1 or 2 extremities.	Responds to verbal commands. Has no sensory deficit which would limit ability to feel or voice pain or discomfort.	
Mositure	**1. Constantly Moist**	**2. Very Moist**	**3. Occasionally Moist**	**4. Rarely Moist**	
Degree to which skin is exposed to moisture	Skin is kept moist almost constantly by perspiration, urine, etc. Dampness is detected every time patient is moved or turned.	Skin is often, but not always, moist. Linen must be changed at least once a shift.	Skin is occasionally moist, requiring an extra linen change approximately once a day.	Skin is usually dry. Linen only requires changing at routine intervals.	
Activity	**1. Bedfast**	**2. Chairfast**	**3. Walks Occasionally**	**4. Walks Frequently**	
Degree of physical activity	Confined to bed.	Ability to walk severely limited or non-existent. Cannot bear own weight and/or must be assisted into chair or wheelchair.	Walks occasionally during day, but for very short distances, with or without assistance. Spends majority of each shift in bed or chair.	Walks outside the room at least twice a day and inside room at least once every 2 hours during waking hours.	
Mobility	**1. Completely Immobily**	**2. Very Limited**	**3. Slightly Limited**	**4. No Limitations**	
Ability to change and control body position	Does not make even slight changes in body or extremity position without assistance.	Makes occasional slight changes in body or extremity position but unable to make frequent or significant changes independently.	Makes frequent though slight changes in body or extremity position independently.	Makes major and frequent changes in position without assistance.	
Nutrition	**1. Very Poor**	**2. Probably Adequate**	**3. Adequate**	**4. Excellent**	
Usual food intake pattern	Never eats a complete meal. Rarely eats more than 1/3 of any food offered. Eats 2 servings or less of protein (meat or dairy products) per day. Takes fluids poorly. Does not take a liquid dietary supplement. OR is NPO and/or maintained on clear liquids or IVs for more than 5 days.	Rarely eats a complete meal and generally eats only about 1/2 of any food offered. Protein intake includes only 3 servings of meat or dairy products per day. Occasionally will take a dietary supplement. OR receives less than optimum amount of liquid diet or tube feeding.	Eats over half of most meals. Eats a total of 4 servings of protein (meat, dairy products) each day. Occasionally will refuse a meal, but will usually take a supplement if offered. OR is on a tube feeding or TPN regimen which probably meets most of nutritional needs.	Eats most of every meal. Never refuses a meal. Usually eats a total of 4 or more servings of meat and dairy products. Occasionally eats between meals. Does not require supplementation.	
Friction and Shear	**1. Problem**	**2. Potential Problem**	**3. No Apparent Problem**		
	Requires moderate to maximum assistance in moving. Complete lifting without sliding against sheets is impossible. Frequently slides down in bed or chair, requiring frequent repositioning with maximum assistance. Spasticity, contractures or agitation lead to almost constant friction.	Moves feebly or requires minimum assistance. During a move, skin probably slides to some extent against sheets, chair restraints, or other devices. Maintains relatively good position in chair or bed most of the time, but occasionally slides down.	Moves in bed and in chair independently and has sufficient muscle strength to lift up completely during move. Maintains good position in bed or chair at all times.		

NOTE: Patients with a total score of 16 or less are considered to be at risk of developing pressure ulcers.
(15 or 16 = low risk; 13 or 14 = moderate risk; 12 or less = high risk)

Total Score:

APPENDIX B: Faces Pain Scale – Revised*

In the following instructions, say "hurt" or pain," whichever seems right for a particular child.

"These faces show how much something can hurt. This face [point to left-most face] **shows no pain. The faces show more and more pain** [point to each from left to right] **up to this one** [point to right-most face] **– it shows very much pain.**

Score the chosen face 0, 2, 4, 6, 8, 10, counting left to right, so "0" = "no pain" and "10" = "very much pain". Do not use words like "happy" and "sad." This scale is intended to measure how children feel inside, not how their face looks.

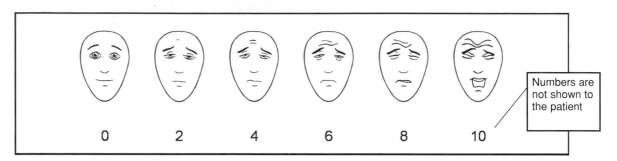

| 0 | 2 | 4 | 6 | 8 | 10 |

Numbers are not shown to the patient

Source: From PAIN, 2001, 93, 173-183 "The Faces Pain Scale – Revised. Toward a Common Metric in Pediatric Pain Measurement," by C.L. Hicks, C.L. von Baeyer, P.A. Spafford, I. van Korlaar, & B. Goodenough. Reprinted with permission of the International Association for the Study of Pain®.

*Note: This is a smaller sample of the actual scale. For further instructions and translations on the correct use of the scale in order to get valid responses, please go to www.painsourcebook.ca

APPENDIX C: Canadian Credible Sources of Nutritional Information

Canadian credible sources of health and nutrition information include professional health organizations, government health agencies, volunteer health agencies, and consumer groups.

Professional health organizations, especially:
- Dietitians of Canada—http://www.dietitians.ca/
- Nutrition Resource Centre— http://www.nutritionrc.ca/about.html
- Canadian Medical Association (CMA)— http://www.pslgroup.com/dg/735a.htm

Government health agencies:
- Health Canada (HC)—http://www.hc-sc.gc.ca/
- Public Health Agency of Canada (PHAC)— http://www.phac-aspc.gc.ca/new_e.html
- Canadian Health Network (CHN)— http://www.canadian-health-network.ca/
- Canadian Food Inspection Agency (CFIA)— http://www.inspection.gc.ca/english/toce.shtml
- Natural Health Products Directorate (NHPD)— http://www.hc-sc.gc.ca/dhp-mps/prodnatur/index_ e.html
- Office of Nutrition Policy and Promotion— http://www.hc-sc.gc.ca/ahc-asc/branch-dirgen/hpfb- dgpsa/onpp-bppn/index_e.html
- Agriculture and Agri-Food Canada (AAFC)— http://www.agr.gc.ca/
- Canadian Nutrient File 2005— http://www.hc-sc.gc.ca/fn-an/nutrition/fiche-nutridata/ index_e.html

Volunteer health agencies such as:
- The Heart and Stroke Foundation of Canada— http://ww2.heartandstroke.ca/Page.asp?PageID=24
- Canadian Diabetes Association—http://www.diabetes.ca/
- Canadian Cancer Society— http://www.cancer.ca/ccs/internet/niw_splash/ 0%2C%2C3172%2C00.html

Reputable Industry and consumer groups such as:
- Canadian Council of Food and Nutrition (CCFN)— http://www.cancer.ca/ccs/internet/niw_splash/ 0%2C%2C3172%2C00.html
- National Council Against Health Fraud (NCAHF)— http://www.ncahf.org/
- Quackwatch—http://www.quackwatch.org/
- Consumers Association of Canada— http://www.consumer.ca
- Food and Consumer Products of Canada— http://www.fcpmc.com/home.asp

Source: Piché, L.A. & Garcia, A.C. (2008). *Canadian supplemental information (CSI) document to accompany nutrition concepts and controversies* (10th ed.). Toronto, ON: Thomson/Nelson.

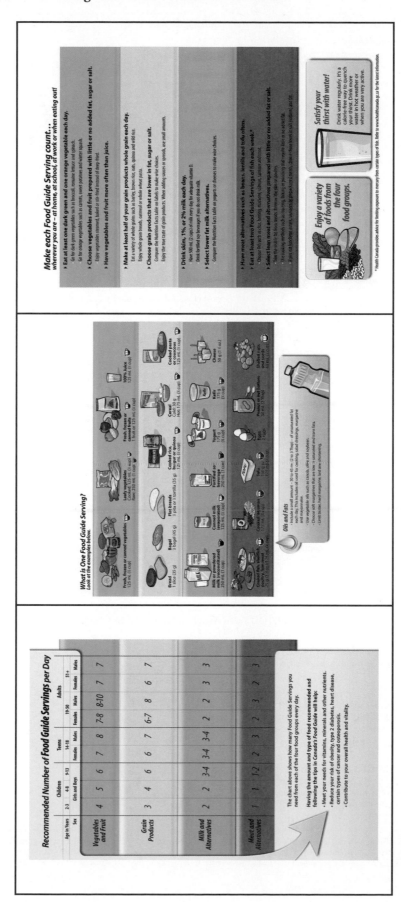

Source: Health Canada. (2007). *Eating Well With Canada's Food Guide.* © Her Majesty the Queen in Right of Canada, represented by the Minister of Health Canada. Cat. No. H164-38/1-2007E. Retrieved June 6, 2008, from http://www.hc-sc.gc.ca/fn-an/alt_formats/hpfb-dgpsa/pdf/food-guide-aliment/print_eatwell_bienmang_e.pdf

APPENDIX E: The Canadian Neurological Scale

SECTION A		MENTATION			*SCORE*
	Level of consciousness			Alert Drowsy	3.0 1.5
	Orientation Place: city or hospital Time: month and year Patient can speak, write or gesture a response.	*Score:* If patient is oriented (can correctly state both place and correct month and year) score 1.0. If patient cannot state both (disoriented), score 0.0.		Oriented Disoriented/NA	1.0 0.0
	Speech *Receptive:* As patient the following separately (do not prompt by gesturing): 1. Close your eyes 2. Point to the ceiling *Expressive:* 1. Show patient 3 items separately, and ask patient to name each object 2. Ask patient what each object is used for, while holding each one up again	*Score:* If patient is unable to do both (Receptive Deficit), score 0.0 and go to Section A2. If patient obeys commands, leave blank and assess expressive speech. *Score:* If patient is able to state the name and use of all 3 objects (Normal Speech), score 1.0 If patient is not able to state the name and use of all 3 objects (Expressive Deficit), score 0.5.		Normal Expressive Deficit Receptive Deficit	1.0 0.5 0.0
				TOTAL:	

SECTION A1		MOTOR FUNCTIONS: WEAKNESS		**WEAKNESS**	
NO COMPREHENSION DEFICIT	**Face** Ask patient to smile/grin, note weakness in mouth or nasal/labial folds.	*Score:* None (no weakness) = 0.5; Present (weakness) = 0.0		None Present	0.5 0.0
	Arm: Proximal Ask patient to lift arm 45-90 degrees. Apply resistance between shoulder and elbow.	*Score:* None (no weakness present) = 1.5; Mild (mild weakness, full ROM, cannot withstand resistance) = 1.0; Significant (moderate weakness, some movement, not full ROM) = 0.5; Total (complete loss of movement; total weakness) = 0		None Mild Significant Total	1.5 1.0 0.5 0
	Arm: Distal Ask patient to make a fist and flex wrist backwards, apply resistance between wrist and knuckles.	*Score:* None (no weakness present) = 1.5; Mild (mild weakness, full ROM, cannot withstand resistance) = 1.0; Significant (moderate weakness, some movement, not full ROM) = 0.5; Total (complete loss of movement; total weakness) = 0		None Mild Significant Total	1.5 1.0 0.5 0
	Leg: Proximal In supine position, ask patient to flex hip to 90 degrees; apply pressure to mid-thigh	*Score:* None (no weakness present) = 1.5; Mild (mild weakness, full ROM, cannot withstand resistance) = 1.0; Significant (moderate weakness, some movement, not full ROM) = 0.5; Total (complete loss of movement; total weakness) = 0		None Mild Significant Total	1.5 1.0 0.5 0
	Leg: Distal Ask patient to dorsiflex foot; apply resistance to top of foot	*Score:* None (no weakness present) = 1.5; Mild (mild weakness, full ROM, cannot withstand resistance) = 1.0; Significant (moderate weakness, some movement, not full ROM) = 0.5; Total (complete loss of movement; total weakness) = 0		None Mild Significant Total	1.5 1.0 0.5 0
				TOTAL:	

SECTION A2		MOTOR FUNCTIONS: MOTOR RESPONSE			
COMPREHENSION DEFICIT	**Face** Have patient mimic your smile. If unable, note facial expression while applying sternal pressure.			Symmetrical Asymmetrical	0.5 0.0
	Arms Demonstrate or lift patient's arms to 90 degrees; score ability to maintain raised arms; apply nail-bed pressure to assess reflex response.			Equal Unequal	1.5 0.0
	Legs Lift patient's hip to 90 degrees; score ability to maintain equal levels (>5 seconds). If unable to maintain raised position, apply nail-bed pressure to assess reflex response.			Equal Unequal	1.5 0.0
				TOTAL:	

Sources: Côté, R., Hachinski, V.C., Shurvell, B.L., Norris, J.W., & Wolfson, C. (1986). The Canadian Neurological Scale: A preliminary study in acute stroke. *Stroke*, 17(4), 731-737; Côté, R., Battista, R.N., Wolfson, C., Boucher, J., Adam, J., & Hachinski, V.C. (1989). The Canadian Neurological Scale: Validation and reliability assessment. *Neurology*, 39, 638-643; Bushnell, C.D., Johnston, D.C.C., & Goldstein, L.B. (2001). Retrospective assessment of initial stroke severity: Comparison of the NIH Stroke Scale and the Canadian Neurological Scale. *Stroke*, 32, 656.

APPENDIX F: Nipissing District Developmental Screen™

Nipissing District Developmental Screen™

The Nipissing, Nipissing District Developmental Screen, and NDDS are trademarks of NDDS Intellectual Property Association, used under license. All rights reserved.

ACTIVITIES FOR YOUR CHILD...

↻ Emotional ✋ Fine Muscle 🏋 Large Muscle 📚 Learning/Thinking
✋ Self-Help 👥 Social 💬 Speech/Language

The following activities will help you play your part in your child's development.

👁 Sing songs with me throughout the day and repeat them often. This helps me learn to sing them on my own. Leave out parts of the song or rhyme for me to finish.

👁 Help me learn new words. Talk to me during bathing, feeding, dressing and doing daily chores. Name my clothing and body parts. Let me help set the table, sort the laundry, and put groceries away.

🏋 Let's play a game. Use two shoeboxes and two toys. We each get a box and a toy. Let's take turns putting our toy in the box, over, under, behind, and on. Talk to me about what we are doing.

🏋 Provide me with toys that allow me to push or pedal with my feet. This will help me learn to climb on and off and to pedal. Make sure I have lots of room. Praise my efforts.

🏋 Let's practice climbing and jumping. I love to get in and out of a box or jump from a bottom step. We can have fun together.

🏋 Let's sing Old MacDonald and move our bodies like the animals: hop like a frog or bunny, squat or waddle like a duck or jump up and down like a kangaroo; etc.

📚 I like to play sorting games with you. We can sort objects by shape, touch, colour, and size. Use spoons, blocks, toys, and clothing.

✋ Let me open and close plastic containers by twisting and turning the lids. Help me find the right lid to put on each container.

✋ I love to pour water from containers during my bath.

✋ I enjoy stringing beads or buttons on a shoelace, string or pipe cleaner. Talk to me about the colour and count the beads as I lace them. Remember, I may still put things in my mouth – so watch me.

✋ I want to become independent. Encourage me to get dressed and undressed, do household tasks, turn lights on and off, and open and close doors.

↻ I am learning about my feelings. Give me words for my feelings and show that you understand.

🏋 I love sharing storybooks with you. Cuddle me while we read together.

I am learning to make decisions. Offer me simple choices throughout the day. For example, "Do you want juice or milk?"

Always talk to your health care or child care professional if you have any questions about your child's development or well being. See reverse side for instructions, limitation of liability, and product license.

2 YEARS

Nipissing District Developmental Screen™

The Nipissing, Nipissing District Developmental Screen, and NDDS are trademarks of NDDS Intellectual Property Association, used under license. All rights reserved.

The Nipissing District Developmental Screen™ is a checklist designed to help monitor your child's development.

Child's Name _____
Birth Date _____ Today's Date _____

By *Two Years* of age, does your child...

Yes No

1. Usually have healthy ears and seem to hear well?
2. Point to at least two familiar objects when asked (e.g. car, bowl)?
3. Ask for help using words or actions?
4. Learn and use one or more new words a week (may only be understood by family)?
5. Join two words together like "want cookie", "more milk", "my hat"?
6. Eat most foods without coughing and choking?
7. Eat with a utensil with little spilling?*
8. Take off own shoes, socks or hat?*
9. Try to run?
10. Play in a squat position? (Picture A)
11. Walk backwards or sideways pulling a toy?
12. Make scribbles and dots on paper or in sand?
13. Put objects into a small container? (Picture B)
14. Like to watch and play near other children?
15. Say "no", and like to do some things without help?*
16. Recognize the use of familiar objects (e.g. drink from cup, hug doll)?
17. Use skills already learned and develop new ones (i.e. no loss of skills)?
18. Copy your actions (i.e. you clap your hands and he/she claps hands)?

A

B

* item may not be common to all cultures

Always talk to your health care or child care professional if you have any questions about your child's development or well being. See reverse side for instructions, limitation of liability, and product license.

2 YEARS

Source: From The Nipissing District Developmental Screen™. Reprinted with permission. The Nipissing, Nipissing District Developmental Screen, and NDDS are trademarks of NDDS Intellectual Property Association, used under license. All rights reserved.

Credits

Inside Back Cover

"Key Laboratory Values" listing: Excerpted from Lewis, S. M., Heitkemper, M. M., Dirksen, S. R., O'Brien, P. G., Giddens, J. F., Bucher, L., et al. (2006). *Medical-surgical nursing in Canada* (1st Canadian ed., pp. 1880–1892). Toronto, ON: Elsevier Canada.

Chapter 1

Figure 1-2: From Alfaro-LeFevre, R. *Critical thinking in nursing: a practical approach* (2nd ed.). (1999). Philadelphia, PA: Saunders.

Figure 1-3: From Alfaro-LeFevre, R. *Critical thinking in nursing: a practical approach* (2nd ed.). (1999). Philadelphia, PA: Saunders.

Figure 1-4: From Potter, P.A., & Perry, A. G. (2005). *Fundamentals of nursing* (6th ed.). St Louis, MO: Mosby.

Chapter 2

Figure 2-1: From Gorrie T. M., McKinney, E. S., Murray, S.S. (1998). *Foundations of maternal-newborn nursing* (2nd ed.). Philadelphia, PA: Saunders.

Figure 2-6: From Rick Brady, Riva, MD.

Figure 2-10: From Rick Brady, Riva, MD.

Figure 2-13: From Rick Brady, Riva, MD.

Chapter 3

Figure 3-1: © Colleen Varcoe.

Figure 3-2: © Annette J. Browne.

Figure 3-3: © Mary Zhang.

Figure 3-4: © Colleen Varcoe.

Figure 3-5: © Colleen Varcoe.

Box 3-1: Adapted from Office of Minority Health. (2001). *National standards for culturally and linguistically appropriate services in health care. Final report.* Washington, DC: Office of Minority Health, Department of Health and Human Services, USA.

Figure 3-6: © Annette J. Browne.

Figure 3-7: © Access Alliance Multicultural Health and Community Services, Toronto, Ontario. Reprinted with permission.

Figure 3-8: © Karol Ghuman.

Figure 3-9: From Kirby, M. J. L. (2002). *The health of Canadians— The federal role. Final report. Volume Six: Recommendations for Reform* (Chapter 13). Retrieved March 10, 2008, from http://www.parl.gc.ca/37/2/parlbus/commbus/senate/Com-e/soci-e/rep-e/repoct02vol6part5-e.htm. Reprinted with permission.

Figure 3-10: From *The Georgia Straight* (March 6-13, 2008, p. 13). Reprinted with permission.

Figure 3-11: From *Special 2006 Run of Statistics Canada Data Using the Statistics Canada CANSIM Tables Generation System, 2006* (Table 202-0802). Toronto, ON: D. Raphael. As reproduced in Raphael, D. (2007). *Poverty and policy in Canada: Implications for health and quality of life* (p. 61). Toronto, ON: Canadian Scholars' Press. Reprinted with permission.

Figure 3-13: © Annette J. Browne.

Figure 3-14: © Health Employees Union, British Columbia. Reprinted with permission.

Figure 3-15: © Mark Richards/PhotoEdit.

Figure 3-16: © Colleen Varcoe.

Chapter 4

Figure 4-2: From Potter, P. A., & Perry, A. G. (2005). *Fundamentals of nursing* (6th ed.). St Louis, MO: Mosby.

Figure 4-6: © Tony Freeman/PhotoEdit.

Chapter 5

Figure 5-1: Adapted from The American Society of Human Genetics, www.ashg.org, 2004.

Figure 5-2: From Goldenring J. M., & Rosen, D.S. (2004). Getting into adolescent heads: an essential update. *Contemp Pediatr* 21(1): 64–90.

Chapter 6

Table 6-2: © M. S. Jellinek and J. M. Murphy. Massachusetts General Hospital. (http://psc.partners.org). English PSC. Reprinted with permission.

Chapter 7

Box 7-1: From Department of Justice Canada. (2007a). *Child abuse fact sheet.* Retrieved April 17, 2008, from http://www.justice.gc.ca/en/ps/fm/childafs.html

Table 7-1: From Public Health Agency of Canada. (2001). *The Canadian incidence study of reported child abuse and neglect highlights.* Retrieved June 6, 2008, from http://www.phac-aspc.gc.ca/cm-vee/cishl01/

Figure 7-1: © Colleen Varcoe.

Figure 7-2: From Cory, J., & Dechief, L. (2007). *Safety and Health Enhancement (SHE) framework for women experiencing abuse: A toolkit for health care providers and planners.* Vancouver, BC: BC Women's Hospital and Health Centre. Retrieved June 6, 2008, from http://www.bcwomens.ca/Services/HealthServices/WomanAbuseResponse/Resources.htm. Reprinted with permission.

Figure 7-3: From Department of Health. (2000). *Framework for the assessment of children in need and their families.* Norwich, UK: Her Majesty's Stationery Office. Available at http://www.dh.gov.uk/en/Publicationsandstatistics/Publications/PublicationsPolicyAndGuidance/DH_4003256. © Crown copyright material is reproduced with the permission of the Controller of HMSO and Queen's Printer for Scotland.

Figure 7-4: Courtesy Daniel J. Sheridan, PhD, RN, CNS, Hanover, MD.

Figure 7-5: Courtesy Daniel J. Sheridan, PhD, RN, CNS, Hanover, MD.

Figure 7-6: Courtesy Daniel J. Sheridan, PhD, RN, CNS, Hanover, MD.

Figure 7-7: Courtesy Jacquelyn C. Campbell, PhD, RN © 1985, 1988, 2001.

Figure 7-8: © Colleen Varcoe.

Chapter 8

Table 8-2: Adapted from Health Canada. (1999). Infection control guidelines: Routine precautions and additional precautions for preventing the transmission of infection in health care. *Canada Communicable Disease Report, 25S4,* 1–148. Retrieved April 16, 2008, from http://www.phac-aspc.gc.ca/publicat/ccdr-rmtc/99pdf/cdr25s4e.pdf

Figure 8-13: Courtesy of *The Pantagraph,* Bloomington, IL, August 10, 1998.

Chapter 9

Figure 9-1: From Health Canada. (2003). *Canadian guidelines for body weight classifications in adults* (Catalogue No. H49-179 /2003E; p. 37). Ottawa, ON: Health Canada. Retrieved June 6, 2008, from http://www.hc-sc.gc.ca/fn-an/alt_formats/hpfb-dgp-sa/pdf/nutrition/weight_book-livres_des_poids_e.pdf

Figure 9-4: Copyright Pat Thomas, 2006.

Figure 9-17: From Rossman, I. (1986). *Clinical geriatrics* (3rd ed.). Philadelphia, PA: Lippincott.

Figure 9-19: From Potter, P. A., & Perry, A. G. (2005). *Fundamentals of nursing* (6th ed.). St Louis, MO: Mosby.

Figure 9-21: From Canadian Hypertension Education Program. (2007). *Assessment of hypertensive patients.* Retrieved April 16, 2008, from http://hypertension.ca/chep/recommendations/diagnosis-assessment/assessment-of-hypertensive-patients/

Art for Table 9-5: (hypopituitary dwarfism) from Hall, R., & Evered, D. C. (1990). *Color atlas of endocrinology* (2nd ed). London, England: Mosby; (gigantism) from Hall, R., & Evered, D. C. (1990). *Color atlas of endocrinology* (2nd ed). London, England: Mosby; (acromegaly [hyperpituitarism]) Reprinted from the Clinical Slide Collection on the Rheumatic Diseases © 1991, 1995, 1997. Used by permission of the American College of Rheumatology; (achondroplastic dwarfism) from Jones, A., & Owen, R. (1995). *Color atlas of clinical orthopedics* (2nd ed). London, England: Mosby; (anorexia nervosa) Courtesy of George, D., Comerci, M. D.; (Marfan's syndrome) from Manusov, E. G., & Martucci, E. (1994). The Marfan syndrome. *Arch Fam Med* 3:824. Copyrighted 1994, American Medical Association; (endogenous obesity—Cushing's syndrome) from Wenig, B. M., Heffess, C. S., & Adair, C. F. (1997). *Atlas of endocrine pathology.* Philadelphia, PA: Saunders.

Chapter 10

Figure 10-3: From McCaffery, M., & Pasero, C. (1999). *Pain: clinical manual* (2nd ed.). St Louis, MO: Mosby.

Figure 10-4: From McCaffery M., & Pasero, C. (1999). *Pain: clinical manual* (2nd ed.). St Louis, MO: Mosby.

Table 10-2: From Gelians, C., et al. (2006). Validation of the critical care observation tool in adult patients. *American Journal of Critical Care, 15,* 420–427. Reprinted with permission.

Table 10-3: From Stevens, B., Johnston, C., et al. (1996). Premature infant pain profile: Development and initial validation. *Clinical Journal of Pain, 12*(1), 13–22.

Chapter 11

Figure 11-1: Courtesy of *The Pantagraph,* Bloomington, IL, July 15, 2001.

Figure 11-2: From Nutrition Screening Initiative. (1993). *Implementing nutrition screening and intervention strategies.* Washington, DC: Nutrition Screening Initiative. (Reprinted with permission by the Nutrition Screening Initiative, a project of the American Academy of Family Physicians, the American Dietetic Association, and the National Council on Aging, Inc., and funded in part by a grant from Ross Products Divisions, Abbott Laboratories.)

Figure 11-3: From Health Canada. (2007). *Eating Well With Canada's Food Guide.* © Her Majesty the Queen in Right of Canada, represented by the Minister of Health Canada. Cat. No. H164-38/1-2007E. Retrieved June 6, 2008, from http://www.hc-sc.gc.ca/fn-an/alt_formats/hpfb-dgpsa/pdf/food-guide-aliment/print_eatwell_bienmang_e.pdf

Art for Table 11-5: (marasmus) from Hall, R., & Evered, D. C. (1990). *Color atlas of endocrinology* (2nd ed.). London, England: Mosby.

Art for Table 11-6: (pellagra) from Latham, M. C., et al. (1980). *Scope manual on nutrition.* Kalamazoo: The Upjohn Company. Copyright by Thomas Spies, MD; (follicular hyperkeratosis) from Taylor, K. B., & Anthony, L. E. (1983). *Clinical nutrition.* New York, NY: McGraw-Hill. Copyright by Harold H. Sandstead; (scorbutic gums) from Taylor, K. B., & Anthony, L. E.: *Clinical nutrition.* New York, NY: McGraw-Hill. Copyright by The Upjohn Company; (kwashiorkor) from Hall, R., & Evered, D. C. (1990). *Color atlas of endocrinology* (2nd ed.). London, England: Mosby; (Bitot's spots) from Taylor, K. B., & Anthony, L. E.: *Clinical nutrition.* New York, NY: McGraw-Hill. Copyright by Helen Keller International, Inc; (rickets) from Latham, M. C., et al. (1980). *Scope manual on nutrition.* Kalamazoo: The Upjohn Company. Copyright by Rosa Lee Nemir, MD; (magenta tongue) from McLaren, D. S. (1981). *Color atlas of nutritional disorders.* London, England: Wolfe Medical. Copyright by C.E. Butterworth, Jr; (HIV infection discordant twins) from Friedman-Kien, A. E. (1989). *Color atlas of AIDS.* Philadelphia, PA: Saunders.

Table 11-8: From Canadian Diabetes Association Clinical Practice Guidelines Expert Committee. (2003). Canadian Diabetes Association 2003 clinical practice guidelines for the prevention and management of diabetes in Canada. *Canadian Journal of Diabetes, 27*(Suppl. 2). Retrieved from http://www.diabetes.ca/cpg2003/chapters.aspx. Reprinted with permission.

Chapter 12

Figure 12-3, B: From Lookingbill, D. P., & Marks, J. G. (1993). *Principles of dermatology* (2nd ed). Philadelphia, PA: Saunders.

Figure 12-4, A: From Hurwitz, S. (1993). *Clinical pediatric dermatology: a textbook of skin disorders of childhood and adolescence* (2nd ed.). Philadelphia, PA: Saunders.

Figure 12-4, B: From Hurwitz, S. (1993). *Clinical pediatric dermatology: a textbook of skin disorders of childhood and adolescence* (2nd ed.). Philadelphia, PA: Saunders.

Figure 12-4, C: From Lookingbill, D. P., & Marks, J. G. (1993). *Principles of dermatology* (2nd ed). Philadelphia, PA: Saunders.

Figure 12-6: From Lookingbill, D. P., & Marks, J. G. (1993). *Principles of dermatology* (2nd ed). Philadelphia, PA: Saunders.

Figure 12-9: From Callen, J. P., et al. (1993). *Color atlas of dermatology.* Philadelphia, PA: Saunders.

Figure 12-10: From Hurwitz, S. (1993). *Clinical pediatric dermatology: a textbook of skin disorders of childhood and adolescence* (2nd ed.). Philadelphia, PA: Saunders.

Figure 12-12: Courtesy Jane Deacon, RNC, MS, NNP, The Children's Hospital, Denver, CO.

Figure 12-13: From Bowden, V. R., Dickey, S. B., & Greenburg, C. S. (1998). *Children and their families: the continuum of care.* Philadelphia, PA: Saunders.

Figure 12-14: From Hurwitz, S. (1993). *Clinical pediatric dermatology: a textbook of skin disorders of childhood and adolescence* (2nd ed.). Philadelphia, PA: Saunders.

Figure 12-15: From Hurwitz, S. (1993). *Clinical pediatric dermatology: a textbook of skin disorders of childhood and adolescence* (2nd ed.). Philadelphia, PA: Saunders.

Figure 12-16: From Gorrie, T. M., McKinney, E. S., & Murray, S.S. (1998). *Foundations of maternal-newborn nursing* (2nd ed.). Philadelphia, PA: Saunders.

Figure 12-17: From Hurwitz, S. (1993). *Clinical pediatric dermatology: a textbook of skin disorders of childhood and adolescence* (2nd ed.). Philadelphia, PA: Saunders.

Figure 12-18: From Gorrie, T. M., McKinney, E. S., & Murray, S.S. (1998). *Foundations of maternal-newborn nursing* (2nd ed.). Philadelphia, PA: Saunders.

Figure 12-19, A: From Habif, T. P., et al. (2005). *Skin disease: diagnosis and treatment* (2nd ed.). St Louis, MO: Mosby.

Figure 12-19, B: From Habif, T. P., et al. (2005). *Skin disease: diagnosis and treatment* (2nd ed.). St Louis, MO: Mosby.

Figure 12-20: From Lookingbill, D. P., & Marks, J. G. (1993). *Principles of dermatology* (2nd ed). Philadelphia, PA: Saunders.

Figure 12-21: From Lookingbill, D. P., & Marks, J. G. (1993). *Principles of dermatology* (2nd ed). Philadelphia, PA: Saunders.

Figure 12-22: From Lookingbill, D. P., & Marks, J. G. (1993). *Principles of dermatology* (2nd ed). Philadelphia, PA: Saunders.

Figure 12-23: From Lookingbill, D. P., & Marks, J. G. (1993). *Principles of dermatology* (2nd ed). Philadelphia, PA: Saunders.

Figure 12-24: From Callen, J. P., et al. (1993). *Color atlas of dermatology*. Philadelphia, PA: Saunders.

Art for Table 12-4: (urticaria [hives]) from Fireman, P. (1996). *Atlas of allergies* (2nd ed.). London, England: Mosby.

Art for Table 12-7: (port-wine stain [nevus flammeus]) from Hurwitz, S. (1993). *Clinical pediatric dermatology: a textbook of skin disorders of childhood and adolescence* (2nd ed.). Philadelphia, PA: Saunders; (strawberry mark [immature hemangioma]) from Lookingbill, D. P., & Marks, J. G. (1993). *Principles of dermatology* (2nd ed). Philadelphia, PA: Saunders; (cavernous hemangioma [mature]) from Habif, T. P., et al. (2005). *Skin disease: diagnosis and treatment* (2nd ed.). St Louis, MO: Mosby; (spider or star angioma) from Hurwitz, S. (1993). *Clinical pediatric dermatology: a textbook of skin disorders of childhood and adolescence* (2nd ed.). Philadelphia, PA: Saunders; (venous lake) from Habif, T. P., et al. (2001). *Skin disease: diagnosis and treatment* (2nd ed.). St Louis, MO: Mosby; (petechiae) from Dockery, G. L. (1997). *Cutaneous disorders of the lower extremity*. Philadelphia, PA: Saunders; (purpura) from Hurwitz, S. (1993). *Clinical pediatric dermatology: a textbook of skin disorders of childhood and adolescence* (2nd ed.). Philadelphia, PA: Saunders.

Art for Table 12-8: (diaper dermatitis) from Hurwitz, S. (1993). *Clinical pediatric dermatology: a textbook of skin disorders of childhood and adolescence* (2nd ed.). Philadelphia, PA: Saunders; (intertrigo [candidiasis]) from Hurwitz, S. (1993). *Clinical pediatric dermatology: a textbook of skin disorders of childhood and adolescence* (2nd ed.). Philadelphia, PA: Saunders; (impetigo) from Hurwitz, S. (1993). *Clinical pediatric dermatology: a textbook of skin disorders of childhood and adolescence* (2nd ed.). Philadelphia, PA: Saunders; (atopic dermatitis [eczema]) from Hurwitz, S. (1993). *Clinical pediatric dermatology: a textbook of skin disorders of childhood and adolescence* (2nd ed.). Philadelphia, PA: Saunders; (measles [rubeola] in dark skin) from Feigin, R. D., & Cherry, J. D. (1998). *Textbook of pediatric infectious diseases* (4th ed.). Philadelphia, PA: Saunders; (measles [rubeola] in light skin) from Hurwitz, S. (1993). *Clinical pediatric dermatology: a textbook of skin disorders of childhood and adolescence* (2nd ed.). Philadelphia, PA: Saunders; (German measles [rubella]) from Hurwitz, S. (1993). *Clinical pediatric dermatology: a textbook of skin disorders of childhood and adolescence* (2nd ed.). Philadelphia, PA: Saunders; (chickenpox [varicella]) from Callen, J. P., et al. (1993). *Color atlas of dermatology*. Philadelphia, PA: Saunders.

Art for Table 12-9: (primary contact dermatitis) from Lookingbill, D. P., & Marks, J. G. (1993). *Principles of dermatology* (2nd ed). Philadelphia, PA: Saunders; (allergic drug reaction) from Lookingbill, D. P.,

& Marks, J. G. (1993). *Principles of dermatology* (2nd ed). Philadelphia, PA: Saunders; (tinea corporis [ringworm of the body]) from Hurwitz, S. (1993). *Clinical pediatric dermatology: a textbook of skin disorders of childhood and adolescence* (2nd ed.). Philadelphia, PA: Saunders; (tinea pedis [ringworm of the foot]) from Feigin, R. D., & Cherry, J. D. (1998). *Textbook of pediatric infectious diseases* (4th ed.). Philadelphia, PA: Saunders; (psoriasis) from Lookingbill, D. P., & Marks, J. G. (1993). *Principles of dermatology* (2nd ed). Philadelphia, PA: Saunders; (tinea versicolor) from Lookingbill, D. P., & Marks, J. G. (1993). *Principles of dermatology* (2nd ed). Philadelphia, PA: Saunders; (labial herpes simplex [cold sores]) from Hurwitz, S. (1993). *Clinical pediatric dermatology: a textbook of skin disorders of childhood and adolescence* (2nd ed.). Philadelphia, PA: Saunders; (herpes zoster [shingles]) from Hurwitz, S. (1993). *Clinical pediatric dermatology: a textbook of skin disorders of childhood and adolescence* (2nd ed.). Philadelphia, PA: Saunders; (erythema migrans of Lyme disease) from Swartz, M. H. (2002). *Textbook of physical diagnosis: history and examination* (4th ed.). Philadelphia, PA: Saunders.

Art for Table 12-10: (basal cell carcinoma) from Lookingbill, D. P., & Marks, J. G. (1993). *Principles of dermatology* (2nd ed). Philadelphia, PA: Saunders; (squamous cell carcinoma) from Lookingbill, D. P., & Marks, J. G. (1993). *Principles of dermatology* (2nd ed). Philadelphia, PA: Saunders; (malignant melanoma) from Lookingbill, D. P., & Marks, J. G. (1993). *Principles of dermatology* (2nd ed). Philadelphia, PA: Saunders.

Art for Table 12-11: (epidemic Kaposi's sarcoma: patch stage) from Friedman-Kien, A. E. (1989). *Color atlas of AIDS*. Philadelphia, PA: Saunders; (epidemic Kaposi's sarcoma: advanced disease) from Friedman-Kien, A. E. (1989). *Color atlas of AIDS*. Philadelphia, PA: Saunders; (epidemic Kaposi's sarcoma: plaque stage) from Friedman-Kien, A. E. (1989). *Color atlas of AIDS*. Philadelphia, PA: Saunders.

Art for Table 12-12: (anthrax) from Ishak, K. G., et al. (2001). *Tumors of the liver, atlas of tumor pathology, third series*. Washington, DC: Armed Forces Institute of Pathology/American Registry of Pathology; (smallpox [variola major]) from Fenner, F., et al. (1988). *Smallpox and its eradication*. Geneva, Switzerland: World Health Organization.

Art for Table 12-13: (seborrheic dermatitis [cradle cap] from Hurwitz, S. (1993). *Clinical pediatric dermatology: a textbook of skin disorders of childhood and adolescence* (2nd ed.). Philadelphia, PA: Saunders; (tinea capitis [scalp ringworm]) from Lookingbill, D. P., & Marks, J. G. (1993). *Principles of dermatology* (2nd ed). Philadelphia, PA: Saunders; (toxic alopecia) from Hurwitz, S. (1993). *Clinical pediatric dermatology: a textbook of skin disorders of childhood and adolescence* (2nd ed.). Philadelphia, PA: Saunders; (alopecia areata) from Hurwitz, S. (1993). *Clinical pediatric dermatology: a textbook of skin disorders of childhood and adolescence* (2nd ed.). Philadelphia, PA: Saunders; (traumatic alopecia: traction alopecia) from Hurwitz, S. (1993). *Clinical pediatric dermatology: a textbook of skin disorders of childhood and adolescence* (2nd ed.). Philadelphia, PA: Saunders; (trichotillomania) from Callen, J. P., et al. (1993). *Color atlas of dermatology*. Philadelphia, PA: Saunders; (pediculosis capitis [head lice]) from Callen, J. P., et al. (1993). *Color atlas of dermatology*. Philadelphia, PA: Saunders; (hirsutism) from Wenig, B. M., Heffess, C. S., & Adair, C. F. (1997). *Atlas of endocrine pathology*. Philadelphia, PA: Saunders; (furuncle and abscess) from Lookingbill, D. P., & Marks, J. G. (1993). *Principles of dermatology* (2nd ed). Philadelphia, PA: Saunders.

Art for Table 12-14: (koilonychias [spoon nails]) from Callen, J. P., et al. (1993). *Color atlas of dermatology*. Philadelphia, PA: Saunders; (paronychia) from Lookingbill, D. P., & Marks, J. G. (1993). *Principles of dermatology* (2nd ed). Philadelphia, PA: Saunders; (Beau's line) from Callen, J. P., et al. (1993). *Color atlas of dermatology*. Philadelphia, PA: Saunders; (splinter hemorrhages) from Callen, J. P., et al. (1993). *Color atlas of dermatology*. Philadelphia, PA: Saunders; (late clubbing) Reprinted from the Clinical Slide Collection on the Rheumatic Diseases. ©1991, 1995, 1997. Used by permission of the American College of Rheumatology; (ony-cholysis) from Arndt, K. A., et al. (1997). *Primary care dermatology*. Philadelphia, PA: Saunders; (pitting) from Lookingbill, D. P., & Marks, J. G. (1993). *Principles of dermatology* (2nd ed.). Philadelphia, PA: Saunders; (habit-tic dystrophy) from Hurwitz, S. (1993). *Clinical pediatric dermatology: a textbook of skin disorders of childhood and adolescence* (2nd ed.). Philadelphia, PA: Saunders.

Chapter 13

Figure 13-8: Copyright Pat Thomas, 2006.

Figure 13-16: From Gorrie, T. M., McKinney, E. S., & Murray, S.S. (1998). *Foundations of maternal-newborn nursing* (2nd ed.). Philadelphia, PA: Saunders.

Figure 13-17, A: From Gorrie, T. M., McKinney, E. S., & Murray, S.S. (1998). *Foundations of maternal-newborn nursing* (2nd ed.). Philadelphia, PA: Saunders.

Figure 13-19: From Behrman, R. E., & Vaughn, V.C. (1992). *Nelson textbook of pediatrics* (14th ed.). Philadelphia, PA: Saunders.

Art for Table 13-1: (hydrocephalus) from Bowden, V. R., Dickey, S. B., & Greenburg, C. S. (1998). *Children and their families: the continuum of care*. Philadelphia, PA: Saunders; (Paget's disease of bone [osteitis deformans]) Reprinted from the Clinical Slide Collection on the Rheumatic Diseases. © 1991, 1995, 1997. Used by permission of the American College of Rheumatology; (acromegaly) from Damjanov, I. (1996). *Pathology for the health-related professions*. Philadelphia, PA: Saunders.

Art for Table 13-2: (torticollis [wryneck]) from Zitelli, B. J. & Davis, H. W. (2002). *Atlas of pediatric physical diagnosis* (4th ed.). St. Louis, MO: Mosby; (thyroid—multiple nodules) from Swartz, M. H. (2006). *Textbook of physical diagnosis: history and examination* (5th ed.). Philadelphia, PA: Saunders; (pilar cyst [Wen]) from Callen, J. P., et al. (1993). *Color atlas of dermatology*. Philadelphia, PA: Saunders; (parotid gland enlargement) from Swartz, M. H. (2006). *Textbook of physical diagnosis: history and examination* (5th ed.). Philadelphia, PA: Saunders.

Art for Table 13-3: (fetal alcohol syndrome) Photo from Streissguth, A. P., Landesman-Dwyer, S., Martin, J. C., et al. (1980). Teratogenic effects of alcohol in humans and laboratory animals. *Science, 209*, 353–361. Illustration copyright Pat Thomas, 2006; (congenital hypothyroidism) from Zitelli, B. J., & Davis, H. W. (2002). *Atlas of pediatric physical diagnosis* (4th ed.). St. Louis, MO: Mosby. Courtesy of Dr. Thomas P. Foley, Jr.; (Down syndrome) from Zitelli, B. J., & Davis, H. W. (2002). *Atlas of pediatric physical diagnosis* (4th ed.). St. Louis, MO: Mosby; (atopic [allergic] facies) from Zitelli, B. J., & Davis, H. W. (2002). *Atlas of pediatric physical diagnosis* (4th ed.). St. Louis, MO: Mosby; (allergic salute and crease) from Zitelli, B. J., & Davis, H. W. (2002). *Atlas of pediatric physical diagnosis* (4th ed.). St. Louis, MO: Mosby.

Art for Table 13-4: (Cushing's syndrome) from Zitelli, B. J., & Davis, H. W. (2002). *Atlas of pediatric physical diagnosis* (4th ed.). St. Louis, MO: Mosby; (hyperthyroidism) from Swartz, M. H. (2006). *Textbook of physical diagnosis: history and examination* (5th ed.). Philadelphia, PA: Saunders; (myxedema [hypothyroidism]) from Hall, R., & Evered, D. C. (1990). *Color atlas of endocrinology* (2nd ed.). London, England: Mosby; (Bell's palsy [right side]) from Swartz, M. H. (2006). *Textbook of physical diagnosis: history and examination* (5th ed.). Philadelphia, PA: Saunders; (scleroderma) Reprinted from the Clinical Slide Collection on the Rheumatic Diseases. © 1991, 1995, 1997. Used by permission of the American College of Rheumatology.

Chapter 14

Figure 14-1: Copyright Pat Thomas, 2006.
Figure 14-3: Copyright Pat Thomas, 2006.
Figure 14-4: Copyright Pat Thomas, 2006.
Figure 14-19: Copyright Pat Thomas, 2006.
Figure 14-23: Courtesy Heather Boyd-Monk and Wills Eye Hospital, Philadelphia, PA.

Figure 14-24: Courtesy Heather Boyd-Monk and Wills Eye Hospital, Philadelphia, PA.

Figure 14-29: From Zitelli, B. J. & Davis, H. W. (2002). *Atlas of pediatric physical diagnosis* (4th ed.). St. Louis, MO: Mosby.

Figure 14-30: From Albert, D. M., & Jakobiec, F. A. (1994). *Principles and practice of ophthalmology*. Philadelphia, PA: Saunders.

Figure 14-31: From Friedman, N., & Pineda, R. (1998). *The Massachusetts eye and ear infirmary illustrated manual of ophthalmology*. Philadelphia, PA: Saunders.

Figure 14-32: From Swartz, M. H. (2006). *Textbook of physical diagnosis: history and examination* (5th ed.). Philadelphia, PA: Saunders.

Figure 14-33: From Albert, D. M., & Jakobiec, F. A. (1994). *Principles and practice of ophthalmology* (vol. 3). Philadelphia, PA: Saunders.

Figure 14-34: From Friedman, N., & Pineda, R. (1998). *The Massachusetts eye and ear infirmary illustrated manual of ophthalmology*. Philadelphia, PA: Saunders.

Art in Table 14-1: (A, pseudostrabismus) from Zitelli, B. J. & Davis, H. W. (2002). *Atlas of pediatric physical diagnosis* (4th ed.). St. Louis, MO: Mosby; (B esotropia) from Zitelli, B. J. & Davis, H. W. (2002). *Atlas of pediatric physical diagnosis* (4th ed.). St. Louis, MO: Mosby; (C exotropia) from Zitelli, B. J. & Davis, H. W. (2002). *Atlas of pediatric physical diagnosis* (4th ed.). St. Louis, MO: Mosby.

Art in Table 14-2: (periorbital edema) from Ibsen, O. A. C., & Phelan, J. A. (1992). *Oral pathology for the dental hygienist* (2nd ed.). Philadelphia, PA: Saunders; (exophthalmos [protruding eye]) from Scheie, H. G., & Albert, D. M. (1977). *Textbook of ophthalmology* (9th ed). Philadelphia, PA: Saunders; (ptosis [drooping upper lip]) Courtesy Heather Boyd-Monk and Wills Eye Hospital, Philadelphia, PA; (upward palpebral slant) from Zitelli, B. J. & Davis, H. W. (2002). *Atlas of pediatric physical diagnosis* (4th ed.). St. Louis, MO: Mosby; (ectropion) from Albert, D. M., & Jakobiec, F. A. (1994). *Principles and practice of ophthalmology* (vol. 3). Philadelphia, PA: Saunders; (entropion) from Albert, D. M., & Jakobiec, F. A. (1994). *Principles and practice of ophthalmology* (vol. 3). Philadelphia, PA: Saunders.

Art in Table 14-3: (blepharitis [inflammation of the eyelids]) from Friedman, N., & Pineda, R. (1998). *The Massachusetts eye and ear infirmary illustrated manual of ophthalmology*. Philadelphia, PA: Saunders; (chalazion) Courtesy Heather Boyd-Monk and Wills Eye Hospital, Philadelphia, PA; (hordeolum [stye]) from Albert, D. M., & Jakobiec, F. A. (1994). *Principles and practice of ophthalmology* (vol. 3). Philadelphia, PA: Saunders; (dacryocystitis [inflammation of the lacrimal sac]) from Friedman, N., & Pineda, R. (1998). *The Massachusetts eye and ear infirmary illustrated manual of ophthalmology*. Philadelphia, PA: Saunders; (basal cell carcinoma) from Scheie, H. G., & Albert, D. M. (1977). *Textbook of ophthalmology* (9th ed). Philadelphia, PA: Saunders.

Art in Table 14-6: (conjunctivitis) from Albert, D. M., & Jakobiec, F. A. (1994). *Principles and practice of ophthalmology* (vol. 1). Philadelphia, PA: Saunders; (subconjunctival hemorrhage) Courtesy Heather Boyd-Monk and Wills Eye Hospital, Philadelphia, PA; (iritis [circumcorneal redness]) from Scheie, H. G., & Albert, D. M. (1977). *Textbook of ophthalmology* (9th ed). Philadelphia, PA: Saunders; (acute glaucoma) from Scheie, H. G., & Albert, D. M. (1977). *Textbook of ophthalmology* (9th ed). Philadelphia, PA: Saunders.

Art in Table 14-7: (pterygium) from Albert, D. M., & Jakobiec, F. A. (1994). *Principles and practice of ophthalmology* (vol. 1). Philadelphia, PA: Saunders; (corneal abrasion) Courtesy Heather Boyd-Monk and Wills Eye Hospital, Philadelphia, PA; (hyphema) from Scheie, H. G., & Albert, D. M. (1977). *Textbook of ophthalmology* (9th ed). Philadelphia, PA: Saunders; (hypopyon) from Scheie, H. G., & Albert, D. M. (1977). *Textbook of ophthalmology* (9th ed). Philadelphia, PA: Saunders.

Art in Table 14-8: (central gray opacity—nuclear cataract) from Friedman, N., & Pineda, R. (1998). *The Massachusetts eye and ear infirmary illustrated manual of ophthalmology*. Philadelphia, PA: Saunders; (star-shaped opacity—cortical cataract) from Friedman, N., & Pineda, R. (1998). *The Massachusetts eye and* *ear infirmary illustrated manual of ophthalmology*. Philadelphia, PA: Saunders.

Art in Table 14-9: (optic atrophy [disc pallor]) from Friedman, N., & Pineda, R. (1998). *The Massachusetts eye and ear infirmary illustrated manual of ophthalmology*. Philadelphia, PA: Saunders; (papilledema [choked disc]) Courtesy Heather Boyd-Monk and Wills Eye Hospital, Philadelphia, PA; (excessive cup-disc ratio) from Friedman, N., & Pineda, R. (1998). *The Massachusetts eye and ear infirmary illustrated manual of ophthalmology*. Philadelphia, PA: Saunders.

Art in Table 14-10: (arteriovenous crossing) from Friedman, N., & Pineda, R. (2004). *The Massachusetts eye and ear infirmary illustrated manual of ophthalmology* (2nd ed.). Philadelphia, PA: Saunders; (narrowed arteries) from Friedman, N., & Pineda, R. (2004). *The Massachusetts eye and ear infirmary illustrated manual of ophthalmology* (2nd ed.). Philadelphia, PA: Saunders; (microaneurysms) from Friedman, N., & Pineda, R. (1998). *The Massachusetts eye and ear infirmary illustrated manual of ophthalmology*. Philadelphia, PA: Saunders.

Chapter 15

Figure 15-1: Copyright Pat Thomas, 2006.

Figure 15-8: From Adams, G. L., Bois, L. R., & Hilger, P. A. (1989). *Boies fundamentals of otolaryngology: a textbook of ear, nose, and throat diseases* (6th ed.). Philadelphia, PA: Saunders.

Figure 15-13: Copyright Pat Thomas, 2006.

Art for Table 15-1: (frostbite) Reprinted from the Clinical Slide Collection on the Rheumatic Diseases. © 1991, 1995, 1997. Used by permission of the American College of Rheumatology; (otitis externa—swimmer's ear) from Habif, T. P., et al. (2005). *Skin disease: diagnosis and treatment* (2nd ed.). St Louis, MO: Mosby; (branchial remnant and ear deformity) from Liebert, P. S. (1996). *Color atlas of pediatric surgery* (2nd ed.). Philadelphia, PA: Saunders.

Art for Table 15-2: (sebaceous cyst) from Liebert, P. S. (1996). *Color atlas of pediatric surgery* (2nd ed.). Philadelphia, PA: Saunders; (tophi) Reprinted from the Clinical Slide Collection on the Rheumatic Diseases © 1991, 1995, 1997. Used by permission of the American College of Rheumatology; (chondrodermatitis nodularis helicis) from Habif, T. P., et al. (2005). *Skin disease: diagnosis and treatment* (2nd ed.). St Louis, MO: Mosby; (keloid) from Liebert, P. S. (1996). *Color atlas of pediatric surgery* (2nd ed.). Philadelphia, PA: Saunders; (carcinoma) from Callen, J. P., et al. (1993). *Color atlas of dermatology*. Philadelphia, PA: Saunders.

Art for Table 15-5: (retracted drum) from Adams, G. L., Bois, L. R., & Hilger, P. A. (1989). *Boies fundamentals of otolaryngology: a textbook of ear, nose, and throat diseases* (6th ed.). Philadelphia, PA: Saunders; (serous otitis media) from Swartz, M. H. (2006). *Textbook of physical diagnosis: history and examination* (5th ed.). Philadelphia, PA: Saunders; (acute purulent otitis media—early stage) from Adams, G. L., Bois, L. R., & Hilger, P. A. (1989). *Boies fundamentals of otolaryngology: a textbook of ear, nose, and throat diseases* (6th ed.). Philadelphia, PA: Saunders; (acute purulent otitis media—later stage) from Adams, G. L., Bois, L. R., & Hilger, P. A. (1989). *Boies fundamentals of otolaryngology: a textbook of ear, nose, and throat diseases* (6th ed.). Philadelphia, PA: Saunders; (perforation) from Swartz, M. H. (2006). *Textbook of physical diagnosis: history and examination* (5th ed.). Philadelphia, PA: Saunders; (insertion of tympanostomy tubes) from Fireman, P. (1996). *Atlas of allergies* (2nd ed.). London, England: Mosby; (cholesteatoma) from Swartz, M. H. (2006). *Textbook of physical diagnosis: history and examination* (5th ed.). Philadelphia, PA: Saunders; (bullous myringitis) from Swartz, M. H. (2006). *Textbook of physical diagnosis: history and examination* (5th ed.). Philadelphia, PA: Saunders.

Chapter 16

Figure 16-1: Copyright Pat Thomas, 2006.

Figure 16-2: Copyright Pat Thomas, 2006.

Figure 16-3: Copyright Pat Thomas, 2006.

Figure 16-6: Copyright Pat Thomas, 2006.

Figure 16-9: From Fireman, P. (1996). *Atlas of allergies* (2nd ed.). London, England: Mosby.

Figure 16-15: From Ibsen, O. A. C., & Phelan, J. A. (1996). *Oral pathology for the dental hygienist* (2nd ed.). Philadelphia, PA: Saunders.

Figure 16-16: From Ibsen, O. A. C., & Phelan, J. A. (1996). *Oral pathology for the dental hygienist* (2nd ed.). Philadelphia, PA: Saunders.

Figure 16-17: Copyright Pat Thomas, 2006.

Figure 16-22: From Zitelli, B. J. & Davis, H. W. (2002). *Atlas of pediatric physical diagnosis* (4th ed.). St. Louis, MO: Mosby.

Promoting Health Box: Smokeless Tobacco and Cancer Risk: From Canadian Cancer Encyclopedia. (2007). Oral cancer. Retrieved February 11, 2008, from http://info/cancer.ca/E/CCE/ccedetails; Canadian Cancer Society. (2007). Any tobacco use can hurt your body. Retrieved February 11, 2008, from http://cancer.ca/ccs; Health Canada. (2007). Smokeless tobacco. Retrieved February 11, 2008, from http://www.hc-sc.gc.ca/hl-vs/tobac-tabac/body-corps/smokeless-sansfumee_e.html; Ontario Tobacco Research Unit. (2006). What population surveys say about smokeless tobacco use. Retrieved February 11, 2008, from http://www.otru.org/pdf/updates/update_oct2006.pdf; Walsh, P. M., & Epstein, J. B. (2000). The oral effects of smokeless tobacco. *Journal of the Canadian Dental Association, 66,* 22–25.

Art for Table 16-1: (foreign body) from Fireman, P. (1996). *Atlas of allergies* (2nd ed.). London, England: Mosby; (perforated septum) from Hawke, M. (1998). *Diagnostic handbook of otorhinolaryngology*. London, England: Martin Dunitz; (acute rhinitis) from Fireman, P. (1996). *Atlas of allergies* (2nd ed.). London, England: Mosby; (allergic rhinitis) from Fireman, P. (1996). *Atlas of allergies* (2nd ed.). London, England: Mosby; (polyps) from Fireman, P. (1996). *Atlas of allergies* (2nd ed.). London, England: Mosby; (carcinoma) from Hawke, M. (1998). *Diagnostic handbook of otorhinolaryngology*. London, England: Martin Dunitz.

Art for Table 16-2: (cleft lip) from Ibsen, O. A. C., & Phelan, J. A. (1996). *Oral pathology for the dental hygienist* (2nd ed.). Philadelphia, PA: Saunders; (herpes simplex 1) from Callen, J. P., et al. (1993). *Color atlas of dermatology*. Philadelphia, PA: Saunders; (angular chelitis [stomatitis, perleche]) from Callen, J. P., et al. (1993). *Color atlas of dermatology*. Philadelphia, PA: Saunders; (squamous cell carcinoma) from Hawke, M. (1998). *Diagnostic handbook of otorhinolaryngology*. London, England: Martin Dunitz; (retention "cyst" [mucocele]) from Hawke, M. (1998). *Diagnostic handbook of otorhinolaryngology*. London, England: Martin Dunitz.

Art for Table 16-3: (baby bottle tooth decay) Courtesy of F. Ferguson, Department of Children's Dentistry, School of Dental Medicine, SUNY at Stony Brook, Stony Brook, NY 11733; (dental caries) Courtesy of A. McWhorter, Pediatric Dentistry, Baylor College of Dentistry, The Texas A & M University System, Dallas, TX; (epulis) from Ibsen, O. A. C., & Phelan, J. A. (1996). *Oral pathology for the dental hygienist* (2nd ed.). Philadelphia, PA: Saunders; (gingival hyperplasia) from Ibsen, O. A. C., & Phelan, J. A. (1996). *Oral pathology for the dental hygienist* (2nd ed.). Philadelphia, PA: Saunders; (gingivitis) from Callen, J. P., et al. (1993). *Color atlas of dermatology*. Philadelphia, PA: Saunders; (meth mouth) from Neville, B. W., et al. (2009). *Oral and maxillofacial pathology* (3rd ed.). St. Louis, MO: Saunders (in press).

Art for Table 16-4: (aphthous ulcers) from Sleisinger, M. H., & Fordtran, J.S. (1993). *Gastrointestinal diseases: pathophysiology, diagnosis, and management* (vol. 1, 5th ed.). Philadelphia, PA: Saunders; (Koplik's spots) from Feigin, R. D., & Cherry, J. D. (1998). *Textbook of pediatric infectious diseases* (4th ed.). Philadelphia, PA: Saunders; (leukoplakia) from Sleisinger, M. H., & Fordtran, J.S. (1993). *Gastrointestinal diseases: pathophysiology, diagnosis, and management* (vol. 1, 5th ed.). Philadelphia, PA: Saunders; (candidiasis or monilial infection) from Callen, J. P., et al. (1993). *Color atlas of dermatology*. Philadelphia, PA: Saunders.

Art for Table 16-5: (ankyloglossia) from Ibsen, O. A. C., & Phelan, J. A. (1996). *Oral pathology for the dental hygienist* (2nd ed.). Philadelphia, PA: Saunders; (fissured or scrotal tongue) from Callen, J. P., et al. (1993). *Color atlas of dermatology.* Philadelphia, PA: Saunders; (geographic tongue [migratory glossitis]) from Callen, J. P., et al. (1993). *Color atlas of dermatology.* Philadelphia, PA: Saunders; (smooth, glossy tongue [atrophic glossitis]) from Adams, G. L., Bois, L. R., & Hilger, P. A. (1989). *Boies fundamentals of otolaryngology: a textbook of ear, nose, and throat diseases* (6th ed.). Philadelphia, PA: Saunders; (black hairy tongue) from Callen, J. P., et al. (1993). *Color atlas of dermatology.* Philadelphia, PA: Saunders; (enlarged tongue [macroglossia]) from Zitelli, B. J. & Davis, H. W. (2002). *Atlas of pediatric physical diagnosis* (4th ed.). St. Louis, MO: Mosby. Courtesy of Dr. Christine Williams; (carcinoma) from Wenig, B. M., Heffess, C. S., & Adair, C. F. (1997). *Atlas of endocrine pathology.* Philadelphia, PA: Saunders.

Art for Table 16-6: (cleft palate) from Zitelli, B. J. & Davis, H. W. (2002). *Atlas of pediatric physical diagnosis* (4th ed.). St. Louis, MO: Mosby. Courtesy of Dr. Michael Sherlock; (bifid uvula) from Hawke, M. (1998). *Diagnostic handbook of otorhinolaryngology.* London, England: Martin Dunitz; (oral Kaposi's sarcoma) from Friedman-Kien, A. E.: *Color atlas of AIDS,* Philadelphia, 1989, Saunders; (acute tonsillitis) from Hawke, M. (1998). *Diagnostic handbook of otorhinolaryngology.* London, England: Martin Dunitz.

Chapter 17

Figure 17-6: Redrawn from Tanner, J. M. (1962). *Growth at adolescence.* Oxford, England: Blackwell Scientific.

Figure 17-8: From Callen, J. P., et al. (1993). *Color atlas of dermatology.* Philadelphia, PA: Saunders.

Figure 17-21: From Moore, K. L., & Persaud, T.N. (1998). *Before we are born: essentials of embryology and birth defects* (5th ed.). Philadelphia, PA: Saunders.

Art for Table 17-3: (dimpling) from Evans, A. J., et al. (1998). *Atlas of breast disease management: 50 illustrative cases.* Philadelphia, PA: Saunders; (edema [peau d'orange]) from Mansel, R. (1995). *Color atlas of breast diseases.* London, England: Mosby; (fixation) from Mansel, R. (1995). *Color atlas of breast diseases.* London, England: Mosby; (deviation in nipple pointing) from Mansel, R. (1995). *Color atlas of breast diseases.* London, England: Mosby.

Art for Table 17-6: (mammary duct ectasia) from Mansel, R. (1995). *Color atlas of breast diseases.* London, England: Mosby; (carcinoma) from Evans, A. J., et al. (1998). *Atlas of breast disease management: 50 illustrative cases.* Philadelphia, PA: Saunders; (intraductal papilloma) from Mansel, R. (1995). *Color atlas of breast diseases.* London, England: Mosby; (Paget's disease [intraductal carcinoma]) from Mansel, R. (1995). *Color atlas of breast diseases.* London, England: Mosby.

Art for Table 17-7: (breast abscess) from Mansel, R. (1995). *Color atlas of breast diseases.* London, England: Mosby; (mastitis) from Mansel, R. (1995). *Color atlas of breast diseases.* London, England: Mosby.

Art for Table 17-8: (gynecomastia) from Evans, A. J., et al. (1998). *Atlas of breast disease management: 50 illustrative cases.* Philadelphia, PA: Saunders; (carcinoma) from Haagensen, C. D. (1986). *Diseases of the breast* (3rd ed.). Philadelphia, PA: Saunders.

Chapter 18

Figure 18-11: Copyright Pat Thomas, 2006.

Figure 18-12: From Nichols, F. H., & Zwelling, E. (1997). *Maternal-newborn nursing: theory and practice.* Philadelphia, PA: Saunders.

Promoting Health Box: Environmental Tobacco Smoke: From American Lung Association. (2006). *Secondhand smoke factsSheet.* Retrieved from http://www.lungusa.org; Canadian Lung Association. (2008). *Lung Association to launch Clean Air for Kids Campaign on January 23.* Ottawa, ON: Author; Health Canada. (2006). *Second-hand smoke.* Retrieved February 5, 2008, from http://www.hc-sc.gc.ca/hl-vs/tobac-tabac/second/index_e.html; Health Canada. (2006). *Smoke-free public places: You can get there.* Ottawa, ON: Author.

Chapter 19

Figure 19-2: Copyright Pat Thomas, 2006.
Figure 19-3: Copyright Pat Thomas, 2006.
Figure 19-4: Copyright Pat Thomas, 2006.
Figure 19-8: Copyright Pat Thomas, 2006.
Figure 19-9: Copyright Pat Thomas, 2006.
Figure 19-15: From Lakatta, E. G. (1985). Cardiovascular function in later life. *Cardiovasc Med, 10,* 37-40.
Art for Promoting Health Box: From The Heart Truth: Awareness and Prevention, www.4women.gov/hearttruth.

Chapter 20

Figure 20-7: From Behrman, R. E., & Vaguhn, V. C. (1992). *Nelson textbook of pediatrics* (14 ed.). Philadelphia, PA: Saunders.
Figure 20-20, B: From Bloom, A., Watkins, P. H., & Ireland, J. (1992). *Color atlas of diabetes* (2nd ed.). St Louis, MO: Mosby.
Figure 20-21: Copyright Pat Thomas, 2006.
Art for Table 20-2: (Raynaud's syndrome) from Walker, J. M., & Helewa, A. (1996). *Physical therapy in arthritis.* Philadelphia, PA: Saunders; (lymphedema) from Swartz, M. H. (2006). *Textbook of physical diagnosis: history and examination* (5th ed.). Philadelphia, PA: Saunders.
Art for Table 20-4: (arteriosclerosis—ischemic ulcer) from Dockery, G. L. (1997). *Cutaneous disorders of the lower extremity.* Philadelphia, PA: Saunders; (venous [stasis] ulcer) from Lookingbill, D. P., & Marks, J. G. (1993). *Principles of dermatology* (2nd ed.). Philadelphia, PA: Saunders; (superficial varicose veins) from Dockery, G. L. (1997). *Cutaneous disorders of the lower extremity.* Philadelphia, PA: Saunders; (deep vein thrombophlebitis) from Dockery, G. L. (1997). *Cutaneous disorders of the lower extremity.* Philadelphia, PA: Saunders.

Chapter 21

Figure 21-1: Copyright Pat Thomas, 2006.
Figure 21-2: Copyright Pat Thomas, 2006.
Figure 21-3: Copyright Pat Thomas, 2006.
Figure 21-4: Copyright Pat Thomas, 2006.
Promoting Health Box: Hepatitis Risk. From Canadian Liver Foundation. *Adult liver diseases.* Retrieved from www.liver.ca/Liver_Disease/Adult_Liver_Diseases/; Health Canada. (2007). *Hepatitis fact sheets.* Retrieved from www.hc-sc.gc.ca/dc-ma/hep/index_e.html; Public Health Agency of Canada. (2006). *Canadian immunization guide* (7th ed.). Retrieved from www.phac-aspc.gc.ca/publicat/cig-gci/index-eng.php
Art for Table 21-2: Copyright Pat Thomas, 2006.
Art for Table 21-3: (umbilical hernia) from Zitelli, B. J. & Davis, H. W. (2002). *Atlas of pediatric physical diagnosis* (4th ed.). St. Louis, MO: Mosby. Courtesy of Dr. Thomas P. Foley, Jr.

Chapter 22

Figure 22-2: Copyright Pat Thomas, 2006.
Figure 22-33, C: From Dieppe, P. A., Cooper, C., & McGill, N. (1991). *Arthritis and rheumatism in practice.* London, England: Gower Medical Publishing.
Figure 22-34, B: From Dieppe, P. A., Cooper, C., & McGill, N. (1991). *Arthritis and rheumatism in practice.* London, England: Gower Medical Publishing.
Table 22-1: From Brown, J. P., & Josse, R. G., for Scientific Advisory Council of the Osteoporosis Society of Canada. (2002). 2000 clinical practice guidelines for the diagnosis and management of osteoporosis in Canada. *Canadian Medical Association Journal, 167*(10 Suppl.), S5.
Figure 22-50: From Zitelli, B. J. & Davis, H. W. (2002). *Atlas of pediatric physical diagnosis* (4th ed.). St. Louis, MO: Mosby.
Figure 22-54: Copyright held by DeWayne Dalrymple.
Promoting Health Box: Preventing Osteoporosis: From Brown, J. P., & Fortier, M. (2006). Canadian Consensus Conference on

Osteoporosis, 2006 update. *Journal of Obstetrics and Gynaecology Canada, 172,* S95–S112; Osteoporosis Canada: www.osteoporosis.ca

Art for Table 22-3: (atrophy) from Bunker, T., & Schranz, P. J. (1998). *Clinical challenges in orthopaedics: the shoulder.* London, England: Martin Dunitz; (dislocated shoulder) from Bunker, T., & Schranz, P. J. (1998). *Clinical challenges in orthopaedics: the shoulder.* London, England: Martin Dunitz; (joint effusion) from Bunker, T., & Schranz, P. J. (1998). *Clinical challenges in orthopaedics: the shoulder.* London, England: Martin Dunitz; (tear of rotator cuff) from Polley, H. F., & Hunder, G. G. (1978). *Physical examination of the joints.* (2nd ed.). Philadelphia, PA: Saunders; (frozen shoulder—adhesive capsulitis) from Polley, H. F., & Hunder, G. G. (1978). *Physical examination of the joints.* (2nd ed.). Philadelphia, PA: Saunders.

Art for Table 22-4: (olecranon bursitis) from Dieppe, P. A., Cooper, C., & McGill, N. (1991). *Arthritis and rheumatism in practice.* London, England: Gower Medical Publishing; (gouty arthritis) from Polley, H. F., & Hunder, G. G. (1978). *Physical examination of the joints.* (2nd ed.). Philadelphia, PA: Saunders; (subcutaneous nodules) from Callen, J. P., et al. (1993). *Color atlas of dermatology.* Philadelphia, PA: Saunders; (epi-condylitis—tennis elbow) from Jones, A., & Owen, R. (1995). *Color atlas of clinical orthopedics* (2nd ed.). London, England: Mosby.

Art for Table 22-5: (ganglion cyst) from Callen, J. P., et al. (1993). *Color atlas of dermatology.* Philadelphia, PA: Saunders; (carpal tunnel syndrome with atrophy of thenar eminence) Reprinted from the Clinical Slide Collection on the Rheumatic Diseases. © 1991, 1995, 1997. Used by permission of the American College of Rheumatology; (ankylosis) from Polley, H. F., & Hunder, G. G. (1978). *Physical examination of the joints.* (2nd ed.). Philadelphia, PA: Saunders; (swan-neck and boutonniere deformity) from Clinical Slide Collection on the Rheumatic Diseases, 1991, 1995, 1997; (ulnar deviation or drift) from Walker, J. M., & Helewa, A. (1996). *Physical therapy in arthritis.* Philadelphia, PA: Saunders; (degenerative joint disease or osteoarthritis) from Walker, J. M., & Helewa, A. (1996). *Physical therapy in arthritis,* Philadelphia, PA: Saunders; (syndactyly) from Liebert, P. S. (1996). *Color atlas of pediatric surgery* (2nd ed.). Philadelphia, PA: Saunders; (polydactyly) from Liebert, P. S. (1996). *Color atlas of pediatric surgery* (2nd ed.). Philadelphia, PA: Saunders.

Art for Table 22-6: (mild synovitis) from Dieppe, P. A., Cooper, C., & McGill, N. (1991). *Arthritis and rheumatism in practice.* London, England: Gower Medical Publishing; (prepatellar bursitis) from Dieppe, P. A., Cooper, C., & McGill, N. (1991). *Arthritis and rheumatism in practice.* London, England: Gower Medical Publishing; (swelling of menisci) from Jones, A., & Owen, R. (1995). *Color atlas of clinical orthopedics* (2nd ed.). London, England: Mosby; (Osgood-Schlatter disease) from Zitelli, B. J. & Davis, H. W. (2002). *Atlas of pediatric physical diagnosis* (4th ed.). St. Louis, MO: Mosby.

Art for Table 22-7: (achilles tenosynovitis) from Dieppe, P. A., Cooper, C., & McGill, N. (1991). *Arthritis and rheumatism in practice.* London, England: Gower Medical Publishing; (tophi with chronic gout) from Dockery, G. L. (1997). *Cutaneous disorders of the lower extremity.* Philadelphia, PA: Saunders; (acute gout) from Dieppe, P. A., Cooper, C., & McGill, N. (1991). *Arthritis and rheumatism in practice.* London, England: Gower Medical Publishing; (hallux valgus with bunion and hammertoes) from Walker, J. M., & Helewa, A. (1996). *Physical therapy in arthritis.* Philadelphia, PA: Saunders.

Art for Table 22-8: (scoliosis) from Zitelli, B. J. & Davis, H. W. (2002). *Atlas of pediatric physical diagnosis* (4th ed.). St. Louis, MO: Mosby; (herniated nucleus pulposus) from Polley, H. F., & Hunder, G. G. (1978). *Physical examination of the joints.* (2nd ed.). Philadelphia, PA: Saunders.

Art for Table 22-9: (congenital dislocated hip) from Zitelli, B. J. (2002). *Atlas of pediatric physical diagnosis* (4th ed.). St. Louis, MO: Mosby; (talipes equinovarus [clubfoot]) from A.E. Chudley, MD; (spina bifida) from Walsh, P. C., et al. (1986). *Campbell's urology* (5th ed.). Philadelphia, PA: Saunders.

Chapter 23

Figure 23-1: Copyright Pat Thomas, 2006.
Figure 23-2: Copyright Pat Thomas, 2006.
Figure 23-3: Copyright Pat Thomas, 2006.
Figure 23-4: Copyright Pat Thomas, 2006.
Figure 23-6: Copyright Pat Thomas, 2006.
Figure 23-53, B: From Fenichel, G. M. (1988). *Clinical pediatric neurology.* Philadelphia, PA: Saunders.
Figure 23-59: From Hickey, J. V. (1986). *Neurological and neurosurgical nursing* (2nd ed.). Philadelphia, PA: Lippincott.
Art for Table 23-9: Copyright Pat Thomas, 2006.
Art for Table 23-11: Copyright Pat Thomas, 2006.

Chapter 24

Figure 24-4: Redrawn from Marshall, W. A., & Tanner, J. M. (1970). Variations in the pattern of pubertal changes in boys. *Arch Dis Child, 45,* 22.
Figure 24-5: Courtesy Connie Cooper.
Art for Table 24-1: Adapted from Tanner, J. M. (1962). *Growth at adolescence,* Oxford, England: Blackwell Scientific.
Art for Table 24-2: Courtesy Connie Cooper.
Art for Table 24-3: (genital herpes—HSV-2 infection) Courtesy of Pfizer Laboratories Division, Pfizer Inc, New York, NY. From *A close look at VD: a slide presentation produced as a public service;* (syphilitic chancre) from Emond, R. T., Rowl, H. A. K., & Welsby, P. (1995). *Color atlas of infectious diseases* (3rd ed.). London, England: Mosby; (genital warts) from Habif, T. P., et al. (2005). *Skin disease: diagnosis and treatment* (2nd ed.). St Louis, MO: Mosby; (carcinoma) from Callen, J. P., et al. (1993). *Color atlas of dermatology.* Philadelphia, PA: Saunders; (urethritis [urethral discharge and dysuria]) from Emond, R. T., Rowl, H. A. K., & Welsby, P. (1995). *Color atlas of infectious diseases* (3rd ed.). London, England: Mosby.
Art for Table 24-4: (phimosis) from Liebert, P. S. (1996). *Color atlas of pediatric surgery* (2nd ed.). Philadelphia, PA: Saunders; (hypospadias) from Liebert, P. S. (1996). *Color atlas of pediatric surgery* (2nd ed.). Philadelphia, PA: Saunders; (epispadias) from Zitelli, B. J. & Davis, H. W. (2002). *Atlas of pediatric physical diagnosis* (4th ed.). St. Louis, MO: Mosby; (Peyronie's disease) Courtesy of Dr. Hans Stricker, Department of Urology, Henry Ford Hospital, Detroit, MI.
Art for Table 24-5: Copyright Pat Thomas, 2006.
Art for Table 24-6: Copyright Pat Thomas, 2006.

Chapter 25

Table 25-1: From Canadian Association of Gastroenterology. (2008). Retrieved from http://www.cag-acg.org/
Promoting Health Box: Colorectal Cancer Screening: From Canadian Cancer Society. (2007a). Colorectal cancer: Understanding your diagnosis. Retrieved May 19, 2008, from www.cancer.ca
Promoting Health Box: Screening for Prostate Cancer: From Canadian Cancer Society. (2007c). Prostate cancer: Understanding your diagnosis. Retrieved May 19, 2008, from www.cancer.ca

Chapter 26

Promoting Health Box: New HPV Vaccine: From Canadian Cancer Society. (2007). *Early detection and screening: Facts for women.* Retrieved on May 19, 2008, from www.cancer.ca; Canadian Paediatric Society: Position statement (ID 2007-01): Human papillomavirus vaccine for children and adolescents. *Paediatrics and Child Health, 12,* 599–903. Also available at http://www.cps.ca/english/index.htm; Health Canada. (2006). *Screening for cervical cancer.* Retrieved from www.hc-sc.gc.ca/iyh-vsv/diseases-maladies/cervical-uterus_e.html; Public Health Agency of Canada. (2007). *What everyone should know about human papillomavirus.* Retrieved from www.phac-aspc.gc.ca/std-mts/hpv-vph/hpv-vph-qaqr_e.html; Society of Obstetricians and Gynaecologists of

Canada. (2008). *HPV info.* Retrieved from www.hpvinfo.ca/hpvinfo/home.aspx

Art for Table 26-2: (pediculosis pubis [crab lice]) from Callen, J. P., et al. (1993). *Color atlas of dermatology.* Philadelphia, PA: Saunders; (herpes simplex virus-type 2 [herpes genitalis]) from Callen, J. P., et al. (1993). *Color atlas of dermatology.* Philadelphia, PA: Saunders; (red rash-contact dermatitis) Courtesy of Pfizer Laboratories Division, Pfizer Inc, New York. From *A close look at VD: a slide presentation produced as a public service;* (syphilitic chancre) from Emond, R. T., Rowl, H. A. K., & Welsby, P. (1995). *Color atlas of infectious diseases* (3rd ed.). London, England: Mosby; (genital human papillomavirus [HPV, condylomata, acuminata, genital warts]) from Habif, T. P., et al. (2001). *Skin disease: diagnosis and treatment* (1st ed.). St Louis, MO: Mosby; (abscess of Bartholin's gland) from Emond, R. T., Rowl, H. A. K., & Welsby, P. (1995). *Color atlas of infectious diseases* (3rd ed.). London, England: Mosby; (urethral caruncle) from Rimsza, M. E. (1989). An illustrated guide to adolescent gynecology. *Pediatr Clin North Am, 36*(3), 641.

Art for Table 26-3: (cystocele) from Symonds, E. M., & McPherson, M. B. A. (1997). *Diagnosis in color: obstetrics and gynecology.* London, England: Mosby-Wolfe; (rectocele) from Huffman, J. W.: (1962). *Gynecology and obstetrics.* Philadelphia, PA, Saunders; (uterine prolapse) from Symonds, E. M., & McPherson, M. B. A. (1997). *Diagnosis in color: obstetrics and gynecology.* London, England: Mosby-Wolfe.

Art for Table 26-4: (human papillomavirus (HPV, condylomata)) from Symonds, E. M., & McPherson, M. B. A. (1997). *Diagnosis in color: obstetrics and gynecology.* London, England: Mosby-Wolfe; (polyp) from Symonds, E. M., & McPherson, M. B. A. (1997). *Diagnosis in color: obstetrics and gynecology.* London, England: Mosby-Wolfe; (carcinoma) from Symonds, E. M., & McPherson, M. B. A. (1997). *Diagnosis in color: obstetrics and gynecology.* London, England: Mosby-Wolfe.

Art for Table 26-5: (gonorrhea) Courtesy of Pfizer Laboratories Division, Pfizer Inc, New York. From *A close look at VD: a slide presentation produced as a public service.*

Art for Table 26-8: (ambiguous genitalia) from Moore, K. L., & Persaud, T.N. (1998). *Before we are born: essentials of embryology and birth defects* (5th ed.). Philadelphia, PA: Saunders; (vulvovaginitis in child) from Feigin, R. D., & Cherry, J. D. (1998). *Textbook of pediatric infectious diseases* (4th ed.). Philadelphia, PA: Saunders.

Chapter 28

Art for unn. figure, centre page 819: From Sorrentino, S. A., & Gorek, B. (2007). *Mosby's textbook for long-term care nursing assistants* (5th ed.). St. Louis, MO: Mosby.

Art for unn. figures, bottom page 819: From Sorrentino, S. A., & Gorek, B. (2007). *Mosby's textbook for long-term care nursing assistants* (5th ed.). St. Louis, MO: Mosby.

Chapter 29

Table 29-1: From Health Canada. (2002). *Guidelines for gestational weight gain ranges.* Retrieved from http://www.hc-sc.gc.ca/fn-an/nutrition/prenatal/national_guidelines-lignes_directrices_nationales-06b-table1_e.html

Figure 29-4: From Symonds, E. M., & McPherson, M. B. A. (1997). *Diagnosis in color: obstetrics and gynecology.* London, England: Mosby-Wolfe.

Figure 29-13: From Symonds, E. M., & McPherson, M. B. A. (1997). *Diagnosis in color: obstetrics and gynecology.* London, England: Mosby-Wolfe.

Art for Table 29-3: (pre-eclampsia) from Symonds, E. M., & McPherson, M. B. A. (1997). *Diagnosis in color: obstetrics and gynecology.* London, England: Mosby-Wolfe.

Art for Table 29-4: (fetal macrosomia) from Symonds, E. M., & McPherson, M. B. A. (1997). *Diagnosis in color: obstetrics and gynecology.* London, England: Mosby-Wolfe.

Table 29-6: From Society of Obstetricians and Gynaecologists of Canada. (2007). Fetal health surveillance: Antenatal and intrapartum consensus guideline. *Journal of Obstetrics and Gynaecology Canada, 29*(9 Suppl. 4), S3–S56.

Chapter 30

Figure 30-1: Adapted from Gerontological Society of America, Katz, S., et al. (1970). Progress in the development of the index of ADL. *Gerontologist, 10,* 20–30.

Figure 30-2: From Lawton, M. P., & Brody, E. M. (1969). Assessment of older people: Self-maintaining and instrumental activites of daily living. *Gerontologist, 9,* 179–186. Copyright The Gerontological Society of America.

Figure 30-3: From Sullivan, M. T. (2002). Caregiver Strain Index (CSI). *Try this: best practice in nursing care to older adults: Issue #14.* Retrieved from http://www.hartfordign.org/publication/trythis/issue14.pdf

Box 30-2: Definitions of the Types of Elder Abuse: From Canadian Network for the Prevention of Elder Abuse. (2008). *What is abuse of seniors?* Retrieved April 18, 2008, from http://www.cnpea.ca/

Box 30-3: Canadian Medical Association Screening Questions: From Patterson, C. (1994). Secondary prevention of elder abuse. In: Canadian Task Force on the Periodic Health Examination (Ed.), *Canadian guide to clinical preventive health care* (pp. 922–999). Ottawa, ON: Health Canada.

Box 30-6: The Public Health Agency of Canada's "Keeping Your Home Safe" Checklist: Excerpts from Public Health Agency of Canada. (2005). *The safe living guide—A guide to home safety for seniors* (3rd ed.). Ottawa, ON: Minister of Public Works and Government Services Canada. Retrieved April 18, 2008, from http://www.hc-sc.gc.ca/seniors-aines/pubs/safelive/index.htm

Appendices

Appendix A: Braden Risk Assessment Scale: © Barbara Braden and Nancy Bergstrom, 1988.

Appendix B: Faces Pain Scale—Revised: From Hicks, C. L., von Baeyer, C. L., & Spafford, P. A., van Korlaar, I., & Goodenough, B. (2001). The faces pain scale—Revised. Toward a common metric in pediatric pain measurement. *Pain, 93,* 173–183. Reprinted with permission of the International Association for the Study of Pain®.

Appendix C: Canadian Credible Sources of Nutritional Information: From Piché, L. A. & Garcia, A. C. (2008). Canadian Supplemental information (CSI) document to accompany nutrition concepts and controversies (10th ed.). Toronto, ON: Thomson/Nelson.

Appendix D: Excerpts from *Eating Well With Canada's Food Guide:* From Health Canada. (2007). *Eating Well With Canada's Food Guide.* © Her Majesty the Queen in Right of Canada, represented by the Minister of Health Canada. Cat. No. H164-38/1-2007E. Retrieved June 6, 2008, from http://www.hc-sc.gc.ca/fn-an/alt_formats/hpfb-dgpsa/pdf/food-guide-aliment/print_eatwell_bienmang_e.pdf

Appendix E: The Canadian Neurological Scale: From Côté, R., Hachinkski, V. C., Shurvell, B. L., Norris, J. W., & Wolfson, C. (1986). The Canadian Neurological Scale: A preliminary study in acute stroke. *Stroke, 17*(4), 731–737; Côté, R., Battista, R. N., Wolfson, C., Boucher, J., Adam, J., & Hachinski, V. C. (1989). The Canadian Neurological Scale: Validation and reliability assessment. *Neurology, 39,* 638–643; Bushnell, C. D., Johnston, D. C. C., & Goldstein, L. B. (2001). Retrospective assessment of initial stroke severity: Comparison of the NIH stroke scale and the Canadian Neurological Scale. *Stroke, 32,* 656.

Appendix F: Nipissing District Developmental Screen™: From The Nipissing District Developmental Screen™. Reprinted with permission. The Nipissing, Nipissing District Developmental Screen, and NDDS are trademarks of NDDS Intellectual Property Association, used under license. All rights reserved.

Index

Page numbers followed by f indicate figures; t, tables; b, boxes.

TABLE 1: Serum, Plasma, and Whole Blood Chemistries

TEST	NORMAL VALUES SI UNITS (Conventional Units)	POSSIBLE ETIOLOGY HIGHER	LOWER
Bicarbonate	21–28 mmol/L (21–28 mEq/L)	Chronic use of loop diuretics, compensated respiratory acidosis, metabolic alkalosis	Acute renal failure, compensated respiratory alkalosis, diarrhea, metabolic acidosis
Bilirubin Total Indirect Direct	5.1–17 μmol/L (0.2–1.3 mg/dL) 3.4–12 μmol/L (0.1–1 mg/dL) 1.7–5.1 μmol/L (0.1–0.3 mg/dL)	Biliary obstruction, hemolytic anemia, impaired liver function, pernicious anemia, prolonged fasting	
Blood gases* Artherial pH Arterial PCO_2 Arterial PO_2	7.35–7.45 (Same as SI units) 35–45 mm Hg (Same as SI units) 80–100 mm Hg (Same as SI units)	Alkalosis Compensated metabolic alkalosis, respiratory acidosis Administration of high concentration of oxygen	Acidosis Compensated metabolic acidosis, respiratory alkalosis Chronic lung disease, decreased cardiac output
Carbon Dioxide (CO_2 content)	21–28 mmol/L (21–28 mEq/L)	Same as bicarbonate	
Chloride	95–105 mmol/L (95–105 mEq/L)	Corticosteroid therapy, dehydration, excessive infusion of normal saline, metabolic acidosis, respiratory alkalosis, uremia	Addison's disease, congestive heart failure, diarrhea, metabolic alkalosis, overhydration, respiratory acidosis, SIADH vomiting
Cholesterol HDL (high-density lipoproteins) Male Female LDL (low-density proteins)	3.6–5.2 mmol/L (140–200 mg/dL) age dependent >0.75 mmol/L (>45 mg/dL) >0.91 mmol/L (>55 mg/dL) <3.4 μmol/L (<130 mg/dL)	Biliary obstruction, cirrhosis hypothyroidism, hyperlipidemia, idiopathic hypercholesterolemia, renal disease, uncontrolled diabetes	Corticosteroid therapy, extensive liver disease, hyperthyroidism, malnutrition
Glucose, fasting	4–6 mmol/L (72–108 mg/dL)	Acute stress, cerebral lesions, Cushing's syndrome, diabetes mellitus, hyperthyroidism, pancreatic insufficiency	Addison's disease, hepatic disease, hypothyroidism, insulin overdosage, pancreatic tumour, pituitary hypofunction, postgastrectomy dumping syndrome
Oxygen saturation (arterial)	≥95% (Same as SI units)	Increased inspired oxygen, polycythemia vera	Anemia, cardiac decompensation, decreased inspired oxygen, respiratory disorders
Potassium	3.5–5.5 mmol/L (3.5–5.5 mEq/L)	Acute or chronic renal failure, Addison's disease, dehydration, diabetic ketosis, excessive dietary or IV intake, massive tissue destruction, metabolic acidosis	Burns, Cushing's syndrome, deficient dietary or IV intake, diarrhea (severe), diuretic therapy, gastrointestinal fistula, insulin administration, pyloric obstruction, starvation, vomiting
Prostate-specific antigen (PSA)	<4 μg/L (<4 ng/mL)	Benign prostatic hypertrophy, prostate cancer, prostatitis	
Proteins Total Albumin Globulin	60–80 g/L (6–8 g/dL) 35–50 g/L (3.5–5 g/dL) 20–35 g/L (2–3.5 g/dL)	Burns, cirrhosis (globulin fraction), dehydration	Congenital agammaglobulinemia, increased capillary permeability, inflammatory disease, liver disease, malabsorption, malnutrition
Sodium	135–145 mmol/L (135–145 mEq/L)	Corticosteroid therapy, dehydration, impaired renal function, increased sodium intake in diet or IV, primary aldosteronism	Addison's disease, decreased sodium intake in diet or IV, diabetic ketoacidosis, diuretic therapy, excessive loss from GI tract, excessive perspiration, water intoxication
T_4 (thyroxine), total	64–154 nmol/L (5–12 μg/dL)	Hyperthyroidism, thyroiditis	Cretinism, hypothyroidism, myxedema

TEST	NORMAL VALUES SI UNITS (Conventional Units)	POSSIBLE ETIOLOGY HIGHER	LOWER
T$_4$ (thyroxine), free	10–30 pmol/L (0.8–2.3 ng/dL)		
T$_3$ uptake	0.25–0.35(25%–35%)	Hyperthyroidism, metastatic neoplasms	Hypothyroidism
T$_3$ (triiodothyronine)	1.7–3.5 nmol/L (110–230 ng/dL)	Hyperthyroidism	Hypothyroidism
Triglycerides	0.45–1.69 mmol/L (40–150 mg/dL)	Diabetes mellitus, hyperlipidemia, hypothyroidism, liver disease	Hyperthyroidism, malabsorption syndrome, malnutrition
Urea nitrogen (BUN)	3.6–7.1 mmol/L (10–20 mg/dL)	Burns, dehydration, GI bleeds, increase in protein catabolism (fever, stress), renal disease, shock, urinary tract infection	Fluid overload, malnutrition, severe liver damage, SIADH

* Because arterial blood gases are influenced by altitude, the value for PO$_2$ decreases as altitude increases. The lower value is normal for an altitude of 1 mile.

GI, gastrointestinal; IV, intravenous; SIADH, syndrome of inappropriate ADH

TABLE 2: Hematology

TEST	NORMAL VALUES SI UNITS (Conventional Units)	POSSIBLE ETIOLOGY HIGHER	LOWER
Bleeding time (simplate)	180–570 sec (3–9.5 min)	Aspirin ingestion, clotting factor deficiency, defective platelet function, thrombocytopenia, vascular disease, von Willebrand's disease	Acute renal failure, compensated respiratory alkalosis, diarrhea, metabolic acidosis
Activated partial thromboplastin time (APTT)	24–36 sec* (Same as SI units)	Deficiency of factors I, II, V, VIII, IX and X, XI, XII; hemophilia; heparin therapy; liver disease	
Partial thromboplastin time (PPT)	25–35 sec (Same as SI units)	Deficiency of factors I, II, V, VII, and X; liver disease; vitamin K deficiency; warfarin therapy	
Prothrombin time (Protime, PT)	10–14 sec* (Same as SI units)	Deficiency of factors I, II, V, VII, and X; liver disease; vitamin K deficiency; warfarin therapy	
International Normalized Ratio (INR)	0.81–1.2 (Same as SI units)	Same etiology as for PT	
Erythrocyte count† (altitude dependent)		Dehydration, high altitudes, polycythemia vera, severe diarrhea	Anemia, leukemia, posthemorrhage
Male	4.7–6.1 x 10^{12}/L (4.7–6.1 x 10^6/mL)		
Female	4.2–5.4 x 10^{12}/L (4.2–5.4 x 10^6/mL)		
Hemoglobin (altitude dependent)†		COPD, high altitudes, polycythemia	Anemia, hemorrhage
Male	8.7–11.2 mmol/L (13.5–18 g/dL)		
Female	7.4–9.9 mmol/L (12–16 g/dL)		
Platelet count (thrombocytes)	150–400 x 10^9/L (150–400 x 10^3/μL)	Acute infections, chronic granulocytic leukemia, chronic pancreatitis, cirrhosis, collagen disorders, polycythemia, postsplenectomy	Acute leukemia, cancer chemotherapy, DIC, hemorrhage, infection, SLE, thrombocytopenic purpura